MW01055709

HAND AND UPPER EXTREMITY SPLINTING

Principles & Methods

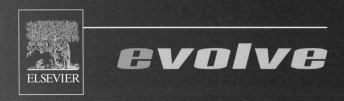

ELSEVIER

evolve

HAND AND UPPER EXTREMITY SPLINTING
Principles & Methods

ELAINE EWING FESS, MS, OTR, FAOTA, CHT
Hand Research
Adjunct Assistant Professor, Indiana University
School of Health and Rehabilitation Sciences
Department of Occupational Therapy
Indianapolis, Indiana

KARAN S. GETTLE, MBA, OTR, CHT
Hand Clinical Specialist
Zionsville, Indiana

CYNTHIA A. PHILIPS, MA, OTR/L, CHT
Hand Clinical Specialist
Back On Track Physical Therapy
Brookline, Massachusetts

J. ROBIN JANSON, MS, OTR, CHT
Lecturer, Part-Time, Indiana University
School of Health and Rehabilitation Sciences
Department of Occupational Therapy
Indianapolis, Indiana

THIRD EDITION
With 4 Contributing Authors

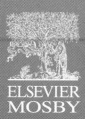

ELSEVIER
MOSBY

ELSEVIER
MOSBY

11830 Westline Industrial Drive
St. Louis, Missouri 63146

Previous editions copyrighted 1981, 1987

International Standard Book Number 0-8016-7522-7

Publishing Director: Linda Duncan
Managing Editor: Kathy Falk
Developmental Editor: Melissa Kuster Deutsch
Editorial Assistant: Colin Odell
Publishing Services Manager: Melissa Lastarria
Project Manager: Joy Moore
Design Manager: Gail Morey Hudson

Printed in the United States of America

Last digit is the print number: 9 8 7 6 5 4 3 2 1

To our unsung heroes—

our families

E.E.F.   K.S.G.   C.A.P.   J.R.J.

Contributors

Joni Armstrong, OTR, CHT
Hand Therapist, Consultant, North Country Peak Performance
Bemidji, Minnesota
University of North Dakota School of Medicine and Health Sciences
Grand Forks, North Dakota

Judith Bell Krotoski, OTR, CHT, FAOTA;
CAPTAIN, USPHS (Ret.)
Private Teaching and Consulting, Hand Therapy Research
Baton Rouge, Louisiana
Former Chief Hand and OT/Clinical Research Therapist
USPHS National Hansen's Disease Programs
Baton Rouge, Louisiana

Alexander D. Mih, MD
Hand Surgeon, The Indiana Hand Center
Indianapolis, Indiana

James W. Strickland, MD
Clinical Professor, Indiana University School of Medicine
Indianapolis, Indiana
Past President, American Academy of Orthopaedic Surgeons
Past President, American Society for Surgery of the Hand

Foreword to First Edition

The emergence of hand surgery as a specialty and the advances in the science and art of hand surgery since World War II have been truly phenomenal. Societies for surgery of the hand have attracted some of the most skillful and dedicated surgeons and have served as a forum for discussion and criticism, new concepts, and the testing and trial of competing ideas.

At first, this exciting advance in hand surgery was not accompanied by a parallel advance in techniques of conservative and nonoperative management of the hand. Not only has this led to a tendency to operate on patients who might have been better treated conservatively, but many patients who have rightly and properly been operated on have failed to obtain the best results of their surgery because of inadequate or poorly planned preoperative and postoperative management.

It is encouraging to note that just in the last decade interest has surged in what is being called "hand rehabilitation." This term is used to cover the whole range of conservative management of the hand. It represents an area in which the surgeon and therapist work closely together, with each bringing their special experience and expertise to the common problem. Hand rehabilitation centers are multiplying, and a new group, the Society of Hand Therapists, has been formed in association with the American Society for Surgery of the Hand to bring together those physical therapists and occupational therapists who specialize in the hand.

Pioneers in the new movement are Elaine Fess, Karan Gettle, and James Strickland, and their work has concentrated on the neglected field of hand splinting. Little research has been done on the actual effect of externally applied forces on joints and tissues of the hand. Experienced surgeons and therapists have developed an intuitive "feel" for what can be accomplished, but there is little in the literature to assist the young surgeon in what to prescribe or to help a young therapist know the hazards that can turn a good prescription into a harmful application. In this situation, Elaine Fess, Karan Gettle, and James Strickland have put their own experience down on paper and made it available to all of us. It is obvious that they have a great deal of experience. It is also clear that they have gone far beyond the "cookbook" stage of previous splinting manuals. They have researched and studied their subject thoroughly, and we are fortunate indeed to have the result of that study presented so clearly and illustrated so well.

What pleases me most about this book is that it deals first with principles and only then with specific design. It begins with an emphasis on anatomy and topography and then with mechanical principles; after chapters on principles of design and fit and construction, the authors discuss specific splints. In addition, there is a good chapter on specific problems and how to handle them.

It is a measure of how far we still have to go in the science of splinting that the authors do not feel able to recommend actual specific forces by numbers to use in dynamic splints. My own feeling is that the boundary between art and science is numbers. Even in hand surgery we are not yet able to say that a specific tendon should be attached with a tension of 200 grams, so why should we expect a therapist to fix a rubber band at a specific level of tension? One day we will take these extra steps toward precision. When data are available, Elaine Fess, Karan Gettle, and James Strickland will be the first to put it into their next book. They have jumped into a clear position of leadership with this book. I am sure they will stay ahead of each new advance as it comes along.

Paul W. Brand, F.R.C.S.*

*Clinical Professor of Surgery and Orthopaedics
Louisiana State University; Chief, Rehabilitation Branch
United States Public Health Service Hospital
Carville, Louisiana*

*Deceased.

Foreword

The opportunity to write the Foreword to this the third edition of *Hand Splinting: Principles and Methods* has special significance to me. Having modestly participated in the writing of the first volume in 1981, I am awestruck by the science and sophistication of today's splinting techniques and applications. Much like hand surgery itself, splinting and hand rehabilitation have progressed from very unscientific, "trial and error" methods to thoughtfully considered, evidence-based techniques for matching the fundamental concepts of anatomy, kinesiology, and biomechanics with the ever increasing body of knowledge on wound healing, tissue remodeling, and adhesion control.

I am old enough to reflect back on my days as an eager orthopaedic resident in the early 1960s. When told by a respected attending physician to splint the hand of an injured patient, I asked, "What kind of splint should I use?" The immediate reply was to ask the therapist to make a "long opponens hand splint with a lumbrical bar," a splint that had been a workhorse for orthopaedists during the polio days when intrinsic muscle paralysis was common. In retrospect, that splint had little practical application to the traumatically altered anatomy of my patient, but I didn't hesitate to request the long opponens splint as I was told. Several days later I had a very different patient with a radial nerve paralysis and queried a different attending physician about the appropriate splinting. He also responded with the same answer: "long opponens hand splint with a lumbrical bar." Over the ensuing weeks I noticed that that splint seemed to be the stock answer regardless of the clinical condition. Like a good resident I just accepted the fact that the long opponens splint seemed to be used for almost all hand conditions. It wasn't until my fellowship in hand surgery that I began to learn that different conditions demanded different splints, but even then our scientific rationale and fabrication techniques were primitive when compared to the technical erudition so eloquently described in this edition.

Early in my hand surgical practice I had the consummate good fortune to hire an extremely bright young therapist who questioned the reasoning behind almost every splint I wanted made for the wide variety of patients and conditions that I was seeing in my fledgling practice. She wanted to understand the underlying biological and biomechanical effects of splints and was particularly inquisitive about the repercussions of applying varying amounts of stress to injured tissues. She challenged the way splints were made and the angles of approach and forces generated by the mobilization slings and rubber bands we were using. She continually questioned existing concepts about moving stiffened joints and repaired tendons. Although initially somewhat annoyed by her constant quest for knowledge and frequent need to dispute and revise the established splinting dictums of the time, I came to appreciate her scientific curiosity. That therapist was Elaine Ewing Fess, OTR, the author of all three volumes of *Hand Splinting: Principles and Methods*, and, in my view, one of the most thoughtful and dedicated students and teachers of hand and upper extremity splinting of our time.

From those modest beginnings, and because of her insatiable curiosity, Elaine Ewing Fess went on to become a brilliant and respected hand therapist, researcher, and teacher. Understandably, she has taught her students to challenge commonly used techniques that lack scientific support and look for better, evidence-based methods. Together with her long-time colleague Karan Gettle and myself, Elaine authored the first truly science-based text on hand splinting, *Hand Splinting: Principles and Methods*, in 1981. An updated second edition written with noted co-author, Cynthia Philips, was published in 1987.

It is no surprise, then, that Elaine Fess, OTR, and Karan Gettle, OTR, together with their outstanding co-authors Cynthia Philips, OTR, and Robin Janson, OTR, have now produced a beautifully updated and markedly expanded third edition that is a true masterpiece. Together with a formidable cadre of distinguished contributors, the authors have extensively revised and supplemented all of the comprehensive sections of the third edition and, even more impressively, they have exhaustively described all splints according to the expanded American Society of Hand Therapists (ASHT) Splint Classification System. In doing so, they have provided clinicians and therapists worldwide with a system that accurately describes almost all known splints and categorizes those splints into a sort-and-search tracking engine, the Splint Sequence Ranking Database Index© (SSRDI). In doing so, they have given us the first orderly tool for easily accessing information about design configuration and clinical application of upper extremity splints.

In my mind, this new work represents the "Bible of Hand Splinting" and should be read, re-read and thoroughly understood by all therapists and physicians engaged in the management of injured, diseased, con-

genitally deformed, and surgically repaired hands and upper extremities.

The authors have taken us a very long way since the "long opponens hand splint with a lumbrical bar" and our patients are much better off because of their dedicated efforts.

James W. Strickland, MD
Clinical Professor of Orthopaedic Surgery,
Indiana University School of Medicine
Indianapolis, Indiana

Preface

Our decision to describe all splints illustrated in this third edition according to the American Society of Hand Therapists (ASHT) Splint Classification System (SCS) has profoundly influenced our own understanding of splinting concepts and subsequently defined the essence of *Hand and Upper Extremity Splinting Principles and Methods, third edition*. Both the original SCS and its updated version, the expanded SCS (ESCS), revolutionize splinting concepts by providing a sophisticated, methodical, and effective language for describing and classifying splints.

From the outset, the original SCS provided a solid basis for naming the substantial number of splint photographs earmarked for the third edition. The opportunity to compare and contrast this vast array of photographs confirmed and honed our expertise in using the SCS. However, as our learning curve advanced, several critical issues became apparent. The first involved our ability to revisit and assess our earlier assigned SCS designations, a key factor to improving our accuracy in naming splints. Tracking nearly 1200 splint illustrations, all of which would eventually have technical ESCS monikers, was rapidly becoming a logistical nightmare. In response, we devised a rudimentary database that over time became increasingly complex as the tasks of making information accessible and manageable became more sophisticated and challenging. What we originally created as a simple tracking device has evolved into a comprehensive, dual-function, sort-and-search engine that automatically rank-orders splints according to their ESCS names and identifies single- or multiple-splint photographs depending on specific input criteria. This sort-and-search engine, the Splint Sequence Ranking Database Index© (SSRDI©) is pivotal to the organization of this book and to its associated interactive website.

The second major issue involved a number of splints that resisted categorization into one or more of the three purpose categories (immobilization, mobilization, and restriction) defined in the original SCS. Naming certain splints was a struggle, and our periodic reassessment of their previously assigned SCS designations revealed serious inconsistencies.

Perplexingly, as the numbers of unnamed splints slowly mounted, it became increasingly apparent that the majority of these splints were simple in design and many fell into a group colloquially dubbed "exercise splints." It was one of those middle-of-the night revelations that finally identified the problem. This group of splints belonged to a heretofore-unidentified fourth purpose category: torque transmission. A trial period was initiated during which we tested this new category and much to our relief the problem of the nonconforming splints was solved. We thank bioengineer David Giurintano, MSME,* for confirming the existence of this fourth splint purpose category and for his assistance in defining its technical designation, as we had originally incorrectly labeled it *force transmission*. Some 135 torque transmission splints are illustrated in this third edition. Ironically, the lowly "buddy strap" was one of the splints that gave us the most trouble until we added the torque transmission category!

A true classification system is not stagnant. Its use begets revision and refinement, allowing the system to grow and evolve. Although not as noteworthy as the addition of a fourth purpose category, other additions, adaptations, and subtleties were incorporated as needed, and we eventually arrived at the current ESCS used in this third edition. For example, the original SCS does not address multipurpose designations, and yet we identified numerous photos in which the splints depicted had two and even three purposes. With identification of SCS deficiencies came the responsibility and challenges of creating the associated representational patterns that would translate our revisions into workable ESCS format.

The ESCS is a technical language by which splints and splint-like devices are classified according to function, not form. Each splint is defined by a mandatory six-section sentence and, as with other languages, section sequence, section connectors, and punctuation are fundamental elements to sentence structure. Careful definition of minute details and consistent

---

*Chief, Rehabilitation Research, Paul Brand Biomechanics Laboratory, Baton Rouge, Louisiana.

implementation of their use was, and continues to be, mandatory for the evolving classification system to work properly, especially in database format. For example, we had to create rules for using "or," "and," and the backslash (/) as connectors between multipurpose or multidirectional ESCS sentence components. Another example, a colon (:) indicates a shift in direction for reciprocal action torque transmission splints such as the design that occasionally is used to improve hand function in radial nerve palsies. In these splints, the task of the "driver" joint alternates between the wrist and finger metacarpophalangeal (MP) joints with wrist flexion producing finger MP extension and finger MP flexion producing wrist extension. A different reciprocal splint design is used to maximize tenodesis hand function of spinal cord injury patients. All reciprocal splints, regardless of their anatomical location, are identified by the presence of a colon in their ESCS names. Uniformity of ESCS sentence pattern structure is key to sorting, searching, and grouping splints in the database. To this end, we developed and put into operation critical structural adjustments and refinements to standardize ESCS sentence format.

One new change to this edition is the use of spacing between the individual parts in a given figure. As many of the figures consist of several parts, it became necessary to differentiate multiple views of one splint from completely different splints that make up a figure. Different views of the same splint are grouped closely together in the layout for ease of the reader. Photos of different splints are spaced farther apart from one another.

Why go to all this trouble? Because for the first time in the history of splinting endeavors, we have a system that accurately describes splints. The ESCS incorporates all design configurations by addressing splint function, a feat accomplished by no other system. An ESCS name tells everyone involved the "what, where, and why" of a splint without getting bogged down in trivial design details. Take for example the ubiquitous "cock-up" splint. Noting in a chart that a patient was fitted with a wrist cock-up splint indicates only that a splint was applied to the wrist, nothing more. In contrast, an ESCS name defines whether the wrist was immobilized, mobilized, restricted, or whether the splint was applied to transmit torque to the finger joints through secondary control of the wrist. In the torque transmission example, the primary focus joints are the twelve finger joints. This is a very different scenario from immobilizing, mobilizing, or restricting the wrist as a single primary focus joint. Likewise, the purposes of wrist immobilization, mobilization, and restriction differ significantly from each other. In addition to defining splint primary joints and purposes,

the ESCS name indicates whether normal joints are included to improve mechanical effect of the splint. In the case of the torque transmission splint, one joint level—the wrist—is included secondarily (type 1) whereas no secondary joint levels (type 0) are included when the wrist is the primary focus joint. Detailed information provided by ESCS names renders retention of colloquial terms (e.g., the "cock-up" splint) woefully inadequate. For even in what should be a difficult challenge, that of differentiating identical-configuration splints, ESCS designations clearly identify distinguishing characteristics of the splints involved. There are many instances throughout this book that parallel this paradigm where same-configuration splints have different ESCS names. It is all about function, not form.

In truth, we could not have anticipated the integrated precision, flexibility, and power of the ESCS when it is used in conjunction with its sort-and-search engine, the SSRDI©. Until we began to see large numbers of splints sorted into their respective categories, we did not realize that we were dealing with an incredibly effective tool with enormous potential. One has only to peruse the Splint Index at the back of this book to recognize the underlying logic and order that these systems working in tandem impart to the splinting knowledge base. The number and kind of splints that may be classified is unlimited. To date, we have not encountered a splint that cannot be classified according to the ESCS. In addition to having positive effects on future patient treatment, research, and professional communication, the near-mathematical precision afforded by the ESCS/SSRDI© makes it an intuitively obvious basis for reimbursement coding and billing. Other nomenclature systems cannot match the precision of the ESCS. Our attempts in earlier editions to organize and name splints now seem primitive in comparison to the preeminence of the ESCS.

We thank Jean Casanova, OTR, and Janet Bailey, OTR, for their insight and vision in bringing together members of the ASHT Splint Nomenclature Task Force for one weekend in 1991 with the directive of putting an end to the entrenched disorder of splinting nomenclature; it was this group of nine therapists who created the original SCS and wrote the manual, *Splint Classification System** (see Chapter 1, A History of Splinting). Three of the four authors of this third edition had the honor of participating on this 1991 Task Force, and although we knew the SCS was important, at the time we did not really understand its potential magnitude.

---

*©American Society of Hand Therapists, 1992.

The ESCS provides the conceptual framework for this third edition, setting the organizational composition of chapters and content. For quick reference, ESCS names of illustrated splints are printed in blue ink at the beginning of the figure captions. Additionally, a comprehensive Splint Index lists all illustrated splints by ESCS designation, in SSRDI© order, starting with articular shoulder splints and ending with nonarticular phalangeal splints. Associated figure numbers are included in the Index to facilitate location of the illustrations in the chapters. With the exceptions of Chapters 17, Splinting for Work, Sports, and Performing Arts; 18, Splinting the Pediatric Patient; and 19, Splinting for Patients with Upper Extremity Spasticity, colloquial splint expressions are not included with ESCS designations. Because the above-referenced chapters do include both ESCS and colloquial nomenclature, they serve as user-friendly learning bridges for readers who are unfamiliar with the ESCS. Abbreviations used throughout this text are listed on the inside back cover.

In addition to extensive updating of existing chapter content and references, this third edition of *Hand and Upper Extremity Splinting: Principles & Methods* includes six new chapters: Chapter 1, History of Splinting; Chapter 14, Splints Acting on the Elbow and Shoulder; Chapter 17, Splinting for Work, Sports, and Performing Arts; Chapter 18, Splinting the Pediatric Patient, by Joni Armstrong, OTR, CHT; Chapter 19, Splinting for Patients with Upper Extremity Spasticity; and Chapter 23, Cast, Splint, and Design Prostheses for Patients with Total or Partial Hand Amputations, by Judith Bell Krotoski, OTR, CHT, FAOTA. We are especially pleased that five of these new chapters provide valuable clinical information about the use of splints in specialized fields. Important new sections are also added to existing classic chapters. Chapter 2, Anatomy of the Hand, Wrist, and Forearm, by James W. Strickland, MD, is expanded to include a new section, Anatomy of the Elbow and Shoulder, by Alexander Mih, MD; and Chapter 3, Biologic Basis for Hand and Upper Extremity Splinting, by Dr. Strickland, includes a new section, Biomechanics, Splinting, and Tissue Remodeling, by Judith Bell Krotoski, OTR, CHT, FAOTA; and a second new section, Soft Tissue Remodeling, that reviews research studies addressing cellular-level mechanical, physiological, and chemical mechanisms of soft tissue responses to stress.

Writing a book is a team effort. The contributions of many individuals who are not listed as authors are as important as the contributions made by the authors of this work. We are especially grateful to our families, who have generously supported us in the preparation of this third edition. For every hour we spent in research, writing, and editing, some 10,000 total hours to date, a family member quietly picked up the slack so that our family lives continued to run smoothly. Special mention goes to Steve Fess who, as Fess Express (self-dubbed), maintained supplies, shuttled reports and items that could not be e-mailed back and forth, ran library searches, and catered our frequent 6 to 10 hour work sessions with carry-in meals. We also thank our many friends who understood and offered their help when we were distracted, late with commitments, and just plain grumpy. Of particular note, Sherran Schmalfeldt launched our work of revising chapters by typing all of the chapters from the second edition onto computer disks. Sherran's generosity and exceptional typing skills allowed us to completely update these chapters instead of just patching them. Family and friends are our unsung heroes to whom we owe so much. We also have strengthened our own long-term friendships, and our continuing capacity to work as an integrated team is especially rewarding. In addition to the pressures of writing this book, we have survived numerous other professional commitments, changing work situations, a Master's thesis, the birth of a child, children in school, two household moves, comings and goings of beloved pets, a husband, children and grandchildren leaving and returning from overseas mission work, long-term parent illnesses, and the deaths of three parents. Friendship and commitment to a common goal are compelling, enduring bonds that are inextricable.

Adding the most essential element of this third edition are the 121 individuals and corporations who kindly shared their photographs of splints, or the splints themselves, with us. Without the marvelous generosity of these individuals and groups from around the world there would be no 3rd edition of this book. Further, it was the sheer numbers and great range of submitted splint photographs that allowed us to develop the ESCS and SSRDI©. It is a privilege to include splint photographs from these international leaders in splint technology in this book. We encourage these individuals, corporations, and others to submit new splint photographs to the website (http://evolve.elsevier.com/Fess/) so that we, and others, may continue to learn from their skills and talents.

Published works reflect the expertise of the professional editorial staff with whom the publications are associated. We are fortunate to have Kathy Falk and her associate, Melissa Kuster, as our editors for this book. As often happens in life, events have a way of coming around full circle. Kathy Falk, as a C. V. Mosby representative attending an early Philadelphia Hand Symposium, initiated the idea of Fess, Gettle, and Strickland writing a new splinting book. She subsequently became primary editor for the project and the first edition of *Hand Splinting Principles and Methods* was published in 1981. We were thrilled and relieved to have Kathy return as primary editor for this third edition. With so many illustrations and associated ESCS names involved, the technical challenges of putting together a book of this scope have been daunting to say the least. Both Kathy and Melissa played pivotal roles in this third edition. They literally restructured and hand-pasted numerous chapters where layout was especially difficult. Were it not for their timely and expert intervention, this book would be hopelessly unwieldy for readers. Thank you, Kathy and Melissa, for your dedication, support, and unflappable good humor throughout this project. Additionally, we are grateful to Diane Schindler who efficiently ensured that all the copyright permissions are in good order.

We also thank medical illustrators Craig Gosling, Chris Brown, Marty Williams, and Gary Schnitz, and photographers Rick Beets and David Jaynes, who employed their considerable artistic talents to make learning easier and more enjoyable for others through their excellent drawings, photographs, and cartoons. John Kirk* has served as our trusted materials expert for all three editions of this book. He openly and honestly shared his considerable knowledge of splinting materials without, even once, touting his own line of materials. Thank you, John, for your wisdom and professionalism over these many years. We are grateful to the many individuals who provided important bits and pieces of information that helped us verify, document, and track text references, splinting resources, and individuals who had submitted photographs to earlier editions. An example of the kindness and professionalism of these individuals is Barbara Lewis, OTR, CHT, who took time out of her busy schedule to assist us in finding a talented contributor to the second edition who we were unable to locate.

As science and the understanding of its principles are an ever-changing landscape, we enthusiastically encourage dialogue, criticism, additions, and updates to this work by all of our colleagues for the advancement of our common base of knowledge!

E. E. F.
K. S. G.
C. A. P.
J. R. J.

---

*WFR Corporation, Wyckoff, NJ.

Acknowledgments

We thank the following individuals and companies for generously contributing photographs, splints, materials, equipment, and ideas:

3-Point Products, Inc.
Aircast
Cheri Alexy, OTR, CHT
Jean-Christophe Arias
Joni Armstrong, OTR, CHT
Norma Arras, MA, OTR, CHT
Sandra Artzberger, MS, OTR, CHT
Janet Bailey, OTR/L, CHT
Rebecca Banks, OTR, CHT, MHS
Jane Bear-Lehman, PhD, OTR, FAOTA
Judith Bell Krotoski, OTR, FAOTA, CHT
Rivka Ben-Porath, OT
Lin Beribak, OTR/L, CHT
Theresa Bielawski, OT (C)
Bledsoe Brace Systems
Christopher Bochenek, OTR/L, CHT
Suzanne Brand, OTR, CHT
Kay Colello-Abraham, OTR, CHT
Diane Collins, MEd, PT, CHT
Ruth Coopee, MOT, OTR, CHT
Lawrence Czap, OTR
Darcelle Decker, OTR, CHT
Carolina deLeeuw, MA, OTR
Shelli Dellinger, OTR, CHT
Lori Klerekoper DeMott, OTR, CHT
Elisha Denny, OTA, PTA
Lisa Dennys, BSc (OT), DCM, Dac
DeRoyal/LMB
dj Orthopedics
Rebecca Duncan, PT
Dynasplint Systems, Inc.
Rachel Dyrud Ferguson, OTR, CHT
Jolene Eastburn, OTR
Susan Emerson, MEd, OTR, CHT
EMPI
Roslyn Evans, OTR, CHT
Expansao
Joan Farrell, OTR, CHT
Bonnie Ferhing, LPT
Sharon Flinn, MEd, OTR/L, CHT
Kenneth Flowers, PT, CHT

Jill Francisco, OTR, CHT
Steven Z. Glickel, MD
Lynnlee Fullenwider, OTR, CHT
Karen E. Gable, EdD
Susan Glaser-Butler, OTR/L, CHT
Patricia Hall, MS, OTR, ATP
Christine Heaney, BSc, OT
Carol Hierman, OTR, CHT
Brenda Hilfrank, PT, CHT
Renske Houck-Romkes, OT
JACE Systems
Jewish Hospital
Caryl Johnson, OTR, CHT
Joint Active Systems, Inc.
Joanne Kassimir, OTR, CHT
Damon Kirk
Kleinert Institute Hand Therapy Center
Jennifer Koryta, OTR
Cheryl Kunkle, OTR, CHT
Elaine LaCroix, MHSM, OTR, CHT
Karen Lauckhardt, MA, PT, CHT
Janet Kinnunen Lopez, OTR, CHT
Daniel Lupo, OTR, CHT
K. P. MacBain, OT
March of Dimes
Helen Marx, OTR, CHT
Karen Mathewson, OTR, CHT
Gretchen Maurer, OTR, CHT
Esther May, PhD, OT
Laura McCarrick, OTR
Conor McCullough, OTR
Peggy McLaughlin, OTR, CHT
Robin Miller, OTR, CHT
Bobbie-Ann Neel, OTR
Jerilyn Nolan, MA, OTR, CHT
North Coast Medical
Orfit Industries
Margareta Persson, PT
Sally Poole, MA, OTR, CHT
Karen Priest-Barrett, OTR, CHT
Barbara Raff, OTR/L, CHT

Donna Reist-Kolumbus, OTR, CHT
Joyce Roalef, OTR/L, CHT
Jill Robinson, PT, CHT
Jean Claude Rouzaud, PT
Sammons Preston Rolyan
Kathryn Schultz, OTR, CHT
Karen Schultz-Johnson, MS, OTR, CHT, FAOTA
Kimiko Shiina, PhD, OTR/L
Linda Shuttleton, OTR
Silver Ring Splint Company
Terri Skirven, OTR, CHT
Barbara Allen Smith, OTR
Smith Nephew Rolyan
Barbara Sopp, MS, OTR, CHT
Donna Breger Stanton, MA, OTR, CHT
Maureen Stark, OTR
Elizabeth Spencer Steffa, OTR/L, CHT
Erica Stern, PhD, OTR, FAOTA
James W. Strickland, MD
Dominique Thomas, RPT, MCMK
David E. Thompson, Ph.D.
Sandra Townsend, OTR, CHT
Linda Tresley, OTR
Stancie Trueman, OT (C)
Regina Roseman Tune, MS, OTR
Ultraflex Systems, Inc.
Paul Van Lede, OT, MS
Griet Van Veldhoven, OT, Orthop. E.
Nelson Vazquez, OTR, CHT
Kilulu Von Prince, OTR
Allyssa Wagner, MS, OTR
Sheila Wallen, OTR/L, MOT
Watts Medical
WFR Corporation
Jill White, MA, OTR
Diana Williams, MBA, OTR, CHT
G. Roger Williams, OTR
Jason Willoughby, OTR
Theresa Wollenschlaeger, OTR, CHT

Contents

PART ONE

History

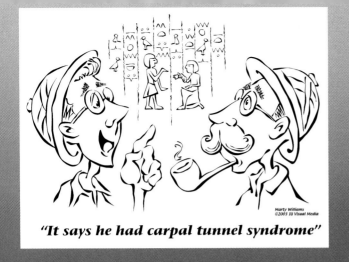

"It says he had carpal tunnel syndrome"

Marty Williams
©2003 IU Visual Media

CHAPTER 1

A History of Splinting

Chapter Outline

Section 1
A History of Splinting:
To Understand the Present, View the Past*

ELAINE EWING FESS, MS, OTR, FAOTA, CHT

The splinting of extremities rendered dysfunctional by injury or disease is not a new concept, and yet clinicians often are not aware of splinting history beyond their own experiences. Delving into the past strengthens the foundation of clinical practice by identifying themes that have persisted over time and by expanding crucial knowledge of the field. It also imparts a heightened appreciation for current methods by providing new insights into the pivotal events that contributed to the development of modern splinting theory and technique.

Those who ignore the past inevitably recreate it.* Both novice and experienced clinicians alike have "invented" revolutionary new splint designs, only to discover later that their highly touted creations have

---

*This section originally was published as an article in the *Journal of Hand Therapy (JHT)*, vol 15:2, 2002, with the understanding that it would later appear in Chapter 1 of this third edition of *Hand and Upper Extremity Splinting: Principles and Methods.* Since the *JHT* publication of this chapter, additional references have been added and some splint nomenclature has changed in response to the expansion and refinement of the ASHT Splint Classification System by the authors of this book.

The perception of history is ever changing, and its documentation is dependent on the information available at the time.

Additional information and resources are openly sought so that this initial study may continue to grow.
*Cf. "Those who cannot remember the past are condemned to repeat it." George Santayana (1863-1952).

been in use for years! Knowledge of history promotes perspective, wisdom, and humility. Historical information also diminishes the odds of recurring mistakes being made by each new generation of clinicians. With experience comes the realization that little is truly new in the world. Ideas beget ideas, eventually creating a wall of knowledge to which many have contributed. Splinting concepts and practices have a rich and, for the most part, undocumented history. In an age abounding in historical treatises, the lack of historical analysis of splinting theory and practice is both surprising and perplexing.

The purpose of this study, which is based on an intensive literature review, is to identify the primary historical factors that shaped the evolution of current splinting technique and practice. With more than 900 references specific to splint design, technique, and application available in the medical literature, individual mention and review of each article is not in the scope of this paper. Instead, published papers, manuals, and books are grouped according to their content and purpose, allowing identification of chronological trends both internal and external to the field.

To more efficiently manage the sheer volume of references, chapters in books are not included in this study unless omission of the work would create a serious deficit in the information base. Publication dates determine the chronological order of events. While a material or technique may have been used several years prior to, or after, its published report, the date of the report is the defining criterion in this study, allowing uniform management of documented events and exclusion of unconfirmed accounts. Splints illustrated in this study are defined according to the American Society of Hand Therapists (ASHT) Splint Classification System as expanded and refined by the authors of this book (ESCS).[10] This allows more accurate description, analysis, and comparison of splints. For the sake of brevity and ease of reading, and because many of the persons mentioned in this article are well known, only the surnames of 20th-century contributors to splinting practice are used in this text. Their full names and credentials are listed in Appendix I.

■ DEFINITION AND PURPOSES OF SPLINTING

The definition of terms provides a foundation from which to work. It also offers insight into past language usage from which contemporary usage has evolved.

Splint, brace, and *orthosis* are often used interchangeably, and *support* is a synonym for all three terms. Webster's *Third International Dictionary* defines *splint* as "a rigid or flexible material (as

wood, metal, plaster, fabric, or adhesive tape) used to protect, immobilize, or restrict motion in a part." Demonstrating the close relationship between noun and verb, *to splint* is "to immobilize (as a broken bone) with a splint; to support or brace with or as if with a splint; to protect against pain by reducing motion."[168]

Stemming from an archaic form meaning "arm" or "armor," *brace* refers to "an appliance that gives support to movable parts (as a joint or a fractured bone), to weak muscles (as in paralysis), or to strained ligaments (as of the lower back)." The verb form of brace means "to prop up or support with braces."

With origins from the Greek *orthosis,* meaning "straightening," an *orthotic device* is "designed for the support of weak or ineffective joints or muscles," and *orthotics* is "a branch of mechanical and medical science dealing with the support and bracing of weak or ineffective joints or muscles."[168]

Despite subtle differences it is apparent that considerable overlap exists among these definitions, and that the definitional criterion focuses on immobilization, support, or restriction purposes. A weak case may be made for the assertion that "support" includes mobilization splints for supple joints but, interestingly, none of these definitions addresses the important concept of splinting to mobilize stiff joints or contracted soft tissues.

Analysis of the reasons cited for splint application in published splinting manuals and books reveals a different scenario, which is more comprehensive in scope. According to noted authors in the field, splints immobilize, mobilize, restrict motion, or transmit torque.[10,71] Listed according to frequency of citation, the purposes of splints are to increase function,* prevent deformity,† correct deformity,‡ substitute for lost motion,§ protect healing structures,‖ maintain range of motion,¶ stabilize joints,** restrict motion,†† allow tissue growth/remodeling,‡‡ improve muscle balance,§§ control inflammation,‖‖ protect normal

---

*References 9, 13, 14, 40, 43, 51, 54, 55, 72, 74, 83, 84, 100, 110, 117, 118, 125, 126, 130, 146, 150, 162, 171, 178, 180.
†References 9, 13, 14, 22, 40, 51, 52, 54, 55, 72, 74, 84, 110, 117, 119, 125, 126, 128, 146, 150, 151, 169, 171, 180.
‡References 13, 14, 22, 40, 43, 44, 54, 55, 72, 74, 84, 100, 117-119, 125, 126, 128, 150, 162, 165, 169, 171, 180.
§References 22, 43, 44, 54, 55, 72, 74, 84, 110, 117, 118, 126, 128, 165, 171, 178, 180.
‖References 40, 43, 44, 72, 74, 84, 117-119, 126, 128, 146, 165, 171, 180.
¶References 13, 14, 43, 44, 54, 55, 74, 117, 119, 128, 162, 169, 180.
**References 13, 14, 72, 74, 84, 100, 117, 118, 126, 128, 146, 178, 180.
††References 13, 14, 40, 44, 72, 74, 124, 165, 180.
‡‡References 24, 27, 40, 72, 74, 84, 117, 146, 165.
§§References 9, 13, 14, 22, 43, 100, 117, 125, 165.
‖‖References 44, 117-119, 126, 128, 165, 180.

structures,¶ allow early motion,[54,55,72,74,165,180] aid in fracture alignment,[14,54,55,83,117,165] decrease pain,[44,52,117,125,171,180] aid in wound healing,[14,54,55,117,171] transmit muscular forces,[24,27,117,128] rest joints,[44,54,55,84] strengthen weak muscles,[13,14,84] influence spasticity,[117,125,126] resolve tendon tightness,[44,165] decrease scar,[119,165] keep paralyzed muscles relaxed,[40,171] encourage predetermined functional stiffness,[40,128] treat infection,[40,117] increase patient independence,[61] and continuously move joints.[126]

From this comprehensive list, six of the cited reasons for splint application each have from 9 to 25 references spanning more than 50 years, indicating lasting affirmation and verification over time. These six rationales are to (1) increase function, (2) prevent deformity, (3) correct deformity, (4) protect healing structures, (5) restrict motion, and (6) allow tissue growth or remodeling. In contrast, three of the last five cited reasons for splinting—keeping paralyzed muscles relaxed, encouraging predetermined functional stiffness, and treating infection—although still appropriate, are more reflective of earlier practice, when polio was prevalent and before antibiotics were available. The final reason cited—continuously move joints—is an obvious newcomer to the list.

■ GENERAL HISTORICAL OVERVIEW

Physical discomfort evokes an instinctive response to immobilize the painful part, and use of extrinsic devices to accomplish the immobilization process is inherently intuitive. In early antiquity, splints were used primarily for treating fractures (Fig. 1-1). Splints of leaves, reeds, bamboo, and bark padded with linen have been dated to ancient Egyptian times, and some mummified remains have been found wearing splints for fractures sustained either before or after death.[5,111]

Copper splints for treating burn injuries were described in 1500 BC.[142] Hippocrates (460-377 BC) used splints, compresses, and bandaging to immobilize fractures. These splints were gutter-shaped split stalks of large plants, wrapped in wool or linen, that were put on separately.[172] Hippocrates also devised a distraction splint for reducing tibial fractures, which consisted of proximal and distal leather cuffs separated by multiple pairs of too-long, springy, narrow wooden slats. When in place on the lower leg, this splint distracted the fracture and brought the bones back into alignment.

In medieval times (1000 AD), use of palm-branch ribs and cane halves for splinting continued. Plaster-like substances were made from flour dust and egg

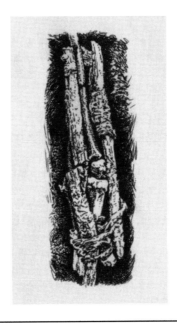

Fig. 1-1   Femur, knee extension immobilization splint, type 0 (1)
This ancient Egyptian splint for a fracture dates from 2750-2625 B.C. (From *British Medical Journal*, March 1908. Reprinted from American Academy of Orthopaedic Surgeons: *Orthopaedic appliances atlas*, vol. 1, JW Edwards, 1952, Ann Arbor, MI.)

whites, and vegetable concoctions were made of gum-mastic, clay, pulped fig, and poppy leaves. The Aztecs (1400 AD) made use of wooden splints and large leaves held in place by leather straps or resin paste.[111] Although most ancient splints were applied to immobilize, Hippocrates' tibial distraction device is a clear example of a mobilization splint.

Moving forward in time, with the introduction of gunpowder in combat, European armor makers were forced to seek other avenues for their armor-fabricating skills. Brace fabrication was a clear alternative for these experts, with their knowledge of metalwork, exterior anatomy, and technicalities of joint alignment. By 1517, joint contractures were treated with turn-buckle and screw-driven metal splints appropriately dubbed "appliances for crooked arms" (Fig. 1-2).

The first one-page splint manual may have been written in 1592, by Hieronymus Fabricius, a surgeon, who devised an illustrated compilation of armor-based splints to treat contractures of all parts of the body (Fig. 1-3). In France and England, from the 1750s to the 1850s, surgeons worked closely with their favorite appliance makers, or "mechanics," to design and build custom braces and splints. A.M. Delacroix, a highly regarded French appliance maker, used thin metal strips as mobilization assists in his braces.

Although plaster of Paris was used in 970 in Persia, it was not accepted until the mid-1800s in Europe or slightly later in America, where it was viewed with

---

¶References 13, 14, 40, 43, 72, 74, 165.

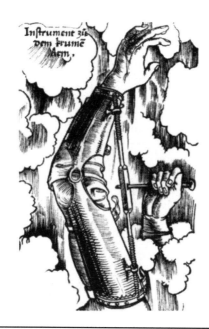

Fig. 1-2   Elbow extension mobilization splint, type 1 (2)
A turnbuckle provides incremental adjustments in this 1517 splint.
(From LeVay D: *The history of orthopaedics*, Parthenon, 1990, Park
Ridge, NJ.)

disfavor by influential surgeons. Early disadvantages included prolonged set-up time and lack of a suitable latticing fabric.

By 1883, surgeons and appliance makers had become fiercely competitive, with surgeons feeling that appliance makers were only "useful if kept in their place." The surgeon/appliance-maker schism deepened and the two parties diverged, becoming independent factions for brace fabrication. Both disciplines had talented devotees.

In 1888, F. Gustav Ernst, an appliance maker, published a book[64] describing and illustrating sophisticated splints for treating upper extremity problems. These included a splint to support a paralyzed arm using a combination of gun-lock and centrifugal springs; a supination splint with ball-and-socket shoulder movement, with a set screw to prevent rotation, rack-and-pinion elbow extension, and a two-piece forearm trough with rotation ratchet movement for supination; a rack-and-pinion elbow and wrist flexion contraction splint with ratchet movement wrist rotation; and a spring-driven wrist splint for wrist paralysis. It also included, for Dupuytren's disease, a

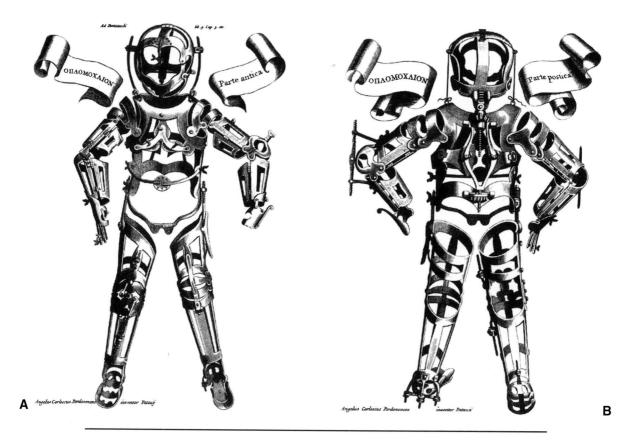

Fig. 1-3   Fabricius' 1592 illustration depicts **(A)** front and **(B)** back of armor-based splints for multiple parts of the body. (From Hieronymus Fabricius: *Opera Chirurgica*, Bolzetti, 1641, Patavii, Italy, in the collection of the Army Institute of Pathology. Reprinted from American Academy of Orthopaedic Surgeons: *Orthopaedic appliances atlas*, vol. 1, JW Edwards, 1952, Ann Arbor, MI.)

rack-and-pinion finger extension splint, a single finger extension flat spring splint, a palmar retention splint, and a pistol-shaped splint for slight cases.

At the same time, Hugh Owen Thomas, a British surgeon, identified principles of treatment and devised, among others, an inexpensive femoral splint and an ambulatory hip splint that allowed rest and outpatient treatment. Sir Robert Jones wrote of Thomas's splint workshop,

> There was a blacksmith at work in a smithy, a saddler finishing off the various splints, and duties of others were the making of adhesive plasters and bandages and the preparation of dressings. There were splints of every size to suit any possible deformity that might appear or for any fracture that might have occurred.[106]

Thomas's successful splinting endeavors spurred on the rapidly developing era of surgeon-fabricated splints and braces. In 1899, Alessandro Codivilla, an orthopedic surgeon in Italy, identified the importance of eliminating contractures prior to rebalancing with tendon transfers, foreshadowing the important contemporary partnership between surgical procedures and splinting.

In America, surgical methods were expanding, and surgeons were moving beyond being just "bone setters," "sprain rubbers," and "bandagists." By the 1880s, the importance of rehabilitation after treatment was beginning to be recognized and orthopedics, as a specialty arena, was gradually assuming autonomy from general surgery. By the early 1900s, plaster of Paris had widespread acceptance as a medium for immobilizing fractures.

■ THE DEVELOPMENT OF SPLINTING PRACTICE IN THE 20TH CENTURY

Many factors combined to shape evolving theory and practice. These included, but were not limited to, disease, political conflict, advancements in medicine and technology, agency and organizational decision-making, centers of practice, and availability of information. Although these factors are discussed separately in the following review of 20th-century events, many overlap and intertwine over time.

Disease and Epidemiology
Infection
Wound infection was a major problem during the first four decades of the 20th century. Seemingly inconsequential trauma to a hand could lead to serious infection, and without the assistance of antibiotics, treatment results were unpredictable. In his 1916 book, *Infections of the Hand*, Kanavel[95] grouped infections into two categories: simple, localized infections;

and grave infections, including tenosynovitis and deep fascial-space abscesses in one subgroup and acute lymphangitis in another. This book of almost 500 pages was important in that Kanavel defined the critical associations between synovial sheaths and fascial spaces. Case studies illustrated the dire consequences of poorly treated hand injuries, including that of a man who died from palmar scratches sustained from rubbing meat; a man who bruised his thumb getting off a streetcar and died of staphylococcus/streptococcus-related pneumonia; and a woman with arthritis who died from undiagnosed wrist infection of unknown etiology. Each of these patients presented with extensive local swelling, redness, and pain; septicemia or toxemia developed; and death occurred within 4 to 5 weeks. Kanavel noted that the age of patients who died averaged 43.8 years.

Differentiating between non-lethal swellings, as with thrombophlebitis or arthritis, was difficult, and failure, by the patient or the physician, to comprehend the potential seriousness of a problem could lead to the patient's untimely death. Although little is mentioned about splinting in his 1916 book, by 1924 Kanavel strongly advocated splinting in the functional position as one of the most important factors in successful treatment of infected hands.[96,97] Because the sequela of extensive infection was substantial restrictive scar, he also employed elastic traction splints to correct soft tissue contractures after infection was resolved.

Poliomyelitis
Identifying the underlying symptomatology and etiology of poliomyelitis spanned nearly two centuries of study. Although they were described by Michael Underwood, a British physician, in 1774,[113] it was not until 1840 that Jacob Heine, a German physician, identified the inconsistent presenting symptoms of poliomyelitis as manifestations of a single disease process. Twenty years later, in 1860, Heine defined standards of treatment management for "spinal infantile paralysis" victims, which were based on his experience. He advocated splinting, baths, and tenotomies, if needed. He also differentiated polio from spastic paralysis.[111]

In 1890, Swedish pediatrician Oscar Medin confirmed that polio was infectious and described anterior horn cell inflammation and tract degeneration as the cause of the weakness and paralysis that accompanied it.

Although the first outbreak of polio in the United States occurred in Louisiana, in 1841, the first epidemic happened in 1894, in Vermont. The first polio pandemic began in Scandinavia in 1905, eventually spreading to New York City and Massachusetts in 1907.

In 1916, the first major epidemic in the United States occurred, with 8,900 new polio cases and 2,400 deaths reported in New York City alone.[145] Epidemics were reported in 1909 and then in 1912, 1916, 1921, 1927, 1931, and 1935. By 1942, there were 170,000 polio victims in the United States. In the majority of these patients, onset occurred between 1906 and 1939.[113]

Frighteningly, the magnitude of the epidemics increased as time passed. The 1933 epidemic resulted in 5,000 new polio cases. Ten years later, in the epidemic of 1943, new cases rose to 10,000. By 1948, 27,000 new cases were reported; in the epidemic of 1950, the number of new cases was 33,000.[145] By the mid-1950s, with a peak of 57,879 new cases of poliomyelitis in the United States in 1952[48] and a 1955 baseline annual morbidity of 16,316,[99] polio had become the major focus of national rehabilitation and research resources.

Development of the iron lung* in 1928 increased polio survival rates and amplified demand for rehabilitative procedures. Large centers like those in Warm Springs, Ga. (1926), Gonzales, Tex., and Rancho Los Amigos, Calif. (1949), became important hubs for research and treatment of poliomyelitis, and their developing orthotic departments were recognized for the splints and braces they created.[113,145,178,179] Some centers were so well known that splints made by these centers were identifiable solely by their configural characteristics (Fig. 1-4). Advancements were also made in tendon transfer theory and technique for rebalancing involved joints and restoring function to paralyzed extremities.

Early on, splinting was a critical factor in the treatment of poliomyelitis. Therapists who worked with patients with upper extremity polio needed in-depth knowledge of anatomy, kinesiology, and the deforming factors of pathology and substitution patterns, since these patients had widely varied patterns of muscle involvement.

During the preparalytic and paralytic stages of polio, splints were used to put muscles in neutral balance to prevent overstretching. Positions favoring maximal return of function were prescribed. For the upper extremity, to protect the deltoid muscles, shoulders were positioned with bed sheets, pillows, and sandbags in the "scarecrow" attitude, with 90° humeral abduction and external rotation and 90° elbow flexion. Splints were used to maintain forearms in 75% supination, wrists in dorsiflexion, fingers in slight flexion, and

*Webster's *Third International Dictionary* defines the iron lung as "a device for artificial respiration in which rhythmic alternations in the air pressure in a chamber surrounding a patient's chest force air into and out of the lungs, especially when the nerves governing the chest muscles fail to function."[168]

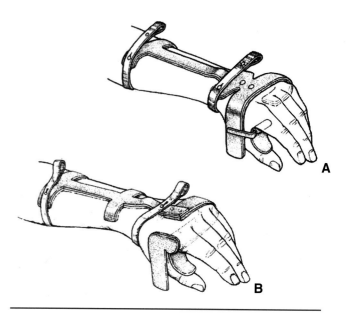

Fig. 1-4   Thumb CMC palmar abduction and MP extension immobilization splint, type 1 (3)
A, Rancho Los Amigos splint, **B,** Bennet splint (Warm Springs). Although they have different configurations, these two splints have the same expanded Splint Classification System designation, because their functions are identical.

thumbs in opposition. Shoulder internal rotation and external rotation positions were alternated to prevent stiffness in either position. Metacarpophalangeal (MP) joints were splinted in extension so that the finger flexors would be used instead of the intrinsic muscles (Fig. 1-5). If proximal interphalangeal (PIP) hyperextension occurred, elastic traction was applied, with attachment to the fingertips by thimbles or woven "Chinese finger-traps."[113,152]

Kendall advocated different shoulder, forearm, and finger MP joint positions, with 75° shoulder abduction (Fig. 1-6), forearm neutral, fingers slightly flexed, and thumb in palmar abduction.[98] Prevention of deformity was so strongly emphasized that the extremities and torsos of some patients were encased in plaster to prevent overstretching of critical muscle groups.

Sister Kenny, a controversial figure in Australia, promoted use of hot packs instead of splints for polio patients. Dismissing completely the traditionally held view that muscle imbalance was the cause of deformity in polio patients, she taught that deformity arose from muscle spasm. In 1935, a royal Australian commission found against Kenny's methods; so in 1940, she moved to the United States, where she found a more accepting climate. Although it is now generally agreed that her methods had no effect on residual paralysis,[111] Sister Kenny was a major influence in polio treatment in the United States. Many polio treatment centers eventually assumed a

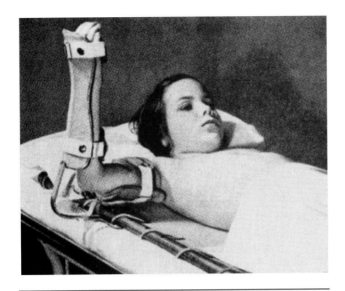

Fig. 1-5   Shoulder abduction and neutral rotation, elbow flexion, forearm supination, wrist extension, index–small finger MP extension, thumb CMC palmar abduction and MP extension immobilization splint, type 0 (10)

This 1942 splint for a patient with polio immobilizes all the joints of the upper extremity except the finger and thumb interphalangeal joints, to provide neutral muscle balance. (From Lewin P: *Orthopedic surgery for nurses, including nursing care,* WB Saunders, 1942, Philadelphia.)

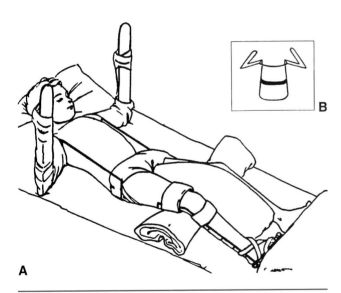

Fig. 1-6   Shoulder abduction and neutral rotation, elbow flexion, forearm neutral, wrist extension, index–small finger flexion, thumb CMC palmar abduction and MP-IP extension immobilization splint, type 0 (19)

A, These 1939 polio splints differ slightly in that they maintain the shoulders in 75° abduction, the forearms in neutral, and the fingers in flexion. **B,** Wire frame for splints. (From Kendall H, Kendall F: *Care during the recovery period in paralytic poliomyelitis,* rev. ed., Public Health Service, 1939, Washington, DC.)

middle-of-the-road approach, using both hot pack and splint interventions.

During the convalescent and chronic stages of polio, as weakness and loss of motion became apparent, splinting goals changed. Maintaining muscle balance and encouraging predetermined joint stiffness to enhance function became the primary focuses of splinting. Positioning was determined by individual patient requirements. If the extrinsic finger extensors were weak, the MP and interphalangeal (IP) joints were splinted in extension. Splints were fabricated from wire or plaster of Paris. Restricted passive range of motion slowed development of joint stiffness. Corrective splinting was used to increase range of motion of stiff joints in order to increase function and improve range of motion for tendon transfers. Therapy often lasted 2 to 4 years.[98]

Jonas Salk's inactivated-virus vaccine, in 1955, and Albert Sabin's oral vaccine, in 1961, resulted in the eventual eradication of poliomyelitis in the United States. By 1960, the incidence of polio had decreased by 90%, and after 1961, the incidence was less than 10%. The last case of polio in the United States from wild virus, not stemming from vaccination, occurred in 1979.[48,145]

Upper extremity splinting continued to play an important role in the treatment of the aftereffects of poliomyelitis:

> Advances in [orthotics] leading to greater functional capacity of the paralyzed upper extremities came after the discovery of the polio vaccine. This came, in part, from a lessening of the demands of acute and convalescent care and the fact that by this time the physician had learned to keep these very severely involved patients alive.[19]

Splints that aided hand and wrist function were often paired with overhead suspension slings, ball-bearing feeders, or walking feeders for shoulder, elbow, and forearm positioning, allowing functional movement of extremities against gravity (Fig. 1-7).[20,61,145] Although leather hand-based splints were used for thumb or isolated finger positioning, most splints were fabricated in metal and had narrow bar configurations. Digital mobilization assists and wrist stop or spring mechanisms were incorporated as needed. Splints often served as bases for activities-of-daily-living (ADL) attachments, and as rehabilitation measures became more sophisticated, vocational activities were emphasized.[20] The intent was to make polio patients as independent as possible.[61]

Political Conflict and War

It has long been acknowledged that declared armed hostile conflict between political states or nations has often accelerated advances in medicine and

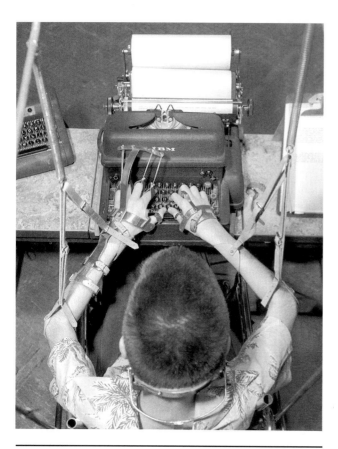

Fig. 1-7 *Left,* Wrist extension, thumb CMC palmar abduction and MP extension immobilization / index–small finger MP-PIP extension mobilization splint, type 0 (11). *Right,* Index-small finger MP flexion restriction / thumb CMC palmar abduction and MP extension immobilization splint, type 0 (6)
Paralysis and weakness aftereffects of polio were often asymmetric, requiring different splints for upper extremity function. (From March of Dimes, archive no. G528.)

development of technology. As medical and technologic changes occur, splinting practice also changes.

Medical Advances Relating to Splinting

Despite the fact that one ninth of all wounds recorded by the Union Army involved the hand and wrist, little attention was given to surgical or rehabilitation procedures for the hand in the official medical and surgical documentation of the Civil War (1861-65). In the official record of surgical procedures for hand injuries in World War I (1917-18), mention was also notably sparse.[8] Gunpowder had forever changed the profile of war injuries, producing wounds that involved massive soft tissue loss and were contaminated with bone fragments and foreign particles. During the Civil War, fear of infection led to the practice of amputating parts

sustaining gunshot wounds that resulted in comminuted fractures.

Joseph Lister's concepts of antisepsis for surgical procedures did not gain universal acceptance until 1877. Infection and the lack of understanding of the need for thorough debridement also plagued wound treatment in World War I. Primary versus secondary closure of wounds was just beginning to be understood by the end of the war, and penicillin would not become available until 1941. Hand injuries were considered minor in comparison with the morbidity-producing problems presented by rampant infection and gangrene.

During the period between the two world wars, general surgical practitioners who had no special knowledge of the hand were treating hand injuries. Flat splinting of fractures was prevalent, traction was often incorrectly applied, and burns were treated without asepsis despite groundbreaking contributions in the treatment of hand infections,[95] reconstructive surgery,[172] tendon repair and grafting,[122] and nerve repair.[37,105]

An important concept that would influence transfer of patients from battlefronts was reported by Trueta, in 1939—namely, that the pressure and immobilization provided by plaster casting promoted wound healing. He also observed that windows in casts caused swelling and edema that could lead to tissue necrosis and infection.[163]

During the early involvement of the United States in World War II, in contrast to previous war experience, the importance of treating hand and upper extremity trauma became apparent as casualties were assessed. Resulting data showed that 25% of all treated wounds involved the upper extremity, with 15% of these affecting the hand.

In 1943-44, at Letterman General Hospital (San Francisco, Calif.), a major debarkation hospital from multiple theaters of operations, delayed wound healing and infection were associated with the long time it took to transport the injured from the Pacific and the China-Burma-India theaters:

> Many patients had been treated with the banjo splint or with flat, straight board splints applied to the hand and wrist in the position of nonfunction. Both methods are equally undesirable and were responsible for many disabled hands.[138]

These difficulties were exacerbated by tropical diseases and metabolic problems.

Since hand and upper extremity injuries required combined knowledge from the surgical fields of orthopedics, plastics, and neurosurgery, a plan was devised to treat patients with hand trauma as a distinct group, to allow focused care. Specialized hand centers in the United States and Europe were established to treat hand and upper extremity trauma.

Appointed special civilian consultant to the Secretary of War in late 1944, Bunnell was given the task of developing and coordinating the Army's hand surgery efforts. His already-published book, *Surgery of the Hand,* became an official Army textbook.[56]

In an early report identifying problems of malunion, joint stiffness, inferior splinting, poor positioning, and ineffective wound coverage, Bunnell described commonly observed, incorrect ways of splinting the hand. He also defined the position of function as forearm neutral, wrist in 20° dorsiflexion and 10° ulnar deviation, fingers in slight flexion, with the index finger flexed the least and the small finger flexed the most, and the thumb in partial opposition with its joints partially flexed. Position of nonfunction was the opposite. He recommended splints for specific problems and emphasized the need for active, as opposed to passive, therapy and active use of the hand as a mainstay of good hand rehabilitation. Splints were constructed of wood, metal, wire, leather, plaster of Paris, and, occasionally, plastic.

In his report, Bunnell opposed "rough manipulation of finger joints," stating that it was more harmful than good.[35] In addition to outlining surgical repair and reconstructive procedures, Bunnell discussed the importance of good splinting and cautioned that improper splinting is harmful, and he dedicated multiple pages to the characteristics of good splints, fitting splints, splinting precautions, immobilizing and mobilizing splints, and splinting for specific problems.[35]

Bricker (March 1945), in the European theater of operations, outlined principles for managing combat injuries of the hand, including:

> Splint purposefully, maintaining the palmar arch and flexion of the metacarpophalangeal joints; use traction only when it is urgently indicated, and then for a minimum length of time; concentrate on maintenance of function as remains; institute active motion as early as possible and supplement by occupational therapy . . .[47]

In July 1945, Hammond listed nine concepts to improve hand care, with one of the nine being that "normal fingers should never be immobilized and should be moved for 10 minutes out of every hour, beginning immediately after the initial operation."[47]

In the United States, in the Zone of the Interior, Frackelton, at Beaumont General Hospital (El Paso, Tex.), noted that "segregation [of hand patients] permitted the proper supervision of corrective splinting and institution of physical and occupational therapy both before and after operation";[77] Hyroop, at Crile

General Hospital (Cleveland, Ohio), reported that "special types of splints were used in contractures, nerve lesions, ankylosed joints, and as part of pre-operative and postoperative therapy." He also noted that nerve repairs under tension were treated postoperatively with splints that allowed progressive motion.[90]

Littler, at Cushing General Hospital (Framingham, Mass.), described MP hyperextension contractures and collateral ligament shortening due to "secondary joint and tendon fixation" that severely hampered reconstructive procedures. These contractures required extensive surgical release "followed by elastic spring splinting with the wrist in extension, and early active exercise." Noting that "deformities of injured hands were common" and that "omission of splinting and improper splinting were very frequent causes," Littler went on to say,

> Corrective splinting was seldom necessary in hands on which protective splinting had been employed and for which persistent active and passive exercise had been undertaken . . . Appropriate protective splinting lessened functional disability and avoided the necessity for weeks of corrective splinting.[114]

Pratt, at Dibble General Hospital (Menlo Park, Calif.), reported that "no difficulty was experienced in combining the two principles of immobilization of the injured part and mobilization of uninvolved joints." He continued with a review of splints frequently used at Dibble, ranging from simple web straps for flexion to wrist immobilization with finger MP flexion assists.[139]

Barsky, at Northington General Hospital (Tuscaloosa, Ala.), also noted the problem of immobilization with the MP joints in extension, which allowed the collateral ligaments to contract. He noted that, to avoid this, the splinting principles of "Koch and Mason were followed with good results, and in the future the universal Mason-Allen splint should be standard equipment for all hand work." He also stated, "Where there was no demonstrable roentgenographic change, elastic splinting accomplished a great deal."[15]

Phalen, at O'Reilly General Hospital (Springfield, Mo.), found Bunnell's splints "very satisfactory," noting that the "spring wrist cock-up splint was particularly effective in relieving flexion contractures of the wrist." A *finger MP flexion, thumb CMC abduction splint* developed at O'Reilly was illustrated (Fig. 1-8).[137]

Graham, at Valley Forge General Hospital (Phoenixville, Pa.), reported that "it was the general rule to institute early motion and mobilization by activity and steady traction. Elaborate mechanical

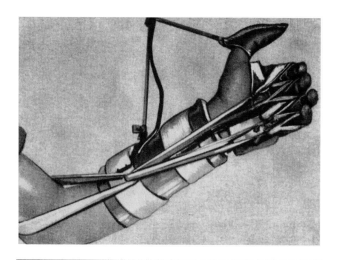

Fig. 1-8   Index–small finger MP flexion, thumb CMC radial abduction and MP-IP extension mobilization splint, type 1 (8), with triceps strap
A triceps strap keeps the MP flexion and thumb abduction / extension directed mobilization forces from pulling the forearm trough distally on the arm. (From Bunnell S: *Surgery in World War II: hand surgery*, Office of the Surgeon General, 1955, Washington, DC.)

splints and appliances were not used for this purpose." Instead, Bunnell knuckle benders, traction gloves, flexion straps, and plaster casts with extension or flexion outriggers were applied. He noted that "traction alone was not adequate in contractures associated with adherent tendons; in these cases surgery was also necessary."[81]

Fowler, at Newton Baker General Hospital (Martinsburg, W.Va.), reported that "mobilization of stiff metacarpophalangeal joints was good" using traction applied by Bunnell knuckle benders or plaster casts with wire outriggers. "If traction succeeded, it was almost always successful within 3 weeks."[78]

Howard, at Wakeman General Hospital (Camp Atterbury, Ind.), stated that

> . . . splinting was a very important procedure in the treatment of hand injuries . . . Splints had to be individualized or they would fail to embody the proper principles to obtain the desired correction. Temporary splints were often made by the ward surgeon with plaster of Paris as a foundation, the attachments consisting of embedded wires or other metallic appliances. The corrective type of splinting consisted of slow, steady traction in the proper direction, with care taken to avoid undue strain on joints not immediately involved.[86]

Howard also cautioned that "forceful manipulation of any small joint of the hand was contraindicated. Prolonged forceful elastic splinting could cause equal damage to small joints."[86]

There is no question that Bunnell set the standard for using hand splints in the treatment of hand trauma. His reports, bulletins, advice, and teaching, in

conjunction with those of other dedicated early hand surgeons, forever changed how hand and upper extremity trauma was managed. Although the splints he advocated may seem antiquated when compared with contemporary ones, most of the principles Bunnell defined nearly 60 years ago continue to be applicable today.

In 1947, on the basis of their experiences in World War II, Allen and Mason described a "universal splint" that they had used with approximately 90% of the hand injuries they treated during the war.[3] Following Kanavel's earlier proposal,[96] this splint maintained the hand in the functional position and could be used for either extremity after initial surgery. They had subsequently employed this "universal splint" in civilian service, and advocated its use for all stages of transport, under pressure dressings, and for a wide range of hand injuries including phalangeal and metacarpal fractures, but excluding tendon and nerve injuries, which require different positioning.

The fabrication of this universal splint was simple. Using a special concrete die, an aluminum sheet was hammered under "blow torch heat" into a molded cup configuration that supported the hand with a trough extension for the forearm. The dome shape was designed to support the arch of the hand, conform to the heel of the hand, and allow the thumb to rest in a "natural grasping position." Following industrial streamlining of fabrication processes, splints were made in two sizes (or three at most). Allen and Mason's "universal splint" became widely accepted as the preferred method for immobilizing the hand when a position of function was required (Fig. 1-9).

A few years later, during the Korean conflict (1950-53), the amputation rate had dropped to 13% (from 49% in World War II) because of improvements in arterial suture technique. "Reconstruction . . . became the treatment of choice for arterial injuries, and these ceased to be a major indication for amputation."[111]

Although more upper extremities were saved, splinting practice did not mirror advances in vascular technique. Problems due to poor splinting methods, similar to those encountered in World War II, arose. In 1952, Peacock wrote:

> Unfortunately, the condition of some of the men from Korea with hand injuries arriving at this Hand Center has re-affirmed the lessons learned in World War II—namely, that improper splinting results in serious deformities which often require months of corrective splinting and operative intervention.[136]

His article on plaster technique for mobilization splinting detailed methods for constructing effective splints that were independent of the services of a

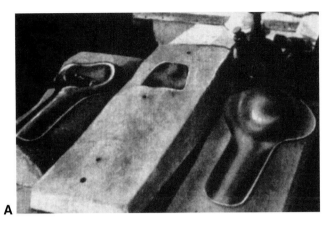

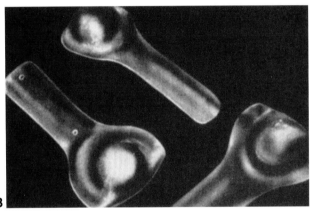

Fig. 1-9   Index, ring–small finger MP abduction, index–small finger flexion, thumb CMC palmar abduction and MP-IP extension immobilization splint, type 1 (16)

A, Cement molds. **B,** Aluminum splints. Allen and Mason's "universal splint" for immobilization of the hand maintained a functional position of the wrist, fingers, and thumb. The dome configuration of the finger pan held the finger MP joints in 30°-40° flexion, and the slight abduction of the fingers helped maintain some extra MP collateral ligament length of the index, ring, and small fingers but not of the centrally located long finger, which was not abducted. (From Allen HS, Mason M: A universal splint for immobilization of the hand in the position of function, *Q Bull Northwest University Med School,* 21:220, 1947.)

brace maker, providing busy community surgeons with viable alternatives.

By the time the United States became involved in the Vietnam conflict (1960-71), vascular repair was routine. With better surgical skill, improvement in antibiotics, more rapid evacuation of the injured, and better equipment, the amputation rate after vascular repair dropped to 8.3%. Internal fixation came into greater use, considerably changing the philosophy of how fractures were treated.[111] Fewer amputations and better fixation of fractures meant that more combat injuries were candidates for rehabilitation. Although splinting concepts defined in World War II and

reinforced in the Korean War remained for the most part unchanged, patients arrived in therapy departments in better condition, with fewer contractures from incorrect positioning.

The Brook Army Hospital Burn Unit contributed critical information on the treatment of burn patients, influencing all hand rehabilitation endeavors with their sophisticated understanding of antideformity position splinting and the importance of MP flexion and IP extension positioning. Progress in upper extremity tendon and nerve repair technique improved results of surgical reconstruction.

Technologic Advances Relating to Splinting

Technologic advances, for the most part, involve improvements in materials used to fabricate splints. Military-generated, high-technology materials eventually found their way into the civilian milieu, enhancing daily life in many arenas, including medicine.

As noted previously, gunpowder prompted the armor makers' precipitous change of vocation from producing suits of armor to creating specialized "appliances," and metal splints came into common usage, a definite improvement over previous fiber-based materials. Plaster of Paris changed how war wounds were treated in World War I, and by World War II and the Korean War, plaster had become an important foundation material for splint fabrication. The use of a given material often overlapped in time that of others. From the 1900s to today, there was no time frame during which only one material was available for splinting purposes (Fig. 1-10).

Beginning with World War I, the aeronautic field has been a major source of technologic development, with its ever-evolving pursuit of materials that reduce structural weight. The first all-metal, aluminum skin airplane flew in World War I. A few years later, in 1924, Kanavel described several aluminum hand splints,[96] introducing an innovative, durable, light-weight splinting material that would reign supreme for more than 40 years.

By 1934, aluminum alloy planes were prevalent and aluminum was commercially available. The relative ease of making aluminum splints facilitated acceptance of the material. Koch and Mason described a wide range of aluminum splints in 1939. Interestingly, because of Koch and Mason's experiences with plaster and leather splints, their aluminum splint designs more closely resembled contemporary splints, with their wide area of applications, than the eventual narrow bar configurations with which aluminum is generally associated.

Later, near European battlefronts during World War II, the military connection came full circle when

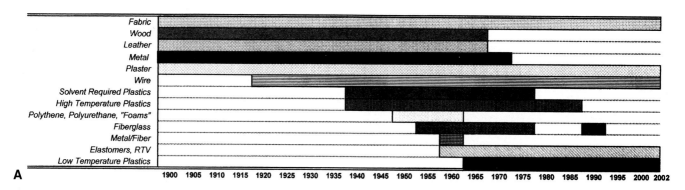

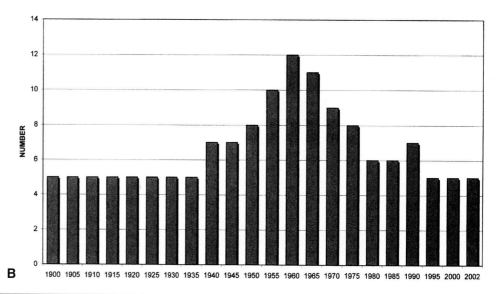

Fig. 1-10   **A,** Splinting materials reported in use between 1900 and 2002, in 5-year increments. The graph shows overlap in time, illustrating the multiple material options available in each 5-year period. **B,** Number of splinting materials reported in use between 1900 and 2002. With the introduction of plastics and the continuing development of material science, the available types of materials increased markedly, beginning in 1940-45 and peaking in 1960-65. After this, a gradual decline of material types occurred as low-temperature thermoplastics prevailed.

aluminum salvaged from downed planes provided a ready source of splinting material for frontline medical units. Aluminum allowed individual fitting and was easily sterilized[2]—both important factors in a war environment.

Aluminum and aluminum alloys were the materials of choice from the late 1940s through the 1960s,* playing a major role in the treatment of polio patients.[20,61] Although few therapists fabricate aluminum splints today, some commercially available components are made of aluminum alloys, and aluminum continues to be a staple for many orthotists.

---

*References 22, 35, 40, 42, 51, 53, 63, 112, 121, 130, 167.

The "plastics" revolution began in the late 1800s and early 1900s with the development of celluloid and Bakelite. The 1930s produced acetylene and ethylene polymers, and the 1950s brought urethanes and silicones.[111] Early plastics were important in the rapidly developing field of aeronautic technology, and a number of aircraft with primitive plastic-wood composite materials were introduced in the late 1930s and 1940s.[62] During World War II, plastics played a role not only in the reduction of airplane and vehicle weight, but also in the creation of parachutes and body armor, in the form of nylon and fiberglass, respectively.

The use of plastics for splinting hand injuries began in the late 1930s and early 1940s. In 1941, Marble described a new plastic material, Thermex, that could be heated and formed and reheated, noting that the surgeon should select the material best suiting the need.[120] Celluloid, when heated, produced simple one-plane-curve splints, but two curves required that the celluloid be cut into strips, heated, and cemented with acetone. Other plastic splint materials of the era included acetobutyrate, cellulose acetate, and Vinylite. In industrial settings, pressure and heat forced these materials to flow conformingly into dies, but the materials could also be shaped by hand using high-temperature heat and molds.

Like later high-temperature plastics, these early materials could not be fitted directly to patients. Bunnell reported that

> A strip of Vinylite softened at one end by immersing in heavy lubricating oil heated over a hot plate to 350°F is quickly laid on a form and pressed about it with a pad of cloth. It hardens at once and can then be trimmed on a bench grinder.[40]

Barsky, in 1945, designed a clear plastic splint to immobilize a thumb 3 weeks after bone and skin grafting procedures (Fig. 1-11). The splint, which was fabricated by the dental department of Northington General Hospital, was designed to protect the thumb until sensation returned.[15] Barsky's plastic splint was unusual, given that most splints were constructed of metal or plaster during World War II.

World War II ended, the Cold War began (1947), and within a few years the United States was involved in the Korean War. Plastics technology continued to evolve in the aeronautic and combat arenas, and new, more sophisticated plastic materials found their way into the commercial market. Although none of these materials was developed specifically for hand splinting endeavors, their considerable allure stemmed from their potential to improve wearability and decrease splint fabrication time in comparison with metal splints.

Celastic, an early plastic composite, was used as a splinting material for about 15 years, beginning in the mid-1950s. It harkened back to celluloid in that it had to be soaked in acetone to initiate curing. Celastic was available in several thicknesses and could be softened again after curing, so corrections and adjustments were feasible. If needed, metal reinforcements could be added as layers were applied. It could be fabricated on a mold or directly on a patient whose skin was protected with several layers of stockinette.[22,42,124,125,130] Although it quickly became obsolete with the introduction of high-temperature thermoplastics, Celastic was important because it was one of the earliest plastic splinting materials readily available to therapists.

Plastic foams of varying levels of rigidity were briefly advocated as splinting materials. At first they were fused to other materials, including elastic wraps[21] and plastics. In 1954, a British physician advocated fused polythene (polyethylene) and

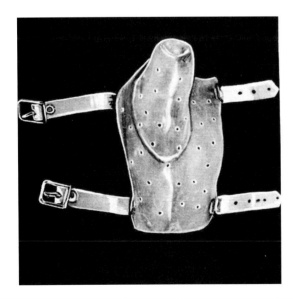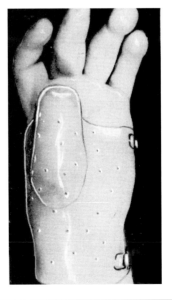

Fig. 1-11   Thumb CMC palmar abduction and MP-IP extension immobilization splint, type 1 (4) This thumb protector splint, circa 1945, is made of a high-temperature thermosetting material. (From Bunnell S: *Surgery in World War II: hand surgery*, Office of the Surgeon General, 1955, Washington, DC.)

polyurethane for hand, foot, neck, and torso splints.[30,31] Beginning as separate sheet materials, the polythene and polyurethane were heated together in a special oven to 120° C, at which time the polythene softened and fused to the polyurethane. The heated fused materials were quickly fitted directly to the patient with the heat-resistant polyurethane side next to the skin, acting as a protective barrier. These splints were lightweight, durable, and impervious to moisture and secretions, but they lacked the close contouring capacity of plaster-of-Paris splints, their greatest market rival.

A few years later, plastic foams were used as freestanding splint materials. Durafoam was a thermosetting plastic substance that, when activated with its catalyst in a special plastic bag, produced a plastic foam that remained malleable for approximately 15 minutes. To form it into a flat sheet, the foam, in its plastic bag, was rolled smooth with a rolling pin and then cut, following a predrawn pattern, while still warm from the catalytic reaction. The cutout splint was then applied directly to the patient and held until it cooled and became rigid.[161] Eventually, in the early 1960s, Durafoam was sold in prefabricated sheets, but it quickly became evident that this material was more appropriate for adapting ADL equipment than for splinting hands.[129]

Illustrating the level of creativity that exemplified the times, Fuchs and Fuchs, in 1954, reported using toy Erector Set parts for splint construction! Providing almost endless adjustment possibilities, these metal pieces were assembled into an array of fitted splint components, including outriggers, forearm bars, connector bars, and palmar bars. The authors noted that a wrist mobilization splint of Erector parts required about 45 minutes to construct. They also thoughtfully provided part numbers of the most frequently used pieces to facilitate ordering from the Erector Set catalogue.[79]

Fiberglass, incorporated in military flak jackets in the late 1940s, found increasing use in automotive components, beginning with the 1953 Corvette with its first-ever plastic composite skin.[62] Fiberglass, in the form of Air-Cast, Orthoply, and Ortho-Bond, was used as a thermosetting splinting material in the mid-1950s to early 1960s.[22,130] It did not gain wider acceptance as a splinting material,[124,125,150] however, until 1964, during the Vietnam conflict, when the U.S. Army Surgical Research Unit, Brook Army Hospital, advocated the use of fiberglass splints for burn patients treated with the open-air (exposure) technique,[166] which was associated with the use of topical antibacterial agents such as sulfamylon cream.[32,33,177]

Fiberglass was lightweight, durable, nontoxic, and resistant to chemicals, and it could be autoclaved, an important feature in decreasing sepsis in burn patients. To make the required negative plaster bandage mold, a normal subject with a similar-size hand first had to be found. Two key measurements were matched between the patient and the normal subject—the breadth of the palm at the distal palmar crease, and the distance between the distal wrist flexion crease and the distal palmar flexion crease over the fifth metacarpal.[177]

A half-shell plaster cast that incorporated the fingers, thumb, wrist, and forearm in the "antideformity position" was prepared on the normal subject. The cured negative plaster cast was removed from the subject's arm, dipped in paraffin, and cooled, providing a separating layer for the fiberglass, which was applied next. After the fiberglass mat was cut to the size of the plaster negative, it was laid on the mold and infused with a thick liquid polyester resin by use of a stiff brush, which pushed the resin into the mat and forced it to contour to the negative cast. When the fiberglass cured, in about an hour, the splint was removed from the plaster negative and hand-sanded to smooth its edges and surfaces. A set of splints was made for each burned extremity, providing a wear-autoclave rotation of sterilized splints.

The combination of open treatment with antibacterial agents and fiberglass splints was adopted by many burn centers throughout the United States during the late 1960s and early 1970s. With the introduction of low-temperature thermoplastics and changing philosophies on burn treatment,[141,169,170] use of fiberglass as a splinting material declined rapidly. Fiberglass was recommended in an updated, "bandage-roll" form in 1990 as a casting material for spasticity management.[67]

During the mid- to late 1950s, at about the same time that Celastic, plastic foams, and fiberglass were finding their way into therapy departments, Plexiglas, Lucite, and Royalite, all high-temperature thermoplastic materials, were well on their way to becoming important additions to therapists' splinting armamentaria.[22,130] Because of the inherent strength of these plastics, the narrow bar designs used with metal splints could also be used with splints fabricated with the new plastics. Dealing with commercial sources meant that sheets of plastic were available only in large sizes (e.g., 52 × 88 inches). Band saws were required for cutting splints from the sheets; edges had to be filed and sanded; therapists had to wear multiple pairs of cotton garden gloves to handle the hot material,[9] and fitting was done on a mold, not on the patient, because of the high temperatures required to make the plastics pliable. Despite all this, these high-temperature plastics were enthusiastically welcomed because of their relative ease of malleability and efficiency of construction in comparison with metal.

Experience determined that Royalite was more resilient than Plexiglas and Lucite, which tended to shatter with the cumulating forces accrued with wearing. At first, cutout splints were heated part by part as the fitting process progressed but this caused somewhat irregular contours as different splint components were heated and reheated.

Eventually it was discovered that an entire splint could be heated at one time in an oven, greatly reducing the heating time required using a heat gun. Therapists fabricating splints invaded ADL kitchens in therapy departments all over the United States, and the phrase "slaving over a hot stove" took on new meaning. Therapists also learned that the time-consuming construction of negative and positive molds could be eliminated entirely by fitting high-temperature thermoplastic splints directly on patients who were first protected with three or four layers of stockinette. Once removed from a patient's hand or arm, a still-warm splint needed only a few key adjustments to quickly obliterate the extra space caused by the multiple layers of protective stockinette.

On the global front, the Cold War had intensified with the successful launching of Sputnik 1 in 1957 and initiation of the space race. In 1959, the Soviet's Luna 1 unleashed the race for the moon, further escalating tensions between the United States and the Soviet Union. By the end of 1966, the United States' Surveyor 1 had landed on the moon; 3 years later, Neil Armstrong and Buzz Aldrin walked on the moon.

Plastics were critical to aerospace research because they lightened rocket payloads, and new developments continued to expand uses for plastics and plastic compounds. Materials became more and more sophisticated as job-specific plastic composites were created.

Splinting materials continued to evolve. Aluminum was relegated to splint reinforcement components, and solvent-requiring materials such as Celastic were abandoned in favor of the more practicable high-temperature thermoplastic materials. Therapists became adept at cutting out intricate bar configuration splints on band saws and decreased edge-finishing time to 3 or 5 minutes with a few well-chosen files. New high-temperature thermoplastic materials were assessed for their splinting potential as soon as they became commercially available, including Kydex, Lexan, Merlon, Boltaron, and high-impact rigid vinyl.[124,125,150] Royalite and Kydex eventually proved superior in their durability and relative ease of fabrication; they were used first as primary splinting resources and later, in the 1980s, for specialized narrow-splint components, such as outriggers, for which strength was essential.[74,162]

Although low-temperature thermoplastic materials were enthusiastically welcomed in the mid- to late 1960s, they had a rocky beginning. Prenyl[125,150] was unattractive, was difficult to conform to small areas of the hand, and required 10 minutes to harden; and the first Orthoplast, a beautiful plastic with a shiny slick surface, flattened with normal body temperature!

Bioplastic,[124,125,150] a thin, pinkish material with a smooth surface, was successful, and the era of low-temperature thermoplastic materials moved forward with smiles of relief. Bioplastic could be fitted directly on patients, and although it had no stretch and little strength, its easy workability made it an instant favorite. Orthoplast, first called Isoprene to differentiate it from the earlier failed material, was a tremendous success.* It emancipated therapists and patients from the protective gloves, stockinette, ADL kitchen ovens, and electric burners required to mold the high-temperature thermoplastic materials efficiently. Therapists quickly discovered that Orthoplast could be heated and held at a constant temperature in a dry skillet throughout an entire clinic day. This unexpected bonus significantly increased treatment efficiency by providing a constant source of heated material for use whenever needed. San Splint, a material similar to Orthoplast, was marketed in Canada.

To provide crucial strength, the low-temperature thermoplastic materials mandated different splint configurations. Of necessity, splint designs changed from narrow bar shapes to the contoured large contact area designs required for low-temperature material strength.

Still in the Cold War race for space, the 1970s brought additional moon landings, and in 1976, two space probes landed on Mars. In the 1980s, probes sent back photographs of Jupiter and Saturn, and the reusable space shuttles served as platforms for space research and deployment of satellites into orbit. Stealth technology, based on carbon-fiber composites and high-strength plastics, reduced radar signatures of combat aircraft.[62] Plastics had become a part of everyday life, both military and civilian, in the United States.

A new type of splinting material based on poly-caprolactones was introduced in the mid- to late 1970s. Providing greater conformability and ease of splint fabrication, the first of these new materials, Polyform and Aquaplast, although different from each other in chemical composition and working properties, were instant successes. Spin-offs from earlier

---

*References 50, 52, 72, 74, 124, 141, 150, 162, 170.

plastics research, these and most of the splint materials that followed were created specifically for the commercial splinting market. Kay Splint, Polyflex, and Orfit joined the ranks of available materials in the mid-1980s. The era of designer splinting materials had arrived.

By the early 1990s, new splinting materials proliferated, saturating the market and creating considerable bewilderment as to splint material properties and uses. Splinting material supply companies developed their own jargons and criteria for describing their individual products, further adding to the confusion. Breger-Lee and Buford's bioengineering studies of viscoelastic properties of 18 popular splint materials provided, for the first time, objective data regarding splinting material characteristics.[28,29] These studies are important in that they furnished factual information about materials, substituting for subjective opinion and vendor enthusiasm.

During the 20th century, major advancements in splinting material technology were accomplished. The rapidly escalating transition of materials—from natural-fiber-based materials such as wood and fabric, through metal and plaster, and eventually to a long line of progressively more sophisticated plastic-based materials—was unprecedented. These advancements were not the consequences of focused splinting-material-specific research but rather were by-products of the rapid developments in combat and aerospace technology through five different wars. It is interesting to notice that while materials changed dramatically, underlying design concepts remained surprisingly constant (Fig. 1-12).

Commercial Products

The link between military and commercial evolution is apparent throughout history. National research resources are first directed at societies' most pressing needs, and few conditions have greater priority than survival in war. Based on civilian need, commercial enterprise is an inexorable part of the natural progression of research development.

As the Cold War came to a close in 1990, a strong commercial contingent of multiple independent rehabilitation product supply companies was already well established, each with unique splinting material lines. Product research and development was, and continues to be, based on therapist feedback. With the exception of Orthoplast, which is an isoprene, or rubber-based material, most contemporary splinting materials are specialized blends of polycaprolactones, providing an almost endless array of potential splinting material properties.[101,164] In addition,

companies offer accessory products, such as strapping materials and fasteners, heating units, die cuts of common splints, prefabricated splints, published resource material, and knowledgeable resource personnel. Smaller companies market a wide range of splint components and prefabricated splints. Increasing accessibility of splinting materials is a key factor in the development and success of splinting endeavors.

Surgical Advances

Discussion of the progress in hand surgery over the last 100 years is a book unto itself and is not within the confines of this study. However, several types of surgical procedures have significantly influenced the course of splinting history during the past 50 years.

Introduced in 1966, Swanson silicone implants quickly became the hope of the future for many patients suffering from arthritis and for some who had sustained certain types of traumatic injuries to hand or wrist joints. Demand for the implants quickly escalated, as did need for the very specific postoperative hand splints that controlled the directional forces affecting joint encapsulation.[154-160]

The early passive motion program for zone II flexor tendon repairs described by Kleinert[45,102-104] was introduced at about the same time; and, later, Duran[60] published a different method for applying passive tension to repaired zone II flexor tendons. Each of these early passive motion programs had its own unique postoperative splint and follow-up routine, as did the two-stage flexor tendon repair described by Hunter in 1971.[87,88] The Kleinert and Duran concepts of early motion for tendon repairs was based on work done by Mason in the 1940s, in which a postoperative splint had also been recommended.[122]

All these surgical procedures depended on sophisticated, well-fitted splints to control the development of scar during the postoperative phases of wound healing. Inexperienced, inept, or unknowledgeable splint fabricators could not be tolerated, since the success of these surgeries relied heavily on correct application of the postoperative splints. Finding a capable and proficient splint maker suddenly became a priority for many hand surgeons.

Advances in Basic Science
Soft Tissue Remodeling

Soft tissue remodeling is a fundamental concept to splinting theory and technique that has been known

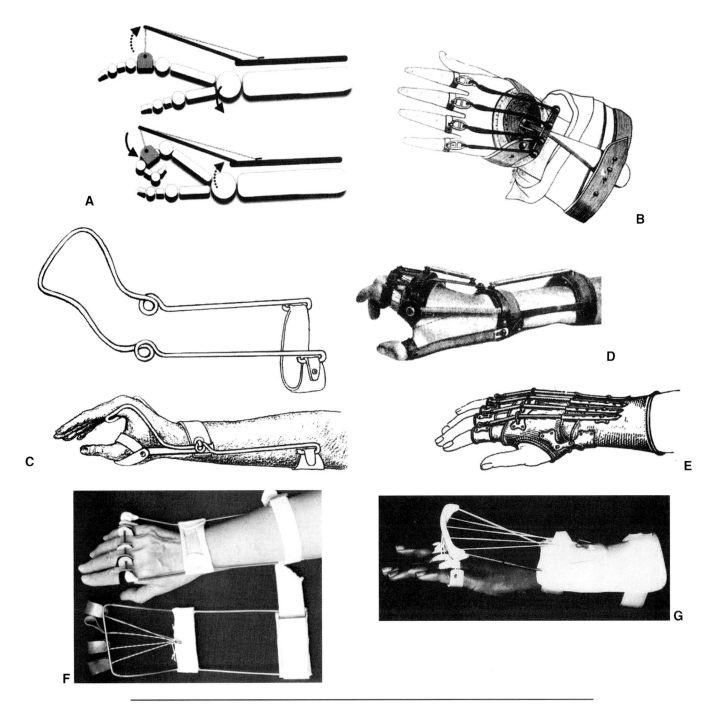

Fig. 1-12   A,B,F,G, Wrist flexion: index–small finger MP extension / index–small finger MP flexion: wrist extension torque transmission splint, type 0 (5) C,E, Wrist flexion: index–small finger MP extension / index–small finger MP flexion: wrist extension torque transmission / thumb CMC radial abduction mobilization splint, type 0 (6) D, Wrist flexion: index–small finger MP extension / index–small finger MP flexion: wrist extension torque transmission / thumb CMC radial abduction and MP extension mobilization splint, type 0 (7)

Splints from 1819 to 1987. Although they have different configurations, all these splints were designed for radial nerve problems, and all have similar Splint Classification names if the thumb is excluded. The splints use a pattern of reciprocal MP finger flexion to achieve wrist extension, and wrist flexion to achieve MP finger extension. Splints A, B (1819), F (1978), and G (1987) have the same Splint Classification System name. Splints F and G are identical except for the addition of a dorsal forearm trough component. Splints C (1916) and E (1919) incorporate the thumb CMC joint, and splint C assists the thumb CMC and MP joints. Splint D is from 1917. (A, B From LeVay D: *The history of orthopaedics*, Parthenon, 1990, Park Ridge, NJ; C-E From American Academy of Orthopaedic Surgeons: *Orthopaedic appliance atlas*, vol. 1, JW Edwards, 1952, Ann Arbor, MI; F From Hollis LI: Innovative splinting ideas. In Hunter JM, Schneider LH, Mackin EJ, Bell JA: *Rehabilitation of the hand*, Mosby, 1978, St. Louis; G From Colditz JC: Splinting for radial nerve palsy, *J Hand Ther* 1:21, 1987.)

empirically since ancient times. Slow, gentle, prolonged stress causes soft tissue to remodel or grow. In discussing treatment of contracted joints, Hippocrates wrote,

> In a word, as in wax modeling, one should bring the parts into their true natural position, both those that are twisted and those that are abnormally contracted, adjusting them in this way both with the hands and by bandaging in like manner; but draw them into position by gentle means, and not violently. . . . This then is the treatment, and there is no need for incision, cautery, or complicated methods; for such cases yield to treatment more rapidly than one would think. Still, time is required for complete success, till the part has acquired growth in its proper position.[172]

In 1517, Hans Von Gersdorff advocated gradual correction of joint contractures using splints with turnbuckles for incremental adjustments; in the mid-1870s, Thomas noted that

> Eccentric forms that cannot be altered in the dead body without rupture of fracture can, during life, be altered by mechanical influences as time and physiological action commode the part to the direction of the employed force.[111]

As marks of beauty, some native tribes insert progressively larger wooden disks into earlobes or lips, and other tribes gradually add rings to lengthen necks. Orthodontic dentistry is founded on soft tissue remodeling, and contemporary plastic surgeons routinely use tissue expansion techniques to cover soft tissue deficits. Bunnell wrote, "The restraining tissues must not be merely stretched, as this only further stiffens the joints by provoking tissue reaction."[36] Nearly all the surgeons who wrote splinting articles between 1900 and 1960 emphasized the need for slow, gentle traction to effect change in soft tissue.

For clinicians, use of soft tissue remodeling concepts seems to have an almost cyclic pattern of dismissal and rediscovery over time, depending on the most alluring treatment du jour. Through experience, clinicians (surgeons and therapists) learn the devastating consequences of forceful manipulation; they abandon these techniques in favor of slow gentle remodeling methods. Then time passes, and a new procedure is advocated for more rapid results. The procedure is applied, experience shows that the procedure either does not work or increases scar formation, and the cycle begins anew.

Bunnell obviously had a dismal encounter with therapy that was too aggressive. Throughout his distinguished career, he extolled the advantages of splinting and active use of the hand and emphatically condemned forceful manipulation,[35,37,38-42] stating that

the best therapist was a bilateral upper extremity amputee!

Knowledge is an ever-evolving process, and remodeling concepts are not relegated to the upper extremity alone. In fact, much of our empirical understanding of soft tissue remodeling is founded historically on experiences dating back to antiquity in the treatment of clubfoot deformity.[172] Over the centuries, while there were those who favored "bandaging" and noninvasive treatment, forceful manipulative and surgical correction of clubfoot deformity became increasingly fashionable with surgeons, and few questioned the results they obtained.

This, however, began to change in the late 1940s. Brand[24,27] has been instrumental in bringing biomechanical principles and soft tissue remodeling concepts and research to the arena of hand and upper extremity surgery and rehabilitation. It is insightful to learn of the pivotal experiences that forever altered his approach for managing soft tissue problems.

In 1948, Brand changed from the technique of treating clubfoot deformity practiced by Sir Denis Browne, a pediatric surgeon in England, to the total-contact plaster cast technique that Brand developed in India. In a recent letter to the author, Brand has elegantly described the early career experiences that led to his interest in soft tissue remodeling and deepened his understanding of this process.

This perceptive transition began when Brand had the opportunity to compare untreated clubfeet in India with feet treated by the Denis Browne manipulation technique in England. Although the feet treated by the English method were "straight," they were capable of little motion, and a noticeable inflammatory response persisted for years. This was in direct contrast to the untreated clubfeet in India, which retained suppleness and showed no inflammation, despite their lack of correct alignment.

Brand developed a method of serially applying total contact plaster casts that slowly and gradually brought a deformed foot into correct alignment by allowing soft tissues to remodel or grow. Brand's narration is fundamental to the tissue remodeling concepts on which splinting endeavors are based.[25] The full text of his important and astute letter appears in Section 2 of this chapter.

By 1949, Brand began applying the same contact casting techniques to the insensitive feet of leprosy patients. Brand's tissue remodeling work became more focused in the mid-1960s with his move to the U.S. Public Health Service Hansen's Disease Center, in Carville, La., where he continued to treat patients with Hansen's disease and where he started the biomechanics laboratory that would eventually receive worldwide acclaim. Brand's investigations into the bio-mechanical reaction of insensate living soft tissue to pressure opened a fountainhead of better understanding of soft tissue remodeling processes.

Others were also interested in soft tissue remodeling. In 1957, Neumann reported on expansion of skin using progressive distention of a subcutaneous balloon.[133] During the late 1960s and early to mid-1970s, Madden and Peacock described the dynamic metabolism of scar collagen and remodeling; and Madden and Arem noted that the response of noncalcified soft tissue to stress is modification of matrix structure, i.e., soft tissue remodeling.[7,116] In 1994, Flowers and LaStayo demonstrated that for PIP joint flexion contractures, the length of time soft tissues are held at their end range influences the remodeling process, with a 6-day time span resulting in statistically better improvement in passive range of motion than a 3-day span.[75]

While investigation continues into the histologic mechanism for remodeling of different soft tissues,* one area of agreement is apparent: application of too much force results in microscopic tearing of tissue, edema, inflammation, and tissue necrosis. Prolonged gentle stress is the key factor in achieving remodeling, and splinting is the only currently available treatment modality that has the ability to apply consistent and constant gentle stress for a sufficient amount of time to achieve true soft tissue growth.[73]

Digital Joint Anatomy and Biomechanics

Digital joint anatomy and biomechanics are better understood today than they were in the early 20th century. Kanavel's 1924 recommendation of the "functional position" for splinting infected hands, with the wrist in 45° dorsiflexion, the MP and IP joints in 45° flexion, and the thumb abducted from the palm and "rotated so that the flexor surface of the thumb is opposite the flexor surface of the index finger," was based on achieving rudimentary use of the hand following injury, "even though only a minimum of motion of the fingers and thumb is retained." He noted that "If such a splint were in universal use, much less would be heard of disability after hand infections."[96,97]

In the same year, Bunnell also advocated the use of the functional position.[36] The position of function subsequently was recommended by leading hand specialists for the next 40 years. During this time, hand surgeons consistently reported problems with MP extension/hyperextension contractures and IP flexion contractures, blaming the deformities on poor

splinting technique while at the same time continuing to recommend the "functional position" for hand injuries excluding tendon and/or nerve damage, which mandated other splint positions.

In 1962, James, discussing fractures of the fingers, reported that

> The metacarpophalangeal joints unless held in 60°-90° flexion during treatment will develop within two to three weeks a permanent extensor contracture, limiting flexion. The interphalangeal joints, particularly the proximal, rapidly develop flexion contractures when held in flexion . . .[92]

Based on empirical experience, Yeakel, in 1964, challenged the use of Allen and Mason's universal splint for "functional position" immobilization of hand injuries, advocating instead the "antideformity position" for the splinting of burn patients.[32,33,82,166,176,177] The University of Michigan Burn Center and Shriner's Burn Center also reported that "antideformity" splinting with burns was preferable to the "functional position."[107,166]

Researchers were also contributing to the growing body of knowledge.[93,94,173] In 1965, Landsmeer and Long published their decisive paper describing effects of a system of two monoaxial joints controlled by either a two-tendon or three-tendon unit, identifying the important interdependent roles of the extrinsic and intrinsic muscle systems.[108] Hand specialists began to regard the intercalated digital joints as functional units in which action at one or two joints affects the remaining joints or joint within the ray. James coined the phrase "safe position" in 1970, noting,

> The metacarpophalangeal joints are safe in flexion and most unsafe in extension; the PIP joints, conversely, are safe in extension and exceedingly unsafe if immobilized in flexion.[91]

The importance of maintaining collateral ligament length by splinting the MP joints in 70° to 90° of flexion and the IP joints in extension[107,170] had not been fully understood by early specialists, hence the earlier recurring problems with MP hyperextension and IP flexion contractures.

Variations of the "antideformity" splint usually involved minor changes in wrist or thumb position. Devised by deLeeuw, dress hooks glued to fingernails and hooked with rubber bands or sutures to the distal end of splint finger pans were important for achieving and maintaining the "antideformity position."[32,57] Advantages of the "antideformity/safe position" splint* quickly became apparent, and use of the "functional position" for patients with acute hand injuries was all but abandoned by the early 1970s.

---

*References 1, 18, 45, 73, 76, 127, 131, 132, 135, 140.

*Also called the "duckbill" or the "clam digger" splint.

Mechanical Systems of Splints

Mechanical systems of splints are alluded to or reviewed briefly by several early-20th-century authors, including Bunnell,[36,40] Kanavel,[96,97] and Koch.[106] Early splint manuals also dealt with basic concepts of leverage, pressure, and 90° angle of pull, but the information was inconsistently presented and sparse in comparison with the wealth of information on splinting materials and fabrication instructions. Despite being a major element of successful splint design and application, the principles of mechanics were addressed only superficially in related literature published prior to 1980.

Beginning in 1974, Fess applied mechanical concepts to common hand splint designs, identifying through trigonometry and simple scale drawings basic forces generated by splints.[10,68,70,72,74] Brand emphasized the importance of understanding splint biomechanics as they relate to critical soft tissue viability, responses to stress and force, inflammation and scar forming process, and tissue remodeling.[26,29] Van Lede and van Veldhoven integrated mechanical principles into a rational and systematic approach to creating and designing splints.[165] Boozer and others identified the important mechanical differences between high- and low-profile splint designs.[23,69,70] Brand[24,27] and Bell-Krotoski[17] emphasize the importance of understanding the transfer of forces in unsplinted joints when a splint is applied.

A thorough knowledge of mechanical concepts of splinting is requisite to treating hand and upper extremity dysfunction from injury or disease. More mechanical principles will be identified as splinting practice continues to evolve.

Agencies

The Office of Vocational Rehabilitation, the Department of Health, Education, and Welfare (DHEW), the U.S. Public Health Service, the National Research Council, the National Academy of Sciences, and the National Academy of Engineering are agencies that have at one time or another influenced the advancement of upper extremity splinting through their support and funding of related grants. The influence of these agencies has far-reaching ramifications, yet few clinicians are aware of the important contributions made by these powerful groups.

It is important to view historical events in context. Beginning at the end of World War I, vocational rehabilitation programs progressively expanded from aiding veterans to assisting civilians with disabilities (1920). By 1940, those who benefited from vocational rehabilitation services included persons in sheltered workshops, the homebound, and workforce personnel.

In 1950, Mary Switzer was named director of the Office of Vocational Rehabilitation. Switzer, an economist, career bureaucrat, and longtime advocate of rehabilitation concepts, demonstrated to Congress the economic advantages of rehabilitating the disabled rather than supporting them in long-term care facilities, noting that rehabilitated adults with disabilities become productive, tax-paying citizens.

During Switzer's 20-year tenure, funding for vocational rehabilitation increased 40-fold. Her vision included education of medical and rehabilitation professionals, research and development in medicine and rehabilitation engineering (Fig. 1-13), in-service training programs, and the establishment of rehabilitation centers and sheltered workshops.[58] While Switzer is acknowledged as the "grandmother" of the independent living movement, Brand notes that she is also the "mother and grandmother of much of the present concept" of hand centers in the United States.[26]

In 1939, in the midst of the devastating poliomyelitis epidemics that were sweeping the United States with ever-increasing virulence, the U.S. Public Health Service published bulletin no. 242, *Care During the Recovery Period in Paralytic Poliomyelitis*, by Kendall, Kendall, Bennett, and Johnson. This 29-cent monograph explained "the line of treatment required during the very long recovery period that follows an acute attack of infantile paralysis." In addition to treatment principles and detailed manual muscle testing instructions, positioning and splinting rationales were clearly defined, and practical shoulder, elbow, hand, and digital splints were described. Simple plaster splints for thumb palmar abduction, MP flexion, and wrist extension were illustrated, and drawings of heavy-wire-based shoulder abduction splints were included.

In a hand-written note, Florence Kendall recalls,

Mr. Kendall and I made (to the best of our knowledge) the first lumbricals cuff. It was made for a polio patient at Children's Hospital School in Baltimore, in 1933 (or 1934). In 1933, Dr. Jean McNamara from Australia showed us how she made an opponens cuff out of papier-mâché.

A training grant from the Office of Vocational Rehabilitation to Milwaukee-Downer College financially underwrote one of the earliest splinting manuals written by a therapist.[22] This important splinting manual, written in 1956 by Dorothy Bleyer, OTR, clearly validates that

the occupational therapist has been called upon professionally to fabricate splints and assistive devices as an aid to the patient for restoration or maintenance of function, correction of dysfunction, or substitution for normal function.

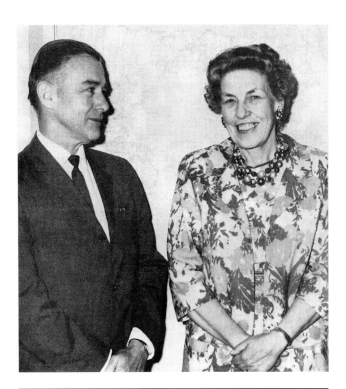

Fig. 1-13   Mary E. Switzer, commissioner of the Vocational Rehabilitation Administration, Department of Health, Education, and Welfare, visited the US Public Health Service Hospital at Carville, LA, on March 9, 1966, to talk to Dr. Paul Brand, Chief Rehabilitation Branch, about the combined research project proposed by the Carville hospital and Louisiana State University School of Electrical Engineering. The project involved three phases: (1) measure forces/pressures exerted to hands and feet by daily tasks; (2) identify a way of teaching patients with Hansen's disease to sense when they are using too much force and are risking injury; and (3) study the pathologic/histologic effects of bruising and damage to soft tissues of the hands and feet. This research was important not only for patients with Hansen's disease but also for patients with other diseases and injuries that resulted in diminished sensibility of the extremities. Switzer and Brand each received the renowned Lasker Award in 1960. Switzer was cited for her "great contributions to the training of rehabilitation personnel, rehabilitation research, and her success in bringing about greater cooperation between government and voluntary rehabilitation efforts." She was described as being the "prime architect of workable rehabilitation services." (*The Star* [Carville, LA], 25(4):1,7, 1966.)

She also warned that "the therapist must be careful not to become known solely as a splint or gadget-maker." The 85-page manual reviewed normal functional upper extremity anatomy, purposes of splinting, and precautions and gave detailed instructions for fabricating splints from a wide range of materials. The U.S. government openly supported this candid affirmation for therapists to actively embrace splinting endeavors.

In March and again in June 1967, the DHEW cosponsored, with Harmarville Rehabilitation Center and the Western Pennsylvania Occupational Therapy Association, a 2-day Institute and Workshop on Hand Splinting Construction[148] for physicians, therapists, and orthotists. Faculty included Edwin Smith, MD, Eleanor Bradford, OTR, Helen Hopkins, OTR, Maude Malick, OTR, Helen Smith, OTR, Major Mary Yeakel, AMSC, and Elizabeth Yerxa, OTR. Among those giving presentations, Yeakel, a research occupational therapist with the Army Medical Biomechanical Research Laboratory at Walter Reed Army Medical Center (Washington, D.C.), introduced the concept of materials science and discussed research in experimental media for splinting.

In 1967, the Committee on Prosthetic-Orthotic Education, National Academy of Sciences-National Research Council published the *Study of Orthotic and Prosthetic Activities Appropriate for Physical Therapists and Occupational Therapists.*[50] This study noted that

> Inasmuch as the total number of certified orthetists and prosthetists in this country (1,103) is relatively low and their distribution inequitable, it is realistic to expect that occupational therapists and physical therapists will frequently be called on to function in an area for which they may not be specifically prepared upon completion of their formal education program.

The report defined criteria that graduates of therapy programs should meet:

- Know the basic principles involved in prosthetics and orthotics, including anatomy, physiology, pathology, biomechanics, and kinesiology.
- Know basic terminology used in identification of prosthetic and orthotic devices and the components thereof.
- Know the mechanical principles on which operation of a device is based as well as the uses and limitations of various devices.
- Know properties and characteristics of materials used in fabrication of devices; know basis of selection of materials for specific purposes.
- Know the basic principles underlying the application of the following clinical activities regarding patients and device use—evaluation, training and patient education, maintenance, adjustments, and checkout performance.
- Appreciate contributions of other disciplines in these areas.

The study also noted that, "where orthotic service is not available, simple orthotic devices may be furnished by occupational therapists and physical therapists." Closing the door to orthotist-controlled splinting practice, this significant 1967 document freed therapists, as long as they were qualified, to provide splinting services to patients.

Funded by the DHEW and the Veterans Administration and compiled by the Committee on Prosthetic-Orthotic Education, National Academy of Sciences-National Research Council, *Braces, Splints and Assistive Devices: An Annotated Bibliography* was published in July 1969. This extensive work classified and briefly described articles about splints and orthoses of the neck and face, upper extremity, and lower extremity that had been indexed in *Index Medicus* from 1956 through 1968. Nearly 500 articles were indexed according to subject matter and author, creating a user-friendly reference document for clinicians interested in splinting.

In 1970, the First Workshop Panel on Upper Extremity Orthotics[51] of the Subcommittee on Design and Development, National Academy of Sciences, National Academy of Engineering, met to review the current status of upper extremity orthotic practice and design and development work and to discuss future design and development needs. The panel consisted of noted physicians, orthotists, therapists, and engineers in the field, including therapists Lois Barber, Kay Bradley (Carl), Clark Sabine, and Fred Sammons. Hand surgeon Mack Clayton was included on this panel. With orthotists from Rancho Los Amigos, Texas Institute for Rehabilitation and Research (TIRR), Rehabilitation Institute of Chicago (RIC), and New York University-Institute of Rehabilitation Medicine (NYU-IRM), a majority of the major orthotic facilities in the United States were represented.

After reviewing upper extremity orthotic practice for hemiplegia, quadriplegia, and arthritis, the panel considered future needs in design and development. Recommendations included the following:

- Initiation of a survey to determine the number of patients with hand disabilities, rehabilitation potentials for specific diagnostic groups (including peripheral nerve and burns), and available treatment.
- More studies on upper extremity/hand kinematics related to functional performance.
- Analysis of effectiveness of current educational programs.
- "Survey training programs for occupational therapists to determine the possible need for intensified or expanded educational efforts."

The DHEW, the Veterans Administration, and the National Academy of Sciences funded this panel.

In 1971, Mayerson's Splinting Theory and Fabrication workshop and accompanying manual were supported by a grant from the National Science Foundation and sponsored by the Department of Occupational Therapy, State University of New York (Buffalo, N.Y.). The introduction to the manual

quotes from the 1967 *Study of Orthotic and Prosthetic Activities Appropriate for Physical Therapists and Occupational Therapists,* indicating that therapy educational programs were taking the National Academy of Sciences study recommendations seriously. Mayerson also stated in the introduction that occupational therapists, in addition to the training they receive in medical subjects, are skilled in the use of equipment and materials needed to fabricate splints. Hand anatomy and kinesiology, materials science, splint checkouts, and detailed information on fabricating splints in various materials were included in this 114-page manual. The 1971 workshop and manual were based on a prior 1969 continuing education workshop on material science and splinting given by Mayerson at the same facility.

The Second Workshop Panel on Upper Extremity Orthotics[52] met in 1971 to review upper extremity orthotic management of rheumatoid arthritis, peripheral nerve injury, and thermal injuries and to discuss future design and development needs in these areas. Hand surgeon William Stromberg attended this meeting. Early discussion identified the important role orthotics play in postsurgical management of rheumatoid arthritis. The Swanson post-MP implant arthroplasty brace was prominently illustrated in the report.

The panel voiced divergent opinions on splint designs and materials for treating other problems in rheumatoid arthritis. Peripheral nerve injury orthotic intervention was also reviewed. Most panelists agreed that patients with unilateral lesions reject functional orthoses, and the long opponens splint was most frequently cited as the splint of choice for positioning in peripheral nerve injury. Many of the panelists opted for wrist-driven or finger-driven prehension orthoses for cases in which nerve regeneration was not possible.

Brook Army Burn Center treatment and splinting procedures were reviewed for thermal burn patients. Finger MP joint extension, IP joint flexion, and thumb adduction contractures were identified as the most common problems in burns. Subsequent panel recommendations included the following:

- Develop a method of evaluating the usefulness of splinting in rheumatoid arthritis
- Create a uniform evaluation system for rheumatoid hand and upper extremity functional status
- Establish a close liaison with the American Society for Surgery of the Hand and the American Academy of Orthopaedic Surgeons Committee on Prosthetics and Orthotics
- Conduct a literature search for information on the functional disabilities secondary to anatomic changes in the rheumatoid hand

- Continue concentrating on functional orthotic intervention for rheumatoid arthritis, peripheral nerve injury, and burns

The DHEW, the Veterans Administration, and the National Academy of Sciences funded this panel, noting that it addressed a problem of national significance.

Hand Centers

The establishment of hand rehabilitation centers advanced splinting practice in several ways. The high expectations of referring hand surgeons, therapist specialization expertise, and the sheer volume of patients treated in hand centers meant that therapists quickly honed their splint-fabricating skills to exceptional levels. With the demands of treating large numbers of complicated hand problems, therapists also became aware of the most efficacious splinting techniques, eliminating those that produced mediocre results. In addition, hand centers provided a forum in which clinicians, both surgeons and therapists, could share their experiences and learn from one another. It is difficult to isolate the sequence of hand center development and the role teaching played in that advancement, since they often serve in combined roles.

The first hand rehabilitation center in the United States—the hand center at the University of North Carolina, Chapel Hill—was started as a result of Erle Peacock's 1961 visit to Brand's New Life Center in Vellore, India, where patients with Hansen's disease were treated. Peacock was so impressed with Brand's specialized rehabilitation team concept that he returned to the United States with hopes of starting a hand center here.

The roots of the Chapel Hill center, however, extend further back in time than Peacock's Vellore visit. In 1960, Brand was in the United States to receive the prestigious Albert Lasker Award given by the International Society for the Rehabilitation of the Disabled.[109] At this time, he met Mary Switzer, Commissioner of the Vocational Rehabilitation Administration (VRA), who also received a Lasker Award. With many polio and war victims needing assistance, Switzer had convinced Congress of the importance of rehabilitation and in so doing had been named the first Commissioner of VRA. Brand and Switzer had the opportunity to discuss rehabilitation concepts at length, and she was impressed with his program in India.[16] After this meeting with Brand, Switzer began encouraging surgeons like Robinson and Peacock to visit Brand in India.[26]

On Peacock's return to the States from India, he met Howard Rusk and Mary Switzer in New York, and they encouraged him to submit a grant to start a hand center. In 1962, a 2-year research and demonstration grant for $10,000 from the Office of Vocational Rehabilitation was awarded for the establishment of a hand center, and the Chapel Hill Hand Rehabilitation Center became a reality.[59]

In 1967, Chapel Hill gave its first major course on upper extremity rehabilitation, followed in 1968 by a second course on hand rehabilitation.[59] In addition to intensive anatomy, physiology of wound healing, biomechanics, and kinesiology concepts, splinting theory and technique played an important role in these two seminars, which were taught by surgeons Peacock and Madden, therapists Hollis,[85] DeVore, Hamilton, and Cummings, and aide Denny. Working primarily in plaster, Hollis, DeVore, and Denny were exceptionally skilled splint fabricators, but more important was their understanding of the biomechanics and the transfer of force moments involved in splint application.

Acceptance criteria for the two Chapel Hill seminars were rigorous, and once accepted, participants faced daunting preconference reading assignments. Already working with hands, Mackin attended the 1967 Chapel Hill conference and Fess attended the 1968 conference. Mackin, with Hunter and Schneider, went on to establish the second hand rehabilitation center in the United States, the world-renowned Philadelphia Hand Rehabilitation Center.

The 1970s were a period of expansion for hand surgery and hand therapy. Although many surgeons constructed their own splints from the 1910s through the 1960s, both experienced and new hand surgeons in the 1970s became part of a different generation; these surgeons no longer made splints themselves. An ability to splint opened doors for therapists. Surgeons and therapists worked together to create better interventions for patients, including splinting procedures. Brand and Bell in Louisiana and Swanson and Leonard in Grand Rapids made important contributions to the rapidly growing splinting knowledge base. New hand centers began to flourish throughout the United States, with Nalebuff, Millender, and Philips in Boston, Strickland and Fess in Indianapolis, Petzolt and Kasch in California, Wilson and Carter in Arizona, Beasley and Prendergast in New York, and Burkhalter and Evans in Florida.

Others set up clinics in university settings or as independent freestanding enterprises; these clinicians included Brown in Atlanta, Olivett in Denver, Fullenwider in Seattle, Pearson in Florida, and Hershman in New Jersey. These surgeons and therapists were in cutting-edge clinical situations. They, along with many others, learned and shared their knowledge in turn, contributing to the evolving splinting technology through publications and teaching seminars.

Knowledge Dissemination and Organizational Leadership

Seminars and Educational Courses

Seminars and educational courses have always been crucial in the dissemination of splinting information. During the first 60 years of the 20th century, surgeons and orthotists presented papers on splinting design and fabrication at their professional conferences.* However, things began to change in the late 1950s, as therapists' contributions to splinting became increasingly acknowledged. Therapists and orthotists at major polio rehabilitation centers throughout the United States took on increasing teaching responsibilities as demand for information about splinting and bracing of polio victims increased.[98,113,145]

Invited at first to serve as faculty for seminars along with surgeons, therapists progressed over time to conducting independent, splinting-specific seminars. Yeakel and Mayerson's material science workshops of the late 1960s were key to disseminating information about new materials, especially plastics.[124,125,150] Malick taught extensively both nationally and internationally, moving from burn splinting to splinting concepts in general. Several generations of therapists grew professionally with Malick as their splinting mentor.

In 1976, the first Hand Surgery and Hand Rehabilitation symposium sponsored by the Philadelphia Hand Center featured the somewhat revolutionary format (for the times) of surgeons and therapists sharing the podium to address hand surgery and hand rehabilitation topics. Over the succeeding 26 years, the success of the Philadelphia seminar has reached unprecedented proportions. Each year, splinting theory, technology, and methods are showcased in lectures and in hands-on workshops. In addition, vendors are available to demonstrate the newest materials, ancillary splinting equipment, and literature resources.

During the second half of the 20th century, universities, professional organizations, other hand centers, individuals, and commercial vendors have all participated at various levels of intensity and frequency in splinting seminars. The demand for learning and improving splinting skills is ever present. At one end of the continuum, surgeons and therapists continue to advance their knowledge, and

new information often translates to new requirements for splinting. At the other end of the continuum, as each generation of therapists enters the clinic environment, practicing and upgrading splinting skills are important for continuing competency.

Professional Organizations

Professional organizations also helped extend splinting practice by supporting continuing education seminars, special interest groups, and informational publications that provided the latest splinting information to practitioners and researchers.[6,11,12] The American Academy of Orthopaedic Surgeons' 1952 *Orthopaedic Appliance Atlas*[5] and the 1982 *Atlas of Orthotics*[4] were important contributions to the standardization of splint language for the extremities.

Organizations also encourage research and define ethics of practice. The previously mentioned 1967 *Study of Orthotic and Prosthetic Activities Appropriate for Physical Therapists and Occupational Therapists,* by the National Academy of Sciences, involved representatives from the American Occupational Therapy Association (Hollis, Zimmerman, Kiburn), the American Physical Therapy Association, and the American Orthotics and Prosthetics Association. This report was an important factor in allowing therapists to fabricate splints for their patients.[50]

Specialty organizations such as the American Society for Surgery of the Hand (ASSH), the ASHT, and the American Association for Hand Surgery (AAHS) provide forums for education and research relating to upper extremity splinting practice. A key factor in defining and maintaining splinting competency, the Hand Therapy Certification Commission (HTCC) assesses therapists' knowledge of splinting theory and practice through carefully researched certification examination questions. While the HTCC certification examination encompasses a much broader scope of practice issues than just splinting, each examination includes a number of splint-related items, depending on representational percentages derived from HTCC's scope of practice research studies.

The ASHT Splint Classification System is an excellent example of how a professional organization can influence a particular body of knowledge. Responding to a member survey that identified wide practice discrepancies in splint terminology and usage, the 1989 Executive Board of the ASHT established the Splint Nomenclature Task Force to create a system that would "conclusively settle the issues regarding splinting nomenclature."[10] This task force, chaired by Jean Casanova, consisted of members of the original splint nomenclature committee and recognized

---

*References 34, 63, 80, 91, 97, 120, 122, 134, 136, 143, 144, 161

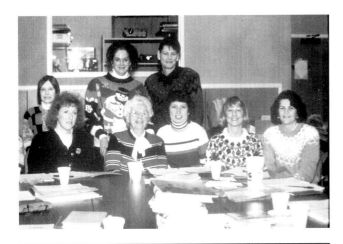

Fig. 1-14   The Splint Nomenclature Task Force members created the ASHT Splint Classification System at a 1991 meeting in Indianapolis, IN. Members attending were (front row, from left) Lori Klerekoper DeMott, OTR, CHT, Maude Malick, OTR, Janet Bailey, OTR, CHT (task force leader), Karan Gettle, MBA, OTR, CHT, and Ellen Ziegler, MS, OTR, CHT; (back row, from left) Cynthia Philips, MA, OTR, CHT, Elaine Fess, MS, OTR, CHT, and Jean Casanova, OTR, CHT (1991 Director, ASHT Clinical Assessment Committee). Nancy Cannon, OTR, CHT, also attended but is not pictured.

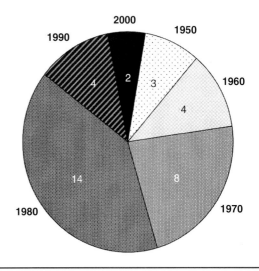

Fig. 1-15   The total number of splinting books and manuals published in each preceding 10-year period. Starting in the 1950s, the number of published splinting manuals and books gradually increased for 30 years, peaking in the 1980s.

splinting authorities in the field of hand rehabilitation* (Fig. 1-14). The task force met in 1991 with all members but one in attendance. The end product of this pivotal meeting was the ASHT Splint Classification System (SCS), published in 1992. Since its original publication, the SCS has been expanded and refined by the authors of this book.

Based on function rather than form, the Splint Classification System uses the terms *splint* and *orthosis* interchangeably. It describes splints through a series of six divisions that guide and progressively refine a splint's technical name, moving from broad concepts to individual splint specifications.

By linking the six required categories, a scientific name "sentence" is created for a given splint, based on its functional purpose. The six required elements in the system include identification of articular/nonarticular status; location; direction; immobilization/mobilization/restriction/torque transmission; type; and total number of joints included. This valuable and innovative classification system provided, for the first time, a true scientific method for categorizing all

upper extremity splints.[71] The Splint Classification System may also be applied to splints or orthoses for the lower extremity.

Publications

Publications define the knowledge base of a field of study. Creation of the *Journal of Hand Therapy* in 1987 was a major advancement for the hand therapy profession. In an almost unprecedented short period of time, this respected professional publication was included, in January 1993, in *Index Medicus,* making splinting and hand rehabilitation information retrievable internationally. The inaugural issue of the *Journal* included a splinting article by Colditz.[49] In addition to scientific articles on splinting, the Practice Forum section of the *Journal* routinely presents short papers on splinting technique.

Tracking publication trends for splinting books, manuals, and articles is crucial to identifying and understanding the evolution of splinting theory and practice. Although the majority of the splinting books and manuals reviewed in this study were written by U.S. authors, the analysis here includes both the 1975 and 1988 editions of the splint book by British therapist Nathalie Barr.[13,14]

A tally of manuals and books devoted exclusively to splinting and published from 1950 to 2001 shows a progressive increase in the number of works published through the 1980s and a distinct reduction in numbers during the 1990s (Fig. 1-15). The numbers for the 2000s are skewed, since only one year is included.

---

*Members of the ASHT Splint Nomenclature Task Force: Jean Casanova, OTR/L, CHT (Director, ASHT Clinical Assessment Committee); Janet Bailey, OTR, CHT (Task Force Leader); Nancy Cannon, OTR, CHT; Judy Colditz, OTR, CHT; Elaine Fess, MS, OTR, FAOTA, CHT; Karan Gettle, MBA, OTR, CHT; Lori (Klerekoper) DeMott, OTR, CHT; Maude Malick, OTR; Cynthia Philips, MA, OTR, CHT; and Ellen Ziegler, MS, OTR/L, CHT.

Analysis of specific information included in these publications indicates that subject matter in the 1950s focused on splint construction, general splinting concepts, and orthotic designs; the 1970s emphasized construction and general splinting concepts; and the 1980s moved away from general splinting to concentrate on diagnosis-specific splinting and principles of splinting (Fig. 1-16). Books and manuals published in the 1990s through 2001 center on general splinting concepts and principles of splinting. Demonstrating progressive development toward more sophisticated levels, the primary motivation for publication changed from how to construct splints in the 1950s, to diagnosis-related splinting in the 1980s and core principles and theory fundamental to splinting in the 1990s and 2000s.

Similar analysis that includes articles in peer-reviewed professional journals as well as books and manuals also shows increasing numbers of splint-specific publications from the 1950s to the 1990s (Fig. 1-17). (Again, the numbers for the 2000s are misleading, since only 1 year of publications is available.) Subject matter analysis indicates a decrease in orthotic and trauma-related publications and a marked increase in subjects relating to tendons, design, materials, fractures, joint/ligaments, and carpal tunnel syndrome/overuse splinting concepts.

It is also interesting to view changes in authorship of publications. With the exceptions of one splinting book of which therapists were first and second authors and a surgeon was third author[72] and one book by a noted hand surgeon, therapists wrote all the splint manuals and books included in the above analysis (journal articles not included). This is in distinct contrast to authorship during the first half of the 20th century, when surgeons authored the majority of splint-related publications (Fig. 1-18).

Two hand rehabilitation books have played strategic roles in disseminating splinting information. The first edition of Wynn Parry's *Rehabilitation of the Hand*, published in 1958, was unique in its time in that its focus was on conservative treatment of the hand, including detailed information on splinting theory and technique.[174] Based on Wynn Parry's extensive military and civilian experience treating hand and upper extremity problems in Great Britain, subsequent editions continued to define and update important splinting and rehabilitation concepts for surgeons and therapists. The fourth edition of this classic work was published in 1981.[175]

The second important book was based on the first Symposium on Rehabilitation of the Hand, sponsored by the Philadelphia Hand Center in 1976. The first edition of the Philadelphia Hand Center's *Rehabilitation of the Hand*, published in 1978, and edited by

Hunter, Schneider, Mackin, and Bell, featured chapters written by therapists and surgeons on a wide variety of topics relating to hand and upper extremity rehabilitation.[89] Indicative of its importance to hand rehabilitation, 10% of the chapters in this first edition were devoted exclusively to splinting, and many other chapters included topic-specific splinting sections. Pulvertaft's prediction in the forward of the first edition was accurate: "There is no need to wish success to the work," he wrote, "for it is assured a special place in the libraries of all who aspire to care for the wounded hand." Now in its fifth edition, *Rehabilitation of the Hand* has no equal, and splinting theory, technique, and application continue to be one of the core components of this great tome.[115]

■ SUMMARY

Splints from the 19th and 20th centuries are shown in Figs. 1-19 through 1-24.

In reviewing events concerning the evolution of splinting theory and practice, several main themes become apparent. From a historical perspective, two parallel lines of splinting practice emerged around the mid- to late 1880s, with both surgeons and orthotists (appliance makers) fabricating splints. This practice continued through the early 1900s, with few instances of cooperative ventures between the two groups.

The great polio epidemics, however, changed this mutually imposed dual autonomy, and surgeons and orthotists worked together for the next four decades, along with practitioners of emerging disciplines—physical medicine physicians and occupational and physical therapists—to combat a powerfully overwhelming common foe, poliomyelitis.

A corollary hand surgical specialty began to develop that, at first, had little effect on the situation, because hand trauma was seen as relatively insignificant in comparison with the ravages imposed by polio and infection. It is apparent that the early hand surgeons in the 1920s and 1930s made their own splints, but the reason for this remains unclear. Two rationales may be advanced: (1) with most orthotic departments fully engaged in treating polio victims, patients with hand trauma were given secondary priority by orthotists, thereby forcing hand surgeons to fabricate their own splints; or (2) orthotists were technically unable to provide the highly individualized type of splinting required by hand surgeons.

Although orthotists fabricated splints during World War II, the relatively few numbers of orthotists meant that surgeons, medical corpsmen, therapists, and nurses also fabricated splints, depending on individual hospital sites and conditions. By the end of

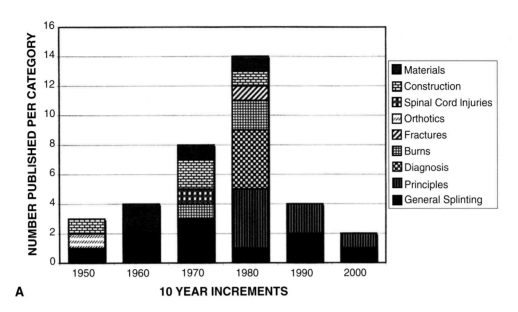

A

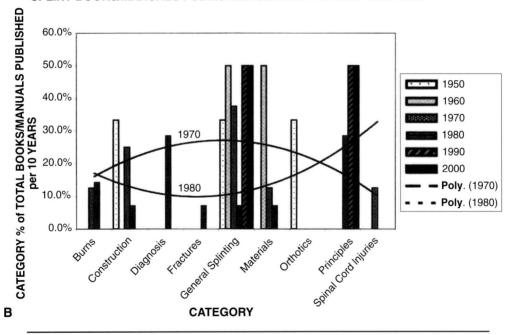

B

Fig. 1-16   Subject matter trends in splint book and manual publishing, 1950 to 2000. **A,** The subject matter of splint books and manuals gradually moved away from detailed particulars of splint fabrication to diagnosis-specific splinting and more sophisticated concepts, including collective guidelines and principles. **B,** Trend lines indicate that a major reciprocal shift in subject matter occurred between the 1970s and 1980s, changing from materials, construction, and general splinting to diagnosis-specific splinting and principles of splinting. While orthotic books and manuals were important during the 1950s, reflecting the emphasis on treating polio patients, orthotic-specific subject matter in splinting books and manuals declined rapidly beginning in the 1960s.

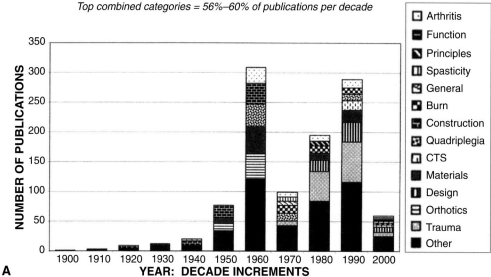

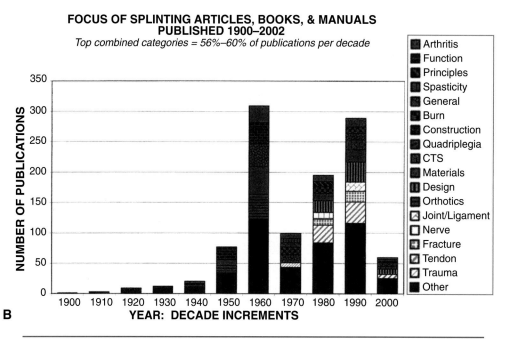

Fig. 1-17   Focus of splinting articles, books, and manuals published from 1900 to 2002. The separate categories at the top of each column represent 56%-60% of publications per decade. **A,** When journal articles were added to books and manuals, splinting publications from 1900 to 2002 showed a steady progressive increase, except in the 1960s, when more splinting publications were produced than in any other decade, before or after. The 1960s were transition years, as the eventual eradication of poliomyelitis resulted in redirection of splinting efforts to other areas, including quadriplegia and arthritis. The pivotal changeover from metal to plastic splinting materials also occurred during this decade. The five most frequent focuses for publications relating to upper extremity splinting during the 1960s included orthotics, splint materials and construction, and splinting quadriplegic and arthritis patients. In contrast, splinting publications in the 1990s revealed an expanding focus. **B,** Publications describing splinting for upper extremity trauma, including tendon, bone, nerve, and joint injuries, increased progressively from the 1970s through the 1990s.

AUTHORSHIP:
SPLINTING ARTICLES & BOOKS PUBLISHED BEFORE 1960

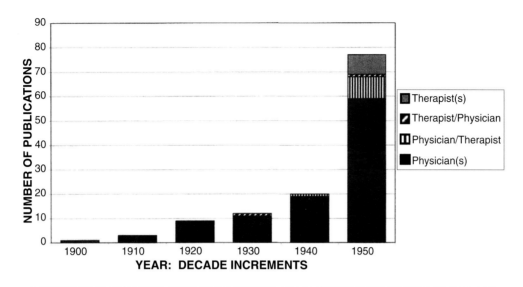

Fig. 1-18   Physicians wrote the majority of splinting articles and books published prior to 1960. By the 1950s, splinting articles and books with therapists as lead authors had increased by 900% from earlier years, but physician-authored splinting publications continued to dominate the decade.

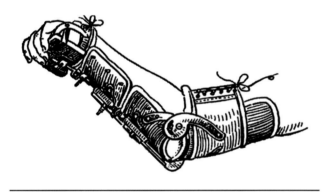

Fig. 1-19   Forearm supination, wrist extension, index–small finger MP extension mobilization splint, type 1 (7)
In this 1905 splint, a series of screw and slide mechanisms allow simultaneous or individual incremental adjustments for forearm supination and wrist and finger MP extension. (From American Academy of Orthopaedic Surgeons: *Orthopaedic appliances atlas*, vol. 1, JW Edwards, 1952, Ann Arbor, MI.)

World War II, most hand surgeons were proficient in splint fabrication, and a few had developed their own commercially available splints.

In the mid to late 1950s, the effectiveness of the polio vaccine was almost immediately apparent in the significant decrease in new cases of polio. The majority of rehabilitative resources, however, continued to be directed to treating the tremendous numbers of polio survivors. These were pinnacle times for orthotists and physical medicine physicians, and the rehabilitation and vocational fields made rapid

advances. Specialized surgical procedures for restoration of function of paralyzed extremities, e.g., tendon transfers or spinal surgery, also underwent major advancements.

A quiet renaissance began in the mid- to late 1950s. Several factors combined to propel this movement forward. Splinting materials were changing, hand surgeons were developing their own field of expertise and were becoming busier with surgical cases, therapists were increasingly interested in splinting activities, and for whatever reason, orthotists were less inclined to be involved in short-term, temporary splinting practice.

The 1960s brought an enormous drop in polio cases, and polio-oriented orthotists and therapists almost literally had to reinvent themselves to find jobs. Looking back, it seems as though therapists were better able to make the transition than were orthotists. There are few clues as to why this occurred, but some articles provide insight. In 1958, Tosberg, a highly respected orthotist, wrote about professional problems of prosthetists and orthotists. He identified poor communication with medical team personnel, the physician in particular, as a commonly encountered problem and urged prosthetists and orthotists to become better acquainted with medical protocol and terminology. He also discussed the need for college-level degrees in prosthetics and orthotics.

In 1963, Engen, also a well-recognized orthotist, presented and later wrote about the technical

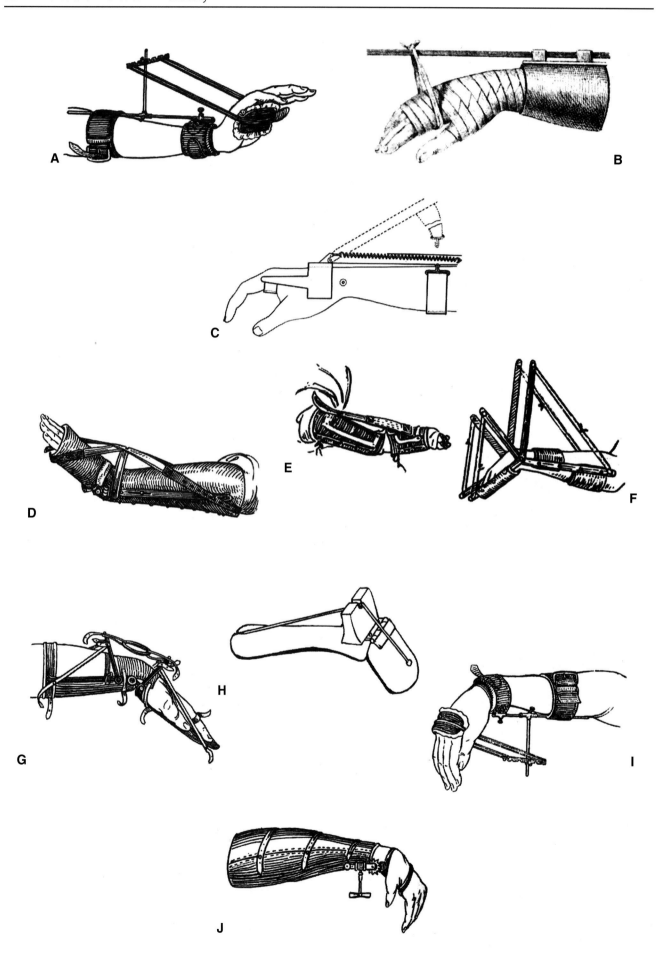

A

B

C

D

E

F

G

H

I

J

Fig. 1-20   A-C, Wrist extension mobilization splint, type 0 (1) D,E, Wrist extension mobilization splint, type 1 (5) F,G, Wrist extension mobilization splint, type 4 (16) H-J, Wrist flexion mobilization splint, type 0 (1)

These wrist mobilization splints span 40 years, from the oldest (splint **H**, 122 years old) to the most recent (splint **C**, 82 years old). Although the materials are old fashioned, the mechanical angles of force application are correct for many of the splints. The expanded Splint Classification System allows similar-functioning splints to be grouped together even though their configurations are different. Splints **A** (1886), **B** (1891), and C (1920) are grouped together; splints **D** and **E** (1908) are grouped together; splints **F** and **G** (1908) are grouped together; and splints **H** (1880), **I** (1886), and **J** (1908) are grouped together. (From American Academy of Orthopaedic Surgeons: *Orthopaedic appliances atlas*, vol. 1, JW Edwards, 1952, Ann Arbor, MI.)

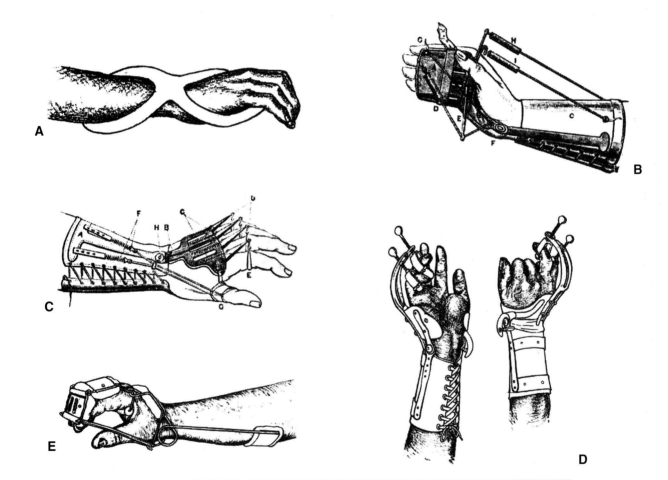

Fig. 1-21   A, Wrist extension, index–small finger MP extension mobilization splint, type 0 (5) B, Wrist extension, index–small finger MP flexion mobilization splint, type 2 (13) C, Wrist extension, index–small finger MP extension, thumb CMC radial abduction and MP extension mobilization splint, type 0 (7) D, Wrist extension, ring–small finger MP-PIP extension mobilization splint, type 0 (5) E, Wrist extension, index–small finger flexion mobilization splint, type 0 (13)

Wrist and finger—or wrist, finger, and thumb—joints are identified as primary joints in these splints from 1869 to 1948. Splint **A**—1943, splint **B**—1869, splint **C**—1869, splint **D**—1927, splint **E**—1948. (From American Academy of Orthopaedic Surgeons: *Orthopaedic appliances atlas*, vol. 1, JW Edwards, 1952, Ann Arbor, MI.)

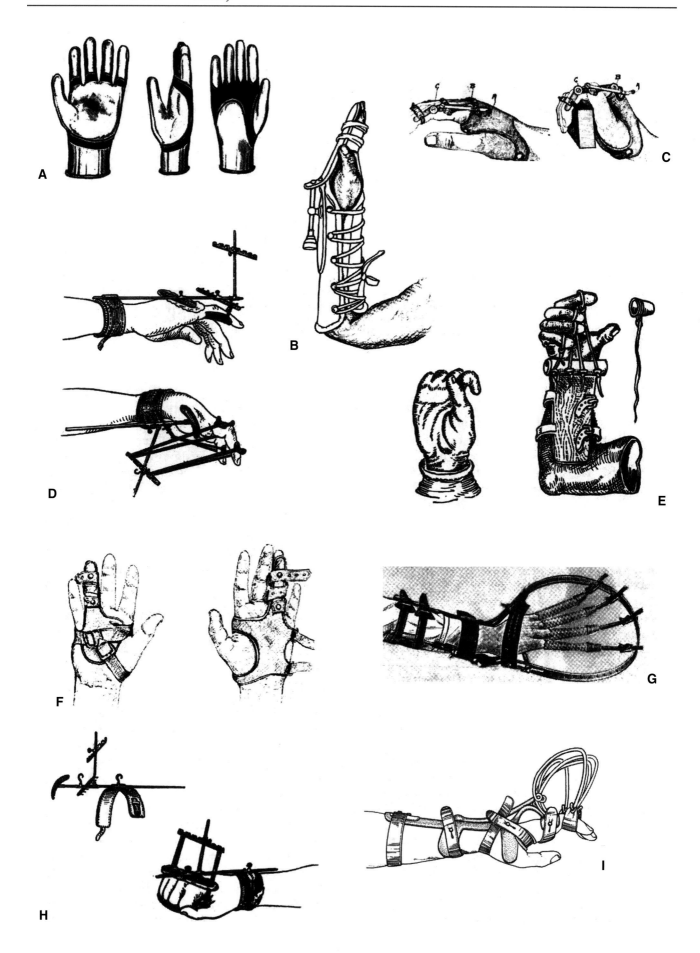

Fig. 1-22   A, Index–small finger MP extension mobilization splint, type 0 (4) B, Index–small finger MP flexion mobilization splint, type 3 (13) C, Index–small finger MP flexion: index–small finger PIP flexion / index–small finger MP extension: index–small finger PIP extension torque transmission splint, type 0 (8) D, Small finger MP-PIP extension mobilization splint, type 1 (3) or Index—long finger MP-PIP flexion mobilization splint, type 1 (5) E, Index–small finger flexion mobilization splint, type 1 (13) F, Ring finger extension mobilization splint, type 0 (3) G, Index–small finger extension and distraction mobilization splint, type 1 (13) H, Index–small finger flexion mobilization splint, type 1 (13) I, Index–small finger PIP extension mobilization splint, type 3 (10).

Of these finger mobilization splints, all but one (splint I) incorporate the metacarpophalangeal (MP) joints as primary joints, either alone or in conjunction with the proximal interphalangeal joints. Problems with MP joint passive motion correlate with the splinting historical review in that understanding the importance of maintaining MP joint collateral ligament length was not widely known until the mid- to late 1960s. With the exception of the one PIP primary joint splint (splint I, 1970), these splints date from 1647 to 1949. Splint A—1949, Splint B—1938, Splint C—1922, Splint D—1908, Splint E—1647, Splint F—1896, Splint G—1934, Splint H—1908, and Splint I—1896. (**A-H** From American Academy of Orthopaedic Surgeons: *Orthopaedic appliances atlas*, vol. 1, JW Edwards, 1952, Ann Arbor, MI, with permission from CRC Press.)

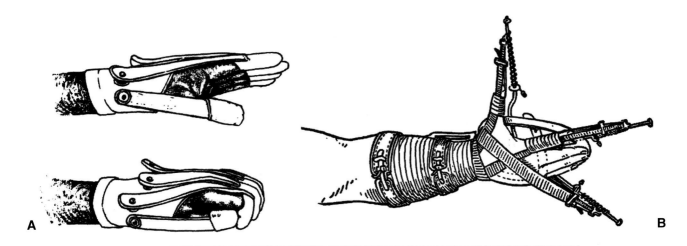

A   B

Fig. 1-23   A, Index–small finger extension, thumb CMC radial abduction and MP-IP extension mobilization splint, type 0 (15) B, Inex finger metacarpal, thumb metacarpal distraction mobilization splint, type 7 (16)
Splint A—1944, Splint B—1889, this splint is fitted to align acute first and second metacarpal fractures. (From American Academy of Orthopaedic Surgeons: *Orthopaedic appliances atlas*, vol. 1, JW Edwards, 1952, Ann Arbor, MI, with permission from CRC Press.)

advances influencing the field of orthotics. The materials he discussed included low-pressure laminates, nylon, dacron, Teflon, Velcro, and anodized aluminum. The high-temperature thermoplastics like Lucite, Plexiglas, and Royalite, with which therapists were learning to make splints, were completely omitted from Engen's discourse, despite the fact that these materials had been available for between 5 and 7 years. Engen also identified patients with arthritis as a potential group of patients who could benefit from better orthotic intervention. Not mentioned were postoperative splinting procedures.

By the late 1960s, therapists were more adept at splinting, and early low-temperature thermoplastic materials were available for clinic use. Surgeons were beginning to do silicone implant arthroplasty and silicon tendon rod grafting procedures, and the importance of early passive motion protocols with flexor tendon repairs were recognized. Powerful government and associated agencies and organizations were actively influencing splinting practice. Between 1967 and 1971, in addition to financially underwriting pivotal splinting publications and seminars, government grants funded several events that significantly

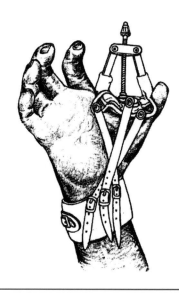

Fig. 1-24   Thumb CMC palmar abduction mobilization splint, type 1 (2)
This splint, which dates from 1946 and was designed to increase thumb CMC joint passive motion, seems overmechanized in comparison with contemporary CMC mobilization splints. (From American Academy of Orthopaedic Surgeons: *Orthopaedic appliances atlas,* vol. 1, JW Edwards, 1952, Ann Arbor, MI, with permission from CRC Press.)

affected splinting practice, including a study that permitted therapists to make splints under certain conditions; an expert panel that made recommendations to ensure that therapist educational programs included appropriate splinting capacities; and efforts directed toward splinting patients with arthritis, burns, and peripheral nerve injuries. Orthotists, at least superficially, participated in early decisions that gave therapists the opportunity to assume responsibility for temporary splinting endeavors, so it seems safe to assume that they were not interested in this rapidly expanding field.

By the 1970s, therapists had enthusiastically embraced the field of upper extremity splinting and were off and running. The art and science of splinting knowledge rapidly expanded, alliances with hand surgeons were forged, professional hand therapy organizations were formed, a professional hand journal was launched, a certification commission was created, and therapists never looked back. Splinting expertise opened so many doors for therapists. While splints were frequently the initial impetus for communication, they provided excellent opportunities for therapists to demonstrate to surgeons that through teamwork they could improve patient care not only by splinting but also by providing the highest quality therapy possible. It may be a long time before such rapid advancement is witnessed again.

The long-range repercussions of today's health care regulations on splinting practice are yet to be determined. Using the expanded Splint Classification System to define splinting terminology and its related costs is a natural step toward standardizing splinting practice and improving reimbursement. The expanded Splint Classification System will also help differentiate between hand therapy professionals and hand therapy pretenders. Unqualified or unskilled health care workers ordering from a commercial catalogue of prefabricated splints will not have the knowledge of anatomy, kinesiology, and biomechanics to procure appropriately designed splints.

Skill is always a highly sought commodity, and regarding splinting endeavors, two additional concepts are certain. Historical review confirms that over the centuries, splints have been, without interruption, an important element in the treatment of bone and soft tissue pathology. History also indicates that surgeons have been inextricably connected with the evolution of splinting concepts. These two entities, surgeons and splints, will most likely continue into the future together. The question is whether therapists will be part of this future.

Splinting is a common denominator for surgeons and therapists so long as both groups continue to advance their knowledge bases in synchrony with each other. For example, a model of synchronous development is the independent creation of splints by both therapists and surgeons for early active motion programs for tendon repairs.[65,66,123,147-148,153] Understanding underlying wound healing physiology and timing, biomechanics of tendon motion on repair sites, and the influences healing processes exert throughout the reparative course allows for the creation of appropriately designed splints and exercise protocols. The point is not who conceives a splint, so long as the splint meets all the technical and individual requisites to reach the objectives for which it was created, and surgeon, therapist, and patient work as a team for the betterment of the patient.

The bottom line is that, when used appropriately and in conjunction with high-quality therapy and surgery, splints make patients better! It will be difficult for health maintenance organizations and third-party payers to ignore this fact so long as surgeons, therapists, and patients continue to work together.

Contemporary therapists must not forget those therapists, surgeons, government officials, and patients who opened the doors of opportunity for our predecessors. Switzer was an essential catalyst, who had both the foresight and the means to effect change. We owe a great deal to her. We must also remember to recognize and thank the early hand therapists like Hollis, Malick, Mackin, Barr, deLeeuw, DeVore, Barber,

Bleyer, Mayerson, Yeakel, Von Prince, Sammons, and many others, who forged the initial paths that now have become multilane highways to the future. Had these talented and dedicated persons "dropped the ball," this history of splinting would have had an altogether different course.

ACKNOWLEDGMENTS

The author thanks Kay Carl and Judy Kiel for having the good sense not to throw out old, moldy splinting manuals and books collected over the years at the Indiana University School of Medicine, Occupational Therapy Program, IUPUI, Indianapolis, Ind.; Karan Gettle and J. Robin Janson for their generous sharing of knowledge, books, articles, and splint resources, and for their unfaltering enthusiasm; and Judy Bell-Kratoski for finding the Brand/Switzer photograph. She also thanks her dedicated husband, Steve Fess, for all the hours he spent tenaciously tracking long-lost references in dusty journals and on eye-blearing microfilm.

REFERENCES

1. Alex JC, Bhattacharyya TK, Smyrniotis C, et al.: A histologic analysis of three-dimensional versus two-dimensional tissue expansion in the porcine model, *Laryngoscope* 111(1):36-43, 2001.
2. Allen HS: Hand injuries in the Mediterranean (North Africa) theater of operations. In Bunnell S: *Surgery in World War II: hand surgery*, Office of the Surgeon General, 1955, Washington, DC.
3. Allen HS, Mason M: A universal splint for immobilization of the hand in the position of function, *Q Bull Northwest U Med School* 21:218-27, 1947.
4. American Academy of Orthopaedic Surgeons: *Atlas of orthotics: biomedical principles and applications*, Mosby, 1982, St. Louis.
5. American Academy of Orthopaedic Surgeons: *Orthopaedic appliances atlas*, vol. 1, JW Edwards, 1952, Ann Arbor, MI.
6. American Occupational Therapy Association, Practice Division: *Orthotics/prosthetics*, AOTA, 1979, Rockville, MD.
7. Arem A, Madden J: Is there a Wolff's law for connective tissue? *Surg Forum* 25:512-4, 1974.
8. Armstrong G: Foreword. In Bunnell S: *Surgery in World War II: hand surgery*, Office of the Surgeon General, 1955, Washington, DC.
9. Arndts L, Lepley M: *Hand splints: a dorsal cock-up and dorsal cock-up cone splint: manual of construction and use*, University of Minnesota Hospitals, Department of Physical Medicine and Rehabilitation, 1965, Minneapolis.
10. Bailey JM, Cannon NM, Fess EE, et al.: *Splint classification system*, American Society of Hand Therapists, 1992, Chicago.
11. Bair J, Gwin C, Hertfelder S, Schafer M: *Hand information packet*, Rev. ed., American Occupational Therapy Association, 1984, Rockville, MD.
12. Bair J, Gwin C, Schafer M: *Orthotics/prosthetics*, Rev. ed., American Occupational Therapy Association, 1984, Rockville, MD.
13. Barr NR: *The hand: principles and techniques of simple splintmaking in rehabilitation*, Butterworth, 1975, Boston.
14. Barr N, Swan D: *The hand: principles and techniques of splintmaking*, ed. 2, Butterworth, 1988, Boston.
15. Barsky AJ: Hand surgery at Northington General Hospital. In Bunnell S: *Surgery in World War II: hand surgery*, Office of the Surgeon General, 1955, Washington, DC.
16. Bell-Krotoski J: Hands, research, amid success, *J Hand Ther* 2(1):5-11, 1989.
17. Bell-Krotoski J: Plaster serial casting for the remodeling of soft tissue: mobilization of joints, and increased tendon excursion. In Fess EE, Gettle K, Philips C, Janson JR: *Hand and upper extremity splinting: principles and methods*, ed. 3, Mosby, 2004, St. Louis.
18. Belohlavek M, Bartleson VB, Zobitz ME: Real-time strain rate imaging: validation of peak compression and expansion rates by a tissue-mimicking phantom, *Echocardiography* 18(7):565-71, 2001.
19. Bennett R: Medical advances influencing the field of orthetics, *Arch Phys Med* 44:531-2, 1963.
20. Bennett R, Driver M: Aims and methods of occupational therapy in the treatment of the after-effects of poliomyelitis, *Am J Occup Ther* 11:145-53, 1957.
21. Bettmann E: Foam rubber techniques of splintage, compression, and traction, *GP* 14:90-5, 1956.
22. Bleyer D: *A manual on the use and construction of splints for the occupational therapist*, Special Committee of the Council on Student Affiliation of the Wisconsin Schools of Occupational Therapy. Milwaukee-Downer College and the Office of Vocational Rehabilitation, Department of Health, Education, and Welfare, 1956, Appleton, WI.
23. Boozer JA, Sanson MS, Soutas-Little RW, et al.: Comparison of the biomedical motions and forces involved in high-profile versus low-profile dynamic splinting, *J Hand Ther* 7(3):171-82, 1994.
24. Brand PW: *Clinical mechanics of the hand*, Mosby, 1985, St. Louis.
25. Brand PW: Lessons from hot feet, *J Hand Ther* 15(2):133-5, 2002.
26. Brand PW, to Fess EE: Written communication, 2002.
27. Brand PW, Hollister A: *Clinical mechanics of the hand*, ed. 2, Mosby, 1993, St. Louis.
28. Breger-Lee DE, Buford Jr, WL: Properties of thermoplastic splinting materials, *J Hand Ther* 5(4):202-11, 1992.
29. Breger-Lee DE, Buford Jr, WL: Update in splinting materials and methods, *Hand Clin* 7(3):569-85, 1991.
30. Brennan J: Moulding polyethelene plastic splints directly to patient: a safe and practical method, *Lancet* 948-51, 1954.
31. Brennan J: Plastic appliances moulded direct to patient, *Lancet* 841-4, 1955.
32. Brook Army Medical Center: *Fingernail hooks and their application*, US Army Surgical Research Unit, Brooke Army Medical Center, 1968, Fort Sam Houston, TX.
33. Brook Army Medical Center: *Physical and occupational therapy for the burn patient*, Motion Picture Section, US Army Surgical Research Unit, Brooke Army Medical Center, 1968, Fort Sam Houston, TX.
34. Browne WE: The necessity for use of splints at certain stages in the treatment of infections of the hand, with demonstration of some of the newer types, *N Engl J Med* 215:743-8, 1936.
35. Bunnell S: Conclusions on the care of injured hand in World II derived from the experiences of the civilian consultant for hand surgery to the Secretary of War. In Bunnell S: *Surgery in World War II: hand surgery*, Office of the Surgeon General, 1955, Washington, DC.
36. Bunnell S: Reconstructive surgery of the hand, *Surg Gynecol Obstet* 39(3):259-74, 1924.

37. Bunnell S: Repair of nerves and tendons of the hand, *J Bone Joint Surg* 10:1-25, 1928.

38. Bunnell S: Splinting the hand. In American Academy of Orthopaedic Surgeons: *Instructional course lectures*, Edwards, 1952. Ann Arbor, MI.

39. Bunnell S: *Surgery in World War II: hand surgery*, Office of the Surgeon General, 1955, Washington, DC.

40. Bunnell S: *Surgery of the hand*, Lippincott, 1944, Philadelphia.

41. Bunnell S: *Surgery of the hand*, ed. 2, Lippincott, 1948, Philadelphia.

42. Bunnell S: *Surgery of the hand*, ed. 3, Lippincott, 1956, Philadelphia.

43. Caldwell H: *Progressive splinting manual using the master template method*, Johnson & Johnson, 1970, New Brunswick, NJ.

44. Cannon NM, Foltz RW, Koepfer JM, et al.: *Manual of hand splinting*, Churchill Livingstone, 1985, New York.

45. Clark N, Saldana M: Kleinert traction: rubber loop to nail fixative method, *J Hand Ther* 3(3):161, 1990.

46. Clase KL, Mitchell PJ, Ward PJ, et al.: FGF5 stimulates expansion of connective tissue fibroblasts and inhibits skeletal muscle development in the limb, *Dev Dyn* 219(3):368-80, 2000.

47. Cleveland M: Hand injuries in the European theater of operations. In Bunnell S: *Surgery in World War II: hand surgery*, Office of the Surgeon General, 1955, Washington, DC.

48. Cohen JL: Enteroviruses and reoviruses. In Braunwald E, Fauci AS Kaspar DL, et al.: *Harrison's principles of internal medicine*, McGraw-Hill, 2001, New York.

49. Colditz JC: Splinting for radial nerve palsy, *J Hand Ther* 1(1):18-23, 1987.

50. Committee on Prosthetic-Orthotic Education, National Academy of Sciences, National Research Council: A study of orthotic and prosthetic activities appropriate for physical therapists and occupational therapists, *Am J Occup Ther* 21(6):404-5, 1967.

51. Committee on Prosthetics Research and Development Department of Energy, National Research Council, National Academy of Sciences, National Academy of Engineering: First workshop panel on upper-extremity orthotics of the Subcommittee on Design and Development. Social and Rehabilitation Service, Department of Health, Education, and Welfare; the National Academy of Sciences; and the Veteran's Administration, 1970, Hillside, IL.

52. Committee on Prosthetics Research and Development, Department of Energy, National Research Council, National Academy of Sciences, National Academy of Engineering: Second workshop panel on upper-extremity orthotics of the Subcommittee on Design and Development. Hillside, IL. Social and Rehabilitation Service, Department of Health, Education, and Welfare; the National Academy of Sciences; and the Veteran's Administration. GPO, 1971, Washington, DC.

53. Convery FR, Conaty J, Nickel V: Dynamic splinting of the rheumatoid hand, *Orthotics Prosthetics* 22:41-5, 1968.

54. Coppard B, Lohman H: Introduction to splinting, Mosby, 1996, St. Louis.

55. Coppard B, Lohman H: *Introduction to splinting*, ed. 2, Mosby, 2001, St. Louis.

56. Cutler CW: The overall picture in the Zone of the Interior. In Bunnell S: *Surgery in World War II: hand surgery*, Office of the Surgeon General, 1955, Washington, DC.

57. deLeeuw C, to Fess FE: Verbal communication on the use of fingernail hooks for positioning burned hands, 1963.

58. Dell Orto AE, Marinelli RP: *Encyclopedia of disability and rehabilitation*, Macmillan, 1996, Basingstoke, UK.

59. DeVore G: Unpublished notes and archival documents on the start of the Hand Rehabilitation Center at Chapel Hill, NC. Property of G. DeVore, 1993, Tucson, AZ.

60. Duran R, Houser R: Controlled passive motion following flexor tendon repair in zones 2 and 3. In Hunter J, Schneider L: *Proceedings of the American Academy of Orthopaedic Surgeons Symposium on tendon surgery in the hand*, Mosby, 1975, St. Louis.

61. Elliott R: Othotics in poliomelitis, *Am J Occup Ther* 11:135-42, 1957.

62. *Encyclopedia Britannica*, Encyclopedia Britannica, Inc, 2001, Chicago.

63. Engen TJ: Technical advances influencing the field of orthotics, *Arch Phys Med* 44:533-6, 1963.

64. Ernst PG: *Orthopaedic apparatus*, Sprague, 1883, London.

65. Evans R: An analysis of factors that support the early active short arc motion of the repaired central slip, *J Hand Ther* 5(4):87-201, 1992.

66. Evans RB: Immediate active short arc motion following extensor tendon repair, *Hand Clin* 11(3):483-512, 1995.

67. Feldman P: Upper extremity casting and splinting. In Glen M, Whyte J: *The practical management of spasticity in children and adults*, Lea & Febiger, 1990, Malvern, PA.

68. Fess EE: Force magnitude of commercial spring-coil and spring-wire splints designed to extend the proximal interphalangeal joint, *J Hand Ther* 2:86-90, 1988.

69. Fess EE: Principles and methods of dynamic splinting. In Hunter J, Schneider L, Mackin E, Callahan A: *Rehabilitation of the hand*, ed. 2, Mosby, 1984, St. Louis.

70. Fess EE: Splints: mechanics versus convention, *J Hand Ther* 8(2):124-30, 1995.

71. Fess EE, Gettle K, Philips C, Janson JR: *Hand and upper extremity splinting: principles and methods*, ed. 3, Mosby, 2004, St. Louis.

72. Fess F, Gettle K, Strickland J: *Hand splinting: principles and methods*, Mosby, 1981, St. Louis.

73. Fess EE, McCollum M: The influence of splinting on healing tissues, *J Hand Ther* 11(2):157-61, 1998.

74. Fess F, Philips C: *Hand splinting principles and methods*, ed. 2, Mosby, 1987, St. Louis.

75. Flowers K, LaStayo P: Effect of total end range time on improving passive range of motion, *J Hand Ther* 7(3):150-7, 1994.

76. Fortune MT, Vassilopoulos C, Coolbaugh MI, et al.: Dramatic, expansion-biased, age-dependent, tissue-specific somatic mosaicism in a transgenic mouse model of triplet repeat instability, *Hum Mol Genet* 9(3):439-45, 2000.

77. Frackelton W: Hand surgery at William Beumont General Hospital. In Bunnell S: *Surgery in World War II: hand surgery*, Office of the Surgeon General, 1955, Washington, DC.

78. Fowler SB: Hand surgery at Newton D. Baker General Hospital. In Bunnell S: *Surgery in World War II: hand surgery*, Office of the Surgeon General, 1955, Washington, DC.

79. Fuchs E, Fuchs R: Corrective bracing, *Am J Occup Ther* 8(2):88, 1954.

80. Glancy J: Technical responsibility of the orthotist, *JAMA* 183:936-8, 1963.

81. Graham WC: Hand surgery at Valley Forge General Hospital. In Bunnell S: *Surgery in World War II: hand surgery*, Office of the Surgeon General, 1955, Washington, DC.

82. Gronley J, Yeakel M, Grant A: Rehabilitation of the burned hand, *Arch Phys Med* 43:508-13, 1962.

83. Hall A, Stenner R: *Manual of fracture bracing*, Churchill Livingstone, 1985, New York.

84. Hogan L, Uditsky T: Pediatric splinting, selection fabrication, and clinical application of upper extremity splints, Therapy Skill Builders, 1998, San Antonio.

85. Hollis LI: Remember? [1979 Eleanor Clarke Slagle lecture], *Am J Occup Ther* 33(8):493-9, 1979.

86. Howard LD: Hand surgery at Wakeman General Hospital. In Bunnell S: *Surgery in World War II: hand surgery*, Office of the Surgeon General, 1955, Washington, DC.

87. Hunter JM, Blackmore SM, Callahan AD: Flexor tendon salvage and functional redemption using the Hunter tendon implant, *J Hand Ther* 2(2):114-21, 1989.

88. Hunter JM, Salisbury RE: Flexor-tendon reconstruction in severely damaged hands: a two-stage procedure using a silicone-Dacron reinforced gliding prosthesis prior to tendon grafting, *J Bone Joint Surg* 53A(5):829-58, 1971.

89. Hunter JM, Schneider LH, Mackin EJ, Bell JA: *Rehabilitation of the hand*, Mosby, 1978, St. Louis.

90. Hyroop GL: Hand surgery at Crile General Hospital. In Bunnell S: *Surgery in World War II: hand surgery*, Office of the Surgeon General, 1955, Washington, DC.

91. James JIP: Common, simple errors in the management of hand injuries, *J R Soc Med* 63:69-71, 1970.

92. James JIP: Fractures of the proximal and middle phalanges of the fingers, *Acta Orthop Scand* 32:401-12, 1962.

93. Johns R, Wright V: An analytical description of joint stiffness, *Biorheology* 2:87-95, 1964.

94. Johns R, Wright V: Relative importance of various tissues in joint stiffness, *J Appl Physiol* 17:824-8, 1962.

95. Kanavel A: *Infections of the hand*, Lea & Febiger, 1916, Philadelphia.

96. Kanavel A: Splinting and physiotherapy in infections of the hand, *JAMA* 83:1984-8, 1924.

97. Kanavel A: The dynamics of the function of the hand with considerations as to methods of obtaining the positions of function by splints, *Med J Aust* Oct. 29, 1927.

98. Kendall H, Kendall F: *Care during the recovery period in paralytic poliomyelitis*, Rev. ed., US Public Health Service, *Bulletin* 242:96, 1939.

99. Keusch G, Bart K: Immunization principles and vaccine use. In Braunwald E, Fauci AS, Kaspar DL, et al.: *Harrison's principles of internal medicine*, McGraw-Hill, 2001, New York.

100. Kiel J: *Basic hand splinting: a pattern-designing approach*, Little, Brown, 1983, Boston.

101. Kirk J, to Gettle K: Written communication on splint material properties, 2001.

102. Kleinert HE, Lubahn JD: Current state of flexor tendon surgery, *Ann Chir Main* 3(1):7-17, 1984.

103. Kleinert HE, Kutz JE, Ashbell S, Martinez E: Primary repair of flexor tendons in no man's land, *J Bone Joint Surg* 49A:577, 1967.

104. Kleinert HE, Kutz J, Cohen M: Primary repair of zone 2 flexor tendon lacerations. In Hunter J, Schneider L: *Proceedings of the American Academy of Orthopaedic Surgeons Symposiom on tendon surgery in the hand*, Mosby, 1975, St. Louis.

105. Koch R, Mason M: Division of nerves and tendons of the hand, with discussion on surgical treatment and its results, *Surg Gynecol Obstet* 56:1-39, 1933.

106. Koch S, Mason M: Purposeful splinting following injuries of the hand, *Surg Gynecol Obstet* 68:1-16, 1939.

107. Koepke G: Splinting the severely burned hand, *Am J Occup Ther* 18:147-50, 1963.

108. Landsmeer JM, Long C: The mechanism of finger control, based on electromyograms and location analysis, *Acta Anat (Basel)* 60(3):330-47, 1965.

109. Lasker Foundation, to Fess EE: Written communication on award to Paul Brand, 2001.

110. Lehneis H: *Upper extremity orthoses*, Rev. ed., Institute of Rehabilitation Medicine, New York University Medical Center, 1971, New York.

111. LeVay D: *The history of orthopaedics*, Parthenon, 1990, Park Ridge, NJ.

112. Levy D, Teasley J, Frackelton W: Splinting the acutely injured hand, *Wisconsin Med J* 64:248-50, 1965.

113. Lewin P: *Orthopedic surgery for nurses, including nursing care*, WB Saunders, 1942, Philadelphia.

114. Littler JW: Hand surgery at Cushing General Hospital. In Bunnell S: *Surgery in World War II: hand surgery*, Office of the Surgeon General, 1955, Washington, DC.

115. Mackin EJ, Callahan AD, Skirven TM, et al.: *Hunter, Mackin & Callahan's rehabilitation of the hand and upper extremity*, ed 5, Mosby, 2002, St. Louis.

116. Madden J, Peacock E: Studies on the biology of collagen during wound healing: dynamic metabolism of scar collagen and remodeling of dermal wounds, *Ann Surg* 174:511-20, 1971.

117. Malick M: *Manual on dynamic hand splinting with thermoplastic materials*, Harmarville Rehabilitation Center, 1974, Pittsburgh.

118. Malick M: *Manual on static hand splinting*, vol. 1, Rev. ed., Harmarville Rehabilitation Center, 1972, Pittsburgh.

119. Malick M, Carr J: *Manual on management of the burn patient*, Harmarville Rehabilitation Center, 1982, Pittsburgh.

120. Marble H: Purposeful splinting following injuries to the hand, *JAMA* 116:1373-5, 1941.

121. Marmor L, Sollars R: Hand splints for traumatic lesions, *J Trauma* 3(6):551-62, 1963.

122. Mason ML: Injuries to nerves and tendons of the hand, *JAMA* 116(13):1375-97, 1941.

123. May EJ, Silfverskiold KL, Sollerman CJ: Controlled mobilization after flexor tendon repair in zone II: a prospective comparison of three methods, *J Hand Surg* 17A(5):942-52, 1992.

124. Mayerson E: Material science and splint workshop, Continuing Medical Education, School of Medicine, State University of New York at Buffalo, 1969, Buffalo, NY.

125. Mayerson E: *Splinting theory and fabrication*, National Science Foundation, Research Foundation of the State University of New York at Buffalo, and School of Health Related Professions, Department of Occupational Therapy. Goodrich Printing, 1971, Clarence Center, NY.

126. McKee P, Morgan L: *Orthotics in rehabilitation: splinting the hand and body*, FA Davis, 1998, Philadelphia.

127. Milner RH: The effect of tissue expansion on peripheral nerves, *Br J Plast Surg* 42:414, 1989.

128. Moberg E: *Splinting in hand therapy*, Thieme-Stratton, 1984, New York.

129. Moore I: Durafoam pre-fabricated sheets, *Am J Occup Ther* 14:256-7, 1960.

130. Moore J: *Adaptive equipment and appliances*, Overbeck, 1962, Ann Arbor, MI.

131. Mostafapour SP, Murakami CS: Tissue expansion and serial excision in scar revision, *Facial Plast Surg* 17(4):245-52, 2001.

132. Mutaf M: Venous changes in expanded skin: a microangiographic and histological study in rabbits, *Ann Plast Surg* 37:75, 1997.

133. Neumann CG: The progressive expansion of an area of skin by progressive distention of a subcutaneous balloon, *Plast Reconstr Surg* 9:121, 1957.

134. Nickel V: Treatment of patients with severe paralysis, *Postgrad Med* 21(6):581-90, 1957.

135. Ohkaya S, Hirata H, Uchida A: Repair of nerve gap with the elongation of Wallerian degenerated nerve by tissue expansion, *Microsurgery* 20(3):126-30, 2000.

136. Peacock E: Dynamic splinting for the prevention and correction of hand deformities, *J Bone Joint Surg* 34A(4):789-96, 1952.

137. Phalen GS: Hand surgery at O'Reilly General Hospital. In Bunnell S: *Surgery in World War II: hand surgery*, Office of the Surgeon General, 1955, Washington, DC.

138. Pratt DR: Hand injuries in a debarkation hospital (Letterman General Hospital). In Bunnell S: *Surgery in World War II: hand surgery*, Office of the Surgeon General, 1955, Washington, DC.

139. Pratt DR: Hand surgery at Dibble General Hospital. In Bunnell S: *Surgery in World War II: hand surgery*, Office of the Surgeon General, 1955, Washington, DC.

140. Raposio E, Cella A, Panarese P, et al.: Quantitative benefits provided by acute tissue expansion: a biomechanical study in human cadavers, *Br J Plast Surg* 53(3):220-4, 2000.

141. Richard R, Staley M, Miller S, Warden G: To splint or not to splint: past philosophy and present practice, part I, *J Burn Care Rehabil* 17(5)444-53, 1996.

142. Robotti EB: The treatment of burns: an historical perspective with emphasis on the hand, *Hand Clin* 6(2):163-90, 1990.

143. Schottstaedt E, Robinson G: Functional bracing of the arm, part I, *J Bone Joint Surg* 38A:477-99, 1956.

144. Schottstaedt E, Robinson G: Functional bracing of the arm: part II, *J Bone Joint Surg* 8A:841-56, 1956.

145. Seavey N, Smith J, Wagner P: *A paralyzing fear: the triumph over polio in America*, TV Books, 1998, New York.

146. Shurr D, Michael J: *Prosthetics and orthotics*, Pearson Education, 2002, Upper Saddle River, NJ.

147. Silfverskiold KL: Splinting tips, *Postgrad Med* 86(6):185-8, 1989.

148. Silfverskiold KL, May EJ: Flexor tendon repair in zone II with a new suture technique and an early mobilization program combining passive and active flexion, *J Hand Surg* 19(1):53-60, 1994.

149. Silfverskiold KL, May EJ, Tornvall AH: Tendon excursions after flexor tendon repair in zone II: results with a new controlled-motion program, *J Hand Surg* 18A(3):403-10, 1993.

150. Smith H, Hopkins E, Bradford F, Malick M: *Institute and workshop on hand splinting construction*, Harmarville Rehabilitation Center, Western Pennsylvania Occupational Therapy Association, and the U.S. Department of Health, Education, and Welfare, 1967, Pittsburgh.

151. Smith L: Orthotics and prosthetics in the United States of America, *Prosth Braces Techn Aids* 8:3-8, 1960.

152. Stevenson J: *Care of poliomyelitis*, Macmillan, 1940, London.

153. Strickland JW, Gettle K: Flexor tendon repair: the Indianapolis method. In Hunter J, Schneider L, Mackin E: *Tendon and nerve surgery in the hand: a third decade*, Mosby, 1997, St. Louis.

154. Swanson AB: A dynamic brace for finger joint reconstruction in arthritis, *NYU Interclinic Inf Bull* 10(8):1, 1971.

155. Swanson AB: A flexible implant for replacement of arthritic or destroyed joints in the hand, *NYU Interclinic Inf Bull* 6:16-9, 1966.

156. Swanson AB: Arthritis finger joint reconstruction: a dynamic post-arthroplasty brace, *Braces Today* 11, 1971.

157. Swanson AB: Flexible implant arthroplasty for arthritic finger joints: rationale, technique, and results of treatment, *J Bone Joint Surg* 54A(3).435-55, 1972.

158. Swanson AB: Finger joint replacement by silicone rubber implants and the concept of implant fixation by encapsulation, *Ann Rheum Dis* 28(5 suppl):47-55, 1969.

159. Swanson AB: Silicone rubber implants for replacement of arthritic or destroyed joints in the hand, *Surg Clin North Am* 48:1113-27, 1968.

160. Swanson AB, Coleman JD: Corrective bracing needs of the rheumatoid arthritic wrist, *Am J Occup Ther* 20(1):38-40, 1966.

161. Swanson J: Durafoam: a new material for rest splints in the prevention of deformity in the chronic rheumatoid diseases, *Can Med Assoc J* 79:638-42, 1958.

162. Tenney C, Lisak J: *Atlas of hand splinting*, Little, Brown, 1986, Boston.

163. Trueta J: *The treatment of war wounds and fractures*, Hamish Hamilton, 1939, London.

164. Van Lede P, to Janson R: Written communication on splint material properties, 2001.

165. Van Lede P, van Veldhoven G: *Therapeutic hand splints: a rational approach*, Provan, 1998, Antwerp, Belgium.

166. Von Prince K, Yeakel M: *The splinting of burn patients*, Charles C. Thomas, 1974, Springfield, IL.

167. von Werssowitz O, Odon F: Biophysical principles in selection of hand splints, *Am J Occup Ther* 9: 77-9, 1955.

168. *Webster's third new international dictionary of the English language*, Unabridged, Merriam-Webster, 1993, Springfield, MA.

169. Willis B: *Splinting the burn patient*, Shriners Burns Institute, 1970, Galveston, TX.

170. Willis B: The use of orthoplast isoprene splints in the treatment of the acutely burned child: preliminary report, *Am Occup Ther* 23(1):57-61, 1969.

171. Wilton J: *Hand splinting: principles of design and fabrication*, WB Saunders, 1997, Philadelphia.

172. Withington E: *Hippocrates*, vol. 3, Harvard University Press, 1999, Cambridge, MA.

173. Wright V, Johns K: Quantitative and qualitative analysis of joint stiffness in normal subjects and in patients with connective tissue diseases, *Ann Rheum Dis* 20:36-46, 1961.

174. Wynn Parry CB: *Rehabilitation of the hand*, ed. 1, Butterworth, 1958, London.

175. Wynn Parry CB, Salter M, Millar D: *Rehabilitation of the hand*, ed. 4, Butterworth, 1981, London.

176. Yeakel MH: Polypropylene hinges for hand splints, *J Bone Joint Surg* 48A(5):955-6, 1966.

177. Yeakel M, Gronley J, Tumbush W: Fiberglass positioning device for the burned hand, *J Trauma* 4(1):57-70, 1964.

178. Young R: *Handbook of hand splints*, Rancho Los Amigos, 1968, Downey, CA.

179. Young R: *Hand splints and their attachments*, Orthotic Department, Rancho Los Amigos Hospital, 1965, Downey, CA.

180. Ziegler F: *Current concepts in orthotics: a diagnosis-related approach to splinting*, Rolyan Medical Products, 1984, Chicago.

Section 2
Lessons From Hot Feet: A Note on Tissue Remodeling

PAUL BRAND, MB, BS, FRCS

Few persons have contributed more to our understanding of biomechanics and soft tissue response to stress then Dr. Paul Brand. Historically, enlightened physicians and brace makers have, for centuries, advocated slow, gentle tension to effect change in soft tissue, but their opinions were based on individual trial-and-error observations. This lack of organization and scientific validation made their teachings vulnerable to contradictory, opposing practices that prompted harsh manipulation to effect soft tissue change. Confusion flourished for centuries. In con-

trast to early practitioners, Dr. Brand transferred his vast clinical experiences and empirical understanding of soft tissue response to stress to the biomechanics laboratory to provide a foundation of knowledge based on scientific inquiry.

His subsequent work has served as a foundation for expanding understanding and investigation into the histologic and biomechanical basis for soft tissue response to stress. Dr. Brand's work is closely entwined with contemporary splinting theory and practice. His straightforward teaching style and exceptional ability to translate difficult biomechanical and physiologic constructs into easily understood concepts facilitate learning for surgeons and therapists alike.

Innovators often are able to identify watershed experiences that forever changed their thinking. Distinguishing the insights that such events bring has twofold importance, in that both truth and process are better appreciated. I had heard Dr. Brand describe the sequence of events that altered his understanding of soft tissue remodeling and asked him if he would write about these experiences for my chapter on the history of splinting. He willingly agreed, and I soon received a beautifully written narrative. On reflection, I realized that it would be a great disservice to bury this important account in the middle of my history chapter.

This letter is not exclusively about correcting clubfoot problems. It is relevant to all those who work with healing tissue and seek to influence the soft tissue remodeling process. It is the base on which splinting endeavors are founded. Read, enjoy, contemplate!—ELAINE EWING FESS, MS, OTR, FAOTA, CHT.

DR. BRAND WRITES: —In 1944, I worked as First Assistant to Sir Denis Browne at the Great Ormond Street Children's Hospital in London. Denis Browne had become quite famous for his management of clubfoot, particularly talipes equinovarus, so we got a very large number of these cases. I was responsible for the follow-up clinic.

Denis Browne was a large man with large hands, and most of the patients he saw were within days of being newborn. His idea was that if the child was seen early, he would correct the deformity completely the very first time the child was seen. His method was to correct the three deformities of each foot, one deformity at a time. First he would correct the metatarsus varus at the level of the mid-foot. Then, when the foot was straight in a length-wise direction, he would correct the varus deformity of the hind foot to bring the os calcis directly under the ankle. Finally, he would correct the equines deformity, and for this correction it was important not to use the foot as a lever to stretch the tendo Achilles, for fear he would break the mid-foot. So Denis Browne would put his large thumb under the full length of the sole of the foot to preserve the arch of the foot while he pushed the foot up into a right angle position or higher.

In all these maneuvers, as I watched him, it was obvious that he was breaking little ligaments and causing at least minor cracks in bones like the talus. The skin on the medial side of the foot had to be stretched, and sometimes little cracks appeared in the skin. I did not like watching this manipulation, because it seemed to me that it was just too violent. However, it did finish up with a foot in a normal relationship to the leg and the sole of the foot in the right position for walking in shoes.

However, at the early stage we did not put shoes on the foot, but we used the Denis Browne splint—which, as you know, has an aluminum soleplate and, at right angles to that, an aluminum sidepiece that goes up to a little above the ankle. The newly manipulated foot was strapped onto the soleplate with adhesive strapping, and then to the lateral upright plate. When both feet had been strapped to their own section of this Denis Browne splint, then the two feet were each attached separately to the crossbar that held the two feet parallel to each other.

Within a week, I had to see the baby at the follow-up clinic and take off the old strapping and reapply it in the same position. The reason for doing the strapping over again was that the foot had swollen grossly inside the first adhesive strapping, and any part that was not covered bulged out.

Anyway, we went on reattaching the splint with fresh strapping every week for a few weeks and then every two weeks until the swelling had gone down.

All this time, the baby had been kicking its legs, as any baby will do, and as one foot kicked downward, the other foot was being withdrawn, and the Denis Browne splint thrust the feet into inversion and eversion because of the bar that connected the two feet. This undoubtedly kept the subtalar joint and the ankle joints in congruity with each other, but these were the only joints that kept moving. The mid-tarsal joints were constantly kept in the same relationship to each other by the soleplate of the splint.

I had to follow these babies up to the stage when they were ready to begin standing and walking, and then they had to be fitted with little boots.

As these young children grew and as they learned to walk freely, they were able to move a little at the ankle joints and some at the subtalar joint, but the foot as a whole remained straight and rather rigid indefinitely.

I was required to keep track of these feet until the children were 12 years old, at which stage I would be seeing them about every 6 months.

Having become very accustomed to observing hundreds and hundreds of these baby clubfeet at all stages of development, my hands became very accustomed to feeling the feet and became aware of those who were doing well and of those who perhaps did not do so well.

When I went to India in 1946 and started a clubfoot clinic, I taught my assistants to do the manipulation and correction just as I had been taught by Denis Browne. I was able to get plenty of aluminum sheathing from the wings of an airplane that had crashed a few miles away from Vellore. I hired a mechanic to use this aluminum sheathing to make Denis Browne splints, and everything seemed to be going well.

However, among the patients who came to my clinic in India (and unlike the patients whom I saw in London), there were several teenagers who had been born with clubfoot, but no attempt had ever been made to correct them. They came to me walking either on the lateral side of the foot or even on the dorsum of the foot. I was interested to know whether one could do manipulation on these late older cases or whether one would have to operate on them.

I began by trying to manipulate the feet, at least part way toward full correction. This meant that I had to handle these feet and feel them and feel the mobility. To my astonishment, I found that these untreated clubfeet of the older children felt cool to the touch and had surprising range of motion of all the joints, even though the range of motion was from a deformed position and was not enough to correct the deformity. I remember being astonished at the contrast between the texture and temperature of the feet I was now seeing in children aged 10 or 12, compared with the feet of children who had been through Denis Browne's treatment, which were corrected in position but so stiff and so hot compared with the untreated feet I was seeing in India.

I felt at once that the Indian feet were better feet than the ones we had treated in England, even though the ones in England were straight and in a better shape. I felt convinced that there was something fundamentally wrong about all those patients in London. I wondered whether we could treat the Indian patients in a way that would not cause the inflammation and the damage to ligaments and to some bones that had been thrust upon the babies in London.

I felt that we had to be *slow*, and we also had to be *gentle*. I hoped that we could achieve this by a gentle contact manipulation keeping within the limits imposed by pain, and then by using total contact plaster casts to hold the partially corrected position for a week or so. Then we would remove the cast, manipulate a little more, and apply a new cast. I hoped that the improvement gained by moderate correction at the beginning of the week would loosen up and allow further improvements that would be maintained by the next cast.

Now, I had several doctors to assist me at the clubfoot clinic, and I taught each of them the technique of little by little manipulation and plaster casts, but I found it very difficult to explain exactly what I meant when I said they had to be gentle. How do you measure gentleness? We were not using anesthetics for the manipulation and plaster casting. So we tried saying that if the baby cried, that meant the manipulation was too strong. However, some babies cried for no reason other than the stranger atmosphere of the clinic and the white coats of the doctors. We had to develop an answer for that as well.

We told the mothers not to feed their babies in the morning before coming to the clinic. So the waiting room where the mothers and the babies were waiting for their turns for treatment was full of screaming babies feeling hungry and not being allowed to go to the breast. As soon as each baby's name was called, the mother would take it to the treatment room and sit herself on a stool opposite the doctor. The old plaster casts had been taken off, and now the baby was allowed to go to the breast and start sucking. For a time the baby's whole interest was to satisfy its hunger. This allowed the doctors to begin feeling the foot and moving it gently into its best new position.

I told the doctors that if the baby remained happy having its meal, that meant that they hadn't pushed hard enough on the foot to correct the position. On the other hand, if they pushed much harder, the baby might let go of the nipple and start to scream, and that meant that they had used too much force. The ideal moment for the manipulation was when the baby showed it recognized that something unpleasant was happening to its foot and it turned its eyes and looked at the doctor without letting go of the nipple. At that moment, the doctor should hold the position and apply the plaster cast.

This resulted in some teasing among the doctors, because when a baby yells, everybody can hear it, and the other doctors would know that the doctor dealing with that baby had gone too far and used too much force.

We used Denis Browne's methods of correcting the three deformities in sequence, and we switched from plaster casts to Denis Browne splints as soon as a full correction had been achieved by serial casting. But the real joy and satisfaction came after a few years, when I was able to compare the feel of the 6-year-old and the 10-year-old feet with my memories of the feel of same-age feet in London. Not only were our feet in India in a normal position (as the London feet had been), but they were mobile and they felt *cool* and soft to the touch.

Appendix: 20th-Century Contributors to Splinting Practice Who Are Cited in the Text

Allen, Harvey S., MD, FACS
Arem, A. J., MD
Bailey, Janet M., OTR, CHT
Barber, Lois M., OTR, FAOTA
Barr, Nathalie B., MBE, FCOT
Barsky, Arthur J., MD
Beasley, Robert W., MD
Bell-Krotoski, Judith A., OTR, FAOTA, CHT
Bennett, George F., MD
Bleyer, Dorothy A., OTR
Boozer, Jeanine A., OTR, CHT
Bradford, Eleanor, OTR
Bradley, T. Kay (Carl), OTR
Brand, Paul W., MB, BS, FRCS
Breger-Lee (Stanton), Donna, MA, OTR, CHT
Bricker, Eugene M., MD
Brown, D. Michael, OTR, CWA
Buford Jr., William L., PhD, BME
Bunnell, Sterling, MD
Burkhalter, William E., MD
Cannon, Nancy M., OTR, CHT
Carter, Margaret S., OTR, CHT
Casanova, Jean S., OTR, CHT
Clayton, Mack, MD
Colditz, Judy, OTR, CHT, FAOTA
Cummings, Johanne, PT
deLeeuw, Carolina F., MA, OTR
Denny, Elisha, PTA, OTA
DeVore, Gloria, OTR
Duran, Robert J., MD
Engen, Thorkild, CO
Evans, Roslyn B., OTR, CHT
Fess, Elaine Ewing, MS, OTR, FAOTA, CHT
Flowers, Kenneth R., PT, CHT
Fowler, S. Benjamin, MD
Frackelton, William H., MD
Fuchs, Ernest M., OTR
Fuchs, Renate L., OTR
Fullenwider, Lynnlee, OTR, CHT
Gettle, Karan S., MBA, OTR, CHT
Graham, Walter C., MD
Hamilton, George, PT
Hammond, George, MD
Hershman, A. Gloria, OTR, FAOTA
Hollis, L. Irene, OTR, FAOTA
Hopkins, Helen L., EdD, OTR, FAOTA
Howard, Lot D., MD
Hunter, James M., MD
Hyroop, Gilbert L., MD
James, J. I. P., MS, FRCS
Johnson, Robert W., MD
Jones, Sir Robert, ChM, FRCSI (Hon)
Kanavel, Allen B., MD, FACS
Kasch, Mary C., OTR, CVE, CHT
Kendall, Florence Peterson, PT

Kendall, Henry Otis, PT
Kenny, Elizabeth, Sister
Kilburn, Virginia, OTR, FAOTA
Kleinert, Harold E., MD
Klerekoper (DeMott), Lori A., OTR, CHT
Koch, Sumner L., MD, FACS
Landsmeer, J. M. F., Prof. Dr.
LaStayo, Paul, PhD, PT, CHT
Leonard, Judy, OTR, CHT
Littler, J. William, MD
Long, Charles, MD
Mackin, Evelyn J., PT
Madden, John W., MD
Malick, Maude, OTR
Marble, H. C., MD
Mason, Michael L., MD, FACS
Mayerson, Edith R., OTR
McNamara, Jean (physician)
Millender, Lewis H., MD
Nalebuff, Edward A., MD
Neumann, C. G., MD
Olivett, Bonnie L., OTR, CHT
Peacock, Erle L., Jr., MD
Pearson, Shirley L., OTR, MS
Petzoldt, Richard L., MD
Phalen, George S., MD
Philips, Cynthia A., MA, OTR, CHT
Pratt, Donald R., MD
Prendergast (Lauckhardt), Karen, MA, PT, CHT
Pulvertaft, R. Guy, CBE, MD, MChir, FRCS
Robinson, David W., MD
Rusk, Howard A., MD
Sabine, Clark L., OTR
Sammons, Fred, OTR, FAOTA
Schneider, Lawrence H., MD
Smith, Edwin M., MD
Smith, Helen D., MOT, OTR, FAOTA
Strickland, James W., MD
Stromberg, William B., MD
Swanson, Alfred B., MD
Switzer, Mary (Commissioner, Vocational Rehab. Admin.)
Tosberg, William A., CO&P
Trueta, Joseph, MD
Van Lede, Paul, OT, MS
van Veldhoven, Griet, OT/OrthopE
von Prince, Maj. Kilulu, MP, OTR, MS
Wilson, Robert Lee, MD
Wynn Parry, Christopher, MBE, MA, DM, FRCP, FRCS, DPhysMED
Yeakel, Lt. Col. Mary H., OTR, BS
Yerxa, Elizabeth J., EdD, OTR, FAOTA
Ziegler, Ellen M., MS, OTR, CHT
Zimmerman, Muriel, MA, OTR, FAOTA

PART TWO

Fundamental Concepts

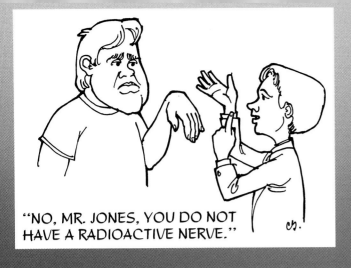

"NO, MR. JONES, YOU DO NOT HAVE A RADIOACTIVE NERVE."

CHAPTER 2

Anatomy and Kinesiology
of the Upper Extremity

Section 1
Hand, Wrist, and Forearm

JAMES W. STRICKLAND, MD

ANATOMY AND KINESIOLOGY OF THE HAND, WRIST, AND FOREARM

One cannot expect to adequately participate in the treatment of disorders of the hand and arm without a solid working knowledge of the intricate anatomic and kinesiologic relationships of the upper extremity. The preparation of externally applied splinting devices to the forearm, wrist, and hand necessitates a thorough understanding of and respect for the underlying anatomic structures. Only through comprehension of the normal anatomy of the human hand can one adequately develop an appreciation for the anatomic alternations that accompany injury and disease. Since it is impossible in this chapter to review in great detail the enormous amount of literature that has been written about the anatomic, kinesiologic, and biomechanical aspects of the hand, readers are directed to the suggested reading list at the end of this chapter for more extensive reading on these subjects.

The anatomy of the hand must be approached in a systematic fashion with individual consideration of the osseous structures, joints, musculotendinous units, blood supply, nerve supply, and surface anatomy. However, it is obvious that the systems do not function independently, but that the integrated presence of all these structures is required for normal hand function. In presenting this material, I stray into the important mechanical and kinesiologic considerations that result from the unique anatomic arrangement of the hand and briefly try to indicate the problems resulting from various forms of pathologic conditions in certain areas. Surface anatomy and a description of the basic patterns of hand function are also included at the end of the chapter.

Osseous Structures

The unique arrangement and mobility of the bones of the hand (Fig. 2-1) provide a structural basis for its enormous functional adaptability. The osseous skeleton consists of eight carpal bones divided into two rows: the proximal row articulates with the distal radius and ulna (with the exception of the pisiform, which lies palmar to and articulates with the triquetrum); the distal four carpal bones in turn articulate with the five metacarpals. Two phalanges complete the first ray, or thumb unit, and three phalanges each comprise the index, long, ring, and small fingers. These 27 bones, together with the intricate arrangement of supportive ligaments and contractile musculotendinous units, are arranged to provide both mobility and stability to the various joints of the hand. Although the exact anatomic configuration of the bones of the hand need not be memorized in detail, it is important to develop a knowledge of the position and names of the carpal bones, metacarpals, and phalanges and an understanding of their kinesiologic patterns to proceed with the management of many hand problems.

The bones of the hand are arranged in three arches (Fig. 2-2), two transversely oriented and one that is longitudinal. The proximal transverse arch, the keystone of which is the capitate, lies at the level of the distal part of the carpus and is reasonably fixed, whereas the distal transverse arch passing through the metacarpal heads is more mobile. The two transverse arches are connected by the rigid portion of the longitudinal arch consisting of the second and third metacarpals, the index and long fingers distally, and the central carpus proximally. The longitudinal arch is completed by the individual digital rays, and the mobility of the first, fourth, and fifth rays around the second and third allows the palm to flatten or cup itself to accommodate objects of various sizes and shapes.

To a large extent the intrinsic muscles of the hand are responsible for changes in the configuration of the osseous arches, and collapse in the arch system resulting from injury to the osseous skeleton or paralysis of the intrinsic muscles can contribute to severe disability and deformity. Flatt[4-6] has pointed out that grasp is dependent on the integrity of the mobile longitudinal arches and when destruction at the carpometacarpal joint, metacarpophalangeal joint, or proximal interphalangeal joint interrupts the integrity of these arches, crippling deformity may result.

Joints

The multiple complex articulations between the distal radius and ulna, the eight carpal bones, and the

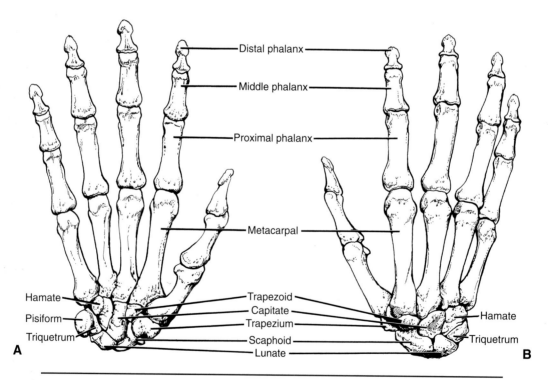

Fig. 2-1   Bones of the right hand. **A,** Palmar surface. **B,** Dorsal surface.

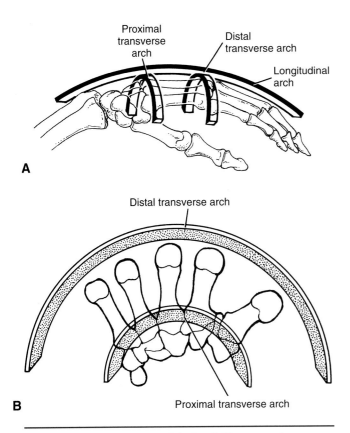

Proximal transverse arch

Distal transverse arch

Longitudinal arch

A

Distal transverse arch

B

Proximal transverse arch

Fig. 2-2   **A,** Skeletal arches of the hand. The proximal transverse arch passes through the distal carpus; the distal transverse arch, through the metacarpal heads. The longitudinal arch is made up of the four digital rays and the carpus proximally. **B,** Proximal and distal transverse arches.

metacarpal bases comprise the wrist joint, whose proximal position makes it the functional key to the motion at the more distal hand joints of the hand. Functionally the carpus transmits forces through the hand to the forearm. The proximal carpal row consisting of the scaphoid (navicular), lunate, and triquetrum articulates distally with the trapezium, trapezoid, capitate, and hamate; there is a complex motion pattern which relies both on ligamentous and contact surface constraints. The major ligaments of the wrist (Fig. 2-3) are the palmar and intracapsular ligaments. There are three strong radial palmar ligaments: the radioscaphocapitate or "sling" ligament, which supports the waist of the scaphoid; the radiolunate ligament, which supports the lunate; and the radioscapholunate ligament, which connects the scapholunate articulation with the palmar portion of the distal radius. This ligament functions as a checkrein for scaphoid flexion and extension. The ulnolunate ligament arises intra-articularly from the triangular articular meniscus of the wrist joint and inserts on the lunate and, to a lesser extent, the triquetrum. The radial and ulnar collateral ligaments are

capsular ligaments, and V-shaped ligaments from the capitate to the triquetrum and scaphoid have been termed the deltoid ligaments. Dorsally, the radiocarpal ligament connects the radius to the triquetrum and acts as a dorsal sling for the lunate, maintaining the lunate in apposition to the distal radius. Further dorsal carpal support is provided by the dorsal intracarpal ligament. These strong ligaments combine to provide carpal stability while permitting the normal range of wrist motion.

The distal ulna is covered with an articular cartilage (Fig. 2-3, *C*) over its most dorsal, palmar, and radial aspects, where it articulates with the sigmoid or ulnar notch of the radius. The triangular fibrocartilage complex describes the ligamentous and cartilaginous structure that suspends the distal radius and ulnar carpus from the distal ulna. Blumfield and Champoux (1984) have indicated that the optimal functional wrist motion to accomplish most activities of daily living is from 10° of flexion to 35° of extension.

Taleisnik[10,11,13,14] has emphasized the importance of considering the wrist in terms of longitudinal columns (Fig. 2-4). The central, or flexion extension, column consists of the lunate and the entire distal carpal row; the lateral, or mobile, column comprises the scaphoid alone; and the medial, or rotation, column is made up of the triquetrum. Wrist motion is produced by the muscles that attach to the metacarpals, and the ligamentous control system provides stability only at the extremes of motion. The distal carpal row of the carpal bones is firmly attached to the hand and moves with it. Therefore during dorsiflexion the distal carpal row dorsiflexes, during palmar flexion it palmar flexes, and during radial and ulnar deviation it deviates radially or ulnarly. As the wrist ranges from radial to ulnar deviation, the proximal carpal row rotates in a dorsal direction, and a simultaneous translocation of the proximal carpus occurs in a radial direction at the radiocarpal and midcarpal articulations. This combined motion of the carpal rows has been referred to as the rotational shift of the carpus. It was once taught that palmar flexion takes place to a greater extent at the radiocarpal joint and secondarily in the midcarpal joint, but since dorsiflexion occurs primarily at the midcarpal joint and only secondarily at the radiocarpal articulation, this now appears to be a significant oversimplification. The complex carpal kinematics are beyond the scope of this chapter, and the reader is referred to the works of Weber,[15] Taleisnik,[12] Lichtman,[7] and Cooney[3] to gain a thorough understanding of this difficult subject.

The articulation between the base of the first metacarpal and the trapezium (Fig. 2-5) is a highly mobile joint with a configuration thought to be similar to that of a saddle. The base of the first metacarpal is

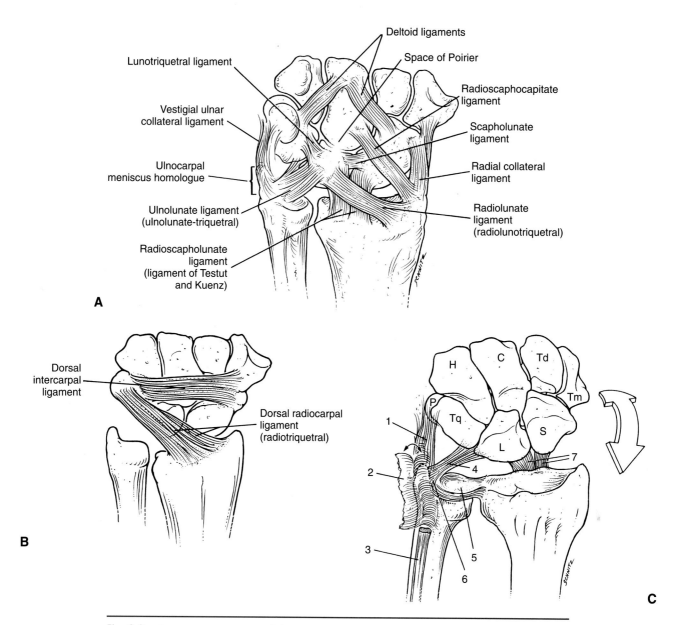

Fig. 2-3   Ligamentous anatomy of the wrist. **A,** Palmar wrist ligaments. **B,** Dorsal wrist ligaments. **C,** Dorsal view of the flexed wrist, including the triangular fibrocartilage. *1,* Ulnar collateral ligament; *2,* retinacular sheath; *3,* tendon of extensor carpi ulnaris; *4,* ulnolunate ligament; *5,* triangular fibrocartilage; *6,* ulnocarpal meniscus homologue; *7,* palmar radioscaphoid lunate ligament. *P,* Pisiform; *H,* hamate; *C,* capitate; *Td,* trapezoid; *Tm,* trapezium; *Tq,* triquetrum; *L,* lunate; *S,* scaphoid.

concave in the anteroposterior plane and convex in the lateral plane, with a reciprocal concavity in the lateral plane and an anteroposterior convexity on the opposing surface of the trapezium. This arrangement allows for the positioning of the thumb in a wide arc of motion (Fig. 2-6), including flexion, palmar and radial abduction, adduction, and opposition. The ligamentous arrangement about this joint, while permitting the wide circumduction, continues to provide stability at the extremes of motion, allowing the thumb to be brought into a variety of positions for

pinch and grasp, but maintaining its stability during these functions. The articulations formed by the ulnar half of the hamate and the fourth and fifth metacarpal bases allow a modest amount of motion (15° at the fourth carpometacarpal joint and 25° to 30° of flexion and extension at the fifth carpometacarpal joint). A resulting "palmar descent" of these metacarpals occurs during strong grasp.

The metacarpophalangeal joints of the fingers are diarthrodial joints with motion permitted in three planes and combinations thereof (Fig. 2-7). The

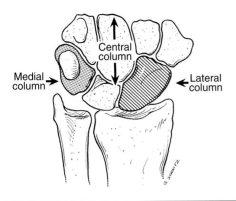

Fig. 2-4   Columnar carpus. The scaphoid is the mobile or lateral column. The central, or flexion extension, column comprises the lunate and the entire distal carpal row. The medial, or rotational, column comprises the triquetrum alone.

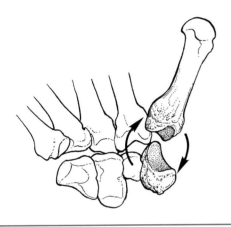

Fig. 2-5   Saddle-shaped carpometacarpal joint of the thumb. A wide range of motion (*arrows*) is permitted by the configuration of this joint.

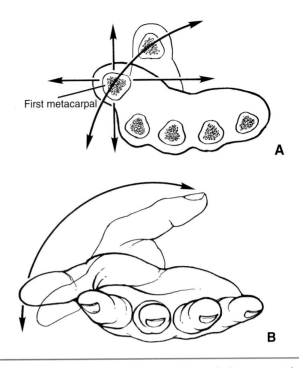

Fig. 2-6   **A,** Multiple planes of motion (*arrows*) that occur at the carpometacarpal joint of the thumb. **B,** The thumb moves (*arrow*) from a position of adduction against the second metacarpal to a position of palmar or radial abduction away from the hand and fingers and can then be rotated into positions of opposition and flexion.

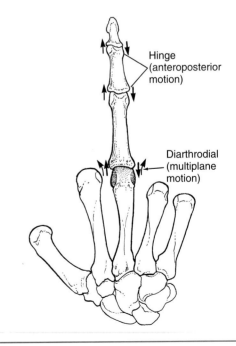

Fig. 2-7   Joints of the phalanges. The diarthrodial configuration of the metacarpophalangeal joint permits motion in multiple planes, whereas the biconcave-convex hinge configuration of the interphalangeal joints restricts motion to the anteroposterior plane.

cartilaginous surfaces of the metacarpal head and the bases of the proximal phalanges are enclosed in a complex apparatus consisting of the joint capsule, collateral ligaments, and the anterior fibrocartilage or palmar plate (Fig. 2-8). The capsule extends from the borders of the base of the proximal phalanx proximally to the head of the metacarpals beyond the cartilaginous joint surface. The collateral ligaments, which reinforce the capsule on each side of the metacarpophalangeal joints, run from the dorsolateral side of the metacarpal head to the palmar lateral side of the proximal phalanges. These ligaments form two bundles, the more central of which is referred to as the *cord portion of the collateral ligament* and inserts into the side of the proximal phalanx; the more palmar portion joins the palmar plate and is termed the *accessory collateral ligament*. These collateral ligaments are somewhat loose with the metacarpophalangeal

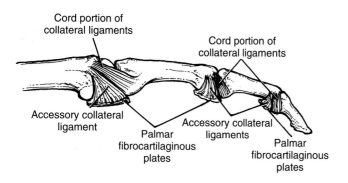

Fig. 2-8   Ligamentous structures of the digital joints. The collateral ligaments of the metacarpophalangeal and interdigital joints are composed of a strong cord portion with bony origin and insertion. The more palmarly placed accessory collateral ligaments originate from the proximal bone and insert into the palmar fibrocartilaginous plate. The palmar plates have strong distal attachments to resist extension forces.

joint in extension, allowing for considerable "play" in the side-to-side motion of the digits (Fig. 2-9). With the metacarpophalangeal joints in full flexion, however, the cam configuration of the metacarpal head tightens the collateral ligaments and limits lateral mobility of the digits. This alteration in tension becomes an important factor in immobilization of the metacarpophalangeal joints for any length of time, since the secondary shortening of the lax collateral ligaments that may occur when these joints are immobilized in extension will result in severe limitation of metacarpophalangeal joint flexion by these structures.

The palmar fibrocartilaginous plate on the palmar side of the metacarpophalangeal joint is firmly attached to the base of the proximal phalanx and loosely attached to the anterior surface of the neck of the metacarpal by means of the joint capsule at the neck of the metacarpal. This arrangement allows the palmar plate to slide proximally during metacarpophalangeal joint flexion. The flexor tendons pass along a groove anterior to the plate. The palmar plates are connected by the transverse intermetacarpal ligaments, which connect each plate to its neighbor.

The metacarpophalangeal joint of the thumb differs from the others in that the head of the first metacarpal is flatter and its cartilaginous surface does not extend as far laterally or posteriorly. Two small sesamoid bones are also adjacent to this joint, and the ligamentous structure differs somewhat. A few degrees of abduction and rotation are permitted by the ligament arrangement of the metacarpophalangeal joint at the thumb, which is of considerable functional importance in delicate precision functions. There is considerable variation in the range of motion present at the thumb metacarpophalangeal joints. The amount

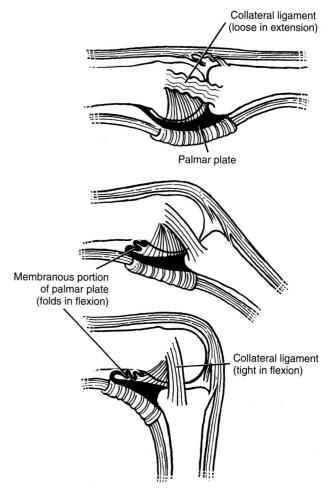

Fig. 2-9   At the metacarpophalangeal joint level, the collateral ligaments are loose in extension but become tightened in flexion. The proximal membranous portion of the palmar plate moves proximally to accommodate for flexion. (Modified from Wynn Parry CB, et al.: *Rehabilitation of the hand*, ed 3, Butterworth, 1973, London.)

of motion varies from as little as 30° to as much as 90°.

The digital interphalangeal joints are hinge joints (Fig. 2-7) and, like the metacarpophalangeal joints, have capsular and ligamentous enclosure. The articular surface of the proximal phalangeal head is convex in the anteroposterior plane with a depression in the middle between the two condyles, which articulates with the phalanx distal to it. The bases of the middle and distal phalanges appear as a concave surface with an elevated ridge dividing two concave depressions. A cord portion of the collateral ligament and an accessory collateral ligament are present, and the collateral ligaments run on each side of the joint from the dorsolateral aspect of the proximal phalanx in a palmar and lateral direction to insert into the distally placed phalanx and its fibrocartilage plate (Fig. 2-10).

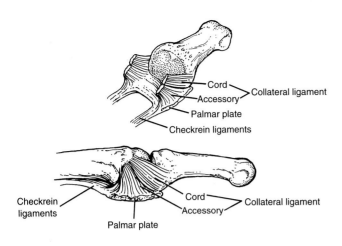

Fig. 2-10 Strong, three-sided ligamentous support system of the proximal interphalangeal joint with cord and accessory collateral ligaments and the fibrocartilaginous plate, which is anchored proximally by the checkrein ligamentous attachment. (Modified from Eaton RG: *Joint injuries of the hand,* Charles C Thomas, 1971, Springfield, IL.)

A strong fibrocartilaginous (palmar) plate is also present, and the collateral ligaments of the proximal and distal interphalangeal joints are tightest with the joints in near full extension.

The stability of the proximal interphalangeal joint is ensured by a three-sided supporting cradle produced by the junction of the palmar plate with the base of the middle phalanx and the accessory collateral ligament structures (Fig. 2-10). The confluence of ligaments is strongly anchored by proximal and lateral extensions referred to as the *checkrein ligaments.* This system has been described as a three-dimensional hinge that results in remarkable palmar and lateral restraint.

A wide range of pathologic conditions may result from the interruption of the supportive ligament system of the intercarpal or digital joints. At the wrist level, interruption of key radiocarpal or intercarpal ligaments may result in occult patterns of wrist instability that are often difficult to diagnose and treat. In the digits, disruption of the collateral ligaments or the fibrocartilaginous palmar plates will produce joint laxity or deformity, which is more obvious. Rupture or attenuation of these supporting structures may result not only from trauma, but may also occur more insidiously with chronic disease processes such as arthritis.

Muscles and Tendons

The muscles acting on the hand can be grouped as extrinsic, when their muscle bellies are in the forearm, or intrinsic, when the muscles originate distal to the wrist joint. It is important to thoroughly understand both systems. Although their contributions to hand function are distinctly different, the integrated function of both systems is important to the satisfactory performance of the hand in a wide variety of tasks. A schematic representation of the origin and insertion of the extrinsic flexor and extensor muscle tendon units of the hand is provided in Figs. 2-11 and 2-15. The important nerve supply to each muscle group is reviewed in this Figure and again when discussing the nerve supply to the upper extremity.

Extrinsic Muscles

The extrinsic flexor muscles (Fig. 2-11) of the forearm form a prominent mass on the medial side of the upper part of the forearm: the most superficial group comprises the pronator teres, the flexor carpi radialis, the flexor carpi ulnaris, and the palmaris longus; the intermediate group the flexor digitorum superficialis; and the deep extrinsics the flexor digitorum profundus and the flexor pollicis longus. The pronator, palmaris, wrist flexors, and superficialis tendons arise from the area about the medial epicondyle, the ulnar collateral ligament of the elbow, and the medial aspect of the coronoid process. The flexor pollicis longus originates from the entire middle third of the palmar surface of the radius and the adjacent interosseous membrane, and the flexor digitorum profundus originates deep to the other muscles of the forearm from the proximal two-thirds of the ulna on the palmar and medial side. The deepest layer of the palmar forearm is completed distally by the pronator quadratus muscle.

The flexor carpi radialis tendon inserts on the base of the second metacarpal, whereas the flexor carpi ulnaris inserts into both the pisiform and fifth metacarpal base. The superficialis tendons lie superficial to the profundus tendons as far as the digital bases, where they bifurcate and wrap around the profundi and rejoin over the distal half of the proximal phalanx as Camper's chiasma (Fig. 2-12). The superficialis tendon again splits for a dual insertion on the proximal half of the middle phalanges. The profundi continue through the superficialis decussation to insert on the base of the distal phalanx. The flexor pollicis longus inserts on the base of the distal phalanx of the thumb.

At the wrist the nine long flexor tendons enter the carpal tunnel beneath the protective roof of the deep transverse carpal ligament in company with the median nerve. In this canal the common profundus tendon to the long, ring, and small fingers divides into the individual tendons that fan out distally and proceed toward the distal phalanges of these digits (Fig. 2-13). At approximately the level of the distal palmar crease the paired profundus and superficialis

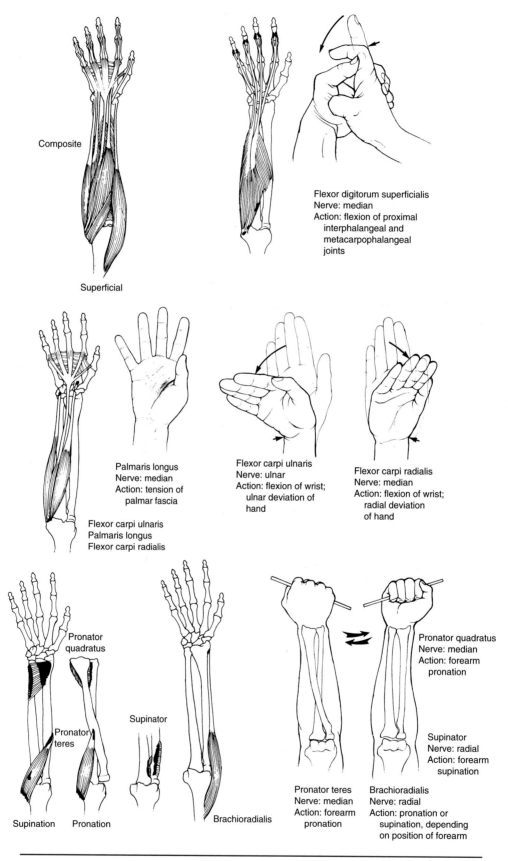

Composite

Superficial

Flexor digitorum superficialis
Nerve: median
Action: flexion of proximal
       interphalangeal and
       metacarpophalangeal
       joints

Palmaris longus
Nerve: median
Action: tension of
       palmar fascia

Flexor carpi ulnaris
Palmaris longus
Flexor carpi radialis

Flexor carpi ulnaris
Nerve: ulnar
Action: flexion of wrist;
       ulnar deviation of
       hand

Flexor carpi radialis
Nerve: median
Action: flexion of wrist;
       radial deviation
       of hand

Pronator
quadratus

Pronator
teres

Supinator

Supination   Pronation

Brachioradialis

Pronator quadratus
Nerve: median
Action: forearm
       pronation

Supinator
Nerve: radial
Action: forearm
       supination

Pronator teres
Nerve: median
Action: forearm
       pronation

Brachioradialis
Nerve: radial
Action: pronation or
       supination, depending
       on position of forearm

Fig. 2-11   Extrinsic flexor muscles of the arm and hand. (Dark areas represent origins and insertions of muscles.) (Modified from Marble HC: *The hand, a manual and atlas for the general surgeon,* Saunders, 1960, Philadelphia.)

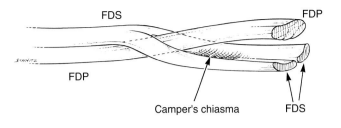

Fig. 2-12   Anatomy of the relationship between the flexor digitorum superficialis *(FDS)*, flexor digitorum profundus *(FDP)*, and the proximal portion of the flexor tendon sheath. The superficialis tendon divides and passes around the profundus tendon to reunite at Camper's chiasma. The tendon once again divides prior to insertion on the base of the middle phalanx.

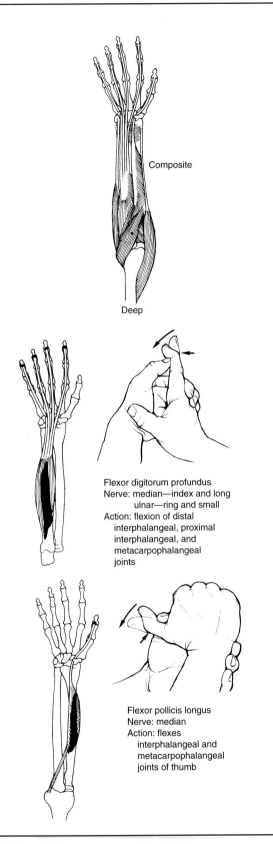

Fig. 2-11, cont'd
For legend see opposite page.

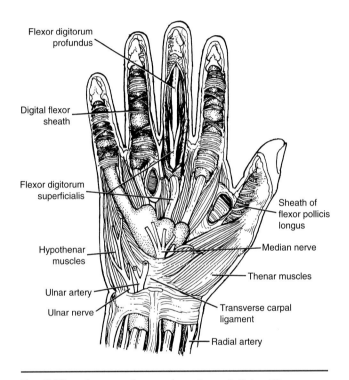

Fig. 2-13   Flexor tendons in the palm and digits. Fibroosseous digital sheaths with their pulley arrangement are shown, as is a division of the superficialis tendon about the profundus in the proximal portion of the sheath.

tendons to the index, long, ring, and small fingers and the flexor pollicis longus to the thumb enter the individual flexor sheaths that house them throughout the remainder of their digital course. These sheaths with their predictable annular pulley arrangement (Fig. 2-14) serve not only as a protective housing for the flexor tendons, but also provide a smooth gliding surface by virtue of their synovial lining and an efficient mechanism to hold the tendons close to the digital bone and joints. There is an increasing recognition that disruption of this valuable pulley system can produce substantial mechanical

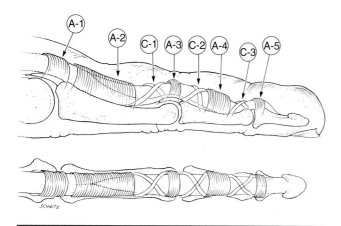

Fig. 2-14   Components of the digital flexor sheath. The sturdy annular pulleys *(A)* are important biomechanically in guaranteeing the efficient digital motion by keeping the tendons closely applied to the phalanges. The thin pliable cruciate pulleys *(C)* permit the flexor sheath to be flexible while maintaining its integrity. (Modified from Doyle JR, Blythe W: The finger flexor tendon sheath and pulleys: anatomy and reconstruction. In American Academy of Orthopaedic Surgeons: *Symposium on tendon surgery in the hand*, Mosby, 1975, St. Louis.)

alterations in digital function, resulting in imbalance and deformity.

Extension of the wrist and fingers is produced by the extrinsic extensor muscle tendon system, which consists of the two radial wrist extensors, the extensor carpi ulnaris, the extensor digitorum communis, extensor indicis proprius and the extensor digiti quinti proprius (extensor digiti minimi) (Fig. 2-15). These muscles originate in common from the lateral epicondyle and the lateral epicondylar ridge and from a small area posterior to the radial notch of the ulna. The brachioradialis originates from the epicondylar line proximal to the lateral epicondyle and, because it inserts on the distal radius, it does not truly contribute to wrist or digit motion. The extensor carpi radialis longus and brevis insert proximally on the bases of the second and third metacarpals, respectively, and the extensor carpi ulnaris inserts on the base of the fifth metacarpal. The long digital extensors terminate by insertions on the bases of the middle phalanges after receiving and giving fibers to the intrinsic tendons to form the lateral bands that are destined to insert on the bases of the distal phalanx. Digital extension, therefore, results from a combination of the contribution of both the extrinsic and intrinsic extensor systems. The extensor pollicis longus and brevis tendons, together with the abductor pollicis longus, originate from the dorsal forearm and, by virtue of their respective insertions into the distal phalanx, proximal phalanx, and first metacarpal of the thumb, provide extension at all three levels. The extensor pollicis longus approaches the thumb obliquely around a small bony tubercle on

the dorsal radius (Lister's tubercle) and therefore functions not only as an extensor but as a strong secondary adductor of the thumb. The extensor indicis proprius also originates more distally than the extensor communis tendons from an area near the origin of the thumb extensor and long abductor. It lies on the ulnar aspect of the communis tendon to the index finger and inserts with it in the dorsal approaches of that digit. The extensor digiti quinti proprius arises near the lateral epicondyle to occupy a superficial position on the dorsum of the forearm with its paired tendons lying on the fifth metacarpal ulnar to the communis tendon to the fifth finger. It inserts into the extensor apparatus of that digit.

At the wrist, the extensor tendons are divided into six dorsal compartments (Fig. 2-16). The first compartment consists of the tendons of the abductor pollicis longus and extensor pollicis brevis and the second compartment houses the two radial wrist extensors, the extensor carpi radialis longus, and brevis. The third compartment is composed of the tendon of the extensor pollicis longus and the fourth compartment allows passage of the four communis extensor tendons and the extensor indicis proprius tendon. The extensor digiti quinti proprius travels through the fifth dorsal compartment and the sixth houses the extensor carpi ulnaris.

Intrinsic Muscles

The important intrinsic musculature of the hand can be divided into muscles comprising the thenar eminence, those comprising the hypothenar eminence, and the remaining muscles between the two groups (Fig. 2-17). The muscles of the thenar eminence consist of the abductor pollicis brevis, the flexor pollicis brevis, and the opponens pollicis, which originate in common from the transverse carpal ligament and the scaphoid and trapezium bones. The abductor brevis inserts into the radial side of the proximal phalanx and the radial wing tendon of the thumb, as does the flexor pollicis brevis, whereas the opponens inserts into the whole radial side of the first metacarpal.

The flexor pollicis brevis has a superficial portion that is innervated by the median nerve and a deep portion that arises from the ulnar side of the first metacarpal and is often innervated by the ulnar nerve. The hypothenar eminence in a similar manner is made up of the abductor digiti quinti, the flexor digiti quinti brevis, and the opponens digiti quinti, which originate primarily from the pisiform bone and the pisohamate ligament and insert into the joint capsule of the fifth metacarpophalangeal joint, the ulnar side of the base of the proximal phalanx of the fifth finger, and the ulnar border of the aponeurosis of this digit. The strong

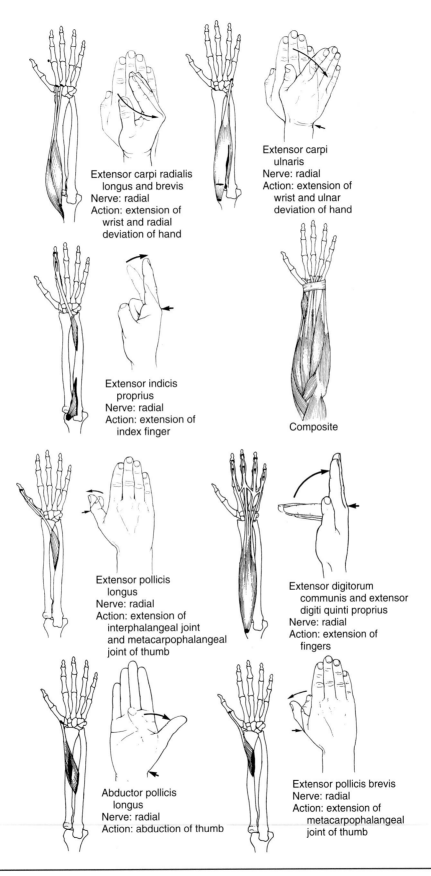

Extensor carpi radialis
longus and brevis
Nerve: radial
Action: extension of
wrist and radial
deviation of hand

Extensor carpi
ulnaris
Nerve: radial
Action: extension of
wrist and ulnar
deviation of hand

Extensor indicis
proprius
Nerve: radial
Action: extension of
index finger

Composite

Extensor pollicis
longus
Nerve: radial
Action: extension of
interphalangeal joint
and metacarpophalangeal
joint of thumb

Extensor digitorum
communis and extensor
digiti quinti proprius
Nerve: radial
Action: extension of
fingers

Abductor pollicis
longus
Nerve: radial
Action: abduction of thumb

Extensor pollicis brevis
Nerve: radial
Action: extension of
metacarpophalangeal
joint of thumb

Fig. 2-15   Extrinsic extensor muscles of the forearm and hand. (Modified from Marble HC: *The hand, a manual and atlas for the general surgeon*, Saunders, 1960, Philadelphia.)

thenar musculature is responsible for the ability to position the thumb in opposition so that it may meet the adjacent digits for pinch and grasp functions, whereas the hypothenar group allows a similar but less pronounced rotation of the fifth metacarpal.

Of the seven interosseous muscles, four are considered in the dorsal group (Fig. 2-18, B) and three as palmar interossei (Fig. 2-18, C). The four dorsal interossei originate from the adjacent sides of the metacarpal bones and, because of their bipennate nature with two individual muscle bellies, have separate insertions into the tubercle and the lateral aspect of the proximal phalanges and into the extensor expansion. The more palmarly placed three palmar interossei (Fig. 2-18, C) have similar insertions and origins and are responsible for adducting the digits together, as opposed to the spreading or abducting function of the dorsal interossei. In addition, four lumbrical tendons (Fig. 2-19, A) arising from the radial side of the palmar portion of the flexor digitorum profundus tendons pass through their individual canals on the radial side of the digits to provide an additional contribution to the complex extensor assemblage of the digits. The arrangement of the extensor mechanism, including the transverse sagittal band fibers at the metacarpophalangeal joint and the components of the extensor hood mechanism that gain fibers from both the extrinsic and intrinsic tendons, can be seen in Fig. 2-19, B,C.

An oversimplification of the function of the intrinsic musculature in the digits would be that they provide strong flexion at the metacarpophalangeal joints and extension at the proximal and distal interphalangeal joints. The lumbrical tendons, by virtue of their origin from the flexor profundi and insertion into the digital extensor mechanism, function as a governor between the two systems, resulting in a loosening of the antagonistic profundus tendon during interphalangeal joint extension. The interossei are further responsible for spreading and closing of the fingers and, together with the extrinsic flexor and extensor tendons, are invaluable to digital balance. A composite, well-integrated pattern of digital flexion and extension is reliant on the smooth performance of both systems, and a loss of intrinsic function will result in severe deformity.

Perhaps the most important intrinsic muscle, the adductor pollicis (Fig. 2-18, A), originates from the third metacarpal and inserts on the ulnar side of the base of the proximal phalanx of the thumb and

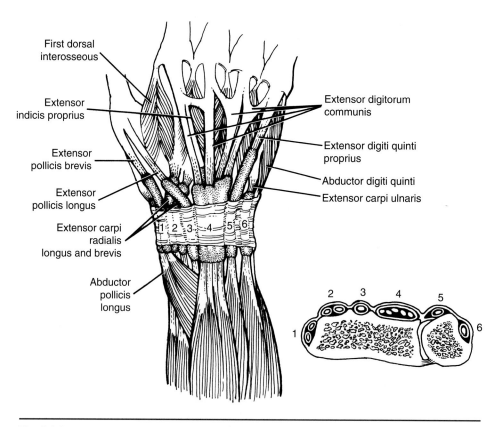

Fig. 2-16   Arrangement of the extensor tendons in the compartments of the wrist.

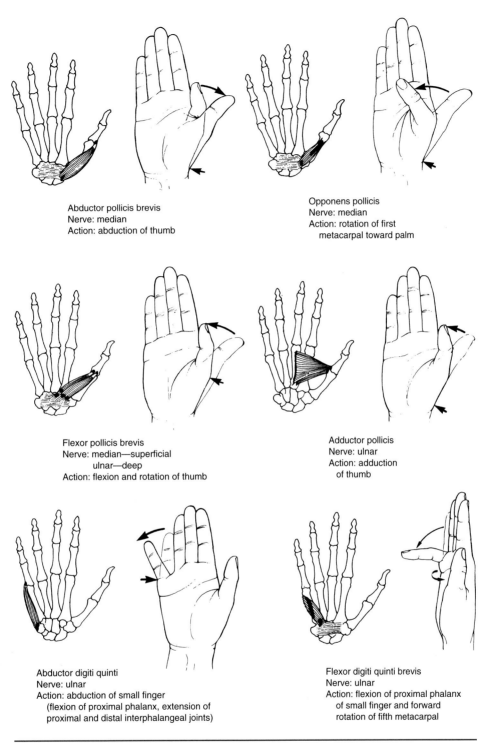

Abductor pollicis brevis
Nerve: median
Action: abduction of thumb

Opponens pollicis
Nerve: median
Action: rotation of first
    metacarpal toward palm

Flexor pollicis brevis
Nerve: median—superficial
        ulnar—deep
Action: flexion and rotation of thumb

Adductor pollicis
Nerve: ulnar
Action: adduction
    of thumb

Abductor digiti quinti
Nerve: ulnar
Action: abduction of small finger
    (flexion of proximal phalanx, extension of
    proximal and distal interphalangeal joints)

Flexor digiti quinti brevis
Nerve: ulnar
Action: flexion of proximal phalanx
    of small finger and forward
    rotation of fifth metacarpal

Fig. 2-17   Intrinsic muscles of the hand. (Modified from Marble HC: *The hand, a manual and atlas for the general surgeon*, Saunders, 1960, Philadelphia.)

into the ulnar wing expansion of the extensor mechanism. This muscle, by virtue of its strong adducting influence on the thumb and its stabilizing effect on the first metacarpophalangeal joint, functions together with the first dorsal interosseous to provide strong pinch. The adductor pollicis, deep head of the flexor pollicis brevis, ulnar two lumbricals, and all interossei, as well as the hypothenar muscle group, are innervated by the ulnar nerve. Loss of ulnar nerve function has a profound influence on hand function.

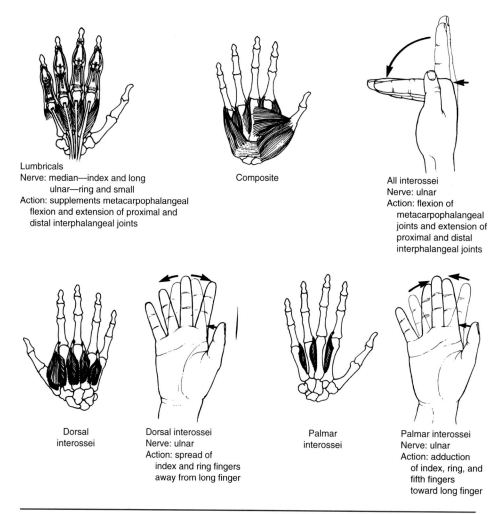

Lumbricals
Nerve: median—index and long
        ulnar—ring and small
Action: supplements metacarpophalangeal
        flexion and extension of proximal and
        distal interphalangeal joints

Composite

All interossei
Nerve: ulnar
Action: flexion of
        metacarpophalangeal
        joints and extension of
        proximal and distal
        interphalangeal joints

Dorsal
interossei

Dorsal interossei
Nerve: ulnar
Action: spread of
        index and ring fingers
        away from long finger

Palmar
interossei

Palmar interossei
Nerve: ulnar
Action: adduction
        of index, ring, and
        fifth fingers
        toward long finger

Fig. 2-17, cont'd
For legend see p. 59.

Muscle Balance and Biomechanical Considerations

When there is normal resting tone in the extrinsic and intrinsic muscle groups of the forearm and hand, the wrist and digital joints will be maintained in a balanced position. With the forearm midway between pronation and supination, the wrist dorsiflexed, and the digits in moderate flexion, the hand is in the optimum position from which to function.

It may be seen that muscles are usually arranged about joints in pairs so that each musculotendinous unit has at least one antagonistic muscle to balance the involved joint. To a large extent the wrist is the key joint and has a strong influence on the long extrinsic muscle performance at the digital level. Maximal digital flexion strength is facilitated by dorsiflexion of the wrist, which lessens the effective amplitude of the antagonistic extensor tendons while maximizing the contractural force of the digital flexors. Conversely, a posture of wrist flexion will markedly weaken grasping power.

At the digital level, metacarpophalangeal joint flexion is a combination of extrinsic flexor power supplemented by the contribution of the intrinsic muscles, whereas proximal interphalangeal joint extension results from a combination of extrinsic extensor and intrinsic muscle power. At the distal interphalangeal joint the intrinsic muscles provide a majority of the extensor power necessary to balance the antagonistic flexor digitorum profundus tendon.

The distance that a tendon moves when its muscle contracts is defined as the amplitude of the tendon and has been measured in numerous studies. In actuality the effective amplitude of any muscle will be limited by the motion permitted by the joint or joints on which its tendon acts. It has been suggested that the amplitude of wrist movers (flexor carpi ulnaris, flexor carpi radialis, extensor carpi radialis longus, extensor carpi radialis brevis, and extensor carpi ulnaris) is approximately 30 mm with the amplitude of finger extensors averaging 50 mm; the thumb flexor,

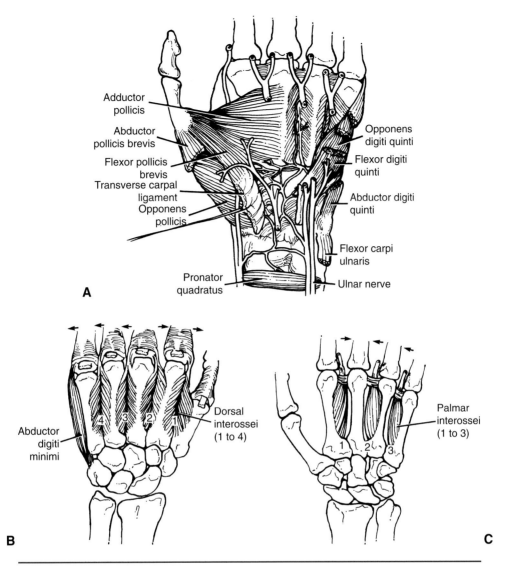

Fig. 2-18   Position and function of the intrinsic muscles of the hand.

50 mm; and the finger flexors 70 mm (Fig. 2-20). Although these amplitudes have been thought to be important considerations when deciding on appropriate tendon transfers, Brand[1,2] has shown that the potential excursion of a given tendon such as the extensor carpi radialis longus may be considerably greater than the excursion that was required to produce full motion of the joints on which it acted in its original position.

Efforts have been made to determine the power of individual forearm and hand muscles and a formula based on the physiologic cross section is generally accepted as the best method for determining this value. The number of fibers in cross section determines the absolute muscle power of a given muscle, whereas the force of muscle action times the distance or amplitude of a given muscle determines the work capacity of the muscle. Therefore a large extrinsic muscle with relatively long fibers such as the flexor digitorum profundus is found to be capable of much more work than is a muscle with shorter fibers such as a wrist extensor. Table 2-1 is an indicator of the work capacities of the various forearm muscles. It can be seen that the flexor digitorum profundus and superficialis have a significantly greater work capacity than do the remaining extrinsic muscles. The abductor pollicis longus, palmaris longus, extensor pollicis longus, extensor carpi radialis brevis, and flexor carpi radialis have less than one fourth the capacity of these muscles.

Several mechanical considerations are important in understanding the effect of a muscle on a given

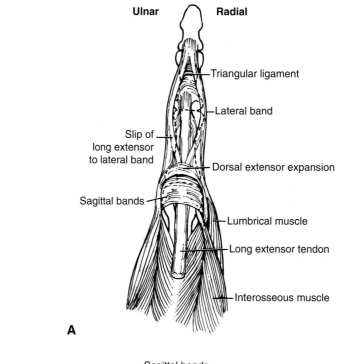

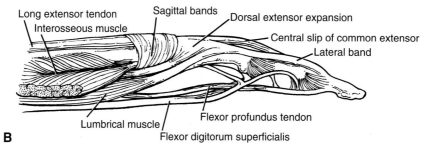

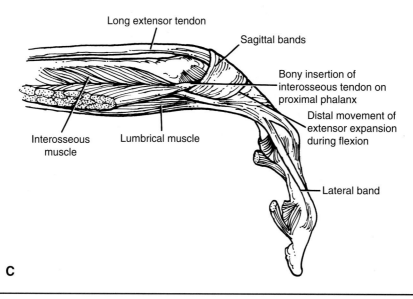

Fig. 2-19   **A,** Extensor mechanism of the digits. **B,C,** Distal movement of the extensor expansion with metacarpophalangeal joint flexion is shown.

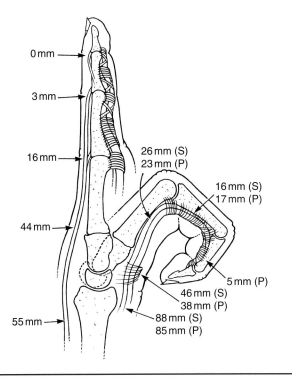

Fig. 2-20   Excursion of the flexor and extensor tendons at various levels. The numbers on the dorsum of the extended finger represent the excursion in millimeters required at each level to bring all distal joints from full flexion into full extension. The numbers shown by arrows on the palmar aspect of the flexed digit represent the excursion in millimeters for the superficialis *(S)* and the profundus *(P)* required at each level to bring the finger from full extension to full flexion. (From Verdan C: An introduction to tendon surgery. In Verdan C: *Tendon surgery of the hand*, Churchill Livingstone, 1979, London.)

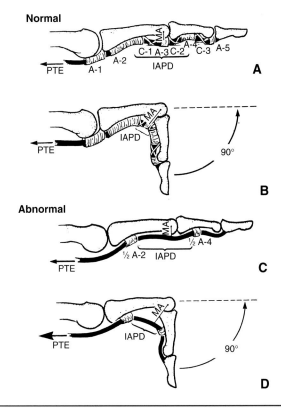

Fig. 2-21   Biomechanics of the finger flexor pulley system. **A.** The arrangement of the annular and cruciate pulleys of the flexor tendon sheath. **A,B,** Normal moment arm *(MA)*, the intraannular pulley distance *(IPD)* between the A-2 and A-4 pulleys, and the profundus tendon excursion *(PTE)*, which occurs within the intact digital fibroosseous canal as the proximal interphalangeal joint is flexed to 90°. Annular pulleys: A-1, A-2, A-3, A-4, and A-5; cruciate pulleys: C-I, C-2, C-3. **C,D,** Biomechanical alteration resulting from excision of the distal half of the A-2 pulley together with the C-1, A-3, C-2, and proximal portion of the A-4 pulley. The moment arm is increased, and a greater profundus tendon excursion is required to produce 90° of flexion because of the bowstringing that results from the loss of pulley support. (From Strickland JW: Management of acute flexor tendon injuries, *Orthopaedic Clinics of North America*, vol 14, Saunders, 1983, Philadelphia.)

TABLE 2-1   Work Capacity of Muscles

Muscle	Mkg
Flexor carpi radialis	0.8
Extensor carpi radialis longus	1.1
Extensor carpi radialis brevis	0.9
Extensor carpi ulnaris	1.1
Abductor pollicis longus	0.1
Flexor pollicis longus	1.2
Flexor digitorum profundus	4.5
Flexor digitorum superficialis	4.8
Brachioradialis	1.9
Flexor carpi ulnaris	2.0
Pronator teres	1.2
Palmaris longus	0.1
Extensor pollicis longus	0.1
Extensor digitorum communis	1.7

From Von Lanz T, Wachsmuth W: Praktische anatomie. In Boyes IH: *Bunnell's surgery of the hand*, ed 5, Lippincott, 1970, Philadelphia.

joint. The moment arm of a particular muscle is the perpendicular distance between the muscle or its tendon and the axis of the joint. The greater the displacement of an unrestrained tendon from the joint on which it acts, the greater will be the angulatory effect created by the increased length of the moment arm. Therefore a tendon positioned close to a given joint either by position of the joint or by a restraining pulley will have a much shorter moment arm than will a tendon that is allowed to displace away from the joint (Fig. 2-21).

In simplifying the biomechanics of musculotendinous function, Brand[1] has emphasized that the "moment" of a given muscle is the power of the muscle to turn a joint on its axis. It is determined by

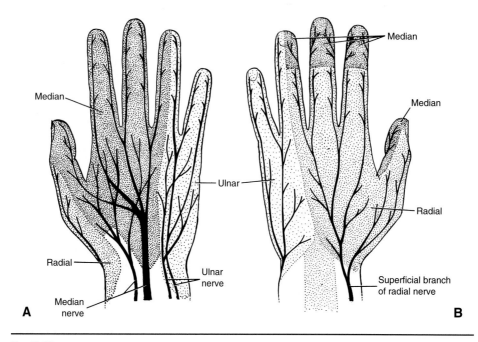

Fig. 2-22   Cutaneous distribution of the nerves of the hand. **A**, Palmar surface. **B**, Dorsal surface.

multiplying the strength (tension) of the muscle by the length of the moment arm. Again, it can be seen that the distance of tendon displacement away from the joint is the critical factor and that it does not matter where the tendon insertion lies. The importance of the various anatomic restraints of the extrinsic musculotendinous units at the wrist and in the digits is magnified by these mechanical factors.

Nerve Supply

In considering the nerve supply to the forearm, hand, and wrist, it is important to realize that these nerves are a direct continuation of the brachial plexus and that at least a working knowledge of the multiple ramifications of the plexus is necessary if one is to fully appreciate the more distal motor and sensory contributions of the nerves of the upper extremity. Injuries at either the spinal cord or plexus level or to the major peripheral nerves in the upper extremity result in a substantial functional impairment for which splinting may be necessary.

The median, ulnar, and radial nerves, as well as the terminal course of the musculocutaneous, are responsible for the sensory and motor transmission to the forearm, wrist, and hand. The superficial sensory distribution is shared by the median, radial, and ulnar nerves in a fairly constant pattern (Fig. 2-22). This chapter is concerned with the most frequent distribution of these nerves, although it is acknowledged that variations are common.

The palmar side of the hand from the thumb to a line passed longitudinally from the tip of the ring finger to the wrist receives sensory innervation from the median nerve. The remainder of the palm as well as the ulnar half of the ring finger and the entire small finger receive sensory innervation from the ulnar nerve. On the dorsal side, the ulnar nerve distribution again includes the ulnar half of the dorsal hand and the ring and small fingers, whereas the radial side is supplied by the superficial branch of the radial nerve. Some innervation to an area distal to the proximal interphalangeal joints is supplied by the palmar digital nerves originating from the median nerve. The area around the dorsum of the thumb over the metacarpophalangeal joint is frequently supplied by the end branches of the lateral antebrachial cutaneous nerve.

The extrinsic and intrinsic musculature of the forearm and hand is supplied by the median, ulnar, and radial nerves (Fig. 2-23). The long wrist and digital flexors, with the exception of the flexor carpi ulnaris and the profundi to the ring and small fingers, are all supplied by the median nerve. The pronators of the forearm and the muscles of the thenar eminence, with the exception of the deep head of the flexor pollicis brevis and the adductor pollicis, which are innervated by the ulnar nerve, are also supplied by the median nerve. All muscles of the hypothenar eminence, all interossei, the third and fourth lumbrical muscles, the deep head of the flexor pollicis brevis, the adductor pollicis brevis, as well as the flexor carpi ulnaris and the ulnar-most two profundi, are supplied by the ulnar nerve. The radial nerve supplies all long extensors of the hand and wrist as well as the long abductor and short extensor of the thumb, the supinator, and the brachioradialis of the forearm.

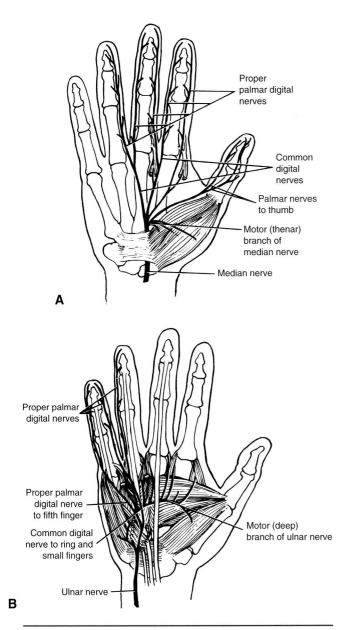

Fig. 2-23   Distribution of the median (**A**) and ulnar (**B**) nerves in the palm.

When considering sensibility, one should remember that the hand is an extremely important organ for the detection and transmission to the brain of information relating to the size, weight, texture, and temperature of objects with which it comes in contact. The types of cutaneous sensation have been defined as touch, pain, hot, and cold. Although most of the nervous tissue in the skin is found in the dermal network, smaller branches course through the subcutaneous tissue following blood vessels. Several types of sensory receptors have been described, and in most areas of the hand there is an interweaving of nerve fibers that allows each area to receive nerve input from several sources. In addition, deep sensibility

from nerve endings in muscles and tendons is important in the recognition of joint position.

The high interruption of the median nerve above the elbow will result in a paralysis of the flexor carpi radialis, the flexor digitorum superficialis, the flexor pollicus longus, the profundi to the index and long fingers, and the lumbricals to the index and long fingers. In addition, pronation will be weakened as a result of the loss of innervation of both the pronator teres and quadratus muscles and, most importantly, the patient will lose the ability to oppose the thumb because of paralysis of the median nerve-innervated thenar muscle group. A more distal interruption of the median nerve at the wrist level produces loss of opposition and both lesions result in a critical impairment of sensation in the important distribution of that nerve to the palmar aspect of the thumb, index, long, and radial half of the ring finger.

High ulnar nerve interruption produces paralysis of the flexor carpi ulnaris, the flexor profundi and lumbricals to the ring and small fingers and, most importantly, the interossei, adductor pollicis brevis, and deep head of the flexor pollicis brevis. The resulting loss of the antagonistic flexion at the metacarpophalangeal joints of the ring and small fingers permits hyperextension at this level by the unopposed long extensor tendons, often resulting in a claw deformity. The loss of the strong adducting and stabilizing influence of the adductor pollicis combined with the paralysis of the first dorsal interosseous muscle results in profound weakness of pinch and produces a collapse deformity of the thumb, necessitating interphalangeal joint hyperflexion for pinch (Froment's sign). More distal lesions of the ulnar nerve usually result in a greater degree of claw deformity due to the sparing of the profundi function of the ring and small fingers. Sensory loss following ulnar nerve interruption involves the palmar ring (ulnar half) and small fingers.

Radial nerve lesions at or proximal to the elbow result in a complete wrist drop and inability to extend the fingers at the metacarpophalangeal joints. It should be remembered that paralysis of this nerve does not result in inability to extend the interphalangeal joints of either the thumb or digits because of the contribution to that function by the intrinsic muscles. The sensory deficit over the dorsoradial aspect of the wrist and hand resulting from radial nerve interruption is of much less significance than are lesions to nerves innervating the palmar side.

Various combinations of paralyses involving more than one nerve of the upper extremity are frequently encountered; those of the median and ulnar nerve are the most common. High lesions of these two nerves produce paralyses of both the extrinsic and intrinsic muscle groups with total sensory loss over the palmar aspect of the hand. More distal combined median

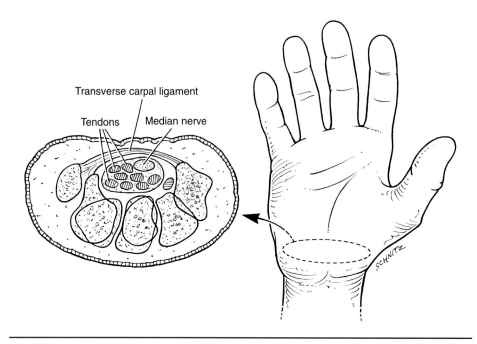

Fig. 2-24 Cross sectional anatomy of the carpal tunnel shows its anatomic boundaries. The carpus and the palmar roof formed by the transverse carpal ligament are shown, as is the position of the median nerve. An increased volume in this passageway most frequently resulting from thickening or inflammation around the nine flexor tendons can result in compression of the median nerve and the condition known as carpal tunnel syndrome.

and ulnar lesions will have their effect primarily on the intrinsic muscles, resulting in the most disabling deformities with metacarpophalangeal hyperextension, interphalangeal flexion, and thumb collapse. An inefficient pattern of digital flexion consisting of a slow distal-to-proximal rolling grasp will result from the loss of the integrated intrinsic participation.

A number of entrapment phenomena are now recognized that may cause complete or partial paralyses, purely sensory deficits, or a combination of these alterations in any of the three major peripheral nerves of the upper extremity. Ulnar nerve compression at the elbow and median nerve compression in the carpal tunnel (Fig. 2-24) are among the more frequent entrapment entities.

Blood Supply

The blood supply to the hand is carried by the radial and ulnar arteries and their branches (Fig. 2-25). The ulnar artery, which can often be palpated just lateral to the pisiform, reaches the wrist in company with the ulnar nerve immediately lateral to the flexor carpi ulnaris tendon. The artery divides at the wrist into a large branch that forms the superficial arterial arch of the hand and a smaller branch that forms the lesser part of the deep palmar arch. As it passes between the pisiform and the hamate (canal of Guyon), the ulnar artery is particularly vulnerable

to repetitive trauma, which may result in thrombosis, giving rise to symptoms of vascular embarrassment and occasionally sensory abnormalities of the ulnar nerve by virtue of its close proximity to this structure.

The radial artery, which may be palpated near the proximal palmar wrist crease, divides into a small superficial branch, which continues distally over the thenar eminence to complete the superficial arterial arch. The larger deep radial branch passes from dorsal to palmar between the heads of the first dorsal interosseous and around the base of the thumb, where it reaches the palm to join the ulnar artery and form the deep palmar arch.

The superficial arterial arch gives off common palmar digital branches that bifurcate into proper digital branches immediately below the central part of the palmar fascia. The palmar metacarpal branches of the deep arch empty into the common palmar digital branches of the superficial arch just proximal to their bifurcation into the phalangeal arteries. It is believed by many that the superficial arterial arch is larger and more important than is the deep arch.

Although little emphasis is placed on the venous drainage of the hand, it is important to remember that the hand, like the remainder of the upper extremity, is drained by two sets of veins: a superficial group located on the superficial fascia and a deep group that travels with the arteries. The superficial venous

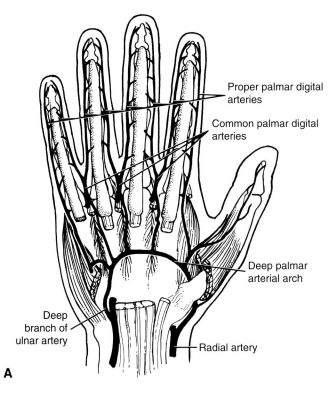

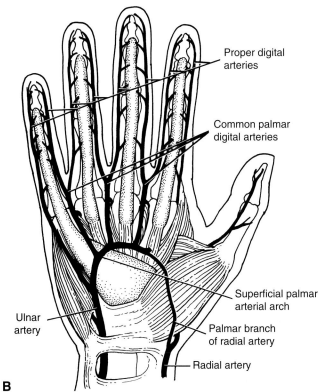

Fig. 2-25   Vascular anatomy of the hand. **A,** The deep arch is supplied by the radial artery. **B,** The superficial arch is supplied by the ulnar artery.

system is the more important, and the majority of these draining vessels form a large network over the dorsum of the hand. The dorsal venous arch receives digital veins from the fingers and becomes continuous proximally with the cephalic and basilic veins on the radial and ulnar borders of the wrist. It is easy to see why injuries over the dorsum of the hand that interrupt or are prejudicial to the flow of venous drainage can result in marked congestion and edema.

Skin and Subcutaneous Fascia

The palmar skin with its numerous small fibrous connections to the underlying palmar aponeurosis is a highly specialized, thickened structure with very little mobility. Numerous small blood vessels pass through the underlying subcutaneous tissues into the dermis. In contrast, the dorsal skin and subcutaneous tissue are much more loose with few anchoring fibers and a high degree of mobility. Most of the lymphatic drainage from the palmar aspect of the fingers, web areas, and hypothenar and thenar eminences flows in lymph channels on the dorsum of the hand. Clinical swelling, which frequently accompanies injury or infection, is usually a result of impaired lymph drainage.

The central, triangularly shaped palmar aponeurosis (Fig. 2-26) provides a semirigid barrier between the palmar skin and the important underlying neurovascular and tendon structures. It fuses medially and laterally with the deep fascia covering the hypothenar and thenar muscles, and fasciculi extending from this thick fascial barrier extend to the proximal phalanges to fuse with the tendon sheaths on the palmar, medial, and lateral aspects. In the distal palm, septa from this palmar fascia extend to the deep transverse metacarpal ligaments forming the sides of the annular fibrous canals, allowing for the passage of the ensheathed flexor tendons and the lumbrical muscles as well as the neurovascular bundles.

Dorsally the deep fascia and extensor tendons fuse to form the roof for the dorsal subaponeurotic space, which, although not as thick as its palmar counterpart, may prove restrictive to underlying fluid accumulations or intrinsic muscle swelling.

Superficial Anatomy

It is particularly important for the person engaged in splint preparation to thoroughly understand the surface anatomy of the forearm and hand, including the various landmarks that represent underlying anatomic structures. Respect for bony prominences and a knowledge of the position of underlying joints will be particularly important if one is to prepare splint devices that are comfortable and either immo-

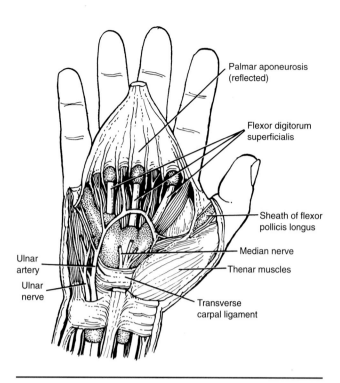

Fig. 2-26   Palmar aponeurosis reflected distally reveals septa and underlying palmar anatomy.

bilize or allow motion at various levels. Figs. 2-27 to 2-29 indicate the various contours of the forearm, wrist, and palm and the underlying structures that are responsible for these contours. In addition, the palmar creases of the surface of the wrist and palm are depicted in relation to their underlying joint structures (Fig. 2-30) to indicate the anatomic borders that must be respected in the preparation of splints designed to allow motion at either the wrist, metacarpophalangeal, or interphalangeal joint level.

Perhaps the most vulnerable of the bony prominences of the wrist and hand are the styloid processes of the radius and ulna. By virtue of their subcutaneous position, these areas are particularly vulnerable to poorly contoured splints. Great care must be taken to avoid appliances that place unequal pressure against these osseous structures.

Functional Patterns

The prehensile function of the hand depends on the integrity of the kinetic chain of bones and joints extending from the wrist to the distal phalanges. Interruptions of the transverse and longitudinal arch systems formed by these structures will always result in instability, deformity, or functional loss at a more proximal or distal level. Similarly, the balanced synergism-antagonism relationship between the long extrinsic muscles and the intrinsic muscles is a requisite for the composite functions required for both

power and precision functions of the hand. It is important to recognize that the hand cannot function well without normal sensory input from all areas.

Many attempts have been made to classify the different patterns of hand function, and various types of grasp and pinch have been described. Perhaps the more simplified analysis of power grasp and precision handling as proposed by Napier[8,9] and refined by Flatt[4-6] is the easiest to consider.

As generally stated, power grip is a combination of strong thumb flexion and adduction with the powerful flexion of the ring and small fingers on the ulnar side of the hand. The radial half of the hand employing the delicate tripod of pinch between the thumb, index, and long fingers is responsible for more delicate precision function.

An analysis of hand functions requires that one consider the thumb and the remainder of the hand as two separate parts. Rotation of the thumb into an opposing position is a requirement of almost any hand function, whether it be strong grasp or delicate pinch. The wide range of motion permitted at the carpometacarpal joint is extremely important in allowing the thumb to be correctly positioned. Stability at this joint is a requirement of almost all prehensile activities and is ensured by a unique ligamentous arrangement, which allows mobility in the midposition and provides stability at the extremes. As can be seen in Fig. 2-31, the thumb moves through a wide arc from the side of the index finger tip to the tip of the small finger, and the adaptation that occurs between the thumb and digits as progressively smaller objects are held occurs primarily at the metacarpophalangeal joints of the digits and the carpometacarpal joint of the thumb.

For power grip the wrist is in an extended position that allows the extrinsic digital flexors to press the object firmly against the palm while the thumb is closed tightly around the object. The thumb, ring, and small fingers are the most important participants in this strong grasp function, and the importance of the ulnar border digits cannot be minimized (Fig. 2-32).

In precision grasp, wrist position is less important, and the thumb is opposed to the semiflexed fingers with the intrinsic tendons providing most of the finger movement. When the intrinsic muscles are paralyzed, the balance of each finger is markedly disturbed. The metacarpophalangeal joint loses its primary flexors, and the interphalangeal joints lose the intrinsic contribution to extension. A dyskinetic finger flexion results in which the metacarpophalangeal joints lag behind the interphalangeal joints in flexion. When the hand is closed on an object, only the fingertips make contact rather than the uniform contact of the fingers, palm, and thumb that occurs with normal grip (Fig. 2-33).

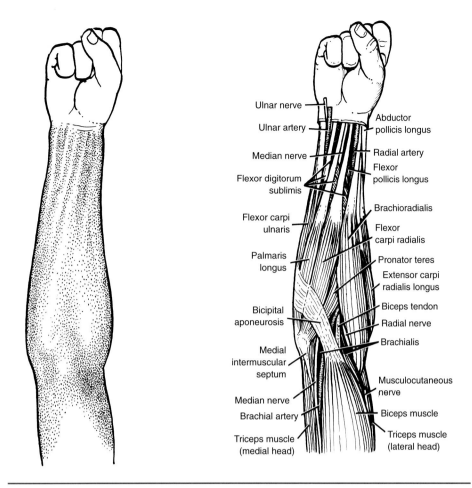

Fig. 2-27   Topographic anatomy of the palmar forearm.

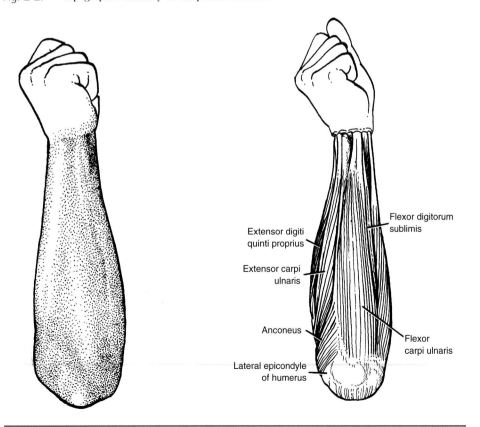

Fig. 2-28   Topographic anatomy of the medial forearm.

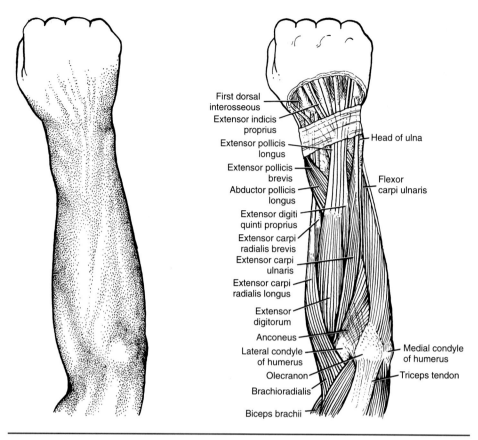

Fig. 2-29 Topographic anatomy of the dorsal forearm and hand.

First dorsal interosseous
Extensor indicis proprius
Extensor pollicis longus
Extensor pollicis brevis
Abductor pollicis longus
Extensor digiti quinti proprius
Extensor carpi radialis brevis
Extensor carpi ulnaris
Extensor carpi radialis longus
Extensor digitorum
Anconeus
Lateral condyle of humerus
Olecranon
Brachioradialis
Biceps brachii

Head of ulna
Flexor carpi ulnaris
Medial condyle of humerus
Triceps tendon

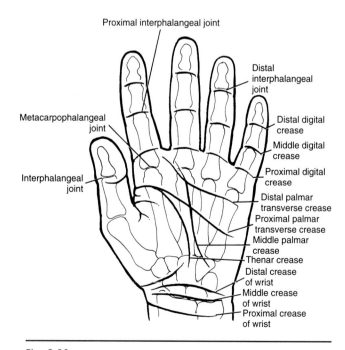

Proximal interphalangeal joint
Distal interphalangeal joint
Metacarpophalangeal joint
Distal digital crease
Middle digital crease
Proximal digital crease
Interphalangeal joint
Distal palmar transverse crease
Proximal palmar transverse crease
Middle palmar crease
Thenar crease
Distal crease of wrist
Middle crease of wrist
Proximal crease of wrist

Fig. 2-30 Relationship of the palmar skin creases to the under-lying wrist and digital joints. Metacarpophalangeal joint motion is delineated by the distal palmar crease.

Certain activities may require combinations of power and precision grips, as seen in Fig. 2-34. Pinching between the thumb and the combined index and long fingers is a further refinement of precision grip and may be classified as either tip grip, palmar grip, or lateral grip (Fig. 2-35), depending on the portions of the phalanges brought to bear on the object being handled. In these functions the strong contracture of the adductor pollicis brings the thumb into contact against the tip or sides of the index or index and long fingers with digital resistance imparted by the first and second dorsal interossei.

The size of the object being handled dictates whether large thumb and digital surfaces, as in palmar grip, or smaller surfaces, as in lateral or tip grasp, are used. Flatt (1974) has pointed out that the dual importance of rotation and flexion of the thumb is often ignored in the preparation of splints, which permit only tip grip because the thumb cannot oppose the pulp of the fingers to produce palmar grip.

The patterns of action of the normal hand depend on the mobility of the skeletal arches, and alterations of the configuration of these arches is produced by the balanced function of the extrinsic and intrinsic

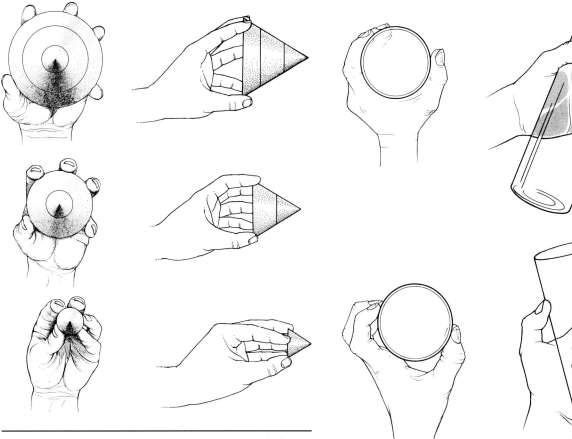

Fig. 2-31   Progressive alterations in precision grasp with changes in object size. Adaptation takes place primarily at the carpometacarpal joint of the thumb and the metacarpophalangeal joints of the digits.

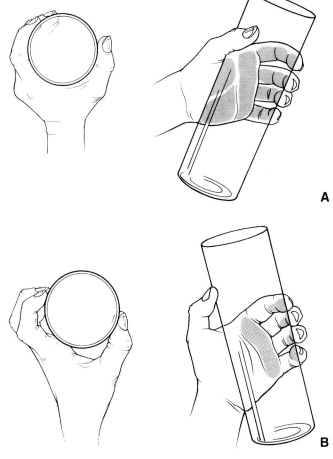

Fig. 2-33   **A**, Normal hand grasping a cylinder. Uniform areas of palm and digital contact are shaded. **B**, Intrinsic minus (claw hand grasping the same cylinder). The area of contact is limited to the fingertips and the metacarpal heads. (From Brand PW: *Clinical mechanics of the hand*, ed 2, Mosby, 1999, St. Louis.)

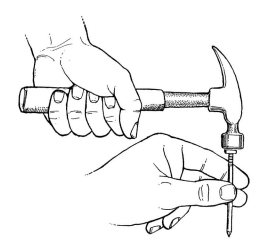

Fig. 2-32   Strong power grip imparted primarily by the thumb, ring, and small fingers around the hammer handle with delicate precision tip grip employed to hold the nail.

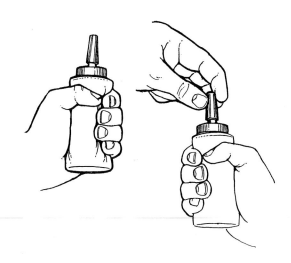

Fig. 2-34   Power grip used to hold the squeeze bottle with precision handling of the bottle top by the opposite hand.

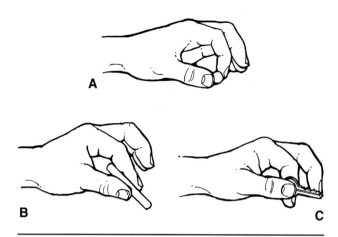

Fig. 2-35   Types of precision grip. **A,** Tip grip. **B,** Palmar grip. **C,** Lateral grip. (Modified from Flatt AE: *The care of the rheumatoid hand,* ed. 3, Mosby, 1974, St. Louis.)

muscles. Whereas the extrinsic contribution resulting from the large powerful forearm muscle groups is more important to hand strength, the fine precision action imparted by the intrinsic musculature gives the hand an enormous variety of capabilities. Although one need not specifically memorize the various patterns of pinch, grasp, and combined hand functions, it is important to understand the underlying contribution of the various muscle-tendon groups, both extrinsic and intrinsic, to these activities. Injuries or diseases that affect the integrity of the arch system or disrupt or paralyze the extrinsic or intrinsic muscles will have a profound impact on hand function.

Section 2
Anatomy of the Elbow and Shoulder

ALEXANDER D. MIH, MD

The wonderful abilities of the hand are intimately related to the function of the shoulder, elbow, and forearm. The extrinsic flexor and extensor tendons of the hand and wrist originate from the forearm bones and/or the distal humerus. Without the proper function of the shoulder, elbow, and forearm, one's ability to use the hand in activities of daily living may be severely compromised. Proper rehabilitation of the hand must, therefore, include attention to the status of these more proximal structures.

Elbow Anatomy

Superficial Anatomy

The abductor muscles (abductor pollicis longus and extensor pollicis brevis) are easily seen in most indi-

viduals, in the distal third of the dorsal forearm. It is at this level that these muscles pass superficial to the wrist extensor tendons. More proximally, the mobile wad of the forearm (brachioradialis, extensor carpi radialis longus and brevis) form the proximal lateral border of the forearm in the anatomical position. In the antecubital fossa, the biceps tendon is easily palpable and serves as a landmark for identifying deeper structures such as the brachial artery. The elbow flexion crease lies approximately 1.5 cm proximal to the joint line with the anatomic elbow extended.

Bone landmarks include the olecranon process of the proximal ulna as well as the lateral and medial humeral epicondyles. The basilic and cephalic veins are visible along the medial and lateral borders of the antecubital fossa, respectively, in most individuals.

Sensory innervation is supplied by the medial antebrachial cutaneous nerve, the lateral antebrachial cutaneous nerve (which is a continuation of the musculocutaneous nerve), and the posterior cutaneous nerve of the forearm. At the level of the elbow, the lower lateral cutaneous nerve of the arm and medial cutaneous nerve of the arm supply sensory innervation.

The radius and ulna exist in a parallel arrangement with proximal and distal articulations to allow forearm rotation. Distally, the sigmoid notch of the radius accommodates the ulnar head while proximally the radial head is covered with articular cartilage allowing rotation on the proximal ulna. The anterior surface of the radius is a site of origin for superficial finger flexors as well as the flexor pollicis longus while the distal surface is the site of insertion of the pronator quadratus. Proximally, just distal to the radial neck lies the radial or bicipital tuberosity that serves as the main site of insertion for the biceps tendon.

The ulna is tapered distally until it slightly enlarges to form the ulnar head, which is covered by articular cartilage. The coronoid process is found at the proximal end of the ulna and becomes larger at this point. The coronoid process serves as a site of insertion for the brachialis muscle as well as the important anterior bundle of the medial collateral ligament. On the lateral side of the coronoid process is the radial notch, which articulates with the cartilage-covered radial head. Proximal to the coronoid process is the trochlear (semi-lunar) notch, which extends from the coronoid process to the olecranon process. The trochlear notch is almost fully covered by cartilage, which articulates with the trochlea of the distal humerus.

The articular surface of the distal humerus consists of the capitellum and trochlea, which articulate with the radial head and proximal ulna, respectively. Along the medial border, the medial epicondyle is quite prominent and from this originates the medial collateral ligament and the flexor pronator muscula-ture of the forearm. The lateral epicondyle is found just proximal to the capitellum and serves as the site of origin for the supinator/extensor muscles as well as the lateral collateral ligament (Fig. 2-36).

Two large fossae are found proximal to the articular surface of the distal humerus and accommodate the coronoid process anteriorly and the olecranon process posteriorly. A very thin membrane of bone separates these two fossae in most individuals.

The radius and ulna are bound together distally by the components of the triangular fibrocartilage com-plex. The interosseous membrane, whose fibers run in an oblique fashion from the ulna distally to the radius proximally, has a stout central band that supplies the majority of resistance to proximal radial migration.

The existence of an ulnohumeral articulation as well as a radiohumeral articulation allows for both elbow flexion/extension and forearm axial rotation.

When viewed from the lateral aspect, the distal humerus has a 30° anterior rotation compared to the axis of the humeral shaft. This is also an average of 5° internal rotation of the distal humerus. Due to the large medial lip of the trochlea, there is 6° of valgus at the articular surface in relation to the humeral shaft.

A 15° angulation exists at the neck of the radius that further accentuates this valgus orientation. A similar angulation is found at the ulna that measures 4° in most individuals.

In the past decade a great deal of research has been carried out to define the ligamentous anatomy at the elbow. The medial collateral ligament is made up of

three components. Of these, the anterior bundle is responsible for the majority of elbow stability. The posterior bundle and the transverse ligament have minor contribution to elbow stability; however, they may be involved in secondary joint contracture. The important anterior bundle of the medial collateral lig-ament originates just inferior to the axis of rotation of the elbow and inserts into the medial aspect of the coronoid process (Fig. 2-37).

The radial side of the elbow has a much more vari-able ligamentous contribution. At least some com-ponent of lateral stability is provided by the lateral musculature.

The radial collateral ligament originates at the axis of rotation at the level of the lateral epicondyle and inserts into the annular ligament. This latter structure firmly connects the proximal radius to the ulna. While additional discreet lateral ligamentous components have been identified, their importance and function are somewhat controversial.

Vascular Anatomy

Proximal to the elbow joint the brachial artery is found slightly medial to the biceps muscle on the surface of the brachialis muscle. It then passes deep to the lacertus fibrosus (the aponeurosis of the biceps that proceeds to insert into the ulna) at the level of the cubital fossa where it divides into both radial and ulnar arteries.

The radial artery passes superficial to the biceps tendon before passing over the surface of the supina-tor and pronator teres muscles respectively. As it con-tinues its course in the forearm, it lies on the surface of the flexor digitorum superficialis and flexor pollicis longus and continues to the level of the wrist where it lies between the tendons of the brachioradialis and flexor carpi radialis, respectively.

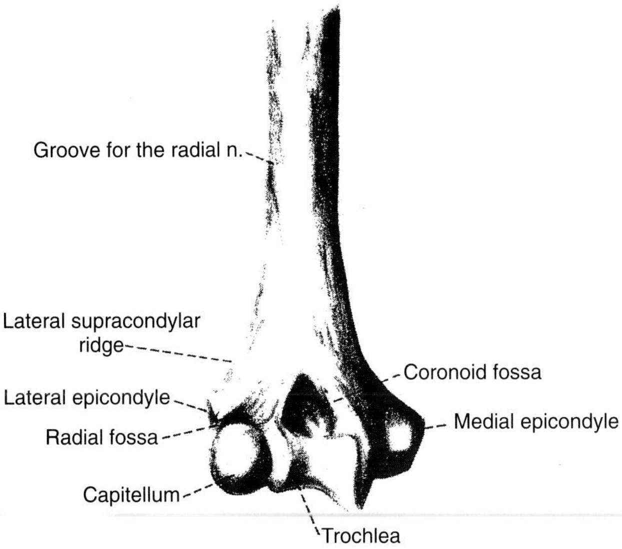

Groove for the radial n.

Lateral supracondylar ridge

Lateral epicondyle

Radial fossa

Capitellum

Coronoid fossa

Medial epicondyle

Trochlea

Fig. 2-36   Bony landmarks at the anterior aspect of the distal humerus. (From Morrey B: *The elbow and its disorders*, ed 2, Saunders, 1993, Philadelphia.)

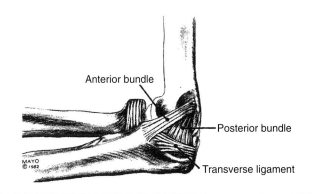

Anterior bundle

Posterior bundle

Transverse ligament

Fig. 2-37   The medial collateral ligament is divided into three separate structures: the anterior bundle, posterior bundle, and transverse ligament. The transverse ligament offers little stability to the elbow joint. (From Morrey B: *The elbow and its disorders*, ed 2, Saunders, 1993, Philadelphia.)

Multiple branches of the radial artery are given off in the proximal forearm, giving both muscular branches as well as communicating branches to similar vessels arising from the ulnar artery.

The ulnar artery has a more complicated description as it passes deep to the pronator teres and the flexor digitorum superficialis muscle belly. In the distal third of the forearm the artery is found directly deep to the flexor carpi ulnaris muscle lying between this muscle and the flexor digitorum profundi. It then continues into the wrist and hand where it forms a superficial palmar arch.

Several important collateral arteries arise from the ulnar artery including the ulnar recurrent artery, which, as its name implies, travels proximally to supply the area around the medial elbow. The common interosseous artery is found more distal and gives rise to both posterior and anterior interosseous arteries.

Nerve Supply

The median nerve consisting primarily of fibers from C6, C7, C8, and T1 is found at the level of the elbow medial to the brachial artery on the surface of the brachialis muscle. As the median nerve crosses to the level of the elbow joint, it passes between the two heads of the pronator teres. At this level it is separated from the brachial artery. It then rejoins the brachial artery distal to the pronator teres; at this level the nerve is found deep to the two heads of the flexor digitorum superficialis and runs in the fascia just dorsal to this muscle. It courses down the remainder of the forearm to emerge deep to the flexor digitorum superficialis tendon to the long finger before passing into the carpal tunnel. Articular branches of the median nerve supply innervation to the joint with all other branches in the forearm supplying muscle innervation.

The anterior interosseous nerve, an important large muscular branch of the median nerve, usually supplies the flexor digitorum profundus to the index finger and, in some people, the long finger. It also provides innervation to the flexor pollicis longus and pronator quadratus muscles. It separates from the main body of the median nerve approximately 5 cm distal to the medial epicondyle. In addition, the anterior interosseous nerve provides a small branch that innervates the wrist joint.

The ulnar nerve continues along the medial border of the triceps muscle and courses posterior to the medial epicondyle. It then enters between the humeral and ulnar heads of the flexor carpi ulnaris muscle where it is then found on the anterior surface of the flexor digitorum profundus. Its course within the forearm is virtually straight. In the middle of the forearm it joins the ulnar artery where they pass together distally beneath the surface of the flexor carpi ulnaris. In the anatomic position, the ulnar nerve is situated medial to the ulnar artery. At the wrist level it is found superficial to the flexor retinaculum, lateral to the pisiform, and medial to the hook of the hamate.

The ulnar nerve is made up of fibers from C8 and T1. Initially it gives off several articular branches to the elbow joint. Multiple muscular branches arise to supply the flexor carpi ulnaris and flexor digitorum profundus of the ring and small fingers.

Various communications may exist between the median and ulnar nerve. The most common one is the Martin Gruber connection that is found in up to 15% of patients. In this relationship, motor fibers from the main body of the median nerve or from the anterior interosseous nerve cross over in the forearm to join the ulnar nerve. These fibers may supply innervation to intrinsic muscles of the hand that are normally innervated by the ulnar nerve. When the Martin Gruber connection exists, a patient with a complete ulnar nerve laceration proximal to the site of the connection may show normal function of their interosseous muscles due to the anomalous innervation supplied by the median nerve.

The radial nerve is located at the level of the elbow between the brachialis and brachioradialis muscles and supplies the motor innervation to these muscles. Just proximal to the radial head the nerve usually divides into a superficial and deep branch. The deep branch is also known as the posterior interosseous nerve. Although the superficial branch of the radial nerve is usually thought of as a sensory nerve only, in a slight majority of people it is found to supply motor innervation to the extensor carpi radialis brevis muscle. The superficial radial nerve continues down the forearm under the brachioradialis muscle, emerging deep to its tendon at the junction of the distal and middle third of the forearm. It travels deep to the cephalic venous system and supplies the radial aspect of the dorsum of the hand.

The deep branch of the radial nerve (posterior interosseous nerve) has no cutaneous distribution. In the proximal forearm it is found to pass deep to the leading edge of the supinator muscle. A superficial and deep lamina of supinator muscle exist and it is between these fibers that the posterior interosseous nerve is found. The posterior interosseous nerve supplies the supinator muscle, extensor digitorum communis, extensor carpi ulnaris, extensor digiti minimi, extensor pollicis longus, abductor pollicis longus, extensor pollicis brevis, and the extensor indicis proprius. The nerve continues on to supply sensory innervation to the wrist joint.

Musculature

Muscles crossing the elbow joint proper affect flexion and extension of the elbow as well as forearm supination and pronation. Muscles whose prime action is to influence elbow motion will be described in this chapter.

The major flexor of the elbow, the biceps brachii, originates at the level of the shoulder with the long head origin from the supraglenoid tubercle and the short head origin from the coracoid process. The confluence of these two heads forms a large single muscle mass that traverses the cubital fossa as a single biceps tendon. This tendon inserts into the posterior aspect of the bicipital tuberosity. An aponeurosis arises from the biceps (also known as the lacertus fibrosus) that forms a thin band of tissue that inserts into the ulna. The musculocutaneous nerve innervates the biceps. In addition to elbow flexion, the biceps is the prime source of supination power.

The brachialis muscle originates from the anterior distal humerus and is made up of 95% muscle fiber as it crosses the elbow joint. It inserts into the base of the coronoid and has the largest cross sectional area of all elbow flexors. The brachialis muscle is unusual in that it has a dual innervation, from both the musculocutaneous nerve and the radial nerve.

The brachioradialis muscle has a broad origin along the lateral column of the distal humerus and forms the radial border of the cubital fossa at the level of the elbow joint (Fig. 2-11). This muscle serves primarily as an elbow flexor and may also affect forearm rotation (Fig. 2-38).

Distal to the brachioradialis muscle is found the extensor carpi radialis longus, also originating from the supracondylar bony column of the distal humerus. It is innervated by the radial nerve. It is weak as an elbow flexor (Fig. 2-15).

Deep to the extensor carpi radialis longus muscle is the origin of the extensor carpi radialis brevis. This is the probable site for muscle degeneration in lateral epicondylitis. Its primary function is that of a wrist extensor (Fig. 2-15).

The extensor digitorum communis originates from the lateral epicondyle. Its primary function is finger extension. It may play a minor role in elbow flexion (Fig. 2-15). The extensor carpi ulnaris muscle is composed of two heads (Fig. 2-15), one originating from the extensor origin of the distal humerus and the other

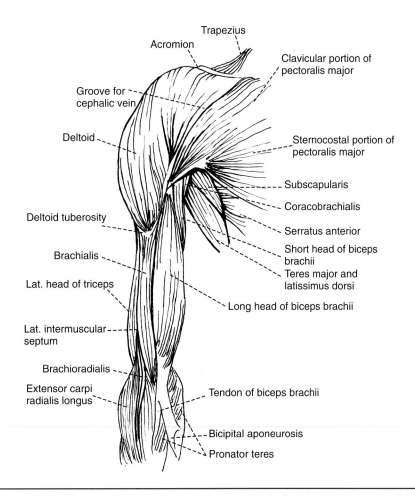

Fig. 2-38 Elbow flexors, such as the brachioradialis, are located on the anterior aspect of the arm. (From Morrey BF: *The elbow and its disorders*, ed 2, Saunders, 1993, Philadelphia.)

from the ulna near the insertion of the anconeus muscle aponeurosis (Fig. 2-39).

The supinator muscle has a three-part origin, the first is the lateral epicondyle, the second the lateral collateral ligament, and the third the proximal crest of the ulna slightly anterior to the anconeus insertion. This rhomboid-shaped muscle has a superficial and deep lamina which encase the posterior interosseous nerve (Fig. 2-15).

The prime elbow extensor is the triceps brachii, which forms the entire muscle mass along the posterior aspect of the elbow. The three-part origin of this muscle includes the long head from the infraglenoid tuberosity of the scapula as well as the lateral and posterior head from the posterior aspect of the humerus. All three heads of this muscle form a confluence at the level of the distal humerus, forming a common tendon attaching to the tip of the olecranon. All three heads are innervated by the radial nerve, with the medial head receiving the most distal innervation (Fig. 2-40).

The anconeus muscle originates from the posterior lateral epicondyle and inserts into the lateral surface of the proximal ulna and receives its radial nerve innervation through the medial head of the triceps. Its primary function is most likely that of a joint stabilizer of the ulna during pronation, although some studies have indicated that it may function as an elbow extensor.

The flexor pronator muscle group lies along the medial aspect of the elbow. The pronator teres consists of two heads, one of which arises from the superior aspect of the medial epicondyle and the other head from the coronoid process. Between these two heads the median nerve passes into the forearm. A broad tendinous insertion at the junction of the middle and distal thirds of the radius is found deep to the brachioradialis. Due to its portion originating above the elbow joint, this muscle functions as an elbow flexor as well as a forearm pronator.

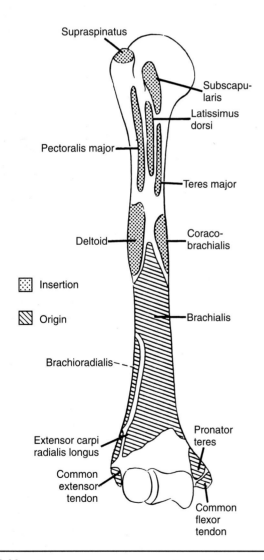

Fig. 2-39   Origins and insertions are indicated for the anterior humerus. (From Morrey BF: *The elbow and its disorders,* ed 2, Saunders, 1993, Philadelphia.)

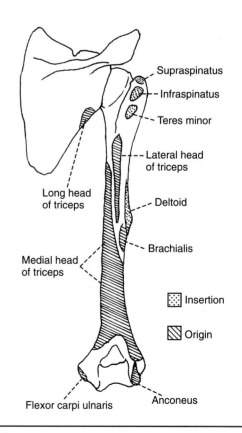

Fig. 2-40   The origins for the triceps long, lateral, and medial heads are found on the anterior humerus and scapula. (From Morrey BF: *The elbow and its disorders,* ed 2, Saunders, 1993, Philadelphia.)

The flexor carpi radialis arises from the anterior aspect of the medial epicondyle and has a minimal ability to pronate the forearm. The palmaris longus muscle likewise originates from the medial epicondyle and functions as a wrist flexor. The flexor carpi ulnaris is composed of two heads, the humeral head from the posterior aspect of the medial epicondyle and the ulnar head from the medial border of the coronoid and proximal ulna. This muscle is a weak elbow extensor and strong wrist flexor (Fig. 2-11).

The flexor digitorum superficialis is composed of two heads with a medial head arising from the medial epicondyle at the level of the common flexor tendon and medial coronoid. A lateral head originates from the proximal radius (Fig. 2-11).

The flexor digitorum profundus origin is entirely distal to the elbow joint proper and has no direct function on elbow motion.

Shoulder Anatomy

The shoulder girdle represents the most proximal aspect of the upper extremity. Movements of the scapula in relation to the chest wall as well as movements of the glenohumeral joint profoundly affect one's ability to place the hand in space. Passing through the region of the shoulder girdle are the nerves and vascular structures that supply the entire upper extremity.

The clavicle, scapula, and proximal humerus form the bony elements of the shoulder girdle. The clavicle is a doubly curved bone that forms a gentle S shape. This bone serves as the site of attachment for pectoralis major, deltoid, trapezius, and sternocleidomastoid muscles. The distal end of the clavicle articulates with the acromion process of the scapula. This articulation forms a synovial joint, which in some individuals is found to be an articular disc. Acromioclavicular ligaments are found along the superior aspect of this joint and prevent posterior translation of the clavicle on the acromion. Medial to the acromioclavicular joint, one finds the coracoclavicular ligaments made up of a conoid and trapezoid portion (Fig. 2-41). The coracoclavicular ligaments' primary function is to prevent superior translation of the clavicle on the scapula. These ligaments are damaged with acromioclavicular joint separations.

The scapula is a thin bone that serves as a site of muscular attachment. It has four major processes: the coracoid, the scapular spine, the acromion, and the glenoid. Two notches are found on the scapula, the suprascapular notch at the base of the coracoid and the spinoglenoid, or greater scapular notch, at the base of the spine.

The coracoid process of the scapula arises from the base of the neck of the glenoid to pass in an antero-

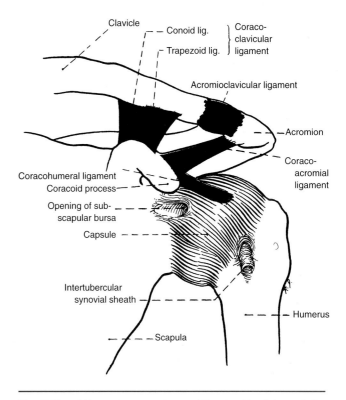

Fig. 2-41   Ligamentous structures of the shoulder joint and the distal clavicle are clearly represented in this Figure. (From Jenkins DB: *Hollingshead's functional anatomy of the limbs and back*, ed 6, Saunders, 1991, Philadelphia.)

lateral position. From this process originates the short head of the biceps and the coracobrachialis tendon. Into this process inserts the pectoralis major and the previously mentioned coracoclavicular ligaments also attach to this process.

The spine of the scapula provides a site of origin for the posterior aspect of the deltoid as well as the insertion of the trapezius muscle. Superior to the scapular spine is found the supraspinatus muscle, while below the spine is the infraspinatus muscle (Fig. 2-42).

At the most lateral edge of the scapular spine, the acromial process is formed. This serves as a site of origin for the deltoid muscle and receives attachment of the coracoacromial ligament, an important structure in the development of shoulder impingement. Several different types of acromial morphology have been identified that represent varying levels of severity of compromise to the supraspinatus outlet. The acromion also is a frequent site of osteophyte formation further adding to rotator cuff impingement.

The glenoid provides the articular surface for the proximal humerus and is covered with articular cartilage. A fibrocartilaginous structure known as the glenoid labrum attaches to the rim of the glenoid and is important in increasing the effective volume

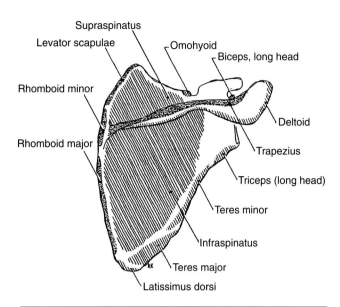

Fig. 2-42   Scapular view showing muscle origins and insertions. Insertions are represented by the darker shaded areas.
(From Rockwood C, Matsen F: *The shoulder*, vol 1, Saunders, 1990, Philadelphia.)

of the glenoid. The glenohumeral ligaments have their origins from the labrum. These ligaments are important in preventing subluxation of the humerus on the glenoid.

Overall, the glenoid averages 7° of retroversion with a 5° superior tilt in the anatomic position. The scapular orientation on the chest wall is found at a 30° anterior orientation.

The humeral articular surface is covered with cartilage. Studies have shown that the thickness of cartilage is greatest at the central portion and thinnest at the periphery. This is in contrast to the cartilage of the glenoid, which is thickest at the periphery and thinnest in the central portion. Overall, only 25% of the humeral head is covered by the glenoid and its accompanying labrum at any single position of humeral rotation.

In the anatomical position, the proximal humerus is retroverted an average of 30° when compared to the humeral condyle alignment. A humeral neck to shaft angle of 130° is also found. The lesser tuberosity of the proximal humerus serves as the site of insertion for the subscapularis muscle with the rotator cuff tendon inserting into the greater tuberosity. Between these tuberosities in the groove rests the biceps tendon. Here the long head of the biceps passes to the superior aspect of the glenoid.

The capsule of the glenohumeral joint holds an average volume of 15 cc and is approximately twice the surface area of the humeral head. This capsule is lined with synovium and extends from the glenoid neck to the level of the outer articular surface of the proximal humerus. Consistent thickenings of the shoulder capsule are identified as ligaments. A coracohumeral ligament arises from the base of the coracoid process to insert into the greater tuberosity. It is felt to have important stabilizing function for the abducted arm.

The important glenohumeral ligaments are the prime stabilizers of the shoulder. The superior glenohumeral ligament, while consistently found, is felt to have minimal importance in maintaining stability of the glenohumeral joint. The middle glenohumeral ligament is variable in size and thickness and has a questionable importance in shoulder stability. The prime stabilizer of the glenohumeral joint is the inferior glenohumeral ligament. This complex structure originates from the glenoid labrum as well as the glenoid neck and inserts into the anatomical neck of the humerus. This ligament is made up of anterior and posterior portions that form a hammock-like structure extending from front to back along the inferior 180° of the glenoid face. This ligament prevents abnormal translation of the proximal humerus during shoulder abduction and rotation (Fig. 2-43).

Musculature

The trapezius muscle originates from the spinous processes from C7 through T12 and inserts into the lateral clavicle, acromion, and scapular spine. This muscle, which is supplied by the spinal accessory nerve, retracts and elevates the scapula (Fig. 2-44).

The rhomboid muscles originate from the lower cervical spinous processes through the fifth thoracic vertebra. These muscles, the minor and major, also act to retract and elevate the scapula. Insertion is into the posterior surface of the medial border at and below the base of the scapular spine. The dorsal scapular nerve, which originates from the fifth cervical root, innervates both muscles (Fig. 2-45).

The levator scapulae muscle originates from the first four cervical vertebrae and inserts onto the superior angle of the scapula. Innervation is from the deep branches of the cervical plexus of the third and fourth cervical nerves and at times the muscle receives a supply from the fifth cervical nerve by way of the dorsal scapular nerve. Its action is to elevate the angle of the scapula and produce a rotation of this flat bone.

The serratus anterior originates from the chest wall and anterolateral ribs to insert onto the inferior angle of the scapula. Its action is to rotate the scapula. The long thoracic nerve made up of contributions of C5, C6, and C7 supplies the serratus anterior (Fig. 2-46).

The pectoralis minor originates from the third through fifth ribs and inserts onto the medial side of

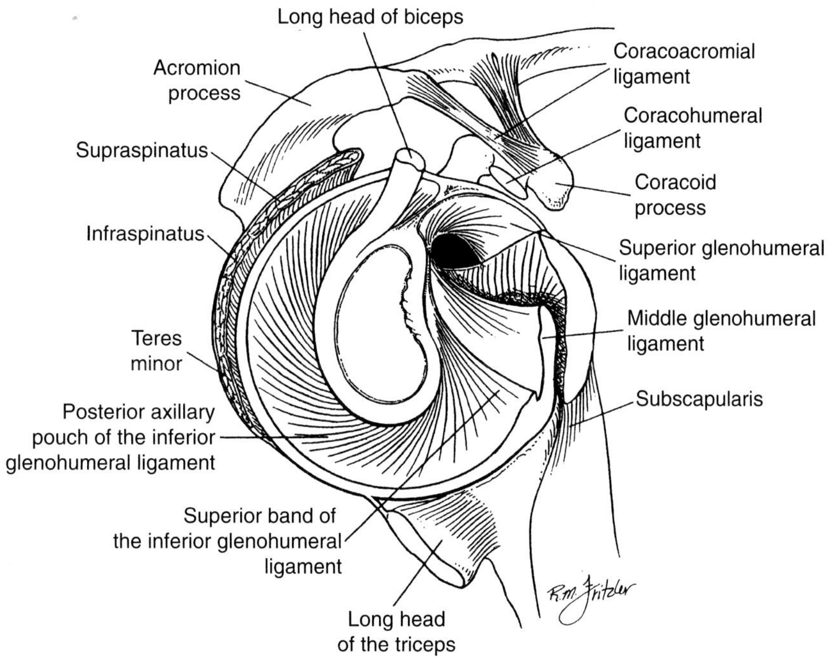

Long head of biceps

Acromion
process

Coracoacromial
ligament

Coracohumeral
ligament

Supraspinatus

Coracoid
process

Infraspinatus

Superior glenohumeral
ligament

Teres
minor

Middle glenohumeral
ligament

Subscapularis

Posterior axillary
pouch of the inferior
glenohumeral ligament

Superior band of
the inferior glenohumeral
ligament

Long head
of the triceps

Fig. 2-43   The inferior glenohumeral ligament is the prime glenohumeral stabilizer. (From Canale
ST: *Campbell's operative orthopaedics*, ed 10, Mosby, 2003, St. Louis.)

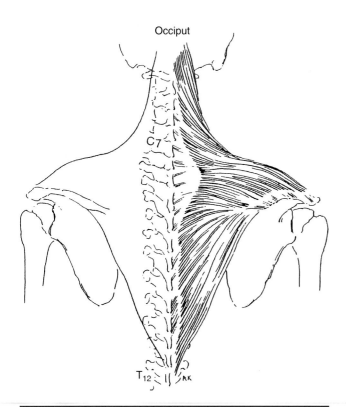

Fig. 2-44   View of the trapezius muscle with origin from the
occiput, nuchal ligament, and the dorsal spines of vertebrae C7
through T12. This muscle inserts onto the acromion, spine of the
scapula, and a portion of the distal clavicle. (From Rockwood C,
Matsen F: *The shoulder*, vol 1, Saunders, 1990, Philadelphia.)

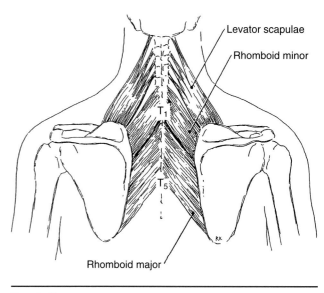

Fig. 2-45   Levator scapulae and rhomboid minor and major
muscles shown with fiber orientation. (From Rockwood C, Matsen
F: *The shoulder*, vol 1, Saunders, 1990, Philadelphia.)

the coracoid process. This muscle, supplied by the medial pectoral nerve, rotates the scapula anteriorly and depresses its lateral angle.

The deltoid muscle is the largest of the gleno-humeral muscles and forms the outer lateral border of

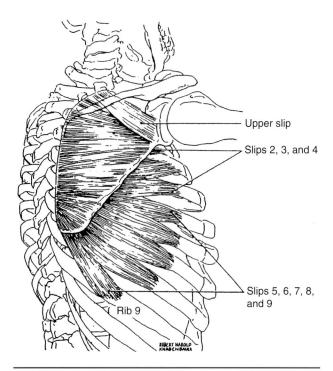

Fig. 2-46   The serratus anterior is divided into three groups of muscles. The upper slip takes origin from the first two ribs and the first intercostal space. The middle portion originates from ribs 2, 3, and 4 with the lower slips originating from ribs 5, 6, 7, 8, and 9. (From Rockwood C, Matsen F: *The shoulder*, vol 1, Saunders, 1990, Philadelphia.)

the shoulder. Three major sections of this muscle exist including the anterior deltoid originating from the lateral one third of the clavicle, the middle third, which originates from the acromion, and the posterior deltoid, which originates from the spine of the scapula, inserting into the deltoid tuberosity on the lateral surface of the humerus. Innervated by the axillary nerve, the prime function of this muscle is to elevate the humerus in the scapular plane. Abduction and flexion of the shoulder are produced by the actions of all three heads of the deltoid (Fig. 2-47).

Muscles of the rotator cuff include the supraspinatus, infraspinatus, teres minor, and subscapularis. The supraspinatus muscle originates from the supraspinatus fossa of the scapula. Prior to insertion onto the greater tuberosity of the humerus, it joins the tendon of the infraspinatus. The supraspinatus muscle is active in all positions of shoulder elevation and is also felt to have an important stabilizing function for the glenohumeral joint. This muscle as well as the infraspinatus and teres minor have an important effect in depressing the humeral head and resisting the sheer force of the deltoid muscle. The supraspinatus is innervated by the suprascapular nerve made up of fibers from C5 and C6.

The infraspinatus muscle originates beneath the scapular spine and infraspinatus fossa and has a common tendon of insertion with the supraspinatus. This muscle is a strong external rotator of the shoulder, supplying approximately 60% of external rotator force, and also functions to depress the humeral head. The infraspinatus is innervated by the suprascapular nerve. The teres minor originates from the lateral part of the scapula and inserts onto the lower

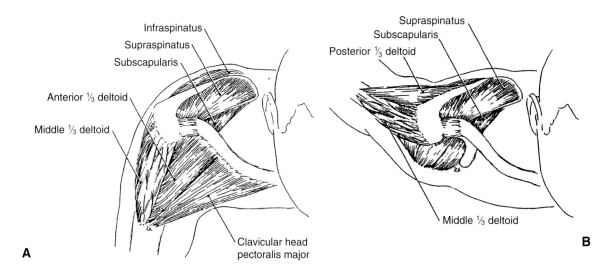

Fig. 2-47   Functional division of the deltoid. **A,** Anterior and middle thirds of the deltoid provide shoulder forward flexion. **B,** Posterior third of deltoid is active during horizontal abduction. The middle third deltoid is active in all motions of the glenohumeral joint. (From Rockwood C, Matsen F: *The shoulder*, vol 1, Saunders, 1990, Philadelphia.)

aspect of the greater tuberosity of the humerus. This muscle serves as an external rotator of the humerus and is supplied by a branch of the axillary nerve (Fig. 2-48).

The subscapularis originates from the subscapularis fossa to insert onto the lesser tuberosity of the proximal humerus. This muscle serves to internally rotate the shoulder and resist anterior subluxation of the glenohumeral joint. The upper and lower subscapular nerves innervate this muscle (Fig. 2-49).

The teres major originates from the posterior aspect of the scapula along its inferior border and inserts along with the latissimus dorsi along the medial lip of the bicipital groove. In traveling to its insertion, the teres major undergoes a 180° spiral rotation and its insertion is slightly posterior to that of the latissimus dorsi. This muscle functions to internally rotate, adduct, and extend the arm and is supplied by the lower subscapular nerve.

The coracobrachialis muscle originates from the coracoid process as a conjoined tendon with the short head of the biceps. Its insertion is the midportion of the humerus and within this muscle lies the musculocutaneous nerve at a point 1.5 to 7 cm distal to the coracoid process. This muscle functions to adduct and flex the glenohumeral joint.

The pectoralis major has three portions: a clavicular portion originating from the medial one half of the clavicle, a middle portion originating from the manubrium and sternum, and an inferior portion originating from the sternum as well as the fifth and sixth ribs. The fibers of all three portions have distinct orientation, with the inferior fibers rotating 180° prior to inserting onto the proximal humerus. The prime function of this muscle is internal rotation and adduction of the glenohumeral joint. This muscle is supplied by the lateral pectoral nerve for the clavicular portion and the medial pectoral nerve to the remainder of the muscle.

The latissimus dorsi originates from the midthoracic spine through the lower lumbar region, the sacrum and the ilium. Connections may also be found from the lower ribs and inferior angle of the scapula. This muscle undergoes a 180° spiral before its insertion onto the medial lip of the bicipital groove. During its course into the axilla it rotates anterior to the teres major at its insertion. It serves to adduct, extend, and internally rotate the shoulder (Fig. 2-50). The thoracodorsal nerve innervates this muscle.

The biceps muscle has a two-part origin, the long head originating from the supraglenoid tubercle and the short head from the coracoid process. While the action of this muscle is at the elbow, its tendons may be involved in shoulder pathology. The long head is frequently involved in shoulder impingement.

The triceps muscle has a single portion that affects the shoulder. The long head, which is found at the level of the glenohumeral joint, originates from the infraglenoid tubercle and the adjacent capsule and labrum. This muscle serves as an important anatomic landmark for major tendon transfers about the shoulder.

Nerve Supply

The brachial plexus supplies innervation for all muscles of the upper extremity and receives contributions from the C5, C6, C7, C8, and T1 nerve roots (Fig. 2-51). The C5 and C6 roots form the upper trunk, the C7 root the middle trunk, and the C8 and T1 roots join to form the inferior or lower trunk. At the level of the clavicle, anterior and posterior divisions sepa-

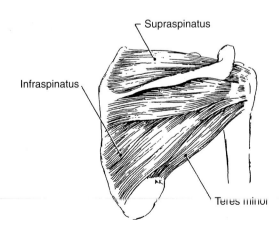

Fig. 2-48 The rotator cuff muscles consist of the supraspinatus, infraspinatus, teres minor, and subscapularis (see also Fig. 2-49). (From Rockwood C, Matsen F: *The shoulder*, vol 1, Saunders, 1990, Philadelphia.)

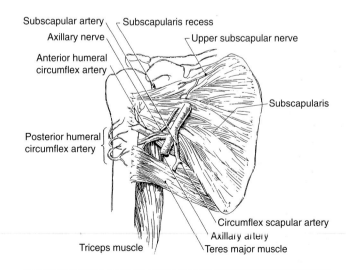

Fig. 2-49 The quadrilateral space conveys the axillary nerve and posterior humeral circumflex artery. The triangular space conveys the circumflex scapular artery. (From Rockwood C, Matsen F: *The shoulder*, vol 1, ed 2, Saunders, 1998, Philadelphia.)

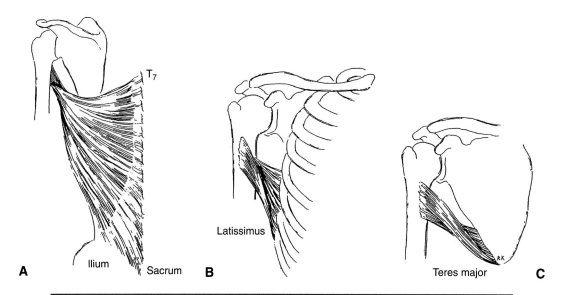

Fig. 2-50   **A,** The latissimus dorsi takes origin from the spinous process of T7 to the sacrum and iliac crest. **B,** It inserts onto the medial lip and floor of the bicipital groove of the proximal humerus. **C,** The teres major has a similar fiber rotation inserting medial to the latissimus dorsi tendon. (From Rockwood C, Matsen F: *The shoulder,* vol 1, Saunders, 1990, Philadelphia.)

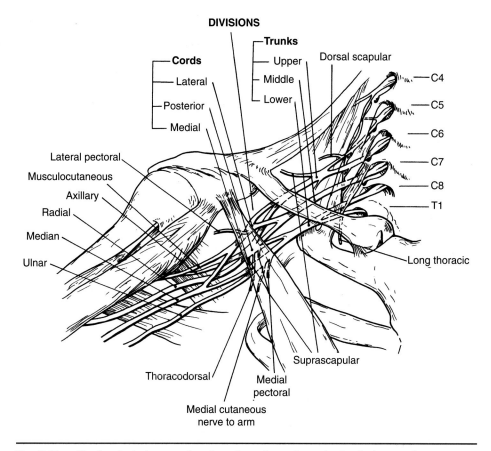

Fig. 2-51   The brachial plexus and its branches, shown from the level of cervical nerve roots, trunks, divisions, and cords. The divisions of the brachial plexus occur at the level of the clavicle. (From Canale ST: *Campbell's operative orthopaedics,* ed 10, Mosby, 2003, St. Louis.)

rate from the trunks to form the lateral, posterior, and medial cords. From these cords the terminal nerves of the brachial plexus arise to form the peripheral nerves of the upper extremity.

The elements of the brachial plexus leave the cervical spine region in between the middle and anterior scalene muscles and are joined by the subclavian artery before passing deep to the clavicle and superficial to the first rib. It is at this level that traumatic injury of the brachial plexus most frequently occurs. For a complete review of the brachial plexus, the reader is referred to standard anatomy textbooks.

Sensation of the Shoulder Girdle

Supraclavicular nerves that originate from the third and fourth cervical nerve roots supply the most superior aspect of the shoulder. The posterior aspect of the shoulder is innervated by the terminal branches of the spinal nerves. The intercostal nerves supply the chest wall and the medial portion of the axilla. The lateral aspect of the shoulder is supplied by the upper lateral brachial cutaneous nerve (a terminal branch of the axillary nerve). The medial brachial cutaneous nerve (originating from the medial cord of the brachial plexus) innervates the medial aspect of the shoulder and axilla. The anterior arm and region over the biceps muscle is supplied by the medial antebrachial cutaneous nerve, also a branch of the medial cord of the brachial plexus (Fig. 2-52).

It is hoped that this chapter will serve as a reference guide (Table 2-2) for the important anatomic and kinesiologic considerations presented in the ensuing chapters on hand splinting.

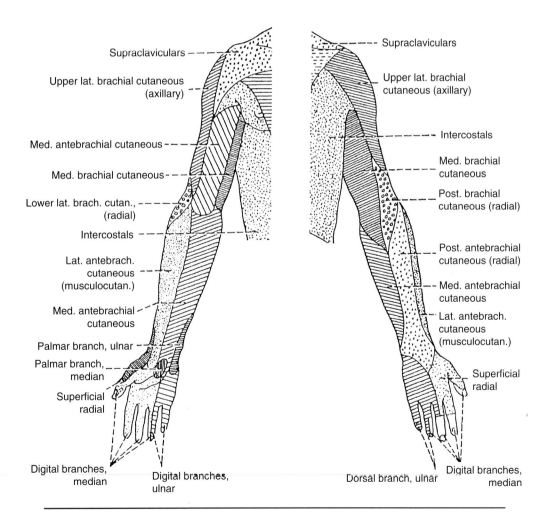

Fig. 2-52   Cutaneous innervation of the upper limb shown on the anterior aspect of the left and the dorsal aspect on the right. (From Flatau E: *Neurologische Schemata für die ärtzliche Praxis,* Springer, 1915, Berlin.)

TABLE 2-2   Reference to the Muscle, Origin, Insertion, and Innervation Described in Chapter 2

Muscle	Origin	Insertion	Innervation
Abductor Digiti Quinti	p. 56, Fig. 2-17	p. 56, Fig. 2-17	p. 64, Fig. 2-17
Abductor Pollicis Brevis	p. 56, Fig. 2-17	p. 56, Fig. 2-17	p. 64, Fig. 2-17
Abductor Pollicis Longus	p. 56, Fig. 2-15	p. 56, Fig. 2-15	p. 64, 74, Fig. 2-15
Adductor Pollicis	p. 58, 59, Fig. 2-17	p. 58, 59, Fig. 2-17	p. 59, 64, 65, Fig. 2-17
Anconeus	p. 76, Fig. 2-40	p. 76	p. 76
Biceps	p. 75, 77, 82, Fig. 2-42	p. 72, 75	p. 75
Brachialis	p. 75, Fig. 2-39, 2-40	p. 74, 75	p. 75
Brachioradialis	p. 56, 75, Fig. 2-11, 2-39	p. 56, Fig. 2-11	p. 64, 74, Fig. 2-11
Coracobrachialis	p. 77, 81	p. 81, Fig. 2-39	p. 82
Deltoid	p. 77, 80, Fig. 2-42, 2-47	p. 77, 80, Fig. 2-39, 2-40, 2-47	p. 80
Extensor Carpi Radialis Brevis	p. 56, 75, Fig. 2-15	p. 56, Fig. 2-15	p. 64, 74, Fig. 2-15
Extensor Carpi Radialis Longus	p. 56, 75, Fig. 2-15, 2-39	p. 56, Fig. 2-15	p. 64, 75, Fig. 2-15
Extensor Carpi Ulnaris	p. 56, 76, Fig. 2-15	p. 56, Fig. 2-15	p. 64, 74, Fig. 2-15
Extensor Digitorum Communis	p. 56, 75, Fig. 2-15	p. 56, Fig. 2-15	p. 64, 74, Fig. 2-15
Extensor Digiti Quinti Proprius	p. 56, Fig. 2-15	p. 56, Fig. 2-15	p. 64, 74, Fig. 2-15
Extensor Indicis Proprius	p. 56, Fig. 2-15	p. 56, Fig. 2-15	p. 64, 74, Fig. 2-15
Extensor Pollicis Brevis	p. 56, Fig. 2-15	p. 56, Fig. 2-15	p. 64, 74, Fig. 2-15
Extensor Pollicis Longus	p. 56, Fig. 2-15	p. 56, Fig. 2-15	p. 64, 74, Fig. 2-15
Flexor Carpi Radialis	p. 53, 77, Fig. 2-11	p. 53, Fig. 2-11	p. 65, Fig. 2-11
Flexor Carpi Ulnaris	p. 53, 77, Fig. 2-11, 2-40	p. 53, Fig. 2-11	p. 64, 65, 74, Fig. 2-11
Flexor Digiti Quinti Brevis	p. 56, Fig. 2-17	p. 56, Fig. 2-17	p. 59, 64, Fig. 2-17
Flexor Digitorum Profundus	p. 53, 77, Fig. 2-11	p. 53, Fig. 2-11	p. 64, 65, 74, Fig. 2-11
Flexor Digitorum Superficialis	p. 53, 77, Fig. 2-11	p. 53, Fig. 2-11	p. 64, 65, Fig. 2-11
Flexor Pollicis Brevis	p. 56, Fig. 2-17	p. 56, Fig. 2-17	p. 56, 59, 64, 65, Fig. 2-17
Flexor Pollicis Longus	p. 53, 72, Fig. 2-11	p. 53, Fig. 2-11	p. 65, 74, Fig. 2-11
Infraspinatus	p. 80, Fig. 2-42, 2-47, 2-48	p. 80, Fig. 2-40, 2-48	p. 80
Interossei	p. 58, Fig. 2-17	p. 58, Fig. 2-17	p. 59, 64, Fig. 2-17
Latissimus Dorsi	p. 82, Fig. 2-50	p. 81, 82, Fig. 2-39, 2-50	p. 82
Levator Scapula	p. 78, Fig. 2-45	p. 78, Fig. 2-42, 2-45	p. 78
Lumbricals	p. 58, Fig. 2-17	p. 58, Fig. 2-17	p. 59, 64, Fig. 2-17
Opponens Digiti Quinti	p. 56	p. 56	p. 59, 64
Opponens Pollicis	p. 56, Fig. 2-17	p. 56, Fig. 2-17	p. 64, 65, Fig. 2-17
Palmaris Longus	p. 53, 77, Fig. 2-11	Fig. 2-11	Fig. 2-11
Pectoralis Major	p. 82, Fig. 2-47	p. 77, 82, Fig. 2-39, 2-47	p. 82
Pectoralis Minor	p. 79	p. 79	p. 80
Pronator Quadratus	p. 75, Fig. 2-11	p. 72, Fig. 2-11	p. 64, 65, 74, Fig. 2-11
Pronator Teres	p. 53, 76, Fig. 2-11, 2-39	p. 76, Fig. 2-11	p. 64, 65, Fig. 2-11
Rhomboid	p. 78, Fig. 2-45	p. 78, Fig. 2-42, 2-45	p. 78
Serratus Anterior	p. 78, Fig. 2-46	p. 78, Fig. 2-46	p. 79
Subscapularis	p. 81, Fig. 2-49	p. 78, 81, Fig. 2-39, 2-49	p. 81
Supinator	p. 73, 76, Fig. 2-11	Fig. 2-11	p. 74, Fig. 2-11
Supraspinatus	p. 80, Fig. 2-42, 2-47, 2-48	p. 80, Fig. 2-39, 2-40, 2-48	p. 80
Teres Major	p. 81, Fig. 2-42, 2-50	p. 81, Fig. 2-39, 2-50	p. 81
Teres Minor	p. 80, Fig. 2-42, 2-48	p. 80, Fig. 2-40, 2-48	p. 81
Trapezius	p. 78, Fig. 2-44	p. 77, 78, Fig. 2-42, 2-44	p. 78
Triceps	p. 76, 82, Fig. 2-40, 2-42	p. 76	p. 76

REFERENCES

1. Brand PW: Biomechanics of tendon transfer, *Orthop Clin North Am* 5:202-30, 1974.
2. Brand PW, Hollister A: *Clinical mechanics of the hand*, ed 3, C.V. Mosby Company, 1999, St. Louis.
3. Cooney W, Linscheid R, Dobyns J: *The wrist diagnosis and operative treatment*, C.V. Mosby Company, 1998, St. Louis.
4. Flatt AE: *The care of minor hand injuries*, C.V. Mosby Company, 1979, St. Louis.
5. Flatt AE: *Care of the arthritic hand*, C.V. Mosby Company, 1983, St. Louis.
6. Flatt AE: *The care of the arthritic hand*, ed 5, Quality Medical Publishing, Inc., 1995, St. Louis.
7. Lichtman D, Alexander A: *The wrist and its disorders*, Philadelphia, W.B. Saunders, 1988.
8. Napier J: The form and function of the carpometacarpal joint of the thumb, *J Anat* 89:362, 1955.
9. Napier J: The precision movements of the hand, *Journal of Bone and Joint Surgery* 36B:902-913, 1956.
10. Taleisnik J: The ligaments of the wrist, *J hand Surg [Am]* 1:110-118, 1976.
11. Taleisnik J: Wrist: Anatomy, function and injury, *American Academy of Orthopaedic Surgeons' Instructional Course Lectures* 27:61, 1978.
12. Taleisnik J: *The wrist*, Churchill Livingstone, 1985, New York.
13. Taleisnik J: Carpal kinematics,. in *The wrist*, Churchill Livingstone, 1985, New York,.

14. Taleisnik J: Soft tissue injuries of the wrist, in Strickland JW, Rettig AR, editors: *Hand injuries in athletes*, W.B. Saunders Company, 1992, Philadelphia.

15. Weber ER: Physiologic bases for wrist function, in Lichtman D, Alexander A, editors: *The wrist and its disorders*, W.B. Saunders Company, 1988, Philadelphia.

SUGGESTED READING

Hollingshead HW: *Anatomy for surgeons*, vol 4, The back and limbs, Harper and Row, 1982, New York.

Matsen FA, Fu FH, Hawkins RJ: *The shoulder: a balance of mobility and stability*, American Academy of Orthopedic Surgeons, 1993, Rosemont, IL.

Morrey BF: *The elbow and its disorders*, ed 2, Saunders, 1992, Philadelphia.

Rockwood CA, Matsen FA: *The shoulder*, Saunders, 1990, Philadelphia.

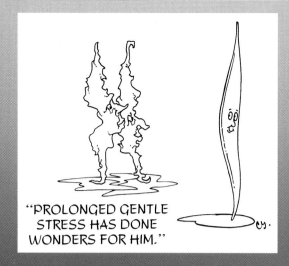

"PROLONGED GENTLE STRESS HAS DONE WONDERS FOR HIM."

CHAPTER 3

Tissue Remodeling

Chapter Outline

Section 1
Biologic Basis for Hand and Upper Extremity Splinting

JAMES W. STRICKLAND, MD

Splints are used to put all or part of the hand at rest so that diseased, injured, or surgically violated tissues can undergo orderly, uninterrupted healing. They are also used to favorably influence tissue healing and minimize the development of restrictive scar tissue, which has a detrimental effect on normal joint and tendon movement. In many clinical situations, there is an appropriate time for the use of immobilizing, mobilizing, restriction, and torque transmission splints to control the essential events of repair. A strong appreciation for the biologic state of the involved tissues will aid in making decisions as to whether the injured part should be managed by rest or stress and the best timing for the use of each type of splint. This chapter provides insight into the nature of normal and abnormal tissue healing in the human hand and upper extremity, and the biologic basis for the use of splints as part of a treatment program designed to restore maximum functional recovery.

Whether secondary to intra-articular destruction, capsular fibrosis, tendon adhesion, or skin and soft tissue scarring, the reduction or cessation of function of the shoulder, elbow, forearm, wrist, or digital joints is profoundly detrimental to hand and upper extremity performance. To proceed with effective therapy to restore function in the involved joints, one must have a thorough understanding of the biologic basis for the underlying pathology. Why is the joint stiffened? Are the articular surfaces damaged? Are the capsular and ligamentous tissues thickened, scarred, or shortened? Are adherent flexor, extensor, or intrinsic tendons preventing motion by a tenodesis checkrein phenomenon? Is the skin, fascia, or subcutaneous tissue scarred or fibrotic? Are there many factors involved in combination to limit joint movement?

Armed with an understanding of the pertinent pathology, one must define the goals of splinting for a particular situation. Is the splint to be used to allow healing, to biologically modify contracted and scarred skin, subcutaneous tissue, fascia, or ligamentous tissues, or is it meant to lengthen tendon adhesions that have become fixed to bone or surrounding tissues? What dangers exist with regard to joint injury or tendon rupture?

Finally, when the pathologic process and the goals of splinting have been defined, consideration is given to the method of splinting that can most effectively impart the desired biologic alteration of the affected tissues. What is the most desirable vector for the appli-

cation of force to a given joint? How much force should be imparted? For how long a period should the force be applied? Through how wide a surface? On what anatomical structures is the force being placed? What measurements will ensure the most effective application of the splint?

To answer these questions and proceed with the design, construction, and application of an effective splint, one must know the necessary sequence of biologic events involved in normal tissue healing and the aberrations in this process that may result in the loss of joint motion. Splinting methods can then be selected to alter and control these events to restore maximum function.

■ TISSUE HEALING

Normal upper extremity function depends on the smooth, friction-free gliding of small cartilaginous articular surfaces and the excursion of stout collagenous tendons unimpeded by restrictive scars and adhesions. The biologic response of tissues to injury results in an alteration of their physical properties and the replacement of normal structures with scar tissue. Therefore a thorough understanding of wound healing and scar formation provides a foundation for the recognition and treatment of problems related to the successful restoration of function following upper extremity injury and surgery.

It must be recognized that scar formation is nonspecific in the sense that the biologic processes and the sequence in which they occur are virtually identical in all organs and tissues. However, the final appearance of the healed scar and the effect it has on function may differ with respect to the specific organ or tissue involved. In the upper extremity and especially the hand, any alteration in the physical characteristics or anatomic arrangement of tissues may prevent relative gliding and reduce function significantly. Although the functional effect varies, the common denominator for the healing of all tissues is scar. The components of the process of tissue healing sequentially include inflammation, fibroplasia, and scar maturation, along with concomitant wound contracture (Fig. 3-1). In the upper extremity, it is particularly relevant that the presence of scar in specialized tissues such as tendon, bone, and joint can result in severe impairment of function. It should also be remembered that the process of wound healing results not only from accidental injury, but also from surgical intervention.

■ INFLAMMATION

Following wounding, the initial biologic response is inflammation (Fig. 3-1, A-C). The open wound,

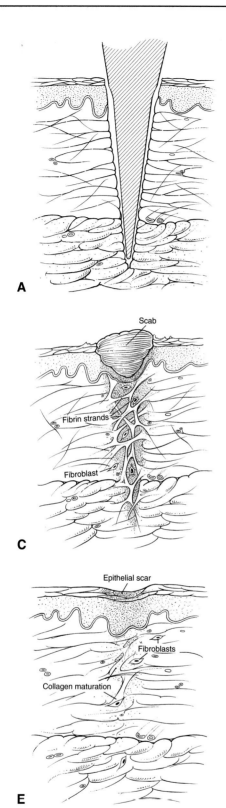

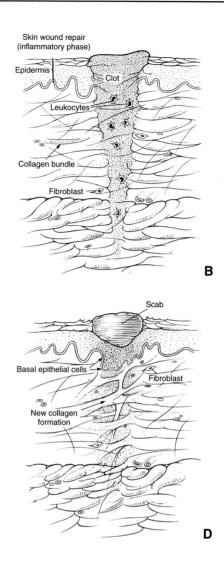

Fig. 3-1   Stages of wound healing. **A,** Initial injury: lacerating object producing injury to the epidermis, dermis, and subcutaneous tissues. **B,** Skin wound repair, inflammatory phase (early). The wound is filled with blood and cellular debris. Clotted blood unites the wound edges. Epithelial cells mobilize and begin migrating across the defect. Serum, plasma, proteins, and leukocytes escape from the venules and enter the wound area. Undifferentiated mesenchymal cells begin transformation to mature fibroblasts. **C,** Late migratory phase. Epithelial cells continue to migrate and proliferate. Debris is removed by leukocytes, and fibroblasts migrate into the wound area along fibrin strands. Capillaries begin regrowth by budding, and the open wound is recognizable as granulation tissue. **D,** Fibroplasia (proliferative phase). Epithelium increases in thickness beneath the scab and forms irregular projections into the dermis. Collagen fibers are laid down in a random pattern. Capillaries continue to invade the wound and fibrin strands, debris, and leukocytes disappear. **E,** Maturation phase. Scab sloughs completely as epithelium resumes normal stratification. Collagen remodels in bulk and form and becomes organized. Wound strength increases and fibroblasts begin to disappear. Vascularity is restored.

containing injured tissues and hemorrhage, is easily contaminated by bacteria and foreign substances. Inflammation is a vascular and cellular response that serves several purposes, including the removal of microorganisms, foreign material, and necrotic tissue in preparation for repair. This inflammatory response is the same regardless of the cause of the injury and is characterized by a transient vasoconstriction, which is followed by vasodilation of local small blood vessels resulting in increased blood flow to the injured area. This phenomenon is associated with local edema and the migration of white blood cells through the walls of the blood vessels.

Phagocytic cells carry out the removal of dead tissue and foreign bodies, including bacteria; when some of the white cells die, their intracellular enzymes and debris are released and become part of the wound exudate. Some of these enzymes facilitate the breakdown of necrotic debris and others dissolve connective tissue. The acute inflammatory response usually subsides within several days except in those wounds that become contaminated with bacteria or retain foreign material; in these cases the wounds continue to have a persistent inflammatory response and remain unhealed for quite some time. A wall of collagen may ultimately be laid down, resulting in the formation of a granuloma.

■ FIBROPLASIA

At the end of the inflammatory phase, migratory fibroblasts enter the wound depths and begin synthesizing scar tissue. This period of scar tissue formation is known as fibroplasia (Fig. 3-1, *D*). It usually begins at the wound site on the fourth or fifth day after injury and continues for 2 to 4 weeks. During this period the wound area becomes recognizable microscopically as granulation tissue with the formation of capillaries or endothelial budding, which results in a characteristic vascularity and redness of the involved tissues.

From the third to the sixth week after injury the number of fibroblasts and blood vessels within the wound slowly diminishes. As the cell population decreases, scar collagen fibers increase and the wound changes from a predominantly cellular structure to predominantly extracellular tissue. It is during this phase that fibroblasts manufacture collagen by a poorly understood mechanism. The collagen molecule is a complex helical structure whose mechanical properties are largely responsible for the strength and rigidity of scar tissue.

Tensile strength is defined as the load per cross-sectional area that can be supported by the wound, and it increases at a rate proportional to the rate of collagen synthesis. During the period of fibroplasia the

tensile strength of the wound increases rapidly. As collagen is produced, the fibroblasts in the wound diminish. The disappearance of fibroblasts marks the end of the fibroblastic phase and the beginning of the maturation phase of wound healing.

■ SCAR MATURATION

The scar tissue formed during the fibroblastic phase is a dense structure of randomly oriented collagen fibers. During the maturation phase of wound healing (Fig. 3-1, *E*), changes in the form, bulk, and strength of the scar occur. Microscopically the weave or architecture of the collagen fibers changes to a more organized pattern, and the strength of the wound continues to increase despite the disappearance of fibroblasts and the reduction in the rate of collagen synthesis. Remodeling is a spontaneous process, and scars may remain metabolically active for years, slowly changing in size, shape, color, texture, and strength. It is during this phase that there is continuous and simultaneous collagen production and breakdown. If the rate of breakdown exceeds the rate of production, the scar becomes softer and less bulky. If the rate of production exceeds the rate of breakdown, then a keloid or hypertrophic scar may result.

Through an unknown mechanism, the surfaces against which scar tissue is deposited influence the nature of the remodeling process. Scar deposited in the presence of cut tendon ends remodels to mimic the organization of tendon bundles. Scar adjacent to an uninjured tendon surface tends to remodel to resemble peritendon. The rate and extent to which a scar remodels vary among individuals and also within the same individual depending on age at the time of injury. Younger animals have been shown to remodel scar tissues more effectively than older animals. In the young, remodeling is rapid and effective and this increased rate of metabolic turnover may be responsible for the excellent restoration of gliding seen in younger patients following injury to bone or tendon. The quantity of scar deposited is directly related to the amount of injured tissue; the larger the scar, the less likely the effective restoration of joint or tendon function.

Because wounds remain metabolically reactive for long periods of time, surgery or a second injury may further increase scar collagen synthesis and lead to more scarring. It may be many months before a wound is sufficiently healed to allow one to proceed with further reconstructive surgical procedures. The physical characteristics of the injured tissues may provide important clues as to the metabolic state of the wound. This prolonged period of metabolic activity may also explain the need for long-term splinting to prevent and overcome joint contractures resulting from wound scar formation.

■ WOUND CONTRACTURE

Open wounds with or without tissue loss undergo wound contraction with dramatic changes in size and shape. The process of contraction begins after a 2- or 3-day latent period, and by 2 to 3 weeks the wounds are often less than 20% of their original area. The forces of contraction will continue to close the wound until balanced by equal tension in the surrounding skin. In the hand this contraction may produce significant functional impairment. Contracture is, of course, beneficial to healing wounds but in the hand it may be functionally detrimental when it involves mobile tissues around or over joints. Splints may be an effective method of minimizing the deleterious effects of wound contracture.

■ SPECIFIC TISSUE HEALING

Although this general scheme is applicable to almost all tissues, hand and upper extremity injuries often involve complex wounding to the deep structures such as bone, joint, tendon, and nerve that must heal so that the unique function of each tissue will be restored. A brief discussion of the unique features of wound healing for each of these tissues is provided next.

Bone and Cartilage Healing

Unlike the healing by the scar formation of soft tissues, bone is capable of limited regeneration. As with the other tissues, the immediate response to injury includes inflammation and edema with associated bleeding in the marrow cavity and surrounding tissues (Fig. 3-2, A). Within a few days the fibroblastic phase of soft tissue healing begins and osteogenic cells from the periosteum and endosteum of the bone begin migration and proliferation at the wound site. These cells lay down callus and a fibrous matrix of collagen to form a bridge between two bony ends at the fracture site (Fig. 3-2, B). The osteogenic cells nearest the bone surface appear to transform directly into osteoblasts and lay down a collagen matrix that calcifies directly into bone (Fig. 3-2, C). The precise mechanism of calcification is not well known, but it appears that the collagen matrix, perhaps in interaction with the surrounding ground substance, initiates crystal formation and deposition.

Remodeling of bone occurs over a prolonged period and appears to be influenced by forces of stress in the healed bone. Although new cartilage formation occurs during bone repair, mature cartilage appears to be incapable of regenerating. Injuries to human articular cartilage appear to be repaired by fibrous union resulting from nonspecific inflammation and fibroplasia.

Tendon Healing

The process of tendon healing (Fig. 3-3) is particularly important because the successful return of function following tendon interruption in the hand results not only from a union of severed tendon ends but also the restoration of gliding. These qualities would seem to be contradictory in that they require both a dense fibrous bond between the severed tendon ends and a free excursion of the tendon in the surrounding tissues. Unfortunately, adhesions resulting from the extrinsic contribution of surrounding tissues to tendon healing frequently restrict the ability of that tendon to glide.

Historically there has been considerable debate with regard to the mechanism of tendon healing,[59,89,90] and investigators have been at odds as to whether a tendon has an intrinsic capability to heal itself or relies exclusively on the cellular response of the tendon sheath and the surrounding perisheath tissues for healing. Upper extremity specialists are well aware that adhesions resulting from the healing process frequently limit tendon excursion, and historically these adhesions have been considered an essential source of reparative cells. Studies on the intrinsic healing capacity of tendons, however, suggest that adhesions may constitute a nonessential inflammatory response at the site of injury. Attention has been focused on attempts to alter the formation of adhesions following tendon repair by biomechanical, biochemical, and biophysical techniques. Until the mechanism of healing is more clearly defined, the restoration of tendon excursion following interruption, repair, and healing will remain an inexact science and a frustrating clinical dilemma.

Nerve Healing

Injury to peripheral nerves necessitates an entirely different type of tissue healing in that the severed nerve fiber must regenerate distally from the point of injury. The injury results in degeneration of the axon and myelin distal to the wound and, for a short distance, proximal to the wound (Fig. 3-4, A). Schwann cells in the distal stump grow toward the proximal stump, and macrophages clear cellular debris from the

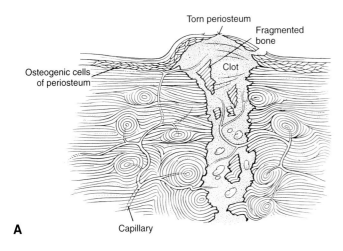

A

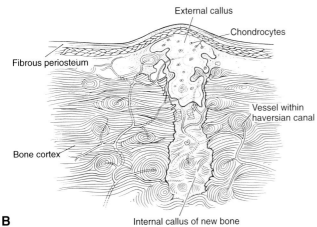

B

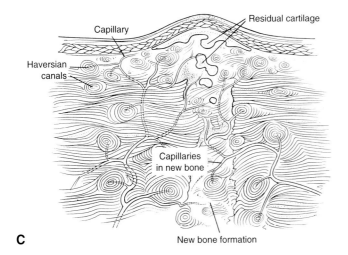

C

Fig. 3-2   Bone healing. **A,** Early stages of bone and fracture repair. Proliferation of osteogenic cells of the periosteum and of endosteal lining of haversian canals and marrow cavity. These cells differentiate into chondroblasts, which form cartilaginous callus. Osteoblasts, which form new bone, and osteoclasts, which resorb dead bone and bone fragments, are present. Periosteal reaction extends beyond the fracture site. **B,** Intermediate phase of bone repair. An external callus of bone or cartilage is formed by osteogenic cells of the periosteum. Cells form bone in areas of high oxygen tension and form cartilage in areas of low oxygen tension. As new capillary growth proceeds, new bone replaces cartilaginous callus. Internal callus is formed by osteogenic cells of the endosteum and is primarily new bone. **C,** Late stage of bone repair. New bone of the external callus extends to join new bone of the internal callus and bridge the fracture defect. Bone is remodeled as osteoclasts resorb callus. Layers of bone laid down around blood vessels form new haversian systems.

---

distal nerve. The cell body and proximal stump of the axon enlarge as the metabolic activity necessary for regeneration commences (Fig. 3-4, *B*). Ultimately, the proximal and distal stumps of the nerve are united, and axon buds migrate distally along the cell column in the endoneural tube (Fig. 3-4, *C*). Finally, Schwann cells envelop the axon and form a new myelin sheath (Fig. 3-4, *D*). The time required for this process varies depending on the nature of the injury, the time of repair, and the proximity of the nerve injury to the central cell.

Repair of a peripheral nerve therefore involves the regeneration of a portion of a highly specialized cell and not of a single tissue. By careful nerve repair the surgeon hopes to provide the optimum setting for successful axonal regrowth. Regenerating axons eventually reach one of several types of receptors or motor endplates, and despite the most careful microscopic repair, distribution of these axons is random. If a sensory axon terminates in a motor endplate or if a motor axon terminates in a sensory endplate, useful function is impossible. Unfortunately, the final performance of even the most meticulous microscopic nerve repair is subject to chance, and normal function is rarely achieved except in extremely young individuals.

◼ JOINT STIFFNESS AND TENDON ADHESIONS

Loss of motion of the shoulder, elbow, forearm, wrist, or small joints of the hand may result from a combination of edema, scar formation, and muscle contracture. These conditions render upper extremity joints stiff by interfering with joint mobility or muscle-tendon excursion. Edema is the first and most obvious reaction of the upper extremity to injury. Although it is reversible in its early stages, persistent edema may result in marked tissue scarring and fibrosis. The amount of edema formation is probably related to the severity of the injury to the involved tissues and results in an alteration in capillary permeability. The protein-rich edema fluid attracts water into the

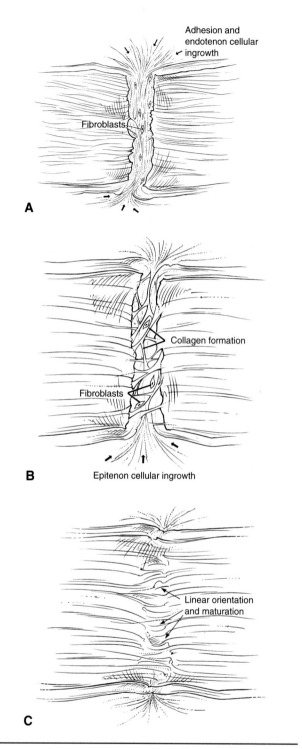

Fig. 3-3   Tendon healing. **A,** At 2 weeks. Following a cellular response of a tendon, tendon sheath, and surrounding perisheath tissues, fibroblasts and collagen fibers are present between the severed tendon ends and are oriented in a plane perpendicular to the long axis of the tendon. **B,** At 4 weeks the fibroblasts have started to become more longitudinally oriented and progressive organization and realignment of collagen fibers occur. **C,** At 8 weeks the collagen is mature and realigned in a linear fashion.

interstitial spaces until normal capillary permeability is reestablished. The fluid fills the interstices of the collateral ligaments and the soft tissue surrounding joints and tendons. Edema is usually most noticeable on the dorsum of the hand because the palmar tissues are fixed and unyielding, whereas the dorsal skin is freely movable and lax. As edema collects on the dorsum of the hand, the metacarpophalangeal joints are forced into hyperextension and the proximal interphalangeal joints assume a flexed position. Collagen is then deposited about the collateral ligaments as well as the flexor and extensor tendons, which become bound to the surrounding immobile structure. Uncontrolled edema comes to involve all the tissues of the hand and/or upper extremity, resulting in restriction of both active and passive movement. The fluid is soon supplanted by scar tissue, which can lead to severe and often permanent contractures. Treatment of reversible edema must be prompt and aggressive because control of the resultant contractures is extremely difficult. Consequently, optimal management of the injured hand includes elevation and early mobilization of joints to minimize edema and limit restrictive scar formation.

Scar tissue can form in almost any area involved in the edema process (Fig. 3-5). This means that not only may the area of injury become the site of scar formation, but also those tissues distant from the injury site may also become involved because of the effects of chronic edema. In addition to the prejudicial effect scar tissue has on joint motion and tendon excursion, muscle tissue may become involved and undergo a process known as myostatic contracture. If the tension within a skeletal muscle is completely removed for a while, the muscle belly shortens at this retracted length. Early on, active and passive exercises or splinting can overcome this contracture; however, if the muscle is allowed to remain in a shortened position for a number of weeks, attempts to promptly restore it to its original length may be impossible or may lead to muscle damage. Denervated or paralyzed muscle does not develop myostatic contracture, which suggests that the normal reflex patterns must be present for the development of this condition. Myostatic contracture apparently involves a change in the compliance of the elastin elements within the muscle fibers and may result in shortening of the muscle's resting length by as much as 40%.

Joint Stiffness

Joint stiffness may result from direct injury or may occur secondarily when afflictions of the skin, fascia, tendon, tendon sheath, muscle, or retinacular

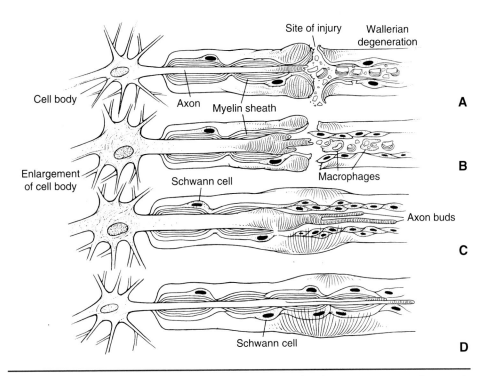

Fig. 3-4   Nerve healing. Axonal regeneration following peripheral nerve severance and repair. **A,** Injury results in degeneration of the axon and myelin distal to the wound and for a short distance proximal to the wound. **B,** A cell body and proximal stump of the axon enlarge as metabolic activity necessary for regeneration commences. The Schwann cells in the distal stump grow forward to the proximal stump and macrophages clear the debris. **C,** Proximal and distal stumps are united by Schwann cells and axonal buds migrate distally along the Schwann cell column in an endoneural tube. **D,** Schwann cells surround the axon and form a myelin sheath.

ligaments prevent joint motion for a prolonged period (Fig. 3-6). This may result in secondary shortening of the joint capsule or collateral ligaments, which limits motion even after the initiating factors have been removed. The vicious triad of injury, edema, and immobilization inevitably leads to restrictive scar tissue, adherent tendons, shortened ligaments, and myostatic muscle contracture. Crushing injuries, lacerations, and burns commonly result in sufficient tissue injury to produce diminished joint motion; various combinations of injury to skin, bone, joint, and tendon may also lead to stiffness. Factors unique to each injury,[21] which will govern the rate of functional recovery and the possibility for permanent joint contracture, include hemorrhage, edema, and prolonged immobilization of a joint in a position favorable to contracture. Infection may also contribute to the development of joint stiffness, and individual variations with respect to collagen maturation will produce different amounts of recovery in different patients with the same injury or surgical procedure.

Common digital contractures and their causes are discussed next. A characteristic combination of findings in the severely stiffened hand includes metacarpophalangeal joint extension, proximal interphalangeal joint flexion, and adduction contracture of the thumb web. A brief review of the factors contributing to the deformity at each joint level will be presented for six types of contracture.

Distal Interphalangeal Joint Contracture

Because of its terminal position on the digit, the distal interphalangeal joint is most vulnerable to crushing injuries, which produce considerable damage to all of the periarticular tissues. Particularly, the joint capsule and collateral ligaments may be damaged by this type of injury, and the edema that results from crushing is often long lasting and results in substantial scarring and limitation of joint motion. Unfortunately, this stiffening is often at least partially permanent and does not respond well to exercise, splinting, or therapy. The degree of functional disability resulting from distal interphalangeal joint contracture is not great because function at the metacarpophalangeal joint and proximal interphalangeal joint is usually retained.

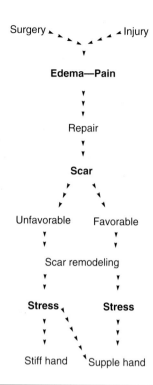

Fig. 3-5   Sequence chart depicting the events following surgery or injury that can terminate in either a stiff hand or a supple, functional hand. Scar that results from injury can be biologically unfavorable or favorable, and its final characteristics can determine the ultimate functional result. (From Weeks PM, Wray RC: *The management of acute hand injuries: a biological approach*, ed. 2, Mosby, 1973, St. Louis.)

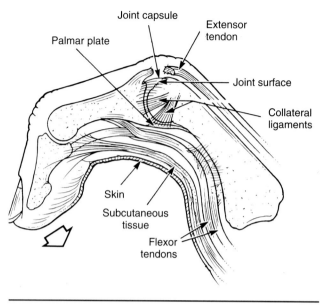

Fig. 3-6   Pathology involving various anatomic structures may result in digital joint stiffness or contracture. This flexion contracture of the proximal interphalangeal joint may result from one or more of the following: (1) disruption of the extensor tendon, (2) fibrosis of the joint capsule, (3) damage to or destruction of the articular surface, (4) injury or secondary shortening of the collateral ligaments, (5) injury or shortening of the palmar plate, (6) adhesions or shortening of the profundus or superficialis tendon, (7) scarring or contracture of the subcutaneous tissue or fascia, and (8) scarring or contracture of the skin.

Proximal Interphalangeal Joint Extension Contracture

These contractures most frequently result from crushing injuries to the joint and involve scarring of the dorsal joint capsule and dorsal-most fibers of the cord portion of the collateral ligament. Adherence of the central extensor tendon with or without involvement of the intrinsic muscle tendons may also result in this deformity, and scarring of the dorsal skin or articular surface damage may also contribute. The outlook for overcoming this contracture by gentle exercise and splinting programs is favorable, although one must be careful not to cause further damage to the extensor tendon or joint.

Proximal Interphalangeal Joint Flexion Contracture

Flexion contractures of the proximal interphalangeal joint most frequently result from direct injury to the joint or from chronic edema and immobilization with the joint in a flexed attitude. Shortening of the palmar plate, with its proximal checkrein extensions, and of the collateral ligaments is the most frequently implicated factor in this deformity, although scarring and adhesion of the palmar skin, flexor tendons, or flexor tendon sheath are often associated components of the contracture. Efforts in extension mobilization splinting may be quite disappointing when this contracture is marked and has become fixed.

Metacarpophalangeal Joint Extension Contracture

The collateral ligaments at the metacarpophalangeal joint are eccentrically placed. Because of the cam configuration of the metacarpal head, the collateral ligaments are lax with the joint in full extension and tight with the joint in flexion. Injury or chronic edema around the joint can result in the deposition of new collagen around the collateral ligaments in their slack position and allow them to shorten. Flexion may rapidly become limited depending on the degree of ligamentous shortening. To a lesser extent, the extension contracture may result from injury or thickening of the dorsal capsule, adherence of the extensor tendon to the metacarpal, scarring of the dorsal skin, obliteration of the palmar synovial pouch, or direct articular damage. Efforts to mobilize this joint by exercise programs or splinting are more successful if initiated early.

Metacarpophalangeal Joint Flexion Contracture

Flexion contractures of the metacarpophalangeal joint are the least frequent of the digital joint deformities and are most frequently associated with ischemic contracture of the intrinsic musculature. Disorders of the palmar skin or palmar fascia or scarring about the palmar synovial pouch may result in this deformity. Adherence or shortening of the flexor tendons or the overlying origin of the fibroosseous canal may also contribute. Efforts at improving function by exercise programs or splinting may not succeed in lengthening the offending structures, and surgical release may be required.

Thumb Web Contracture

Adduction deformity of the first web space can be an extremely disabling contracture and may result from simple scarring of the skin between the thumb and index finger. Scarring of the fascia or musculature of the first web space may also result from direct injury, ischemia, or chronic edema, and secondary stiffening of the carpometacarpal joint may result. Distention of the dorsal first web skin by edema will pull the thumb into adduction, and myostatic contracture of the first dorsal interosseous or adductor pollicis muscles results in further deformity. Efforts at serial web space widening may be successful if the scarring is not extensive, although surgical release of the offending tissues is frequently required.

Tendon Adhesions

Limited excursion may result from direct injury to flexor, extensor, or intrinsic tendons, and the scar resulting from the healing of contiguous tissues may also result in excursion-limiting adhesions to these structures. In particular, fractures of the metacarpals or phalanges, in areas where they have a close anatomic relationship to the digital tendons, may result in the tendons becoming bound in an unyielding fracture callus, which, in addition to reducing the amount of active motion possible, provides a checkrein restriction on the passive ability to flex or extend the involved joints (Fig. 3-7). These limitations of joint motion secondary to tendon adhesions are well recognized and can be determined by careful physical examination. For example, adhesions occurring between the extensor tendon and the metacarpal limit the distal excursion of the extensor mechanism and restrict composite flexion of the digital joints. Although one might be able to fully flex the metacarpophalangeal joint with the proximal interphalangeal joint in extension or fully flex the proximal interphalangeal joint with the metacarpophalangeal joint in full extension, the checkrein phenomenon produced

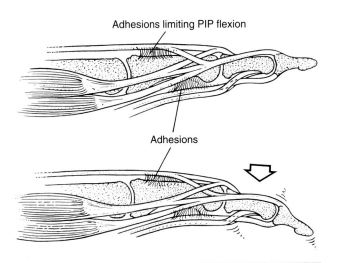

Fig. 3-7   Dorsal adhesions may form between the extensor mechanism and the proximal phalanx or palmarly between the flexor tendons and the proximal phalanx as a result of tendon injury, fracture, or crushing injury. The restricted excursion of the extensor mechanism can limit active extension or active and passive flexion of the proximal interphalangeal (PIP) joint. Flexor tendon adhesions can limit active flexion or active and passive extension.

by the diminished excursion of the extensor tendon does not permit composite flexion at both joints. Similar testing is possible on the palmar side of the involved digits, and this type of careful examination allows one to differentiate motion loss secondary to tendon adhesions from true joint stiffening.

Efforts at improving tendon excursion include early joint motion following fracture, crush injury, or tendon damage. Early active and passive exercise programs have been designed to provide controlled tendon gliding and are felt to have added considerably to the final results following tendon interruption. In addition to providing a beneficial biologic effect on adhesion formation around healing tendons and their adjacent tissues, these motion programs diminish the likelihood of secondary joint stiffening and are probably effective in reducing edema formation.

■ BIOLOGIC RATIONALE FOR SPLINTING
Influence on Scar Remodeling

It is apparent that the scar formation and wound contracture that are an integral part of the orderly healing of hand tissues may have a great influence on tendon gliding and joint movement. Measures designed to prevent digital stiffness include elevation, positioning of joints to lessen the possibility of collateral ligament shortening, implementation of early motion programs, relief of pain, control of edema, elimination of hematoma formation, prevention of infection, and the use of splints. Although very little meaningful scientific information has been provided to indicate at which points during the healing process it is most appropriate to use immobilization, mobilization, restriction, and/or torque transmission splints to favorably control the production and remodeling of scar tissue, a review of the biologic sequence of the reparative process may allow us to draw some reasonably sound conclusions.

Excluding early motion programs for tendon repair, there seems to be little benefit in using mobilizing splints that apply stress to healing wounds during the period of inflammation. Stress at this time might result in separation of repaired structures or a prolongation of the inflammatory phase by inflicting repeated injury to the involved tissues. Therefore it is probably appropriate to use splints that immobilize the involved part during the inflammatory phase and withhold the application of stress for one or more weeks depending on the specific injury or surgical procedure.

During the period of fibroplasia, which usually begins during the second week and continues for 6 weeks, it may be biologically suitable to institute the use of mobilization splinting designed to provide light stress with the hope of returning function as quickly as possible. The decision to apply stress to healing tissues during this phase is mitigated by the condition of injured or repaired structures. Unstable fractures, collateral ligament injuries, extensor tendon repairs, nerve repairs, skin grafts, and some flexor tendon repairs may be vulnerable to further damage or disruption with the premature application of stress. The use of mobilization splinting should be withheld until 3 to 6 weeks have elapsed. If there are no healing tissues that might be jeopardized by the early application of stress, then gentle mobilization efforts may be commenced within the first or second week. Careful observation of splinted areas and measurements of hand edema and motion changes in the involved joints indicate the efficacy of the use of splints on the biology of the healing tissues.

After the sixth week of wound healing, during the period of scar maturation and remodeling, it may be appropriate to increase the amount and duration of application of the force being imparted to the healing structures. Ideally, whatever joint stiffening and loss of tendon excursion may have developed during the inflammatory and fibroplastic stages will have resulted from immature scar that can still be favorably altered and modified by the judicious use of mechanical stress. Mobilization splints applied during this stage are designed to influence the remodeling collagen and ensure the maximum recovery of articular gliding and tendon excursion. The process of wound contracture may also be favorably modified by the use of splints

that resist the contractile influence of wound healing on the movable parts of the injured hand.

Weeks[127] has stated that the only acceptable clinical method we have of accelerating the modification of scar tissue is the application of stress to the scar. Splints may be implemented to assist the conversion of unfavorable scar to favorable scar by controlling the biologic process of synthesis and degradation of collagen. Mobilization splints must be designed to maximize the amount of stress applied to the offending scar while minimizing damage to normal hand tissues. The amount and direction of the force applied by a mobilization splint must be carefully monitored to prevent damage to the skin and subcutaneous tissues and to avoid undue compression or distraction of the involved joints. The force must not be applied too rapidly or the ligaments may not have the capacity to undergo the desired biologic alteration and may rupture.

An important concept emphasized by Brand[19,21,23] is that stretch represents a passive action, which results in elongation of the elastic elements of various tissues. Elongation that is accomplished by stretch inevitably shortens again when the force on the involved tissues is relaxed. If tissues are pulled to the point of rupture, a vicious process of inflammation and scar formation results, and the ultimate effect on healing is worse than if the stretching force had never been applied. Brand also suggests that true lengthening of any living tissue results from an alteration of the activity of living cells as they constantly take up and absorb old tissues and lay down new tissue components. Old collagen is absorbed and new collagen is laid down in new patterns that are responsive to specific tissue requirements. When applying a splint, one hopes to stimulate the living cells to provide the most favorable new tissue[50] rather than to try to break old tissues. This may be accomplished by keeping the tissues in a "physiologic state" that creates the appropriate demands on the new cells to make changes in the configuration of new tissues. Brand stresses that the best method to accomplish this is to keep the involved tissues in a prolonged state of mild tension.

This application of stress to injured hand tissues should be directed toward minimizing the reparative response and maximizing the biologic reorganizational response. Its application may be opposite to that which one normally considers when attempting to modify scar configuration. For instance, in an effort to mobilize an adherent tendon in the palm, stress from a splint must be applied distally rather than relying on the usual proximal stress resulting from muscle contracture. Application of a small constant force has been shown to be much more beneficial than the intermittent application of large forces (Fig. 3-8).[20] Clinically useful information with regard to the behavior of upper extremity scars can be made by observing the response of given tissues to their initial loading while the scar is still immature. Improvements in joint motion and a decrease in edema may indicate a favorable modification of the scar maturation process.

Splints implemented in an effort to provide the most favorable remodeling of scar and adhesions are most effective if they use the entire range of motion that is possible in the joints of the involved extremity. Splints should be designed to hold tension on the restraining tissues and scar for a given period of time.[51] As already pointed out, the tension need not be high, and the hand should be positioned so that joint or tendon scar and adhesions are the limiting factors for movement. Alternating the direction of splinting to gently pull the offending tissues in opposite directions is also important. When sufficient healing of injured or operated tissues has occurred, some increase in the tension of mobilization splints and their period of application can then be allowed, and active muscle contracture by the patient will be beneficial.

Unfortunately, the application of splints often involves little more than trial and error rather than a scientific process involving the direct application of methods for the careful measurement of the amount of force being applied by a particular splint and concerns for the mechanical aspects of force

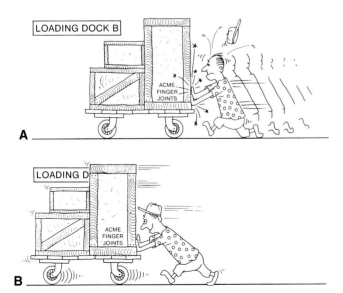

Fig. 3-8   This cartoon demonstrates (**A**) the ineffectiveness of intermittent application of large forces and (**B**) the effectiveness of the application of small constant forces in an effort to move an object (or joint). The same principles apply to the use of splints in an effort to produce a favorable biologic influence on scar tissue.

application. Consideration of the appropriate vector, moment arm, the amount of force applied, and the length of force application is very important and must be carefully correlated with the state of tissue healing in the affected part. Several investigators, including Brand,[17,26,27] Madden[2,3,86-88] and Weeks,[127] have expressed the need for a more scientific approach to the application of external stress and have begun to provide information that will ultimately be useful in the preparation and application of biologically effective splints. A great deal of additional study is necessary to better understand the exact effect of various stress forces being applied to specific areas of scarring, contracture, and adhesions. Data from the writings of Brand, Madden, and Weeks are included in the following discussion.

Splint Biodynamics

It is important that those involved in the preparation and application of splints have an understanding of what tissues are the limiting factors in the diminished movement of a given joint. Is it periarticular scarring or adherent tendons or a combination of both that prevents joint rotation? The injured extremity should be inspected for areas of wounding, edema, inflammation, infection, and the amount of active and passive motion loss. Alterations in joint movement produced by variations in the posture of adjacent joints can also point out which tissues are preventing normal motion. A reasonable assessment can then be made as to whether a particular scar has the biologic potential to undergo favorable remodeling.

Initial considerations for a splinting program should be directed toward determining the immediate mechanical effects of stress on scar tissue so that the clinician can best predict the subsequent biologic course that will follow splint application. As the splinting process proceeds, an observation of the changes in the motion of the involved joints gives an indication of the effectiveness of a particular splinting regimen on the mechanical properties of the remodeling scar. Then appropriate alterations in the splinting program can be made. Again, our clinical skills are directed at most favorably altering the biologic processes of collagen degradation, synthesis, and reorganization.

When applying forces in an effort to improve joint rotation, one must recognize that the direction and amount of force applied by the splint are critical to its biologic efficacy. There must be great concern for the mechanics involved in the various methods of force application and the effect of resultant forces on the injured part. Care must be taken to prevent undue traction or compression, and one must not confuse the manipulation of scar tissue that often leads to rupture with the gentle loading of injured tissues. Brand[17,26,27] has pointed out the effectiveness of to-and-fro tension on adhesions and scar in an effort to alter their configuration and favorably produce tissue lengthening. This may be done either by exercise programs or by alternating flexion and extension splinting.

Force, Area, and Pressure Determinations

The amount of force that can be applied to a given digit to improve joint rotation is limited by the ischemic effects produced by the splint that is in contact with the finger. The pressure exerted on the skin cannot exceed the capillary pressure in the cutaneous vessels for a long time or ischemia will result. Capillary pressure averages about 30-35 mm Hg. To ensure perfusion, forces applied to the skin cannot be excessive. The pressure produced by a well-fitting splint is dissipated over its area of skin contact; measurements of this area can be multiplied by measurements of the force imparted by the splint to determine the exact pressure applied to the contact surface. These simple measurements can be incorporated into the process of splint preparation and fitting to determine how much force they are generating over a given area of application. Because rubber bands are frequently employed to provide the force during mobilization splinting, it is important to determine their exact force. There is little uniformity in the elasticity of these simple rubber rings, which are manufactured without consideration for this exacting biologic use. The force generated by rubber bands can be measured with a simple spring-loaded scale, which determines the tension on the rubber band at the exact length that will be used in a given splint (Fig. 3-9). Combined with measurements of the area of application of the attached slings, one can make a reasonably accurate determination of the amount of pressure imparted to the offending scar tissue and its overlying skin (Fig. 3-10). Serial readings, of course, are necessary to determine changing forces in the rubber bands and altered areas of sling contact as the range of motion of the involved joint improves.

Weeks[127] states that the average person can tolerate 6 oz of force for up to 4 hours and lesser amounts of force for much longer periods (Fig. 3-11). Fortunately, the excessive force that produces ischemia also causes pain, which will serve as an effective warning system. One must therefore be very careful about the use of splints in the anesthetic hand, where this alarm mechanism is not present. Many biologic variables, including the nature of the injury to skin and subcutaneous tissues, the stiffness of tissues that

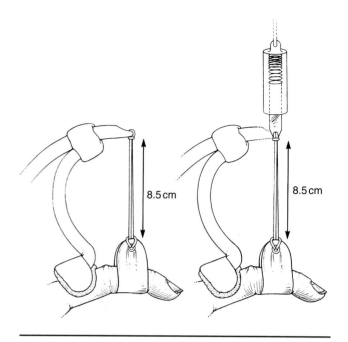

Fig. 3-9   A simple spring-loaded scale can measure the force generated by a rubber band and sling combination attached to an outrigger splint. It is important that the scale measure the force of the rubber band at the exact length it will be used in the splint.

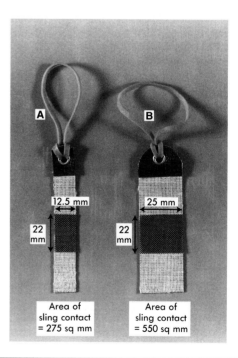

Fig. 3-10   Depicts the varied contact area on the palmar and lateral aspects of a digit created by two slings of varied width. A, The small sling is 12.5 mm wide and has 22 mm of circumferential contact with the digit. It therefore has an area of sling contact of 275 mm. B, The wider sling has 25 by 22 mm of contact with the digit, for an area of sling contact of 550 mm. The amount of force that can be tolerated using the wider sling is significantly greater.

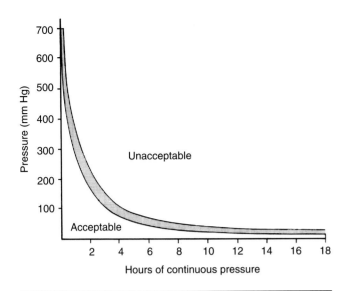

Fig. 3-11   Allowable pressure versus time of application for tissue over bony prominences. This curve gives general guidelines for the application of splinting force, but should not be taken to provide absolute values. (Redrawn from Reswick JB, et al: *Bedsore biomechanics*, McMillan Press, 1976, London.)

TABLE 3-1   Guide to Duration of Pressure Application

Short-Term (less than 2 hours)	Long-Term (continuous for more than 8 hours)
50 mm Hg/mm²	30 mm Hg/mm²
75 gm/cm²	50 gm/cm²
1 lb/in²	12 oz/in²

Modified from Brand PW: *Clinical mechanics of the hand*, Mosby, 1985, St. Louis.

surround small blood vessels, and the temperature of the skin, can alter the veracity of pressure calculations to some extent.

Brand suggests a useful guide with regard to the amount of pressure that can be safely applied by splinting (Table 3-1). He states that in short-term application (less than 2 hours) ischemia should not be a problem, and the numbers in Table 3-1 can be ignored. Actual pressure necrosis is likely only in insensate hands because a patient with normal sensation will discard a splint because of the discomfort produced by ischemia.

Brand condemns the use of typical slings to apply force in mobilization splints because changes in the posture of the finger result in a tilting of the sling and localization of the pressure to a smaller area of contact. He points out that when a sling is in good position with a 90° angle of approach, a contact area of 4 cm² applied with 200 gm of force results in (200 ÷ 4) 50 gm/cm² pressure at the point of application. Changes in joint position that result from this tension alter the contact area of the sling and impart the same force on a much smaller surface area. At 70° the sling takes the force on less than one third of the available sling surface, and the pressure then rises to 150 gm/cm², an unacceptable amount that could cause necrosis within a few hours. Because this amount of pressure is painful, the patient will almost certainly not use the splint, and consequently its effectiveness as an influence on scar remodeling is lost.

This observation indicates the need for a frequent review of the mechanics of each splint with modifications when necessary to ensure that the maximum amount of contact surface of a given sling is being used. Brand also points out that reaction bars such as the dorsal phalangeal bar of an outrigger splint can apply uneven pressure and are likely to cause ischemia and pain. Because of their reciprocal midposition in the three-point system, these bars apply force that is twice that of the proximal and distal ends of the splint. He further states that one must be wary of small tolerable stresses applied repetitively, which result in shearing injuries to underlying tissues. The more the repetition of the stress applications, the more likely are the unfavorable consequences.

We can see that, although we still lack many of the answers to the appropriate application of forces in modifying the biologic healing process and restoring maximum tendon excursion and joint motion, it is possible to provide some scientific measurement of exactly what forces are being imparted by a given splint. At the present time simple measurements of the forces imparted by a rubber band, the area of splint contact, and the mechanics of splint design and application can aid in the preparation of a physiologically safe and a biologically effective splint. Careful clinical monitoring, however, is still paramount, and a simple observation of the appearance of the skin underlying a sling can provide considerable information.

Blanching occurs when there is too much tension, and a good mobilization splint applies constant tolerable tension that can be maintained for long periods. Small increments of improvement of joint motion can be achieved in this manner and are preferable to methods that involve strong forces applied over short periods of time in an effort to make rapid gains. These techniques often rupture scar and underlying tissues and set up a vicious cycle of inflammation, further scarring, and contracture, which are detrimental rather than beneficial to the recovery of function.

Splinting for Tendon Adhesions

The high propensity for injured tendons to develop excursion-limiting adhesions following repair has resulted in a number of techniques designed to impart a controlled amount of tendon motion at an early stage of tendon healing.[92] It is hoped that these methods will favorably modify the quantity, strength, and length of adhesions and permit the maximum recovery of tendon performance. Flexor tendon injuries in the digital canal are particularly prone to the development of adhesions, and programs designed to provide digital joint motion and tendon movement by means of early active,[48,118,122] active extension-passive flexion[74,75] (rubber band), or passive flexion and extension[44] have been employed to produce the desired biologic alteration of the tendon healing process. In some excellent animal studies, Gelberman and associates[59] have demonstrated that these methods are effective in decreasing adhesion formation and increasing the tensile strength of repaired tendons. Boyer reports that more vigorous mobilization methods are not substitutes for modern suture repair techniques.[16]

Efforts to restore tendon gliding are designed to result in biologic modification of the scar around the tendon. At the present time the only effective clinical method for accomplishing this favorable scar remodeling is the application of stress to the offending tissue. Passive joint motion directed to provide stress on peritendinous adhesions may be effective, although it must be recognized that certain scars simply do not yield to stress. The favorable remodeling of the scar around a tendon is best accomplished by applying stress to the tendon, which in turn transmits the stress to the scar. Weeks[127] has demonstrated that small loads impart significant elongation of tendons and that as the load increases, the percentage of elongation rapidly decreases. He plotted his results on a stress-strain curve, which demonstrated that as an initial small load was applied, a significant elongation of the tendon occurred. As the load was increased, the percent of elongation rapidly decreased until further loading resulted in tendon breakage (Fig. 3-12). He felt that these changes correlate with the physical alterations occurring in the tendon as the collagen fibers are changed from their normal wavy pattern to a straightened configuration. He concluded that we could assume that the strain recorded after the application of small forces to a tendon was the result of changes in the restricting scar.

The clinical importance of this information again lies in the need to provide small but continuous forces, whenever possible in opposite directions, in an effort to modify and elongate restrictive tendon adhesions.

Overzealous efforts to achieve rapid gains by the application of large forces will not prove to be biologically effective and may result in tendon attenuation or rupture.

Splinting for Joint Contractures

When collateral ligaments are subjected to increasing load, their response may be somewhat different from that seen in the tendon. Weeks[127] carried out experiments and determined the percentage of elongation of ligaments subjected to various loads. He plotted his information on a stress-strain curve (Fig. 3-12). Ligaments were found to exhibit a much greater elongation with a much smaller load than do flexor tendons. He further noted that when a ligament with predominantly elastic fibers was subjected to a small force, it reached a functional length quite rapidly.

Weeks made further observations regarding the phenomenon known as *creep*, which involves an elongation of a structure when a load is applied and

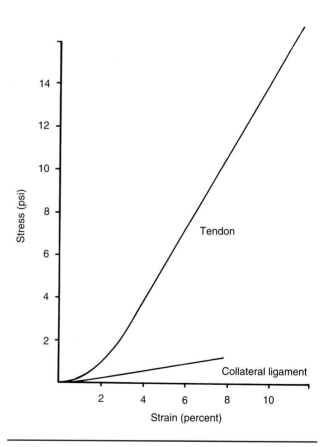

Fig. 3-12   Stress-strain curves for tendon and metacarpophalangeal joints are depicted. (From Weeks PM, Wray RC: *The management of acute hand injuries: a biological approach*, ed 2, Mosby, 1973, St. Louis.)

maintained at a constant level over time. Although in human flexor tendon the amount of creep is very small, a ligament was found to demonstrate considerably more elongation. He does note, however, that when a ligament of predominantly elastic fibers is subjected to a small force, the creep cannot be measured accurately. It was his impression that when the load is applied to a finger, the elongation that occurs actually reflects creep in the scar around the ligament rather than the ligament itself. The load levels that can be applied and tolerated by a finger are far below those, which cause tendon or ligament elongation, and changes that occur are probably the result of physical changes within the scar tissue.

There must be particular concern for the effect of excessive stress on a joint when it is applied for too long a period or with too great a mechanical advantage. The joint quickly reaches the maximum rotation permitted by the scar tissue, and at that point the joint can be forced open like a book. The ligaments do not have a chance to undergo biologic alteration. The forces the splint applies can tend to angulate the finger without true congruous articular gliding (Fig. 3-13).

Articular surface destruction or joint subluxation may result. One must therefore have a realistic understanding that some shortened collateral ligaments simply cannot be sufficiently elongated by splints to result in improved joint motion. Extension contractions at the metacarpophalangeal joint perhaps serve as the most appropriate clinical example of this problem.

Measurements of Biologic Activity

In an effort to determine the effectiveness of splinting programs in modifying the biologic processes involved in tissue healing and scar formation it is important to measure the response of the affected tissues. Hand performance perhaps can best be determined by serially measuring changes in the active and passive range of motion throughout the course of the splinting program (Fig. 3-14). Brand indicates that torque-angle measurements are more objective for passive range of motion and use standard weights or springs applied to a given finger to determine changes in joint angles resulting from the application of these weights (Fig.

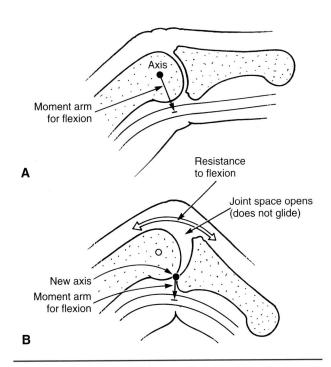

Fig. 3-13   **A,** When the functional axis is the same as the anatomic axis, the flexor tendon has good moment arm for flexion. **B,** When gliding is blocked at the joint surface, the functional axis for flexion moves to a point on the joint surface where the joint now tilts (not glides). The moment arm for flexion is now reduced to the point that the flexor tendon loses its ability to actively flex, and the joint opens like a book. (From Brand PW: *Clinical mechanics of the hand,* Mosby, 1985, St. Louis.)

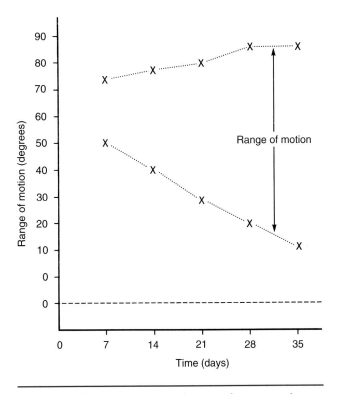

Fig. 3-14   Changes in the range of motion of a contracted proximal interphalangeal joint at standard torque resulting from serial measurements over 1 month. The graph depicts an improved range of motion caused mostly by an increase in the angle of extension. (From Brand PW: *Clinical mechanics of the hand,* Mosby, 1985, St. Louis.)

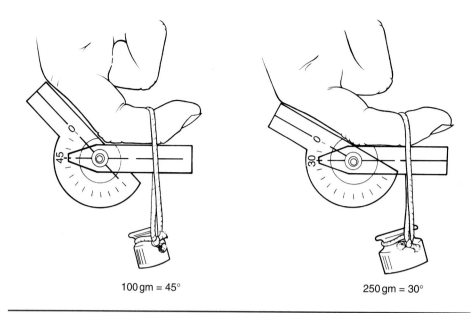

100 gm = 45°   250 gm = 30°

Fig. 3-15   Torque-angle measurements provide a more objective measurement of the passive range of motion. In this way, the passive position of a given joint can be consistently measured with the application of a constant force, and changes in the position of the joint resulting from the application of increased weight can also be observed. In this drawing a 100 gm weight applied to a digit results in a 45° flexed attitude to the proximal interphalangeal joint. Weight of 250 gm increases the extension to 30°. (Modified from Brand PW: *Clinical mechanics of the hand*, Mosby, 1985, St. Louis.)

3-15). Measurements of skin temperature, sensation, strength, and functional performance also describe the efficacy of a given program. Particularly important are tests that evaluate the range of motion of a given joint while changing the position of proximal joints such as the wrist or metacarpophalangeal joint. These tests can provide useful information as to whether the loss of joint motion results from diminished tendon excursion or is the primary result of periarticular fibrosis.

Brand states that, after the removal of compressive dressings, the hand will have been dependent on external support for several weeks and looks almost normal. Within 24 hours edema fluid fills the unsupported hand, particularly if it is allowed to be dependent. It then takes several days of vigorous range of motion exercises and elevation to get the normal pumping action of the hand restored and the hand volume improved. He recommends the regular use of a volumeter to provide measurements of upper extremity edema and feels that this measurement can be used as a rough determinant of the biologic state of the hand (Fig. 3-16). A volume graph based on serial measurements can indicate when the therapeutic effects may have been too vigorous, resulting in tissue strain and inflammation (Fig. 3-17). He emphasizes that exercises for mobilizing the hand and reducing excessive fluid should be simple, frequent, light, and repetitive.

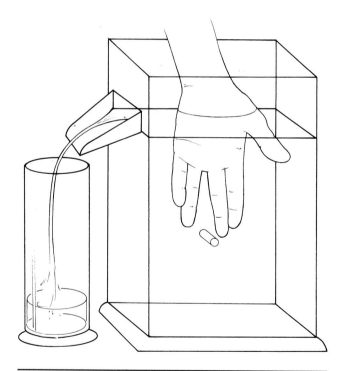

Fig. 3-16   Transparent hand volumeter to determine hand volume. The rim of the overflow spout is wide, level, and flat. The tank is filled to the overflow level, after which the hand is immersed in the tank. A transverse rod ensures immersion to the same level with each measurement. The overflow is measured and often compared with the volume on the opposite, uninjured side to give an indication of the amount of edema present. (Modified from Brand PW: *Clinical mechanics of the hand*, Mosby, 1985, St. Louis.)

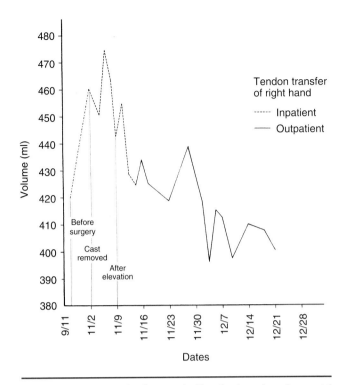

Fig. 3-17   An example of a record of hand volume based on serial measurements with a volumeter. These determinations were used after a tendon transfer. Note comments at different points in the patient's treatment program, such as "before surgery," "cast removed," and "after elevation." (Modified from Brand PW: *Clinical mechanics of the hand*, Mosby, 1985, St. Louis.)

■ SUMMARY

This section emphasizes the importance of a thorough understanding of the biologic changes in the hand as a response to disease, injury, or surgery. Unfortunately, scar tissue is an inevitable and necessary ingredient of the normal healing process, and its presence may be extremely prejudicial to hand function, where it may limit tendon excursion and small joint gliding. Carefully conceived, constructed, and applied hand splints can rest injured tissues or apply gentle stress to the restrictive scar tissue surrounding the normal elastic and gliding tissues and maximize joint performance. One must, however, have an appreciation for the biologic events necessary to satisfactory tissue healing and the effect the application of stress will have on this process. The concept that little is accomplished by the mechanical lengthening of scarred tissues and that by applying a mobilizing splint one hopes to stimulate living cells to provide more favorable new tissue is critical. The application of too much stress over too short a period of time or embarking on ill-conceived or ill-constructed splinting programs may prove to be far more detrimental to the overall performance of the involved joints than if no splinting program had been initiated at all.

Although we are still lacking in good scientific evidence to indicate the most appropriate timing for the application of stress to the injured hand and to date have very little understanding as to the appropriate amounts of force to apply to a given joint and for what period of time, it appears that the application of small loads over a sustained period, using the most advantageous mechanics of application, will lead to the most effective biologic remodeling of restrictive scar and the best long-term performance of the hand.

Section 2
Biomechanics, Splinting, and Tissue Remodeling

JUDITH BELL KROTOSKI, OTR, FAOTA, CHT

The hand is the dynamic precision operating tool of the upper extremity. It has to be splinted with its internal and external capacities for force and movement in mind, and with regard to how these are balanced and interplay for efficient and effective skill in our endless variety of tasks performed in everyday living. Our hands function through critical balance and movement of bony structures. These bony components are motored by muscles acting on tendons crossing multiple mobile joints, restrained by ligaments, sheaths, and opposing muscle systems.[34,46] One joint cannot be treated without consideration of what will be the result at other joints. Just as there can be no flexion of a finger without equal and opposite elongation of its antagonistic extensor tendons, and vice versa, one joint is connected to other joints in a dynamic linkage where one joint cannot act alone without restraint or stabilization of other joints.* Clinicians who grasp the concept that treatment of the hand has to include enhancing, stabilizing, or restricting the biomechanics of the hand are much farther along in ability to successfully treat patients, and certainly to splint the hand for correction and function.

A good understanding of the principles underlying biomechanics of tissue contracture and soft tissue growth and remodeling gives one the ability to take control of and use the body's normal tissue remodeling process and to use it to advantage in preventing contracture and in restoring range of motion. Those who understand the biomechanics underlying deformity can deduce the biomechanics of correction needed to arrest or reverse the process.

---

*References 30, 32, 56, 58, 94, 113.

■ UNDERLYING PRINCIPLES IN THE BIOMECHANICS OF TISSUE

Stiffness and contracture of joints, skin, and muscle tendon units occur when these structures of the hand are no longer asked or required to extend and flex fully within the time frame needed to maintain their normal limits of mobility. Close inspection of a finger interphalangeal joint flexion contracture that is long-standing will reveal not only joint stiffness and increased resistance to extension, but a real and limiting loss of tissue on the volar aspect of the joint, and growth of additional tissue on the dorsum of the joint (Fig. 3-18). Since this has happened gradually, the slow changes often go unnoticed, until a limitation of the joint angle is clearly observed as deformity. It is impossible to emphasize enough the malignant and progressive nature of the contracture from unbalanced force and stress in tissue.

Our skin and soft tissue are not inelastic and unyielding, but living and capable of responding to the internal and external forces which act upon them in an ongoing process. Some stress of tissue is needed in order to maintain normal healthy tissue. Hands that are not used develop thin shiny skin, stiff joints, and muscle atrophy. Joints and other soft tissue range of motion within given limits are maintained by the daily flexion and extension of the joints throughout the ends of their range, and the various stresses encountered on use of the extremities. Force acting on a tissue causes stress in the tissue that is needed and healthy. Too much force will damage any tissue, and too little force can also cause unwanted tissue response.

The clinician using splinting or any treatment for mobilizing stiff joints and reducing soft tissue contracture has to work between a range of what is too little force or stress, which will not be effective, and too much, which can damage tissue (Fig. 3-19). Tissue damage is not always visible; there can be damage at a cellular level that is not detected. Brand found in his soft tissue research that tissue can be damaged and have histological changes from low stress that is repetitive, even without there being a break in the skin.[28] Tissue damage of cells following injury is evidenced through the reaction of tissue to damage, an elevation in temperature that lasts longer than one hour, redness (erythema), or swelling. Damaged tissue can repair itself and recover, but tissue that was previously mobile and elastic in its normal state is replaced by scar tissue, which is less mobile, relatively inelastic, and tends to contract more as a wound heals.[29] Scar is the reparative tissue of the body and binds many structures together in an effort to heal. Scar tissue then can be inhibiting of joint movement and contributes to making joint stiffness permanent.

Swelling of tissue in and around joints exacerbates joint stiffness, limiting mobility by the increased volume and increased viscosity of fluid. These not only restrain tissue movement, but also create a situation in which higher force in the tissue is required

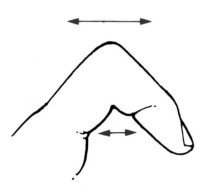

Fig. 3-18   Palmar skin becomes shortened in longstanding joint flexion contractures. These often require skin grafting before other surgery unless remodeled by splinting.

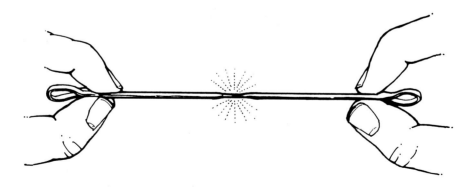

Fig. 3-19   Skin and other soft tissue have viscoelastic properties and will elongate and contract to a predetermined limit. Force beyond this limit deforms the tissue and tears some cells just as it would a rubber band.

for movement. Range of motion of a joint will not be normal either to its ends of range, or in the ratio of movement produced for given stress tension, so long as there is swelling of tissue in and around the joint. This is why it is so important to control and eliminate swelling of the tissue that involves the joints as soon as possible. Any treatment that increases tissue swelling thus works in the opposite direction of improvement in range of motion.

Aggressive range of motion exercise involving actual stretch of the tissue produces more swelling and actual tissue damage that introduces more scar. If scar is constantly stressed with repetitive intermittent forces, it may even become hypertrophic, where there occurs an increase in scar over what is needed for healing and the additional scar also has the tendency to contract even further. The reaction of scar tissue to high or repetitive low or moderate stress can sometimes be observed on the surface of a soft tissue suture line where it crosses a joint. Where there is no joint movement, the suture line may have a normal appearance, while the section of suture line crossing the joint has a wider and thicker band of scar that can be observed to have developed in response to higher tissue stresses on movement.

The ongoing soft tissue remodeling that is active in tissue contracture is active in tissue growth as well. In living tissue, there are cells dying and being replaced by new cells in a constant renewal of tissue. Normal tissue is being replaced and even the scar is being continuously replaced and remodeled. This tissue replacement is accelerated after injury, and continues at an accelerated rate for a long period after injury. This tissue remodeling process can be used to advantage in treatment because tissue is being absorbed where there is less stress in tissue and grows where there is more stress.

Joint and tissue contractures can often be prevented. Contracture is not inevitable if recognized and arrested or reversed at an early stage of development. But contracture is often progressive following disease or injury. This is particularly true when the patient or health care worker does not understand the underlying mechanics of contracture, what is needed for its prevention, minimization, and correction, or the patient does not have access to needed treatment.

It is easiest to prevent tissue contracture and inhibiting aspects of scar initially after injury. Every therapist knows the need for the return of the hand to full joint movement and tendon excursion following injury, as soon as this can be safely accomplished. If the hand moves only in restrictive positions or the joints are not moved throughout their full range of motion, the result will be joint stiffness and contracture of the skin and soft tissue, and this can include contracture of muscle tendon units acting at the joints as well.

Joint and soft tissue contracture can be mild, moderate, or severe. A joint is still mobile if there is joint glide and if passive extension can reduce the joint contracture within the limits of its natural full excursion. For an interphalangeal joint finger flexion contracture, this would be extension of the joint position to full extension (0° of flexion). In the initial period following disuse or injury, reduction of swelling, and gentle, internal or external range of motion exercise by the patient or therapist may be all that is necessary to dissipate excessive fluid and restore the normal forces and stresses in the tissues that act to maintain tissue mobility, joint, and tendon excursion. It is when these other attempts to restore mobility are not enough that splinting for remodeling can apply gentle stress in the tissue where needed and encourage growth of new tissue in order to achieve correction.

There is a direct relationship between the amount of joint stiffness or tissue contracture and the force needed to move the tissue; as mobility decreases, stiffness increases. More and more force is required mechanically in order to move the joint and tissue in the position opposite contracture until tissue disruption occurs.

Long-standing contracture becomes "fixed" contracture. Mechanically speaking, this is an advanced stage of contracture where so much force is required to move the contracted joint or to elongate its soft tissue, that tissue will be torn and injured when it is moved. Aggressive stretching of the tissue with mobilization techniques to reduce fixed contracture can be found suggested in literature and thus tried by therapists, but does not work and should be avoided. The tearing of tissue and subsequent inflammatory tissue reaction from "stretching" creates even more scar and results in even more contracture and inelasticity than there was before correction was attempted. Such damage to the tissues of the joint works in the opposite direction of correction. The use of the tissue remodeling technique can often help restore or improve joint and soft tissue mobility and has been found to be successful where other forms of splinting and other types of treatment often fail.

Joint and soft tissue contractures are usually progressive over time. What at first appears as a mild contracture will continue to progress into moderate and severe contracture unless something is done to restore normal biomechanical balance to the tissue and forces acting on the tissue, either externally through corrective exercise and splinting, or internally through tendon transfers, muscle, and joint restoration.

Deformity is progressive over time. It is not what happens with initial impairment that causes tissue contracture, but the secondary result of impairment disrupting a normal balance of forces acting on the tissue. Time then is also needed in order to reverse deformity. Tissue contracture does not happen overnight and cannot be corrected overnight.

Disability is progressive with deformity. Joint and tissue contractures may not at first be disabling to a patient's life and work, but can easily become progressively disabling with increasing deformity. The degree of severity of disability is directly related to the patient's requirement for use of the hands. What is no disability at all to one patient may prevent another from returning to the same occupation. Finger length is needed to operate and manipulate objects in normal skill activities. Joint stiffness can greatly limit dexterity and time it takes to perform tasks. Some patients become adept at substitutions; these are not improvements but rather adaptations over what would normally be required. Disability is greater where higher skill is needed in the activity such as when playing a musical instrument, tying a rope, and cutting with scissors. Often the portion of the hand with joint stiffness is functionally amputated when the hand must be used with skill, in order that the remaining parts can be used uninhibited.

■ BIOMECHANICS OF TRANSFER OF FORCE* TO PROXIMAL AND DISTAL JOINTS[18,25]

Immobilize one joint and additional force is transferred to another joint or joints when the hand is used. A splint that holds one joint in the same position will in turn transfer force that would normally occur at that joint both proximally and distally to other joints. Those who understand this transfer of force can use it to advantage and apply a splint to one joint specifically for mobilization of other joints. In treatment for joint and soft tissue mobilization, this splinting for transfer of force is used for a limited period and for the specific purpose of facilitating joint motion and tissue remodeling.

Transfer of force can be therapeutic if intentional. Therapists have long used stabilization or restraint of one joint or joints during exercise for the mobilization in therapy treatment of other stiff joints and for increased excursion of tendons caught in scar. This is what happens when a therapist blocks one joint with his/her hand while encouraging free movement of

*Note: In engineering terminology, this is called *torque transmission*.

another. One step further is to apply this concept to splinting. For instance, by holding the proximal interphalangeal joint of a finger in the position of extension with a splint, the force normally exerted at this joint through attachment of the flexor digitorum superficialis muscle tendons is transferred proximally to act in flexion at the metacarpophalangeal joint. The force of the flexor digitorum profundus is similarly transferred to flexion of the metacarpophalangeal joint, but its force for flexion is also increased at the distal interphalangeal (DIP) joint if the DIP joint where it attaches is left free (Fig. 3-20). If there is a condition of joint stiffness or limited flexion at the metacarpophalangeal joint, or the distal interphalangeal joint, splinting the proximal interphalangeal joint can help mobilize these other joints. The transfer of force, which engineers and physicists call moment, occurs whether the joint is held by an internal splint (e.g., a pin placed through the joint) or by an external splint (e.g., restraint by various splinting materials including plaster).

In patients with a peripheral-nerve-injured intrinsic minus hand, surgical intrinsic replacement procedures can internally rebalance and restore flexion of the metacarpophalangeal joints and extension of the proximal interphalangeal joints lost by the muscle paralysis. The balance in operation of the fingers provided by the tendon transfers is critical to success of the surgery. Where preexisting joint contracture exists, splinting the interphalangeal joints before and after surgery can often enhance the balance achieved by surgery. Splinting before surgery allows remodeling of joint contractures and restoration of range of motion for interphalangeal joint extension. At the

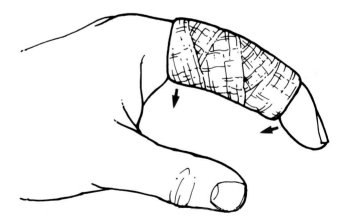

Fig. 3-20   Index finger MP, DIP extension and flexion torque transmission / PIP extension mobilization splint, type 0 (3)
A splint that holds a joint in one position can (1) remodel and mobilize the joint and soft tissue being held, (2) transmit torque to proximal and distal joints, and (3) mobilize the muscle tendon units that act on the joint.

same time, through transfer of flexion moment to the metacarpophalangeal joint, the finger splints provide temporary restoration of metacarpophalangeal joint flexion. Cast splinting after surgery helps establish, reinforce, and enhance the newly transferred tendons in reestablishing metacarpophalangeal joint flexion and interphalangeal joint extension, and also helps maintain the interphalangeal joints in a corrective position (Fig. 3-21).

Unintentional and unrecognized transfer of force can cause joint damage and tissue contracture over time. While transfer of force can be therapeutic when intentional, if unintentional and unrecognized, the long-term effect from unbalanced transfer of force from what is normal can be harmful. For instance, an arthrodesis of the proximal interphalangeal joint serves as an internal splint for this joint and additional force of finger flexor tendons is transferred proximally and distally. A therapist or surgeon not understanding the transfer of moment for flexion muscle force may be surprised to later find flexion contractures have developed at the two other joints from increased flexion force acting at these joints. The potential for joint contracture is even worse if the antagonistic extension of the finger has been disrupted by the surgery, as often happens, and the increased joint flexion is left unopposed.

▓ BIOMECHANICS OF MUSCLE TENDON UNITS

The muscle systems acting on the hand and upper extremity not only make it possible for the hand to fully flex and extend fingers at joints, these balanced systems also provide selective positioning for the fingers and thumb in a wide variety of postures and degrees of contact with objects. It is the selective variation in force, positioning, and timing of the fingers' movements as they work with objects that enables the dexterity and skill of hand function.

Muscle tendon units will shorten and lose excursion when not routinely required to extend fully. It is not the muscle tendons that contract, but the muscle fibers attaching to the tendons. There is evidence that the muscle has the capacity to increase its number of sarcomeres for lengthening, and that muscle loses sarcomeres when it becomes contracted; thus, even for the muscle, the objective of contracture reduction is one of growth of tissue in order that excursion can be restored.

An interruption in movement or excursion of muscles in certain directions for extended periods of time results in loss of joint flexibility and pliability and the inevitable skin and soft tissue contracture. Multiple situations arise with disease and injury of the hand where muscle tendon units acting on the joints become damaged or imbalanced and limit wrist and finger tendon excursion and joint movement, which in turn secondarily result in joint contractures.

Since the tendons of the extrinsic muscles originating in the forearm cross several joints, extrinsic muscle tendon unit shortening can lead to contracture of several joints. It is not an easy task to control all of the joints of the fingers and wrist in a splint that will allow full tendon excursion of the extrinsic flexor or extensor tendon units that originate in the forearm but act on the fingers and thumb. With full-length finger splints on the fingers, active finger extension at the metacarpophalangeal joint increases extension tension on the extrinsic finger flexor muscle tendon units and helps maintain or restore excursion length

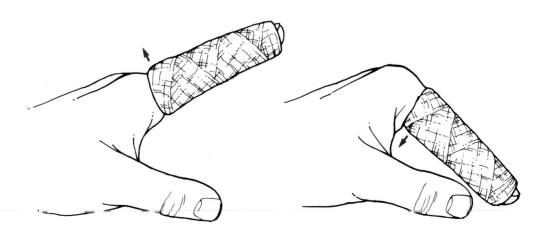

Fig. 3-21   Index finger MP extension and flexion torque transmission splint, type 2 (3)
The stabilization of the finger's normal interphalangeal joints transfers extension and flexion forces proximal to the metacarpophalangeal joint.

(Fig. 3-22). In conditions of mild extrinsic finger flexor muscle tendon unit contracture, the increase in force for metacarpophalangeal and interphalangeal extension made possible by the splint may be all that is needed to encourage restoration of normal excursion and resting tension.

In mild cases of extrinsic finger flexor muscle tendon unit contracture, a serially adjusted volar *wrist extension, finger extension mobilization splint, type 0* can be used to remodel the fingers and wrist into extension.[1,13] When there is extrinsic flexor muscle tendon unit tightness, it is easy to underestimate the amount of pressure occurring at the fingertips, and it is very easy to have a patient develop ischemic tissue damage from volar splints that do not dis-tribute pressure throughout the length of fingers. Splinting the fingers individually and then applying a volar splint is a safer way to attempt the tissue remodeling for flexor muscle tendon unit tightness. (See Chapter 22: Plaster Casting for Remodeling of Soft Tissue.)

Where there is moderate to severe muscle contracture, splinting the fingers in extension first, and then adding a *wrist extension, finger extension, thumb extension mobilization splint* can result in a large increase in tension in the forearm, fingers, and thumb flexor muscle tendon units. It is often necessary to place the wrist and/or metacarpophalangeal joints in flexion initially. The corrective position of the wrist is decided by the amount of wrist extension (starting from full flexion) that can be achieved while the fingers and wrist are maintained under mild, gentle tension. This positioning is progressively changed into full finger and wrist extension through serial splints

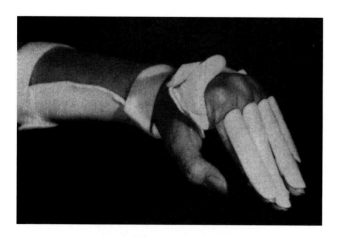

Fig. 3-22   Finger MP extension and flexion torque transmission splint, type 1 (5) \\ Finger MP extension and flexion torque transmission splints, type 2 (3); 4 splints @ finger separate These torque transmission splints prohibit motion of secondary wrist and IP joints to transfer moment to the MP joints, increasing MP extension and flexion motion.

applied every 3-4 days, depending on how the splints are tolerated. It is far better to start with a gentle extension tension that is gradually increased, than to apply too much force and have tissue damage requiring delay or cessation of treatment.

■ CORRECTION OF JOINT DEFORMITY AND STIFFNESS

A digital mobilization splint, individually, or in combination with mobilization splinting of the wrist and forearm, can be used successfully to correct and rebalance externally what has become imbalanced internally.

In the Paul W. Brand Biomechanics Laboratory,[1] formerly located at the United States Public Health Service Hospital, Carville, La., transfer of moment and soft tissue mechanics have been studied extensively with engineers. The in-depth anthology of his work beginning in the 1960s is in the book *Clinical Mechanics of the Hand*.[24,28,29,31,35] Unique tensiometers designed and created by engineers working with Brand were used to measure the force potential during surgery of transferred tendons. Torque range of motion devices were invented and reported for measuring the resultant change in angle and joint resistance to movement after surgery.[12,31] This same torque range of motion measurement technique is described for measuring the changes in angle and joint resistance following treatment with splinting or casting for remodeling (Fig. 3-23, A-C).

That there is increased resistance to joint or other soft tissue movement with stiffness and contracture can be demonstrated and quantified by the recording of joint-angle and mechanical measurement of resistance to finger extension (or flexion). Measurement technique for grading joint and soft tissue contracture, stiffness, and resistance to tissue movement has been described in detail and is available in several references, as is technique for determining if stiffness is related to joint versus tendon excursion.[31,37,52] Suffice it to say that successful treatment of contracture can be documented and quantified by objective measures of improvement in joint-angles, decreased resistance to joint and tissue movement, and growth of tissue where there has been contracture.

Mobilization splints with rubber band traction or restriction splints can be used for correction of some of the same problems as plaster cast remodeling, because it is not the plaster that results in success but the mechanics introduced by the splint. In early

[1]Paul W. Brand Biomechanics Laboratory, United States Public Health Service Hospital, Summit Medical Center, Baton Rouge, La.

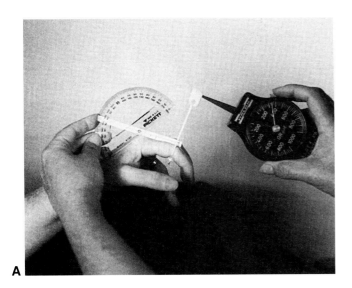

A

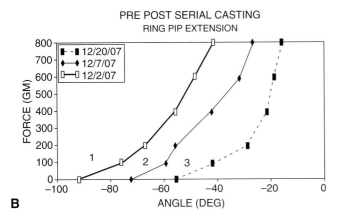

PRE POST SERIAL CASTING
RING PIP EXTENSION

B

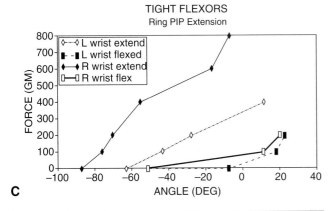

TIGHT FLEXORS
Ring PIP Extension

C

Fig. 3-23 A, Instrument technique for measuring torque range of motion (TQROM). Haldex strain gauge and goniometer adaptation for clinic measurements. B, Stress versus strain torque-angle curve measurements precasting and two measurements postcasting for right ring finger proximal interphalangeal joint. C, Stress versus strain torque-angle curve measurements precasting and postcasting for extrinsic flexor digitorum superficialis muscle tendon unit tightness. (From Breger-Lee DE, Bell-Krotoski J, Brandsma JW: Torque range of motion in the hand clinic, *J Hand Ther* 3:7-13, 1990.)

stages of joint stiffness and tissue contracture, elastic traction splinting might be equally as effective, and can possibly be more effective by allowing less restriction of joint movement. But these splints have their limits and do not always work for patients with moderate to severe tissue contractures. This is understandable when one considers that the constant tension needed to encourage tissue remodeling is difficult to obtain and maintain using elastic traction splints. Additionally, mobilization splints utilizing elastic traction can be more costly, and they can be more cumbersome and less cosmetic. These splints can also be injurious to the tissue under the traction cuffs if not checked frequently by both the therapist and the patient, whereas plaster mobilization splints conform precisely, do not constrict tissue, and hold an exact tension throughout the length of a finger or hand (do not create pressure in small areas of high tension when applied correctly).

Surgical correction for joint contractures is another often tried alternative to tissue remodeling. As compared with splint remodeling, surgical correction often additionally requires a skin graft to replace missing skin tissue, a collateral ligament release, and correction of the original cause of the contracture. All of these cannot be done very well together and the additional scar formed from a skin graft in a first-stage procedure may only lessen the chance of a successful repair. If the joint is remodeled with splinting, the skin graft and collateral ligament release often are unnecessary, and surgery can focus on correcting other problems, e.g., tendon transfers for restoring normal finger balance. Where needed, surgical correction such as collateral ligament release can be combined with casting for remodeling to enhance surgical results.

■ MAINTAINING IMPROVEMENT

Improvement achieved by progressive tissue remodeling may only be temporary unless attention is also given to maintaining improvements achieved in the long range or reversing an underlying muscle imbalance. Correction can become permanent with restoration of damaged muscles, peripheral nerve reinnervation of muscles which provide balance to the fingers, and when tissue remodeling and mobilization are otherwise combined with reconstructive surgery to correct underlying muscle imbalance.

■ TIMING

Remodeling for all joint contracture and extrinsic muscle tendon unit shortening, in particular, needs to be done before surgery if at all possible rather than after. This is particularly true where there is concurrent muscle tendon unit tightness. After surgery, it is often not possible to progressively put the wrist and fingers in the complete full wrist and finger extension position needed for correction of extrinsic flexor muscle tendon unit contracture. Such positioning after tendon transfers for the intrinsic minus hand, for example, would reduce or obliterate the tension-producing capacity of the transferred tendons. And when tendon transfers must act against resistance to movement from joint stiffness and contracted soft tissue they cannot be as effective. Attempts at joint contracture correction after tendon repair or transfer correction of the fingers does not allow for the matching of tendon tension required for correction with the best achievable joint positions and tendon excursions. Still, although it is harder, additional gains may be able to be made by splinting for remodeling following surgical correction and the technique is sometimes needed to further improve and enhance correction achieved by surgery.

■ INTRINSIC MINUS HAND AND TENDON TRANSFERS

The functional operation of the fingers of the hand depends upon a balanced interaction and stabilization between intrinsic and extrinsic muscle systems in the hand, not just finger flexors and extensors. The intrinsic muscles, which originate in the hand, stabilize the joints in order that power from the extrinsic muscles originating outside of the hand can flex and extend the fingers in various positions between full opening and closing of the hand in order to hold and manipulate objects. Without the intrinsic muscles of the hand the fingers and thumb collapse when attempting to hold an object, there is inability in opening the fingers at the distal joints, and the fingers primarily flex at the metacarpophalangeal joints, without selective positioning of the fingers for pinch and grasp.

In any patient with impairment of ulnar and/or median peripheral nerves of the hand and upper extremity, interphalangeal contracture and eventual joint deformity is usually the result. The underlying causes are the muscle imbalances created by the selective loss of the intrinsic muscles, which support, control, and help the extrinsic muscles position the fingers, with retention of strong and healthy extrinsic muscles, which act to fully open and close the fingers. Without the translational forces of the intrinsics on the dorsal hood needed to fully extended the fingers at the interphalangeal joints, there is an overpull in extension of the fingers at the metacarpophalangeal joints by the extensor digitorum communis that has its primary insertion at the proximal phalanx, not the

interphalangeal joints. Without the intrinsics, the metacarpophalangeal joints have lost their primary flexor, and these joints flex only after full flexion of the interphalangeal joints by the flexor digitorum superficialis and profundus (Fig. 3-24, A). Splinting the interphalangeal joint into extension allows the finger to be brought into full extension by the extensor digitorum communis and into flexion at the metacarpophalangeal joint by the flexor digitorum superficialis and profundus (Fig. 3-24, B).

Torque transmission of extrinsic muscle power may also be used to splint proximal joints in order to improve distal joint motion. For example, if MP joints are splinted in flexion for a prolonged period of time, stiff IP joints will remodel over time, increasing both their passive and active range of motion. Transmission of moment (also called torque transmission) concepts are not new. They date back to the turn of the century, perhaps earlier. Brand has long been an advocate of these concepts since the early 1960s[18] and is credited with popularizing these concepts in hand rehabilitation circles.[25,41]

If surgically transferred tendons have enough excursion in the right directions, and are powered

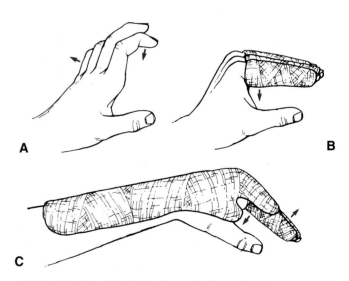

Fig. 3-24   B, Finger MP extension and flexion torque transmission / finger IP extension mobilization splint, type 0 (3); 4 splints @ finger separate. C, Index–small finger MP extension restriction / thumb CMC palmar abduction mobilization splint, type 1 (6) \\ Finger MP extension and flexion torque transmission splint, type 2 (3); 4 splints @ finger separate
Correction of finger extrinsic muscle imbalance caused by loss of intrinsic musculature. A, Without casting, the fingers primarily extend at the metacarpophalangeal joint, and primarily flex at the distal interphalangeal joint and interphalangeal joints. B, Preoperative casting transfers flexion of the superficialis and profundus to the metacarpophalangeal joint restoring primary flexion. B,C, Postoperative casting and metacarpophalangeal extension restriction helps augment desired action of the intrinsic transfers at the metacarpophalangeal joint.

with sufficient muscle contraction, balance of the fingers can be restored for flexion at the metacarpophalangeal joints and extension at the proximal interphalangeal joints. This correction can totally arrest any tendency for further contracture at these joints. A splint can be helpful to hold proximal and distal interphalangeal joints in extension in the initial stage of recovery. The splint helps support these joints (which have lost their physiologic extension by the nerve injury) during the initial stages of recovery until they can be fully supported by the new tendon transfers. The splinting of the interphalangeal joints does transfer some additional extension force to the metacarpophalangeal joint from the interphalangeal joint dorsal hood finger extensor mechanism. This transfer of force might be of concern, were it not that with the other finger joints splinted, hyperextension does not usually occur. The physiological limits in excursion of the finger flexors restrict metacarpophalangeal hyperextension, and after surgery, restraint is added by the routing and tension of the newly transferred tendons.[33]

If the tendon transfers are attached to lateral bands at the dorsal interphalangeal joint with too much tension or if they become embedded in scar during the surgical recovery period, the result can be severe metacarpophalangeal flexion contracture and interphalangeal joint swan neck deformity (hyperextension at the proximal interphalangeal joints). Once established, this contracture is maliciously progressive and can be a worse deformity than the intrinsic minus hand the tendon transfers were intended to correct. Swan neck deformities can mechanically limit the fingers in making a fist when the hand is used and are not cosmetically pleasing. In the early stages of surgical recovery when the tendency of the fingers to swan neck is first observed, splinting the proximal interphalangeal joints in slight flexion can help transfer the force moment for finger extension to the metacarpophalangeal joints. This is combined with positioning the metacarpophalangeal joints just short of complete extension (15° flexion) in a resting splint worn between exercises. Splinting for a few days or weeks is not likely to result in increased length of the tendons transferred, but promotes maximal mobilization of the soft tissue and scar around the tendons transferred and helps provide enough tendon excursion to balance their action at the fingers.

If there is too little tension and too much excursion in the new tendon transfers, they will not balance the movement of the fingers and the fingers will have a tendency to still hyperextend at the metacarpophalangeal joint and flex at the metacarpophalangeal joint upon attempts to actively extend the fingers. If this is observed during the initial stages of recovery,

splinting of the interphalangeal joints in extension and the metacarpophalangeal joints in 90° of flexion, with limited extension of the metacarpophalangeal joints during exercise, can be tried to encourage helpful restraining scar form around the transferred tendons and "desired" flexion contracture and stiffness at the metacarpophalangeal joints. This sometimes restores acceptable balance of the fingers on extension. If not, additional surgery to adjust the tension of the transfers is needed to restore the finger balance for use of the fingers.

Postsurgery, because of the strong mechanical ability of the extensor digitorum communis to provide finger extension at the metacarpophalangeal joints, the patient with intrinsic replacement surgery must be guarded against early full extension and any hyperextension at the metacarpophalangeal joints for at least 6 weeks. Since the patient must be guarded in this fashion, casts can be used in lieu of other forms of splinting. A dorsal *MP extension restriction / MP flexion torque transmission splint* not allowing the metacarpophalangeal joint to fully extend is often used in conjunction with finger IP extension mobilization casts* for the first few weeks, but the finger casts alone by their slight weight and by their holding the fingers in full extension are sometimes all that is needed (Fig. 3-24, *B,C*).

■ WOUND HEALING

Brand never intended his soft tissue remodeling technique using plaster to be used other than for mobilization. Employing a different concept, Brand also recommends plaster immobilization casts to protect wounds held in immobilized positions to enhance healing. He actually cautions against splinting for mobilization at the same time it is necessary to immobilize a part for wound healing. When treating a wound or infection, the integrity of the tissue is of first concern and movement can prolong and expand infection and tissue inflammation, thereby delaying tissue healing. In these cases, plaster has much to offer and is underused to help immobilize a part while allowing a wound to breathe. It can absorb exudates away from the wound, and may be a splinting material of choice for immobilization of wounds. But plaster casting of wounds is a different concept than casting for tissue remodeling, and requires immobilization or restriction splints.

---

*Depending on the specific surgery and if full IP joint extension is present, the IP extension casts may be considered *MP flexion torque transmission splints, type 2 (3)*.

It is important to note that even a splint intended for immobilization may have the same effect on the hand as a mobilization splint, as the biomechanics of the hand remain the same. The splint used for immobilization or restriction of one joint will have some effect on the proximal and distal joints not splinted, unless these joints are also included in the splint; this is important to keep in mind when making an immobilization splint. When immobilizing a severe infection of the hand, for instance, it is often advisable to include the distal joint(s) below the wound and at least one joint more proximal to avoid any movement at these joints until infection has somewhat subsided.

■ SUMMARY

Understanding the intricate nuances and interrelationships of normal and abnormal biomechanics of the hand/upper extremity allows clinicians to positively influence the tissue remodeling process through application of astutely designed splints. Splints may be used to immobilize, mobilize, restrict, or transfer moment (torque transmission) depending on individual patient needs. All splints affect tissue remodeling in one form or another. Splinting is not just the laying on of an external device on an extremity; rather it is the rational, premeditated thought process behind the design selection and application of a splint that renders it an efficacious instrument for influencing soft tissue healing and remodeling.

Section 3
Soft Tissue Remodeling

FESS, GETTLE, PHILIPS, JANSON

Hand/upper extremity specialists know from experiential knowledge derived from years of clinical practice that splinting is the most efficacious method currently available for improving joint motion limited by soft tissue contracture and/or fibrosis. Unfortunately, a paucity of research studies documenting the efficacy of splinting endeavors exists in current medical literature. Sometimes that which is most evident is the last to be researched formally. While the daily gains of splinting endeavors have been documented for many years in clinics throughout the world, perhaps the inherent simplicity and unmistakableness of these gains has created the false assumption that changes accomplished through splint application do not require investigation. Through developing empirical practice, splint designs that

succeed are continued and those that fail are discarded, providing an ever-evolving, highly sophisticated armamentarium of splint options from which clinicians may select the designs that best meet their patient needs. This progressive advancement of splint designs has served clinicians well over many years with few clinicians stopping to question the underlying basis for the achieved improvements in motion. As third-party insurers challenge the value of using splints to correct joint stiffness, clinicians are faced with proving the obvious. Fortunately, splinting is not the only treatment modality founded on soft tissue remodeling concepts. Research generated by other fields often provides insight and understanding on topics of mutual interest. The disciplines of hand/upper extremity rehabilitation and orthopedic surgery, plastic surgery, dentistry, bioengineering, biochemistry, and cellular biology share common interests in regard to understanding the underlying mechanism of tissue remodeling.

The concept of soft tissue remodeling is not new. Native tribes have used tissue remodeling for centuries[14,39,126] to increase ear, lip, or neck size as signs of beauty. In the field of medicine, Hippocrates (460-377 BC) described correction of clubfoot through gentle serial adjustments over time[49,131] and Celsus, in AD 20, wrote that skin flaps could be stretched and approximated.[14] Turnbuckle braces that corrected contracted joints through incremental adjustments were reported in the early 1500s,[80] with variations on this concept used without interruption up to and including current times.[49,80]

Twentieth-century medical practice significantly advanced understanding of tissue remodeling with many clinicians and researchers contributing to a rapidly expanding knowledge base. In 1915, Morestin noted that skin could be slowly increased through serial stretches.[130] Brand recognized the importance of soft tissue remodeling in the late 1940s, developed the total contact plaster cast method for remodeling soft tissue, and by the 1960s had established a biomechanics laboratory to investigate the reaction of living soft tissue to pressure.[9,20,22,49] In 1957, Neumann reported successfully expanding skin using a subcutaneous balloon[96] and in 1969 Ilizarov began documenting his extensive work using distraction forces[67] to increase bone length. Madden[86,87] and Madden and Peacock[88] described the dynamic metabolism of scar and collagen remodeling and Madden and Arem noted that the response of noncalcified soft tissue to stress is modification of matrix structure.[2,3] Matev, in 1970, recommended bone distraction lengthening for thumb reconstruction. However, it was not until 1976 that the usefulness of tissue expansion for reconstructive surgeries began to be appreciated fully when Radovan[107,108] reported successfully using a temporary tissue expander for breast reconstruction. Later that same year Austad, Pasyk, and McClatchey[5] described the results of their investigation of the mechanism of soft tissue expansion in animal models. The 1980s and 1990s produced important advances in the clinical application of tissue expansion techniques and in research to identify the biomechanical and biochemical mechanisms underlying tissue remodeling. Tissue expansion is now an accepted treatment technique that has been used with multiple types of tissues including skin, bone, skeletal muscle, nerves, blood vessels,[93] cardiac tissue, smooth muscle, lung, urogenital structures,[77,116] and bowel.[43,72]

Because control of soft tissue response is the common denominator for splinting and tissue expansion methods, similarities exist. For example, expanders typically are adjusted on a biweekly or weekly schedule, as are splints, especially serial mobilization splints applying inelastic tension. Also, pressure and magnitude of force application constraints must be respected, allowing sufficient tension to remodel and concomitantly avoiding damage to involved soft tissue cellular structures. Capillary perfusion drops when pressure exceeds 20-30 mm Hg.[55,97,135] Whether a splint or an expander exceeds this parameter is irrelevant; the result is injurious tissue damage. Further, Slavin notes that if the stimulus for growth is removed, cellular attrition commonly occurs.[120] Although referring to operative tissue expansion procedures, his prophetic words are applicable to splinting endeavors, underscoring the importance of maintaining both active and passive joint motion once splints achieve passive joint motion. Experienced clinicians are well aware of how quickly joint deformity can recur if retention splints, usually in the form of night splints, are not used. While authors agree that prolonged gentle tension results in soft tissue remodeling, the exact biologic mechanism that generates these tissue changes is better, but not completely, understood, even with today's sophisticated research equipment and methods.

■ STRESS INFLUENCES ON SOFT TISSUE

Two types of soft tissue deformation exist: (1) mechanical creep and (2) biologic creep. These two types of tissue changes are differentiated by the length of time the deforming force is applied. Mechanical creep involves acute or transient application of tension-stress as with some manual joint mobilization techniques, while biologic creep occurs with chronic or prolonged application of tension-stress. Most

splinting efforts rely on biologic creep to influence soft tissue remodeling.

Mechanical creep, a limited increase in length when tissue is stretched under constant load, involves a plastic deformation of the collagen network and displacement of ground substance and fluid.[17,26,27,60] This type of tissue alteration "occurs when water is displaced from type I and III collagen in skin and also when associated elastic fibers undergo microfragmentation."[120] With mechanical creep, collagen fibers are reorganized from a relaxed random pattern to orienting longitudinally in the direction of the applied force. Once collagen fibers are realigned in parallel fashion, further change is limited without causing tissue damage.[42,83] While acute tissue expansion methods are used in surgical reconstruction procedures,* this technique does not provide as much surface area gain as does chronic tissue expansion.[54] Mechanical creep also may involve recruitment of adjacent tissue.[83,96,114] Splints that are worn for short periods of time several times a day probably attain soft tissue change through mechanical creep.

Biologic creep involves generation of new tissue secondary to application of a persistent stretching force,[60,120] as evidenced by increased cellular mitotic activity.* An increase in mitotic activity is reported to occur within 24-48 hours[6,76] and mitotic activity is noted to persist in response to persistent force.[82] DNA synthesis and cell proliferation occur.[5,70,82,121,123] Interestingly, even cells in culture respond to longitudinal stretching with increased mitotic rate and realignment shape with the direction of force.[38,129]

Applying a biomechanical model, cell shape seems to be critical to this tissue growth process.[53] As cells deform from an applied stretch, a mechanotransduction phenomenon causes cell spread, which is then followed by cell proliferation until spaces are filled and equilibrium is restored (Fig. 3-25).[68] Prolonged strain seems to affect various signaling pathways, which are highly integrated[103] as mechanical tension is converted into growth promoting signals.[40,68,110,112] Referring to this stretch-induced signal-transduction pathway, De Filippo and Atala† note in their special topic article in *Plastic and Reconstructive Surgery*, "The mechanisms behind the principle of stretch-induced cellular growth involve a network of several integrated cascades that include growth factors, cytoskeletal structures, and protein kinases."[43] Although the mechanism by which cells respond to mechanical stretch is described in various ways, mild cell hypoxia is thought to be involved in the process,[85]

*References 17, 20, 26, 27, 42, 83, 102.
†From Children's Hospital and Harvard Medical School, Boston, Mass.

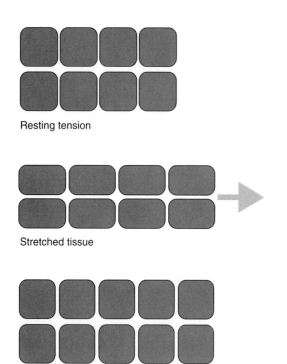

Resting tension

Stretched tissue

Growth restores resting tension

Fig. 3-25 Mechanical stress-tension initiates tissue remodeling. (From De Filippo RE, Atala A: Stretch and growth: the molecular and physiologic influences of tissue expansion, *Plast Reconstr Surg* 109(7):2450-62, 2002; adapted from www.plasticsurgery.org.)

as identified through tissue oxygen tension measurements.[4,91] In short, expansion causes mild ischemia, which stimulates growth factors that, in turn, stimulate angiogenesis and cell synthesis.[78]

The following account published in *Plastic and Reconstructive Surgery* highlights a long-standing but rapidly dwindling debate as to whether expanded soft tissue gains are due to mechanical or biologic creep. Noting that "Tissue expansion is a phenomenon whereby skin, mucosa, nerves, and muscles progressively expand over an underlying enlarging space-occupying lesion," Zambacos et al. describe a massive prepatellar bursa on the knee of a 47-year-old male carpet layer as being the longest case of tissue expansion ever reported. Development of the bursa lasted more than 20 years! Emphatically reporting that the histologic appearance of the expanded tissues were identical to those of normal skin, they continue, "This finding not only shows that in the long term there is no significant change in the quality of the skin, but also suggests that long-term tissue expansion leads to new skin formation rather than merely stretching of existing structures."[137]

In its earliest phase, biologic creep involves mechanical creep deformation, but this situation changes as time progresses and mitotic activity takes place. Also, tissues bordering expanded tissue may undergo increments of mechanical creep, forming transitional connections between biologic creep expanded tissues and nonexpanded tissues. Both types of deformation occur as the tissue remodeling process progresses.[6]

SPECIFIC TISSUES

While prolonged low-load mechanical strain induces tissue growth, differing tissue responses are unique to individual tissue types. Tissue growth is associated with angiogenesis, dermal thinning and epidermal thickening,[120] increased fibroblastic collagen synthesis,[95] increased myofilaments, increased mitotic activity,[6,36,76,82,106] and increased neovascularization.[1,5,6,14,60]

Conflicting reports may be found in the medical literature regarding specific tissue responses to stress. These disparities are often attributable to the type of expansion used, human versus animal models, and/or to dissimilar levels of cellular analysis. For example, expanded tissue may seem unperturbed when viewed with light microscopy but electron microscopy of the same expanded tissue may find evidence of cell degeneration. Few clinicians and researchers debate that tissue growth occurs but the exact mechanism for remodeling of different tissues continues to be investigated. A quick review of current tissue expansion literature is important to identifying and understanding the issues and processes involved in tissue remodeling.

Skin

Expanded epidermis undergoes cellular hyperplasia[115] and thickens,[1] returning to normal or near normal thickness in 1-4 years.[115] No qualitative or quantitative change in melanocyte, Merkel cell, or Langerhans cell populations[115] are noted and rete ridges flatten and return to normal by 2 years.[115] The dermis exhibits a collagen synthesis increase after 4 days of expansion[71,81,95,104,105] and collagen and elastic bundles thicken and reorient.[115] At 6 to 12 weeks, the dermis thins[115] and may not return to original thickness.[115] In contrast, two investigators report dermal thickening.[1,95] The question as to whether or not permanent biomechanical, biochemical, and physical changes occur in expanded dermis seems to be open to further inquiry.[10,128,132] Investigators agree that the size and number of pilosebaceous structures do not change in expanded tissues. While the distance between these structures increases, no new hair follicles are created.[1,7,99,115]

Muscle

Expanded muscle tissues exhibit increased mitochondrial activity including size and number,* increased number of sarcomeres,[73] and increased number of blood vessels[73] with no vascular changes and no damage.[125] A reduction in individual muscle fiber size[63] and thinning and decreased mass are also reported.† Inflammation is reported to be absent[6,106] and function remains normal.[108] Skeletal muscle grows with tension[66,73] and musculocutaneous flaps may be expanded without problems.[64,109,111]

In an intriguing study of expanded pectoralis major muscle for breast reconstruction, Gur et al. found consistent evidence of cell loss and degeneration in biopsies of postexpansion pectoralis muscle when examined with an electron microscope, although tissues from the same biopsies appeared normal under light microscopic examination. Interestingly, all subjects (n = 19) reported normal function with no muscle weakness and no problems carrying out daily activities. "There was no clinical evidence of a decrease in muscle strength or function in this group of patients."[63]

Bone

Mechanical tension-stress produces osteogenesis[117] in bone and once trabecular alignment is established during bone growth, it is not altered by disuse.[15] Multiple studies report that gradual distraction grows bone and associated soft tissues,[62,65,66,124,136] and growth is even along the distracted area.[102] Khouri et al note that "Ilizarov demonstrated in the laboratory and in the clinic that distraction is the only means of inducing true tissue regeneration."[72]

Nerve

Most nerve expansion studies involve animal models. At 18 months after nerve expansion, no differences in nerve conduction velocity (NCV) and muscle contraction force between nerve grafting and nerve expansion/repair procedures were found, although muscle weight was significantly greater with grafting[133]; in skin that was expanded 110%, no change in nerve function was noted.[134] Expanded/repair nerve compares favorably with traditional nerve repair results.[119] Using electron microscope evaluation, although degenerative changes were present beginning at 8% limb lengthening up to 33% of limb lengthening, nerves in an animal model recovered normal structure within 2 months postexpansion.[69] Another electron microscopic study found that nerves elongated by 88% retained their intraneural cytoskeleton components despite some loss of myelin.[47] Expanded Wallerian degenerated nerve exhibits increased Schwann cell proliferation and increased vascularity at the expander site.[57,100,101]

■ VASCULAR AND LYMPHATIC SYSTEMS

Most vascular volume and/or lengthening procedures involve acute intraoperative expansion. Studies on the affects of intravascular volume expansion with stents indicate that adaptive vessel remodeling occurs after stent placement with endothelial and smooth muscle cell hyperplasia taking place. Expanders have been used intraoperatively to increase arterial length.[56] Studies involving influences of tissue expansion on the lymphatic system are rare. Ercocen found that the expander itself reduces lymphatic flow.

■ DEVICES THAT REMODEL SOFT TISSUES

Soft tissue expansion devices may be two-dimensional or three-dimensional depending on the direction(s) of applied force. Surgery is required to insert noninflatable or inflatable force-transducing devices or to incorporate bone pins/screws as links to distraction frames.[72] Producing more dermal thickening than three-dimensional expanders,[1] two-dimensional expanders operate in one plane by pulling wound boundaries together.[1] This type of expander stimulates biological tissue gain, maintains mechanical creep, prevents stretchback.[1,98] Three-dimensional expanders push/compress tissue away from fixed boundaries, stretching tissues in all directions.[1] Tissue gain is five times more than that for two-dimensional expanders.[1] Tissue deformation, via biologic creep, assumes the configuration of the expansion device.

In contrast, splints apply noninvasive mobilization forces that are unidirectional, or sometimes bidirectional, to in vivo soft tissues surrounding three-dimensional bone and joint structures that comprise a multiarticulated open kinematic chain. Mobilization splinting to remodel soft tissues limited by adhesion, stiffness, or contracture is efficacious because splint-generated biologic creep or tissue remodeling occurs in the plane(s) of normal joint function. It is important to remember that associated normal and abnormal anatomical structures also apply remodeling forces in addition to those applied by splints. Knowing how to effectively control and harness these

---

*References 4, 5, 63, 70, 73, 79, 106, 109, 115.
†References 4, 5, 78, 79, 106, 115.

multiple forces is a key factor to successful splinting outcomes (Fig. 3-26).

SUMMARY

Soft tissue remodeling is inherent to life. As we move from infancy to adulthood our soft tissue structures continuously adapt to keep pace with our lengthening skeletal frames. Through pregnancy, weight changes, skeletal pathology, disease, or injury our soft tissues continue to adapt, sometimes for the better and sometimes for the worse. It is only when life leaves that tissue remodeling ceases.

The remodeling process can be positively influenced to correct deformity caused by disease or injury through the judicious use of externally or internally applied devices that apply prolonged, sustained, controlled, gentle forces. Understanding the biomechanical and biochemical processes involved in tissue remodeling allows therapists and surgeons to better treat their patients. Extensive investigation into the causative factors underlying cellular growth is already well underway. We all need to be a part of this exciting and challenging frontier. Knowledge derived from other disciplines provides therapists with an important step up into the future. Splints apply forces externally and expanders apply forces internally. Each is used to affect tissue remodeling. Although an assumption of parallel influences and results is self evident, considerable splinting research is needed to conclusively connect the bridge between splinting and tissue expansion frames of knowledge.

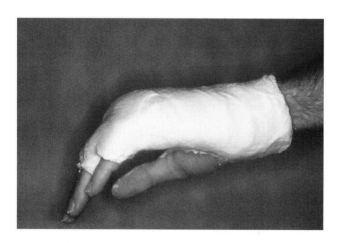

Fig. 3-26   Index–small finger DIP extension and flexion torque transmission splint, type 3 (13)
As described by Brand in the 1950s, joints beyond the physical boundaries of a splint may be remodeled over time by controlling secondary joints and allowing active motion at primary joints. This splint encourages DIP active motion by controlling the secondary wrist, MP, and PIP joints.

REFERENCES

1. Alex JC, Bhattacharyya TK, Smyrniotis G, et al: A histologic analysis of three-dimensional versus two-dimensional tissue expansion in the porcine model, *Laryngoscope* 111(1):36-43, 2001.
2. Arem A, Madden J: Is there a Wolff's law for connective tissue? *Surg Forum* 25:512-4, 1974.
3. Arem AJ, Madden JW: Effects of stress on healing wounds: I. Intermittent noncyclical tension, *J Surg Res* 20(2):93-102, 1976.
4. Argenta L, Marks M, Pasyk K: Advances in tissue expansion, *Clin Plast Surg* 12(2):159-71, 1985.
5. Austad E, Pasyk K, McClatchey K: Histomorphologic evaluation of guinea pig skin and soft tissue after controlled tissue expansion, *Plast Reconstr Surg* 70:704-10, 1982.
6. Austad E, Thomas S, Pasyk K: Tissue expansion: dividend or loan? *Plast Reconstr Surg* 78(1):63-8, 1986.
7. Baker S, Swanson N: Clinical applications of tissue expansion in head and neck surgery, *Laryngoscope* 100:313-9, 1990.
8. Baker S, Swanson N: Rapid intraoperative tissue expansion in reconstruction of the head and neck, *Arch Otolaryngol Head Neck Surg* 116:1431-4, 1990.
9. Bauman JH, Brand PW: Measurement of pressure between foot and shoe, *Lancet* p. 629-32, 1963.
10. Beauchene J, et al: Biochemical, biomechanical, and physical changes in the skin in an experimental animal model of therapeutic tissue expansion, *J Surg Res* 47:507, 1989.
11. Bell JA: Plaster cylinder casting for contractures of the interphalangeal joints. In Hunter J, et al: *Rehabilitation of the hand*, ed 1, Mosby, 1978, St. Louis.
12. Bell-Krotoski J, Breger DE, Beach RB: Biomechanics and evaluation of the hand. In Mackin E, et al: *Rehabilitation of the hand*, ed 5, Mosby, 2002, St. Louis.
13. Bell-Krotoski JA: Plaster cylinder casting for contractures of the interphalangeal joints. In Mackin E, et al: *Rehabilitation of the hand*, vol 2, ed 5, Mosby, 2002, St. Louis.
14. Bennett R, Hirt M: The history of tissue expansion: concepts, controversies and complications, *J Dermatol Surg Oncol* 19(12):1066-73, 1993.
15. Biewener AA, Fazzalari NL, Konieczynski DD, et al: Adaptive changes in trabecular architecture in relation to functional strain patterns and disuse, *Bone* 19(1):1-8, 1996.
16. Boyer MI, Gelberman RH, Burns ME, et al: Intrasynovial flexor tendon repair. An experimental study comparing low and high levels of in vivo force during rehabilitation in canines, *J Bone Joint Surg* [Am] 83-A(6):891-9, 2001.
17. Brand PW: *Clinical mechanics of the hand*, Mosby, 1985, St. Louis.
18. Brand PW: Deformity in leprosy. In Cochrane RG, Devey TF: *Leprosy in theory and practice*, Wright & Sons, LTD, 1964, Bristol, England.
19. Brand PW: Hand rehabilitation: management by objectives. In Hunter JM, Schneider LC, Mackin E: *Rehabilitation of the hand*, ed 2, Mosby, 1984, St. Louis.
20. Brand PW: Lessons from hot feet: a note on tissue remodeling. In Fess E, et al: Hand and upper extremity splinting principles and methods, ed 3, Mosby, 2004, St. Louis.
21. Brand PW: Mechanical factors in joint stiffness and tissue growth, *J Hand Ther* 8(2):91-6, 1995.
22. Brand PW: Personal communication from Paul Brand: soft tissue remodeling for club foot deformity, 2001, Seattle, WA.
23. Brand PW: The forces of dynamic splinting: ten questions before applying a dynamic splint to the hand. In Hunter JM, Schneider LC, Mackin E: *Rehabilitation of the hand*, ed 2, Mosby, 1984, St. Louis.

24. Brand PW, Beach RB, Thompson DE: Relative tension and excursion of muscles in the forearm and hand, *J Hand Surg [Am]* 6(3):209-29, 1981.

25. Brand PW, Bell J, Buford Jr WL: *Biomechanics of deformity and correction of the insensitive hand, annual seminar,* Gilles W. Long Hansens Disease Center, 1984, Carville, LA.

26. Brand PW, Hollister A: *Clinical mechanics of the hand,* ed 2, Mosby, 1993, St. Louis.

27. Brand PW, Hollister A: *Clinical mechanics of the hand,* ed 3, Mosby, 1999, St. Louis.

28. Brand PW, Hollister A: External stress: effect at the surface. In Brand PW, Hollister A: *Clinical mechanics of the hand,* ed 3, Mosby, 1999, St. Louis.

29. Brand PW, Hollister A: Hand stiffness and adhesions. In Brand PW, Hollister A: *Clinical mechanics of the hand,* ed 3, Mosby, 1999, St. Louis.

30. Brand PW, Hollister A: Mechanics of individual muscles at individual joints. In Brand PW, Hollister A: *Clinical mechanics of the hand,* ed 3, Mosby, 1999, St. Louis.

31. Brand PW, Hollister A: Methods of clinical measurement in the hand. In Brand PW, Hollister A: *Clinical mechanics of the hand,* ed 3, Mosby, 1999, St. Louis.

32. Brand PW, Hollister A: Muscles: the motors of the hand. In Brand PW, Hollister A: *Clinical mechanics of the hand,* ed 3, Mosby, 1999, St. Louis.

33. Brand PW, Hollister A: Operations to restore muscle balance to the hand. In Brand PW, Hollister A: *Clinical mechanics of the hand,* ed 3, Mosby, 1999, St. Louis.

34. Brand PW, Hollister A, Agee JM: Transmission. In Brand PW, Hollister A: *Clinical mechanics of the hand,* ed 3, Mosby, 1999, St. Louis.

35. Brand PW, Hollister A, Thompson D: Mechanical resistance. In Brand PW, Hollister A: *Clinical mechanics of the hand,* ed 3, Mosby, 1999, St. Louis.

36. Brandy D: The principles of scalp extension, *Am J Cosmetic Surg* 11:245-54, 1994.

37. Breger-Lee DE, Bell-Krotoski J, Brandsma JW: Torque range of motion in the hand clinic, *J Hand Ther* 3:7-13, 1990.

38. Brunette DM: Mechanical stretching increases the number of epithelial cells synthesizing DNA in culture, *J Cell Sci* 69:35, 1984.

39. Burnett W: Yank meets native, *Natl Geogr* 88:105, 1945.

40. Chen C, et al: Geometric control of cell life and death, *Sci* 276:1425, 1997.

41. Colditz JC: Preliminary report on a new technique for casting motion to mobilize stiffness in the hand. In Proceedings, American Society of Hand Therapists 22nd annual meeting, *J Hand Ther* 13(1):68-73, 2000.

42. Concannon MJ, Puckett CL: Wound coverage using modified tissue expansion, *Plast Reconstr Surg* 102(2):377-84, 1998.

43. De Filippo RE, Atala A: Stretch and growth: the molecular and physiologic influences of tissue expansion, *Plast Reconstr Surg* 109(7):2450-62, 2002.

44. Duran R, et al: Management of flexor tendon lacerations in Zone 2 using controlled passive motion postoperatively. In Hunter J, Schneider L, Mackin E: *Tendon surgery in the hand,* Mosby, 1987, St. Louis.

45. Ehlert TK, Thomas JR: Rapid intraoperative tissue expansion for closure of facial defects, *Arch Otolaryngol Head Neck Surg* 117(9):1043-9, 1991.

46. Elfman H: Biomechanics of muscle, *J Bone Joint Surg [Am]* 48A:363-77, 1966.

47. Endo T, Nakayama Y: Histologic examination of peripheral nerves elongated by tissue expanders, *Br J Plast Surg* 46(5):421-5, 1993.

48. Evans R, Thompson D: Immediate active short arc motion following tendon repair. In Hunter J, Schneider L, Mackin E: *Tendon and nerve surgery in the hand, a third decade,* ed 3, Mosby, 1997, St. Louis.

49. Fess EE: A history of splinting: to understand the present, view the past, *J Hand Ther* 15(2):97-132, 2002.

50. Fess EE, McCollum M: The influence of splinting on healing tissues, *J Hand Ther* 11(2):157-61, 1998.

51. Flowers K, LaStayo P: Effect of total end range time on improving passive range of motion, *J Hand Ther* 7(3):150-7, 1994.

52. Flowers K, Pheasant S: Use of torque angle curves in the assessment of digital joint stiffness, *J Hand Ther* 1(2):69-75, 1988.

53. Folkman J, Moscona A: Role of cell shape in growth control, *Nature* 273:345, 1978.

54. Foster JA, Scheiner AJ, Wulc AE, et al: Intraoperative tissue expansion in eyelid reconstruction, *Ophthalmology* 105(1):170-5, 1998.

55. Frantz RA, Xakellis GC: Characteristics of skin blood flow over the trochanter under constant, prolonged pressure, *Am J Phys Med Rehabil* 68(6):272-6, 1989.

56. Freehafer AA, Peckham PH, Keith MW: Determination of muscle-tendon unit properties during tendon transfer, *J Hand Surg [Am]* 4(4):331-9, 1979.

57. Fujisawa K, et al: Elongation of wallerian degenerating nerve with a tissue expander: a functional, morphometrical, and immunohistochemical study, *Microsurgery* 16(10):684-91, 1995.

58. Garcia-Elias M, An KN, Berglund L: Extensor mechanism of the fingers. I. A quantitative geometric study, *J Hand Surg [Am]* 16(6):1130-6, 1991.

59. Gelberman RH, Manske PR: Factors influencing flexor tendon adhesions, *Hand Clin* 1(1):35-42, 1985.

60. Gibson T, Kenedi R: Biomechanical properties of skin, *Surg Clin North Am* 47(2):279-94, 1967.

61. Greenbaum SS: Intraoperative tissue expansion with the Foley catheter, *J Dermatol Surg Oncol* 19(12):1079-83, 1993.

62. Gugenheim J: The Ilizarov method: orthopedic and soft tissue applications, *Clin Plast Surg* 25(4):567-78, 1998.

63. Gur E, Hanna W, Andrighetti L, et al: Light and electron microscopic evaluation of the pectoralis major muscle following tissue expansion for breast reconstruction, *Plast Reconstr Surg* 102(4):1046-51, 1998.

64. Homma K, Ohura T, Sugihara T, et al: Prefabricated flaps using tissue expanders: an experimental study, *Plast Reconstr Surg* 91(6):1098-107, 1993.

65. Ilizarov G: Clinical application of a tension-stress effect for limb lengthening, *Clin Orthop* 250:8-26, 1990.

66. Ilizarov G: The tension-stress effect on the genesis and growth of tissue. Part I. The influence of stability of fixation and soft-tissue preservation, *Clin Orthop* 238:249-81, 1989.

67. Ilizarov GA, Lediaev VI, Shitin VP: [The course of compact bone reparative regeneration in distraction osteosynthesis under different conditions of bone fragment fixation (experimental study)], *Eksp Khir Anesteziol* 14(6):3-12, 1969.

68. Ingber D: Tensegrity: the architectural basis of cellular mechanotransduction, *Annu Rev Physiol* 59:573, 1997.

69. Ippolito E, et al: Histology and ultrastructure of arteries, veins, and peripheral nerves during limb lengthening, *Clin Orthop* (308):54-62, 1994.

70. Johanson TM, Lowe L, Brown MD, et al: Histology and physiology of tissue expansion, *J Dermatol Surg Oncol* 19(12):1074-8, 1993.

71. Johnson P, Kernahan D, Bauer BS: Dermal and epidermal response to soft-tissue expansion, *Plast Reconstr Surg* 81(3):390-7, 1988.

72. Khouri RK, Schlenz I, Murphy BJ, et al: Nonsurgical breast enlargement using an external soft-tissue expansion system, *Plast Reconstr Surg* 105(7):2500-12; discussion 2513-4, 2000.

73. Kim K, Hong C, Futrell J: Histomorphologic changes in expanded skeletal muscle in rats, *Plast Reconstr Surg* 92(4): 710-6, 1993.

74. Kleinert HE, et al: Primary repair of flexor tendons in no-man's land, *J Bone Joint Surg* 49A:577, 1967.

75. Kleinert HE, Kutz J, Cohen M: Primary repair of zone 2 flexor tendon lacerations. In Hunter J, Schneider L: *American Academy of Orthopaedic Surgeons symposium on tendon surgery in the hand*, Mosby, 1975, St. Louis.

76. Knight K, McCann J, Vanderkolk C: The redistribution of collagen in expanded pig skin, *Br J Plast Surg* 43(5):565-70, 1990.

77. Lailas N, Cilento B, Atala A: Progressive ureteral dilation for subsequent ureterocystoplasty, *J Urol* 156(3):1151-3, 1996.

78. Lantieri LA, Martin-Garcia N, Wechsler J, et al: Vascular endothelial growth factor expression in expanded tissue: a possible mechanism of angiogenesis in tissue expansion, *Plast Reconstr Surg* 101(2):392-8, 1998.

79. Leighton WD, Russell RC, Feller AM, et al: Experimental pretransfer expansion of free-flap donor sites: II. Physiology, histology, and clinical correlation, *Plast Reconstr Surg* 82(1):76-87, 1988.

80. LeVay D: *The history of orthopaedics*, Parthenon, 1990, Park Ridge, NJ.

81. Lew D, Fuseler J: The effect of pulsed expansion of subfascially placed expanders on the extent and duration of mitosis in the capsule and rat integument, *J Oral Maxillofac Surg* 51(2):154-8, 1993.

82. Lew D, Fuseler J: The effect of stepwise expansion on the mitotic activity and vascularity of subdermal tissue and induced capsule in the rat, *J Oral Maxillofac Surg* 49(8):848-53, 1991.

83. Liang M, Briggs P, Heckler FR, et al: Presuturing—a new technique for closing large skin defects: clinical and experimental studies, *Plast Reconstr Surg* 81(5):694-702, 1988.

84. Machida B, Liu-Shindo M, Sasaki G: Immediate versus chronic tissue expansion, *Ann Plast Surg* 26(3):227-32, 1991.

85. MacLennan SE, Corcoran JF, Neale HW: Tissue expansion in head and neck burn reconstruction, *Clin Plast Surg* 27(1):121-32, 2000.

86. Madden J: Wound healing: biologic and clinical features. In Sabiston J: *Davis-Christopher textbook of surgery*, Saunders, 1981, Philadelphia.

87. Madden J: Wound healing: the biological basis of hand surgery, *Clin Plast Surg* 3(1):3-13, 1976.

88. Madden J, Peacock E: Studies on the biology of collagen during wound healing: dynamic metabolism of scar collagen and remodeling of dermal wounds, *Ann Surg* 174(3):511-20, 1971.

89. Manske PR, Gelberman RH, Lesker PA: Flexor tendon healing, *Hand Clin* 1(1):25-34, 1985.

90. Manske PR, Lesker PA, Gelberman RH, et al: Intrinsic restoration of the flexor tendon surface in the nonhuman primate, *J Hand Surg* [Am] 10(5):632-7, 1985.

91. Marks M, Burney RE, Mackenzie JR, et al: Enhanced capillary blood flow in rapidly expanded random pattern flaps, *J Trauma* 26(10):913-5, 1986.

92. Mason ML, Allen HS: The rate of healing of tendons: an experimental study of tensile strength, *Ann Surg* 113:424-59, 1941.

93. Meland N, Smith A, Johnson C: Tissue expansion in the upper extremities, *Hand Clinics* 13:303, 1997.

94. Micks JE, Reswick JB: Confirmation of differential loading of lateral and central fibers of the extensor tendon, *J Hand Surg* [Am] 6(5):462-7, 1981.

95. Mustoe T, Bartell T, Garner W: Physical, biomechanical, histologic and biochemical effects of rapid versus conventional tissue expansion, *Plast Reconstr Surg* 83:687-91, 1989.

96. Neumann CG: The progressive expansion of an area of skin by progressive distention of a subcutaneous balloon, *Plast Reconstr Surg* 9:121, 1957.

97. Newson T, Pearcy M: Skin surface PO_2 measurement and the effect of externally applied pressue, *Arch Phys Med Rehabil* 62(390), 1981.

98. Nordstrom R: "Stretch back" in scalp reductions for male pattern baldness, *Plast Reconstr Surg* 73:422-6, 1984.

99. Nordstrom R, Divine J: Scalp stretching with a tissue expander for closure of scalp defects, *Plast Reconstr Surg* 75:578-81, 1985.

100. Ohkaya S, Hibasam H, Hirata H, et al: Nerve expansion in nerve regeneration: effect of time on induction of ornithine decarboxylase and Schwann cell proliferation, *Muscle Nerve* 20(10):1314-7, 1997.

101. Ohkaya S, Hirata H, Uchida A: Repair of nerve gap with the elongation of Wallerian degenerated nerve by tissue expansion, *Microsurgery* 20(3):126-30, 2000.

102. Olenius M, Dalsgaard C, Wickman M: Mitotic activity in expanded human skin, *Plast Reconstr Surg* 91:213, 1993.

103. Osol G: Mechanotransduction by vascular smooth muscle, *J Vasc Res* 32:275, 1995.

104. Pasyk K, Argenta L, Hassett C: Quantitative analysis of the thickness of human skin and subcutaneous tissue following controlled expansion with a silicone implant, *Plast Reconstr Surg* 81:516, 1988.

105. Pasyk K, Austad E, Cherry G: Intracellular collagen fiber in capsule around silicone expanders in guinea pigs, *J Surg Res* 36:125, 1984.

106. Pasyk K, Austad E, McClatchey K: Electron microscopic evaluation of guinea pig skin and soft tissues expanded with a self-inflating silicone implant, *Plast Reconstr Surg* 70:37-45, 1982.

107. Radovan C: *Adjacent flap development using expandable silatic implant*, Presented at the Annual Meeting of the American Society of Plastic and Reconstructive Surgeons, 1976, Boston.

108. Radovan C: Breast reconstruction after mastectomy using a temporary expander, *Plast Reconstr Surg* 69:195-206, 1982.

109. Rowsell A, Godfrey A, Richards M: The thinned latissimus dorsi free flap: a case report, *Br J Plast Surg* 39:210, 1986.

110. Ruoslahti E: Stretching is good for a cell, *Science* 276:1345, 1997.

111. Russell R, Khouri RK, Upton J, et al: The expanded scapular flap, *Plast Reconstr Surg* 96(4):884-95, 1995.

112. Sachs F: Biophysics of mechanoreception, *Membr Biochem* 6:173, 1986.

113. Sarrafian S, et al: Strain variations in the components of the extensor apparatus of the finger during flexion and extension, *J Bone Joint Surg* [Am] 52A(5):980-90, 1970.

114. Sasaki G: Intraoperative sustained limited expansion as immediate reconstructive technique, *Clin Plast Surg* 14:63-573, 1975.

115. Sasaki G: *Tissue expansion in reconstructive and aesthetic surgery*, Mosby, 1998, St. Louis.

116. Satar N, Yoo JJ, Atala A: Progressive dilation for bladder tissue expansion, *J Urol* 162(3 Pt 1):829-31, 1999.

117. Sato M, Ochi T, Nakase T, et al: Mechanical tension-stress induces expression of bone morphogenetic protein (BMP)-2 and BMP-4, but not BMP-6, BMP-7, and GDF-5 MRNA, during distraction osteogenesis, *J Bone Miner Res* 14(7):1084-95, 1999.

118. Silfverskiold KL, May EJ: Flexor tendon repair in zone II with a new suture technique and an early mobilization program combining passive and active flexion, *J Hand Surg* [Am] 19(1):53-60, 1994.

119. Skoulis TG, Lovice D, von Fricken K, et al: Nerve expansion. The optimal answer for the short nerve gap. Behavioral analysis, *Clin Orthop* 314:84-94, 1995.

120. Slavin SA: Nonsurgical breast enlargement using an external soft-tissue expansion system, *Plast Reconstr Surg* 105(7):2513-4, 2000.

121. Squier C: The stretching of mouse skin in vivo: effect on epidermal proliferation and thickness, *J Invest Dermatol* 74:68, 1980.

122. Strickland JW, Gettle K: Flexor tendon repair: the Indianapolis method. In Hunter J, Schneider L, Mackin E: *Tendon and nerve surgery in the hand—a third decade*, Mosby, 1997, St. Louis.

123. Takei T, Rivas-Gotz C, Delling CA, et al: The effect of strain on human keratinocytes in vitro, *J Cell Physiol* 173(1):64-72, 1997.

124. Tsuchiya H, Tomita K, Shinokawa Y, et al: The Ilizarov method in the management of giant cell tumors of the proximal tibia, *J Bone Joint Surg Br* 78(2):264-9, 1996.

125. Twigg SM, Chen MM, Joly AH, et al: Advanced glycosylation end products up-regulate connective tissue growth factor (insulin-like growth factor-binding protein-related protein 2) in human fibroblasts: a potential mechanism for expansion of extracellular matrix in diabetes mellitus, *Endocrinology* 142(5):1760-9, 2001.

126. Weeks G: Into the heart of Africa, *Natl Geogr* 110:257, 1956.

127. Weeks PM, Wray RC: *The management of acute hand injuries: a biological approach*, Mosby, 1973, St. Louis.

128. Wieslander J, Wieslander M: Prefabricated (expander) capsule-lined transposition and advancement flaps in reconstruction of lower eyelid and oral defects: an experimental study, *Plast Reconstr Surg* 105:1399, 2000.

129. Wilson E, Mai Q, Sudhir K, et al: Mechanical strain induces growth of vascular smooth muscle cells via autocrine action of PDGF, *J Cell Biol* 123(3):741-7, 1993.

130. Wilson J: Serial excision, *Br J Plast Surg* 1:117-8, 1948.

131. Withington E: *Hippocrates*, vol III, Harvard University Press, 1999, Cambridge, MA.

132. Wollina U, Berger U, Stolle C, et al: Tissue expansion in pig skin: a histochemical approach, *Anat Hist Embryol* 21(2):101-11, 1992.

133. Wood RJ, Adson MH, VanBeek AL, et al: Controlled expansion of peripheral nerves: comparison of nerve grafting and nerve expansion/repair for canine sciatic nerve defects, *J Trauma* 31(5):686-90, 1991.

134. Wood FM, McMahon SB: The response of the peripheral nerve field to controlled soft tissue expansion, *Br J Plast Surg* 42(6):682-6, 1989.

135. Xakellis GC, Frantz RA, Arteaga M, et al: A comparison of changes in the transcutaneous oxygen tension and capillary blood flow in the skin with increasing compressive weights, *Am J Phys Med Rehabil* 70(4):172-7, 1991.

136. Yashi N, Kojimoto H, Shimomura Y: The effect of distraction upon bone, muscle, and periosteum, *Orthop Clin North Am* 22:563, 1991.

137. Zambacos GJ, Shroff N, Newman PL, et al: Massive prepatellar bursa: a case of natural tissue expansion: anatomic and histologic implications, *Plast Reconstr Surg* 108(1):267-8, 2001.

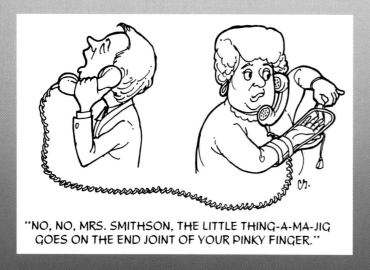

"NO, NO, MRS. SMITHSON, THE LITTLE THING-A-MA-JIG
GOES ON THE END JOINT OF YOUR PINKY FINGER."

CHAPTER 4

Classification and Nomenclature of Splints and Splint Components

Chapter Outline

Good communication, an essential to efficacious patient intervention, is dependent upon a precise and accurate professional vocabulary. A clear and specialized language improves clinical knowledge and understanding. In contrast, poorly defined professional terminology stymies clinical judgment and insight, limiting patient rehabilitative potential. The purpose of this chapter is to provide the reader with a solid foundation for professional communication in the splinting domain by (1) reviewing seven historical methods for classifying splints, (2) describing and applying the American Society of Hand Therapists' Splint Classification System, as expanded and refined by the authors of this book, and (3) providing a common vocabulary of splint component terminology.

■ HISTORICAL SPLINT CLASSIFICATIONS

The product of convoluted development over several centuries, previous description and classification of splints were fraught with confusion, redundancy, and omission. By its very nature, the field of upper extremity splinting embraces a profusion of devices and terminology. This, coupled with the fact that similar splints are often used for dissimilar purposes, led to the inevitable evolution of a mismatched and awkward colloquial splinting jargon that was both pervasive and widespread. Demonstrating the profundity of the problem, historically, splints have been categorized via a multitude of differing systems, the most common of which include grouping according to purpose, configuration, mechanical properties, power source, material, anatomic site, and descriptive phrase. Each method possessed distinct advantages and disadvantages. While some classification systems were more precise than others, none effectively provided clear definition and separation of individual splints and splint components. The need for common descriptive splint terminology has been apparent to clinicians, students, and patients for years.

Familiarity with historical splint classifications provides a foundation for understanding the origins of current splinting methods and basic splinting nomenclature. The following is a brief review of seven of the more well-known splint classifications from the past.

Purpose of Application

Splints may be designed to prevent deformity by substituting for weak or absent muscle strength, as in peripheral nerve injuries, spinal cord lesions, and neuromuscular diseases. They may be used to support, protect, or immobilize joints, allowing healing to occur after bone, tendon, vascular, nerve, joint, or soft tissue injury or inflammation. Correction of existing deformity represents another commonly encountered reason for splint application. To achieve full active joint motion potential, remodeling of joint capsular structures, tendon adhesions, or soft tissues often requires prolonged slow, gentle, passive traction that is best provided by splinting. Splints also may provide directional control for coordination problems and serve as a base for attachment of specialized devices that may facilitate and enhance hand function.

External Configuration

External configuration has often served as a basis of categorization of upper extremity splints and includes

the subcategories of bar splints, spring splints, contoured splints, and combinations thereof.

Bar Splints

Bar splints, because of their narrow component design, must be fabricated in strong inelastic materials such as stainless steel, aluminum, and the thicker high-temperature plastics (Fig. 4-1). With the introduction of low-temperature thermoplastics, bar splint designs have all but disappeared in the treatment of upper extremity problems, with the exception of some chronic injuries or disease processes that require more permanent splinting solutions.

Spring Splints

Spring splints, as exemplified by many of the DeRoyal/LMB, Bunnell, Capener, and Wynn Parry, and other commercial and custom splints, rely on three-point pressure and spring-action forces to provide constant force application to mobilize joints (Fig. 4-2).

Contoured Splints

Because of their ease of fabrication with low-temperature materials that allow direct fitting on patients, contoured splints have revolutionized upper extremity splinting techniques, moving splint

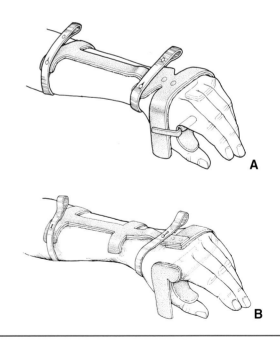

Fig. 4-1   A, Wrist extension, thumb CMC palmar abduction immobilization splint, type 0 (2) B, Wrist extension, thumb CMC palmar abduction immobilization splint, type 0 (2)
These examples of bar splints, (**A**) Rancho Los Amigos and (**B**) Bennett (Warm Springs), both function to immobilize the wrist and maintain thumb CMC palmar abduction while allowing thumb MP and IP motion.

fabrication out of the realm of orthotists and into therapy clinics and physician's offices (Fig. 4-3). Since low-temperature materials lack required rigidity, splint designs of necessity have become wider. Fortuitously, this generates greater patient comfort because of decreased splint pressure from an increased area of force application (see Chapter 6).

Combinations

Combinations of bar, spring, and contoured splints comprise the fourth subcategory. Engen, Bailor, and

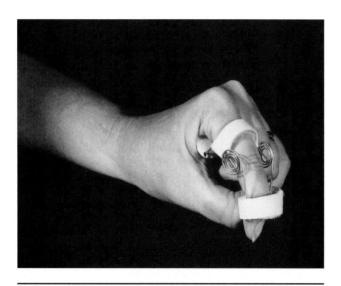

Fig. 4-2   Index finger PIP extension mobilization splint, type 1 (2)
This Capener splint generates forces through bilateral springs and a three-point pressure system to provide extension mobilization forces to the PIP.

DeRoyal/LMB splints (Fig. 4-4) are examples of how the strength of metal may be coalesced with the close-fitting capabilities of plastics.

Mechanical Characteristics

Upper extremity splints have also been grouped according to mechanical characteristics of their components, resulting in two major subdivisions: static splints and dynamic splints. Static splints have no moving components and provide support and immobilization, while dynamic splints employ traction devices such as rubber bands, springs, cords, or Velcro strips to alter the range of passive motion of a joint or joints. Confusion arises with this classification method, when "static" splints are used to improve motion of stiff joints by serially altering a splint or by fitting new splints every 2 to 3 days to maintain slight tension on the joint(s) being mobilized as range of motion increases. The phrase "static progressive splint" was introduced in an attempt to clarify this discrepancy but this created further confusion. While there is no mechanical difference in the application of force to soft tissue between a technique such as serial casting and a "static progressive splint," the fact that there is no difference is not readily perceived by those who are novices to splint design and fabrication.

Source of Power

The source of power is another categorical method that divides control splints into those that use internal power and those that provide external power. These splints are often associated with long-term

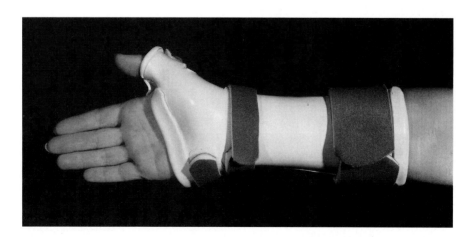

Fig. 4-3   Wrist extension, thumb CMC radial abduction and MP flexion immobilization splint, type 0 (3)
Contoured splints are often more comfortable to wear because of increased surface contact of the splint with the extremity. An indication for this splint design includes deQuervain's stenosing tenosynovitis, in which all joints included within the splint are considered primary for resting the extensor pollicis brevis and abductor pollicis longus tendons.

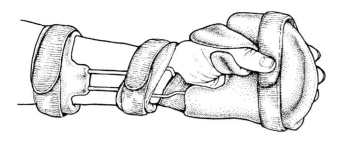

Fig. 4-4   Index–small finger 20° flexion, thumb CMC palmar abduction and MP extension immobilization splint, type 1 (15) This Wire-Foam splint combines metal and plastic to produce a durable, close-fitting, adjustable splint.

disability, providing more permanent splinting solutions than their relatively temporary splint counterparts that are used with more acute problems. Durable materials, mechanical joints, and specialized tension adjustment systems are the hallmarks of these splints, which are often employed to provide gross hand function in cases of severe upper extremity paralysis. Internally powered splints rely on a patient's residual muscle power to produce motion of nonfunctional joints following various paralytic conditions (Fig. 4-5). Externally powered splints are driven by an external source such as a battery or artificial muscle. Generally, both the internal and external power splints facilitate gross grasp through wrist extension, or tenodesis effect.

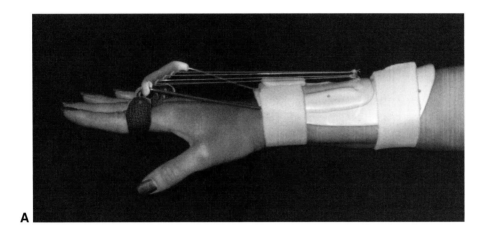

A

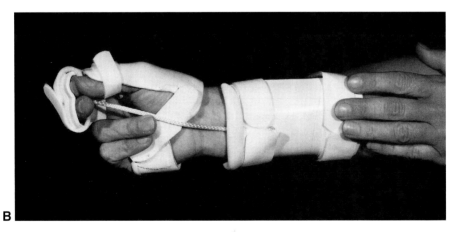

B

Fig. 4-5   A, Wrist flexion: index–small finger MP extension / index–small finger MP flexion: wrist extension torque transmission splint, type 0 (5). B, Wrist extension: index–long finger flexion / wrist flexion: index–long finger extension torque transmission / thumb CMC palmar abduction and MP-IP extension immobilization splint, type 2 (10)
A, Originally designed by Irene Hollis, OTR, this splint may be used as a substitute for lack of active wrist and MP joint extension as seen in radial nerve palsy. Motion is created through transmission of torque generated through active wrist flexion to create passive MP extension and inversely, to create passive wrist extension through active MP flexion. B, Digital grasp and release patterns are controlled by active wrist extension and gravity-assisted flexion in this tenodesis splint. [Courtesy (A) Peggy McLaughlin, OTR, CHT, San Bernadino, Calif.]

Materials

A fifth means of classification is based on the materials from which splints are fabricated. Categories include metal, plaster, plastic, and soft splinting materials; subcategories within this classification system change as technology advances and new products are introduced. This is especially true of plastics, where newer or improved substances frequently make established materials obsolete.

Anatomic Part

Yet another classification method relates to the anatomic part splinted, as in wrist splints, finger splints, thumb splints, shoulder splints, etc. These subcategories are grouped according to the anatomic focus of a given splint but do not describe the presence of secondary joints that may also be affected by the splint.

Descriptive Phrase

Introduced in the first edition of this book in 1981, the descriptive phrase approach to categorizing splints was the first method to recognize the important role of secondary joints, which are included in splints for mechanical control purposes, but are not the primary target joints of splints.[3] An important prelude to the development of the ASHT Splint Classification System (SCS), this method lacked the power, extensiveness, and refinement of the SCS.

■ ASHT SPLINT CLASSIFICATION SYSTEM (SCS)

Responding to an earlier extensive survey of its members that identified wide practice discrepancies in splint terminology and usage, the 1989 Executive Board of the ASHT established a Splint Nomenclature Task Force to create a splint nomenclature system that would "conclusively settle the issues regarding splinting nomenclature."* This Task Force consisted of members of the original splint nomenclature committee who conducted the earlier survey and recognized splinting authorities in the field of hand

rehabilitation.* Following important plenary meetings in preceding years, the Task Force met in January 1991 in Indianapolis, Ind. With all Task Force members but one attending the meeting, debate was intense and thorough. Each member contributed major concepts to the development of the Classification System and, because of the critical interlacing of knowledge, had even one of those at the Indianapolis meeting been absent, the mission would have failed. The end product of this pivotal meeting was the 1992 publication of the ASHT Splint Classification System, in book format.[†] Special credit must be given to Jean Casanova for her vision of what could be done, to Janet Bailey for her organizational skills, and to Nancy Cannon for her insightful pre-meeting task assignments to Task Force members.

The ASHT Splint Classification System is based on splint function rather than splint form, and the terms "splint" and "orthosis" may be used interchangeably, allowing more universal application. All splints have inherent mechanical characteristics that combine to a series of predictable patterns.[2-4] The integration of these mechanical patterns with accepted anatomic and kinesiologic terminology produces a logical and precise approach to describing splints.

The SCS describes splints through a series of six predefined divisions that guide and progressively refine splints' technical names, working from broad concepts to individual splint specifications (Fig. 4-6). Just as grammatical sentences in languages are comprised of various required elements, Splint Classification sentences are also constructed of required elements. Linking of the six required categories or elements forms a scientific name "sentence" for a given splint based on its functional purpose. The six required SCS elements include identification of articular/nonarticular; location; direction; purpose (immobilization, mobilization, restriction, torque transmission); type; and total number of joints.

Articular/Nonarticular

The first division separates splints into two groups: (1) those that affect articular structures and (2) those that affect an anatomic segment or structure but do not affect joint motion or cross a joint. Comprising the vast majority of splints, articular splints use three-point pressure systems to affect a joint or joints by immobilizing, mobilizing, restricting, or transmitting torque. Since most splints are articular in nature, the term "articular" is assumed and is not included as part of the technical name. In contrast, nonarticular

*ASHT Splint Nomenclature Task Force Members: Jean Casanova, OTR/L, CHT (Director, ASHT Clinical Assessment Committee); Janet Bailey, OTR, CHT (Task Force Leader); Nancy Cannon, OTR, CHT; Judy Colditz, OTR, CHT; Elaine Fess, MS, OTR, FAOTA, CHT; Karan Gettle, MBA, OTR, CHT; Lori (Klerekoper) DeMott, OTR, CHT; Maude Malick, OTR; Cynthia Philips, MA, OTR, CHT; and Ellen Ziegler, MS, OTR/L, CHT.

†ASHT, 401 North Michigan Avenue, Chicago, IL 60611.

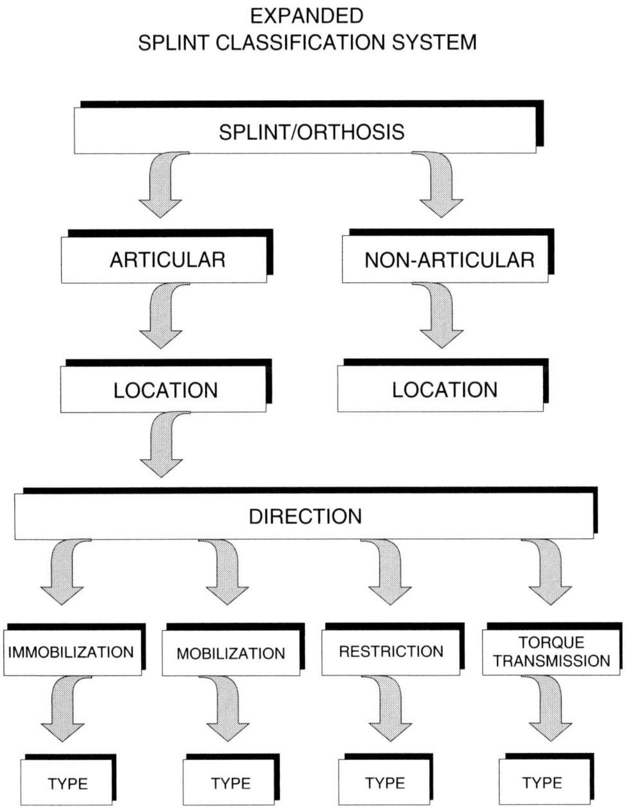

EXPANDED
SPLINT CLASSIFICATION SYSTEM

SPLINT/ORTHOSIS

ARTICULAR   NON-ARTICULAR

LOCATION   LOCATION

DIRECTION

IMMOBILIZATION   MOBILIZATION   RESTRICTION   TORQUE TRANSMISSION

TYPE   TYPE   TYPE   TYPE

Fig. 4-6   Expanded Splint Classification System (ESCS) divisions.

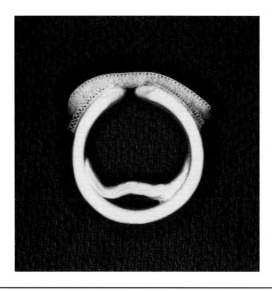

Fig. 4-7   Nonarticular finger proximal phalanx splint
This "pulley ring" splint is an example of a nonarticular splint designed to provide external support to a healing structure without inclusion of a joint. (Courtesy Diane Collins, MEd, PT, CHT, New Canaan, Conn.)

splints employ coaptational, two-point pressure forces to stabilize or immobilize isolated body segments. These splints do not include joints and to differentiate them from articular splints, the term "nonarticular" is always included in the technical name. Splints that are classified in the nonarticular group include "pulley rings" for protection of healing digital pulleys (Fig. 4-7), "tennis elbow" cuffs, and some fracture braces.

Location

Both articular and nonarticular splints are divided further into location of the primary anatomic part(s) included in the splint. For articular splints, location involves identification of the joints that are the key focus of the splint, e.g., *shoulder, index–small finger MP, thumb CMC,* etc. For nonarticular splints, location identifies long bones (humerus, radius, ulna, metacarpal, phalanx) or soft tissue anatomic structures such as digital pulleys. With the first two required elements in place, splints begin to take shape based solely on their partially finished technical

names. For example, a humeral fracture splint would be classified as a *nonarticular humerus splint* and an articular splint affecting the elbow is classified as an *elbow splint.*

Nonarticular splints are coaptational in design with their two-point counter forces directed inward. Since these splints all work in the same manner mechanically, there is no need to define their direction, the next required element. The only exception to the six required elements in an SCS name, nonarticular splints use only the first two categories. Nonarticular splint definition stops here, with location.

Direction

Applicable only to articular splints, direction is the next division after location. Direction uses existing kinematic terminology to define the primary kinematic function of splints, e.g., extension, flexion, abduction, opposition, internal rotation, distraction, compression, coaptation, etc. With this third element in place, splint definition is more refined. For example, a splint designed to extend the finger MP joints is called an *index–small finger MP extension splint.* If this splint includes extension and radial deviation as its prime kinematic function, as with splints used with postoperative MP arthroplasty patients, it is defined as an *index–small finger MP extension and radial deviation splint.*

Purpose: Immobilization/Mobilization/ Restriction/Torque Transmission‡

The fourth element in building an SCS splint name divides articular splints into one of four groups according to the primary objective of the splint: immobilization, mobilization, restriction, or torque transmission. Does the splint immobilize, mobilize, restrict motion of, or transmit torque to the primary focus joint(s)? By describing intended anatomic joint motion rather than splint component motion, the SCS eliminates past confusion encountered when "static" splints—splints with no moving parts—were used to mobilize joints. It also gets rid of the uncertainty of how to classify splints that possess both moving and nonmoving parts. The SCS makes the ambiguous terms "static," "dynamic," and "static-progressive" out-of-date and irrelevant. This fourth part of the sentence tells how a splint works. For example, a splint applied to the long finger distal interphalangeal (DIP) joint to allow healing of a ruptured terminal extensor tendon is a *long finger DIP hyperextension immobilization splint*. Splints can have more than one purpose. A splint that allows the extrinsic long extensors to extend the ulnar two finger IP joints by limiting MP extension after an ulnar nerve injury is a *ring–small finger MP extension restriction / IP extension torque transmission splint*.

Torque transmission purpose includes those splints that intentionally (1) create motion of primary joints situated beyond the boundaries of the splint itself or (2) harness secondary "driver" joint(s) to create motion of primary joints that may be situated longitudinally or transversely to the "driver" joint(s). While all splints transmit torque to adjacent joints not included in the splints, torque transmission splints are applied with the specific intent of transferring moment/transmitting torque to designated, predetermined primary joints. Often considered "exercise splints," torque transmission splints may seem exceedingly simple in design but, in truth, many of these splints are founded on sophisticated biomechanical and kinesiological concepts. For example, a splint that secondarily limits IP motion in order to facilitate motion of a primary MP joint is called a *finger MP extension and flexion torque transmission splint* (Fig. 4-8, *A*). Another example, the ubiquitous "buddy tape splint," is a torque transmission splint in that one or more secondary joints are harnessed as "driver" joints to create motion at one or more designated primary joints (Fig. 4-8, *B*). The first

example splint works longitudinally and the second splint example works transversely.

Type

Unlike the first four elements, which are intuitively obvious, the fifth element, type, requires some thought to understand its critical role in the classification hierarchy. The four previous categories define how splints affect primary target joints. In contrast, type identifies the secondary joint level included in

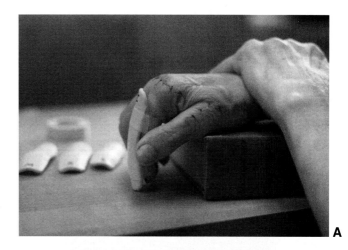

A

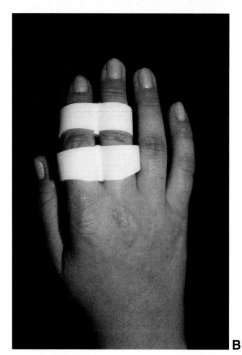

B

Fig. 4-8   A, Index finger MP extension and flexion torque transmission splint, type 2 (3) B, Long finger MP-PIP extension and flexion torque transmission splint, type 2 (4)
Torque transmission splints may create motion of primary joints situated **(A)** longitudinally or **(B)** transversely to secondary joints.

---

‡Identified by the authors of this book, *torque transmission* is a new, fourth purpose category that is added to the three purpose categories originally defined in the SCS.

splints. Secondary joints are those joints incorporated in splints to provide biomechanical control of joints proximal, distal, and/or adjacent to the primary joints (Fig. 4-9). Control of secondary joints mechanically optimizes and focuses splint forces on the primary joints. When secondary joints are not controlled, splint forces are often misdirected allowing unwanted force dissipation at nonprimary joints. Type is often diagnosis specific, separating similar looking splints into different categories to comply with dissimilar diagnostic requirements.

There are a total of ten joint levels in the upper extremity. These include the shoulder, elbow, forearm, wrist, finger MP, finger PIP, finger DIP, thumb CMC, thumb MP, and thumb IP levels. The type element requires counting the secondary joint levels (Fig. 4-10). It is critical to understand that only the joint levels are counted, not the individual joints. For example, if the MPs and wrist are included as secondary joints in a splint designed to improve index–small PIP extension, type is defined as "2" (index–small MPs = 1 level; plus wrist = 1 level; for a total of 2 levels), *not* 5 (5 = sum of all secondary individual joints). The technical name for this splint is *index–small finger PIP extension mobilization splint, type 2*. If no secondary joint levels are included in a splint, the type is "0," as with a *wrist extension immobilization, type 0*; if one secondary joint level is included, it is a *type 1*, and so on.

Do not count individual secondary joints separately when defining type. Count only the joint levels. If secondary joints are erroneously totaled individually rather than as joint levels, the entire classification system falls apart, allowing absurd situations where mechanically identical splints are classified into different categories based on the number of

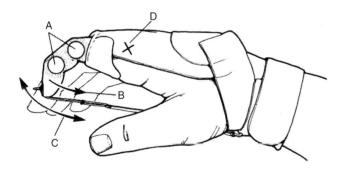

Fig. 4-9   Index finger IP flexion mobilization splint, type 1 (3) Illustrating the ESCS, this drawing identifies the main components used to "name" a splint: **(A)** anatomic focus (IP joints), **(B)** kinematic direction (flexion), **(C)** primary purpose (mobilization), **(D)** number of secondary joint levels (type 1), and the final element of the ESCS delineates the total number of joints incorporated within this splint (3). (From Fess EE, Kiel JH: Upper extremity splinting. In Neistadt M, Crepeau E, *Willard & Spackman's Occupational Therapy*, ed 9, Lippincott, 1998, Philadelphia.)

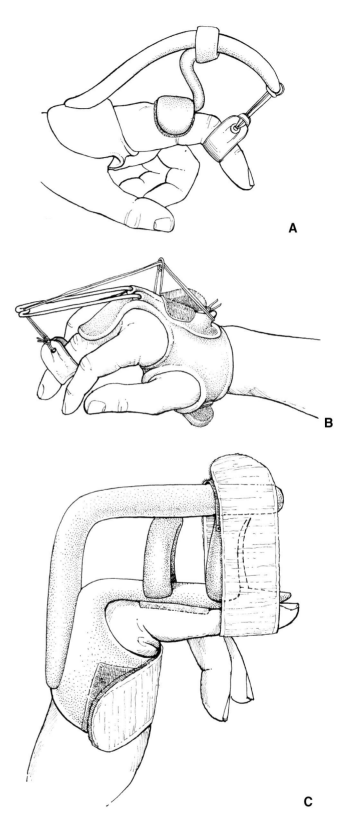

Fig. 4-10   **A,** Index finger PIP extension mobilization splint, type 1 (2) **B,** Long finger PIP extension mobilization splint, type 1 (2) **C,** Small finger PIP extension mobilization splint, type 2 (3) Although their designs and types of traction differ, these PIP extension mobilization splints have the same function. Note that two secondary joints are incorporated in **(C)** to increase the splint's mechanical advantage.

fingers included in the splints, e.g., an index finger MP extension splint is incorrectly put in a different classification category from an index–long finger MP extension splint!

Type is a fundamental and essential element for accurately defining splints and its inherent intricacy produces an unexpected consequence. Type, in effect, separates those individuals with "just-passing knowledge" from true upper extremity rehabilitation professionals. Understanding of type is the difference between seat-of-the-pants intervention and true science. Accurate identification of type requires a thorough understanding of upper extremity anatomy, biomechanics, and pathology, which is beyond the grasp of those functioning with minimal proficiency. For example, knowing the differences between an *IP flexion splint, type 0,* an *IP flexion splint, type 1,* and an *IP flexion splint, type 2* and when to apply each is key to providing the most efficacious treatment possible and to fully optimizing patient potential. No matter how beautiful their splints may be, those who lack the required knowledge base to identify the type category accurately and to use it to its optimum are limited in their abilities to produce splints that truly work for their patients.

Total Number of Joints

The sixth and final required element of the ESCS delineates the total number of individual joints incorporated in splints. This element, like the first four, is intuitively obvious. Following the type designation, the sum of all the individual joints, primary and secondary, included in the splint is placed in parentheses at the end of the name sentence. For example, a shoulder abduction splint that incorporates the elbow, forearm, and wrist as secondary joints is a *shoulder abduction splint, type 3 (4),* while the PIP extension splint mentioned in a previous example is an *index–small finger PIP extension mobilization splint, type 2 (9).* There are a total of four joints in the shoulder splint and nine individual joints in the PIP splint.

Design Options

Not a requirement of the ESCS method of describing splints, design options such as specific materials, component specification (dorsal, volar, low-profile, high-profile), etc., may be added at the end of the ESCS splint name, but only in situations where it is important to communicate specific fabrication or design information.

The expanded and refined Splint Classification System (ESCS) allows upper extremity specialists to communicate information about splints and their application via a logical and consistent scientific language (Table 4-1) for the first time. Positive ramifications of using the ESCS include the following:

1. The ESCS allows accurate definition of splints because it is both specific and extensive in nature. Clinicians have considerable range in defining their splints according to ESCS criteria. Knowing why splints are applied and understanding their inherent mechanical patterns are strategic to using the ESCS.

2. Splint referrals and prescriptions using the ESCS appropriately allow clinicians the freedom to choose the design options they feel best meet the needs of their patients. With the ESCS, it is no longer suitable for physicians and other referral sources to say, "I want a splint that looks like the one on page 251 for this patient." Instead, ESCS-based referrals specify, "I want a splint that protects this patient's intrinsic transfer by keeping the MPs and wrist in 30° of flexion." The look of the splint is left to the informed judgment of the clinical specialist treating the case.

3. Reimbursement for splints is facilitated because the ESCS groups splints consistently and accurately. Less involved splints are easily differentiated from more complicated splints.

4. The ability to accurately define splints based on their function rather than on their looks provides a critical foundation for advancement of our upper extremity rehabilitation knowledge base. Similar and dissimilar functional splint designs may be compared and contrasted to identify the most efficacious choices for given situations. Opinion regarding what kind of splint is best must now be backed with scientific data.

5. In providing a specialized technical language, the ESCS also is a key factor in ascending the specialty of upper extremity rehabilitation to the status of a legitimate profession. To be a true profession in the technical sense, a field of knowledge must have its own language that is specific to the field. The ESCS is unique to upper extremity rehabilitation and no other classification system currently available competes with its completeness, accuracy, and power.

It is important to understand that similar or identical looking splints may be classified in different categories according to their intended purposes and way in which they function mechanically (Table 4-2). This is one of the ESCS's strongest features in that clinicians are able to describe exactly why each splint is applied without the confusion encountered from past methods of classification.

Throughout this third edition, all illustrated splints are classified and indexed according to the expanded Splint Classification System. This index is located at the end of this book. Accompanying figure and page numbers are provided for all splints, facilitating location of the splints.

SPLINT COMPONENT TERMINOLOGY

A splint is no more than a series of specialized parts that perform specific functions. Some parts directly affect extremity position, while others maintain alignment and spatial interrelationships between various splint components. When assessing an extremity for splint application, rather than considering the intended splint as a whole, it is important to think of the splint as interconnected parts with each part meeting a specific need for a given clinical problem. There is no standard splint that may be prescribed for a given pathologic situation. There is no decree that similarly functioning splint parts must look alike or may be used only with certain diagnoses. Each patient presents different problems, even though the specific injury or disease may be similar to those of others. Patients must be approached without preconceived ideas, to allow for the creation of splints, part by part, that meet not only physical but also emotional and socioeconomic requirements. An inability to accommodate to these individual factors is the main cause for failure of many commercial splints. Remember that patients and their hands do not come in small, medium, and large, nor are their lifestyles identical!

To effectively accomplish component splint designing, a sound knowledge of the basic splint parts and their purposes is essential. As was noted earlier in this chapter, each splint part has a task for which it has been designed. It may vary in shape from splint to splint, but its purpose will remain constant. Some parts immobilize, some support, others stabilize, and still others provide attachment sites. Following is an alphabetical listing of common splint parts, their purposes, and pertinent information concerning each component. This list is meant to provide a basic foundation of common language for further communication. It should not be viewed as definitive, but rather should be added to, elaborated upon, and deleted from as the splint maker accumulates experience and expertise.

C Bar

This component (Fig. 4-11) is fitted in the first web space for the purpose of maintaining or increasing the distance between the first and second metacarpal bones. Its presence affects motion at the car-

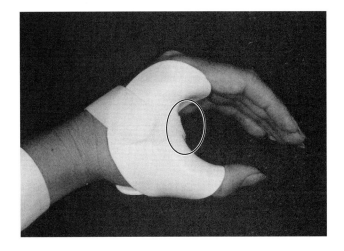

Fig. 4-11   Thumb CMC palmar abduction immobilization splint, type 2 (3)
The C bar component of a splint functions to preserve and/or increase soft tissue length of the first web space.

pometacarpal (CMC) joint of the thumb. A C bar is often elongated to incorporate a thumb post or an index finger palmar phalangeal bar. The width of a C bar should not impede movement of the mobile fourth and fifth metacarpals. Because extension of this component with a palmar phalangeal bar blocks MP flexion, care should be taken to maintain full MP flexion of the index finger through exercise.

Connector Bar

This component (Fig. 4-12) maintains alignment and position of other splint parts. Depending on specific location and purpose in regard to the overall splint design, connector bars may or may not be constructed of materials homologous to the main body of the splint.

Crossbar

This transverse medial or lateral extension (Fig. 4-13), in combination with similar bars, provides splint stability on the extremity. Crossbars may work in pairs, singly in three-point configurations with the most distal point serving as deviation bars, or in the case of highly contoured splints, with the proximal and distal bars molded together to form continuous lateral borders of segmental troughs, e.g., as in a forearm trough.

Cuff or Strap

Designed to hold the splint in place on the extremity, this splint part (Fig. 4-14) is usually constructed of a softer, more pliable material. Cuffs tend to be wider

TABLE 4-1 Expanded Splint Classification System (ESCS)

Combinations of Primary and Secondary Joints

When a primary joint is linked with its potential secondary joint partners, a predictable linear pattern emerges (see specific examples at bottom of table). For this exercise, only joints proximal to the primary joints are considered. Joints distal to primary joints may also function as secondary joints. However, for ease of demonstration, these less common scenarios are not included in this chart. *Forearm and thumb joints are not included.*

| Primary Joints | | Secondary Joints | | | | | | Type | Total Joints |
		DIP	PIP	MP	Wrist	Elbow	Shoulder		
DIP	1								(1)
PIP	1								(1)
MP	1								(1)
Wrist	1								(1)
Elbow	1								(1)
Shoulder	1								(1)
DIP	2								(2)
PIP	2								(2)
MP	2							TYPE "0"	(2)
DIP	3								(3)
PIP	3								(3)
*MP	3								(3)
DIP	4								(4)
PIP	4								(4)
MP	4								(4)
DIP	1		1						(2)
PIP	1			1					(2)
MP	1				1				(2)
**Wrist	1					1			(2)
Elbow	1						1		(2)
DIP	2		2						(4)
PIP	2			2					(4)
MP	2				1			TYPE "1"	(3)
DIP	3		3						(6)
PIP	3			3					(6)
MP	3				1				(4)
DIP	4		4						(8)
PIP	4			4					(8)
MP	4				1				(5)
DIP	1		1	1					(3)
PIP	1			1	1				(3)
MP	1				1	1			(3)
Wrist	1					1	1		(3)
DIP	2		2	2					(6)
PIP	2			2	1				(5)
MP	2				1	1		TYPE "2"	(4)
DIP	3		3	3					(9)
PIP	3			3	1				(7)
MP	3				1	1			(5)
DIP	4		4	4					(12)
PIP	4			4	1				(9)
MP	4				1	1			(6)

TABLE 4-1   Continued

Primary Joints		Secondary Joints						Type	Total Joints
		DIP	PIP	MP	Wrist	Elbow	Shoulder		
DIP	1		1	1	1				(4)
PIP	1			1	1	1			(4)
MP	1				1	1	1		(4)
DIP	2		2	2	1				(7)
***PIP	2			2	1	1			(6)
MP	2				1	1	1		(5)
DIP	3		3	3	1			TYPE "3"	(10)
PIP	3			3	1	1			(8)
MP	3				1	1	1		(6)
DIP	4		4	4	1				(13)
PIP	4			4	1	1			(10)
MP	4				1	1	1		(7)
DIP	1		1	1	1	1			(5)
PIP	1			1	1	1	1		(5)
DIP	2		2	2	1	1			(8)
PIP	2			2	1	1	1		(7)
DIP	3		3	3	1	1		TYPE "4"	(11)
PIP	3			3	1	1	1		(9)
****DIP	4		4	4	1	1			(14)
PIP	4			4	1	1	1		(11)
DIP	1		1	1	1	1	1		(6)
DIP	2		2	2	1	1	1	TYPE "5"	(9)
DIP	3		3	3	1	1	1		(12)
DIP	4		4	4	1	1	1		(15)

EXAMPLES:

* *Primary joints* = 3 MPs
   Secondary joints = [none] = Type 0
   Total joints = [3 MPs] = (3)

** *Primary joints* = Wrist
   Secondary joints = [elbow level] = Type 1
   Total joints = [wrist + elbow = 2 joints] = (2)

*** *Primary joints* = 2 PIPs
   Secondary joints = [MP level + wrist level + elbow level = 3 levels] = Type 3
   Total joints = [2 PIPs + 2 MPs + 1 wrist + 1 elbow = 6 joints] = (6)

**** *Primary joints* = 4 DIPs
   Secondary joints = [PIP level + MP level + wrist level + elbow level = 4 levels] = Type 4
   Total joints = [4 DIPs + 4 PIPs + 4 MPs + 1 wrist + 1 elbow = 14 joints] = (14)

TABLE 4-2   Possible Diagnoses Associated with a Single Splint Design

Because the ESCS defines splint function rather than form, classification of splints using this system is diagnosis specific. As illustrated here, the splint form may be identical but its function differs according to its purpose of application. In providing a splint with its ESCS "name," clinicians convey exactly why the splint was applied.

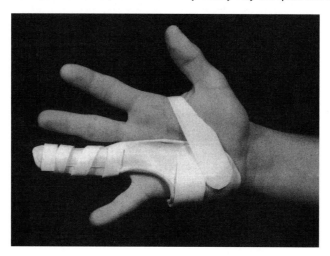

Location	ESCS Name	Secondary Joints	Indication for Splinting
RING FINGER	**Immobilization**		
	PIP & DIP extension immobilization splint, type 1 (3)	MP joint	Intraarticular fracture of PIP & DIP joints
	DIP extension immobilization splint, type 2 (3)	MP & PIP joints	Pediatric fracture of distal phalanx
	PIP extension immobilization splint, type 2 (3)	MP & DIP joints	Intraarticular fracture of PIP joint
	MP extension immobilization splint, type 2 (3)	PIP & DIP joints	Dupuytren's contracture
	MP & PIP extension immobilization splint, type 1 (3)	DIP joint	Fractures of proximal and middle phalanges
	MP, PIP, DIP extension immobilization splint, type 0 (3)	All three joints are primary	Dupuytren's contracture
	PIP lateral deviation immobilization splint, type 2 (3)	MP & DIP	PIP collateral ligament repair
	Mobilization		
	PIP & DIP extension mobilization splint, type 1 (3)	MP joint	PIP & DIP joint contracture
	DIP extension mobilization splint, type 2 (3)	MP & PIP joints	DIP joint contracture
	PIP extension mobilization splint, type 2 (3)	MP & DIP joints	PIP joint contracture
	MP extension mobilization splint, type 2 (3)	PIP & DIP joints	MP joint contracture
	MP & PIP extension mobilization splint, type 1 (3)	DIP joint	MP & PIP joint contractures
	MP, PIP, DIP extension mobilization splint, type 0 (3)	All joints are primary	Flexor tendon scar / adherent in palm

Adapted from Splint Classification System, Chicago, 1992, American Society of Hand Therapists.

than straps, dispersing pressure over half the lateral width of the extremity segment. In addition, they increase the area of force application, resulting in greater patient comfort (see also discussion of finger cuff).

Deviation Bar

A deviation bar (Fig. 4-15) is an immobile component that positions a body segment, usually the elbow, wrist, or fingers, in the coronal plane. It controls undesirable or detrimental abduction/adduction movements of the segment to which it is fitted, and is often used to protect unstable or healing joints. To be fully effective, the height of this ulnarly or radially based bar should be no less than half the thickness of the segment to which it is fitted and no greater than the full segment thickness. These bars are usually continuations of the splint itself, thus providing contoured strength in addition to positioning.

Mobilization Assist or Traction Device

This splint part (Fig. 4-16) creates a mobilizing force on a segment, resulting in passive or passive-assisted motion of a joint or successive joints. Traction devices

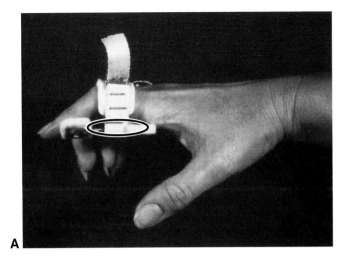

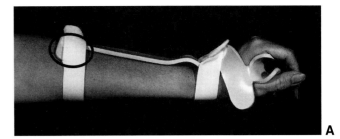

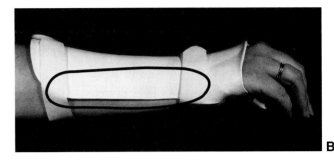

Fig. 4-13   A, Thumb CMC palmar abduction mobilization splint, type 3 (4) B, Wrist extension immobilization splint, type 0 (1)
A, Crossbars often provide the basis for strap attachments. B, Fused crossbars increase splint strength in contour designs.

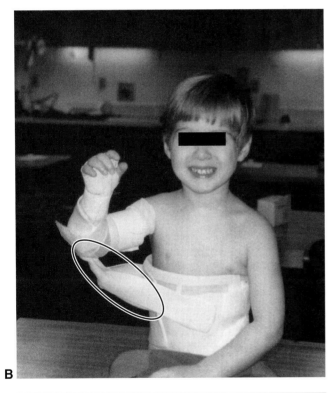

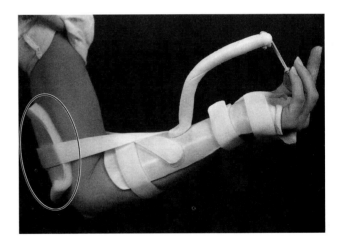

Fig. 4-12   A, Index finger PIP extension mobilization splint, type 0 (1). B, Shoulder abduction and external rotation immobilization splint, type 3 (4)
A, These connector bars maintain the distance between the proximal and distal crossbars of this splint. B, Acting as a strut between the trunk and upper extremity, the connector bar functions to position the shoulder in abduction and external rotation.

Fig. 4-14   Long finger MP flexion mobilization splint, type 1 (2); with triceps cuff
A triceps cuff provides a proximal stabilizing force to counteract this splint's tendency toward distal migration.

Finger Cuff

may be made of self-adjusting resilient or elastic materials such as rubber bands or spring wire, or they may be fabricated from more rigid, inelastic materials such as fishing line, unwaxed dental floss, Velcro, cording, or leather. The more rigid materials often rely on the wearer for adjustment.

Whether circumferential or U-shaped in design, this splint component (Fig. 4-17, A,B) attaches a traction assist to the finger. Finger cuffs may be closed or open, and are usually made of a flexible but inelastic material (Fig. 4-17, A). With extension traction, cuffs must be cut to allow full flexion of proximal and distal finger joints. Designed by Paul Brand, MD, low-profile cuffs of plaster (Fig. 4-17, B) provide excellent con-

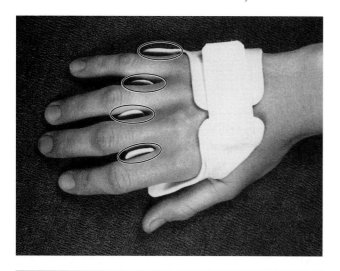

Fig. 4-15   Index–small finger MP flexion and ulnar deviation restriction splint, type 0 (4)
The deviation bars of this splint function to maintain normal alignment of the MP joints by preventing ulnar deviation. (Courtesy K. P. MacBain, OTR, Vancouver, BC.)

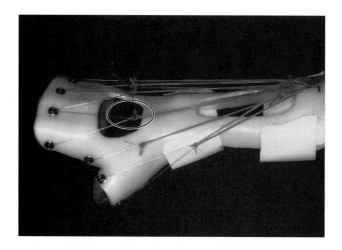

Fig. 4-16   Wrist extension, index–small finger MP extension, thumb CMC radial abduction and MP extension mobilization splint, type 0 (7)
This splint for radial nerve palsy employs a combination of elastic rubber band and inelastic filament traction. Elastic traction glides proximal to the outrigger while the inelastic component is situated distally. (Courtesy Dominique Thomas, RPT, MCMK, Saint Martin Duriage, France.)

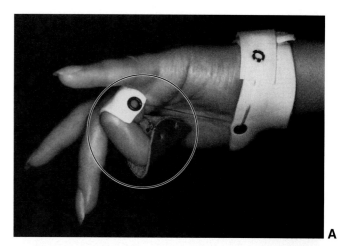

A

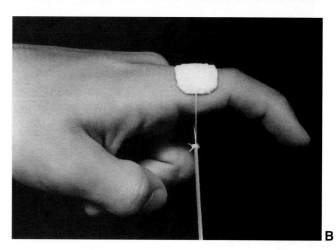

B

Fig. 4-17   A, Ring finger flexion mobilization splint, type 0 (3)
A, Two open slings provide the base for traction in this composite flexion splint. A perpendicular pull is provided between the proximal and distal phalanx. B, A contiguous fit of this cuff on the dorsum of the finger is provided even in the absence of a 90° angle of approach of the mobilization assist. [Courtesy (A) Dominique Thomas, RPT, MCMK, Saint Martin Duriage, France; (B) Design by Paul W. Brand, MB, BS, FRCS.]

tiguous fit, shorten the cuff moment arm, and position the axis of rotation of the traction assist nearer to the phalanx. These modifications effectively combine to decrease soft tissue shear by the cuff, making this innovative design ideal for hands with diminished sensibility.

Fingernail Attachment

A fingernail attachment (Fig. 4-18) is any device that, when fastened to the fingernail, provides an attachment site for a traction assist. It may be adhered to the nail with a fast-setting ethyl cyanoacrylate glue or, in the case of a suture loop, tied through the distal free edge of the nail body. The innovative idea of gluing dress hooks to fingernails was conceived by Carolina F. deLeeuw, MA, OTR, while working on the burn unit of Brooke Army Hospital in the early 1960s. At that time, fingernail hooks were a major factor in successfully positioning digits of burn patients treated with topical antibacterial agents, where dressings were kept to a minimum.[5] Today, fingernail hooks and Velcro continue to be excellent adjuncts for treating acute hand injuries.

Forearm/Humerus Bar or Trough

This longitudinal splint part (Fig. 4-19) rests proximal to the wrist (for a forearm bar/trough) or the elbow

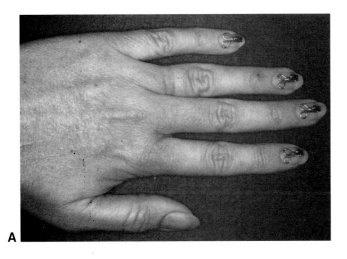

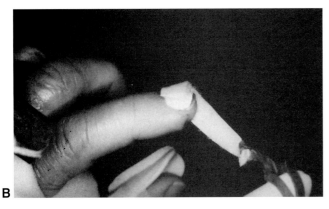

Fig. 4-18   Fingernail attachment devices are generally secured with ethyl cyanoacrylate glue. Application of the device to the proximal nail creates less stress on the nail bed attachment from distal pull. **A,** Dress hooks. **B,** Velcro hook tabs.

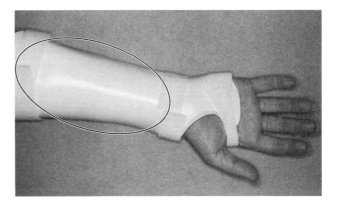

Fig. 4-19   **Wrist neutral immobilization splint, type 0 (1)** A forearm trough allows the surface area to disperse the hand weight. A trough two-thirds the length of the forearm will comfortably support the proximally transferred weight of the hand.

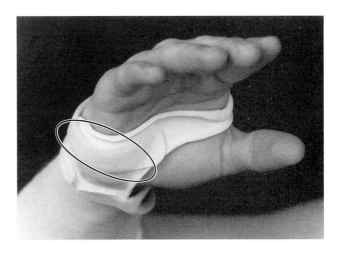

Fig. 4-20   **Wrist neutral immobilization splint, type 0 (1)** A hypothenar bar supports the mobile fourth and fifth metacarpals and allows MP flexion while not impeding the distal palmar flexion crease.

(for a humerus bar/trough), on one or more surfaces of the forearm or upper arm. Forearm and humerus bars/troughs provide counterforce leverage to support the weight of the hand or forearm, and for maximum efficiency and comfort should be at least two-thirds the length of the forearm or humeral segment to which it is fitted.

Hypothenar Bar

The bar that palmarly supports the ulnar aspect of the transverse metacarpal arch is called a hypothenar bar (Fig. 4-20) and is frequently the continuation of a deviation bar or a dorsal or palmar metacarpal bar. A hypothenar bar should not inhibit flexion of the ring and small MP joints and should be contoured carefully to provide a contiguous fit. Poor molding of this bar may result in excessive pressure as the hand is used.

Joint

Mechanical overlapping of splint components (Fig. 4-21) results in either an axis of rotation or a solid

immobile bond. When an axis of rotation is required to allow anatomic joint motion, either a commercially available joint may be used or a joint may be constructed using one or, in special cases, two strategically placed rivets. Use of two rivets allows excellent "seating" on the extremity by components proximal and distal to the articulations.

Metacarpal Bar

This splint component (Fig. 4-22) supports the transverse metacarpal arch dorsally or palmarly. A correctly fitted metacarpal bar should allow full motion of the second through fifth MP joints. The ulnar and radial extensions of a metacarpal bar frequently include a hypothenar bar or an opponens bar, respectively.

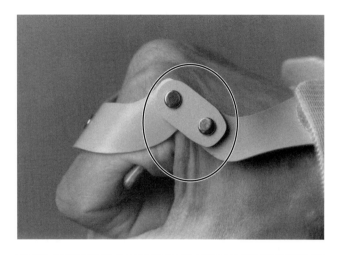

Fig. 4-21   Index–small finger MP ulnar deviation restriction splint, type 0 (4)
Two mobile splint joints have been utilized to allow MP flexion and restrict ulner deviation. The distal splint joint should be centered at the MP joint axis of rotation. (Courtesy Julie Belkin, OTR, CO, MBA, Annapolis, Md.)

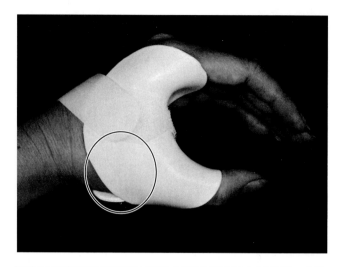

Fig. 4-23   Thumb CMC palmar abduction immobilization splint, type 2 (3)
An opponens bar maintains the position of the first metacarpal. Fabrication may necessitate a longer lever arm for the first and second metacarpal to maintain palmar abduction.

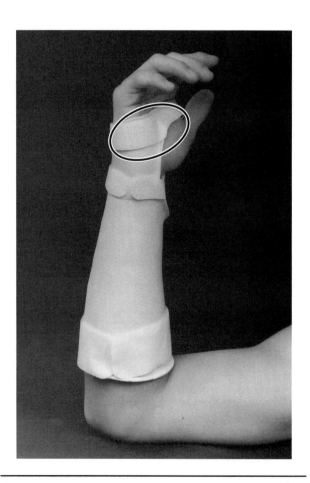

Fig. 4-22   Wrist extension immobilization splint, type 0 (1)
Wrist immobilization splints may be fitted palmarly providing support to the transverse metacarpal arch via a metacarpal bar.

Opponens Bar

Usually designed in conjunction with a C bar, an opponens bar (Fig. 4-23) positions the first metacarpal in various degrees of abduction and opposition while preventing radiodorsal motion of the metacarpal. This bar should be long enough to fully control the first metacarpal bone but should not be so long that it interferes with placement of the hand.

Outrigger

This splint part (Fig. 4-24) is extended out from the main body of a splint for the purpose of positioning mobilization assists or traction devices. To maintain correct alignment of traction devices, outrigger length must be adjusted as change occurs in passive range of motion of the joint(s) being mobilized. Because magnitude of the mobilizing forces will be abated with outrigger instability or material weakness, outriggers should furnish a rigid or near-rigid foundation for mobilization assists.

Phalangeal Bar or Finger Pan

Fitted dorsally or palmarly, a phalangeal bar (Fig. 4-25) positions the phalangeal segments and maintains the transverse arch. Because of the fragility of the dorsal skin, the magnified forces of a mobilizing splint, and the often narrow design of the bar itself, a dorsal phalangeal bar (once called a lumbrical bar) often requires padding to disseminate splinting forces on the underlying soft tissue. The ulnar and radial sides of a dorsal or palmar bar should enclose at least one-half the width of the phalanx to prevent lateral displacement of the finger or fingers from the bar. Longitudinally, a phalangeal bar should extend a minimum of two-thirds the length of the phalangeal segment(s) included in the splint. A palmar phalangeal bar should not limit flexion of the IP joints. When the full length of the finger(s) is included, the phalangeal bar is called a finger pan. Finger pans may be fitted dorsally or palmarly.

Prop

A prop (Fig. 4-26) is an attachment that places the splinted extremity away from a supporting surface to position or to prevent pressure from prolonged resting of the extremity on a rigid or semi-rigid surface.

Reinforcement Bar

This adjunctive splint component (Fig. 4-27) increases splint strength/durability. Although an occasional reinforcement bar may be appropriate, persistent use of reinforcement bars is frequently indicative of poor splint design or material choice.

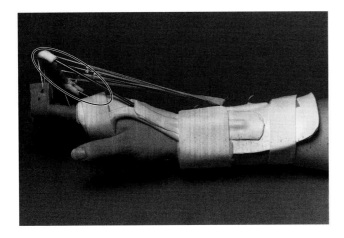

Fig. 4-24   Index–small finger IP extension mobilization splint, type 2 (13)
Outrigger configurations vary in style according to purpose and must be adjusted to accommodate changes in PROM (passive range of motion). (Courtesy Lisa Dennys, BSc, OT, London, Ont.)

Fig. 4-25   A, Ring–small finger MP extension restriction / IP extension torque transmission splint, type 0 (6) B, Index–small finger PIP extension mobilization splint, type 2 (9) C, Index–small finger MP 20° flexion and IP extension immobilization splint, type 1 (13)
A, Used for an ulnar nerve injury, this splint incorporates a dorsal phalangeal bar to restrict MP joint extension protecting the volar plates. This splint is fabricated from one long narrow single or double rectangular piece of plastic twisted into an 8 providing strength for MP positioning. B, The mobilization splint restricts MP joint extension with a dorsal phalangeal bar and stabilizes traction to the PIP joints. C, A phalangeal bar that includes all of the fingers either volarly or dorsally is called a finger pan. In this picture a lateral splint border prevents ulnar digital displacement. The transverse arch is well supported in the palm as seen in the higher second and third metacarpal as well as the lower fourth and fifth metacarpal. [Courtesy (A) Brenda Hilfrank, PT, CHT, South Burlington, Vt.; (C) Lin Beribak, OTR/L, CHT, Chicago, Ill.]

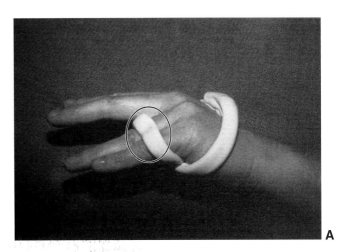

A

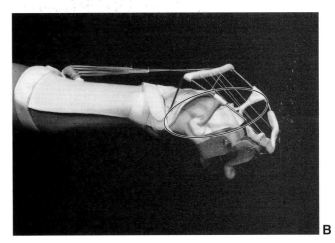

B

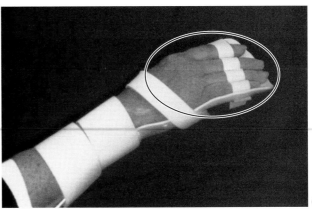

C

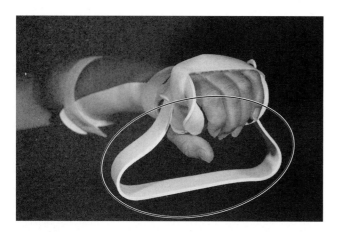

Fig. 4-26 A prop may be of assistance in positioning or preventing soft tissue injury of the upper extremity. Props are especially helpful for positioning paralytic extremities.

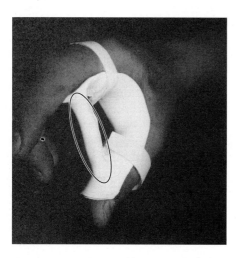

Fig. 4-27 **Thumb CMC palmar abduction immobilization splint, type 3 (4)**
A reinforcement bar may be used to add strength to a splint, e.g., for maintaining this first and second metacarpal position. (Courtesy Cynthia Philips, MA, OTR, CHT, Framingham, Mass.)

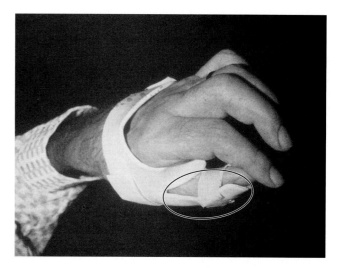

Fig. 4-28 **Thumb CMC palmar abduction and opposition mobilization splint, type 0 (3)**
This thumb post positions the thumb in palmar abduction and opposition while allowing IP flexion for prehension. See also Fig. 4-3: A thumb post fitted circumferentially increases stability in positioning. (Courtesy Patricia Hall, MS, OTR, ATP, Fortville, Ind.)

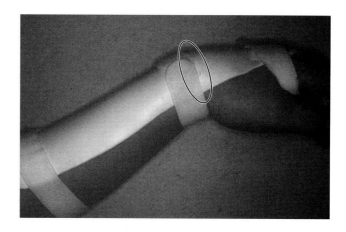

Fig. 4-29 **Index–small finger extension torque transmission splint type 1 (13)**
A wrist bar placed in flexion will augment active extrinsic finger extension. Caution must be taken to not create median nerve compression with wrist flexion positioning.

Correctly contoured material and incorporation of sound mechanical principles is far more effective in providing splint strength than is retrospective trussing with extra layers of materials.

Thumb Phalangeal Bar or Post

Positioning the proximal and distal phalanges of the thumb, this component (Fig. 4-28) is usually a distal extension of a C bar. When only the proximal thumb phalanx is immobilized, full IP joint motion should not be inhibited by overextension of the thumb post distally. Since configuration of this bar is often long and narrow, contouring of the material to half of the thick-

ness of the splinted segment will increase component stability. When the immobile thumb is to be used in functional activities, it is preferable to design the thumb post to fit dorsally, allowing sensory areas of the thumb to be free for grasping.

Wrist Bar

Whether fitted palmarly, dorsally, ulnarly, or radially, any splint part that supports the carpal area of the extremity may be considered a wrist bar (Fig. 4-29). This bar frequently connects the forearm bar/trough

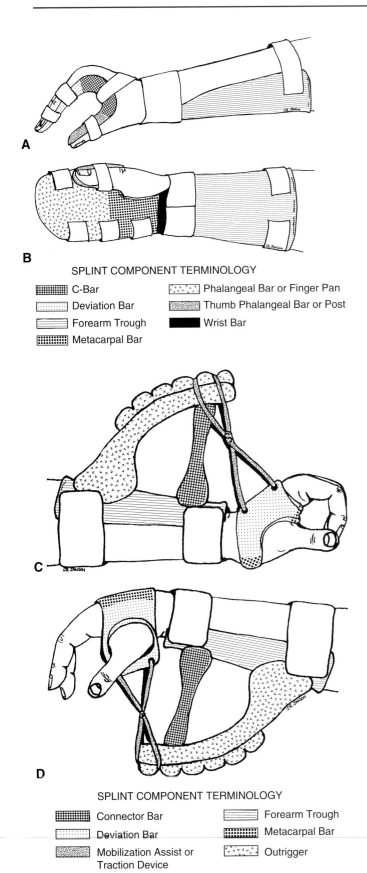

SPLINT COMPONENT TERMINOLOGY

C-Bar		Phalangeal Bar or Finger Pan	
Deviation Bar		Thumb Phalangeal Bar or Post	
Forearm Trough		Wrist Bar	
Metacarpal Bar			

SPLINT COMPONENT TERMINOLOGY

Connector Bar		Forearm Trough	
Deviation Bar		Metacarpal Bar	
Mobilization Assist or Traction Device		Outrigger	

Fig. 4-30   A,B, Index–small finger MP 70° flexion and IP extension, thumb CMC palmar abduction immobilization splint, type 3 (16) C, Wrist extension mobilization splint, type 0 (1). D, Wrist flexion mobilization splint, type 0 (1)

A,B, A splint represents the coalescence of many individual components to form the whole of the splint. **C,D,** Anatomy of a splint: individual components within this splint are identified via different graphic patterns. This wrist mobilization splint (a.k.a. "dinosaur") design uses the same forearm trough base and outrigger for extension and flexion, **(C)** but requires individually fitted thermoplastic metacarpal bars to support the palmar arch volarly with wrist extension mobilization splinting **(D)** and dorsally with wrist flexion mobilization splinting.

proximally and the metacarpal bar distally. Positional attitude of this bar in the sagittal plane exerts substantial influence on the kinetic interrelationships of distal anatomical structures. As a result, the wrist bar must be positioned advantageously and with deliberation.

Splint Component Integration

Individual splint components combine to allow a splint to function in the manner for which it was designed to operate, with each part providing an integral task toward achieving the overall goal of the splint (Fig. 4-30). Those who see only the external configurations of splints miss critical nuances that make splinting endeavors successful. The astute upper extremity specialist knows how component parts function individually, understands how they relate to each other, and is able to manipulate each component as it relates to the whole, in order to achieve the best possible splinting advantage for upper extremity patients.

■ SUMMARY

Clinicians involved in splint preparation should have a thorough knowledge of the nomenclature of the entire spectrum of splint components, their capabilities, and indications. A creative flexibility must be developed that allows the clinician to draw from a large assortment of splint components in the preparation of a splint that will best suit the requirements of a particular upper extremity problem. Although one must be cognizant of splint classification systems employed in the past, it is important to avoid the confusion that results from the intrinsic limitations of these out-of-date methods. Adherence to a limited classification system narrows splint fabrication options and fails to adequately respond to the almost unlimited assortment of individual situations that exist in the diseased or injured hand/upper extremity. This chapter reviews the important expanded and refined Splint Classification System and sets the stage for its use throughout the entire spectrum of this book. We hope that this approach will best allow for more accurate descriptions of splints, thereby aiding all upper extremity rehabilitation specialists in the difficult area of communication.

REFERENCES

1. ASHT: *American Society of Hand Therapists Splint Classification System*, ed 1, The Society, 1992, Chicago.

2. Fess EE: *Splint Mechanical Patterns©*, presented to the ASHT Splint Nomenclature Task Force, January, 1991, American Society of Hand Therapists Splint Classification System, 1991, The Society.

3. Fess EE, Gettle KS, Strickland JW: *Hand splinting: principles and methods*, ed 1, Mosby, 1981, St. Louis.

4. Fess EE, Philips CA: *Hand splinting: principles and methods*, ed 2, Mosby, 1987, St. Louis.

5. Von Prince KMP, Yeakel MH: *The splinting of burn patients*, Thomas, 1974, Springfield, IL.

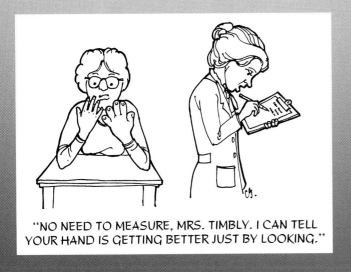

"NO NEED TO MEASURE, MRS. TIMBLY. I CAN TELL YOUR HAND IS GETTING BETTER JUST BY LOOKING."

CHAPTER 5

Upper Extremity Assessment and Splinting

Chapter Outline

Thorough and unbiased assessment procedures furnish essential foundations for splinting programs by delineating baseline pathology from which splint designs may be created and patient progress and splinting methods may be evaluated. Assessment information also assists in predicting the rehabilitation potential of the diseased or injured upper extremity and provides data to which subsequent measurements may be compared. Conclusions gained from evaluation procedures aid in ordering treatment priorities, promote both patient and staff incentive, and define functional capacity when rehabilitative efforts culminate. Through analysis and integration, assessment also serves as the vehicle for professional communication, eventually increasing and validating the comprehensive body of rehabilitation knowledge.

The design and configuration of upper extremity splints are significantly influenced by the evaluation process, which involves gathering and integrating data derived from various sources, including physician referral, direct observation, and precise measurements. A finished splint must not only meet the more obvious requirements of physical condition, it should also take into account the patient's psychological and socioeconomic capacities. Additionally, experience, preference, and philosophy of the members of the rehabilitation team are important aspects in dictating splinting programs. Therefore these factors must be considered in the overall assessment process. The purpose of this chapter is to review upper extremity assessment theory and techniques as applied to upper extremity splinting concepts.

■ INSTRUMENT CRITERIA

A splinting assessment involves the use of a variety of evaluation techniques and instruments whose resultant data is integrated to produce a clearly defined picture of composite upper extremity function. Assessment tools range in sophistication from simple observational methods to highly complex standardized tests. While observational skills provide the initial basis for identifying pathology, specific measurements provide concrete numerical information about specialized components of hand and upper extremity function such as motion, sensibility, mass, temperature, strength, coordination, and dexterity. Both observation and measurement play vital roles in evaluating a diseased or injured extremity for application of a splint.

Much of the initial impression of pathology may be gleaned from an astute interview, observation, and careful inspection and palpation of the extremity.[56] A detailed history; observation of posturing and use of the extremity; identification of skin and soft tissue condition, skeletal and joint stability, composite motion, general strength, musculotendinous continuity, pain, and neurovascular status; and a subjective appraisal of the patient's attitude toward his or her disability provide the examiner with the source and general parameters of the problem.

Once the patient's overall condition is understood, measurements should be taken to further delineate the problem. Directly influencing the interpretation and understanding of upper extremity dysfunction, both the quality of the instruments and the effects of the procedures used in the assessment process must be identified.

Because the caliber of information in a splinting assessment is dictated by the sophistication, predictability, and accuracy of the measurement instruments used, it is critical to choose evaluation tools with care and forethought. Dependable, precise instruments provide data that is minimally skewed by extraneous factors or biases, thereby diminishing

subjective error and facilitating objective and accurate definition. Instruments that measure diffusely produce undelineated and nonspecific data. Those proven to measure with precision yield more reliable and selective information. In an age of consumer awareness and accountability, it is no longer sufficient to rely on homemade nonvalidated evaluation tools, which almost universally produce meaningless splinter data.

Equally important to the identification of instrument standards is understanding how the testing process can affect resultant data. Position of the extremity, fatigue, physiologic adaptation, length of the test, and motivation are but a few of the factors that can influence test results. Also, instruments that are used to measure upper extremity dysfunction should not have been used as practice tools in therapy. Evaluation tools that have been used in the training process produce skewed data and render subsequent testing information invalid and meaningless. Selection criteria must therefore reflect understanding of testing protocol as well as instrumentation requirements.

Standardized tests, the most sophisticated of measurement instruments, are statistically proven to be both reliable and valid. They measure consistently between instruments, examiners, and from trial to trial (reliability) and they measure what they purport to measure (validity). To date, the few truly standardized tests available for measuring upper extremity dysfunction are limited to instruments that evaluate coordination, dexterity, and work tolerance. Surprisingly, most of the currently used assessment tools lack many of the primary elements of good instrumentation.[24] When choosing upper extremity testing instruments, selection should be guided by how closely inherent properties of the instrument coincide with those of standardized tools.

To qualify as a standardized test, an instrument must have all of the following elements: (1) a statement that defines the purpose or intent of the test, (2) correlation statistics or other appropriate measure of instrument reliability (not mean or average values), (3) correlation statistics or other appropriate measure of instrument validity (not mean or average values), (4) detailed descriptions of the equipment used in the test, (5) normative data, drawn from a large population sample, which is divided into subcategories according to appropriate variables such as hand dominance, age, sex, or occupation, and (6) specific instructions for administering, scoring, and interpreting the test. Of these criteria, reliability and validity are the two most important factors and the remaining criteria are dependent on their presence. Because relatively few upper extremity evaluation tools fully meet standardization criteria, instrument selection should be predicated on satisfying as many of the standardization requisites as possible, ensuring an identifiable level of quality control. Because a universal upper extremity assessment instrument is nonexistent, a variety of tools are needed to measure the various parameters of condition and performance, including range of motion (ROM), strength, sensation, volume, dexterity and coordination, vascular status, and patient satisfaction.[2-4,24,56]

RECORDING AND TIMING OF ASSESSMENT EXAMINATIONS

Not all patients who are evaluated for splints require all of the tests within an upper extremity assessment battery. Most upper extremity specialists use a few quick tests to check function initially and add the more sophisticated testing procedures as dictated by the patient's condition. Generally, initial and final evaluations are more comprehensive, whereas intervening evaluations are less extensive, concentrating on assessing progress in specific areas, such as active and passive range of motion, volume, or muscle strength. The frequency of reevaluation depends on diagnosis, physiologic timing, and the patient's response to the application of the splint. For example, because they often respond quickly to splinting measures, early postoperative patients require more frequent measurements than do those individuals who have been splinted to correct longstanding deformities.

The actual recording of assessment data varies according to the specific test and to the amount of change observed. Motion values may be recorded on a daily, thrice weekly, or weekly basis while strength measurements may require notation each month. The important concept is that change in status is documented with appropriate objective measurements with each visit to the clinic. Standardizing clinical treatment in hand therapy is frequently accomplished through use of SOAP notes. Short-term and long-term goals must be stated and objective data is recorded to justify treatment and document changes.

Although evaluation data dictate the design of a splint, knowledge obtained from reevaluation sessions directs alterations in splint configuration and wearing schedule. Splinting is a dynamic, ever-changing process that is intimately interwoven with and directed by information gleaned from assessment procedures. With the designing, constructing, and fitting of a splint comes the all-important responsibility of maintaining and updating its efficiency. This is done through

vigilant reassessment of the hand/extremity and constant reevaluation of the exercise routine, wearing schedule, and the splint itself (Box 5-1).[34] Failure to attain anticipated goals requires reassessment of the splinting and exercise programs.

CLINICAL EXAMINATION OF THE UPPER EXTREMITY

Referral and Interview Information

The information provided in the signed referral and ensuing initial interview is paramount because it directly influences the eventual splint design and subsequent treatment. In addition to the patient's name, age, sex, hand dominance, hospital number, and designation of involved extremity, the referral should include diagnosis, date and circumstances of injury and/or onset of medical problem, purpose and timing of splint application, and specific instructions and precautions. The patient interview provides pertinent medical history (with dates), including associated conditions that may influence splint-wearing tolerance such as diabetes, use of corticosteroid medications, past chemotherapy, etc. Without this minimum baseline information the initiation of a splinting program should not be undertaken. In this age of litigation it is preferable to have the information in writing. Operative notes, radiographic reports, vascular studies, and the results of pertinent testing procedures such as nerve conduction velocity studies (NCVs) and electromyograms (EMGs) are also essential for evaluating and treating upper extremity dysfunction.

Identification of the etiology, diagnosis, rehabilitation potential, physiologic timing, and physician's treatment philosophy allows early triage of possible therapy and splinting options. Because their associated splinting theories differ considerably, it is important to differentiate upper motor neuron lesions from the often more acute peripheral lesions associated with upper extremity trauma. It is also necessary to identify organic or systemic diseases, which follow chronic courses from acute or subacute situations. For example, a proximal interphalangeal (IP) joint hyperextension deformity is treated differently in a spastic hand, a rheumatoid arthritic hand, and a young athlete's hand. When dealing with postoperative patients, it is essential to know which structures were involved, which structures were repaired, quality of repairs, method of repair, type of fixation, passive range of motion (PROM) and active range of motion (AROM) at surgery, and precautions including amount of tension permitted on the repair and amount of range of motion allowed. These are critical factors that

BOX 5-1   Splint Evaluation Criteria[1]

NEED
1. Is application of splint necessary on initial examination?
2. Does it continue to be necessary on reevaluation?

DESIGN
Given the diagnostic requirements, does the splint meet general design concepts, including adaptation for the following:
1. Individual client factors (age, motivation, intelligence, vocation/avocation, clinic proximity)
2. Cost (appropriate to individual client factors and third-party payers)
3. Duration of time splint is to be used (temporary, semipermanent, permanent)
4. Simplicity (no irrelevant parts; splint is applicable and pertinent to the need)
5. Optimal function (splint allows usage and performance without unnecessary reduction of motion)
6. Optimal sensation (splint permits as much sensory input as possible)
7. Efficient fabrication (no extraneous parts or procedures, such as the use of reinforcement parts instead of curving contour, bonding instead of uninterrupted coalescing of components, straps instead of contiguous fit, inappropriate use of padding)
8. Application and removal (appropriate to individual client factors)
9. Client suggestions (requested adaptations that would not alter or jeopardize splint function)
10. Influencing primary and secondary joints (motion allowed or restricted appropriately; components accomplish intended functions)
11. Attaining purpose (immobilize, mobilize, restrict motion, or transmit torque)
12. Effect on joints not included in splint; kinetic effects (avoids application of contraindicated forces to nonsplinted joints)
13. Anatomical variables (surface of application appropriate, healing structures protected as necessary, external hardware considered)
14. Exercise regimen (permits efficient execution of prescribed therapeutic exercises)

MECHANICS
Given the diagnostic requirements, does the splint meet mechanical criteria, including adaptation for the following:
1. Reduction of pressure and shear (length and width of components appropriate; edges flanged as required; contiguous fit of components present)
2. Immobilization or stabilization forces (90° angle of approach to involved segment or joint)
3. Mobilization forces (90° angle of approach to segments mobilized, perpendicular to joint axes)
4. Magnitude of mobilization forces (supple joint: force sufficient to position segment; stiff joint: force does not exceed safe limits)
5. Difference of passive mobility of successive joints (relative stiffness of joint considered; mobilizing force is not abated at less stiff or normal joints)
6. Components (provide optimum mechanical benefit)
7. Material strength (properties of material correlates with strength requirement; curving contour present at potential weak areas)
8. Elimination of friction and shear (joint axes aligned with splint articulations; contiguous fit present)

CONSTRUCTION
Given the diagnostic requirements, does splint fabrication and workmanship provide the following:
1. Good overall aesthetic appearance
2. Corners rounded, edges and surfaces smooth and flanged appropriately
3. Joined surfaces stable and finished (bonds solid, securing devices of sufficient number and correctly applied; internal edges smoothed, securing devices finished)
4. Ventilation (appropriately placed, splint strength not jeopardized)
5. Padding and straps secured

FIT
Given the diagnostic requirements, has the splint been fitted appropriately to adapt to the following:
1. Anatomical structure (bony prominences, arches, dual obliquity, skin creases)
2. Ligamentous stress (immobilization, mobilization, restriction, or torque transmission forces correctly applied to avoid damage or attenuation)
3. Joint alignment (anatomical axes aligned with splint articulation; splint does not shift inappropriately on extremity)
4. Kinematic changes (splint does not inappropriately inhibit motion of unrestricted or partially restricted joints; splint does not inappropriately transmit torque)
5. Contiguous fit of components on extremity

CLIENT EDUCATION
Given the diagnostic requirements, does the splinting program include consideration of and instructions for the following:
1. Wearing times and exercise regimen (reflects physiological timing; is adapted to client routine; is understood by client)
2. Donning and doffing (process explained and demonstrated, understood by client)
3. Wearability (client gadget tolerance not exceeded; interfaces such as stockinette or powder used appropriately; acceptable to age and personality characteristics)
4. Precautions (written and verbal instructions provided, understood by client)

Note: Although an attempt has been made to provide a complete listing, these criteria should not be considered all-inclusive.
[1]Adapted from Fess E, Kiel J: Upper extremity splinting. In Neistadt M, Crepeau E: *Willard & Spackman's Occupational Therapy*, ed 9, Lippincott, 1998, Philadelphia.

directly influence splint design. Postoperative timing is also critical. A splint that is appropriate 8 weeks after repair may be detrimental at an earlier time because wound tensile strength is insufficient to withstand splinting forces. Differing philosophies as to when and how certain injuries may be splinted during the early postoperative phase also make it imperative to know the preferences of the referring physician before embarking upon a course of splinting and therapy. A surgeon who prefers to use early passive motion postoperatively would be more than alarmed to discover that an early active motion splinting and exercise program had been initiated for a patient with newly repaired flexor tendons!

Posture

The normal hand at rest assumes a consistent posture with the wrist in 10-15° of dorsiflexion, the thumb in slight extension/abduction with the metacarpophalangeal and interphalangeal joints flexed approximately 15-20°, and the fingers exhibiting progressively greater composite flexion to the ulnar side of the hand. The thumbnail lies in a plane perpendicular to that of the index finger, and at rest, the extended longitudinal attitudes of the four fingers converge on a small area at the base of the thumb near the thenar crease. When the wrist is brought into full extension, finger adduction and flexion increase, the transverse metacarpal arch flattens slightly, the extended longitudinal point of convergence moves proximally onto the forearm, and the thumb pad approximates the lateral aspect of the proximal phalanx of the index finger. Conversely, wrist flexion produces a passive attitude of finger abduction and extension, and although the thumb metacarpophalangeal and interphalangeal joints assume a nearly full extension posture, the thumb web space narrows as passive tension on the extensor pollicis longus tendon increases and the first metacarpal is adducted. Changes from the normal resting posture or from normal tenodesis effect are strong indicators of pathology such as joint contracture, nerve paralysis, or tendon adherence, and merit further investigation before splint design may commence.

When splinting the hand, it is especially important to understand that normal finger convergence points change when the fingers are flexed individually and when they are flexed simultaneously. Individual finger flexion most often results in convergence points at the base of the thumb. In contrast, simultaneous finger flexion points most often converge in the radial middle third of the forearm (Fig. 5-1). Additionally, specific patterns of convergence points differ between individuals for both independent and simultaneous

finger flexion.[23] Splints must be designed to reflect the effect of these different convergence locations according to specific patient anatomy and splinting requirements.

Skin and Subcutaneous Tissue

Thorough examination of the surface condition and contours of the extremity helps define pathology and influences splint configuration. Closely correlated with neurovascular status, tissue viability, and the inflammatory process are skin color, temperature, texture, and moisture. These should be carefully noted. Alterations from normal extremity size and contour should also be identified, including areas of atrophy, tissue deficit, scarring, local swelling, generalized edema, and abnormal masses or prominences. In addition to providing important information regarding condition of soft tissue and how the extremity is used, skin creases serve as anatomical guides for splint application. Absence of wrinkles or creases at or near joints may indicate loss of motion or inflammation, and callus formation or embedded surface grime are excellent clues as to how the extremity is used. Because the application of any splinting device, no matter how well fitted, produces pressure and shear to the underlying cutaneous surface, tissue friability, especially in scarred or grafted areas, must be carefully evaluated. Splints should be designed such that they do not jeopardize normal structures, healing structures, or tissue of questionable viability. Circumferential or narrow components should be avoided in borderline cases. Whenever possible, pressure should be minimized by increasing the area of application of strategic splint parts.

Bone

When splinting patients who have sustained injury to the skeletal structures of the upper extremity, operative notes are essential. In addition to obtaining a current x-ray and identifying the site and type of fracture, it is critical to know how stable the reduction is, the methods used to obtain and maintain good alignment, other related injuries and repairs, and the amount of time elapsed since reduction. Complications including rotational deformity, delayed union, pseudoarthrosis, and malunion must be assessed, and the presence of fixation equipment such as K-wires, tension band wires, compression plates, screws, or external fixation devices should be noted (Fig. 5-2). Portions of a splint may be designed to support and protect the fracture site while others mobilize stiffened adjacent joints. With closed reductions, follow-up x-rays are helpful after splint fabrication to insure

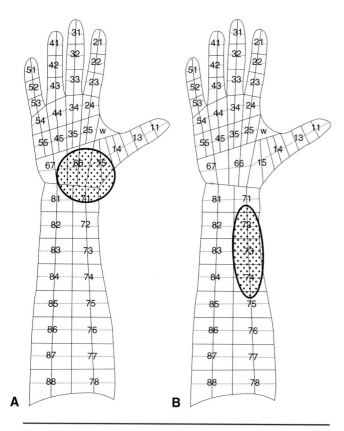

A, **B**,

Fig. 5-1   **A,** Individual finger flexion convergence points occur most often in areas 15, 66, and 71 at the base of the thumb. **B,** Simultaneous finger flexion convergence points occur most often in the radial middle third of the forearm in areas 72, 73, and 74.

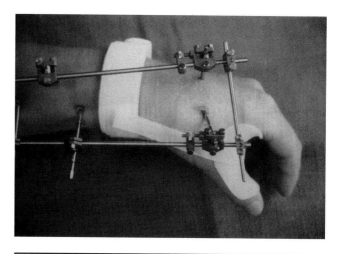

Fig. 5-2   **Thumb CMC palmar abduction immobilization splint, type 2 (3).**
External fixation device placement creates changes in a splint's design and fabrication. (Courtesy Brenda Hilfrank, PT, CHT, South Burlington, Vt.)

that reductions are not altered. Splint components must be positioned to avoid encroachment on pins or external fixation devices. Splinting should be knowledgeably integrated with the pace of physiologic healing and should not unduly stress the mending fracture site. Wound healing principles and how they are affected by the application of external forces must be clearly understood. A splint that is appropriate 6 to 8 weeks after reduction may actually be detrimental if applied at an earlier time. Rigid fixation devices allow early motion to those joints of the extremity that do not require immobilization to stabilize fractures. It is important that both therapist and patient understand the inherent forces involved and their physiologic repercussions before splint application may begin. Additionally, upgrading from immobilization splinting to mobilization splinting must be carefully coordinated with the referring physician. Incorrect splinting or timing of splinting may result in poor or failed outcome. Close communication between members of the rehabilitation team is therefore essential to obtain optimal functional results.

Joint

Joint stability, passive motion, etiology, and elapsed time since injury and repair are important when evaluating articular function. For the hand, with the exception of the five-ligament complex of the thumb carpometacarpal joint, each digital articulation achieves stability through a consistent configuration of three ligaments. A pair of collateral ligaments provides lateral stability, and a dense palmar plate allows a full arc of flexion while preventing excessive hyperextension of each joint. Wrist, elbow, and shoulder ligamentous structures are intricate and, like the ligaments of the hand, are essential to normal upper extremity function. Attenuation or disruption of key ligaments at these joints results in predictable patterns of pathology. Continuity, relative length, and glide of upper extremity ligaments must be carefully assessed, since unstable joints, subluxation, dislocation, and limited passive motion directly influence the purpose of splint application, resulting in numerous splint designs, each created to meet specific requirements. Depending on physiologic timing, splints may be used to protect healing ligamentous structures and limit motion until tensile strength is sufficient to tolerate normal motion and resistance. Joints whose supporting ligaments have been attenuated by disease or trauma may be improved functionally through the application of immobilization or restriction splints. Mobilization and torque transmission splints may be used to correct passive joint deformity through remodeling of soft tissues surrounding stiffened joints.

Differentiating pathology at the capsular or articular level from pathology involving the musculotendinous system is imperative to achieving efficacious splint design. For example, a hand-based splint that does not incorporate the wrist may be used for joint motion limitations resulting from shortened or fibrosed periarticular structures or intra-articular adhesions. In contrast, presence of extrinsic musculotendinous pathology requires a splint design that controls the wrist in addition to providing corrective forces to more distal digital joints. Both the tenodesis effect on passive joint motion (Fig. 5-3) and the relative tightness of the intrinsic muscles (Fig. 5-4) must be identified before the final splint configuration may be reached. According to Lister, "if adjustment of the position of the joints proximal to an apparently contracted joint results in its full extension, then the limitation is due either to tendon shortening or to tendon adhesions proximal to the joints adjusted."[38] When extrinsic structures are involved, regardless of whether the primary focus joint is shoulder, elbow, wrist, or a digital joint, incorporation of secondary adjacent joints in the splint, to direct mechanical focus to primary joints, is required almost universally.

Muscle and Tendon

Diminished or absent active motion in the presence of normal passive articular motion may indicate loss of muscle tendon continuity, impaired contractile capacity, or limitation in tendon glide. The effect is observable in the resting hand when the normal cascading posture of the digits is altered, and pathology is assessed through measurement of active motion of those joints spanned by the involved musculotendinous units and through manual muscle testing procedures.[35] Again, relating diagnosis, surgical intervention, and physiologic timing is critical to designing upper extremity splints that affect muscle tendon function. Because healing tendon needs differ according to site of injury, designing splints requires thorough knowledge of tendon healing physiology, biomechanics, and tendon excursion at each joint. For example, a Zone VIII extensor digitorum communis tendon laceration does not need immobilization of IP joints because IP joint motion exerts minimal tension on the repair site. Tensile strength dictates splinting and exercise routines, and regardless of whether the purpose of application is for immobilization, mobilization, restriction, or torque transmission, if extrinsic muscle tendon units are involved, position of adjacent joints is a significant factor. For the hand, not only is the influence of tenodesis effect on distal joints important, the point at which involved tendons cross the wrist should also be identified. At the crossing point, controlling wrist attitude may alter tension on specific tendons. Especially significant during early wound healing, the effect wrist posture has on injured or healing structures influences the selection of splint components and determines splint length and configuration. For example, postoperative splinting is employed to reduce tension on repaired or transferred tendons of the shoulder, elbow, wrist, or hand. When splinting to increase tendon excursion and active joint range of motion, it is also important to consider the position of adjacent, usually proximal, key joints. As noted previously, the underlying cause for limitation in joint range of motion must be carefully analyzed. Capsular or articular pathology often requires less

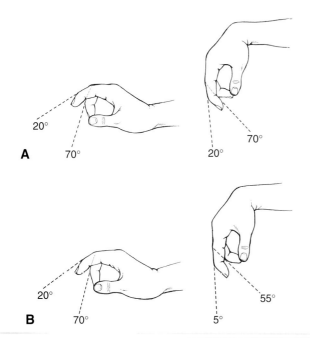

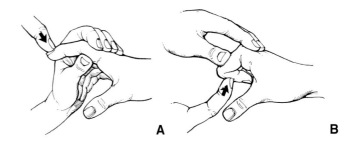

Fig. 5-3   **A,** If stiffness is limited to the joint and periarticular structures, both the range and arc of motion will be unaffected by altered wrist position. **B,** However, if extrinsic musculotendinous units are involved, the arc of motion will remain constant, but range of motion measurements will change as wrist posture is altered.

Fig. 5-4   **A,** If the intrinsic muscles have become tight, full passive flexion of the proximal interphalangeal joint will be absent when the metacarpophalangeal joint is held in extension. **B,** Full passive proximal interphalangeal flexion is possible with the metacarpophalangeal joint in flexion.

complicated splint designs that are classified as ESCS *type 0,* whereas involvement of extrinsic tendons usually necessitates more complicated splints that control adjacent joints and are classified as greater than "0" ESCS types (Fig. 5-5).

Nerve

Both motor and sensory aspect of nerve function must be evaluated when assessing upper extremities for splints. Nerves have predictable patterns of innervation, and disruption of these patterns indicates pathology or anomalous innervation, each of which must be identified and analyzed before a splinting program may begin (Fig. 5-6). The motor capacity of a nerve may be evaluated through EMGs and manual muscle testing procedures. Identifying areas of diminished or absent sensibility is also important to the design and fitting of upper extremity splints, for these areas are especially vulnerable to damage from pressure and friction. Although a splint may be fitted correctly, the lack of sensory feedback from the extremity often results in an absence of the frequent unconscious adjustments normally made by the patient. This leads to tissue breakdown through pressure necrosis, rendering the splint unwearable and useless. Forewarned, the upper extremity specialist may incorporate into the design of the splint wider and longer components, thereby distributing splinting forces

over a greater area and decreasing the potential for pressure and shear. The patient or family must be judicious in visual inspection of the skin several times daily to prevent skin breakdown. NCVs and the Semmes-Weinstein calibrated monofilaments tests are useful tools for identifying areas of sensibility dysfunction (Fig. 5-7). Areas of pain, dysesthesia, and hyperesthesia also should be noted and recorded.

As with tendons, tension on healing neurovascular structures may be controlled through application of splints, allowing minimal tension during early healing stages and progressing to normal joint motion as physiologic timing permits. Careful monitoring and documentation of nerve function are critical to successful splinting regimens. Decreased sensibility or increased pain requires immediate reassessment of the splinting program.

Vascular Status

In addition to vascular studies, volumetric measurements, circumferential measurements, thermal imaging, and biofeedback may be used to assist in monitoring upper extremity vascular status. Skin temperature and color and composite mass of the extremity provide essential clues to understanding the vascular status of a diseased or injured hand or arm. Areas with questionable tissue viability should be

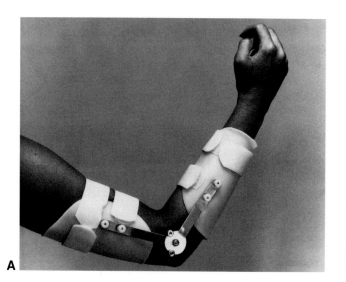
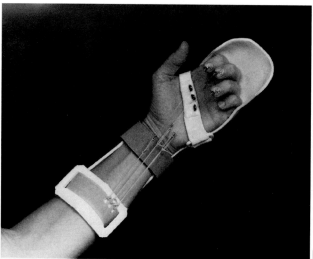

Fig. 5-5   A, Elbow Flexion and Extension restriction splint, type 0 (1) B, Index–small finger extension restriction / index–ring finger flexion mobilization splint, type 1 (13)
Type 0 splints may be indicated for an articular problem that does not involve extrinsic tendons. Injuries involving extrinsic tendons require incorporation of secondary joints as seen in this postoperative splint for a Zone II flexor tendon repair. In this splint, all joints are primary except the wrist. [Courtesy **(A)** Helen Marx, OTR, CHT, Wickenburg, Ariz.; **(B)** Barbara Smith, OTR/L, CHT, Edmond, Okla.]

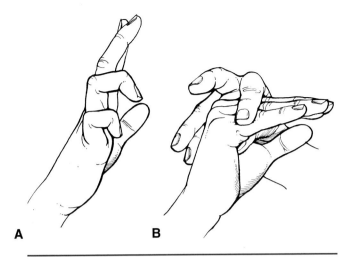

Fig. 5-6 **A,** Lack of innervation of the intrinsic muscles results in an inability to actively extend the interphalangeal joints of the ring and small fingers in ulnar nerve paralysis. **B,** This is due, however, to loss of intrinsic flexion at the metacarpophalangeal joint and concomitant zigzag collapse, rather than pathology of the extrinsic extensor muscle group.

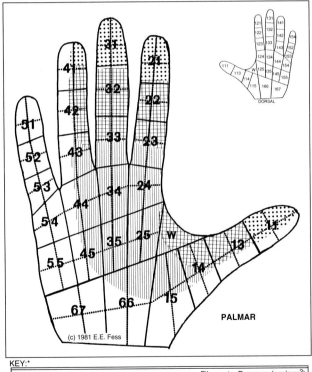

KEY:*

	Filament	Pressure (gm/mm²)
Normal	1.65–2.83	1.45–4.86
Diminished light touch	3.22–3.61	11.1–17.7
Diminished protective sensation	3.84–4.31	19.3–33.1
Loss of protective sensation	4.56–6.65	47.3–439.0
Untestable	6.65	439.0

*Levine, S., Pearsall, G., & Ruderman, R.: J Hand Surg., 3:211, 1978.

Fig. 5-7 Areas of sensibility disruption should be identified before a splinting program is initiated.

carefully defined. Care should be taken to prevent obstruction of venous return and arterial flow with application of a splint. By increasing the area of force application of splint components and by achieving a contiguous fit, splint pressure on the extremity is reduced. Additionally, factors that may affect splint fit, such as local swelling or generalized edema, should be noted and recorded. Splint designs that employ circumferential components or forces that may jeopardize tissue viability should be avoided in extremities that exhibit signs of vascular instability. Areas that depend on newly established collateral circulation and lymphatic drainage should be treated with extreme caution, and splinting measures should be undertaken only after close consultation with the referring physician. As time progresses, the sensitivity of these areas to pressure decreases and splinting and exercise routines may be gradually graded in intensity. Once a splint is fitted, an increase from baseline temperature or volume readings may indicate that too much force is being utilized and an inflammatory reaction is taking place. Conscientious monitoring of alterations in extremity size, temperature, and color provides guidelines as to the physiologic response of the extremity to treatment methods, allowing timely intervention and adjustment of splinting and exercise techniques.

Function

Careful observation of the patient during evaluation sessions assists the examiner in discovering how the patient views his disability and how he uses the extremity. Is the hand/extremity protected or guarded by the patient? Is there reluctance to remove it from a pocket, glove, or dressing? Does he willingly allow examination and touching of the extremity? Is the extremity used spontaneously? Are normal use patterns apparent or are certain parts of the hand avoided as objects are grasped and released? Are proximal joints of the extremity used to substitute for lost or limited distal joint range? Is the manner in which the extremity used altered when vision is occluded? Are callus formations and embedded surface grime noticeable? Does pain seem to be a limiting factor? Are motions smooth and coordinated?

Queries about difficulties encountered during ADL vocational, or avocational tasks may also be illuminated during assessment of general extremity function. Is the patient independent in self-care? Is he employed? Are there tasks he can no longer accomplish at work or at home? If the patient is being considered for a splint, how will its presence affect extremity function on the job and at home? Are the patient's expectations for rehabilitation realistic?

Information gleaned from observation and interviews helps form a general concept of how the extremity is used and the patient's attitude toward the disability. Handedness, dexterity, and coordination tests, ADL and vocational tests, and patient satisfaction surveys further refine understanding through generation of numerical data, which may then be compared to the noninvolved extremity, to scores of normal subjects, or to scores of diagnosis-specific patient populations.

UPPER EXTREMITY ASSESSMENT INSTRUMENTS

Upper extremity evaluation instruments are divided into six basic categories: condition, motion, sensibility, pain, function, and patient satisfaction.

Condition Assessment Instruments

Condition involves the neurovascular system as it pertains to tissue viability, nutrition, inflammation, patency of vessels, and arterial, venous, and lymphatic flow. In addition to observation of the extremity, noninvasive measurement of extremity volume, skin temperature, and arterial pulses more clearly defines the status of skin, subcutaneous tissues, and neurovascular function.

Volume

Based on the principle of water displacement, commercially available volumeters measure composite extremity mass (Fig. 5-8). In 1981 Waylett and Seibly reported the commercial hand volumeter to be accu-

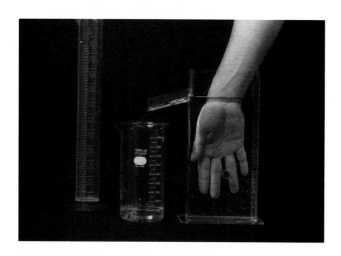

Fig. 5-8   The volumeter measures composite hand mass and has been shown to be accurate to within 10 ml when used according to specifications.

rate to within 10 ml when used according to the manufacturer's specifications.[57] It is important to remember a few basic concepts: (1) volumeters should be newly filled for each patient measurement; (2) use of an aerated hose to fill the tank decreases accuracy; and (3) routine precautions must be taken to avoid patient cross contamination from infected wounds. Although less accurate in assessing extremity mass, circumferential measurements may be taken at predetermined levels using a weighted tape measure or, for smaller joints, external calipers. Reliability of these instruments depends on consistency of placement and tension of the tape or calipers. They provide a quick means of assessment that may be applicable in situations where immersion in water is contraindicated or when only one joint is involved. It should be documented in the chart if jewelry is worn, if compressive dressings are removed immediately before volumeter measurements are taken, or if circumferential measurements are done over dressings, since these circumstances skew measurements, rendering subsequent comparisons invalid. Generally, normal comparison values for either volumetric or circumferential measurements may be obtained from the contralateral extremity so long as it is understood that size differences may preexist (see form on p. 635).

Vessel Patency

The Doppler scanner may be used to map arterial flow through audible ultrasonic response to arterial pulsing; and because of its direct relationship to digital vessel patency, skin temperature may be used to assess tissue viability of the extremity. Temperature biofeedback may also be used to compare cutaneous temperature between the involved and noninvolved extremity.

Motion Assessment Instruments

The measurement of motion involves muscle/tendon continuity, contractile and gliding capacity, neuromuscular communication, and voluntary control. Techniques for evaluating upper extremity motion include goniometric measurements and the determination of isolated muscle strength.

Range of Motion

Goniometric evaluation of the upper extremity is essential to monitoring articular motion and musculotendinous function. Both passive and active motion should be recorded using an appropriate size goniometer with a 0° neutral starting position, as recommended by the American Academy of Orthopaedic Surgeons (AAOS). Digital motion may be measured

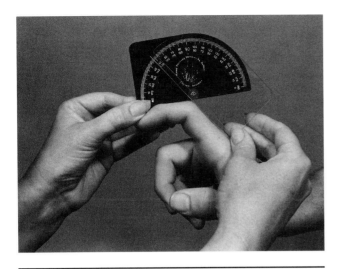

Fig. 5-9   Either lateral or dorsal placement of the goniometer is appropriate, provided that consistency is maintained for subsequent examinations.

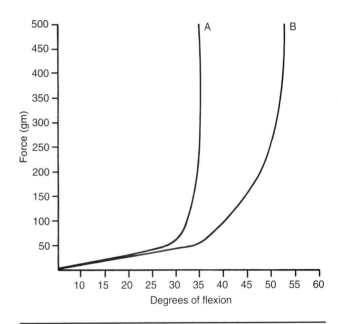

Fig. 5-10   A shortened goniometer arm allows accurate measurement of distal interphalangeal (DIP) joints when assessing composite digital flexion.

Fig. 5-11   This torque range of motion graph indicates that the proximal interphalangeal joint of the long finger (B) has more passive "give" than that of the index finger (A), indicating that the long finger may respond more readily to mobilization splinting.

from either the lateral or dorsal aspect of the joint, provided that consistency of placement is maintained throughout the examination and during subsequent tests. Most upper extremity specialists use dorsal placement of goniometers unless considerable swelling around the joint is present (Fig. 5-9). Proximal joints should be maintained in neutral position with a neutral wrist position especially important due to its effect on digital joint position. Deviation from established ROM measurement protocol must be documented. Normal motion values are obtained from measurement of the contralateral extremity or from norms developed by the AAOS.[1] Although goniometric measurement is not technically a standardized assessment tool, its reliability and validity have been studied extensively.* Composite digital motion values may be computed as total active motion and total passive motion.[3,4] Total active motion (TAM) equals the summation of active flexion measurements of the metacarpophalangeal, proximal interphalangeal, and distal interphalangeal joints of a digit, minus the active extension deficits of the same three joints. Total passive motion (TPM) is computed in a similar manner using passive motion values (Fig. 5-10). Total motion reflects both the extension and flexion capacities of a single digit and is expressed as a single numeric value (see Figures 2-5 in Appendix B, and Figures 1-3 in Appendix C).

Brand's technique of torque range of motion (TQROM) refines passive range of motion measurement by applying predetermined, consistent, and incremental amounts of force to stiffened joints and

measuring resultant passive joint motions with a goniometer.[12,13] Once measured, a torque/length curve may be constructed for each joint by plotting coordinates on a graph, and the relative degree of stiffness of the joints may be visualized (Fig. 5-11). An electronic device for measuring joint stiffness has also been developed.[41]

Muscle Strength

Isolated muscle strength through manual muscle testing is used to define effects of peripheral nerve

---

*References 11, 22, 27, 29, 30, 42, 43, 51, 52.

or musculotendinous dysfunction in the upper extremity. It is also used to identify potential donor muscles for tendon transfers. Although criteria for grading muscle strength have been improved, portions of the test are subject to examiner interpretation. Patient substitution patterns also decrease test reliability. To enhance inter-rater reliability, it is important that all members of the team use the same method of conducting and interpreting manual muscle examinations. Numerous grading systems currently exist, but the two most frequently used are Seddon's numerical system of 0 through 5 and the ratings of zero, trace, poor, fair, good, and normal recommended by the Committee on After-Effects, National Foundation of Infantile Paralysis, Inc. The latter is further refined by a plus-minus system for accomplishment of partial ranges (see Appendix B-8).

Sensibility Assessment Instruments

Sensibility relies on neural continuity, impulse transmission, receptor acuity, and cortical perception. Assessment of sensibility may be divided into sudomotor/sympathetic response and the abilities to detect, discriminate, quantify, and recognize stimuli (see Appendix B-9).

Sympathetic Response

Moberg's ninhydrin test and the wrinkle test identify areas of disturbance of sweat secretion after peripheral nerve disruption. The involvement of sympathetic fibers in a peripheral nerve injury results in areas of dry denervated skin that do not react to environmental warmth (dry or wet) by sweating or wrinkling. The ninhydrin and wrinkle tests measure physiologic reactions that cannot be controlled by the patient. Onne (1962) and Phelps and Walker (1977) have shown that these sympathetic responses correlate positively with sensibility return only in early, completely transected peripheral nerves.[45,47] This significantly reduces the validity and reliability of these tests. While inclusion of a sympathetic response test in an assessment battery for use with specific patients, e.g., children, patients with language problems, or patients whose motivation may be suspect, the inclusion criterion of early complete transected nerve is paramount. If this criterion is met, sympathetic response tests are helpful, but they should not be relied on as a primary sensibility assessment instrument.

Detection

Detection, the most fundamental level on the sensibility continuum, requires the patient to perceive a single-point stimulus from normally occurring atmospheric background stimuli. Based on von Frey's work

in the late 1800s, the Semmes-Weinstein calibrated monofilaments are available in a 20-filament set or a minikit of five filaments. The S-W nylon filaments are graded in diameter and individually attached to handles. The amount of force transmitted by each monofilament is directly related to its length and diameter (Fig. 5-12). As gradually increasing pressure is applied, each filament bends at a specific force, thereby controlling and limiting the magnitude of the touch/pressure stimulus. This results in a spectrum of calibrated light to heavy forces that assess cutaneous touch capabilities in patients who exhibit peripheral sensory dysfunction. The smallest diameter filament perceived by the patient within a designated area of the upper extremity is recorded. As testing instruments the monofilaments are unique in their ability to control the amount of force applied (see Appendix B-10).[2,6-9]

Another instrument, the vibrometer, is advocated by some. Unfortunately, nearly all currently available vibrometry instruments, including computerized vibrometers, lack stimulus pressure control. Concentrated instrumentation research is needed before vibrometry may be used with confidence in clinical situations.

Discrimination

Discrimination, the second level in the sensibility assessment continuum, assesses a patient's capacity to perceive stimulus A from stimulus B. This requires detection of each stimulus as a separate entity and the ability to distinguish between the two. Discrimination requires finer reception acuity and more

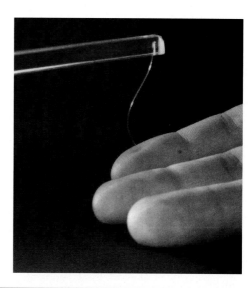

Fig. 5-12 Depending on the diameter of the filament, the Semmes-Weinstein calibrated monofilaments control the amount of force applied as light touch/pressure.

judgment on the part of the patient than first-level detection does.

Weber's two-point discrimination test is the most commonly used method of assessing sensibility of the upper extremity. Affording better accuracy and consistency, specialized commercial, handheld, two-point instruments have replaced the once used unfolded paperclip. With the instrument tips oriented longitudinally on the digit, the examiner randomly applies one or two points to the hand, relying on absence of skin blanching to control the amount of force applied. Following each stimulus, the patient reports whether he feels one or two points. The narrowest tip width at which the patient makes 7 of 10 correct responses is the distance reported. (Note: The number of correct responses required may vary slightly from examiner to examiner.) Bell and Buford reported that, even with experienced examiners, the amount of force applied between one and two points easily exceeds the resolution or sensitivity threshold for normal sensation.[6,8] They also noted that the tremendous variance in pressures applied resulted in poor levels of interrater reliability. This perhaps explains some of the lack of agreement in reporting discriminatory function.

Quantification

Quantification is the third level on the sensory capacity hierarchy. This requires grading stimuli according to their perceived level of density. A patient may be asked which of several alternatives is roughest, most irregular, or smoothest; or she might be required to rank the items from smoothest to roughest. Although there are no tests specific to this area currently available, some of the sensory reeducation techniques incorporate the basic concepts of quantification. For example, Barber's dowel textures have reliability studies on normal subjects, representing an important initial step toward standardization.[58]

Recognition/Identification

Recognition, the final and most complicated sensibility level, is based on the patient's ability to identify objects. Seddon's coin test and Porter's letter test are examples of instruments that use identification of items or shapes to assess functional sensibility. The picking-up test described by Moberg may also be adapted to include identification of picked-up objects when vision is occluded.

Pain Assessment Instruments

Pain often determines patient compliance for splint wearing. Although subjective in nature, measurement of pain is important to helping patients achieve their maximum rehabilitation potential. Visual analogue scales (VAS) and numerical rating scales (NRS) have been shown to have good reliability for a wide range of diagnoses. The McGill Pain Questionnaire is also frequently used to define pain. These self-ratings are easy to administer and are viewed positively by patients. Incorporation of a pain assessment test allows clinicians to better understand their patients and more appropriately design, fit, and adapt splints to meet the special circumstances of individual patients.* Additionally, high reliability has been reported for several patient satisfaction questionnaires that assess symptom severity, including pain (see Appendix B-11).

Function Assessment Instruments

Hand function reflects the integration of all systems and is measured in terms of handedness tests, grip/pinch, coordination and dexterity, and ability to participate in activities of daily living and vocational and avocational tasks.

The Waterloo Handedness Questionnaire (WHQ) is a 32-item self-administered questionnaire that has high reliability[46,53] and has been shown to be more specific and accurate than the traditional self-report for determining handedness.[36,40] Further, when the WHQ is correlated with grip strength, it was found that in individuals with greater polarization of hand preference (i.e., always right or always left) there was a statistically significant greater difference between their dominant and nondominant grip strengths than in individuals who were less polarized (i.e., ambidextrous or nearly ambidextrous).[39] Use of the WHQ has far-reaching ramifications for future clinical and research investigation in that it refines understanding of hand preference as it relates to function.

Grip Strength

A commercially available hydraulic dynamometer (Fig. 5-13) may be used to measure grip strength. In a study of reliability of grip assessment instruments by the California Medical Association, the Jamar dynamometer was recommended because of its validity and consistency of measurement. Studying the effect of wrist position on grip, Pryce reported the strongest grip measurements occurred with the wrist in 0-15° extension.[48] The American Society for Surgery of the Hand and the American Society of Hand Therapists recommend that the second handle

---

*References 14, 25, 28, 33, 44, 50, 55.

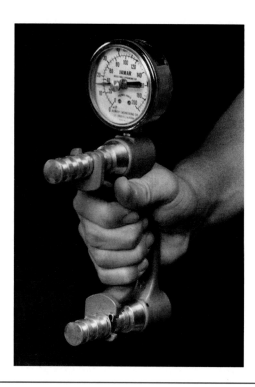

Fig. 5-13   Maximum grip strength depends on the size of the object being grasped. Normal values for the five handle positions form a bell-shaped curve.

position be used in determining grip strength and that the average of three trials be recorded.[3,4] AMA guidelines require that grip be recorded in kilograms.[2] Normal adult grip strength changes according to the size of the object being grasped. Therefore grip scores for the five consecutive Jamar handle positions create a bell curve, with the first position being the least advantageous for strong grip, followed by the fifth and fourth positions. Strongest normal adult grip values occur at the second and third handle positions. It is important to understand that inconsistent handle position or inaccurate dynamometer calibration may be erroneously interpreted as advances or declines in patient progress (see Appendix B-7).[24]

Pinch Strength

Using a commercially available pinchometer, three types of pinch may be assessed. These include (1) prehension of the thumb pulp to the lateral aspect of the index middle phalanx[31] (key, lateral, or pulp-to-side); (2) pulp of the thumb to pulps of the index and long fingers (three-jaw chuck, three-point chuck); and (3) thumb tip to tip of index finger (tip-to-tip). The mean or average value of three trials is recorded as recommended by the American Society for Surgery of the Hand, and comparisons may be made with scores from the opposite hand. Standardized terminology is needed for describing pinch. After identifying more

than 200 terms for pinch in the medical literature, Casanova and Grunert developed a logical descriptive system based on digital contact.[16]

Coordination and Dexterity

Standardized tests that measure upper extremity dexterity and coordination are available in several levels of difficulty.

The Jebsen hand function test[32,49] assesses gross coordination and dexterity and is inexpensive to assemble and easy to administer and score. It consists of seven subtests: (1) writing, (2) card turning, (3) picking up small objects, (4) simulated feeding, (5) stacking, (6) picking up large lightweight objects, and (7) picking up large heavy objects. Jebson norms are categorized according to maximum time, hand dominance, age, and sex. The Jebson has been used in several studies to determine effectiveness of various types of splints[54] and appropriateness of splint application.[15]

Another example of a standardized test that measures gross coordination and dexterity is the Minnesota Rate of Manipulation Test (MRMT). Five functions are included in the MRMT: (1) placing, (2) turning, (3) displacing, (4) one-handed turning and placing, and (5) two-handed turning and placing. Norms of this instrument are based on more than 11,000 subjects.

The Purdue Pegboard evaluates finer coordination than the previously discussed instruments. It requires prehension of small pins, washers, and collars. Measurement categories are divided into (1) right hand, (2) left hand, (3) both hands, (4) right, left, and both, and (5) assembly. Normative data are defined according to gender and type of job.

The Crawford Small Parts Dexterity Test adds a more difficult dimension to measurement of upper extremity coordination and dexterity. This test requires subjects to control not only their hands but also small tools, such as tweezers and a screwdriver, and correlates positively with vocational activities that demand very fine coordination skills.

Other upper extremity coordination and dexterity tests are available. These should be carefully evaluated according to the criteria for standardized tests discussed earlier in this chapter to ensure that they measure accurately and consistently. Although many tests claim to be standardized, few actually meet the requisites.

Activities of Daily Living, Vocation, and Avocation

Observation and interviews identify specific tasks related to activities of daily living and vocational and avocational skills the patient is not able to perform or has difficulty performing. Once identified, each task must be carefully analyzed to discover why the patient is experiencing problems. Is range of motion sufficient? Does lack of strength influence performance, or is there a problem with coordination? Eventually a pattern of deficit becomes apparent, and the direction and emphasis of a treatment program begin to emerge. According to individual patient requirements, splints may be designed to increase range of motion, to restrict motion, to substitute for absent muscle power, to transmit torque, or to serve as a base of attachment for adapted equipment.

The Flinn Performance Screening Tool (FPST) is a self-administered functional test consisting of more than 300 laminated photographs in two volumes detailing ADL, vocational, and avocational tasks.[26] This test is important in that it has high reliability and represents an early bridge toward accurate documentation of function. The Valpar Work Samples are standardized with independent reliability and validity for the different tests. Both the FPST and the Valpar upper extremity work samples are excellent test instruments for determining how application of splints affects upper extremity function.

Other tests, including computerized tests, are available but most have not been studied for instrument reliability. One, the BTE Work Simulator, has been shown to produce inconsistent resistance in the dynamic mode both within and between machines, rendering it inappropriate for assessments requiring consistency of stimulus.[17,20,21]

Patient Satisfaction

Testing of patient satisfaction has become an integral part of rehabilitation endeavors. Just as other test instruments must meet instrumentation criteria, so too must patient satisfaction assessment tools meet these criteria. Satisfaction surveys are often in the form of patient-completed questionnaires. Current symptom/satisfaction tools that are used in evaluating patients with upper extremity injury or dysfunction include the Medical Outcomes Study 36-Item Health Survey (SF-36),[10] the Upper Extremities Disabilities of Arm, Shoulder, and Hand (DASH),[5] the Michigan Hand Outcomes Questionnaire (MHQ),[18,19] and the Severity of Symptoms and Functional Status in Carpal Tunnel Syndrome questionnaire.[10,37]

■ OTHER CONSIDERATIONS

Additional factors that must be evaluated to create splint designs that meet the unique requirements of each individual include the patient's age, motivation, ability to understand and carry out directions,

response to injury, and probable response to the application and wearing of a splint. For example, splinting materials or designs for adult patients may not be appropriate for a thumb-sucking toddler whose hand is frequently moist. A complicated splint could further confuse a forgetful geriatric patient, and a shy teenager may not comply with a schedule that requires wearing a splint to school.

Because splinting materials and procedures are often expensive, economic variables should also be taken into consideration. Is the patient able to bear the burden of these expenses? Are there less costly alternatives? Will the patient be able to schedule return visits for splint adjustments around family and occupational responsibilities? Will third-party payers authorize follow-up visits for splint adjustments?

The preferences and philosophic orientation of the members of the rehabilitation team significantly influence splint design. Although often taken for granted and overlooked, these factors must also be identified and evaluated. Why is a given splint design "traditionally" applied? Can a more efficacious splint be designed? Does this splint design really meet the needs of this patient, or is it simply more expedient for those involved in the construction and fitting process?

Finally, third-party reimbursement factors are increasingly playing greater and greater roles in upper extremity rehabilitation intervention. How is managed care affecting splint selection and use? Are there splints that consistently produce good results at less cost?

■ SUMMARY

Formal assessment procedures provide data upon which splinting and exercise programs are created and tailored to meet the unique requirements of individual patients. Assessment also identifies and directs the need for adjustments as changes occur and assigns numerical value to treatment results. Without the use of evaluation tools that measure consistently and accurately, definition of pathology and identification of change are often nebulous and indistinct. This may cause splint application to be more harmful than beneficial to the patient. Splint designs should not only reflect the physical requirements of a diseased or injured upper extremity, they should also satisfy individual patient variables. Assessment data are the foundation on which splints are created and used; without this essential information splints should not be designed, constructed, or fitted. The expanded Splint Classification System, the Waterloo Handedness Questionnaire, and the Flinn Performance Screening Tool are important instruments that, along with traditional measurement tools, will assist clinicians in providing splinting solutions that truly meet individual patient requirements.

REFERENCES

1. AAOS: *Joint motion: method of measuring and recording*, The Academy, 1965, Chicago.
2. American Medical Association: The upper extremities. In Cocchiarella L, Andersson G: *Guides to the evaluation of permanent impairment*, AMA Press, 2000, Chicago.
3. American Society for Surgery of the Hand: *The hand: examination and diagnosis*, Churchill Livingstone, 1983, New York.
4. American Society of Hand Therapists: *American Society of Hand Therapists Clinical Assessment Recommendations*, American Society of Hand Therapists, Chicago, 1992.
5. Amadio PC: Outcomes assessment in hand surgery. What's new? *Clin Plast Surg* 24(1):91-4, 1997.
6. Bell-Krotoski J, Buford W: The force/time relationship of clinically used sensory testing instruments, *J Hand Ther* 1:76, 1988.
7. Bell-Krotoski J, Tomancik E: The repeatability of testing with Semmes-Weinstein monofilaments, *J Hand Surg* [Am] 12(1):155-61, 1987.
8. Bell-Krotoski J, Buford WL, Jr.: The force/time relationship of clinically used sensory testing instruments, *J Hand Ther* 10(4):297-309, 1997.
9. Bell-Krotoski J, Fess EE, Figarola JH, Hiltz D: Threshold detection and Semmes-Weinstein monofilaments, *J Hand Ther* 8(2):155-62, 1995.
10. Bessette L, Keller RB, Lew RA, et al: Prognostic value of a hand symptom diagram in surgery for carpal tunnel syndrome, *J Rheumatol* 24(4):726-34, 1997.
11. Boone DC, Azen SP, Lin CM, et al: Reliability of goniometric measurements, *Phys Ther* 58(11):1355-90, 1978.
12. Brand PW, Hollister A: *Clinical mechanics of the hand*, ed 2, Mosby, 1993, St. Louis.
13. Breger-Lee D, Voelker E, Giurintano D, et al: Reliability of torque range of motion: a preliminary study, *J Hand Ther* 6(1):29-34, 1993.
14. Carey SJ, Turpin C, Smith J, et al: Improving pain management in an acute care setting. The Crawford Long Hospital of Emory University experience, *Orthop Nurs* 16(4):29-36, 1997.
15. Carlson JD, Trombly CA: The effect of wrist immobilization on performance of the Jebsen Hand Function Test, *Am J Occup Ther* 37(3):167-75, 1983.
16. Casanova J, Grunert B: Adult prehension: patterns and nomenclature for pinches, *J Hand Ther* 2:231-44, 1989.
17. Cetinok EM, Renfro RR, Coleman EF: A pilot study of the reliability of the dynamic mode of one BTE Work Simulator, *J Hand Ther* 8(3):199-205, 1995.
18. Chung KC, Hamill JB, Walters MR, et al: The Michigan Hand Outcomes Questionnaire (MHQ): assessment of responsiveness to clinical change, *Ann Plast Surg* 42(6):619-22, 1999.
19. Chung KC, Pillsbury MS, Walters MR, et al: Reliability and validity testing of the Michigan Hand Outcomes Questionnaire, *J Hand Surg* [Am] 23(4):575-87, 1998.
20. Coleman EF, Renfro RR, Cetinok EM, et al: Reliability of the manual dynamic mode of the Baltimore Therapeutic Equipment Work Simulator, *J Hand Ther* 9(3):223-37, 1996.
21. Dunipace KR: Reliability of the BTE work simulator dynamic mode [letter], *J Hand Ther* 8(1):42-3, 1995.
22. Eliasziw M, Young SL, Woodbury MG, et al: Statistical methodology for the concurrent assessment of interrater and intrarater reliability: using goniometric measurements as an example, *Phys Ther* 74(8):777-88, 1994.
23. Fess EE: Convergence points of normal fingers in individual flexion and simultaneous flexion, *J Hand Ther* 2:12-9, 1989.
24. Fess EE: Documentation: essentials of an upper extremity assessment battery. In Mackin EJ, Callahan AD, Skirven TM, et al: *Rehabilitation of the hand*, ed 5, Mosby, 2001, St. Louis.
25. Flaherty SA: Pain measurement tools for clinical practice and research, *AANA J* 64(2):133-40, 1996.
26. Flinn S: *The Flinn Performance Screening Tool*, Functional Visions, Inc. 1997.
27. Gajdosik R, Bohannon R: Clinical measurement of range of motion: review of goniometry emphasizing reliability and validity, *Phys Ther* 67(12):1867-72, 1987.
28. Goossens PH, Heemskerk B, van Tongeren J, et al: Reliability and sensitivity to change of various measures of hand function in relation to treatment of synovitis of the metacarpophalangeal joint in rheumatoid arthritis, *Rheumatology* (Oxford) 39(8):909-13, 2000.
29. Grohmann JE: Comparison of two methods of goniometry, *Phys Ther* 63(6):922-5, 1983.
30. Hillenbrandt F, Duval E, Moore M: The measurement of joint motion: III reliability of goniometry, *Phys Ther Rev* 29:302, 1949.
31. Ho RW, Chang SY, Wang CW, et al: Grip and key pinch strength: norms for 15- to 22-year-old Chinese students, *Chung Hua I Hsueh Tsa Chih* (Taipei) 63:21-7, 2000.
32. Jebsen RH, Taylor N, Trieschmann RB, et al: An objective and standardized test of hand function, *Arch Phys Med Rehabil* 50:311-9, 1969.
33. Joos E, Peretz A, Beguin S, et al: Reliability and reproducibility of visual analogue scale and numeric rating scale for therapeutic evaluation of pain in rheumatic patients, *J Rheumatol* 18(8):1269-70, 1991.
34. Kagel EM, Rayan GM: Thumb digital neuropathy caused by splinting, *J Okla State Med Assoc* 93(9):435-6, 2000.
35. Kendall H, Kendall F, Wadsworth G: *Muscle testing and function*, ed 4, Williams & Wilkins, 1993, Baltimore.
36. Kersten K, Zichella D, Bear-Lehman J, et al: *A correlational study between self-reported hand preference and results of the Waterloo Handedness Questionnaire; Occupational Therapy*, Columbia University, 1995, New York.
37. Levine DW, Simmons BP, Koris MJ, et al: A self-administered questionnaire for the assessment of severity of symptoms and functional status in carpal tunnel syndrome, *J Bone Joint Surg Am* 75(11):1585-92, 1993.
38. Lister G: *The hand: diagnosis and indications*, ed 2, Churchill Livingstone, 1984, New York.
39. Lui P, Fess EE: *Comparison of dominant and nondominant grip strength: the critical role of the Waterloo Handedness Questionnaire*, Submitted for publication.
40. Lui P, Fess EE: *Establishing hand dominance: self-report versus the Waterloo Handedness Questionnaire*, Submitted for publication.
41. Luster S, Patterson P, Cioffi W, et al: An evaluation device for quantifying joint stiffness in the burned hand, *J Burn Care Rehab* 11(4):312-7, 1990.
42. MacDermid JC, Chesworth BM, Patterson S, et al: Intratester and intertester reliability of goniometric measurement of passive lateral shoulder rotation, *J Hand Ther* 12(3):187-92, 1999.
43. Mayerson NH, Milano RA: Goniometric measurement reliability in physical medicine, *Arch Phys Med Rehabil* 65(2):92-4, 1984.
44. Miller MD, Ferris DG: Measurement of subjective phenomena in primary care research: the Visual Analogue Scale, *Fam Pract Res J* 13(1):15-24, 1993.

45. Onne L: Recovery of sensibility and sudomotor activity in the hand after severe injury, *Acta Chir Scand* [Suppl] 1:300, 1962.

46. Peters M, Murphy K: Cluster analysis reveals at least three, and possibly five distinct handedness groups, *Neuropsychologia* 30:373-80, 1992.

47. Phelps P, Walker E: Comparison of the finger wrinkling test results to established sensory tests in peripheral nerve injury, *Am J Occup Ther* 31:565, 1977.

48. Pryce J: The wrist position between neutral and ulnar deviation that facilitates maximum power grip, *J Biomech* 13(6):505-11, 1980.

49. Rider B, Linden C: Comparison of standardized and non-standardized administration of the Jebsen Hand Function Test, *J Hand Ther* 1:121-6, 1988.

50. Roach KE, Brown MD, Dunigan KM, et al: Test-retest reliability of patient reports of low back pain, *J Orthop Sports Phys Ther* 26(5):253-9, 1997.

51. Rothstein J, Miller P, Roetiger R: Goniometric reliability in a clinical setting. Elbow and knee measurements, *Phys Ther* 63(10):1611-5, 1983.

52. Sabari JS, Maltzev I, Lubarsky D, et al: Goniometric assessment of shoulder range of motion: comparison of testing in supine and sitting positions, *Arch Phys Med Rehabil* 79(6):647-51, 1998.

53. Steenhuis RE, Bryden MP, Schwartz M, et al: Reliability of hand preference items and factors, *J Clin Exp Neuropsychol* 12(6):921-30, 1990.

54. Stern EB: Grip strength and finger dexterity across five styles of commercial wrist orthoses [published erratum appears in *Am J Occup Ther* 50(3):193, 1996], *Am J Occup Ther* 50(1):32-8, 1996.

55. Triano JJ, McGregor M, Cramer GD, et al: A comparison of outcome measures for use with back pain patients: results of a feasibility study, *J Manipulative Physiol Ther* 16(2):67-73, 1993.

56. Tubiana R, Thomine J, Mackin E: *Examination of the hand and wrist*, Mosby, 1996, St. Louis.

57. Waylett-Rendal J, Seibly D: A study of the accuracy of a commercially available volumeter, *J Hand Ther* 4:10-3, 1991.

58. Yerxa EJ, Barber LM, Diaz O, et al: Development of a hand sensitivity test for the hypersensitive hand, *Am J Occup Ther* 37(3):176-81, 1983.

PART THREE

Principles

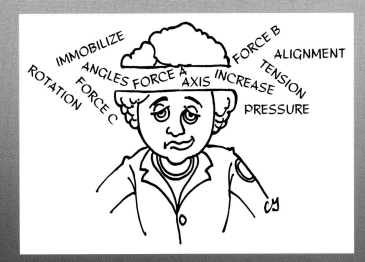

CHAPTER 6

Mechanical Principles

Chapter Outline

Splinting requires the application of external forces to the extremity; therefore it is essential to understand the basic mechanical principles involved in the design, construction, and fitting of all upper extremity splints. Mechanical concepts provide the framework upon which splints function. Splints are ineffective and may be harmful when mechanical principles are ignored or misunderstood. Many therapists have learned the basic concepts of mechanics through trial and error, deductively choosing an approach that yields the most favorable result. Few, however, have the opportunity, expertise, or time to specifically analyze the differences among the many available options. Physicians, although usually possessing a more formal understanding of biomechanics, frequently do not apply this knowledge to splinting in clinical situations and may accept without question a poorly functioning splint that will ultimately produce less favorable results.

The purpose of this chapter is to integrate material from the field of mechanical engineering with the fundamental knowledge of the medical specialist as it pertains to splinting. To clarify the mechanical concepts involved, scale diagrams, force arrows, and simple formulas illustrate the basic principles. For a more in-depth explanation, additional mathematics equations are presented in Appendix E. Gravitational forces and multiple splint components have not been included in the scale diagrams included in this chapter so that fundamental principles may be emphasized and further clarified.

■ PRINCIPLES

Understand Basic Force Systems

Mechanically, splints operate on one of two force systems regardless of their external configurations.

161

Most splints used in upper extremity clinical practice apply consistent, linear oriented, three-point pressure systems to affect joint motion. These splints incorporate three parallel reciprocal forces with the proximal and distal forces oriented in the same direction and the middle reciprocal force oriented in the opposite direction (Fig. 6-1, *A,B*).[9-12,14] Designated as "articular" by the ESCS,[1] three-point pressure splints influence joint motion through immobilization, mobilization, restriction, or torque transmission forces. In contrast, systems of multiple opposing two-point pressures characterize coaptation splints (Fig. 6-1, *C*).[21,22] Coaptation splints are circumferential in design and are usually, but not always, classified as nonarticular splints because they do not influence joint motion. Defined by the segments upon which they act, coaptation splints provide specialized support to healing structures including repaired digital pulleys, stable fractures, and soft tissues damaged from overuse or repetitive stress. Understanding the elemental foundation for splint function is absolutely essential to all splinting endeavors.

Increase the Area of Force Application

Since splinting materials are, to varying degrees, rigid, their improper application to the extremity may cause damage to the cutaneous surface and underlying soft tissue as a result of excessive pressure. Problems from pressure occur most often in areas where there is minimal subcutaneous tissue to disperse pressure, such as over bony prominences, or in areas where the inherent structure of the splint predisposes to increased pressure of mechanical counterforces.

The formula

$$\text{Pressure} = \frac{\text{Total force}}{\text{Area of force application}}$$

indicates that a force of 25 gm applied over an area of 1 cm by 1 cm would result in a pressure of 0.25 gm per square millimeter. If, however, the same 25 gm of force were distributed over an area of 5 cm by 5 cm, the pressure per square millimeter would be decreased to 0.01 gm, or $\frac{1}{25}$ the pressure per square millimeter. In other words, increasing the area of force application decreases the pressure.

Clinically, this has the following implications: (1) wider, longer splints are more comfortable than short, narrow splints (Fig. 6-2); (2) rolled edges on the proximal and distal aspect of a palmar splint and the distal aspect of a dorsal splint cause less pressure than do straight edges (Fig. 6-3); (3) continuous uniform pressure over a bony prominence is preferable to unequal pressure on the prominence (Fig. 6-4); and (4) a contiguous fit is of paramount importance (Fig. 6-5, *A*).

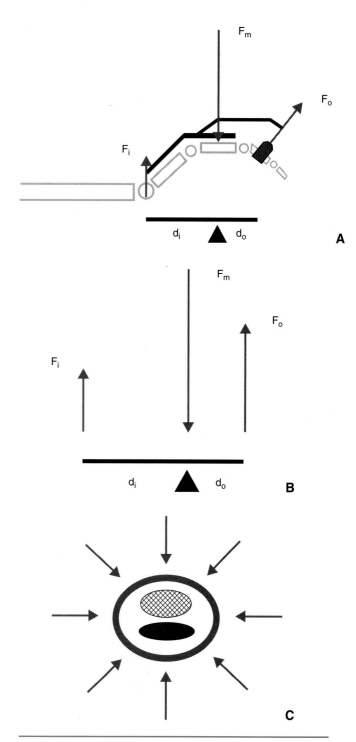

Fig. 6-1   **A,B,** Splints with three-point pressure systems have a middle reciprocal force, the magnitude (F_m) of which is the sum of the opposing proximal (F_i) and distal (F_o) forces. d_i = input distance; d_o = output distance. **C,** With circumferential configurations, coaptation splints do not have a middle reciprocal force. (From Fess EE: Splints: mechanics versus convention, *J Hand Ther* 8(2):124-30, 1995.)

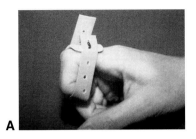

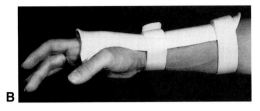

Fig. 6-2 **A, Index finger IP flexion mobilization splint, type 0 (2) B, Wrist extension mobilization splint, type 0 (1)**
A, A dorsal phalangeal bar of thermoplastic disseminates pressure over the dorsum of the phalanx. **B,** With minimized pressure forces and improved mechanical factors, patient comfort is enhanced by splints with greater contact area.

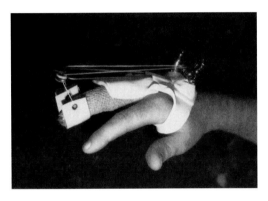

Fig. 6-3 **Long–ring finger PIP extension mobilization splint, type 2 (6)**
Rolled edges allow for dissemination of pressure over a greater area, as illustrated on the distal edges of this splint. (Courtesy Kathryn Schultz, OTR, CHT, Orlando, Fla.)

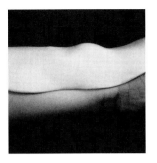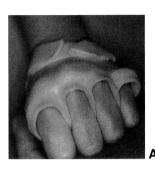

Fig. 6-4 **B, Index–small finger MP flexion restriction splint, type 0 (4)**
A congruous fit over bony prominences will reduce the possibility of soft tissue damage by evenly dispersing pressure forces over a larger area.

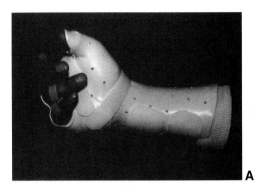

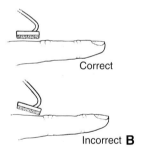

Fig. 6-5 **A, Index–small finger MP flexion, thumb CMC radial abduction and MP flexion immobilization / thumb IP extension restriction splint, type 1 (8) \\ Small finger MP supination, PIP extension and flexion torque transmission splint, type 2 (4)**
A, Designed to facilitate adjustments as edema diminishes, this two-piece metacarpal fracture splint has excellent contiguous fit. **B,** To reduce pressure, the full surface area of a dorsal phalangeal bar should contact the dorsum or the proximal phalanx. This is one of the few components where padding is almost always mandatory. [Courtesy (**A**) Lin Beribak, OTR/L, CHT, Chicago, Ill.]

While this applies to all parts of a splint that are in contact with soft tissue, it is especially important where splint components are narrow and the resultant force is great (Fig. 6-5, *B*). Generally, a continuous force applied to the extremity should not exceed 50 gm per square centimeter.[6-8] Pressure on underlying soft tissues is decreased by attaining contiguous fit of splint components that are both wide and long (Fig. 6-6, *A,B*), but hand and upper extremity function is contingent on freedom of joint motion. While longer, wider splints decrease pressure, a judicious balance must be attained between diminishing pressure to splinted

areas and allowing full, unencumbered motion to unsplinted joints and segments.

The addition of an elastomer lining to a splint helps provide a close-fitting support surface for the hand and diminishes pressure through excellent contiguous

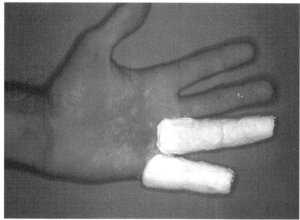

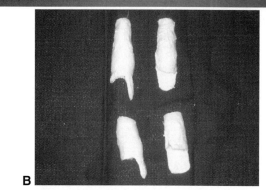

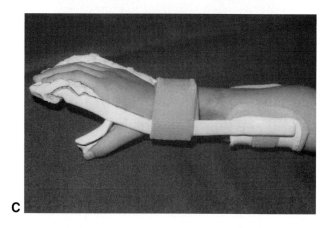

Fig. 6-6   A, B, Ring finger IP extension mobilization splint, type 0 (2) \\ Small finger IP extension mobilization splint, type 0 (2). C, Index–small finger extension, thumb CMC palmar abduction and MP-IP extension mobilization splint, type 1 (16)
A,B, The proximal palmar extension on these IP mobilization splints increases splint mechanical advantage and decreases pressure. **C,** Providing a contiguous fit, an elastomere lining may be used to decrease splint pressure in a difficult-to-fit extremity. [Courtesy **(A,B)** Christopher Bochenek, OTR/L, CHT, Cincinnati, OH; **(C)** Kimiko Shiina, PhD, OTR/L, Yokohama, Japan.]

fit (Fig. 6-6, *C*). Padded materials such as heavy felt or foam rubber also give uniform pressure distribution because of their inherent properties and are valuable in reducing pressure in areas where the forces are great and splint components are narrow. Padding may

be appropriate in such instances, but the zealous use of padding is never a substitute for care in designing, fabricating, and fitting splints.

Using an increased area of application to disperse the forces causing pressure is also important in the construction of a splint. Rounded corners and smooth splint edges not only increase splint cosmesis, they diminish the effects of force on the splint material (Fig. 6-7) and help decrease excessive pressure on underlying skin.

Increase Mechanical Advantage

The design and construction of splints should be adapted to include use of favorable force systems. Many splints fail because of patient discomfort or because of fractured components. These problems may result from inattention to the lever systems at play between the splint and the extremity or between individual splint parts.

Mechanically, splints are simple machines, levers, that work in equilibrium. Incorporating forces, axis of rotation, moment arms, and resistances, splints are predictable and balanced systems. For example, if a splinted forearm, wrist, and hand are viewed as a parallel force system with the wrist being the axis (A), the hand being the weight or resistance (F_i), and the forearm providing the counterforce to the force (F_o) of the proximal end of the forearm trough of the splint, the splint itself is considered a first-class lever (Fig.

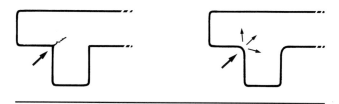

Fig. 6-7   Rounded internal corners increase splint durability by dissipating forces.

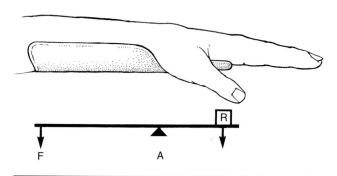

Fig. 6-8   **Wrist neutral immobilization splint, type 0 (1)**
Many splints may be functionally classified as first-class levers. *F,* Force; *A,* axis; *R,* resistance.

6-8) and may be further analyzed as to force lines of action, moment arms, and resultant forces. When the wrist is in neutral position, the forearm trough works as a force arm (FA), the perpendicular distance between the axis and the force line of action (FLA). The palmar metacarpal bar functions as the resistance arm (RA), the perpendicular distance between the axis and resistance line of action (RLA) (Fig. 6-9). If the weight of the average adult hand is approximately 0.9 pound, and if lengths of the forearm trough (d_i) and palmar support (d_o) are 8 inches and $2\frac{1}{2}$ inches, respectively, the resultant force at the proximal end of the splint may be computed using the formula

$$F_i \times d_i = F_0 \times d_0$$
$$F_i = \frac{F_0 \times d_0}{d_i}$$
$$= \frac{0.9 \times 2.5}{8}$$
$$= \frac{2.25}{8}$$
$$= 0.28 \text{ pound}$$

If, however, the forearm trough (FA) were only 4 inches in length and the palmar support and resistance remained unchanged, the force at the proximal end of the splint would be twice as great (Fig. 6-10), resulting in patient discomfort and considerably magnifying the chances for pressure problems of the underlying soft tissue:

$$F_i = \frac{F_0 \times d_0}{d_i}$$
$$= \frac{0.9 \times 2.5}{4}$$
$$= 0.56 \text{ pound}$$

To simplify the concepts of parallel forces, the splints in Figures 6-9 and 6-10 are shown in neutral position. Similar concepts apply to any rigid support regardless of shape (Fig. 6-11). If the weight of the hand, its direction of force, and the length of the palmar support are constant, lengthening the forearm trough decreases the resulting force at the end of the splint. This concept may be further generalized to include other types of splints and splint components. Given a constant resistance, resistance line of action, and resistance arm, the amount of force at

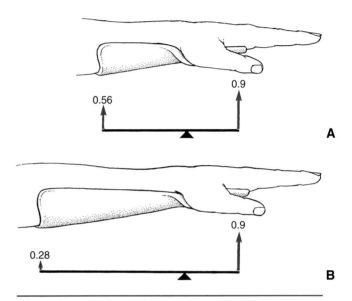

Fig. 6-10   A, Wrist neutral immobilization splint, type 0 (1) B, Wrist neutral immobilization splint, type 0 (1)
As shown in these scale drawings, the transferred weight of the hand is more comfortably supported by the leverage of a long forearm bar.

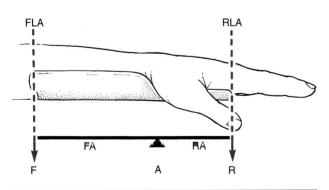

Fig. 6-9   Wrist neutral immobilization splint, type 0 (1)
Identification of mechanical terminology as it relates to a first-class lever system expedites subsequent force analysis. *FLA*, Force line of action; *FA (di)*, force arm (perpendicular between axis and FLA); *A*, axis; *RA (do)*, resistance arm (perpendicular between axis and RLA); *RLA*, resistance line of action.

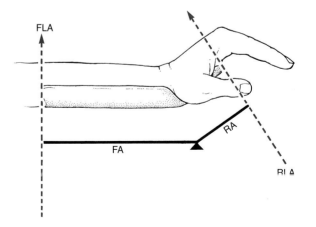

Fig. 6-11   Wrist extension immobilization splint, type 0 (1)
With the wrist bar placed in extension, the splint continues to act as a first-class lever, but the direction of the resistance line of action is altered. *FLA*, Force line of action; *FA (di)*, force arm; *RA (do)*, resistance arm; *RLA*, resistance line of action.

the opposite end of the first-class lever may be decreased by increasing the length of the force arm (Fig. 6-12).

The preceding examples indicate the relative relationship between the length/distance of the force arm and the length/distance of the resistance arm, which is designated mechanical advantage (MA):

$$MA = \frac{\text{Force arm}}{\text{Resistance arm}} = \frac{d_i}{d_0}$$

In the previous examples, when the force arm was 8 inches, the mechanical advantage was 3.2, but the mechanical advantage was decreased to 1.6 when the forearm trough was shortened to 4 inches. Splints with greater mechanical advantage produce less proximal force, resulting in diminished pressure and increased comfort.

Strap placement is critical to achieving optimum mechanical function of splints. A good design may be rendered less effective if straps are not placed strategically at maximum lengths of splint lever arms. For example, a forearm trough may be of sufficient length to reduce pressure and increase wearing comfort, but if the proximal strap is placed incorrectly at a point 2 inches distal to the proximal end of the splint, the

length of the forearm trough is mechanically shortened by 2 inches, to the point where the strap is attached! To accrue maximum benefit of splint lever systems, straps must be attached as far distally and proximally on a splint as possible.

Careful control of the force system between splint components will also augment the durability of splints. For example, consider the lever action of an outrigger on the proximal bond or rivet attaching the outrigger to the forearm trough. If the outrigger is viewed as a rigid first-class lever system, the amount of force generated on the proximal attachment may be computed for progressively increased attachment lengths when the resistance, resistance line of action, and resistance arm remain unchanged (Fig. 6-13). A longer force arm will result in a longer attachment bar and increased mechanical advantage, producing less force on the proximal bond and a stronger, more durable union of the two splint parts.

The combination of the first three mechanical principles supports collective experiential findings that long, wide splints are more comfortable and more durable than are short, narrow ones. When a segment is being splinted, the splint should extend approximately two-thirds its length and be contoured to half its width.

Use Optimum Rotational Force

The mobilization of stiffened joints through traction requires a thorough understanding of the resolution of forces to obtain optimum splint effectiveness. This must be achieved without producing patient frustration or increased tissue damage through joint compression or separation.

Theoretically, any force applied to a bony segment to mobilize a joint may be resolved into a pair of concurrent rectangular components acting in definite directions. These two components consist of a rotational element producing joint rotation and a translational element producing joint distraction or compression (Fig. 6-14). As a force approximates a perpendicular angle to the segment being mobilized, the translational element is lessened and the rotational component increases until at 90° the full magnitude of the force is applied in a rotational direction (Fig. 6-15, A). In practical terms this means that mobilization traction should be applied at a 90° angle to harness the force potential of the traction device without producing an unwanted pushing or pulling force on the articular surfaces of the involved joint (Fig. 6-15, B). This also means that, as the passive range of motion of the joint begins to improve, the outrigger to which the traction device is attached must be adjusted to maintain the 90° angle (Fig. 6-16). In

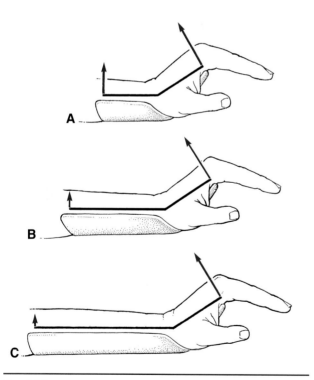

Fig. 6-12   A, Wrist extension immobilization splint, type 0 (1) B, Wrist extension immobilization splint, type 0 (1) C, Wrist extension immobilization splint, type 0 (1)
As illustrated in these scale drawings, a longer forearm bar or trough decreases the resultant pressure caused by the proximally transferred weight of the hand to the anterior forearm.

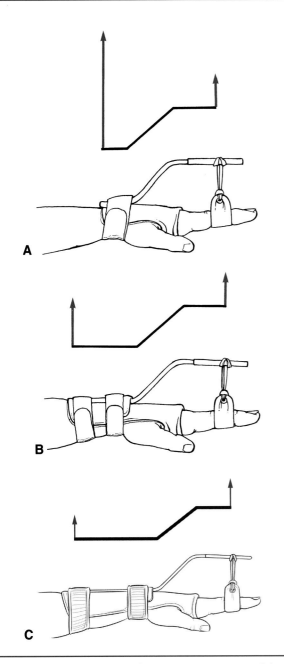

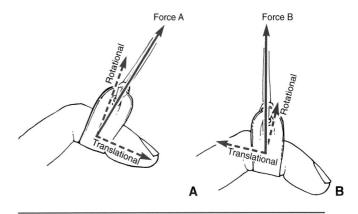

Fig. 6-14   Any force may be analyzed according to rotary and nonrotary components.

Fig. 6-13   A, Index–small finger MP extension mobilization splint, type 1 (9) B, Index–small finger MP extension mobilization splint, type 1 (9) C, Index–small finger MP extension mobilization splint, type 1 (9)
An extended outrigger attachment length produces less leverage on the proximal bond or rivet (drawings to scale).

the case of multiple joint splinting, when motion limitations may not be the same, it may be necessary to provide one or more outrigger extensions for adjacent fingers to maintain the required 90° angle of pull (Fig. 6-17). Careful attention to the patient's complaints about the splint provides useful clues as to its mechanical function. If the patient observes that the finger cuffs tend to migrate distally or proximally on the

fingers, a 90° angle probably has not been achieved or maintained.

In splint designs that incorporate secondary joints, two or more rotational forces affect digital joint motion. For example, in a *finger PIP extension mobilization splint, type 1,* while the mobilization assist applies force in one direction, the dorsal phalangeal bar applies force in an opposite direction to control the secondary MP joint(s). Just as the mobilization assist must have a 90° angle of approach to the segment being mobilized, so too must the dorsal phalangeal bar, but its force is instead directed to the proximal segment. Providing inelastic traction, the connector bar/dorsal phalangeal bar unit must have a 90° angle of approach to the segment being stabilized to be fully effective (Fig. 6-18). If a 90° angle of approach is not present, the dorsal phalangeal bar moves distally or proximally when the mobilization assist is attached to the finger and the patient uses his hand.

Achieving a 90° angle of force application in splints whose dorsal phalangeal bars are solid extensions of the dorsal metacarpal bars, as opposed to separate dorsal phalangeal bars, can be challenging and is also difficult to monitor visually. A properly fitted separate dorsal phalangeal bar automatically adjusts to changes in proximal phalanx position, remaining firmly seated and in contiguous contact with the dorsum of the phalanx. In contrast, a dorsal phalangeal bar that is a solid continuation of a dorsal metacarpal bar cannot self-adjust to positional changes of the proximal phalanx, increasing the potential for uneven pressure distribution over the dorsum of the phalanx, which may lead to unwarranted soft tissue injury.

An analysis of the interaction between rotational and translational elements may also provide insight as to why some three-point pressure splints such as *finger PIP extension mobilization splints* like the "safety pin" and "joint jack" become clinically less

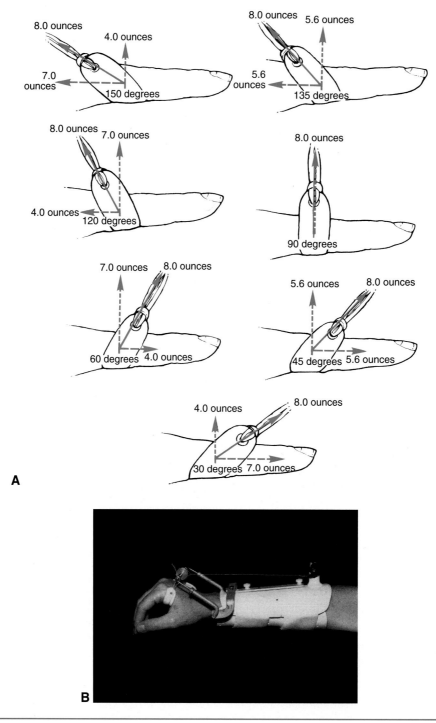

A

B

Fig. 6-15   B, Wrist extension mobilization splint, type 0 (1)
A, At 90° the translational force is zero, resulting in no element of joint compression or distraction. *Small-dashed lines,* rotational force; *large-dashed lines,* translational force; *solid arrows,* mobilization assist force. **B,** Eliminating translational forces, a 90° angle of pull allows the full magnitude of this mobilization assist to be focused on the wrist joint. [Courtesy **(B)** Shelli Dellinger, OTR, CHT, San Diego, Calif.]

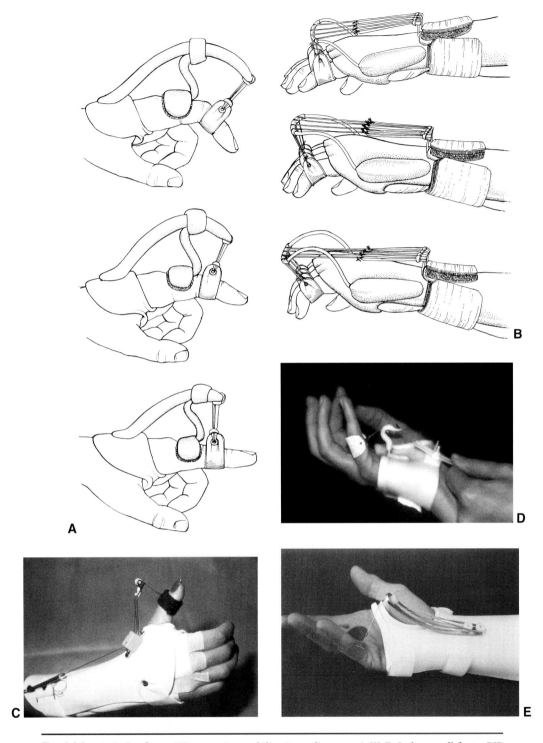

Fig. 6-16   **A,** Index finger PIP extension mobilization splint, type 1 (2) **B,** Index–small finger PIP extension mobilization splint, type 2 (9) **C,** Thumb MP-IP extension mobilization splint, type 2 (4) **D,** Small finger MP flexion mobilization splint, type 0 (1) **E,** Small finger MP flexion mobilization splint, type 1 (2)

A,B, A 90° angle of the mobilization assist to the mobilized segment must be maintained as passive joint motion changes. **A,** High profile. **B,** Low profile. **C,** The thumb outrigger is easily adjustable by loosening the allen set screws in the retaining block, sliding the outrigger proximally or distally as needed, and retightening the screws. **D,** This innovative outrigger self-adjusts as MP joint flexion improves. **E,** A slotted outrigger facilitates adjustments as MP flexion increases. [Courtesy **(C)** Jean Claude Rouzaud, Montpellier, France; **(D)** Nelson Vazquez, OTR, CHT, Miami, Fla., and Damon Kirk, WFR Corporation, Wyckoff, N.J.; **(E)** Helen Marx, OTR, CHT, Human Factors Engineering of Phoenix, Wickenburg, Ariz.]

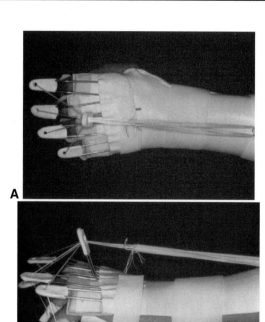

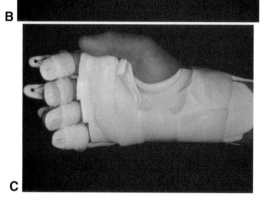

Fig. 6-17   A-C, Index–small finger PIP extension mobilization splint, type 2 (13) \\ Finger PIP extension torque transmission splint, type 1 (2); 4 splints @ finger separate

Adaptation of the outrigger is often necessary to maintain a perpendicular pull on segments whose passive joint motions are dissimilar. A-C, Different length outriggers provide correct 90° angle of force application to each finger PIP joint. B,C, The separate PIP torque transmission splints assist in remodeling stiff PIP joints. (Courtesy Jill Francisco, OTR, CHT, Cicero, Ind.)

effective as the flexion angle of the joint is increased (Fig. 6-19). Once again, clinical experience is verified by mechanical force assessment. Since the proximal and distal translational elements produce joint compression with resulting abatement of the rotational components, *finger PIP extension mobilization splints* like the "joint jack" and "safety pin" splints are more appropriately employed for flexion contractures of 35° or less.

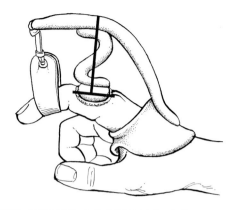

Fig. 6-18   Index finger PIP extension mobilization splint, type 1 (2)

A 90° angle of approach of a dorsal phalangeal bar to the proximal phalanx prevents proximal or distal migration of the bar.

In addition to the requisite 90° angle of approach to the length of the segment being mobilized, it is also important that the mobilizing force be perpendicular to the joint axis of rotation to ensure that equal tension is placed on both of the joint's collateral ligaments (Fig. 6-20). If a 90° angle of force application is not achieved and maintained, a discrepancy in force magnitude is placed on the collateral ligaments with one ligament receiving more mobilizing force than its mate, creating differential remodeling between the two ligaments, which leads to joint instability.

Consider the Torque Effect

Torque equals the product of the force times the length of the arm on which it acts ($T = F_i \times d_i$). This concept is important in splinting because the amount of pull from a mobilization assist is not equal to the amount of rotational force or torque at the joint. The amount of torque depends on the distance between the joint axis and the point of attachment of the mobilization assist. The torque increases as the distance between the two increases if the applied force is held constant (Fig. 6-21). This explains why a patient may be able to tolerate a given amount of traction at one location but cannot tolerate the same amount when the attachment device is moved distally. Patients may be taught to use the torque phenomenon advantageously by advancing their finger cuffs distally as their pain tolerance permits. This must be done judiciously, however, since too much distal advancement may result in an inferior angle of the traction device or in attenuation of ligamentous structures.

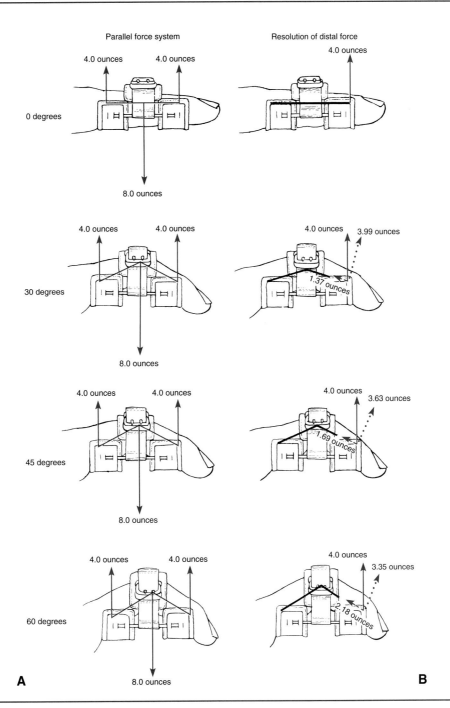

Parallel force system   Resolution of distal force

0 degrees

30 degrees

45 degrees

60 degrees

A   **B**

Fig. 6-19   Finger PIP extension mobilization splint, type 0 (1)

A, While the magnitude of the parallel forces of a three-point pressure splint remain constant with the proximal interphalangeal joint in various degrees of flexion **(B)** the rotational and translational components of the proximal and distal forces (only distal end illustrated for simplicity) change until at 60° the compression force (translational) on the joint is nearly two-thirds that of the rotational force **B,** Clinically this means that the greater the flexion deformity the less effective the splint becomes in its ability to correct the deficit. (Key: Dotted arrow = rotational force; dashed arrow = translational force; solid arrow = traction force.) (Special recognition to Kenneth Dunipace, PhD retired, former Chairman of the Division of Engineering, Purdue University School of Engineering and Technology at Indianapolis for his assistance with the analysis of this splint.)

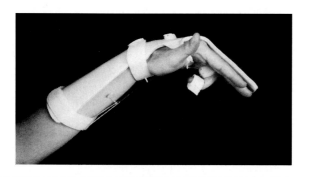

Fig. 6-20   Index–small finger extension restriction / ring finger flexion mobilization splint, type 1 (13)
A creative sling system and palmar pulleys maintain correct force alignment on ring finger joints in this splint used to treat repaired flexor tendons in Zone II. [Courtesy Stancie Trueman, Missiauga, Ontario, Canada.]

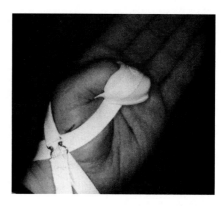

Fig. 6-22   Thumb MP-IP flexion mobilization splint, type 0 (2)
A *type 0* splint is appropriate when all joints involved have a similar passive range of motion. In this particular splint, the thumb CMC joint has full mobility.

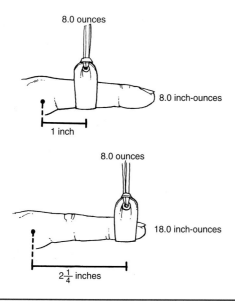

8.0 ounces

8.0 inch-ounces

1 inch

8.0 ounces

18.0 inch-ounces

$2\frac{1}{4}$ inches

Fig. 6-21   As the distance between the joint axis and the point of attachment of the mobilization assist increases, the amount of torque on the joint increases.

Consider the Relative Degree of Passive Mobility of Successive Joints

When a force is exerted on a proximally based, multiarticular segment, all parts of the segment are moved in the direction of the force if motion of the successive joints is unimpaired. When motion is limited or stopped at a given articulation, the remaining mobile joints are moved in the direction of the force with minimal motion occurring at the restricted

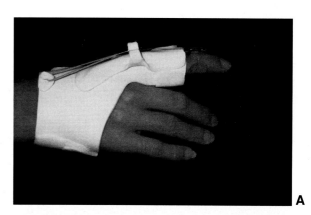

A

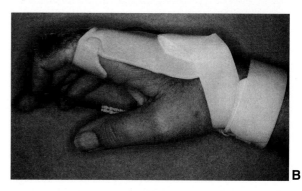

B

Fig. 6-23   A, Index finger PIP extension mobilization splint, type 1(2) B, Index finger PIP flexion mobilization splint, type 2 (3)
These splints control motion at the normal secondary MP joints, allowing optimum mechanical purchase when joint motion is unequal within the longitudinal ray. The proximal phalanx is stabilized and the middle phalanx receives the mobilizing force in each splint, although the direction of pull is different. [Courtesy **(A)** Peggy McLaughlin, OTR, CHT, San Bernadino, Calif.]

joint. In other words, when all joints within a longitudinal ray exhibit stiffness, they may be splinted in unison (Fig. 6-22). If an inequality of passive motion exists, the splint must be adapted to stabilize the normal, secondary joints within the segment, allowing the full magnitude of the traction to be directed toward the less mobile primary joints (Fig. 6-23). If these changes are not made, the rotational force is dissipated in unwanted motion at the secondary mobile joints, resulting in potential damage to these normal joints and ineffective traction on the stiffened primary joints.

Control Reaction Effect at Secondary Joints

If the discrepancy in amount of stiffness between primary and secondary joints within the same longitudinal segment is marked, as a mobilization force is directed to a stiff joint and reciprocal force secondary joint motion is controlled, the end of the stabilized segment may have a tendency to displace or sublux at the level of the secondary joint (Fig. 6-24). Reaction displacement is especially problematic when secondary finger MP joints, with their imbricated palmar plates, are not held in full flexion, allowing the collateral ligaments to slacken and increasing the potential for the base of the proximal phalanx to sublux. Although reaction displacement forces occur at other digital joints, their immediate consequences are less obvious due to the presence of tighter palmar plates and collateral ligaments than those at the finger MP joints. If, however, prolonged tension is placed on these ligaments, they may remodel, allowing incremental displacement of the segment involved and joint instability. Dorsal phalangeal bars that are solid continuations of dorsal metacarpal bars must be fitted with great care and they must be monitored vigilantly to ensure that reaction displacement does not create narrow, tissue-damaging fulcrums at the distal edges of the dorsal phalangeal bars, with resultant magnifi-

cation of displacement torque. Properly fitted, separate (not attached to metacarpal bars) dorsal phalangeal bars have fewer tendencies to create edge fulcrums because of their abilities to maintain contiguous contact on the phalanx through minute self-adjustments. Reaction effect is best controlled by adapting critical splint components, e.g., phalangeal bars, to provide circumferential support or through strategic placement of straps (Fig. 6-23).

Consider the Effects of Reciprocal Parallel Forces

As noted earlier, the use of three parallel forces in equilibrium as exemplified by a first-class lever system is basic to splinting of the hand, with the splint acting as the proximal and distal counterforces to the forces of the hand and forearm and a strap at the axis of the splinted segment providing the reciprocal middle force. In an analysis of the interrelationships of forces in a first-class lever system in equilibrium, the combined downward weights must be opposed by an equal upward force at the axis: A + B = C (Fig. 6-25). This means that the middle opposing force is of greater magnitude than the force at either the proximal or distal end of the splint. These reciprocal parallel forces form the basis for what is frequently termed three-point fixation. Since the middle force in splinting is frequently placed over a joint (Fig. 6-26), care should be taken to minimize the amount of pressure exerted on the underlying soft tissue. This can be accomplished by widening the area of force application.

Understanding parallel force systems also allows the accurate prediction of high-stress areas within the splint itself. Because the summation of the proximal and distal forces equals the middle opposite direction

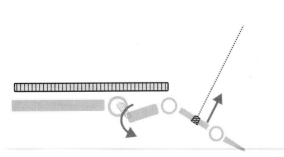

Fig. 6-24   When mobilization traction is applied to primary joints, reaction displacement may occur at secondary joints if the amount of stiffness is markedly different between primary and secondary joints.

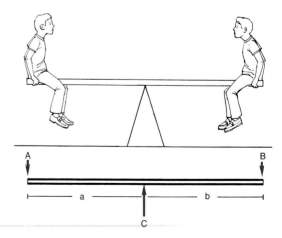

Fig. 6-25   A balanced teeter-totter provides an easily visualized representation of a first-class lever in equilibrium. The combined downward weights (A and B) must be opposed by an equal opposite force (C).

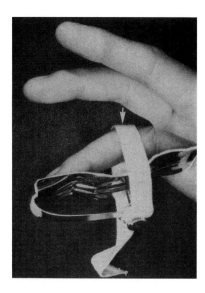

Fig. 6-26   Ring finger PIP extension mobilization splint, type 1 (2)
If not monitored carefully, excessive pressure at the site of the middle opposing force *(arrow)* may cause soft tissue damage.

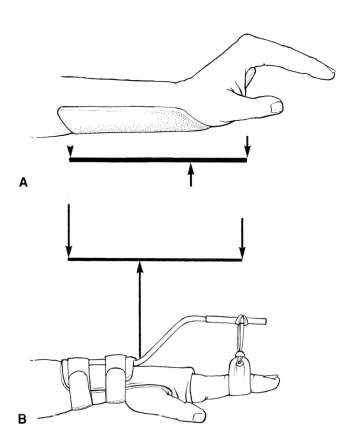

Fig. 6-27   A, Wrist extension mobilization splint, type 0 (1) B, Index–small finger MP extension mobilization splint, type 1 (9)
Analyses of the parallel force systems present in a *type 0 wrist extension mobilization splint* (**A**) and a *type 1 finger MP extension mobilization splint* (**B**) indicate the areas of greatest stress to be at the wrist and the proximal bend of the outrigger, respectively.

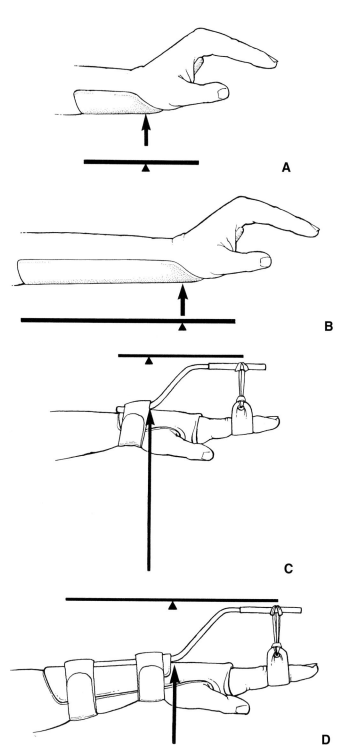

Fig. 6-28   A, Wrist extension mobilization splint, type 0 (1) B, Wrist extension mobilization splint, type 0 (1) C, Index–small finger MP extension mobilization splint, type 1 (9) D, Index–small finger MP extension mobilization splint, type 1 (9)
An increased mechanical advantage (MA) results in a decrease in the magnitude of the middle opposing force. The MA is greater in **B** and **D**.

force, it becomes readily apparent why splints with narrow wrist bars frequently become fatigued and fracture at the wrist, and outriggers break at the level of the proximal bend (Fig. 6-27). When the mechanical advantage (MA) is increased, the magnitude of the middle opposing force is decreased (Fig. 6-28). Anticipation of the greater magnitude of the middle force allows preventive measures to be taken during splint design and construction phases. The forearm bar may be lengthened to decrease the force and the vulnerable area may be contoured or reinforced to increase the mechanical strength of the material.

Another example of reciprocal parallel forces is the force interrelationships within a dorsal outrigger with a dorsal phalangeal bar. The dorsal phalangeal bar provides a reciprocal middle force to the upward force at the proximal and distal ends of the splint (Fig. 6-29). The resulting downward force at the dorsal phalangeal bar is greater than the forces at either end of the splint, further explaining the clinical finding that pressure is consistently a problem under dorsal phalangeal bars and must be dealt with by good fit and dissemination of pressure through padding.

The concept of three-point reciprocal forces may be of further assistance in attempts to eliminate splint pressure over a given area. For example, the middle opposing force on a dorsal outrigger without a dorsal phalangeal bar occurs at the distal aspect of the dorsal metacarpal bar, resulting in downward force on the back of the hand (Fig. 6-30, A,C). If splint pressure in this area were contraindicated due to edema, poor

skin quality, or underlying metacarpal fractures, the addition of a dorsal phalangeal bar would change the position of the middle reciprocal force to the dorsum of the proximal phalanx, resulting in rotation upward, away from the back of the hand by the dorsal metacarpal bar (Fig. 6-30, B,D).

A related concept, assuming an extension mobilization splint applies consistent torque over time, as joint extension increases, the mechanical advantage increases and the force on the proximal end of the splint decreases (Fig. 6-31). If the scenario is reversed, the more flexion that is present, the smaller is the MA and the greater is the force at the proximal end of the splint. Clinically, this means that extension mobilization splints with shorter moment arms, e.g., hand-based splints, are more uncomfortable, especially at the proximal strap, when the joints they affect have flexion deformities of 60° or more. When more than one digit is included in a splint, it is important to remember that the proximal force is multiplied by the number of digits in the splint.[14]

Use Appropriate Outrigger Systems

With unique force systems, outriggers provide the foundations from which mobilization assists are attached or through which they are guided. It is outrigger placement and positioning that permits 90° angle of force application of mobilization assists. Because outrigger force systems differ depending on the height of the outrigger, outrigger design must be coordinated with individual patient requirements. For mobilization splints, high-profile outrigger designs require fewer adjustments than do low-profile outrigger designs.[4,12,13] If, however, joints are supple and the splint is fitted to substitute for absent active motion, the issue of number of sequential adjustments is moot and a low-profile outrigger design may be more acceptable to patients due to less overall bulk.

High-profile outriggers also require less patient strength to oppose outrigger forces and they provide greater joint stability through translational forces as fingers are flexed than do low-profile outriggers (Fig. 6-32).[14] Another consideration is the additional factor of drag or friction from mobilization assists as they are pulled over the fulcrum of a low-profile outrigger. This adds to forces resisting finger motion opposite to that of the assists and must also be considered.[15] For example, a high-profile outrigger often is preferable for a post–MP arthroplasty patient with weak grip strength, requiring less strength to flex the MP joints while simultaneously providing greater joint stability as MP joints are flexed. If grip strength and joint stability are not problematic, either a high- or low-profile outrigger design may suffice.

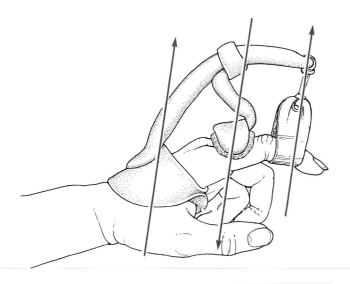

Fig. 6-29   Index finger PIP extension mobilization splint, type 1 (2)

Reciprocal parallel forces may be identified in this *type 1 finger PIP extension mobilization splint.*

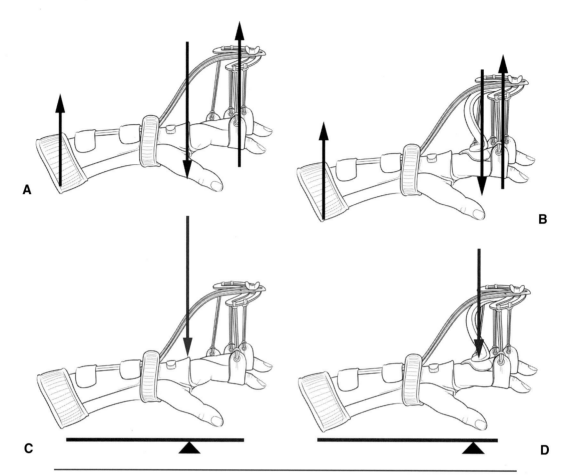

Fig. 6-30   A, Index–small finger MP-PIP extension mobilization splint, type 1 (9) B, Index-small finger PIP extension mobilization splint, type 2 (9) C, Index-small finger MP-PIP extension mobilization splint, type 1 (9) D, Index-small finger PIP extension mobilization splint, type 2 (9) Addition of a dorsal phalangeal bar changes the site of application of the middle opposing force (**A** and **B**). Because of an increased mechanical advantage, the force at the dorsal phalangeal bar is less than the force at the dorsal metacarpal bar (**C** and **D**).

The sometimes-heard justification for inappropriate choice of outrigger design, "But the patient insisted on a low-profile outrigger," is ludicrous in the extreme, inadvertently identifying poor splinting knowledge on the part of the therapist who makes such a statement. The wholesale use of only one outrigger design is as inappropriate and detrimental to good therapeutic intervention as is use of only one modality, treatment approach, splint material, or splint design! Comparable to using a wide range of splinting methods and materials, wisely choosing from a range of outrigger options increases patients' chances to attain their full rehabilitative potential.

Incorporate Articulated Components Appropriately

Concomitantly providing elements of control and motion, articulated splints protect healing soft tissue structures (Fig. 6-33, *A,B*) and improve function (Fig. 6-33, *C,D*). Articulated splint components must be accurately aligned with anatomical joint axes. If a splint articulation is not aligned with its anatomical joint, the splint tends to "piston" on the extremity as active movement occurs, causing shear forces and friction.

Increase Material Strength by Providing Contour

The time-honored engineering principle of strength through contour is directly applicable to the design and construction of hand splints and is in many instances a concept that is concomitant with the previous consideration of force dissemination and use of leverage.

When a large force is placed on a flat, thin piece of material, the counterforce produced by the material is insufficient, and the material bends. If, however, the

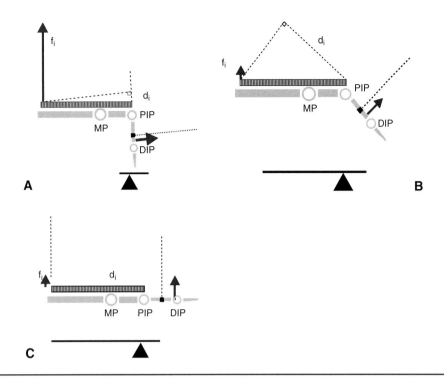

Fig. 6-31   In a *type 1 PIP extension mobilization splint*, the force at the proximal end of a splint decreases and the mechanical advantage increases as joint extension motion increases. (From Fess EE: Splints: mechanics versus convention, *J Hand Ther* 8(2):124-30, 1995.)

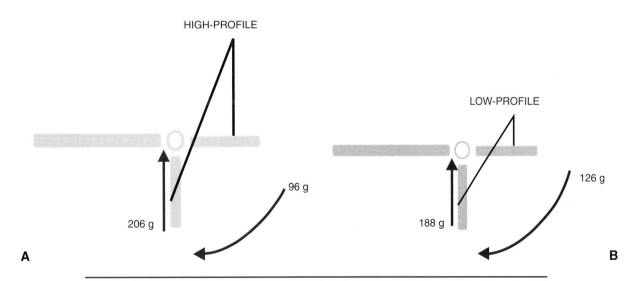

Fig. 6-32   As a joint is actively moved in a direction opposite to the pull of the mobilization assist, high-profile outriggers (A) provide better joint stabilization and require less strength to initiate and maintain motion than do low-profile designs (B). (From Fess EE: Splints: mechanics versus convention, *J Hand Ther* 8(2):124-30, 1995.)

material is contoured into a half-cylinder shape, the material has, in mechanical terms, become stiffer (Fig. 6-34) and produces a greater counterforce, enabling the material to withstand greater forces without bending (Fig. 6-35).

In considering the design of a splint and the materials to be used, one must take care to match the design to the material properties. The low-temperature materials commonly used in physicians' offices and therapy departments for splint fabrication

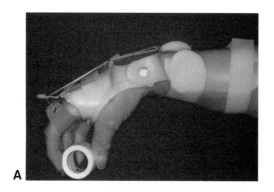

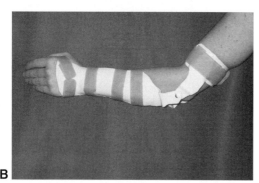

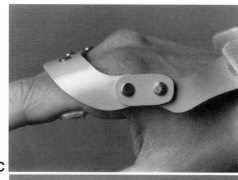

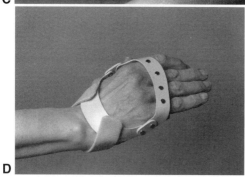

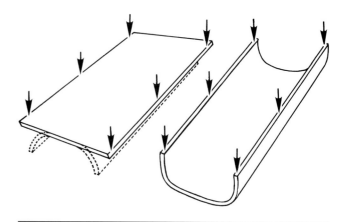

Fig. 6-34   Contour mechanically increases material strength.

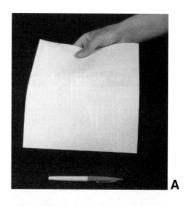

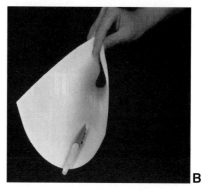

Fig. 6-35   A flat sheet of paper cannot hold the weight of a pen, but, when the paper is contoured into a partial cylinder shape, the pen is supported.

Fig. 6-33   A, Wrist flexion: index–small finger MP extension / index–small finger MP flexion: wrist extension torque transmission splint, type 0 (5) B, Forearm neutral immobilization splint, type 2 (3) C,D, Index–small finger MP ulnar deviation restriction splint, type 0 (4)
Articulated splints allow controlled motion to diseased or injured joints and enhance function. [Courtesy (A) Jill Francisco, OTR, CHT, Cicero, Ind.; (B) Rebecca Banks, OTR, CHT, MHS, Blackburn, Australia; (C,D) Julie Belkin, OTR, CO, MBA, 3-Point Products, Annapolis, Md.]

are easily bendable in sheet form, requiring splint designs that provide strength through contour. The thicker high-temperature plastics and specific metals conversely do not need the additional strength attained through material contour and are appropriate for the narrower bar type of splints. Outriggers may be constructed of either kind of material, but, if low-temperature plastic substance is chosen, mechanical thickness is essential for strength in the form

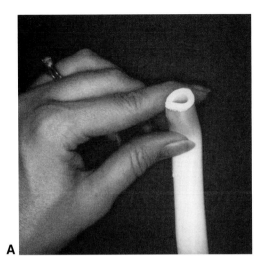

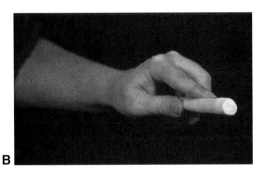

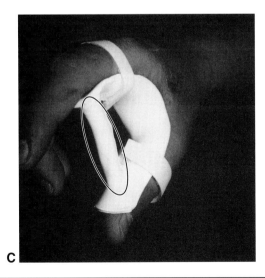

Fig. 6-36   C, Thumb CMC palmar abduction mobilization splint, type 3 (4)
Depending on the specific properties of the low-temperature plastic, outrigger strength may be increased by forming a **(A)** tube or **(B)** solid coil. **C,** Placed at a 90° angle, a tubed connector bar reinforces this CMC mobilization splint. (C Courtesy Cynthia Philips, MA, OTR, CHT, Boston, Mass.)

of either a hollow tube or solid coil (Fig. 6-36). Reinforcement bars are stronger when they are contoured.

Eliminate Friction

Kinetic friction occurs when surfaces in contact with each other move relative to one another. If a difference in density exists between the surfaces, the harder surface may begin to erode the softer, less dense surface. If the surfaces are similar, damage may occur on either side or on both sides.

Clinically kinetic friction may occur between the splint and the extremity or between contiguous cutaneous surfaces. In either case it may result in skin irritation, blistering, and eventual breakdown. Friction caused by a splint usually indicates poor fit, improper joint alignment, or inefficient fastening devices. Friction between cutaneous surfaces, such as adjacent digits, may often be abated by interposing a layer of gauze bandage between the two surfaces. Steps should be taken to alleviate the frictional problem at the first sign of cutaneous embarrassment because, if the splint is left unattended, prolonged trauma to the skin may render the extremity unsatisfactory for further splinting efforts until healing occurs. Good contiguous fit, proper joint alignment, strategic placement of straps, and use of Dycem help stabilize a splint and minimize friction on an extremity.

Avoid High Shear Stress*

To begin, it is necessary to define a few important terms that describe the material behavior of soft tissues.
1. *Force* is a vector and therefore has a magnitude, direction, and point of application. It changes the direction and/or velocity of objects, and when applied to a surface, forces result in deformation of solid or semisolid substances.
2. *Strain* is a measure of the deformation of a material. It is defined as a ratio of the change in a reference length (gauge length) to the original length. Overall, or average, strain can be measured as can local strain (Fig. 6-37). These two are equal only in special circumstances. If the two points defining the gauge length are extremely close, strain can be thought of as varying from point to point within a material. Because it is a ratio, it is used instead of absolute displacement.
3. *Stress* describes the distribution of forces on the surface or within a material (Fig. 6-38). Force

*Written and researched by David E. Thompson, Ph.D., Dean of Engineering, University of Idaho, Moscow, Idaho.

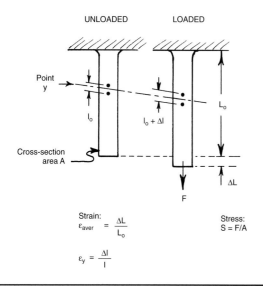

Fig. 6-37   Pictorial definition of strain in materials.

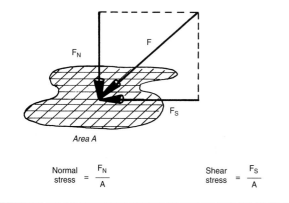

Fig. 6-38   Pictorial definition of normal and shear stress at a surface.

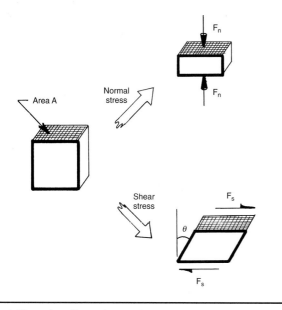

Fig. 6-39   The effects of normal and shear stress on an internal element within a material.

can be thought of as having both a normal component (perpendicular to the surface) and a shear component (parallel to or tangent to the surface). If these components are divided by the area over which they act, the ratios define normal and shear stresses. Although stress is defined at the surface of an object, stresses can be thought of as existing within the material as well.

Stress is a more meaningful term than just *force*. For example, if one pushes a finger onto the point of a tack with a force of 5 pounds, it will puncture the skin. However, the same force applied over 1 square inch will cause only a small indentation.

Normal stresses are usually termed *pressure* or *tensile stresses*. At a point within a substance, these stresses act equally in all directions. In a simple diagram of stress applied to a rectangular element (Fig. 6-39), the elements remain rectangular, even though they deform. High normal stresses are required to cause damage to soft tissues. Brand[5] states that pressures in excess of 200 pounds per square inch (psi) are required for single loads to cause damage to soft tissues, but in all probability the real damage to the tissues comes from shear and not pressure effects.

Modulus of Elasticity

By plotting the normal stress within a test sample (Fig. 6-40) versus the resulting overall strain, engineers learn a great deal about the test material. For materials like steel, the slope of this curve is termed its modulus of elasticity. It is a measure of the stiffness of the material. Other materials, like aluminum, collagen fibers, and skin, have no linear relationship or may or may not be so simply characterized. In this case, engineers use the term *apparent modulus of*

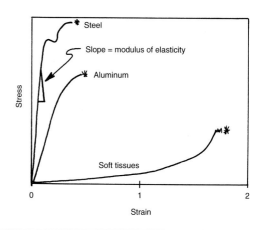

Fig. 6-40   Stress–strain relationships for steel, aluminum, and soft tissues. The vertical scale for the steel and aluminum curves has been altered to allow them to be included. Typical maximum stresses for steel are around 150,000 psi, compared with 300 psi for soft tissues.

elasticity, defined as the stress divided by the total strain. For soft tissues, there is a large region where the material deforms readily at very low stresses.[17,19] The apparent elastic modulus is very low in this region. As the tissues reach high strains, however, the stress required to achieve additional strain rises markedly, and the apparent elastic modulus rises concomitantly.

Shear stresses, unlike normal stresses, are directional. Within a two-dimensional slice of material, their direction of action is defined in terms of the rotational direction of an element. As shown in Fig. 6-39, the rectangular elements have deformed in a clockwise manner into diamond shapes, and the resulting forces within the material are high. For soft tissues, this results in damage at much lower stress levels than for pure normal stress acting alone.

Shear Modulus

There is an equivalent modulus to the elastic modulus, which defines a material's ability to resist shear stress instead of normal stress. This is the shear modulus, defined in terms of the shear stress divided by the angle of deformation of the rectangular elements (Fig. 6-39).

Stress Concentrations (Scar, Changes in Elastic Modulus)

A critical factor that is often overlooked in managing soft tissues relates to the mechanical properties of the tissues and any factors that cause dramatic variations in these properties. Scar tissue is extremely rigid and noncompliant in comparison with normal, healthy soft tissue. When tissue is loaded in the presence of either an internal or external scar, property variation results in a concentration of stresses where there are dramatic spatial variations in the strain or deformation in the region of the scar. An identical effect occurs where the applied loads change rapidly across a surface and large strain gradients result. Murphy[18] discusses these and other effects.

An Experimental Demonstration

To illustrate the behavior of soft tissues, three simple experiments are included here. They use a 5 × 12 × 2–inch foam test sample mounted in an Instron materials testing machine. A sample was ruled with horizontal and vertical lines spaced $\frac{1}{4}$ inch apart to produce a grid of squares on the entire face. A piece of $\frac{3}{4}$-inch plywood was glued to the bottom of the specimen to distribute the loading uniformly along this edge (Fig. 6-41).

In the first test a smaller piece of wood was placed on the top surface, and the sample was loaded as shown in Fig. 6-42. At high loads the resulting strains and the distribution of shear and normal stresses are depicted graphically in their effects on the small squares on the specimen. In region A, the deformation of the squares is due to pure normal stress. The diamond-shaped squares in region B attest to the high shear produced in this region. It must be noted that this region is below the surface of the specimen and even outside of the area beneath the upper plywood-loading bar. The shear in this region is due to the sudden change in the pressure at the surface of the specimen. Bennett[3] demonstrated this edge effect mathematically.

When loaded uniformly in a second test (Fig. 6-43), no shear is produced anywhere within the specimen.

In the third test a small piece of harder rubber was inserted into the foam (Fig. 6-44). This was done to simulate a scar deep within the tissues. When the load was applied, the elements nearer the surface deformed more than the deeper structures. This is characteristic of soft tissues because of their nonlinear stress–strain relationship. Shear production can be seen around the edge of the loading bar and also around the edges of the simulated scar.

Discussion

According to Brand,[5] the human body responds to mechanical stress in one of three ways. If the stress is within acceptable limits, the tissues hypertrophy and become more robust in tolerating additional stress. If the stresses are very low, the tissues atrophy and become more fragile. If the loads are excessive, however, the tissues break down and may ulcerate. If the tissues are then rested so they can heal, scarring results. Scar tissues create an environment where stresses are concentrated and further breakdown is more likely. It is therefore more appropriate to prevent scar altogether than to attempt to protect tissues after they have failed.[5,16]

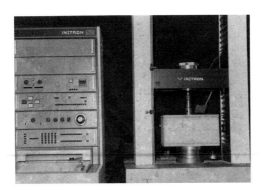

Fig. 6-41 The experimental setup showing the Instron testing machine with the foam test specimen in place.

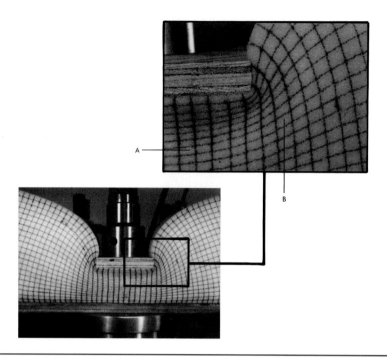

Fig. 6-42   Close-up of the test specimen at a strain of 0.5 with an inset depicting the localized effects of shear stress resulting in diamond-shaped elements.

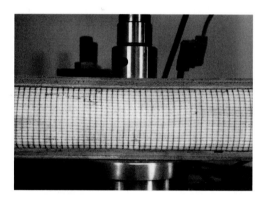

Fig. 6-43   Close-up of the test specimen with uniform loading at the same strain as in Fig. 6-42.

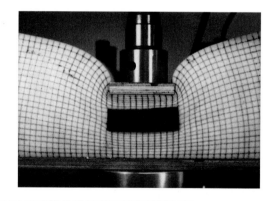

Fig. 6-44   Close-up of the test specimen with a simulated scar consisting of a hard rubber insert located deep within the specimen. The overall strain is the same as in Figures 6-42 and 6-43.

If one examines the skin around the border of the heel and great toe, it is possible to see the body's response to shear stress resulting from a sudden change in normal stress. The pressures arising during gait are high in the regions immediately under the heel and great toe,[2] but they fall to zero as one moves around and out from under the weight-bearing areas. This rapid variation in pressure gives rise to shear, much the same as in the test shown in region B of Fig. 6-42. The buildup of callus in these regions is a direct response to shear stress and underscores its importance in the care and management of soft tissues.

The general principles of the application of mechanical stress to soft tissues are summarized as follows:

1. Avoid high-pressure areas by spreading the stresses in space. This involves large surface areas. In all cases, the splint and/or padding should conform as closely as possible to the contours of the surface of the hand to afford the greatest possible contact area.
2. Avoid high shear effects by rounding sharp edges and keeping pressures low. In Fig. 6-5, B, the "incorrect" method shown not only produces large pressures, it creates extremely large shear stresses. The shear effects are amplified by any motion of the bar relative to the finger. The rolled edges of the splint shown in Fig. 6-3 reduce the shear effects

caused by the sudden change in pressure at the edge of the splint.

3. Reduce the peak levels by spreading them out in time. Using protective materials has the effect of ameliorating pressure peaks caused by accidental bumping of splints on solid immovable objects. Increasing the thickness of the protective material will continue to spread the stresses in both space and time, but above a certain thickness this is impractical because it also causes instability and allows misalignment of the splint.

4. Beware of the effects of repetitive stresses. The damage to soft tissues is cumulative, and breakdown will occur more rapidly in regions already involved in an inflammatory response to mechanical trauma.[20]

The experimental work for this section on shear was done at the National Hansen's Disease Center, Carville, La., and the analysis of the results was accomplished in the Computer Graphics Research and Applications Laboratory at Louisiana State University, Baton Rouge. The funding for this research was provided by the U.S. Public Health Service, Department of Health and Human Services, under research contract 240-83-0060.

▓ SUMMARY

Initially the clinician engaged in the preparation of upper extremity splints may consider the mechanical principles of splinting to be technically difficult and not truly germane to the clinical situation. Nonetheless, it is extremely important that the general principles be learned and reviewed to ensure that the finished product is more than an accumulation of the splint maker's experience through numerous inefficient, nonproductive trials. The mathematic details of mechanical engineering or bioengineering are not essential to the basic conceptual understanding of the mechanics of splint design and preparation. A concentrated effort to understand the principles described in this chapter combined with periodic review as experience is gained will pay large dividends in the ultimate performance of a splint.

REFERENCES

1. ASHT: *American Society of Hand Therapists Splint Classification System*, ed 1, The Society, J. Bailey, et al, 1992, Chicago.
2. Bauman JH, Brand PW: Measurement of pressure between foot and shoe, *Lancet* p. 629-32, 1963.
3. Bennett L: Transferring load to flesh, Part II. In *Bull Prosthet Res*, Veterans Administration, 1971, Washington, DC.
4. Boozer JA, Sanson MS, Soutas-Little RW, et al: Comparison of the biomedical motions and forces involved in high-profile versus low-profile dynamic splinting, *J Hand Ther* 7(3):171-82, 1994.
5. Brand PW: *Repetitive stress on insensitive feet*, United States Public Health Service Hospital, 1975, Carville, LA.
6. Brand PW: *Clinical mechanics of the hand*, Mosby, 1985, St. Louis.
7. Brand PW, Hollister A: *Clinical mechanics of the hand*, ed 2, Mosby, 1993, St. Louis.
8. Brand PW, Hollister A: *Clinical mechanics of the hand*, ed 3, Mosby, 1999, St. Louis.
9. Fess E, Philips C: *Hand splinting: principles and methods*, ed 2, Mosby, 1987, St. Louis.
10. Fess E, Gettle K, Strickland J: *Hand splinting: principles and methods*, Mosby, 1981, St. Louis.
11. Fess EE: *Mechanical concepts in splinting*, Kinesiology class instructor notes, Indiana University Medical School, Occupational Therapy Program, 1974: Indianapolis.
12. Fess EE: Principles and methods of dynamic splinting. In Hunter J, et al: *Rehabilitation of the hand*, ed 2, Mosby, 1984, St. Louis.
13. Fess EE: Principles and methods of splinting for mobilization. In Hunter J, et al: *Rehabilitation of the hand*, ed 3, Mosby, 1989, St. Louis.
14. Fess EE: Splints: mechanics versus convention, *J Hand Ther* 8(2):124-30, 1995.
15. Gyovai J, Howell J: Validation of spring forces applied in dynamic outrigger splinting, *J Hand Ther* 5(1):8-15, 1992.
16. Hampton GH: Therapeutic footwear for the insensitive foot, *J Phys Ther* 52(1):23-9, 1979.
17. Markenscoff X: I.V. Yannas, on the stress-strain relation for skin, *J Biomech* 12:127-9, 1979.
18. Murphy EF: Transferring load to flesh, Part I. In *Bull Prosthet Res*, Veterans Administration, 1971, Washington, DC.
19. Sakata K, Parfitt G, Pinder KL: Compressive behavior of a physiological tissue, *Biorheology* 9(3):173-84, 1972.
20. Thompson D: The pathomechanics of soft tissue damage. In Levin MA, O'Neal LW: *The diabetic foot*, Mosby, 1983, St. Louis.
21. Van Lede P: Personal communication.
22. Van Lede P, van Veldhoven G: *Therapeutic hand splints: a rational approach*, vol 1, Provan, 1998, Antwerp, Belgium.

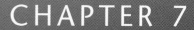

"NO, MR. ADAMS, I DON'T
THINK AN INNER TUBE
WOULD WORK BETTER."

CHAPTER 7

Principles of Using Outriggers and Mobilization Assists

Chapter Outline

OUTRIGGERS
Select Appropriate Design Configuration
Select Appropriate Material
Establish and Maintain Correct Directional Orientation
   Platform for Application of Mobilizing Force(s)
MOBILIZATION ASSISTS
Identify Optimum Force Magnitude Parameters
Therapists' Abilities to Select Rubber Band Tensions
Appropriate Boundaries

Identify Optimum Torque Magnitude Parameters
Correlate Physical Properties of the Mobilization Assist
   with Patient Requirements
Correlate Physical Properties of the Mobilization Assist
   and Interface Material with the Design of the Splint
Consider the Principles of Mechanics and Fit
Control Direction and Maintain Force Magnitude
SUMMARY

S plints that are designed to increase or to substitute for motion use carefully directed forces to correct or control joints limited by stiffness or loss of active power. Regardless of their external configuration, these splints must have a means of generating forces sufficient to apply prolonged gentle pull to stiffened joints in order to influence collagen alignment or to move passively supple joints through arcs of functional motion. Excluding serial splints, which rely on frequent alterations or replacements to improve articular motion, splinting mobilization forces are produced by specialized two-component units consisting of an *outrigger* and one or more *mobilization assists*. These two-component units function together to supply predetermined stable and accurate force application for correction of joint deformity or for substitution of weakened or lost muscle power.

Outriggers have dual purposes: (1) they provide strategically placed attachments or fulcrums for

mobilization assists and (2) they control mobilization assist alignment. Overall outrigger configuration is defined by specific patient parameters, while outrigger size, location, and orientation are determined by the angular position of the individual joint being moved, providing a simultaneous 90° angle of pull (a) to its mobilized segment and (b) to its joint axis of rotation (Fig. 7-1, *A-Q*).

Mobilization assists provide either elastic or inelastic traction. They may be constructed of a variety of materials with different physical properties (Fig. 7-2, *A-Q*). A well-functioning mobilization assist should generate a consistent and controlled force, should conform to the splint design, and should be adapted to meet the unique requirements of the patient. Mechanical and fit principles, including angle of approach, torque, pressure, friction, and ligamentous stress must also be considered when fitting these components to an extremity. Mobilization assists are the fuel or power for mobilization splints; therefore it is

184

essential that the criteria for and ramifications of using these components be thoroughly understood by all those involved in the rehabilitation process. Lack of knowledge may result in either an ineffective splint or a splint that actually causes damage to the extremity. Too much force, torque, or pressure may cause additional inflammation, scarring, and deformity. Conversely, too little force or a poorly chosen material or design may actually prevent the patient from reaching full rehabilitative potential.

The purpose of this chapter is to discuss those principles that govern the use of outriggers and mobilization assists. These principles include outrigger design concepts, identification of optimal force or torque

magnitudes, physical properties of outrigger and assist materials, correlation to patient requirements and splint design, and concepts involving principles of mechanics and fit.

■ OUTRIGGERS
Select Appropriate Design Configuration

The type of outrigger used in a mobilization splint should be reflective of individual patient needs. The number of primary joints being mobilized, their specific range of motions, and the number and positions of secondary joints included in the splint all influence the shape of an outrigger. The purpose of the splint is also important to outrigger design. Is the splint intended to correct joint deformity or to substitute for loss of muscle power? Although specific outrigger configurations and materials vary, a common feature

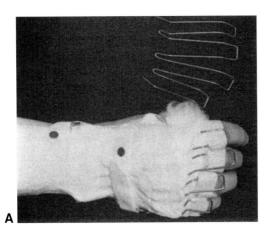

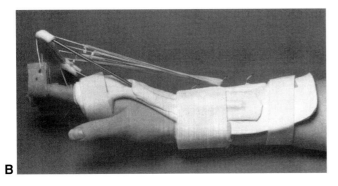

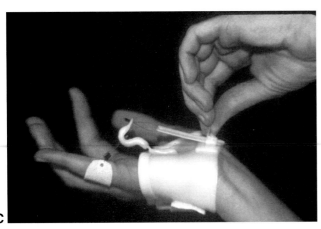

Fig. 7-1   A, Index–small finger MP extension and radial deviation mobilization splint, type 1 (5) B, Index–small finger IP extension mobilization splint, type 2 (13) C, Small finger MP flexion mobilization splint, type 0 (1) D-G, Ring finger MP flexion mobilization splint, type 0 (1) H,I, Index–small finger MP extension mobilization splint, type 1 (5) J,K, Index–small finger MP extension and radial deviation mobilization splint, type 2 (6) L, Index–small finger MP extension and radial deviation mobilization splint, type 1 (5) M, Index–small finger DIP extension and flexion torque transmission splint, type 2 (12) N, Small finger middle phalanx distraction, PIP distraction and extension or flexion mobilization splint, type 2 (3) P, Wrist extension mobilization splint, type 0 (1) Q, Shoulder abduction and external rotation mobilization splint, type 3 (4)

A,B, Outrigger configurations and materials vary considerably, reflecting individual patient needs. A number of outrigger designs allow easy adjustment and refinement of mobilizing force direction and application: C-G, a Click-strip allows incremental adjustments and its "cobra" design outrigger automatically adjusts to maintain a 90° angle to the proximal phalanx; H,I, Digitec, J,K, Allieu-Rouzaud, and L, Swanson outriggers facilitate transverse and longitudinal adjustments; M, aligned but separate outriggers allow individual adjustments to secondary finger MP and PIP joints; N,O, a wire "hoop" outrigger permits application of a distraction force and joint extension or flexion forces; P, this "dinosaur" outrigger design maintains placement of the mobilization assist and eases adjustments; and Q, exchanging progressively longer outrigger dowel rods increases shoulder motion in this splint designed by McClure and Flowers. [(A) from Hollis I: Innovative splinting ideas. In Hunter JM, et al: *Rehabilitation of the hand*, Mosby, 1978, St. Louis; Courtesy (B) Lisa Dennys, BSc, OT, London, Ontario; (C-G) Nelson Vazquez, OTR, CHT, Miami, Fla., and Damon Kirk, WFR Corporation, Wyckoff, N.J.; (H,I) Helen Marx, OTR, CHT, Human Factors Engineering of Phoenix, Wickenburg, Ariz.; (J,K) Jean Claude Rouzaud, Montpellier, France; (L) from Leonard J, Swanson A, Swanson G: *Postoperative care for patients with Silastic finger joint implants [Swanson design]*, Orthopaedic Reconstructive Surgeons P.C. of Grand Rapids, Mich., 1984; (M) from Rose H: MP/PIP adjustable digit blocking splint, *J Hand Ther* 9(3):247-8, 1996; Courtesy (N,O) Christopher Bochenek, OTR / L, CHT, Cincinnati, Ohio]

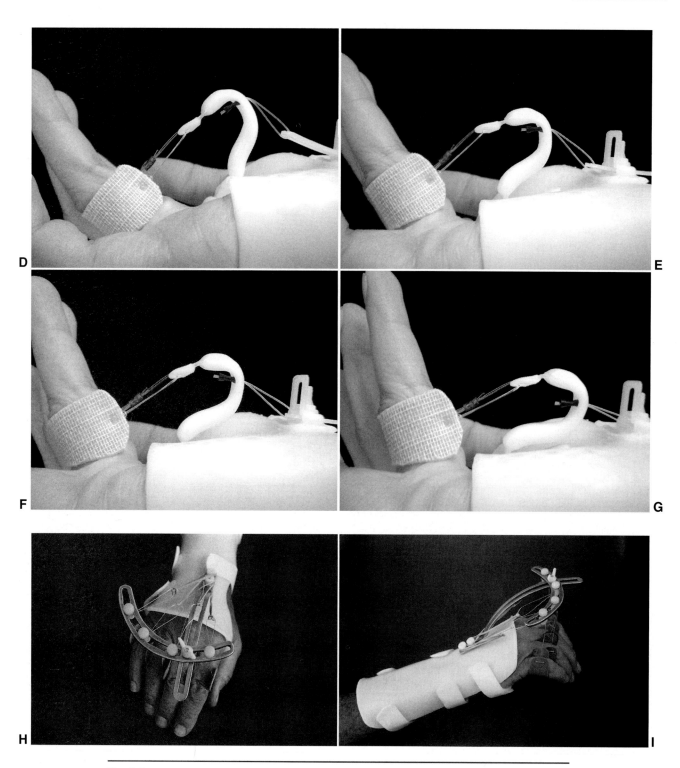

Fig. 7-1, cont'd
For legend see p. 185.

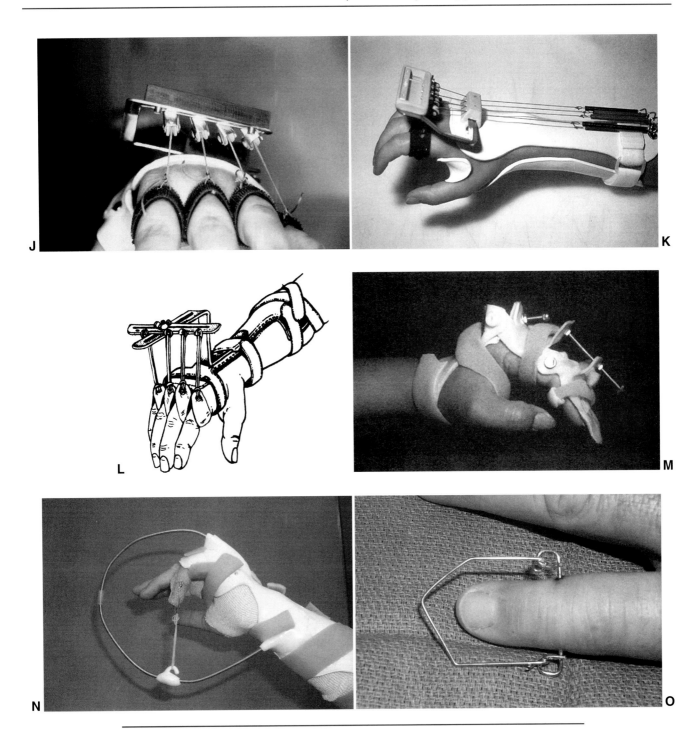

Fig. 7-1, cont'd
For legend see p. 185.

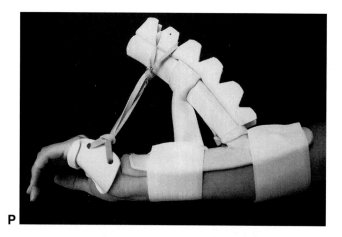

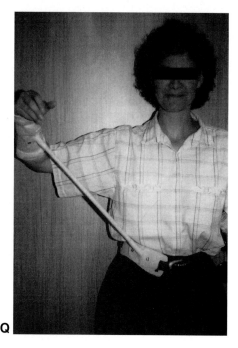

Fig. 7-1, cont'd
For legend see p. 185.

high-profile outrigger also requires less opposite-direction strength than does a low-profile design. Conversely, if the splint is to be worn while the patient works in a confined area, or if the splint substitutes for lost muscle power by mobilizing passively supple joints, a low-profile design is preferable. It is important to remember that mechanical suitability always takes priority over design cosmesis and/or ease of fabrication.[1,7-10,12,14] Once optimum mechanical requirements are achieved, other factors such as configuration mass or construction ease may be considered. Outrigger selection based solely on relative mass or quick availability is inappropriate if it fails to provide required stability and control of mobilizing forces.

Select Appropriate Material

Outrigger material selection must correspond to the purpose for splint application. If a splint is applied to mobilize stiffened joints, its outrigger must be fabricated from a material strong enough to provide a solid foundation for controlling the direction of pull of the mobilizing assists and ensuring that mobilization forces are not abated due to outrigger instability. If a splint moves passively supple joints through a functional arc of motion, its outrigger may be rigid or it may be made of a material that gives slightly, thereby providing a measure of extra "spring" to the mobilization assists through the inherent material properties of the outrigger itself.

Outrigger materials include stainless steel, high-temperature plastics, heavy-gauge wire, and tubed or rolled low-temperature plastics. Commercially available plastic tubing for outriggers must be stabilized to eliminate tube rotation within the reinforcement tunnels that bond them to their respective splints, thus avoiding rotational instability in the longitudinal plane.

Establish and Maintain Correct Directional Orientation Platform for Application of Mobilizing Force(s)

Two mechanical axes must be aligned for each joint that is mobilized. A mobilization force should provide a 90° angle of approach to the longitudinal axis of the segment being mobilized and at the same time the force must also be perpendicular to the axis of rotation of that same joint. In other words, both the segment and the joint must be considered when mobilization forces are employed. Failure to achieve correct force application results in dissipation of the amount of force applied through harmful joint attenuation or compression translational forces and/or an inequality of force application to the lateral aspects of

prevails for outriggers used for remodeling soft tissue in that they must be strong enough to provide a solid unchanging base for controlling the direction of pull of mobilization assists. In contrast, splints designed to substitute for loss of muscle power that move supple joints through predefined arcs of motion may not need outriggers that are as rigid as those of their soft tissue remodeling counterparts. Mechanical principles also play an important role in deciding outrigger configuration.[1,14,16] For example, if it is difficult for a patient to return for follow-up visits, a high-profile outrigger is preferable because, as joint motion improves, the high-profile design maintains an angle of pull closer to 90° than does a low-profile outrigger; if muscle weakness opposite the pull of the splint is a problem, a

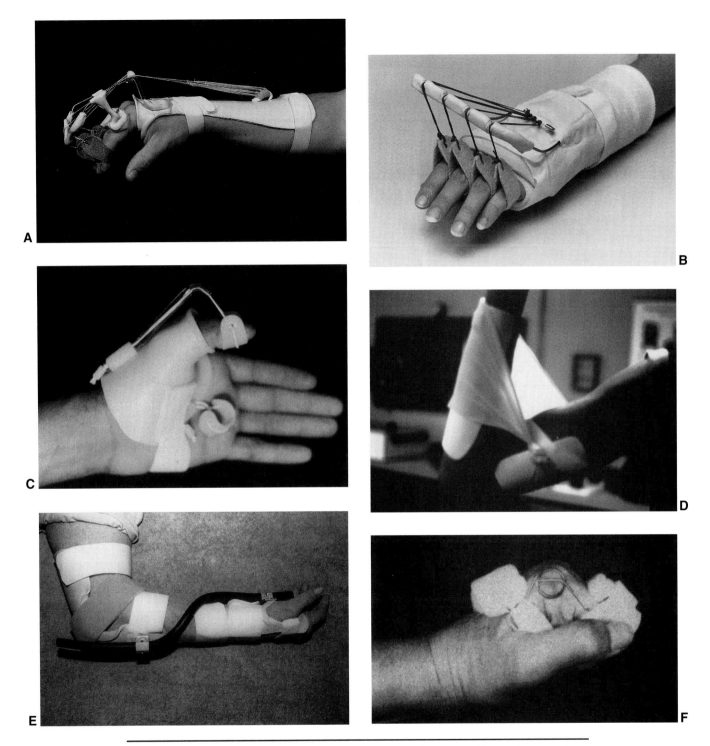

Fig. 7-2   A, Index–small finger PIP extension mobilization splint, type 2 (9) B, Index–small finger MP extension and radial deviation mobilization splint, type 1 (5) C, Thumb IP extension or flexion mobilization splint, type 2 (3) D, Elbow flexion mobilization splint, type 0 (1) E, Forearm supination mobilization splint, type 2 (3) F, Index–small finger MP extension restriction / IP extension torque transmission splint, type 0 (12) G, Wrist extension, index–small finger MP extension, thumb CMC radial abduction and MP extension mobilization splint, type 0 (7) H, Index finger PIP extension mobilization splint, type 2 (3) I, Long finger PIP extension mobilization splint, type 0 (1) J,K, Small finger PIP extension mobilization splint, type 2 (3) L,M, Thumb IP extension mobilization splint, type 0 (1) N,O, Wrist extension, index–small finger extension mobilization splint, type 0 (13) P, Long–ring finger PIP extension mobilization splint, type 1 (4) Q, Thumb CMC palmar abduction mobilization splint, type 3 (4)

Mobilization assists may be fabricated from a wide variety of materials: **A,** rubber band and dental floss, **B,C,** elastic thread, **D,** exercise band, **E,** rubber tubing, **F,** spring coil, **G,** spring wire, **H,I,** springs, **J-M,** Velcro, **N,O,** heavy gauge wire, **P,** string/monofilament, and **Q,** turnbuckles. [Courtesy **(B)** Barbara Allen, OTR/L, Oklahoma City, Okla.; **(C,P)** Kathryn Schultz, OTR, CHT, Orlando, Fla; **(D)** Robin Miller, OTR/L, CHT, Ft. Lauderdale, Fla.; **(G)** Jean-Christophe Arias, Saint-Etienne, France; **(I)** Renske Houck-Romkes, Rotterdam, Netherlands; **(J,K)** Janet Bailey, OTR/L, CHT, Columbus, Ohio; **(L,M)** Susan Glaser-Butler, OTR/L, CHT, Virginia Beach, Va.; **(N,O)** Dominique Thomas, RPT, MCMK, Saint Martin Duriage, France; **(Q)** Daniel Lupo, OTR, CHT, Ventura, Calif.]

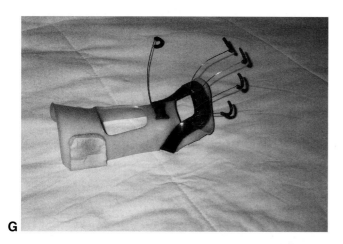

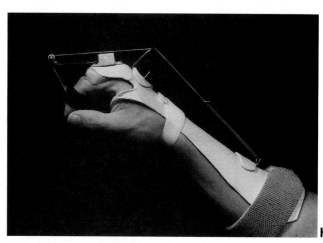

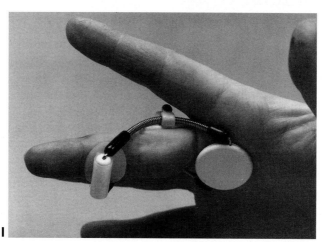

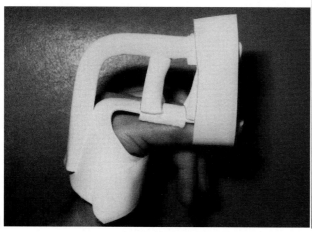

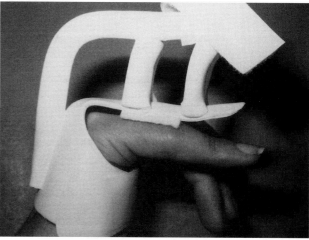

Fig. 7-2, cont'd
For legend see p. 189.

the joint capsule, which produces joint instability. Outrigger position is the key factor in controlling mobilization assist position and therefore the angle of application of each mobilizing force (see Chapter 10: Principles of Fit).

As joint angulation changes through soft tissue remodeling or growth, outrigger position must be altered to keep pace with the soft tissue changes, thus maintaining correct alignment of the mobilizing assist directional forces. Some outrigger designs provide a

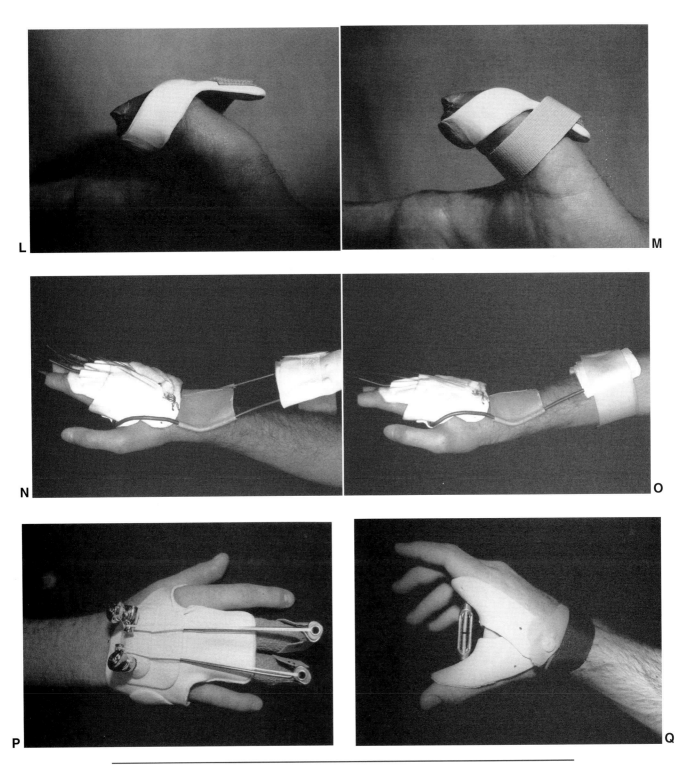

Fig. 7-2, cont'd
For legend see p. 189.

constant 90° angle of pull through their innovative designs (Fig. 7-3).[6]

■ MOBILIZATION ASSISTS
Identify Optimum Force Magnitude Parameters

When discussing mobilization assists and the forces they impart, it is important to understand the funda-mental differences between a splint designed to sub-stitute for absent or weak active motion and a splint that corrects passive motion limitations. Both of these splints are classified as mobilization splints, but the mobilizing forces employed by each splint differ. A substitution splint is applied to a passively supple joint, requiring a force that is just sufficient to pull or push the splinted segment into predetermined align-

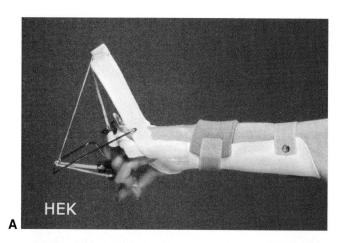

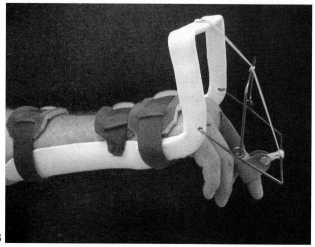

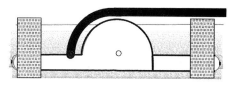

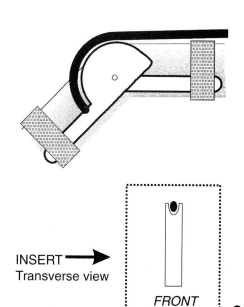

INSERT →
Transverse view

FRONT

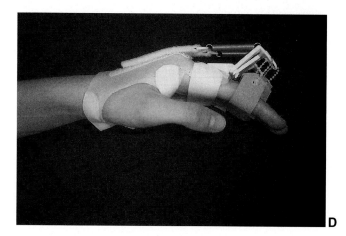

Fig. 7-3   A, Long–ring finger PIP extension mobilization splint, type 2 (5) B, Long finger PIP extension mobilization splint, type 2 (3) C, Finger PIP extension mobilization splint, type 0 (1) D, Index–small finger PIP extension mobilization splint, type 1 (8) A, A crane outrigger automatically adjusts, via the top rubber band, to maintain a 90° angle of pull as joint range of motion changes. Incorporation of a second crane outrigger to an existing crane out-rigger decreases considerably the amount of strength a patient needs to move opposite to the pull of the outrigger. Both the (C) Dunipace and the (D) OSSY outrigger designs maintain constant 90° angle of pull regardless of joint position. [Courtesy (A) From Christine M. Kleinert Institute for Hand and Microsurgery, Inc. (B) Jason Willoughby, OTR, Richmond, Ky.; (D) from Srinivasan MS, Knowles D, Wood J: The OSSY splint, a new design of dynamic extension splint, *Br J Hand Ther* 5(3):72-4, 2000, and splint cour-tesy Barbara Boling, North Coast Medical, Morgan Hill, Calif.]

ment. Due to the presence of normal passive motion, determination of the amount of force to use is not imperative. The mobilization assist is simply adjusted until the desired joint position is achieved (Fig. 7-4). This, however, cannot be done with splints designed to correct fixed articular deformities. Knowledge of the magnitude of the force generated by the mobilization assist is critical when applying a corrective splint when a joint *lacks* normal passive motion. Regardless of the force used, the segment cannot readily be brought into alignment without disrupting tissue continuity. The key, therefore, is to provide enough tension to control collagen alignment and to stimulate tissue growth while not tearing soft tissue. Too much force will cause damage, escalating the inflammatory response and scar formation. Conversely, too little force will not affect tissue remodeling and joint motion will remain unchanged or diminish further.

Just how much force is required to influence growth and collagen alignment without causing additional tissue damage? Although this question seems elemental, and a few researchers and hand specialists have tried to define the parameters of splinting forces, quantitative statistical data are almost nonexistent in the literature. Some authors have correlated lack of skin blanching or no increase in joint inflammation with appropriate splinting forces, and others have attempted to apply numerical values to better define force magnitude. Delineating the important interrelationship between magnitude and time, Kosiak (1959) found that the amount of pressure causing damage in

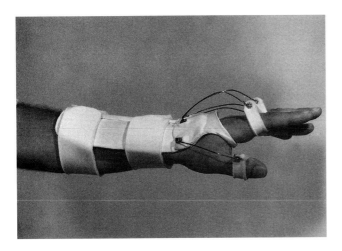

Fig. 7-4   Wrist extension, index–small finger MP extension, thumb CMC radial abduction and MP extension mobilization splint, type 0 (7)
Mobilization assist force measurements are not necessary for substitution splints because normal passive range of motion is present. (Courtesy Christine Heaney, BSc, OT, Ottawa, Ontario.)

laboratory animals was related to a combination of force and duration. Based on experience, Malick[15] suggested 0.5 pounds of force and Brand[2-5] recommended splinting forces ranging from between 100 and 300 gm. Pearson[19] noted that joint deformity could be corrected with as little as 3 ounces of rubber band traction, and Fess, Gettle, and Strickland[12] used 8 ounces of force to describe resolution of forces and the need for a 90° angle of approach of traction used in hand splinting. Based on these early contributions, others have agreed with the general concept of using 100 to 300 gm of force to remodel digital soft tissues.[7-10,12-14,18,21,22] Despite this, most clinicians currently rely on feel to judge the amount of force they apply to the hand.

Therapists' Abilities to Select Rubber Band Tensions

Recognizing that most splints are fitted without measuring assist force, Fess[11] assessed the abilities of 47 therapists (36 Registered Occupational Therapists, 3 Registered Physical Therapists, and 8 Occupational Therapy Students) to select rubber band tensions. Clinical experience of the therapists ranged from none to more than 40 years and 24 of the 47 subjects reported that they considered themselves hand specialists. The average number of splints made per subject ranged from 0 to more than 20 per week and of total patient loads, the percent of hands treated ranged from 0-100%. Of those who considered themselves specialists in hands, experience ranged from 0 to 17 years in hand rehabilitation.

Using a standard set of instructions, subjects selected rubber band tensions appropriate to two case histories from two tension adjustment frames (Fig. 7-5). The case histories involved two PIP joint flexion deformities of 50/90° of left index fingers, one acute (6 weeks) and one chronic (6 months). The splints pictured in the two case histories were of identical design (Fig. 7-6). To ascertain the reliability of the therapists' skills, subjects chose their rubber band tensions from two frames, which were identical except for the color of the top surface and the number of rubber band choices. The blue frame allowed nine options of randomly weighted rubber bands in 50 gm increments; the yellow frame had five options of randomly arranged bands in 100 gm increments (Fig. 7-7). Band tensions were obtained by attaching standardized brass weights to high-quality no. 33 rubber bands (Fig. 7-8) that had been checked for consistency of length. Tensions in both frames ranged from 100 to 500 gm.

Subjects were asked to read the first case history, select and record the number of an appropriate tension from the blue frame, and then (without

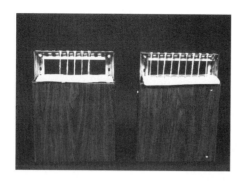

Fig. 7-5   In accord with two case histories, therapists selected rubber band tensions from two tension adjustment frames.

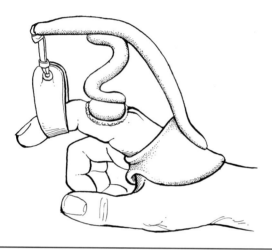

Fig. 7-6   Index finger PIP extension mobilization splint, type 1 (2)
The splints described in the case histories were identical for both the chronic and acute injury.

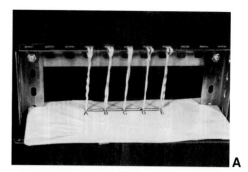

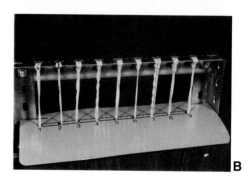

Fig. 7-7   To test selection reliability, rubber bands were randomly arranged in (A) 100 gm and (B) 50 gm increments.

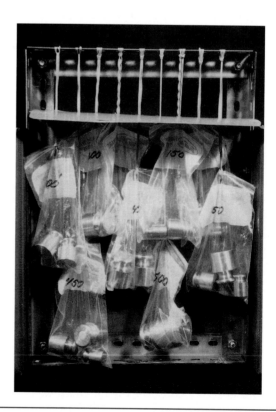

Fig. 7-8   Standard brass weights were attached to no. 33 high-quality rubber bands and suspended from the tension adjustment frames.

returning to the blue frame) select and record the same tension on the yellow frame. The same format was then used for the second case history.

Results indicated that of the four major groups tested—(1) students, (2) not specialists in hands, (3) specialists in hands but not members of the ASHT, and (4) members of ASHT—no statistical differences were found between the 50 gm increment frame and the 100 gm increment frame for both flexion deformities. Therapists at all levels of experience were capable of identifying a rubber band tension and replicating that tension in a second set of rubber band options ($p < .05$).

For three of the four groups tested, therapists applied less force to the acute flexion deformity than they did to the chronic deformity. This was found to be statistically significant in the ASHT group and the "not specialized" group. Students did not alter the forces when treating the acute and chronic cases.

Variables correlated positively with lighter tension selections (Fig. 7-9) included (1) a 91% to 100% case load of hand patients, (2) six or more hand splints made per week, (3) six or more years specializing in hands, and (4) member of ASHT. Of this group, mean tension selections ranged from 164.3 to 197.5 gm (5.8 to 7.0 ounces) for the acute proximal interphalangeal flexion deformity, and 265.0 to 293.8 gm (9.4 to 10.4 ounces) for the chronic proximal interphalangeal flexion deformity.

Those variables that did not correlate with lighter tension selections included years of experience other than hands, hours spent in academic splint class, a case load of up to 30% hand problems, not specializing in hands, and students. Interestingly, students and less experienced therapists almost universally selected greater tensions than did the more experienced hand specialists. In other words, if a mistake was made, it was most often made in the direction of applying too much tension rather than too little.

This investigation indicates that experienced hand specialists alter their rubber band tensions according to diagnosis. These selections are not haphazard, but instead can be replicated at a statistically significant level. And, verifying some of the parameters suggested in the literature, the overall magnitude of tension used ranged from 164 to 294 gm, depending on the acuteness of the injury.

Appropriate Boundaries

Although the research just cited needs to be further correlated with clinical studies, a general concept of the "safe boundaries" of the force magnitude required to influence tissue growth and collagen alignment, as identified by highly experienced hand specialists, begins to emerge. These parameters may be used as a standard with which any type of mobilization assist component affecting the small joints of the hand may be compared and evaluated, whether possessing elastic or inelastic properties. Further investigation needs to be undertaken to determine whether this tension range is effective for larger joints whose moment arms are greater such as the elbow or for more complicated articulations such as those found in the wrist.

Identify Optimum Torque Magnitude Parameters

While knowledge of force magnitude is fundamental to good splint fabrication and fit, it is not the only important factor in understanding the complex mechanical interrelationships involved in mobilizing a joint through prolonged gentle traction. The point on the finger at which the rotational force is applied is also an essential factor. In the previous section, optimal ranges of forces were identified, but are these parameters applicable to all splinting situations? What happens when these forces are applied at different

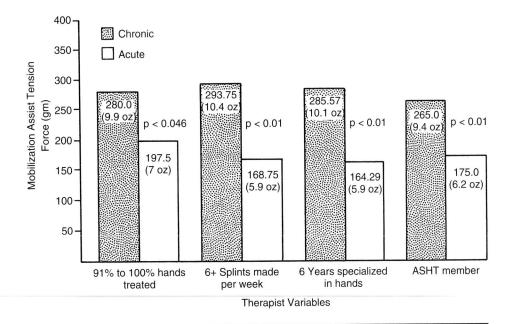

Fig. 7-9   Statistically significant positive differences were found between four variables and lighter rubber band tension selections.

distances from the joint axis of rotation? The answer requires an understanding of torque. Torque (see Chapter 5) is defined as the product of the amount of rotational force and the perpendicular distance between the axis of joint rotation and the force line of action, or torque equals force times distance (T = FD). For example, a force of 200 gm placed 2 cm, 4 cm, and 6 cm away from a joint would result in torque measurements of 400 gm/cm, 800 gm/cm, and 1200 gm/cm, respectively. A splinting force that is appropriate at one distance may not be appropriate at another. The "safe boundaries" of force described in the previous section were derived from a study involving deformities at the PIP joint and an application of rotational force to the midportion of the middle phalanx, a distance of approximately 1 cm from the joint axis. What then, are appropriate forces proximal and distal to this point, and what are force parameters for the MP and DIP joints? To date, there are no published research studies specifically addressing these issues, but if one assumes that forces similar to those defined for the PIP joint would be applicable to the MP and DIP joints, "safe boundaries" of force may be deduced through torque parameters for each joint of a finger. Torque acts as a common denominator for interpreting the mechanical stresses of rotational force placed on a given joint at different levels of a digit. The previously defined force range of 164-294 grams may be converted into torque by multiplying each 1 cm away from the joint axis, resulting in a torque margin of safety of 164 cm/gm to 294 cm/gm. Using these torque parameters as standards, safe force magnitudes may be equated for various distances from a joint axis by applying the basic torque formula (164 cm/gm = F × D; 294 cm/gm = F × D);

Distance from axis (cm)	"Safe force boundaries" (gm)
1	164-295
2	84-147
3	55-98
4	41-74
5	33-59
6	27-49
7	23-42
8	21-37

Notice that the further away from the joint a mobilizing force is applied, the less amount of force is required to remain within the "safe boundary" range for remodeling digital soft tissue structures. These forces may in turn be applied to each of the three joints of a finger (Fig. 7-10). Although these force parameters may not be considered absolute without further research, it is graphically apparent that there is no single force or force range that is appropriate for

all splinting needs. Forces for correction of joint deformity are directly related to the distance between the point of force application and the axis of rotation of the joint being mobilized: the greater the distance, the less the force required. Torque also allows comparison of forces imparted by prefabricated splints of differing sizes (Fig. 7-11).[7] Representing the actual amount of stress applied to a joint, the determination of torque magnitude is essential to understanding and using prolonged gentle traction for mobilization of stiffened digital joints.

Mobilization splints must be monitored carefully to ensure that force/torque application is effective and at the same time not harmful to soft tissue. Increased redness, swelling, and/or pain are indicative of too much force/torque being applied. If patient wearing tolerance is less than 30 minutes due to vascular insufficiency or numbness, mobilization assist force/torque must be adjusted.

Correlate Physical Properties of the Mobilization Assist with Patient Requirements

Mobilization splinting is dependent upon a series of interrelated variables that describe joint condition, the most important of which include, but are not limited to, time/duration, degree of angulation, and end feel. When aligned, these variables form a series of separate but parallel condition continuums, each of which ranges from minor to major level of involvement. Selection of a mobilization assist depends on the amount of joint involvement as it relates to duration of the problem over time, the degree of joint angulation, and the hardness of end feel or give as the joint is passively moved to its end range of motion. Generally speaking, the greater are the time, angulation, and hardness of end feel, the greater is the need for inelastic traction (see illustration, front inside cover).

The physical properties of the material making up a mobilization assist regulate the range of forces it generates. For example, rubber bands of a given size and quality produce a fairly predictable force spectrum,[17] whereas spring coil assists produce another range of forces. Unfortunately, however, not all coil splints create similar tensions, nor do rubber band components. Even among assists made of similar substances, variables such as shelf life and quality may alter the amount of force created. Durability must also be considered. An assist that requires frequent adjustments to keep it within the required force parameters creates more work for the therapist and unnecessary inconvenience and expense for the patient. Those responsible for fabricating mobilizing splints should be well acquainted with the basic similarities and differences of the many materials currently used for mobilization

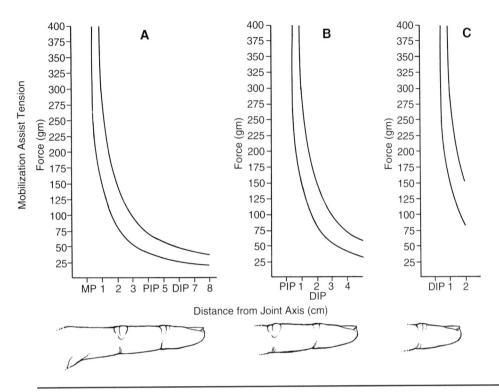

Fig. 7-10   Using torque parameters, "safe boundaries" for different levels of force application may be computed for the (**A**) metacarpophalangeal, (**B**) proximal interphalangeal, and (**C**) distal interphalangeal joints.

assist components in order to increase patients' opportunities to achieve their full rehabilitative potential.

The concepts described by Brand[4,5] help identify the conditions under which mobilization assists produce optimal ranges of tension by plotting their reactions to progressive loading on length-tension curves. These graphic representations are invaluable in understanding why, when, and how mobilization splints work.

Rubber band tensions are directly influenced by length and thickness of the bands. If two rubber bands of the same length but with differing thicknesses are subjected to similar loads, the narrower of the two bands elongates more quickly with less tension but is not as durable in splinting situations (Fig. 7-12). Force ranges are also influenced by the quality of the rubber bands (Fig. 7-13).

The forces produced by spring-coil or spring-wire splints are regulated by the thickness and resiliency of the wire, the size and number of coils, and the distance from the coil to the distal end of the splint. Larger wire diameters, tighter coils, and longer distances generate greater forces. Longer and larger diameter spring wire splints follow a similar pattern. Like those for rubber bands, length tension curves for springs vary according to the properties of the materials from which the springs are made. Tracking a more linear pattern than rubber bands, some springs may double or triple their resting length with minimal to moderate increases in force, while others quickly exceed safe force parameters with very little change in length (Fig. 7-14). Springs are often more durable than rubber bands and shelf life is excellent. Caution is needed when using spring-coil or spring-wire mobilization assists because they often produce narrowly appropriate force ranges, quickly exiting the boundaries of "safe force parameters" for remodeling soft tissues.[7]

Other materials such as elastic thread, exercise tubing, orthodontic elastics, Velcro, and cotton webbing exhibit widely differing force tension curves (Fig. 7-15).

Since the physical properties of a mobilization assist influence durability and regulate the amount of tension produced, the choice of material comprising the assist is extremely important and should be carefully coordinated to meet the individual needs of the patient. For example, if a splint is needed to correct a 30° flexion contracture of a proximal interphalangeal joint, none of the spring coil splints illustrated in Fig. 7-11 would produce appropriate forces, but elastic traction in the form of rubber bands or

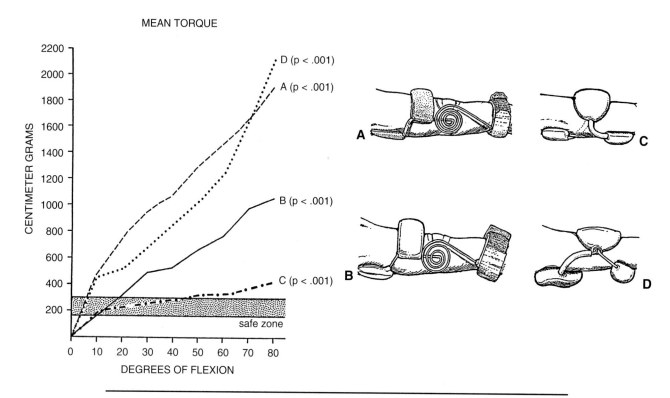

MEAN TORQUE

Fig. 7-11   A,B, Finger PIP extension mobilization splint, type 1 (2) C,D, Finger PIP extension mobilization splint, type 0 (1)

Although not representative of all splints of this design, these commercially available spring coil splints produced excessive force measurements. Splints A and B apply force 3 cm from the proximal interphalangeal joint axis of rotation and C and D, 2 cm from the axis. Splint B meets "safe force" criteria (gray area between solid horizontal parallel lines) for a flexion deformity ranging between 10° and 15°; A and D have even less applicable range. Splint C stays within the "safe force" boundaries between 10° and 45°. (From Fess EE: Force magnitude of commercial spring-coil and spring-wire splints designed to extend the proximal interphalangeal joint, *J Hand Ther* 1:86-90, 1988.)

exercise tubing cut to given lengths could be used. Cotton webbing or Velcro could provide inelastic traction when tightened to specific tensions and should also be considered.

It is important to remember that a "static progressive" mobilization assist is yet another form of inelastic traction, just as is a mobilization assist made of Velcro or some other non-stretchy/springy material. Due to its inherent lack of elastic/spring physical properties, inelastic mobilization of soft tissues requires incremental adjustments of the mobilization assists over time to have an effect on tissue remodeling. This gentle unchanging tension applied by inelastic mobilization assists is one of splinting's most effective techniques for remodeling upper extremity soft tissues. Because inelastic mobilization assists are not "self-adjusting," most patients must return to the clinic every 3-4 days for tension adjustments to the assists, although some patients are able to adjust their own inelastic mobilization assists.

Correlate Physical Properties of the Mobilization Assist and Interface Material with the Design of the Splint

Splint design also influences the type of mobilization assist that may be used. Because of their physical properties, some materials may not be compatible with certain splint designs. For example, a mobilization assist that requires length to generate appropriate force parameters would probably have limited effectiveness with a hand-based splint design simply because of the relative shortness of the splint. Because of inherent mechanical bias, some splints and assist components are more effective under specific conditions. For example, a three-point pressure splint, such as the commercially available "safety pin" splint that utilizes a Velcro or webbing assist to generate force, would not be effective in correcting a 45° flexion deformity. In this instance it is not the material from which the assist is made that is the problem, but rather

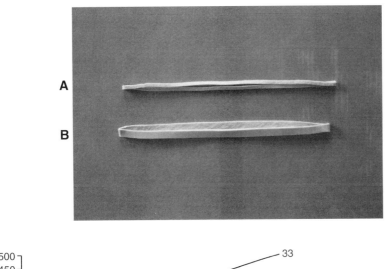

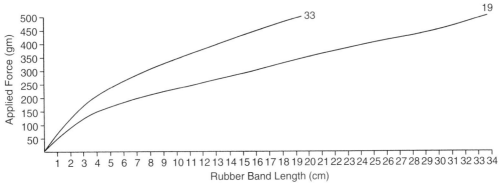

Fig. 7-12   Rubber band thickness influences length tension and durability. Comparison of rubber bands with identical resting length **(A)** indicates that the thinner bands (19) elongate more quickly with less force than do the heavier bands (33) **(B)**.

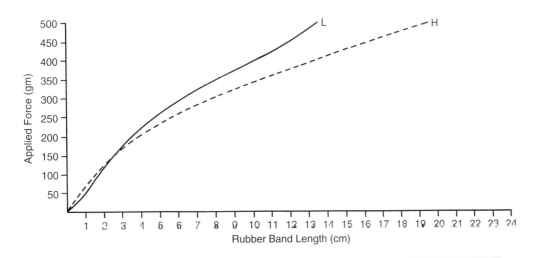

Fig. 7-13   High-quality rubber bands *(H)* stretch more with less force than do lower-quality bands of the same size *(L)*.

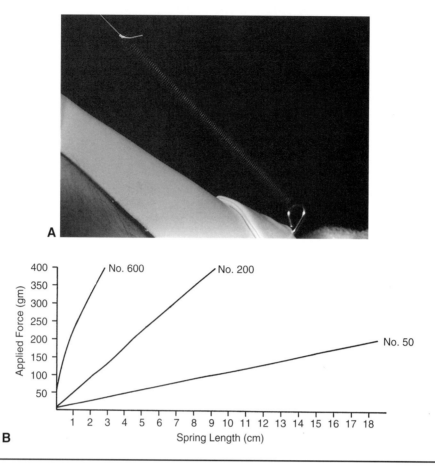

Fig. 7-14   **A,** Scomac spring lengths change with different weights. **B,** These no. 50, no. 200, and no. 600 Scomac springs respond differently to the application of increasingly greater forces. A small amount of force lengthens a no. 50 spring, while considerable force minimally lengthens a no. 600 spring.

the design of the splint itself. Mechanically, three-point pressure splints are ineffective when used to correct deformities greater than 35° (see Chapter 6). Velcro, however, could be used as a mobilization assist to correct a 45° flexion deformity if it were attached to an outrigger to provide a 90° angle of approach.

If a low-profile outrigger design is used, the interface material between the rubber band and the finger cuff should be constructed of an inelastic material that glides smoothly over the outrigger fulcrum. Interface materials often include nylon fish line (Fig. 7-16) or nylon cording. In the early 1970s, Philips introduced the technique of using unwaxed dental floss as an interface material because of its durability and its easy knot tying and knot retention properties.[20] Occasionally interfaces are made of rigid materials, e.g., strong wire, to ensure force application is directed accurately and proportionately as required.

Outrigger height influences the design of mobilization assists. If the outrigger is a high-profile design, or if a low-profile outrigger is used on a hand-based splint (Fig. 7-17), the length at which the assist produces an optimal force range is critical. Too much elasticity in the assist requires an excessively tall outrigger to generate an appropriate force range. Conversely, an assist should be long enough to prohibit forces from grossly exceeding the upper limits of the acceptable force range when the finger is actively moved in a direction opposite to that of the assist. Since an elastic assist may increase in length by as much as 6 cm as a finger moves away from the direction of pull of the assist, it is important also to identify the forces generated by the assist in its elongated position (Fig. 7-18). Although active compression is beneficial to the nutrition of articular surfaces by stimulating synovial fluid infusion as objects are grasped, care should be taken to avoid excessive resistance to the digits as mobilization assists are stretched through functional motion patterns. These concepts are also applicable to forearm-based low-profile outrigger designs but the criteria are often easier to attain because of the additional length of the splints. The acceptable force range

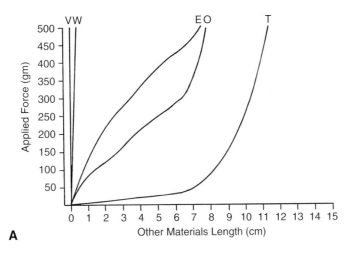

A

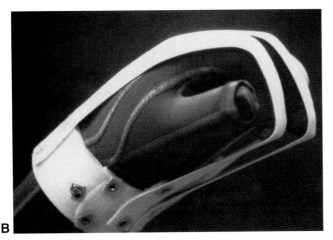

B

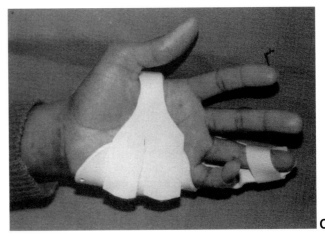

C

Fig. 7-15   B, Index–small finger flexion mobilization splint, type 0 (12) C, Ring finger, small finger MP-PIP extension mobilization splint, type 0 (5) D, Elbow flexion mobilization splint, type 0 (1) E, Index–small finger MP flexion and IP extension, thumb CMC radial abduction and MP-IP extension immobilization splint, type 1 (16) F, Thumb IP flexion or extension mobilization splint, type 2 (3)
Mobilizing assist materials elongate as tension or force is applied. A, Providing a wide range of options for use as mobilization assists, the length tension curves for Velcro (V), cotton webbing (W), exercise tubing (E), orthodontic rubber band (O), and elastic thread (T) differ considerably. Splint designs differ according to mobilization assist materials used: B, Velcro, C, cotton webbing, D, exercise tubing, E, orthodontic rubber band, and F, elastic thread. [Courtesy (**B,C**) Lin Beribak, OTR/L, CHT, Chicago, Ill.; (**D**) Sally Poole, MA, OTR, CHT, Dobbs Ferry, N.Y.; (**F**) Kathryn Schultz, OTR, CHT, Orlando, Fla.

does not change but assists with greater elastic properties may be used to facilitate adjustment.

Consider the Principles of Mechanics and Fit

Outrigger-mobilization assist units should apply a force that is 90° to the longitudinal axis of the segment being mobilized. This eliminates joint compression and distraction and allows the full magnitude of the force to be directed toward correcting the deformity or moving a passively supple joint through an arc of motion. To avoid unequal stress to ligamentous struc-tures surrounding the immediate joint and those more proximal in the ray, the angle of traction should also be perpendicular to the axis of the joint being mobilized. Providing final increments of refinement, guides, or pulleys can control the direction of force (Fig. 7-19).

Pressure applied by the finger attachment device should also be carefully monitored. Finger cuffs should be as wide as possible without impeding adjacent joint motion to distribute forces over a larger area and decrease pressure. Generally, cuffs should be con-structed of a strong but pliable material, because the

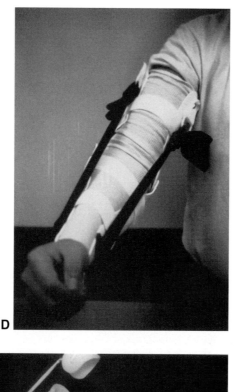

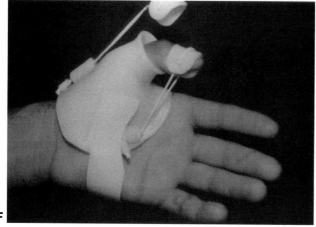

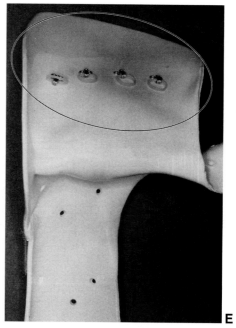

Fig. 7-15, cont'd
For legend see p. 201.

combination of a rigid finger cuff and lack of a 90° angle of approach may create an unfavorable situation (Fig. 7-20). A low-profile finger cuff designed by Brand (Fig. 7-21) eliminates the potentially dangerous leverage effect produced by conventional cuffs. This cuff design is especially helpful when dealing with a hand that lacks sensibility. If hooks, suture loops, or Velcro are attached to the fingernails, the amount of traction should not jeopardize the vascular status of the nail bed or surrounding tissue.

Friction between a finger cuff and the underlying cutaneous surface often indicates lack of a 90° angle of approach of the traction, allowing the cuff to migrate proximally or distally. By altering the length of the outrigger as joint motion changes, this friction may

be controlled. Friction may also occur between the surfaces of the mobilization assist and the outrigger at the fulcrum point in low-profile splint designs. As the portion of the assist that comes in contact with the outrigger moves back and forth, friction is created, eventually undermining the strength of the assist. An interface of nylon line or unwaxed dental floss between the elastic assist and the finger attachment device increases durability (Fig. 7-22), as do pulleys on the outrigger (Fig. 7-23). Another site of friction that may jeopardize the longevity of a mobilization assist component is the junction of the elastic assist and the interface. As stress is applied, the harder interface material (nylon line, dental floss, etc.) cuts into the softer elastic assist. Protective liners

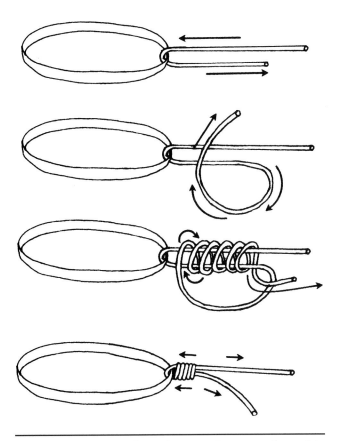

Fig. 7-16   When nylon fishing line is used as an interface, a fisherman's knot keeps the connection from loosening.

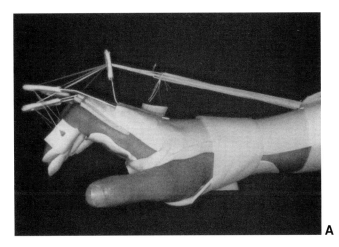

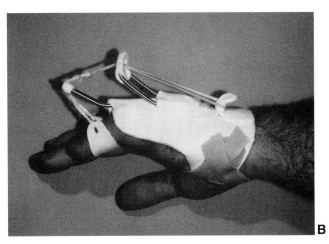

Fig. 7-17   A, Index–small finger PIP extension mobilization splint type 2 (9) \\ Finger PIP torque transmission splint, type 1 (2); 4 splints @ each finger separate B, Small finger PIP extension mobilization splint, type 1 (2)
A, A mobilization assist that requires more distance to generate a force range necessary for splinting stiff joints requires a longer splint design. B, A relatively short splint may be used with a soft/medium end-feel joint where extrinsic tendons are not involved. [Courtesy **(A)** Jill Francisco, OTR, CHT, Cicero, Ind.; **(B)** Susan Emerson, MEd, OTR, Dover, N.H.]

or special looping techniques may alleviate this problem.

Control Direction and Maintain Force Magnitude

Once correct tensions are set (Fig. 7-24), corrective splints require careful monitoring and frequent readjusting to maintain their effectiveness (Fig. 7-25). An elastic assist may lose some of its rebound ability, creating excessive length and a concomitant inability to generate mobilizing forces within the desired range. These types of assists may require adjustment or replacement as often as every 2 or 3 days, depending on physical properties and use. The optimum range of forces for a spring coil splint occurs at very specific joint ranges. These ranges differ from one type of coil splint to another, resulting in splints of limited use if they cannot be readily adjusted. Inelastic traction must be adjusted frequently as joint motion changes, as must the length of an outrigger to maintain a constant 90° angle of approach of the mobilizing force.

Although outrigger height does not influence force magnitude of mobilization assists, it does influence adjustment schedules. Low-profile outriggers lose the

required 90° angle of approach more quickly than do their high-profile counterparts (Fig. 7-26). This, however, is a concept applicable only when working with correctional forces. If the purpose of a splint is to substitute for weak or absent active motion, full passive joint motion is a prerequisite, and the need for sequential adjustments to accommodate motion improvements is nonexistent. Low-profile outriggers are appropriate design options for control or substitution splints because they do not need sequential adjustments. Conversely, high-profile outriggers provide longer increments of near 90° angle of pull than do the low-profile designs, indicating that for correctional splints the higher design option requires fewer

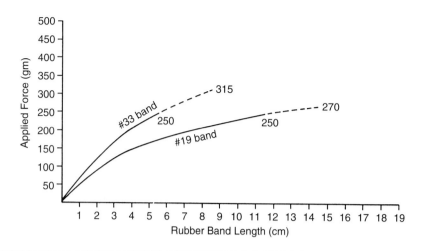

Fig. 7-18 Forces increase as a finger is moved in a direction opposite to the pull of the mobilization assist. Greater force is required to elongate a no. 33 rubber band by 3 cm than is required to elongate a no. 19 rubber band by the same 3 cm distance. To stretch the additional 3 cm, the original 250 gm force is increased by 20 gm for the no. 19 rubber band as compared to a 65 gm increase for the no. 33 band.

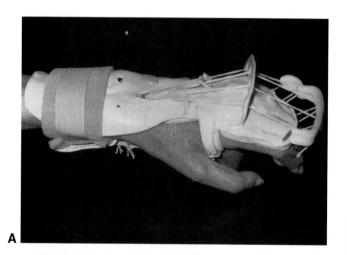

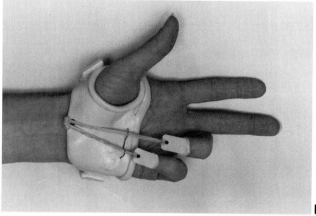

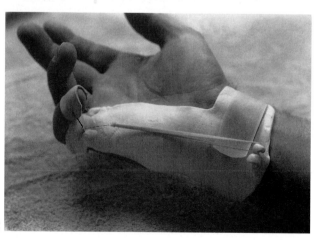

Fig. 7-19 **A,** Index–small finger PIP extension mobilization splint, type 2 (9) **B,** Ring–small finger flexion mobilization splint, type 0 (6) **C,** Small finger IP flexion mobilization splint, type 2 (4) **D,** Index–long finger IP, small finger PIP flexion mobilization splint, type 1 (9) **E,** Index finger MP extension and radial deviation mobilization splint, type 1 (2)
Pulleys and guides refine the direction of pull of mobilization assists. [Courtesy **(A)** Diana Williams, MBA, OTR, CHT, Macon, Ga.; **(B)** Barbara Allen Smith, OTR/L, Edmond, Okla.; **(C)** Carolina deLeeuw, MA, OTR, Tacoma, Wash.; **(D)** Shelli Dellinger, OTR, CHT, San Diego, Calif.; **(E)** Peggy McLaughlin, OTR, CHT, San Bernadino, Calif.]

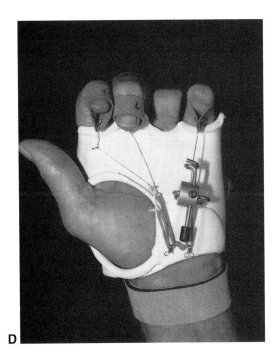

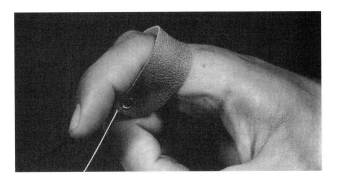

Fig. 7-20   In the absence of a 90° angle of pull, the area of force application of a rigid-material finger sling decreases and resultant pressure increases.

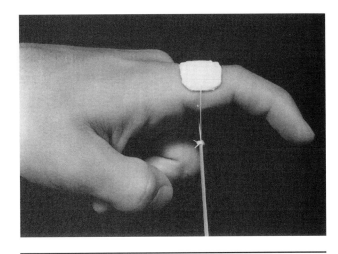

Fig. 7-21   Designed by Paul Brand, MB, BS, FRCS, this low-profile finger cuff allows the full width of the cuff to remain in contact with the dorsum of the finger even if a 90° angle of pull is not present.

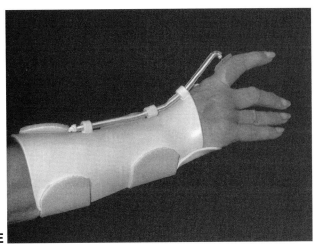

E

Fig. 7-19, cont'd
For legend see opposite page.

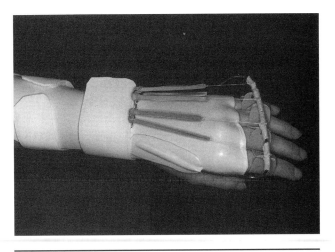

Fig. 7-22   Index–small finger MP extension mobilization splint, type 1 (5)
Using an inelastic material as an interface between a mobilization assist and a finger cuff diminishes friction at the outrigger fulcrum. (Courtesy Barbara Raff, OTR, Lake Zurich, Ill.)

adjustments as improvements in motion are gained. High-profile outrigger splints also require less patient strength to volitionally oppose mobilization assist pull and they provide greater joint stability to joints being mobilized than do low-profile outrigger splint designs. Whether these concepts are important in designing correctional splints depends entirely on the patients' individual needs, including their abilities to return to the clinic for adjustments and the time demands of the therapists' caseloads.

With the creation of a splint comes the responsibility for maintaining its effectiveness. To set only the initial force is not sufficient. Target joints and mobi-

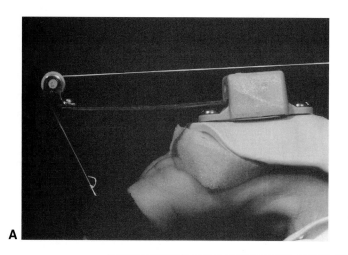
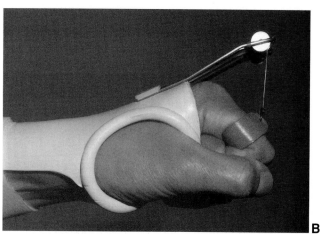

Fig. 7-23   B, Index–long finger MP extension mobilization splint, type 1 (3)
By decreasing friction, outrigger pulleys increase the durability of the assist unit and ease active finger motion as seen in **A** and **B**. (**B** Courtesy Ester May, PhD, OT, Adelaide, South Australia.)

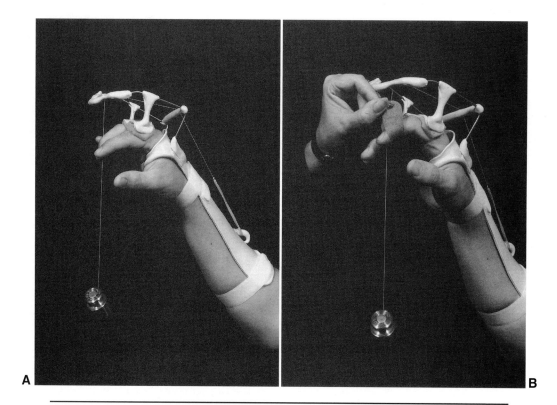

Fig. 7-24   Index–small finger PIP extension mobilization splint, type 2 (9)
A simple method of setting tension, an appropriate size standard brass weight is attached to the untrimmed end of the assist unit and is suspended from the outrigger at a 90° angle (**A**). The finger is then pulled gently into position and a mark is placed on the fishing line at the point where the cuff will be attached (**B**).

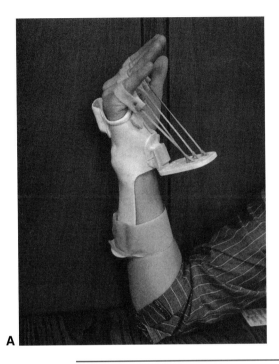
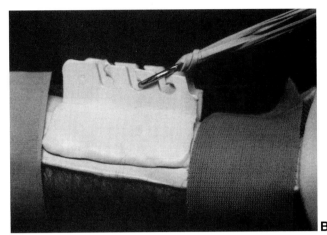

Fig. 7-25   A, Index–small finger MP flexion mobilization splint, type 1 (5)
A, Constructed of a solid piece of material in which multiple holes have been drilled, this "slab" outrigger facilitates maintenance of a 90° angle of pull. B, A series of attachment sites in the form of progressive notches eases tension adjustment. [Courtesy (A) Joyce Roalef, OTR /L, CHT, Dayton, Ohio; (B) Karen Schultz-Johnson, MS, OTR, FAOTA, CHT, Edwards, Colo.]

lization assists change with time, making previously set tensions ineffective and obsolete. To date, no mobilization assist component exists that maintains optimal force parameters throughout the full arc of joint motion without adjustments. Frequent measurements of joint motion, tension checks, and monitoring of the traction angle of approach identify the need for alterations.

BOX 7-1   Clinical Hints

1. Maintain a 90° angle to segment being moved and to joint axis of rotation. Adjust length of outrigger and angle of mobilizing assist as joint deformity changes.
2. Use pulleys to reduce drag over outrigger in low-profile outriggers.
3. If mobilization assist has an inelastic interface material distal to pulley, ensure that the knot connecting the rubber band/spring to the interface does not move through the pulley creating friction or binding.
4. Include mechanism to ease tension adjustment by patient for night/day tension adjustments.
5. Connector bars may be molded in different shapes and secondarily strengthen and stabilize outriggers.
6. Mobilization assists may be marked with ink, a knot, or a blocking tether to indicate the amount of joint excursion allowed during exercise or use.
7. A fisherman's knot provides a reliable connection when attaching a nylon line interface to parts of a mobilization assist.
8. If splinting material is coated, remove the coating before bonding separate components such as outriggers.

■ SUMMARY

Influencing splint designs, outriggers are platforms from which mobilization assists work. Providing the power source for splints, mobilization assists are constructed from elastic or inelastic materials. They are influenced by the physical properties of the materials from which they are made and therefore generate different ranges of forces. It is the upper extremity specialist's responsibility to determine optimum force and torque parameters, to set the mobilization assist at an appropriate tension, and to maintain its adjustment according to the individual needs of each patient (Box 7-1). Angle of approach, pressure, friction, and ligamentous stress also must be carefully monitored so that the patient reaches full rehabilitative potential as quickly as possible. If these factors are not attended to, expensive and disappointing delays may occur.

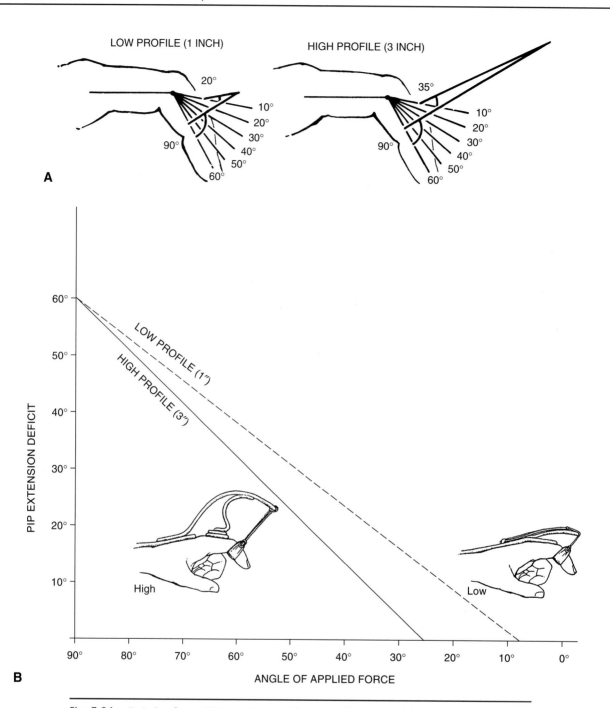

LOW PROFILE (1 INCH)

HIGH PROFILE (3 INCH)

A

PIP EXTENSION DEFICIT

ANGLE OF APPLIED FORCE

High

Low

B

Fig. 7-26 **B,** Index finger PIP extension mobilization splint, type 2 (3)
A, As passive motion improves, the high-profile design maintains a better angle of pull without adjustment than does the low-profile design. **B,** Comparison of low-profile outriggers and high-profile outriggers. (From Fess EE: Principles and methods of splinting for mobilization of joints. In Mackin E, et al: *Rehabilitation of the hand,* ed 5, Mosby, 2001, St. Louis.)

REFERENCES

1. Boozer JA, Sanson MS, Soutas-Little RW, et al: Comparison of the biomedical motions and forces involved in high-profile versus low-profile dynamic splinting, *J Hand Ther* 7(3):171-82, 1994.
2. Brand P: The forces of dynamic splinting: ten questions before applying a dynamic splint to the hand. In Hunter JM, Schneider LC, Mackin EJ, Callahan AD: *Rehabilitation of the hand*, ed 1, Mosby, 1978, St. Louis.
3. Brand P: The forces of dynamic splinting: ten questions before applying a dynamic splint to the hand. In Mackin EJ, Callahan AD, Skirven TM, et al: Rehabilitation of the hand, ed 5, Mosby, 2002, St. Louis.
4. Brand PW: *Clinical mechanics of the hand*, Mosby, 1985, St. Louis.
5. Brand PW, Hollister A: *Clinical mechanics of the hand*, ed 2, Mosby, 1993, St. Louis.
6. Dunipace K: Constant 90° pull outrigger, Unpublished personal communication, 1999.
7. Fess EE: Force magnitude of commercial spring-coil and spring-wire splints designed to extend the proximal interphalangeal joint, *J Hand Ther* 2:86-90, 1988.
8. Fess EE: Principles and methods of dynamic splinting. In Hunter J, Schneider L, Mackin E, et al: *Rehabilitation of the hand*, ed 2, Mosby, 1984, St. Louis.
9. Fess EE: Principles and methods of splinting for mobilization. In Hunter J, Schneider L, Mackin E, et al: Rehabilitation of the hand, ed 3, Mosby, 1989, St. Louis.
10. Fess EE: Principles and methods of splinting for mobilization. In Schneider L, Mackin E, Callahan A: *Rehabilitation of the hand*, ed 4, Mosby, 1995, St. Louis.
11. Fess EE: Rubber band traction: physical properties, splint design and identification of force magnitude. Proceedings American Society of Hand Therapists, *J Hand Surg* 9A:610, 1984.
12. Fess E, Gettle K, Strickland J: *Hand splinting principles and methods*, ed 1, Mosby, 1981, St. Louis.
13. Fess EE: Splints: mechanics versus convention, *J Hand Ther* 8(2):124-30, 1995.
14. Fess EE, McCollum M: The influence of splinting on healing tissues, *J Hand Ther* 11(2):157-61, 1998.
15. Malick M: *Manual on dynamic hand splinting with thermoplastic materials*, Harmarville Rehabilitation Center, 1974, Pittsburgh.
16. Marx H: Comparison of the biomechanical motions and forces involved in high-profile versus low-profile dynamic splinting, *J Hand Ther* 8(1):41, 1995.
17. Mildenberger LA, Amadio PC, An KN: Dynamic splinting: a systematic approach to the selection of elastic traction, *Arch Phys Med Rehabil* 67(4):241-4, 1986.
18. Murray KA, McIntyre FH: Active traction splinting for proximal interphalangeal joint injuries, *Ann Plast Surg* 35(1):15-8, 1995.
19. Pearson SO: Dynamic splinting. In Hunter J, Schneider L, Mackin E, et al: *Rehabilitation of the hand*, ed 1, Mosby, 1978, St. Louis.
20. Philips CA: Unwaxed dental floss for rubber band interface in dynamic splinting, Personal communication, 1973.
21. Prosser R: Splinting in the management of proximal interphalangeal joint flexion contracture, *J Hand Ther* 9(4):378-86, 1996.
22. Schenck RR: Dynamic traction and early passive movement for fractures of the proximal interphalangeal joint, *J Hand Surg* [Am] 11(6):850-8, 1986.

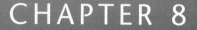

CHAPTER 8

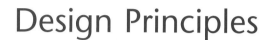

Design Principles

Chapter Outline

The principles of splint design evolve from the integration of the principles of fit, mechanics, construction, and using outriggers and mobilization assists. The most important consideration in splint design is the exact function expected of the splint for a specific patient. A thorough understanding of the particular problem and therapeutic goals for which a splint is required is essential to the design process. Armed with this knowledge, one can determine the ultimate configuration of the splint to be constructed. Twenty-two fundamental principles must be considered in the designing of a given splint. These principles range from general to specific and result in a series of decisions that lead to the final splint design.

The principles of design may be divided into two categories. Nine general principles based on individual patient characteristics form a framework for the overall designing process of upper extremity splints. The consideration and incorporation of these broad principles implements the creation of a splint that is practical for the patient. Adherence to the remaining thirteen specific principles concerned with the particular pathologic situation allows the clinician to create a splint that ensures optimum functional benefit for the patient. The specific principles of design also increase patient tolerance and compliance of the splint. It should be emphasized that the principles discussed in this chapter are used only after there has been an appreciation of all factors unique to each patient. Decisions are made based on personal, technical, and medical considerations. The result is often substantially different splint configurations for patients with similar therapeutic needs but different logistic or personal requirements. With experience, these decisions can be made automatically, without the need to review a detailed checklist of the principles listed here. Consultation with all persons involved in the rehabilitative effort must precede the actual design process, for this information strongly influences decisions as to splint configuration.

All of these principles are integrated and considered by the upper extremity specialist almost simultaneously as assessment of the patient progresses, eventually leading to a splint design that is unique to the situation. Astute observation and careful objective measurement provide the foundation on which critical decisions are made, allowing design creation "from the inside out," rather than haphazard application of a preconceived or standard configuration without regard to important individual variables.

■ GENERAL PRINCIPLES OF DESIGN

The basic considerations for splint design are discussed in the following principles.

Consider Individual Patient Factors

The individual requirements of each patient are the most influential factors in determining the ultimate size and configuration of a given splint. After the functional requirements of the splinting program are established, additional individual factors must be addressed: How much of the pathologic condition and rehabilitation program does the patient understand, and how much of the program can he intelligently accomplish for himself? How accessible is the splinting facility, and how often will he be able to return for splint adjustments or changes? To what extent will his family be able to assist him in splint application and exercises? What are the age, occupational, and motivational factors involved?

All these factors come into careful consideration at the onset of a splinting program. Serial mobilization splints that must be changed every 3 or 4 days may present a hardship to a patient located many miles from the therapy department; the use of an elaborately designed splint for a patient with poor motivation or an inadequate understanding of proper splint application will almost certainly result in improper use of the splint (Fig. 8-1). Modifications also may be dictated by patient age. Splints designed for use on adults may be poorly tolerated by or inappropriate for

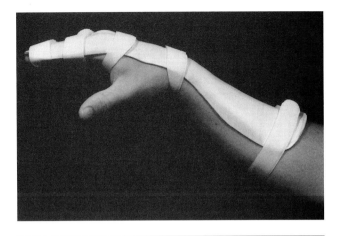

Fig. 8-1   Index–small finger extension restriction splint, type 1 (13)
This finger restriction splint used in early passive range of motion of flexor tendon repairs would be contraindicated for a young child because of its ease of removal.

a child; for children, creative approaches often help with wearing compliance (Fig. 8-2). It is important to remember that an injured hand or arm is not an autonomous entity requiring treatment. Injured extremities are attached to individual beings, each with his/her own set of physical and emotional parameters. Psychological factors including, but not limited to, peer pressure, secondary gain, dysfunctional family life, pending legal action, or substance abuse may negatively influence splint compliance. Identifying and adapting to patient emotional issues may be more challenging than dealing with the physical injury.

Economic factors may influence splint design. A patient may not be able to return to the clinic for frequent adjustments to a mobilization outrigger or a commercial splint may be too expensive. The influence of managed care and third party payment providers is omnipresent in the rehabilitation arena, often dictating the number of visits and procedures that may be performed. Before incurring time and cost expenses to patients, it is prudent to check with the associated medical insurers to discern those splinting procedures that will be reimbursed and those that will not (Fig. 8-3).

Consideration of specific circumstances such as these allows for the appropriate creation of a design that is more likely to be successful.

Consider the Length of Time the Splint Is to Be Used

In general, the shorter the anticipated need of a splint, the simpler its design, material type, and construction

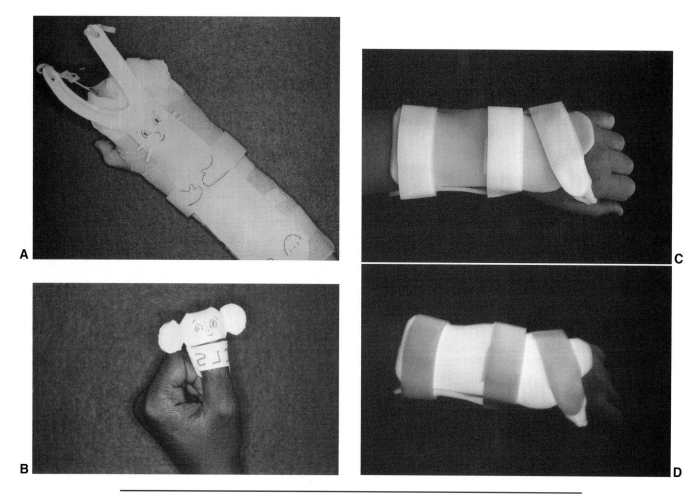

Fig. 8-2   A, Index–long finger extension mobilization splint, type 1 (7) B, Nonarticular thumb distal phalanx splint C,D, Wrist extension immobilization splint, type 0 (1)
A,B, Imagination and humor can entice a child to cooperate in the splinting program. C,D, Glow-in-the-dark splinting material (Reveals™ Nite-Lite™, WFR Corporation, Wyckoff, N.J.) improves splint compliance for children and teenagers. [Courtesy (C,D) Damon Kirk, WFR Corporation, Wyckoff, N.J.]

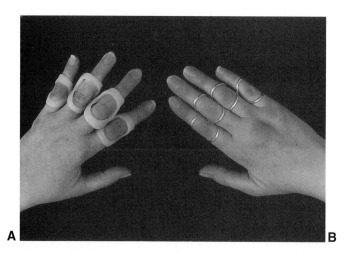

Fig. 8-3   A,B, Finger PIP extension restriction splint, type 0 (1); 4 splints @ finger separate
Different standards may exist for custom splints (left) and commercially available splints (right), depending on third-party insurers' criteria. (Courtesy Cindy Garris, OTR, Silver Ring Splint Company, Charlottesville, Va.)

should be. An elaborately designed splint that requires numerous hours to design, construct, and fit and is expected to be discarded or replaced within a few days can rarely be justified to cost- and efficiency-conscious consumers, hospital administrators, and third-party insurers. However, if the same splint were to be worn for 2 or 3 months, its preparation would certainly be more appropriate. Similarly, if the device is expected to be used for several years or more, a more durable, long-lasting splint should be considered. For special circumstances, consultation with an orthotist may be indicated to allow for splint construction with more resilient materials such as aluminum, steel, and some of the polyester resins.

Strive for Simplicity and Pleasing Appearance

Attempts should be made to keep the overall design as simple and cosmetically pleasing as possible. At best, an upper extremity splint is a strange-looking device, attracting attention to its wearer and further emphasizing the deformity. A poorly designed splint becomes even more obvious, lessening patient acceptance, increasing frustration, and possibly decreasing the potential for successful rehabilitation. Sometimes only a large, somewhat cumbersome splint will accomplish the desired objectives, but in many instances a simple adaptation functions equally well (Fig. 8-4, A-G). Above all, consideration for the wearer should take precedence over any impulse to design a complicated and elaborate masterpiece that may serve only as a monument to its creator!

Allow for Optimum Function of the Extremity

The upper extremity has the unique ability to move freely in a wide range of motions, which allows for the successful accomplishment of a tremendous variety of daily tasks. The segments of the arm and hand function as an open kinematic chain, with each segment of the chain dependent on the segments proximal and distal to it. Compensation by normal segments when injury or disease limits parts of the chain often provides for the continued functional use of the extremity. Because of this adaptive ability, splinting of the upper extremity should be carefully designed to prevent needless immobility of normal joints. Often simple in design, splints that substitute for lost motion (Fig. 8-5, A,B) or control deforming substitution patterns (Fig. 8-5, C-G) enhance function by positioning specific joints in more advantageous positions. If digital joint limitation is caused by capsular pathology condition alone, the wrist may not require

incorporation in the splint design. If, however, wrist position, by virtue of its effect on the osseous chain or the extrinsic musculotendinous units, directly influences distal joint motion, secondary immobilization of the wrist may be required to obtain maximum splint efficiency. Although the mechanical purchase on a stiff joint may be enhanced by stabilization of normal secondary joints proximal or distal to the primary joint, care should be taken to apply this concept in appropriate circumstances only. If similar results can be obtained by leaving these adjacent joints free, the kinetic chain will have the advantage of added motion.

Splinting literature is replete with descriptions of "functional" splints but few research studies actually validate these claims. Further, exceedingly divergent splint purpose categories often are touted for the same diagnosis. More research is needed to identify the most efficacious splints for commonly treated upper extremity pathology. This is not with the intent of creating splinting "cookbook" methodology, but rather to distinguish options that truly are functional. An example of what is needed is Hannah and Hudak's study[16] that compared three splints commonly used to treat radial nerve paralysis, a *wrist extension mobilization splint, type 0 (1)* (Fig. 8-6, A), a *wrist flexion: index–small finger MP extension / index–small finger MP flexion: wrist extension torque transmission / thumb CMC radial abduction and MP extension mobilization splint, type 0 (7)* (Fig. 8-6, B), and a *wrist extension, finger MP extension, thumb CMC radial abduction and MP extension mobilization splint, type 0 (7)* (Fig. 8-6, C). The authors found statistically higher patient functional ability and compliance with the third splint, the *wrist extension, finger MP extension, thumb CMC radial abduction and MP extension mobilization splint, type 0 (7)*. Raising new questions, the authors noted that the thumb was included in the torque transmission splint and the MP extension mobilization splint; it was not included in the wrist mobilization splint. Interestingly, the authors also described one subject who preferred the wrist mobilization splint because it was easier to put on and it was less conspicuous, voicing the subjectivity clinicians have long noted with their patients!

Allow for Optimum Sensation

Without sensation, the hand is perceptively blind[20] and functionally limited. Because cutaneous stimuli provide feedback for activity, splint designs should leave as much of the palmar tactile surface areas and the radial and ulnar borders of the hand as free from occlusive material as possible (Fig. 8-7).

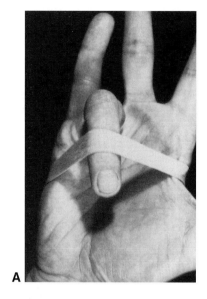

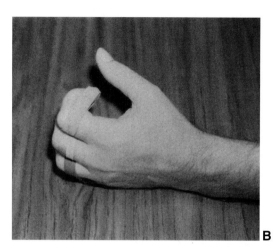

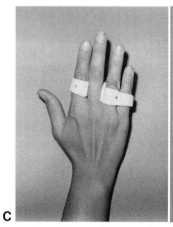

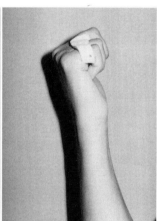

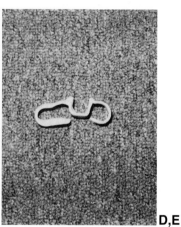

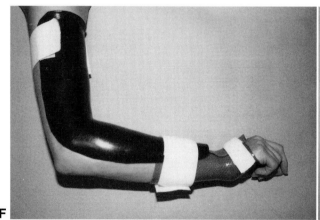

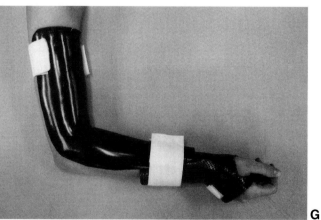

Fig. 8-4   A, Ring finger PIP flexion mobilization splint, type 1 (2) B, Finger IP flexion mobilization splint, type 0 (2); 4 splints @ finger separate C-E, Long finger MP extension and flexion torque transmission splint, type 1 (4) F,G, Forearm pronation or supination mobilization splint, type 2 (3) G, Forearm supination or pronation mobilization splint, type 2 (3)

Although differing in size, all of these splints have a common element of simplicity. A,B, A wide rubber band can be an effective splint for increasing proximal interphalangeal joint flexion. C-E, This innovative splint incorporates a simple design to transmit torque to the long finger MP joint. F,G, Inelastic traction is used in this two-piece splint designed to increase pronation or supination. [Courtesy (B) Darcelle Decker, OTR, CHT, Danville, Pa.; (C-E) Regina Roseman Tune, MS, OTR, Richmond, Va.; (F,G) Paul Van Lede, OT, MS, Orfit Industries, Wijnegem, Belgium.]

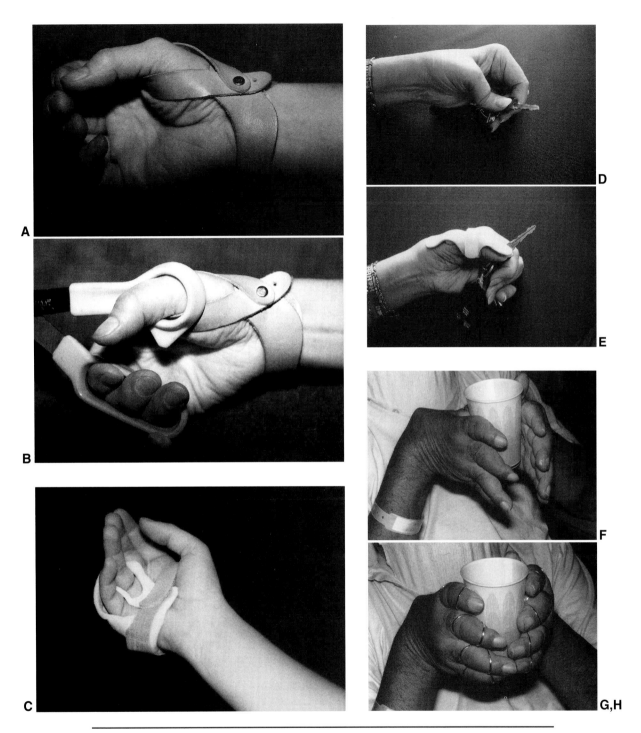

Fig. 8-5   A,B, Thumb CMC palmar abduction mobilization splint, type 0 (1) C, Ring–small finger MP extension restriction / IP extension torque transmission splint, type 0 (6) E, Thumb MP extension immobilization / IP extension restriction splint, type 0 (2) G,H, Finger PIP extension restriction splint, type 0 (1); 4 splints @ finger separate
A,B,D-G, Splints position key joints to improve hand function. C, Restricting full MP extension and generating IP extension through torque transmission of the extrinsic extensors, this splint for ulnar nerve paralysis allows full flexion of the fourth and fifth digits. [Courtesy **(A,B)** Elizabeth Spencer Steffa, OTR / L, CHT, Seattle, Wash.; **(C)** Sandra Artzberger, OTR, CHT, Milwaukee, Wis.; and Bonnie Ferhing, LPT, Fond du Lac, Wis.; **(F,G,H)** Cindy Garris, OTR, Silver Ring Splint Company, Charlottesville, Va.]

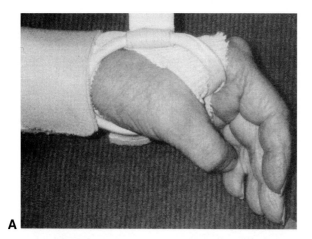

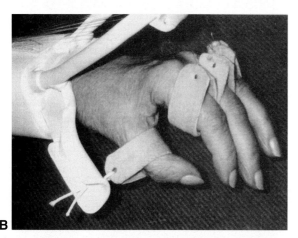

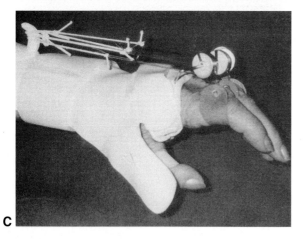

Fig. 8-6   A, Wrist extension mobilization splint, type 0 (1) B,
Wrist flexion: index–small finger MP extension / index–small finger
MP flexion: wrist extension torque transmission / thumb CMC
radial abduction and MP extension mobilization splint, type 0 (7)
C, Wrist extension, finger MP extension, thumb CMC radial
abduction and MP extension mobilization splint, type 0 (7)
A single-subject research design study found that splint C provided
better hand function for patients with radial nerve paralysis.
(From Hannah S, Hudak P: Splinting and radial nerve palsy: a single-
subject design, *J Hand Ther* 14(3):216-8, 2001.)

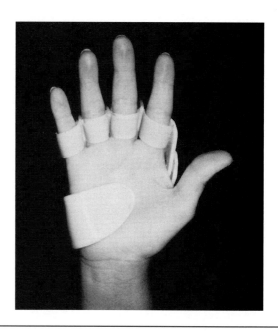

Fig. 8-7   Index–small finger MP ulnar deviation restriction
splint, type 0 (4)
Splints designed to leave large palmar tactile surface areas of the
hand free from splint material enhance functional use. (Courtesy
Joan Farrell, OTR, CHT, Punta Gorda, Fla.)

Allow for Efficient Construction and Fit

The splint design should also allow for quick, efficient
construction. With increasing concern for medical
costs, long construction and fit times are, for the
most part, inappropriate. Proper design can expedite
construction and fit and decrease expense. Because
each part that must be bonded or jointed increases
the construction time, the incorporation of multiple
components into the main body of the splint at the
design stage results in improved efficiency. For
example, providing contour at the time of designing
eliminates the need for separate reinforcing strips that
must be cut, formed, and bonded during the splint
preparation phase. However, at times the addition of
a separate piece, such as a dorsal phalangeal bar, can
facilitate future splint adjustments without the need
to modify the entire splint. Anticipation of the fit and
construction factors at the design level also eliminates
much of the need for time-consuming experimen-
tation and innovation during patient contact (Fig.
8-8, A-E).[21]

Commercial splint mechanisms, including articulated joints, springs, coils, and outrigger components,
may speed fabrication time. If commercially available
splint parts are used, they must perform equal to or
better than their custom-made counterparts. There is
never any excuse for using commercial components

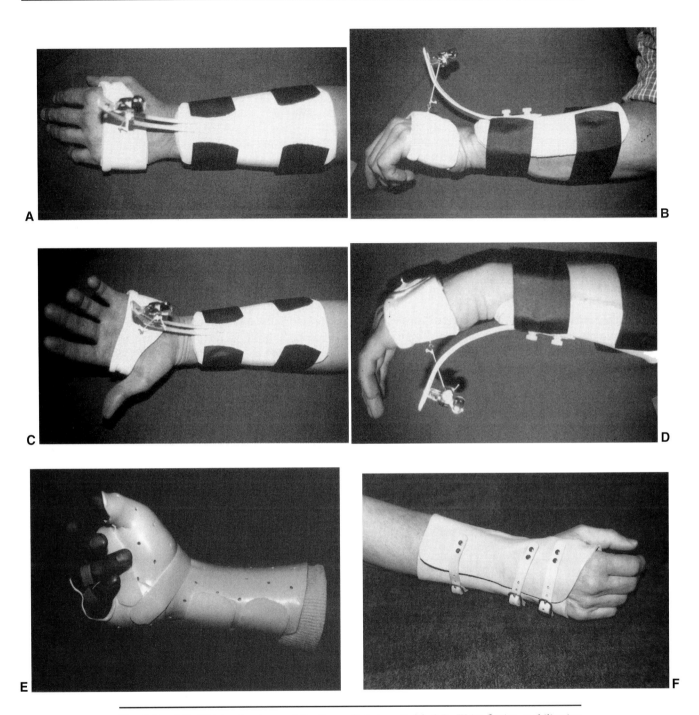

Fig. 8-8   **A,B,** Wrist extension mobilization splint, type 0 (1) **C,D,** Wrist flexion mobilization splint, type 0 (1) **E,** Small finger MP supination, PIP extension and flexion torque transmission splint, type 2 (4) \\ Index–small finger MP flexion, thumb CMC radial abduction and MP flexion immobilization / thumb IP extension restriction splint, type 1 (8) **F,** Wrist extension immobilization splint, type 0 (1)
A-D, A combination of custom and commercial components allows efficient splint construction and fitting. **E,** Two-piece splint design facilitates adjustments as edema decreases **F,** If it meets all the individual criteria and if a good fit can be obtained, a commercially available splint may save time and expense. **[(A-D)** from Mullen TM: Static progressive splint to increase wrist extension or flexion, *J Hand Ther* 13(4):313-5, 2000; Courtesy **(E)** Lin Beribak, OTR/L, CHT, Chicago, Ill.; **(F)** Elizabeth Spencer, OTR, and Lynnlee Fullenwider, OTR, CHT, Seattle, Wash.]

that fail to meet the unique requirements of a given situation.

On occasion, a commercially available splint may seem to meet the requirements of a given upper extremity problem (Fig. 8-8, *F*). If the splint satisfies all the individual variables, if a good fit is obtained, and if the cost does not exceed that of a similar design custom-made splint, the use of a prefabricated commercial splint may actually be more expedient in regard to overall time and expense.

Provide for Ease of Application and Removal

Whenever possible, patients should be able to apply and remove their splints independently. Dependence on others for assistance may lead to frustration of both patient and family, resulting in poor wearing habits or discarding of the splint. To allow for ease of wear and removal, the splint should be designed for simple hand and forearm insertion with straps provided that can be tightened or loosened without great difficulty. Individual adaptations in the splint design, fastening devices, or method of splint application may be necessary to further facilitate patient independence (Fig. 8-9, *A-D*). Patients should be able to demonstrate independence in applying and removing their splints before leaving the clinic.

Postoperative splinting tasks for rheumatoid arthritis patients and others with poor bilateral finger dexterity may be especially demanding. Combining postsurgery requisites for multiple digital joints with realistic methods for splint donning and doffing requires innovative creativity (Fig. 8-9, *E,F*).[5]

Consider the Splint/Exercise Regimen

In some instances, designing several functions into one splint may lessen patient confusion and simplify the wearing and exercise routines. For example, amalgamation of purposes[4] (e.g., a mobilization and immobilization system) (Fig. 8-10, *A-C*), directions, as with a digital flexion and extension system (Fig. 8-10, *D,E*), or several joint levels (Fig. 8-10, *F-H*) into a single splint eliminates the need for a more complicated alternating two-splint routine. Efficient design considerations such as these are more clearly understood by the patient, allowing him to direct his attention more fully to rehabilitation. Written instructions for splint application and use are essential.

Take into Account Patient-Associated Risk Factors

Variables that extend duration of wound healing stages, cause skin or soft tissues to be friable, or pre-dispose tissue to scarring or nerve damage must be taken into consideration when designing splints and splint wearing schedules. These variables may include, but are not limited to, therapeutic intervention factors, such as medication or radiation; systemic diseases like peripheral vascular disease, poor nutritional status, diabetes mellitus, rheumatoid arthritis, scleroderma, or Raynaud's disease; use of tobacco, alcohol, other substances including the effects of many widely available herbal supplements that may effect coagulation or wound healing; and the possibility or presence of infection. Patients with associated risk factors that undermine tissue nutrition or viability require splints that disperse pressure and minimize shear through contiguous fit over large contact areas. Narrow splint components and constricting circumferential straps are to be avoided. If used, mobilizing forces should be cautiously monitored to ensure that force magnitude is gentle and force angle of application is 90° both to the segments being mobilized and to the axes of rotation of the involved joints. Plaster serial casting (a form of inelastic mobilization splinting) with its wide contact area, intricate capacity for conforming fit, and minimal, controlled force application over several days may be more appropriate for these patients than are single-surface splints that apply elastic or inelastic traction. Avoidance of pressure injuries to skin is paramount when using splints, and neurovascular status must be frequently and carefully monitored. The predominant criterion is that splint application does not cause additional trauma to tissues whose viability already may be tenuous.

■ SPECIFIC PRINCIPLES OF DESIGN

The individual considerations, including age, intelligence, location, economic status, general health, and lifestyle, of the particular patient are important aspects of the general principles of design, with primary emphasis directed toward splint function, appearance, economy, safety, and patient acceptance. The remaining 13 specific principles of design stress the accomplishment of predetermined goals as defined by the unique pathologic condition being treated. The questions to which the specific design principles pertain are as follows:

- What is the exact disease, injury, or deformity for which splinting is needed?
- What are the immediate and long-term goals of the splinting regimen?
- What is the most efficient and effective means of reaching these goals?
- What anatomic and material variables must be considered?

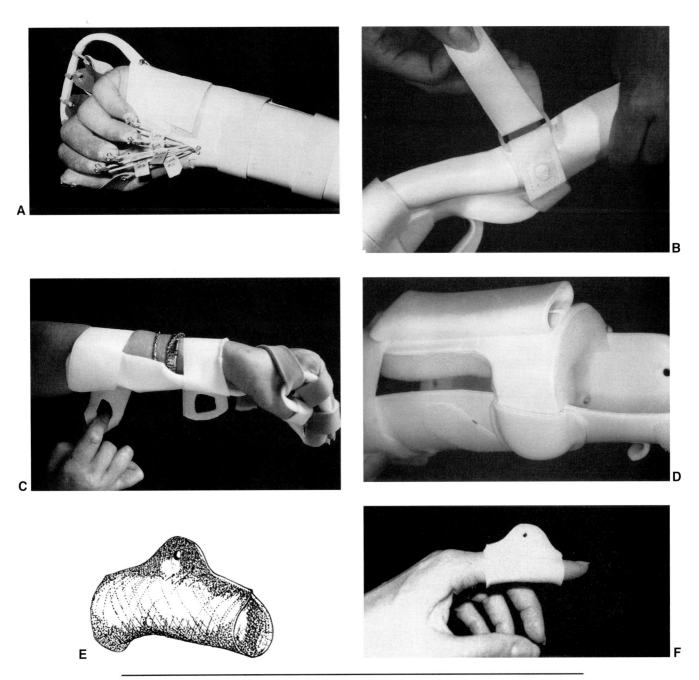

Fig. 8-9   **A,** Index–small finger flexion, thumb CMC palmar abduction and MP flexion mobilization splint, type 1 (15); or index–small finger MP extension mobilization splint, type 1 (5) **C,** Index–small finger flexion, thumb CMC palmar abduction immobilization splint, type 3 (16) **E,F,** Finger MP extension and flexion torque transmission / PIP extension immobilization splint, type 1 (3)

A, Numbered rubber band "tags" ensure correct application of traction. Tags also may be color-coded. **B,C,** Adapted straps facilitate application and removal of bilateral finger and thumb immobilization splints. **D,** When the outrigger is not in use, a dorsal "pocket" allows easy detachment from the splint. **E,F,** A "splint-sling" stabilizes postoperative procedures and facilitates splint donning and doffing. [Courtesy **(A)** Joan Farrell, OTR, CHT, Punta Gorda, Fla.; **(E,F)** from Emerson S: The rheumatoid hand: postoperative splint options, *J Hand Ther* 6(3):214, 1993.]

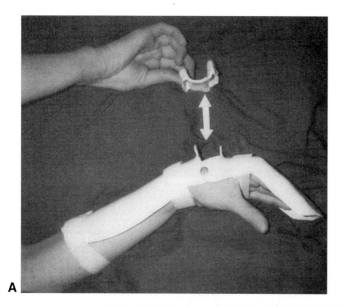

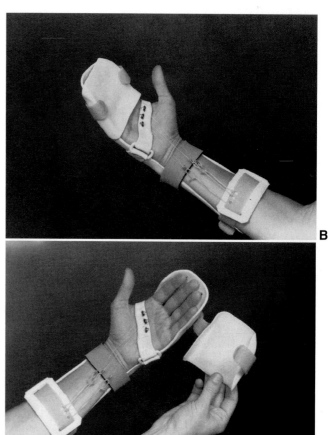

Fig. 8-10   **A,** Wrist extension restriction: finger flexion mobilization / finger extension restriction / wrist flexion: finger extension restriction splint, type 0 (13); with wrist locking device **B,C,** Index–small finger extension restriction / index–ring finger flexion mobilization splint, type 1 (13) **D,** Thumb IP flexion or extension mobilization splint, type 2 (3) **E,** Index–small finger MP extension or flexion mobilization splint, type 1 (5) **F,** Wrist extension mobilization splint, type 0 (1) **G,** Wrist extension, finger MP extension, thumb CMC radial abduction and MP extension mobilization splint, type 0 (7)

Splints that combine several functions facilitate wearing and exercise schedules for patients. **A,** A removable wrist lock. **B,C,** Removable finger restriction component. **D,E,** Flexion and extension outriggers. **F-H,** Detachable finger and thumb outriggers. [**(A)** from Dymarczyk M: A locking mechanism for the tenodesis splint for flexor tendon repairs, *J Hand Ther* 14(3), 2001; Courtesy **(B,C)** Barbara Smith, OTR, Edmond, Okla.; **(D)** Kathryn Schultz, OTR, CHT, Orlando, Fla.; **(E)** K. P. MacBain, OTR, Vancouver, BC; **(F-H)** Jean-Christophe Arias, Saint-Etienne, France.]

Because of the often highly complicated pathology and physiology involved in treatment and reconstructive procedures of a diseased or injured hand or upper extremity, close communication between the surgeon and the therapist is absolutely imperative. Misunderstood, misdirected, or poorly timed intervention to healing tissue could seriously jeopardize the rehabilitation potential of a hand or upper extremity. The referring physician's evaluation, rehabilitative goals and prognosis, operative notes, x-rays, and arteriograms are essential data on which splinting and exercise programs are based. Once these data are

obtained, splints may be designed to impart controlled forces to identified upper extremity segments or to immobilize, mobilize, restrict, or transmit torque to predetermined primary joints. Upper extremity injuries frequently involve multiple anatomic structures, requiring multifaceted splinting solutions.

A careful evaluation of the extremity with regard to existing and potential joint mobility is perhaps the single most important consideration in determining the ultimate configuration of an upper extremity splint. Specific recorded data obtained from active and passive range of motion measurements provide the

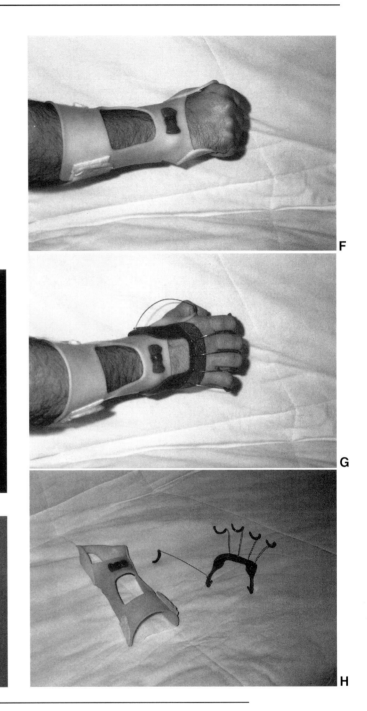

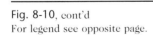

Fig. 8-10, cont'd
For legend see opposite page.

examiner with an accurate assessment of motion discrepancies and allow for splint design that effectively targets the problem areas.

Identify Primary Joint Segments

The first step in splint design is to identify which anatomical structures the splint will influence. Splints that do not affect joints, nonarticular splints, concentrate on individual segments of the upper extremity open kinematic chain (e.g., humerus, forearm, metacarpal, or phalanx). Nonarticular splints usually employ conforming, two-point coaptation forces to support or reinforce healing tissues; splint design is determined by the length and circumference of the segment to which the splint is applied.

In contrast, upper extremity articular splints influence a joint or series of joints and are more complicated in design. Primary joints are those specific joints upon which the splint will focus. These joints may have adjacent or surrounding healing tissues, lack volitional active and/or passive motion, be painful, lack alignment, have diminished or absent sensibility, or they may exhibit diminished functional capacity due to upper motor neuron problems.

When dealing with a particularly difficult situation in which numerous joints are involved, it is sometimes helpful to mark the primary joints with a water-soluble felt-tip pen (Fig. 8-11, *A*). This method or other graphic techniques that allow clear visualization of the splinting objectives are important to accurate splint design, especially when students and other novice splint fabricators are involved.

According to the expanded SCS, only primary joints incorporated in a splint are specifically named. If the ESCS name is known for a given splint, the primary joints included in the splint are easily recognized because they are the only joints that are individually identified (Fig. 8-11, *B*).

Determine Kinematic Direction

After careful identification of the primary problem joints, the next step in designing a splint is to define the force direction(s) to be applied to the primary joint(s). Force direction may include abduction, adduction, extension, flexion, internal rotation, external rotation, ulnar deviation, radial deviation, pronation, supination, palmar abduction, radial abduction, circumduction, distraction, or compression depending on the primary joint(s) involved. Different directions may be incorporated into a splint to achieve separate goals at other involved joints (Fig. 8-12).

Review Purpose: Immobilization, Mobilization, Restriction, Torque Transmission

Once key joints are determined, direction of forces and splint purpose are defined almost simultaneously. Purpose identifies the functional objective(s) of a given splint. Are joints to be immobilized to allow healing? Is it desirable to increase or to maintain the passive range of motion or to substitute for absent active motion? Should articular motion be allowed within predefined limitations? Is the splint applied to transfer moment or torque to joints outside the boundaries of the splint? It is imperative that the designer of the proposed splint clearly understands the reason for the application of the splint and adapts the splint design accordingly.

Immobilization splinting allows rest, protects healing structures, or strategically positions the part when motion loss is expected. Including one or multiple joints (Fig. 8-13, *A*), immobilization splints are commonly used to promote healing of osseous,

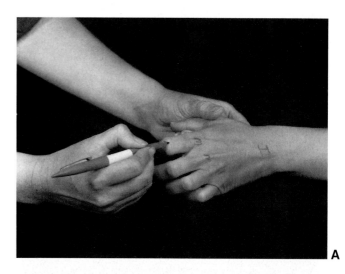

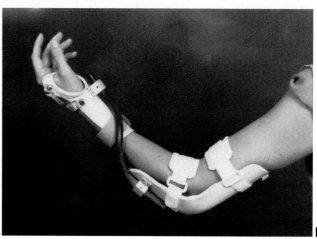

Fig. 8-11   **B,** Forearm supination mobilization splint, type 2 (3) **A,** In complicated cases, graphic identification of primary joints may aid the novice in splint design. **B,** In this supination splint, the forearm is the only primary joint. Both the wrist and elbow are included in the splint as secondary joints to provide better control of forearm position. [Courtesy **(B)** Barbara Smith, OTR, Edmond, Okla.]

capsular, ligamentous, or tendonous structures and to provide rest to inflamed joints with the goal of lessening or preventing deformity. A badly damaged joint with no expectation of functional salvage may be splinted to allow stiffening in the most favorable position. Often worn for relatively short periods, the more pliable plastic materials or plaster are more suitable for fabricating these splints. Immobilization splints may also be used in conjunction with splints that have different purposes of application (Fig. 8-13, *B*).

Mobilization splints may substitute for absent active motion in supple joints or they may be used to improve passive range of motion of stiff joints through soft tissue remodeling. Mobilization splints that substitute for lost motion are traditionally applied to

CHAPTER 8   Design Principles   **223**

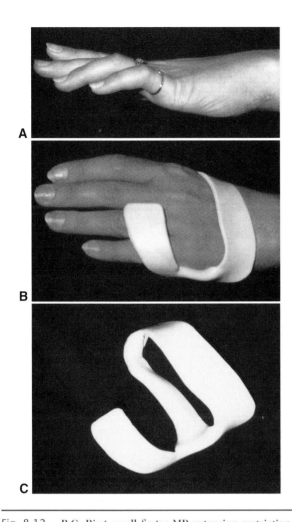

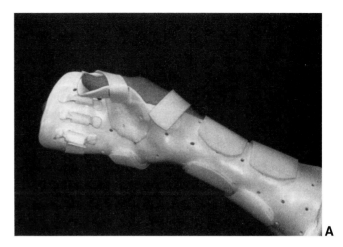

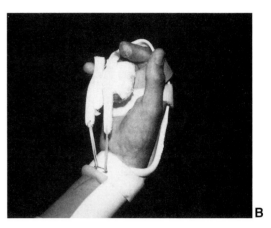

Fig. 8-12   B,C, Ring–small finger MP extension restriction / IP extension torque transmission splint, type 0 (6)
A-C, Combining MP extension restriction and IP extension torque transmission, this splint improves hand function by counteracting the typical MP hyperextension and IP flexion deforming forces associated with ulnar nerve paralysis. (Courtesy Peggy McLaughlin, OTR, CHT, San Bernadino, Calif.)

Fig. 8-13   A, Index–small finger MP flexion and IP extension immobilization splint, type 4 (16) B, Index–small finger MP extension restriction / long–ring finger PIP flexion mobilization splint, type 1 (7) \\ Finger DIP extension immobilization splint, type 0 (1): 2 splints long and ring finger separate
A, Individual finger straps ensure correct positioning in this finger immobilization splint. The thumb joints and wrist are included in the splint as secondary joints. **B,** Circumferential casts immobilize the distal joints of the long and ring fingers to allow fracture healing while the MP and PIP joints are mobilized for early passive mobilization of flexor tendon repairs. [Courtesy **(A)** Lin Beribak, OTR / L, CHT, Chicago, Ill.; **(B)** Robin Miller, OTR, CHT, Ft. Lauderdale, Fla.]

improve hand or extremity function and may be fabricated of more durable, less adjustable materials because of their expected length of use. An example of a substitution splint is the use of a *wrist and MP extension mobilization splint* to provide wrist and finger MP extension in radial nerve paralysis (Fig. 8-10, *F-H*). To be effective, this group of mobilization splints requires full passive joint motion. If full joint excursion is not present, a different mobilization splint that uses elastic or inelastic traction to remodel shortened or adherent soft tissues is first required to decrease the existing deformity. Splints designed to increase passive range of motion are often temporary and should be easily adapted because configurative alterations must be made as the arc of joint motion changes (Fig. 8-14).

Restriction splints limit a joint's normal arc of motion to allow healing or to improve function. Depending on the physical characteristics of the materials from which they are made, restrictive splints prohibit motion on a continuum ranging from minimal restraint of joint motion using soft materials (Fig. 8-15, *A*) to exacting control of motion with thermoplastics or metals (Fig. 8-15, *B*). Splints that restrict joint motion are often used postoperatively to protect repairs while allowing partial active range of motion.

Torque transmission splints (Fig. 8-16, *A-D*) transfer movement longitudinally or transversely to sel-

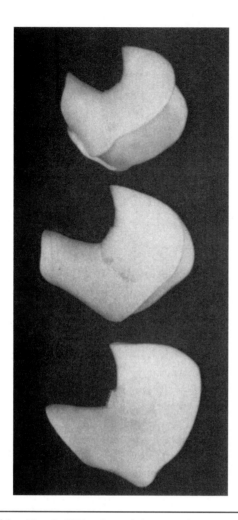

Fig. 8-14 **Thumb CMC palmar abduction splint, type 1 (2)** Thermoplastic thumb CMC mobilization splints are used serially to increase carpometacarpal joint passive motion.

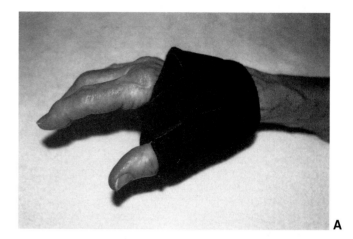

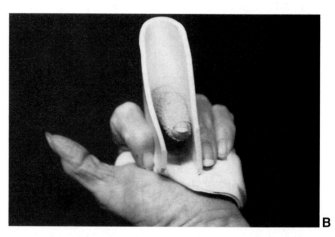

Fig. 8-15 **A, Thumb CMC circumduction restriction splint, type 1 (2) B, Long finger PIP radial and ulnar deviation restriction splint, type 2 (3)** **A,** A neoprene splint provides gentle restrictive forces to a thumb CMC joint. **B,** PIP lateral motion is prohibited in this "bowling alley" splint design. [Courtesy **(A)** Joni Armstrong, OTR, CHT, Bemidji, Minn.]

ected joints to provide motion to supple joints or to remodel stiff joints and effect a corresponding improvement in passive and active joint motion. Used autonomously or in conjunction with mobilization (Fig. 8-16, C) or restriction splints, torque transmission splints include one or more joints in order to augment motion at other joints by allowing an increase or decrease of tension on musculotendinous units. Torque transmission splints require sophisticated knowledge of anatomy, biomechanics, and the principles of splinting.

Drawing on the ingenuity and creativity of those responsible for creating splints, it is not unusual to have primary joints with different purpose requirements in the same hand. Splints may be designed to include various combinations of the above four purposes, e.g., restriction / torque transmission (Fig. 8-16, D) or restriction / mobilization / immobilization (Fig. 8-16, E,F).

Identify Secondary Joints

Maximum mechanical benefit of splinting forces may be obtained by controlling joints proximal and/or distal to injured or diseased primary joints. Secondary joints are normal or less involved joints that are included in a splint to focus immobilization, mobilization, restriction, or torque transmission forces to primary joints (Fig. 8-17, A). When secondary joints are controlled, dissipation of desired forces at the more mobile secondary joints is avoided. Secondary joints may also be included in a splint to decrease pressure and to gain increased mechanical advantage on adjacent joints (Fig. 8-17, B).

Splints fail to achieve their purposes when the importance of controlling secondary joints is not understood or disregarded. For example, when a stiff

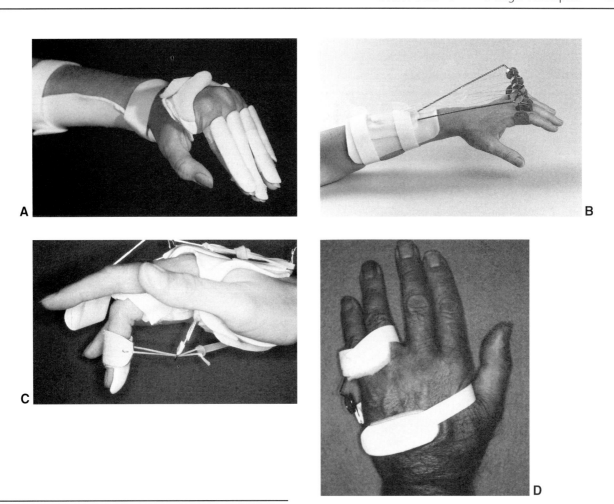

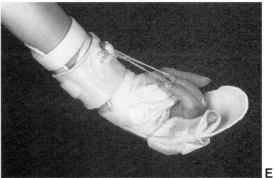

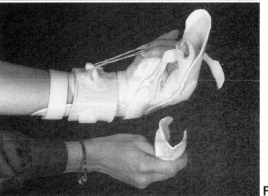

Fig. 8-16   A, Index–small finger MP extension and flexion torque transmission splint, type 1 (5) \\ Finger MP extension and flexion torque transmission splints, type 2 (3); 4 splints @ finger separate B, Wrist flexion: index–small finger MP extension / index–small finger MP flexion: wrist extension torque transmission splint, type 0 (5) C, Long finger PIP flexion or extension torque transmission splint, type 1 (2) \\ Long finger PIP flexion or extension mobilization splint, type 1 (2) D, Ring–small finger MP extension restriction / IP extension torque transmission splint, type 0 (6) E,F, Index–long finger extension restriction / index–long finger flexion mobilization / ring–small finger MP flexion IP extension immobilization splint, type 1 (13)

Splints may have single or multiple purposes. Single purpose: A, One proximal and four distal MP torque transmission splints combine to facilitate active motion at the finger MP joints. B, A splint used with radial nerve paralysis patients transmits torque to achieve finger MP extension through active wrist flexion and wrist extension through active finger MP flexion. C, A PIP flexion mobilization splint and a PIP torque transmission splint are used together to improve PIP joint flexion or extension. Multipurpose: D, Restriction and torque transmission splint. E,F, Restriction, mobilization, and immobilization splint: because of associated injuries to the ring and small fingers, this splint, designed to be used for early passive mobilization of index and long flexor tendon repairs, has a removable component (F) that immobilizes the fourth and fifth digits in extension. [Courtesy (B) Helen Marx, OTR, CHT, Human Factors Engineering of Phoenix, Wickenburg, Ariz.; (C) Jill Francisco, OTR, CHT, Cicero, Ind.; (E,F) Joanne Kassimir, OTR, CHT, photography by Owen Kassimir, Huntington Station, N.Y.]

middle joint (e.g., finger PIP or thumb MP) is situated between adjacent proximal and distal normal joints in an intercalated digital ray, mobilization traction applied distally on the ray results in dispersion of forces to the normal joints with little effect on the stiff primary middle joint. When all joints of a digital ray are equally impaired, the necessity of immobilizing proximal or distal joints is less important (Fig. 8-17, *C*).

The technical ESCS name of a splint does not indicate how many individual secondary joints are included in a splint, nor are the secondary joints specifically named. The SCS type designation describes how many joint levels are incorporated (e.g., a type 1 splint has one secondary joint level; a type 2 has two secondary joint levels, etc.).

Determine if the Wrist, Forearm, and/or Elbow Should Be Included

Deciding whether a finger or thumb splint should be hand-based or forearm-based is a major step in the design process. An incorrect choice may needlessly immobilize the wrist or result in a splint that is ineffective in increasing range of motion or providing protection to healing structures. The key question concerns wrist position and whether it alters or affects the motion or stability of more distal structures. If wrist posture does influence articular motion or changes the tension on vulnerable structures (Fig. 8-18, *A,B*), the wrist must be incorporated in the splint. If, however, wrist motion does not influence articular motion or inappropriately stress tissue, a hand-based splint design may be considered (Fig. 8-18, *C,D*).

If the forearm is a primary joint and the splint purpose is immobilization or mobilization, both the wrist and elbow must be included in the splint as secondary joints to fully influence motion of the forearm (Fig. 8-4, *F,G*; 8-11, *B*). Shoulder splints frequently include the elbow as a secondary joint to control shoulder rotation and the forearm and wrist may be incorporated as secondary joints in shoulder splints to prevent dependent positioning of the hand and to decrease pressure from the splint on the arm. In instances where concomitant pathology also exists at the wrist, forearm, or elbow for which splinting is required, the impaired joints are designated as primary joints instead of secondary joints. For example, in a forearm neutral immobilization splint, the wrist usually is included as a secondary joint; but if wrist pathology is also present, requiring extension immobilization, the wrist becomes a primary joint and the splint is designated a *forearm neutral, wrist*

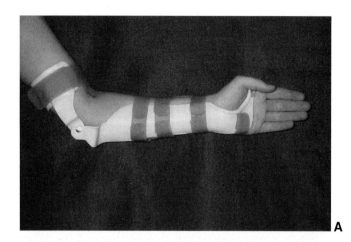

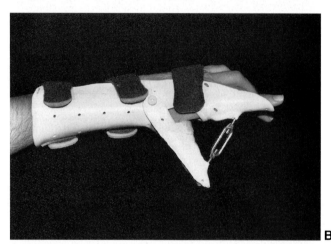

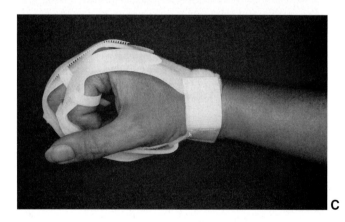

Fig. 8-17 **A,** Forearm neutral immobilization splint, type 2 (3) **B,** Thumb CMC palmar abduction mobilization splint, type 6 (7) **C,** Index–small finger flexion mobilization splint, type 0 (12) **A,** The elbow and wrist are secondary joint levels in this forearm immobilization splint. **B,** To improve mechanical advantage and disperse pressure over a wider area, this thumb CMC joint mobilization splint incorporates six secondary joint levels: wrist, finger MP, PIP, DIP, and thumb MP, IP levels. **C,** This *type 0* finger flexion splint includes no secondary joint levels. [Courtesy **(A)** Rebecca Banks, OTR, CHT, MHS, Blackburn, Australia; **(B)** Daniel Lupo, OTR, CHT, Ventura, Calif.]

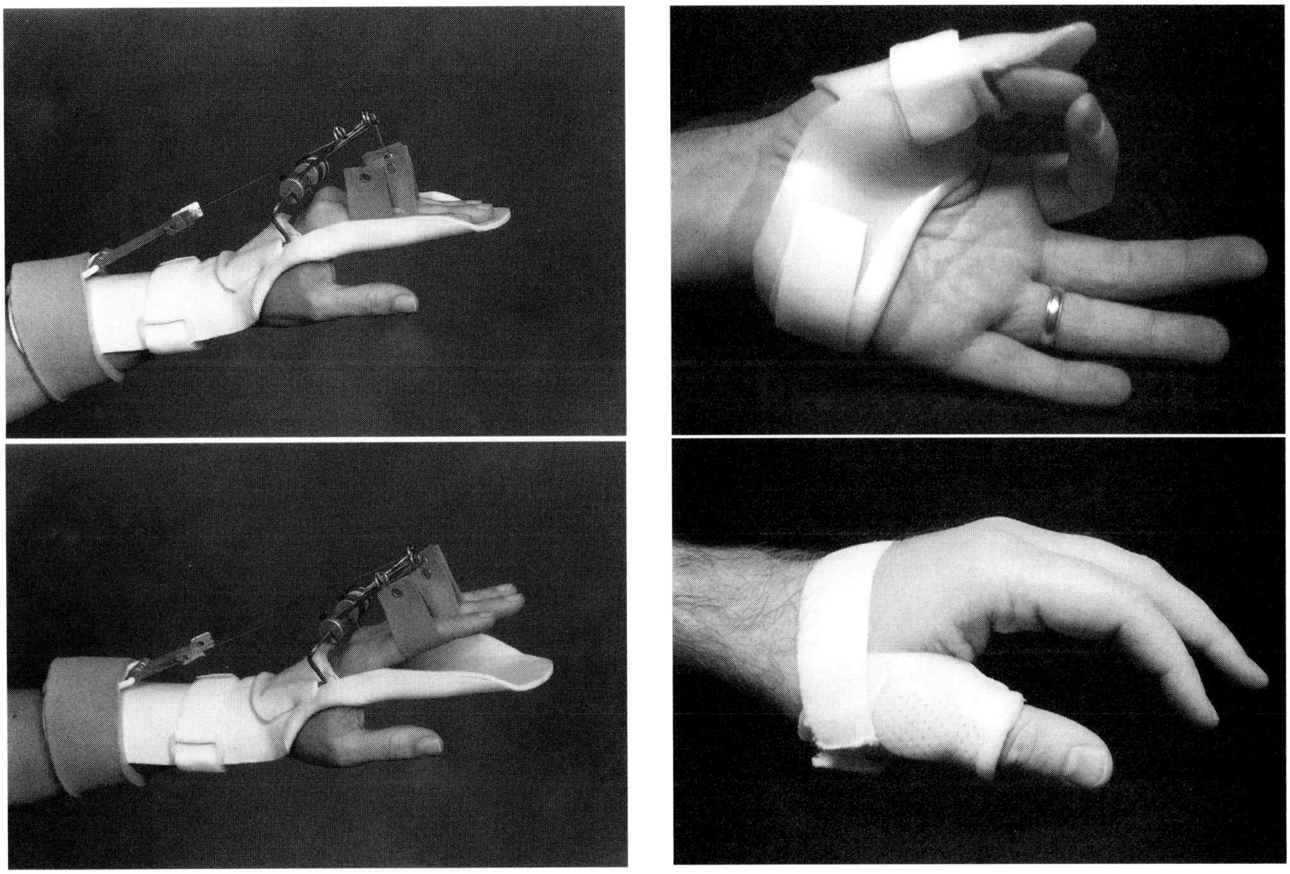

Fig. 8-18   A,B, Index–small finger MP extension mobilization / index–small finger flexion restriction splint, type 1 (13) C, Thumb MP flexion immobilization / IP extension restriction splint, type 1 (3) D, Thumb MP flexion immobilization splint, type 2 (3)
A,B, The wrist is included as a secondary joint level in this splint designed to allow early restricted motion of extensor tendon repairs. C, Restriction of thumb IP extension allows increased stability to the arthritic MP joint. D, A thumb MP flexion splint immobilizes the MP joint and provides protection to the fixation pin while allowing motion of the CMC and wrist joints. [Courtesy (A,B) Barbara Smith, OTR, Edmond, Okla.]

extension immobilization splint, type 1 (3). In this example, only the elbow is considered a secondary joint.

The option of including the wrist, forearm, or elbow in a splint influences fabrication and fit time, splint cost, splint effectiveness, and patient comfort and acceptance. Although larger splints that incorporate these joints as secondary joints require more preparation time, are less acceptable to patients, and are more expensive, the function they provide in controlling the effects of musculotendinous units on more distal joint motion cannot be attained with smaller splints that contain no secondary joints. Conversely, if a smaller splint that includes only primary joints will suffice, economy of cost and time is achieved and the potential for patient acceptance is enhanced.

Adapt for Anatomic Variables

Individual anatomic variables, abnormal structures, soft tissue defects, or skin friability may also influence the design of the splint and are important in the choice of surface on which the proposed splint will be based. The presence of significant dorsal synovial swelling over the carpus may preclude dorsal application and a prominent radial styloid process is a frequent problem in palmarly applied splints that incorporate the wrist. Widening the area of splint application and contiguous fit decrease splint pressure on the extremity, lessening the potential for damaging friable cutaneous surfaces. Avoidance of nerve distribution areas where nerves are prone to become hypersensitive with pressure from splints, as with the superficial branch of the radial nerve, is important.

Also, excessive tension on nerves may occur when splints hold joints at or near their normal limits of motion, increasing potential for nerve compression problems. The median nerve is especially susceptible when the wrist is splinted in flexion.

Integrate Medical/Surgical Intervention Variables

Design and configuration alterations ensure that splints do not interfere with medical and/or surgical interventions. For example, splints must be adapted to accommodate for the presence of surgical fixation or distraction hardware (Fig. 8-19, A), dressings, surgical drains, and possibly the occasional intravenous or hemodialysis access site. Postoperative splints must be configured so that they do not impinge on suture lines, incorrectly stress repairs, or jeopardize tissue viability of tissue grafts, flaps, replants, or transplants. Upper extremity wounds being treated with open technique also require splint design alterations, and splints must be created so that they facilitate edema reduction and avoid creating additional swelling to healing upper extremities.

It is not unusual for a new treatment technique to instigate the development of a new and unique-to-the-procedure splint design or splint component. In the 1960s, a new outrigger design was created to position postoperatively patients' hands that had Swanson MP arthroplasty implants[27]; the open technique for treating burn patients with topical antibiotic agents generated development of fingernail hooks that allowed positional traction to be applied to digits without using digital slings or cuffs (Fig. 8-19, B).[2] Advances in tendon repair techniques have also influenced splint designs (Fig. 8-19, C-E).*

Use Mechanical Principles Advantageously

The employment of mechanical principles adds detail and dimension to the development of the upper extremity splint. These principles determine the length and width of the splint, regulate splint position, define the angles of attachment of traction devices (Fig. 8-20, A-C), and may help identify additional splint components and their configurations (Fig. 8-20, D). Failure to consider and adapt to these principles may result in an ineffective or uncomfortable splint that may have otherwise been designed appropriately.

Consider Kinetic Effects

Because the upper extremity functions as an open kinematic chain, the inclusion of a joint in a splint can

*References 1, 3, 6–14, 17, 19, 23–26, 30.

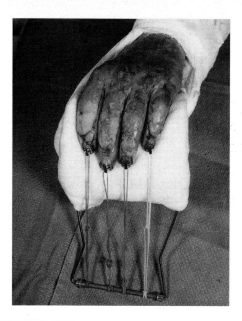

A

B

Fig. 8-19   A, Thumb CMC palmar abduction immobilization splint, type 2 (3) B, Index–small finger MP flexion and IP extension, thumb CMC palmar abduction and MP-IP extension mobilization splint, type 1 (16) C,D, Index–small finger MP-PIP extension mobilization / index–small finger flexion restriction splint, type 1 (13) E, Index–long finger extension restriction / index–long flexion mobilization splint, type 1 (7)
Medical or surgical treatment techniques can influence splint design. **A,** A splint maintains thumb CMC mobility as an external fixator stabilizes a fracture. **B,** Dress hooks glued to the fingernails connect elastic traction mobilization assists to the fingers in this splint that mobilizes finger and thumb joints into an antideformity position. **C,D,** Designed to permit early passive mobilization to extensor tendon repairs in Zone V, this splint allows active flexion and passive extension of the metacarpophalangeal joints within a predetermined limited arc of motion. **E,** For Zone II flexor tendon repairs, this splint allows restricted active finger extension and passive finger flexion. Two palmar pulleys act as fulcrums and control the direction of the flexion mobilization assists. [Courtesy **(A)** Brenda Hilfrank, PT, CHT, South Burlington, Vt. **(B)** Kilulu Von Prince, OTR, MS, Clovis, Calif.; **(C,D)** Roslyn Evans, OTR, CHT, Vero Beach, Fla.; **(E)** Jean Claude Rouzaud, PT, Montpellier, France.]

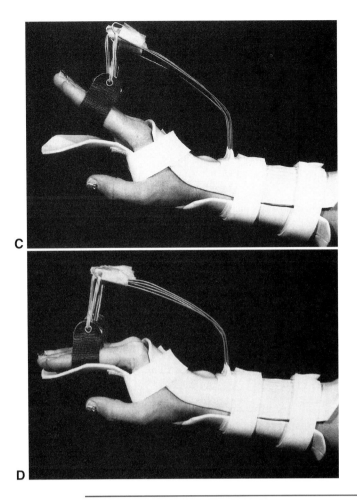

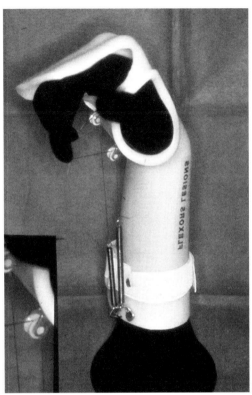

Fig. 8-19, cont'd
For legend see opposite page.

alter external and internal forces to proximal or distal joints. Recognition of the potential problems and understanding how to positively control and use these altered forces are important factors in the astute upper extremity specialist's armamentarium. For example, if a thumb metacarpophalangeal joint is immobilized, the stresses of normal use of the first ray are increased at both the CMC and IP joints. A splinted wrist may create a greater demand for shoulder and elbow motion to substitute for the impeded wrist movement. Increased force on unsplinted joints becomes a significant factor in designing splints when adjacent joints cannot tolerate the extra stress, necessitating the creation of splints that produce minimal compensatory effects to proximal or distal structures.

Kinetic concepts may also be used advantageously to enhance motion or to prevent deformity. By secondarily immobilizing the wrist and interphalangeal joints of the fingers in *MP torque transmission splints*, the specialist may harness the full power of the extrinsic digital flexors and extensors to produce

metacarpophalangeal joint motion in a postoperative MP replacement arthroplasty patient (Fig. 8-16, *A*). A flexed wrist enhances finger extension and abduction, and an extended wrist requires greater proximal excursion of the extrinsic extensors to produce full simultaneous digital extension. Flexed metacarpophalangeal joints in an intrinsic minus hand facilitate interphalangeal extension via the intact extrinsic extensors. Postoperative tendon transfer splints implement kinetic concepts to protect healing transfers[15] (Fig. 8-21) and, later, to facilitate volitional use of transfers. A thorough understanding of upper extremity anatomy and kinesiology are prerequisites to identifying and using kinetic concepts to their full potential in splint designs.

Decide Whether to Employ Inelastic or Elastic Mobilization Forces

The kind of traction a mobilization splint uses has major influence on the final design of the splint.

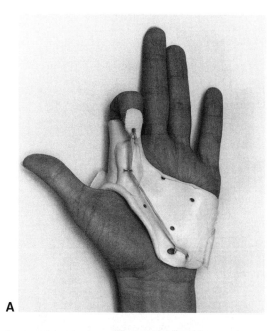

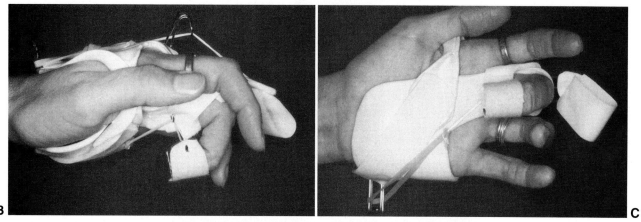

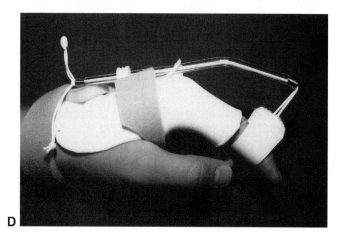

Fig. 8-20   A, Index finger IP flexion mobilization splint, type 1 (3) B,C, Long finger IP flexion or extension mobilization splint, type 1 (3) D, Index finger PIP extension mobilization splint, type 1 (2)

Mechanical principles are crucial to successful splint designs. Combined dorsal and palmar proximal phalanx components provide excellent stabilization of the metacarpophalangeal joints in these splints, allowing elastic traction mobilizing forces to be directed to the interphalangeal joints. [Courtesy **(A)** Barbara L. (Allen) Smith, OTR, Edmond, Okla.; **(B,C)** Jill Francisco, OTR, CHT, Cicero, Ind.]

Mobilization splints use either inelastic (Fig. 8-22) or elastic traction (Fig. 8-23) to generate joint motion of primary supple joints or to effect tissue remodeling of primary stiff joints. Traditionally, inelastic traction splints were viewed as being simpler in design than were their elastic traction counterparts. However, the abundance of exceptions now makes this perception passé. Elastic traction splints may be very simple in design and, conversely, inelastic traction splints may involve mechanically sophisticated methods for applying and changing tension.

Selection of traction is dependent on individual patient factors including age; acuteness of the injury and motivation; splinting criteria, including complexity of altering outrigger length, adjusting mobilization assist tension, availability and cost of materials; and, not to be disregarded, therapist expertise. Providing all other factors are equal, most experienced therapists correlate type of traction with (1) acuteness or chronicity of the injury and (2) the inherent characteristics of specific joints. For example, an acute PIP joint flexion deformity responds readily to elastic traction extension torque, but the same elastic traction applied to a chronic PIP joint flexion deformity with no end-range give is relatively useless. Experience teaches that chronic PIP flexion deformities with no end-range give respond best to inelastic traction in the form of serially applied plaster casts. Another example, serially applied inelastic traction in the form of progressively wider *thumb CMC palmar abduction mobilization splints*, often produces better results for increasing motion at the thumb carpometacarpal

joint than do mobilization splints using elastic traction (Fig. 8-14).

It makes sense that chronically stiff joints respond better to inelastic traction when one considers what is happening at the cellular level. Assuming both types of traction are adjusted appropriately, inelastic traction maintains consistent mobilizing tension on remodeling soft tissues for longer periods of time than does elastic traction, which allows tension to fluctuate. In contrast, the magnitude of force may be more

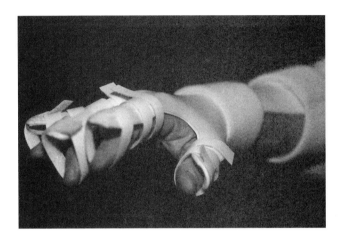

Fig. 8-22   Index–small finger extension, thumb CMC radial abduction and MP-IP extension mobilization splint, type 1 (16) Inelastic traction is used to increase finger and thumb extension and thumb CMC radial abduction. (Courtesy Elizabeth Spencer Steffa, OTR / L, CHT, Seattle, Wash.)

Fig. 8-21   Thumb IP flexion and extension torque transmission splint, type 12 (13)
Facilitating simultaneous index finger extension and thumb IP extension, this innovative splint helps reeducate an extensor indicis proprius transfer to restore extensor pollicis longus function. (From Goloborod'ko S: Training splint for EIP to EPL transfer, *J Hand Ther* 10(1):48, 1997.)

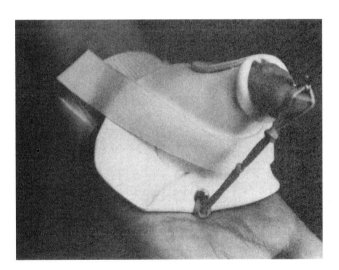

Fig. 8-23   Thumb CMC palmar abduction and IP flexion mobilization splint, type 1 (3)
Splints may incorporate both inelastic and elastic traction. Thumb CMC joint motion is improved using inelastic traction through serial splint adjustments as the IP joint is mobilized using elastic traction. (From Fess EE: Splinting for mobilization of the thumb. In Hunter J: *Rehabilitation of the hand*, ed 1, Mosby, 1984, St. Louis.)

finely adjusted and controlled with elastic traction, a factor that is especially useful when splinting to mobilize supple joints or to correct acute joint stiffness.

Both inelastic and elastic traction must be adjusted as joints remodel and range of motion improves. Because of this, the type of traction and corresponding splint design often reflect ease of adjustment of outriggers and mobilization assists (Fig. 8-24, *A-H*).[22] Decisions at this point in the design process result in major changes in the final configuration of the splint.

Determine the Surface for Splint Application

The decision as to what surface or surfaces of the hand, forearm, or upper arm a splint is to be applied is the next step in the progression through the hierarchy of design principles. This decision is influenced by the interrelationships of anatomic and mechanical factors. Although pressure is usually tolerated better on the anterior surface of the upper extremity, one must be aware that this side makes the greatest contribution to function and sensation. A finger extension mobilization splint using elastic traction is mechanically more efficient when based dorsally, and a palmar elastic traction splint provides a stable base for digital flexion mobilization forces. Ulnar deviation of the wrist may be controlled from either the ulnar or radial surface, but if passive ulnar deviation is to be increased using elastic traction, the splint should be based on the ulnar aspect of the forearm. Serial elbow extension splints are best applied anteriorly (Fig. 8-25, *A*) to avoid pressure on the ulnar nerve. Because of the size and weight of the arm, the surface of splint application for shoulder immobilization splints depends on the amount of shoulder abduction and internal or external rotation needed. Restriction splints are more effective when restriction components correspond to the direction of the restricted motion (Fig. 8-25, *B*); e.g., an MP ulnar deviation splint should incorporate an ulnar deviation bar, regardless of whether the splint base is situated on the dorsal or palmar aspect of the hand. Splints applied to the internal side of the angle of a deformity (e.g., a palmar-based PIP extension mobilization splint) have an added variable of friction at the proximal and distal points of splint contact that splints applied to the exterior side of the angle of deformity (for this example, a dorsally based splint) do not have.[28] The greater the angle of deformity, the greater is the friction. Many other variables influence the determination of surface of splint application, including the presence of wounds, poor sensibility, fixation hardware, skin grafts, hand dominance, dexterity, and occupation.

Identify Areas of Diminished Sensibility

It is important to identify areas of decreased or absent sensibility before finalizing a splint design. Because of the increased possibility for pressure necrosis, special care should be taken to create splints that prevent or minimize forces over those areas where sensibility is impaired. Widening of narrow components, contiguous fit, and the judicious use of padding are effective methods of decreasing splint forces on insensitive portions of the extremity.

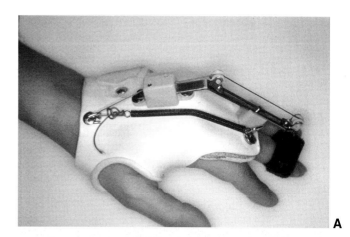

A

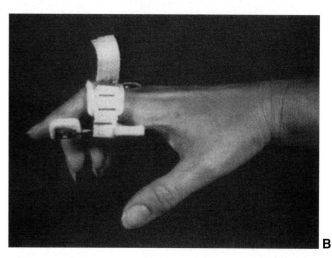

B

Fig. 8-24   A, Long finger PIP extension mobilization splint, type 2 (6) B, Index finger PIP extension splint, type 0 (1) C,D, Index finger IP flexion mobilization splint, type 0 (2) E, Small finger MP flexion mobilization splint, type 0 (1) F-H, Index–small finger IP flexion mobilization splint, type 2 (13)
All of these splints incorporate different methods to facilitate adjustment of outrigger (**A,E**) or mobilization assists (**A-H**). [Courtesy (**A**) Jean Claude Rouzaud, PT, Montpellier, France; (**E**) Nelson Vazquez, OTR, CHT, Miami, Fla., and Damon Kirk, WFR Corporation, Wyckoff, N.J.; (**F-H**) from Schanzer D: Static progressive end-range proximal interphalageal / distal interphalangeal flexion splint, *J Hand Ther* 13(4):310-2, 2000.]

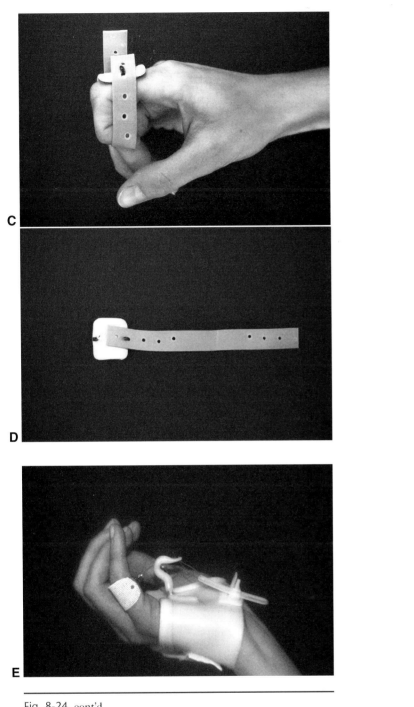

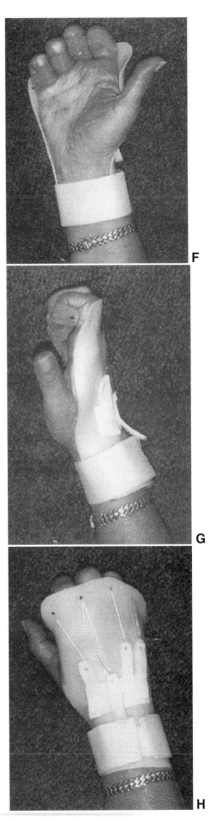

Fig. 8-24, cont'd
For legend see opposite page.

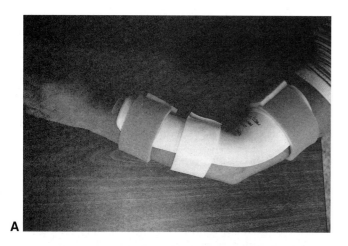

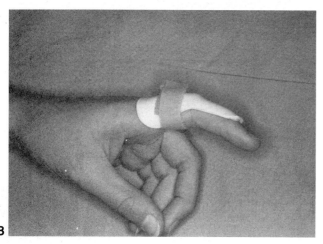

Fig. 8-25   A, Elbow extension mobilization splint, type 0 (1)
B, Index finger PIP extension restriction splint, type 0 (1)
Splint surface of application takes into consideration most of the
design principles reviewed in this chapter. While anatomical
and mechanical concepts predominate decisions as to surface of
splint application, patient-specific variables must not be ignored.
(Courtesy (B) Lori Klerekoper DeMott, OTR, CHT, Columbus, Ohio)

Choose the Most Appropriate Materials

The wide variety of splinting materials currently
available allows the upper extremity specialist to
selectively match materials to meet the specific
requirements of individual patients. Each material has
idiosyncratic properties that are advantageous or less
advantageous to given situations. Some are stronger
or more durable (Fig. 8-26, A), while others mold so
closely and evenly that fine skin creases are dupli-
cated on the internal surface of the splint. The property of becoming translucent during the malleable
stage may help with hard-to-fit anatomic variables,
and the ability to form a rapid and strong bond econ-
omizes construction time. Some materials are soft
(Fig. 8-26, B,C), some are less expensive, and others

withstand the high temperatures required for certain
types of sterilization techniques. Although not all
problems may be anticipated (Fig. 8-26, D), understanding patients' lifestyles helps define splint material selection.

The more familiar upper extremity specialists
become with the multitude of available materials, the
better opportunities they have for selecting materials
that best meet the special needs of their patients. The
day of the universal splint material ended more than
three decades ago. Contemporary specialists understand the implications of the differing material properties as they apply to treatment situations and use
them to their advantage.[29]

Adaptation of design to incorporate the properties
of available materials is also an important consideration in the fabrication of hand splints. Many of the
low-temperature materials require splint designs that
provide strength and support through increased
contour of the material to the hand. A bar design
splint constructed from these materials would be an
inappropriate design choice because of the inherent
weakness of the material. Technical difficulties in
splint fabrication must also be considered to avoid
poor results when working with a particular material.
If the material has a high cohesive or bonding factor,
a circumferential design may increase fit problems
when overlapping ends bond together unexpectedly,
and the choice of a rigid material for a design whose
success depends on a close fit may lead to frustration
and failure.

■ SUMMARY

Therapist experience and motivation play major roles
in splint design. Because of this, it is important that
therapists attentively and routinely upgrade their
splinting knowledge and skills. Those new to the
splinting arena must remember that even the most
experienced splint fabricators at some time had to
make their first splints; if asked, these experts smil-
ingly relate that their first splints were difficult and a
long way from perfect! Therapists are not born into
the world knowing how to make splints. Proficiency
comes with practice fueled by an internal desire to
improve for the sake of the patient and an acute discomfort with mediocrity. The more knowledgeable
therapists care about splinting theory, technique, and
materials, the better the opportunities they provide
for patients to achieve their full rehabilitative potential. An emerging adage, "Those with only hammers in
their toolboxes will treat everything with a hammer,"
is applicable to therapist splinting expertise. Indicative of a poor knowledge base, wholesale application

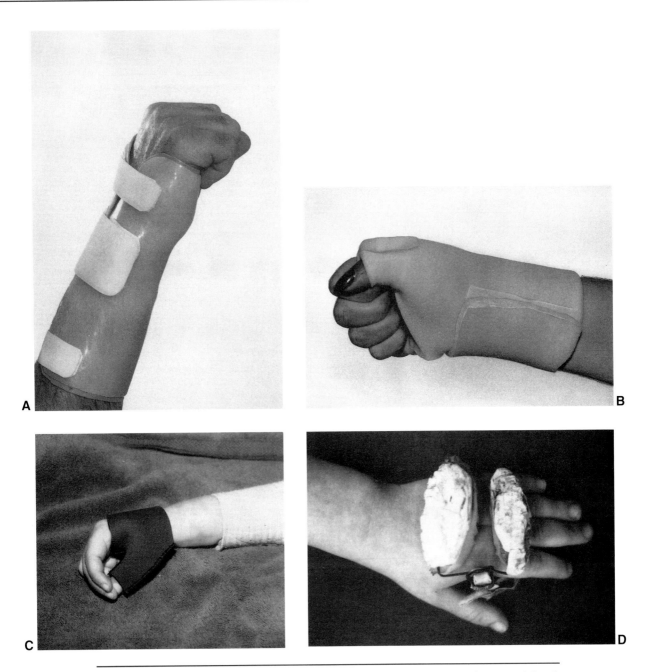

Fig. 8-26   A, Wrist extension immobilization splint, type 0 (1) B, Wrist circumduction and thumb CMC circumduction restriction splint, type 1 (3) C, Thumb CMC palmar abduction and MP-IP extension mobilization splint, type 0 (3) D, Index–small finger MP extension restriction / IP extension torque transmission splint, type 0 (12)

A, Bonding polyethylene to Plastazote produces a comfortable and extremely durable wrist immobilization splint that may be used with early return to work patients. A polyurethane foam splint (B) permits protected motion of the wrist and thumb carpometacarpal and metacarpophalangeal joints and a neoprene splint (C) positions the thumb to improve hand function. D, Splinting materials used in children's splints should be durable and nontoxic. The plastic portion of this Orthoplast and spring-wire splint is almost unrecognizable because of the patient's habit of chewing on it! [Courtesy (A) Theresa Bielawski, OT(C), Toronto, Ont., and Jane Bear-Lehman, PhD, OTR, FAOTA, New York, N.Y.; (B) Rivka Ben-Porath, OT, Jerusalem, Israel; (C) Joni Armstrong, OTR, CHT, Bemidji, Minn.]

of prefabricated splints or poorly done custom splints, without regard to basic splinting principles, is not therapeutic splinting and, in truth, may be detrimental to patients. Splinting is an important and integral part of treating upper extremity dysfunction. Remember, splinting skills are acquired, not bestowed!

The general principles of design provide the basic framework on which the fabrication of any upper extremity splint must be based; whereas the specific principles, altered by individual patient variables and functional requirements, influence the final configuration of the splint. The experienced specialist does not employ these principles one by one in checklist fashion but considers them simultaneously, adding, eliminating, and supplementing them with innovation and creativity. The challenge is to create a splint that not only meets the functional objectives but also is acceptable and well tolerated by the patient.

REFERENCES

1. Cooney W, Lin G, An KN: Improved tendon excursion following flexor tendon repair, *J Hand Ther* 2(2):102-6, 1989.
2. deLeeuw C: Personal communication from Carolina deLeeuw: fingernail hooks for positioning burned hands, 1963, Tacoma, WA.
3. Duran R, et al: Management of flexor tendon lacerations in Zone 2 using controlled passive motion postoperatively. In Hunter J, Schneider L, Mackin E: *Tendon surgery in the hand*, Mosby, 1987, St. Louis.
4. Dymarczyk M: A locking mechanism for the tenodesis splint for flexor tendon repairs, *J Hand Ther* 14(3), 2001.
5. Emerson S: The rheumatiod hand: postoperative splint options, *J Hand Ther* 6(3):214, 1993.
6. Evans R: A study of the zone 1 flexor tendon injury and implications for treatment, *J Hand Ther* 3(3):133-48, 1990.
7. Evans R: An analysis of factors that support the early active short arc motion of the repaired central slip, *J Hand Ther* 5(4):187-201, 1992.
8. Evans R, Thompson D: Immediate active short arc motion following tendon repair. In Hunter J, Schneider L, Mackin E: *Tendon and nerve surgery in the hand, a third decade*, Mosby, 1997, St. Louis.
9. Evans R, Hunter J, Burkhalter W: Conservative management of the trigger finger: a new approach, *J Hand Ther* 1(2):59-68, 1988.
10. Evans RB: Clinical application of controlled stress to the healing extensor tendon: a review of 112 cases, *Phys Ther* 69(12):1041-9, 1989.
11. Evans RB: Immediate active short arc motion following extensor tendon repair, *Hand Clin* 11(3):483-512, 1995.
12. Evans RB, Burkhalter WE: A study of the dynamic anatomy of extensor tendons and implications for treatment, *J Hand Surg* [Am] 11(5):774-9, 1986.
13. Evans RB, Thompson DE: The application of force to the healing tendon, *J Hand Ther* 6(4):266-84, 1993.
14. Fess EE: Splinting flexor tendon injuries, *Hand Surg* 7(1):101-8, 2002.
15. Goloborod'ko S: Training splint for EIP to EPL transfer, *J Hand Ther* 10(1):48, 1997.
16. Hannah S, Hudak P: Splinting and radial nerve palsy: a single-subject design, *J Hand Ther* 14(3):216-8, 2001.
17. Hunter JM, Salisbury RE: Flexor-tendon reconstruction in severely damaged hands. A two-stage procedure using a silicone-dacron reinforced gliding prosthesis prior to tendon grafting, *J Bone Joint Surg Am* 53(5):829-58, 1971.
18. Kleinert HE, et al: Primary repair of flexor tendons in no-man's land, *J Bone Joint Surg* 49A:577, 1967.
19. May EJ, Silfverskiold KL, Sollerman CJ: Controlled mobilization after flexor tendon repair in zone II: a prospective comparison of three methods, *J Hand Surg* [Am] 17(5):942-52, 1992.
20. Moberg E: Aspects of sensation in reconstructive surgery, *J Bone Joint Surg* 46A:817-25, 1964.
21. Mullen TM: Static progressive splint to increase wrist extension or flexion, *J Hand Ther* 13(4):313-5, 2000.
22. Schanzer D: Static progressive end-range proximal interphalageal / distal interphalangeal flexion splint, *J Hand Ther* 13(4):310-2, 2000.
23. Silfverskiold KL, May EJ: Flexor tendon repair in zone II with a new suture technique and an early mobilization program combining passive and active flexion, *J Hand Surg* [Am] 19(1):53-60, 1994.
24. Silfverskiold KL, May EJ, Tornvall AH: Tendon excursions after flexor tendon repair in zone. II: Results with a new controlled-motion program, *J Hand Surg* [Am] 18(3):403-10, 1993.
25. Strickland JW, Glogovac SV: Digital function following flexor tendon repair in Zone II: a comparison of immobilization and controlled passive motion techniques, *J Hand Surg* [Am] 5(6):537-43, 1980.
26. Strickland JW, Gettle K: Flexor tendon repair: the Indianapolis method. In Hunter J, Schneider L, Mackin E: *Tendon and nerve surgery in the hand, a third decade*, Mosby, 1997, St. Louis.
27. Swanson AB: A flexible implant for replacement of arthritic or destroyed joints in the hand, *NYU Interclin Inform Bull* 6:16-9, 1966.
28. Van Lede P, van Veldhoven G: *Therapeutic hand splints: a rational approach*, vol 1, Provan, 1998, Antwerp, Belgium.
29. van Veldhoven G: Creativity in splinting, *Br J Hand Ther* 5(3):77-9, 2000.
30. Cannon NM, Strickland JW: Therapy following flexor tendon surgery, *Hand Clin* 1(1):147-65, 1985.

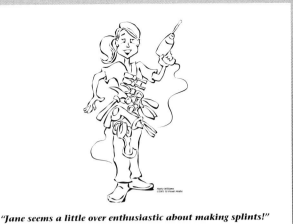

"Jane seems a little over enthusiastic about making splints!"

CHAPTER 9

Construction Principles

Once a splint has been designed and a pattern prepared,* construction of the splint is technically not as difficult as are the preceding stages and those to follow. The principles of construction represent concepts that are directly related to the durability, cosmesis, and comfort of the finished product. Adherence to the principles listed at the beginning of this chapter should produce a splint that will be well tolerated, durable, and visually acceptable.

Construction of a thermoplastic splint may be divided into five phases: (1) transfer of the pattern to the material, (2) heating of the material, (3) cutting of the material, (4) joining of separate parts, and (5) finishing details of the splint. Because fitting of unassembled parts of the splint usually occurs after the cutting

phase, there is an obligatory time separation between the initial construction phases and the final phases of joining and finishing. Many of the principles of construction are applicable to more than one phase and should be considered as overall guidelines rather than as techniques specific to a single phase.

STRIVE FOR GOOD COSMETIC EFFECT

Since a splint is an unusual-looking, extraneous piece of equipment, it has little inherent cosmetic value however well-designed, constructed, or fitted it may be. It is therefore important that all efforts be directed toward making the external appearance of a splint as pleasing as is possible. Splints that resemble an aberrant assortment of discarded junk have no place in today's therapeutic armamentarium. Material or fabrication expense should not significantly influence

---

*Refer to Chapter 21, Patterns, and Chapter 18, Splinting the Pediatric Patient, for pattern information.

237

splint cosmesis. Inexpensive materials may be neatly assembled into a functional splint, and, conversely, more costly materials may be poorly constructed and assembled with resultant splint discoloration, fatigue, and irregular surfaces. Good splint appearance is achieved through careful attention to detail during the various phases of construction. Materials should not be overworked. Bubbles and burn spots from overheating are unacceptable, as are rough edges, sharp corners, pen marks, fingerprints, and dirty smudges. Isopropyl alcohol pads are helpful for removing pen marks used for tracing patterns onto splint material. Use of a fingernail to mark patterns on splinting materials is even better because pen marks are eliminated altogether. Fingerprints are less likely to occur when quick light strokes are used, and by delaying working with the material for a few seconds, its contact surface area is allowed to become more resilient to unintentional marring. For increased cosmesis, the number of different materials used in a splint should be kept to a minimum. When joining pieces of a material whose opposing surfaces differ in texture, take care to align the surfaces so that the external surface textures match. Also, remember that the type of thermoplastic material chosen contributes to the overall cosmetic effect of the splint.

■ APPROPRIATELY MATCH MATERIAL TO CONSTRUCTION CIRCUMSTANCES

Splint material choice is reflective of many factors ranging from physical limitations of workspace and availability of equipment, to patient specific requirements involving anatomic and physiologic condition, age, and ability to cooperate in the fabrication and fit processes. Therapist experience is also a major factor in material selection. As therapists gain experience, they often acquire personal preferences for certain splinting materials. For example, an inexperienced therapist may prefer materials with moderate drape and easy conformability properties, while an experienced therapist may opt for materials that require more skill in handling but have faster bonding and remolding capabilities, allowing greater efficiency of fabrication. Appraisal of splinting material requirements as they relate to construction conditions is an ever-evolving process. The more knowledgeable therapists are about material properties, the better they are at selecting the most suitable materials for the construction tasks they face. Working with splinting company representatives is a quick way to learn to efficiently and accurately match materials to specific client requirements. Also, consider doing an Internet search using the key words "splinting material" or

"low-temperature thermoplastics" to learn more about available splinting products.

Low-temperature thermoplastics may be separated into material content categories that help define their conformity and stretch properties. Plastic and/or rubber are common components in most thermoplastic splinting materials. Plastics contain a polycaprolactone synthetic and synthetic rubbers contain isoprene. Plastic and elastic splint materials are often described according to the subjective categories of minimal, moderate, and maximum resistance to stretch. The more plastic content a material has, the greater its conformability and drape are; and the more rubber content a material has, the more it resists stretch. Although conformability and resistance to stretch are on opposite relative ends of the materials continuum, their respective positions do not connote that one is better than the other. It simply means that their physical properties are different.

It is important to identify main factors that will influence splint construction prior to initiating the actual fabrication process. Questions that help match appropriate materials to specific circumstances include the following: Is the material better suited for small, medium, or large splints? And, does the material permit ease of reheating and refitting without overstretching or loss of overall physical integrity? Generally speaking, materials with high plastic/elastic content that conform effortlessly are often better matched to small- or medium-sized splints. High-conformability materials are easily stretched and are therefore less applicable to large area splint designs because of their tendency to "grow" in size with heating and handling. Materials that can be overhauled again and again yet remain devoid of stretching usually include elastic or rubber-like materials. These materials are well suited for circumstances where multiple serial adjustments are anticipated.

Many excellent splinting materials are available commercially. Some better-known materials are grouped according to their key intrinsic properties. The vast diversity of therapist preference and opinion regarding splinting materials makes it difficult to identify consistently agreed upon material handling properties. Although a few independent studies have been done regarding splint material properties,[1-3] more research is needed. Readers are encouraged to peruse available product information and to talk with other therapists and manufacturer representatives to learn specific tips and methods for working with various materials. Just as one chooses one's own clothing to be compatible with outside temperature, so should splinting materials be chosen to correspond to the requirements of individual situations. Blind adherence to only one material unfairly limits patient potential.

While each material has unique characteristics, its rudimentary composition establishes its general handling qualities.

When ordering splinting materials, it is good policy to always investigate local and national suppliers for competitive prices and selection. Remember, available splinting materials change with time and equivalent characteristics are often discovered within a range of similar but competing materials. Request samples and use them to create frequently made splints. Look for memory, conformability, and ease of bonding and finishing. Does the material return to its original dimension? How do the edges appear when cut? How difficult are they to smooth? How much working time is allowed before the material hardens? When the splint material is positioned on the extremity does it conform smoothly and easily?

Materials may be purchased in different thicknesses, in solid or perforated form, and in colors. Once comfort level is reached with a given material's basic handling properties, experiment with the material in different thicknesses and in different perforation patterns. Material thickness and perforation absence, presence, and configuration directly influence material working properties and alter indications for use. Material color helps patient acceptance, especially with children and teenagers, and allows therapists more creative latitude.

Age of splinting material is also an important factor in defining handling properties. Some materials deteriorate more quickly than others, increasing splint potential for breaking or other problems. It is important to identify the specific shelf life for each material from the purchasing company. Mark date of delivery or expiration date on material boxes or containers as they arrive in the clinic.

USE EQUIPMENT APPROPRIATE TO MATERIAL

The availability of a wide variety of splinting materials helps meet the unique splinting needs of patients. It is vital that the hand specialist be thoroughly versed in the idiosyncrasies of the physical properties and the specific equipment requirements of these materials. The use of dissimilar substances mandates that construction methods be carefully adapted to meet specific criteria of the materials. This is especially important when switching between low- and high-temperature forming substances. Although metal files and electric sanders are appropriate tools for smoothing edges on high-temperature material splints, these devices cause friction gumming and exaggerate roughness on low-temperature material edges. Power saws produce burrs on the edges of cold, low-temperature forming materials, whereas cutting the same material with scissors after it is warmed produces a continuous, smooth-finished splint edge. If the material piece is too large to fit in a heating unit, a utility knife may be used to score the sheet, providing strategically placed groove-lines for breaking the piece into smaller sections. An indelible marking device or fingernail indentation should be used when transferring a pattern to a material that requires wet heat for cutting and forming; whereas the use of a water-soluble pen with a dry heat material is preferable, since the pen marks can be washed off when no longer needed.

When working with wire, it is important to understand the purpose of the component being constructed and the stresses to which it will be subjected, for the type of wire selected will dictate the tools required for shaping. Ordinary coat hanger wire may be molded with the aid of pliers, or a bending bar may be necessary to shape more resilient wire, such as the steel-welding rod frequently used in outriggers. To produce smoothly contoured, tightly coiled springs from heavy-gauge piano wire, other specialized bending jigs are required (Fig. 9-1).

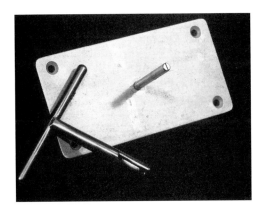

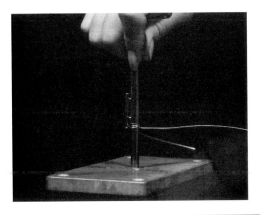

Fig. 9-1   Special equipment such as this adapted Wynn Parry jig is necessary when shaping heavy-gauge wire.

■ USE TYPE OF HEAT AND TEMPERATURE APPROPRIATE TO MATERIAL

The reaction of splinting materials to heat varies with the type of material, but temperature extremes in either direction (too much heat or not enough) directly influence construction techniques. Overheating causes blistering, stretching, and surface irregularities, and underheating may produce rough-cut edges and uneven pliability. Bonding of low-temperature materials is also not as reliable when temperature is not optimum. Splint construction is not only influenced by temperature; the type of heat used also influences the process. Two types of heat are used in splint constructing and fitting—wet heat and dry heat.

Wet Heat

Electric fry pans, splint heat pans, or hydrocollators are used to heat water to requisite levels for splint fabrication. Immersion for approximately one minute in water heated to 150-170° Fahrenheit is adequate to render most low-temperature thermoplastics pliable, depending on material thickness and presence/configuration of perforations. Although most thermoplastic materials remain opaque when heated, white Aquaplast, Encore, and Reveal become transparent when ready to form, providing helpful see-through materials that ease difficult construction or fit situations. It is often difficult to focus wet heat to small areas of an already formed splint, but this may be solved through the use of equipment that provides narrow directional control of hot water (Fig. 9-2).

Accessory equipment aids splint construction process. Pan liners prevent material from sticking to heat pan surfaces and large spatulas facilitate removal of thermoplastic material from hot water. Wrapping spatula handles in pipe insulation lets spatulas float to the surface when they are inadvertently dropped into hot water pans, easing retrieval.

When multiple pieces of thermoplastic are heated simultaneously, paper towels may be used to separate pieces as they are heated, preventing adherence to one another. In a similar concept, large surface area splints, such as full-length arm splints, may be fitted slowly into electric fry pans by gradually folding their extra material lengths over paper towels to form multiple imbricated layers of immersed splinting material. Each successive fold requires its own sheet of paper toweling to prevent facing surfaces from adhering to each other. Another helpful technique for preventing thermoplastic materials from sticking together during heating involves coating material with liquid soap to give nonstick surface coatings. The liquid soap may be added to the water in a heat pan, or it may be smeared on the countertop next to the heat pan so that as warm materials are removed, they are placed on the soapy countertop and turned to coat both sides. Some materials have a tendency to stick to the fingers of those making the splints. To prevent these sticky-surface materials from adhering, coat hands with cold cream or mineral oil, or immerse hands in cold water prior to handling the materials.

Dry Heat

Knowledge of splint material properties is important to improving efficiency. Using dry heat alone, some materials, such as Orthoplast, may be heated to malleable stage in a dry heat pan and held for prolonged periods of time at a constant warm temperature, providing splint material that is immediately ready for cutting and fitting throughout the day (Fig. 9-3). Also, when working in environments where water sources are remote or cumbersome (e.g., hospital bedside or surgery), use of dry heat and these specific heat-suspension materials eliminates time-consuming and inefficient transporting and heating of water.

Dry heat is unique in that it eliminates surface contamination introduced by minerals and other impurities contained in water-based wet heat, making bonding of components more durable. Materials such as Orthoplast bond more readily to themselves when dry heat is employed and the need for additional surface cleaning with chemical solvents is also eliminated. Scraping prebond surfaces to roughen them and heating one surface to a higher temperature increases strength of dry heat bonds. The type of heat also influences the speed at which materials become malleable. Most low-temperature materials respond

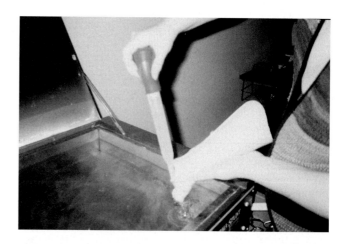

Fig. 9-2   If a thermoplastic material requires wet heat, a turkey baster is helpful in directing hot water to small areas on a splint. (Courtesy Joni Armstrong, OTR, CHT, Bemidji, Minn.)

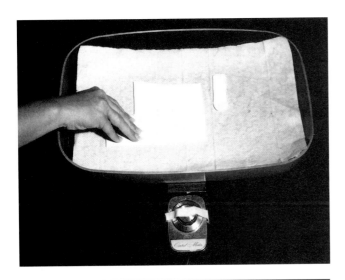

Fig. 9-3   Large pieces of Orthoplast may be heated in a dry skillet lined with a paper towel to prevent sticking and surface impregnation. Use of a dry skillet allows the material temperature to be consistently maintained over many hours, providing malleable plastic whenever it is needed throughout the day. To ensure that skillet temperature is consistent, the temperature gauge is taped.

more quickly and uniformly to wet heat, especially if they have been contoured previously. However, if only a small section of a splint needs heating, the use of dry heat from a heat gun allows adjacent structures to remain unaltered.

Whether wet or dry heat is used, it is critical that patients are protected from hot splint materials during fabrication and fitting of splints. Cotton or elastic stockinette protects patients from inadvertently being burned by hot materials as they are fitted to extremities. Burn patients with skin grafts or patients with hypersensitivity to heat require special care and attention, as do pediatric patients and patients with fragile skin such as those taking corticosteroid medications.

■ USE SAFETY AND ERGONOMIC PRECAUTIONS AND WORK EFFICIENTLY

Incorporation of sound safety and ergonomic techniques during the construction phase of splint fabrication is essential for protecting therapists and patients from accidental injury and for generating efficient use of time. Exposure to a large volume of hand trauma and overuse injuries results in therapists' awareness of the potential dangers of working with both manual and power tools and an appreciation of the need for high safety standards.

Eyes should be protected, rings removed, and loose hair and clothing secured before any piece of power

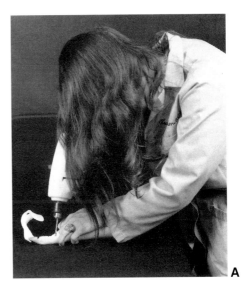

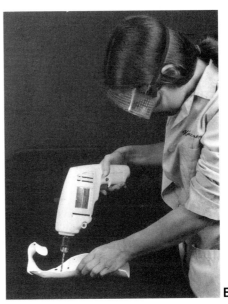

Fig. 9-4   Safety precautions should be carefully observed when working with hand tools or power equipment. A, Incorrect. B, Correct.

equipment is turned on (Fig. 9-4). When working with power drills, secure the material being drilled to prevent its sudden movement or rotation. Since studies show that dull or poorly maintained tools cause accidents, both hand and power tools should be inspected and repaired routinely. Careful attention should be directed to the wiring of wet-heat electrical appliances, and water temperature consistency should be routinely monitored for accuracy. Protection of both patient and therapist from potential harm by hot or sharp materials during splint formation and construction stages is of utmost importance. Materials warmed with wet heat should be dried thoroughly before handling and application. Gloves and stockinette provide a heat barrier when working with high-temperature substances, and sharp edges of metal and wire should be taped to prevent inadvertent injury. When cutting wire, eliminate potentially dangerous bits of flying debris by cutting with a towel draped over the therapist's hand, wire cutters, and wire. Sewing machines are often required in construction of neoprene soft splints and adapted straps. It is advisable to replace the machine needle when starting a new project or when the needle starts to stick.

Therapists' use of good body ergonomics is fundamental to reducing fatigue and work-related injuries. Avoid awkward postures that create back, neck, or arm strain. It is easy for therapists to become engrossed in splint construction tasks, forgetting uncomfortable stances until insidious muscle aches and pains are felt. Analyze workspace and work habits. Identify problems and incorporate ergonomically sound solutions. Therapists routinely do this for their patients; therapists should also do it for themselves!

Additionally, it is imperative that therapists protect their own hands from injury that may occur from prolonged, cumulative stress to digital joints. Thumb CMC joints may be susceptible to injury if improper tools and/or techniques are used in splint fabrication. Stress to the thumb CMC joint is needlessly magnified when thermoplastic materials are not heated sufficiently. Splint materials must be soft and malleable before they are cut with scissors (Fig. 9-5). Also, large, short-blade scissors with good mechanical advantage lessen transferred cutting forces to the thumb CMC joint. Scissors may be padded to prevent tendonitis and tool handle size should be chosen to assure optimum ergonomic fit. If tool handles irritate the area of the A1 pulley or interfere with extensor pollicis brevis (EPB) or abductor pollicis longus (APL) function, inflammation may occur, potentially precipitating pain, tendon triggering or deQuervain's. Viscolas or other shock-prevention material applied to tools may be helpful in prevention of these problems. Using tools instead of fingers to accomplish tasks that stress digital joints extends hand health. For example, when splint adjustments are needed, rather than pulling Velcro off by hand, remove it with pliers. Scissors, pliers, and drive and rotary punches need to be sharpened routinely to decrease the effort required for their use.

Incorporation of safety and ergonomic standards throughout splint construction promotes work efficiency. Other tactics also speed the construction stage. For example, using precut dies condenses fabrication time by decreasing the amount of time required to make patterns and cut splints out of sheet

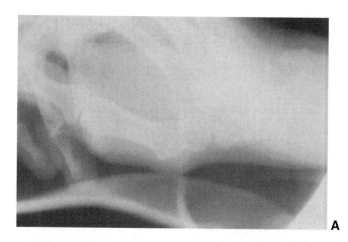

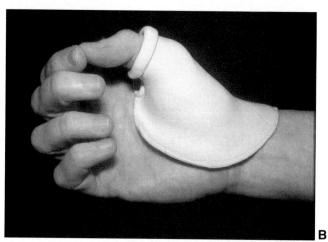

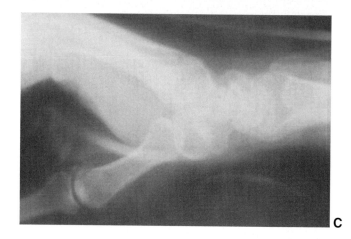

Fig. 9-5   **B, Thumb CMC palmar abduction and MP flexion immobilization splint type 1 (3)**
Cutting thermoplastic splint material that has not been heated sufficiently puts stress on the thumb CMC joint. **A,** Thumb CMC joint subluxes as splinting material is cut without splint. **B,** Thumb CMC, MP immobilization splint. **C,** CMC joint is stabilized by splint as splint material is cut. (Courtesy Caryl Johnson, OTR, CHT, New York, N.Y., and Steven Z. Glickel, MD, New York, N.Y.)

material. Precuts are available in many commonly fabricated splints and materials. Although precuts are more expensive, they may increase construction efficiency provided they approximate fairly closely patients' hand sizes. If precuts are too small or too large, saved cut-out time is negated in time-consuming adaptations. As a positive side effect, precuts also decrease stress on the therapists' thumb CMC joints because splint cut-out time is reduced.

■ CONSIDER INFORMATION DATA ON MATERIAL SAFETY DATA SHEETS (MSDS)

Chemical products that are routinely used in the clinic setting include, but are not limited to, solvents, glues, cold sprays, etc. It is vital that therapy staffs be informed about potential hazards of these and similar products. To find out whether or not a product is hazardous, consult the product's material safety data sheet (MSDS) obtained by request from the vendor selling the product or the product's manufacturer, or access the information via the Internet. "The MSDS lists the hazardous ingredients of a product, its physical and chemical characteristics (e.g., flammability, explosive properties), its effects on human health, the chemicals with which it can adversely react, handling precautions, the types of measures that can be used to control exposure, emergency and first aid procedures, and methods to contain a spill."[4] It should also be noted that the Occupational Safety and Health Administration's (OSHA) Hazard Communication Standard (29 CFR 1910.1200) "requires all employers (including those in the health care industry) to develop a written hazard communication program that ensures that employees are formally trained in the hazards associated with exposure to chemical agents, and in the methods and procedures designed to protect them from those hazards."[5] Therapists should be aware of their own safety as well as that of staff and patients whenever hazardous chemical products are used in the clinic. General precautionary measures include, but are not limited to, provision of adequate ventilation during use of chemical products and eye and skin protection as indicated. In addition to safe use of chemical products, these substances should be properly stored and disposed of as advised by the product's MSDS. In some cases, weighing potential risks against the benefits of using some chemical products may affect use of safer alternative methods.

Watch for patients with medical conditions that are reactant to products, including allergy, toxicity, asthma, or respiratory disorders. Another common condition seen among patients and staff alike is an allergy to rubber. Patients, and sometimes staff, are often unaware of their allergy until neoprene or elastic stockinette, or in the case of staff personnel, rubber gloves, are donned frequently or for extended periods of time.

■ ROUND CORNERS AND SMOOTH EDGES

Both inside and outside corners of a splint should be rounded for increased strength, durability, cosmesis, and comfort. Novice splinters may find that drawing around a coin at each corner during the pattern transfer phase of splint construction is helpful in attaining uniformity of these curved regions. To enhance the overall cosmetic effect and to prevent pointed edges from causing damage to clothing or injury to the patient, corners should also be rounded on straps and accessory splint parts such as outriggers and finger cuffs (Fig. 9-6). Splint edges should be smoothed and slightly rounded. To finish the edges, trim with scissors while the splint is in the cool-down stage, reheat the edges with a heat gun or dip the splint edge in water. Smoothing heated edges with a moist finger eliminates unsightly edge imperfections. Edge nicks and points jeopardize patient comfort, diminish splint cosmesis, and decrease splint strength.

When cutting low-temperature materials, edge imperfections are reduced/eliminated by using smooth, easy, long cutting strokes, and by avoiding complete closure of the scissor blades. Good cutting technique also saves time by decreasing the need for finishing details such as spot heating and smoothing

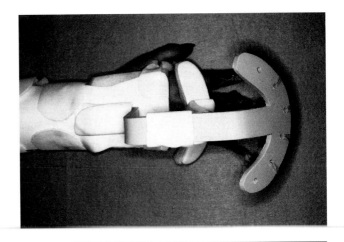

Fig. 9-6   Index–small finger PIP extension mobilization splint, type 2 (9)
Corners should also be rounded on accessory components such as outriggers, dorsal phalangeal bars, finger cuffs, and straps.

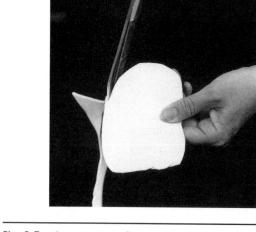

Fig. 9-7   Improper use of scissors results in rough, uneven splint edges.

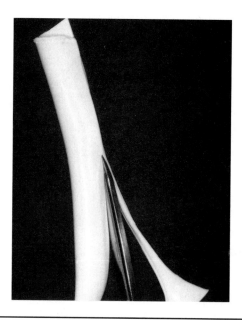

Fig. 9-8   Simultaneous cutting of bonded pieces creates a smooth single edge.

(Fig. 9-7). A quick method for obtaining smooth finished edges on separate tube or doubled splint components involves combining the bonding and cutting steps into one. Gently tube (or double) the heated material and then cut off the excess material along the cut edge(s) with scissors. The cutting force of the scissors simultaneously fuses the newly cut edges together in a smooth unbreakable bond (Fig. 9-8).

High-temperature materials, wire, and metals require files, sandpaper, emery cloth, or steel wool to finish edges. Novices to these materials may spend prolonged periods of time finishing edges, but with experience most high-temperature splints or splint components can be finished in a maximum of 3 to 5 minutes of filing and sanding. When smoothing edges, care should be taken to avoid marring the wider, adjacent surfaces of the material. Finger cuffs or slings also require smooth edges. A resourceful method for constructing custom-made finger slings involves affixing moleskin to cotton stockinette and then cutting out slings according to the sizes needed. Punching holes in the ends of the slings completes the procedure. Dycem may be glued to the inner surface of slings to increase traction on cutaneous finger surfaces.

■ ANALYZE AND INTEGRATE EFFECTIVE MECHANICAL PRINCIPLES

Mechanical principles may be used to enhance strength and durability of splints through integration of advantageous leverage systems and increasing area of force application as splints are constructed. Appropriate choice of the thicknesses and low-temperature thermoplastic materials contributes directly to the mechanical strength of splints. Splint strength is also increased with circumferential designs. Rounding inside corners increases the area of force application, diminishing chances of material fatigue and fracture at more vulnerable corner sites. Rolling edges of inside cuts also disperses pressure by widening the area of force application. A rolled edge at the first web space internal cut also increases the area of force application (Fig. 9-9). Area of force application is also a factor when attaching a wire component to a splint. Creation of a "position impression" in the thermoplastic splint base by lightly pressing the heated wire component into the splint increases base material conformity around the wire (increased area of force application) and subsequently strengthens the attachment site as a second layer of material is bonded over the wire, sandwiching it securely between two layers of bonded splint material.

Use of efficacious mechanical advantage also assists the fabrication process itself. For example, with wire, application of the bending force at a point 12 or 15 cm away from the actual site of the bend creates a long lever arm and decreases the force required to bend the wire, thus making the shaping process easier (Fig. 9-10, A). Bending wire takes practice. Generally one pair of pliers is held at the point where a bend is desired as a second pair of pliers is used to bend the wire to the appropriate angle or shape (Fig. 9-10, B,C).

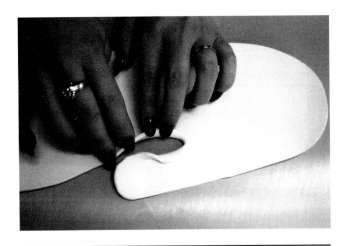

Fig. 9-9   Rolled edges at the terminal end of an inside cut will disseminate cracking forces and increase splint durability.

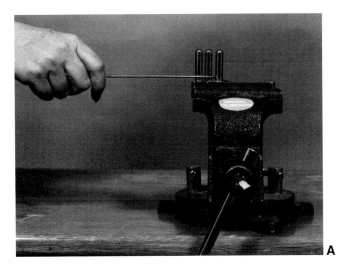

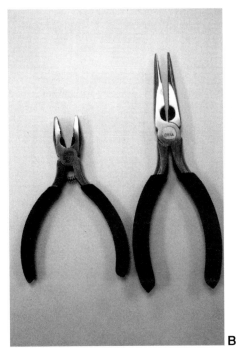

When joining splint parts, one rivet or screw post allows axial rotation, whereas two or more rivets or screw posts afford a solid and stable splint joint. Providing longer sites of attachment for outriggers (Fig. 9-11) increases the durability of the bonded or riveted interface by increasing the ratio between the lengths of the resistance arm and the force arm of the outrigger.

A careful analysis of a broken splint or splint part is an important step in determining why a splint has failed. The resulting evaluation of the force systems involved in the splint should facilitate repair and aid future splint preparation through technique improvement.

■ STABILIZE JOINED SURFACES ACCORDING TO PURPOSE: FIXED BOND OR ARTICULATED LINK

With the many self-bonding splinting materials on the market today, the need for riveting splint components together has diminished considerably. However, occasions arise when the extra strength afforded by a rivet is useful, if not mandatory. When a separate part is attached to a splint, consideration of the function of the part and its requirements with regard to joint stability or mobility is important. An understanding of mechanical principles and the use of equipment appropriate to the material selected will ensure a more favorable result. It is important to reemphasize that, although one rivet allows motion between the joined surfaces, two or more rivets, surface bonding, or gluing results in a secure coupling of splint components.

Surface bonding and gluing require careful observance of methods specific to individual materials. A

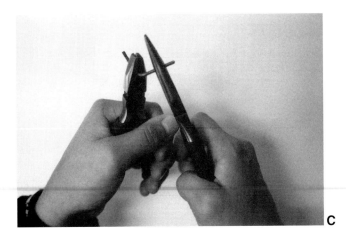

Fig. 9-10   **A,** Applying force at a point distal to the intended bend provides a longer lever arm with which to shape wire. **B,C,** Different types of pliers ease bending wire to specific angles or curves.

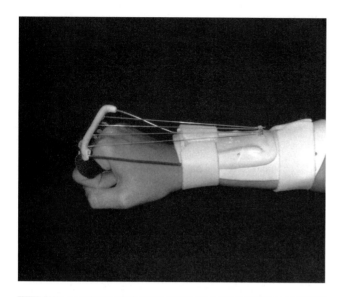

Fig. 9-11   Wrist flexion: index–small finger MP extension /
index–small finger MP flexion: wrist extension torque transmission splint, type 0 (5)
The increased mechanical advantage (MA) afforded by a long
attachment site allows for a stronger bond at the proximal end of
the outrigger. (Courtesy Peggy McLaughlin, OTR, CHT, San
Bernardino, Calif.)

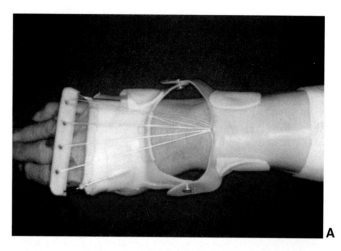

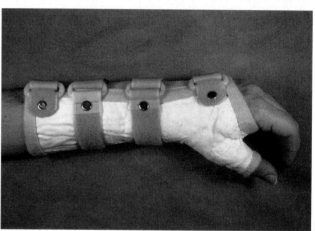

Fig. 9-12   A, Wrist flexion: index–small finger MP extension /
index–small finger MP flexion: wrist extension torque transmission splint, type 0 (5) B, Wrist extension, thumb CMC palmar
abduction and MP flexion restriction splint, type 0 (3)
A, This wrist joint is constructed with metal screw posts allowing
transfer of moment to the wrist. B, Rivets permanently position
straps on a splint. [Courtesy (A) Jill Francisco, OTR, Cicero, Ind.;
(B) Jennifer L. Henshaw, OTR, Santa Rosa, Calif.]

successful bond depends on proper cleaning and
heating of the contiguous surface areas for optimum
results. Surfaces must be completely dry to achieve a
secure bond. When bonding coated thermoplastic
materials, coatings must be removed in order to
achieve successful adherence of the joined surfaces.
Scraping or application of a solvent removes surface
coatings, providing the clean surfaces required for
forming solid bonds between thermoplastic components. A word of caution: If care is not taken, warm
uncoated materials can accidentally self-adhere to
other splint components or material scraps, creating
unwanted bonding of assorted pieces!

The choice of metal fastener type depends on the
specific parts to be joined and the characteristics of
the materials used (Fig. 9-12, A,B). If motion is desired
in a splint, a metal rivet or screw post is more durable
than a self-rivet of thermoplastic material. If a rivet is
used, placement of a paper spacer between the two
surfaces to be joined allows smoother rotation of the
joint after the setting of the rivet and removal of the
paper. Different types of screw posts may also be used
for joint motion or stabilization. If joint motion
restrictions are needed, blocks may be added to the
splint to limit unwanted joint motion. Plastic rivets of
a homologous low-temperature material provide a
stable bond but may fracture with constant stress. A
Silastic or elastomer insert may incorporate a unique
series of self-rivets that coincide exactly with holes in

the splint, allowing consistently accurate placement of
the insert on the splint. Fabrication of the insert is relatively easy. One to three holes are punched in the
splint where the Silastic insert is to be formed. As the
Silastic is setting up, it flows into the holes in the base
splint as it simultaneously conforms to the patient's
hand, forming self-rivet protrusions wherever the rivet
holes are located.

For comfort and a more pleasing appearance, rivets
and screw posts should be flush with the material
surface, particularly when they will contact the
patient's skin. This is accomplished by countersinking
high-temperature materials or, in the case of the
softer, low-temperature materials, by heating and
molding of the rivet or the surrounding surface area.

Tape or moleskin placed over an "internal" metal rivet or screw post prevents deterioration and rusting of the rivet and decreases chances of producing skin irritation. External rivet or screw post parts should be smooth and unobtrusive, providing good appearance, comfort, and function.

When adding a wire component to a splint, it is important to provide a durable and solid union. The combination of the smoothness and narrow diameter of wire, plus the torque created from the distally applied forces of mobilization assists, makes it difficult to stabilize a wire component such as an outrigger to the supporting body of the splint. A secure union of plastic and wire parts is accomplished by forming a zigzag, open loop, or 90° angle on the proximal end(s) of the wire component at the point(s) of attachment (Fig. 9-13, A). The configured end(s) prevents dislodging once thermoplastic reinforcement strips are bonded over the wire, onto the body of the splint. To ensure a solid bond without air pockets, the shaped wire must also closely duplicate the external contour of the component to which it is bonded (Fig. 8-16, B, 9-13, B). Some commercial outriggers such as the Phoenix provide specifically designed screw posts for attaching the outrigger to the splint base, eliminating bonding.

PROVIDE VENTILATION AS NECESSARY

The ventilation of a splint should be executed judiciously and prudently, depending on the patient, the patient's lifestyle, splint configuration, the materials employed, and the environment. Splints with large skin contact areas more often require adaptation to improve air circulation. Ventilation holes should be small enough to prevent tissue protrusion and should be randomly positioned away from splint edges to eliminate weakening of the material (Fig. 9-14, A). With the exception of microperforated materials such as Orfit, ventilation holes should not be situated over bony prominences, near edges, across narrow components, or in areas of high stress forces that require close material contact to decrease pressure. Ventilation holes in microperforated materials are so small and closely distributed that many of these materials can be closely fitted over bony prominences without causing soft tissue breakdown (Fig. 9-14, B). A word of caution, however: Not all microperforated materials maintain their small perforations with heating and stretching. Unfortunately, perforations in some "microperforated" materials enlarge slightly with heat, creating an irregular textured surface that does not distribute pressure as evenly as is required for contouring over problematic areas. If in doubt about

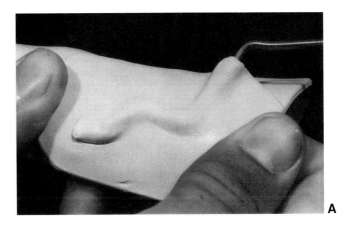

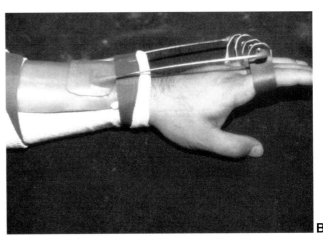

Fig. 9-13 B, Wrist flexion: index–small finger MP extension / index–small finger MP flexion: wrist extension torque transmission splint, type 0 (5)
Curling, zigzagging, or forming right angles at the ends of wire components provides a more stable attachment site. [Courtesy (B) Kathryn Schultz, OTR, CHT, Orlando, Fla.]

a material, fabricate a *wrist immobilization splint, type 0 (1)* and wear it for a day. If the perforations are large enough to inhibit pressure distribution over the radial styloid or ulnar head, the problem will be readily apparent. As a matter of policy, always check patients wearing ventilated splints within an hour or so of initial splint application.

Low-temperature splint materials may be ventilated with a hand tool such as an all-purpose drive punch or rotary punch. The use of an electric drill, although suitable for high-temperature materials, with softer materials causes friction melting around the holes, resulting in rough burred edges. Perforations should be made from the inside out to give a smoother inner splint surface; heating or sanding, depending on material type, should smooth external and internal edges of all ventilation holes.

Commercially available perforated materials may produce poor finished products because of the preset

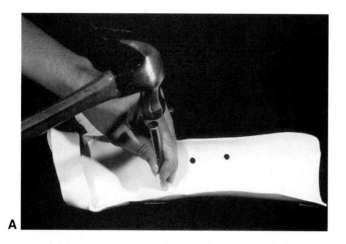

A

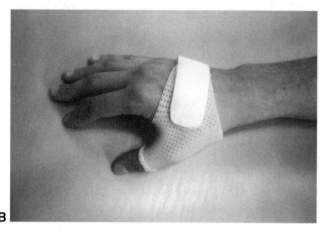

B

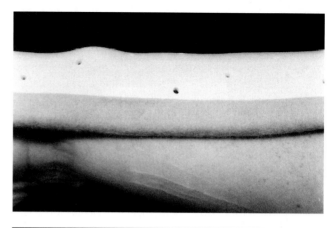

Fig. 9-15   To achieve a smooth, protected edge on splints constructed from materials with larger perforations, a narrow band of self-adhesive moleskin may be adhered over splint edges.

Fig. 9-14   **B, Thumb CMC palmar abduction and MP flexion immobilization splint, type 0 (2)**
A, Ventilation holes should be made from the inside of the splint to ensure a comfortable inner surface. **B,** The small microperforations in materials such as Orfit are not problematic on most splint edges since the edges are easily smoothed when warm. The material may also be rolled to decrease edge pressure as demonstrated at the thumb IP joint.

perforation pattern and the inevitable enlargement that occurs with heating and stretching during fit. Multiple, large stretched openings, rough edges, and structural weakness are often the result of poor planning and fitting.

If perforated material is used, extra attention to detail must be taken during the pattern transfer and molding stages of splint construction. Careful placement of the pattern on the material diminishes the chance of cutting through perforations. The avoidance of overheating lessens the potential for overstretching and enlarging of the preset holes. If the perforation pattern is such that it is impossible to eliminate edge imperfections, it is important to ensure that the edges of the splint are finished in a manner that prevents injury to the patient and destruction of clothing (Fig. 9-15).

Tubed cotton stockinette splint liners coupled with nonperforated materials are an excellent alternative to perforated materials. These interface liners absorb perspiration, are easy to doff and don, and are washable. Patients are given two or three stockinette liners and are instructed to rotate wearing and washing schedules of the liners, ensuring that they always have a clean splint interface available.

■ SECURE PADDING AND STRAPS

Padding should be used prudently and appropriately and it should never serve as a correction of a poorly fitted splint. Although splint padding is available in a range of materials, foam padding is most often used in splint fabrication. Foam padding is categorized into two basic groups: closed or open cell foam. For most splinting purposes, closed cell foam padding is preferable in that it does not absorb moisture, odors, or bacteria. Padding should be anchored securely to the splint, allowing ease of splint application and removal. Increased comfort is provided when the padding material is cut slightly larger than the part to which it is to be adhered, allowing it to curl around splint edges, disseminating pressure (Fig. 9-16).

If padding is used as a spacer between a splint and bony prominence, with the goal of decreasing splint pressure and increasing comfort, the padding should be applied over the prominence before splint fabrication is begun. Be aware that some padding materials may stubbornly adhere to skin and hair, making removal of the padding difficult. An alternate technique is to use therapeutic putty molded directly over the bony prominence to provide a spacer as the splint is fitted. Once the splint cools, the putty is easily

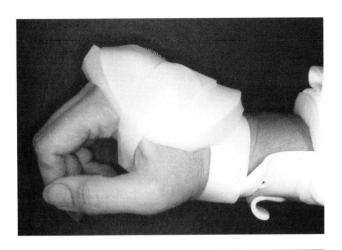

Fig. 9-16   Padding cut slightly larger than the splint part will help disseminate edge pressure.

removed, whereas padding may, in some cases, permanently adhere to the thermoplastic. A stockinette may also serve as an interface between padding and heated thermoplastic, preventing adherence of padding to the warm material.

Materials for scar management should be in position on the hand/extremity prior to fitting the splint. Lining splints is not recommended except in very special circumstances. It is advisable to place a layer of moleskin in the splint before applying foam if future splint adjustments are dependent on application of wet heat. Foam adhered to splint surfaces can accumulate water as wet heat adjustments are carried out unless it is removed prior to splint adjustment. Some adhesive-backed foam paddings are difficult to remove in one piece, tearing into chunks and leaving residues. To alleviate this problem, moleskin may be used as an interface material between the splint and foam padding. When used in this manner, both moleskin and foam are easily removed from the splint without tearing or fragmenting and may be reused after wet heat adjustments are completed. An alternative to the moleskin and foam padding combination is to use soft strapping material for splint padding and adhere it to the inside of the splint with hook Velcro.

Padding may also be fixed to the dressing and the warm splint material may in turn be applied over the padding. After the material cools, remove the pad from the dressing and apply it to the splint. For ease of removal and cleaning, Velfoam strapping may be attached with hook Velcro in lieu of foam padding.

Straps should be strategically placed to provide splint stability on the extremity and should facilitate independent splint application and removal. Generally, straps should be placed at the far distal and proximal limits of the splint and over strategic joints; this allows the full mechanical advantage of the splint design to be used. Strapping materials are available in sticky-backed (self-adhesive) or plain-backed. Both hook and loop Velcro come in assorted widths and colors. One-inch and two-inch widths are most commonly used in hand/upper extremity splinting. Soft strapping provides comfort and conformity but is not as resilient as Velcro. Cost of soft strapping also may be prohibitive for some clinics. Straps can be attached to the splint with (metal or plastic) rivets, screws, commercial D-rings, glue, or Velcro. A heat gun may be used to spot heat the placement areas of Velcro prior to attachment to the splint to increase adherence. Being careful not to burn the Velcro, the back of Velcro strapping may also be heated to improve adherence. When refitting a splint, remove the Velcro hook before warming because it does not stretch during the remolding process.

Patients should easily be able to accomplish strap fastening and unfastening procedures. To prevent fraying, strap ends should be treated and corners should be rounded for a more pleasing appearance and increased durability (Fig. 9-17, *A,B*). Overlapping soft materials should lie flat and be joined securely, as should fastening devices such as Velcro, buckles, and snaps.

With pressure-sensitive interlocking materials such as Velcro, the hook portion should be used sparingly because of its abrasiveness to skin and clothing. Hook material should not comprise the length of the straps themselves, but it serves as a durable fastening device when used in single lengths rather than multiple, smaller buttons (Fig. 9-18, *A,B*). Velcro loop straps should be long enough to provide complete coverage of the portion of the hook that has been adhered to the splint, to prevent snagging and tearing of clothing, and to provide tabs that are easier to grasp.

Straps may be adapted to facilitate use through the addition of loops or tabs (Fig. 9-19, *A,B*) and may be converted to adjustable straps by increasing the length and pulling through a D-ring. When applying a hook to a contoured area, small cuts in each corner allows the Velcro to smooth out and better conform to the area. Hook Velcro may be secured to a splint by heating the Velcro and embedding it into the thermoplastic. Hint: Save scissor wear and tear by designating one pair of scissors to be the "gummy" Velcro scissors!

■ SUMMARY

The principles of splint construction provide strategic guidelines for the actual fabrication of a given splint after the design and pattern-making stages have been

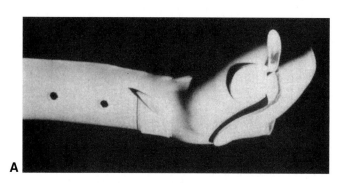

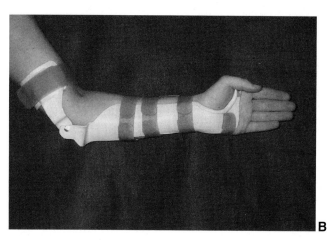

Fig. 9-17   A, Index finger MP extension restriction / thumb CMC radial abduction and MP extension immobilization splint, type 1 (4) B, Forearm neutral immobilization splint, type 2 (3)
A, With repeated closures, pointed corners on fastening strips pull away and curl, eventually resulting in detachment of the entire strip. **B,** Rounding the ends of Velcro straps and fastening strips
improves appearance and increases durability. [Courtesy **(B)** Rebecca Banks, OTR/L, CHT, Blackburn, Australia.]

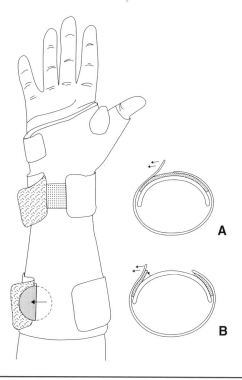

Fig. 9-18   Wrist extension, thumb CMC radial abduction and
MP extension immobilization splint, type 0 (3)
A single Velcro fastening strip **(A)** that directs unlocking forces to
the center of the strip is more durable than are small button-Velcro
fastening strips **(B)** that direct unlocking forces at structurally
weaker edges.

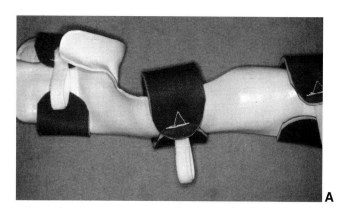

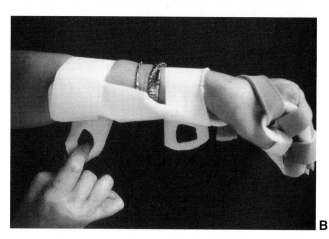

Fig. 9-19   A, Index–small finger flexion, thumb CMC palmar
abduction and MP-IP extension immobilization splint, type 1 (16)
B, Index–small finger flexion, thumb CMC palmar abduction and
MP-IP flexion immobilization splint, type 1 (16)
A slight overlap of strap ends facilitates opening and closing and
provides complete protection from hook snagging. Loops ease strap
manipulation for patients with limited grasp.

completed. When combined with the important principles of splint fit, the creation of a comfortably fitting, durable, and cosmetically satisfactory splint should be ensured. Failure to adhere to these principles as they pertain to the sometimes-trivial details of splint manufacture may result in splint disuse because of patient discomfort, splint breakage, or, more important, failure of the splint to correct the problem for which it was originally designed. To this end, meticulous attention to detail is the overriding consideration; attempts to "short-cut" these construction principles to speed splint preparation inevitably result in failure.

REFERENCES

1. Breger-Lee DE, Buford WL: Update in splinting materials and methods, *Hand Clin* 7(3):569-85, 1991.
2. Breger-Lee DE, Buford WL, Jr.: Properties of thermoplastic splinting materials, *J Hand Ther* 5:202-11, 1992.
3. Breger-Lee DE: Objective and subjective observations of low-temperature thermoplastic materials, *J Hand Ther* 8(2):138-43, 1995.
4. Occupational Safety & Health Administration's website, Standard Interpretations 01/18/1995; The need for Material Safety Data Sheets (MSDSs). http://www.osha.gov/pls/oshaweb/owadisp.show_document?p_table=INTERPRETATIONS&p_id=21676
5. Occupational Safety & Health Administration's website, Standard Interpretations 06/24/1994-MSDSs must be distributed to customer with shipment of chemical. http://www.osha.gov/pls/oshaweb/owadisp.show_document?p_table=INTERPRETATIONS&p_id=21524

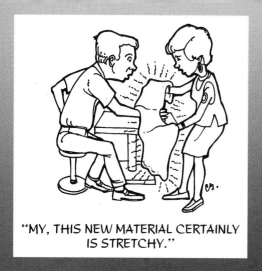

"MY, THIS NEW MATERIAL CERTAINLY IS STRETCHY."

Principles of Fit

Chapter Outline

The accurate fitting of upper extremity splints to accommodate the individual anatomic variations of patients with a wide variety of clinical diagnoses is a necessary and demanding process. Prefabricated splints designed for universal wear or poorly contoured splints created without a thorough knowledge of the principles of proper splinting are uncomfortable and result in pressure problems or noncompliance, often with substantial functional loss to the patient.

With the availability of a wide spectrum of fabrication materials that may be individually adapted to each patient's needs, no excuse is ever appropriate for the use of splints that do not fit comfortably and are poorly tolerated. The basic principles of splint fitting should be thoroughly understood by anyone engaged in the management of upper extremity problems. Well-designed and well-fitted splints not only positively affect patient rehabilitation; they often have a secondary effect of increasing physician referral because they reflect the high-level expertise of their fabricators.

Following the design and construction phases, the principles of fitting comprise the next major step in the production of a well-functioning splint. These principles encompass mechanical, anatomic, kinesiological, and technical factors. Fit concepts relating to anatomic structures include consideration of bone, skin, soft tissue, joint, tendon, ligament, nerve, and vascular structures; skeletal architecture; and the mechanical principles that are directly applicable to the shaping of splints. Kinesiological concepts deal with the extremity in motion and with the forces that implement this motion, and technical principles incorporate techniques based on practical application and efficiency. The mechanical principles described in Chapter 6 and the outrigger and mobilization assist principles in Chapter 7 must be applied to the fitting of a splint in order to attain ultimate design effectiveness.

MECHANICAL CONSIDERATIONS
Use Principles of Mechanics Effectively

Employment of the principles of mechanics during the fitting of a hand splint is paramount, because the use of improper forces can damage cutaneous, ligamentous, or articular structures. Mechanical principles that must be considered in splint fitting include dissemination of applied force to reduce pressure, elimination of shear and friction, and leverage (Fig. 10-1) as applied to the placement of straps, finger cuffs, and fingernail attachment devices such as hooks or Velcro. When mobilizing stiff joints, mobilizing

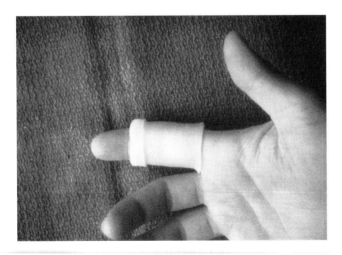

Fig. 10-1   Index finger DIP flexion torque transmission splint, type 1 (2)
This splint increases the mechanical advantage of the flexor digitorum profundus. (Courtesy Brenda Hilfrank, PT, CHT, South Burlington, Vt.)

forces should be directed perpendicular to both the segment being moved and to the rotational axis of the joint. If traction is applied simultaneously to several joints of the same digital ray, a perpendicular pull must be attained at each rotational axis. Care should be taken periodically to reevaluate the immobilization, mobilization, restriction, or torque transmission effects as a splint is fitted and in follow-up treatment sessions. It is imperative that splint alterations are made as the condition of the hand changes; otherwise, the effectiveness of the splint is compromised.

Mechanical concepts influence nearly all phases of the splint fitting process to some degree. Anatomic considerations of splinting and mechanical concepts are closely intertwined in that solutions for many anatomically related splinting problems are based on application of mechanical principles. Because of this, specific anatomic factors and their related mechanical concepts are presented in tandem in the following discussion of anatomic splinting considerations.

ANATOMIC CONSIDERATIONS
Skin/Soft Tissue

Adapt for Skin/Soft Tissue Alterations

Poor fitting splints can jeopardize the healing process by causing further damage through application of unwarranted destructive shear or pressure forces. Splints fitted over portions of an extremity where skin or soft tissue is of questionable viability or where soft tissue defects exist present serious challenges. Depending on specific individual circumstances, avoidance of splinting material around and over problematic areas, including major soft tissue deficits, open wounds, burns, skin grafts, or revascularized areas, is often an appropriate and workable solution (Fig. 10-2). While soft tissue defects and areas of questionable viability are relatively obvious, it is also important to identify and monitor patients who are at risk to develop skin/soft tissue problems, including those with diagnoses associated with decreased sensibility and/or poor vascularity such as diabetes, or those patients taking medications such as corticosteroids that may produce tissue friability. These patients often require special splint design adaptations and rigorously careful splint fit because their tolerance to splinting forces may be less than that of other individuals.

Use Skin Creases as Boundaries

Because the dorsal and palmar skin creases correspond directly to the underlying joints (Fig. 10-3, A,B), their presence graphically indicates the areas at which motion takes place in the hand/extremity, providing tangible boundaries for splint preparation. If the MP

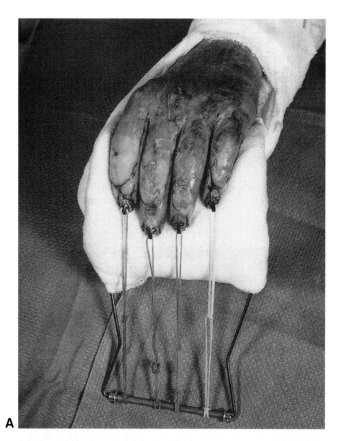

A

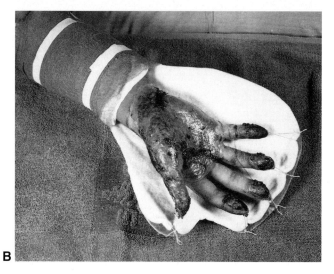

B

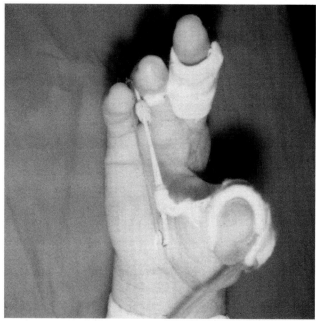

C

Fig. 10-2   A, Index–small finger MP flexion and IP extension, thumb CMC palmar abduction and MP-IP extension mobilization splint, type 1 (16) B, Wrist extension, index–ring–small finger MP abduction, index–small finger extension, thumb CMC radial abduction and MP-IP extension mobilization splint, type 0 (16) C, Long finger PIP extension mobilization splint, type 0 (1) \\ Ring finger MP extension, thumb CMC palmar abduction and MP extension mobilization splint, type 1 (3)

A, Allowing healing of dorsal cutaneous surfaces, this splint uses fingernail hooks to position the MPs in flexion and IPs in extension without the aid of dorsal straps. B, For palmar burns, this splint uses fingernail attachments to mobilize the wrist, fingers, and thumb into extension and radial abduction, eliminating the need for finger cuffs. Both (A) and (B) are made of fiberglass and may be sterilized. C, These two splints work together to increase motion of the thumb CMC joint and digital longitudinal arch. [Courtesy (A,B) Kilulu Von Prince, OTR, MS, Clovis, Calif.; (C) Carol Hierman, OTR, CHT, Cedar Grove, N.C., Elisha Denny, PTA, OTA, Pittsboro N.C., ©UNC Hand Rehabilitation Center, Chapel Hill, N.C.]

joints are to be unencumbered by a splint, the distal aspect of the splint must be applied proximal to the distal palmar flexion crease; if the thumb is to retain full mobility, the splint material should lie ulnar to the thenar crease; and full mobility of a PIP joint may be achieved by terminating the splint slightly proximal to the middle flexion crease of the digit. Conversely, if a joint is to be immobilized, the splint should be extended as close as possible to the next segmental crease, both proximally and distally, to provide

maximum mechanical purchase (Fig. 10-4, A-D). A restriction splint for a worker, athlete, or musician and may require a shorter lever arm, allowing partial joint motion.

Use Principles of Mechanics to Protect Skin/Soft Tissue

Reduce Pressure. The dissemination of pressure is an important concept in the design and fitting of splints. Excessive pressure, regardless of good splint

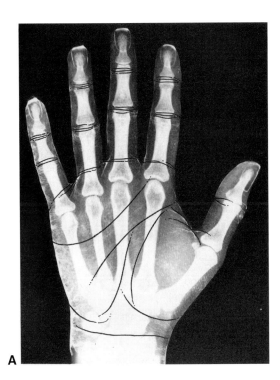

A

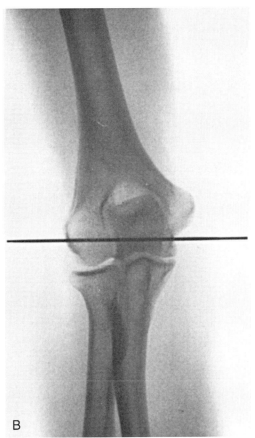

B

Fig. 10-3   A, Most skin creases correspond directly to underlying joints indicating the boundaries of motion for each segment. (NOTE: Although this is a palmar view, the dye outlines the fingernails and shows through from the dorsum.) Exceptions: The proximal digital flexion creases and the distal palmar flexion creases (A) are located distally and proximally to the finger MP joints, respectively, and the elbow flexion crease lies approximately 1 centimeter proximal to the anatomical joint space of the elbow (B). (B from Morrey BF: *The elbow and its disorders*, ed 3, Philadelphia, 2000, Saunders.)

design and construction, may render the splint intolerable and unwearable. Increasing the area of force application decreases pressure. This should be considered in the original design of the splint and may be augmented at the time of fitting by achieving good contiguous fit of the material on the extremity, by contouring the material nearly the full length of the segment being fitted without limiting motion,[7,8] and by rolling the proximal and distal ends of the splint (Fig. 10-5, A,B). It is important that the splint material follows the contours of the extremity as closely as possible. If full wound coverage is not present, the splint may be applied over an appropriate dressing. In some instances, application of a splint may be detrimental to specific local tissue viability. The splint should then be designed and fitted to avoid the problematic area and any adjacent tissue that may be of questionable viability. Splint borders encroaching on soft tissue defects should be contoured outward to increase the area of force application and to decrease edge pressure (Fig. 10-6, A,B).

Padding may be used appropriately to decrease the influence of splint parts that cannot be widened because of their specific functions or place of application. It may also be used to disseminate pressure over especially difficult areas where contouring of the splint material and achievement of a contiguous fit are insufficient to prevent underlying soft tissue damage. When using padding within a contoured space, it is important to achieve a fit that will accommodate the addition of the padding without effectively diminishing the area of the concavity and compromising the fit of the splint (Fig. 10-7, A-C). However, one should beware of overuse of padding because, in addition to its eventual contamination by moisture and dirt, it is frequently indicative of a poorly fitted splint. Adherence of padding to splint material prior to fitting is an easy method of insuring that sufficient space has been allowed to accommodate the added bulk of the padding.

A word of caution: Cutting holes in splints in hopes of alleviating pressure is a common mistake that often creates greater pressure around the circumferential border of the cutout. Cutout holes in large surface area components, especially if components are circumferential or nearly circumferential, can result in extrusion of edematous soft tissue into the open cutouts. It is preferable either to circumvent a problematic area or to provide a close contiguous fit that disseminates pressure. When external fixators or k-wires are present, cutouts in the splint may be required to accommodate external hardware (Fig. 10-8, A-C). Patients should be monitored closely to ensure that cutout borders adjacent to pins or fixators do not impinge underlying soft tissue.

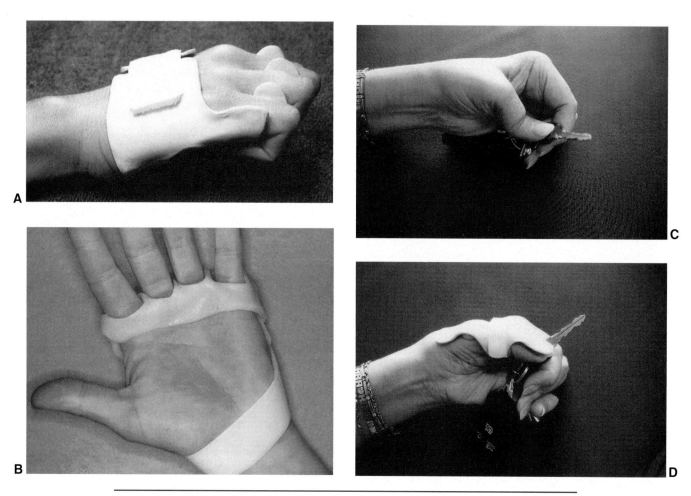

Fig. 10-4   A, Index–small finger MP flexion and ulnar deviation restriction splint, type 0 (4) B, Index–small finger MP flexion and ulnar deviation restriction splint, type 0 (4) D, Thumb MP extension immobilization / IP extension restriction splint, type 0 (2)
Immobilization or blocking components should be extended to include at least two thirds of the length of the proximal and distal segments that the splint incorporates. A, Flexion of the metacarpophalangeal joints is blocked because the palmar phalangeal bar is of sufficient length. B, This palmar phalangeal bar was not fitted far enough distally and thus allows more metacarpophalangeal flexion. C, This rheumatoid thumb with boutonniere deformity demonstrates collapse of the articular segments during pinch. D, With the splint in place, the weakened and unstable joints are positioned and supported, allowing functional use of the thumb. [Courtesy (A) KP MacBain, OTR, Vancouver, BC; (C,D) J. Robin Janson, OTR, CHT, Indianapolis, Ind.]

Eliminate Shear and Friction. The elimination of shear and friction is fundamental to well-fitting splints. Friction/shear of splint material against skin or friction caused by skin against skin, as with adjacent fingers, often is the result of an improperly designed or poorly fitted splint. The splint may be too large, the angle of pull incorrect, or the splint axis may not correspond to the anatomic joint axis. Careful observation of the area of friction and a reevaluation of the various principles of fitting hand splints helps identify problems and direct corrective measures. When shear occurs between two cutaneous surfaces, placement of an appropriate material between two surfaces helps alleviate troublesome contact areas (Fig. 10-9). If a splint with both dorsal and volar components is needed to increase stability of internal fixation or closed reduction, padding selected components helps increase comfort as positional stability is reinforced. Additionally, application of Dycem to the internal forearm trough of a volar splint decreases distal splint migration.

Use Optimum Leverage. Fingernail attachment devices such as dress hooks or Velcro buttons should be applied to the proximal and center aspect of the nail. Distal attachment results in considerable discomfort because of the leverage effect of the nail away

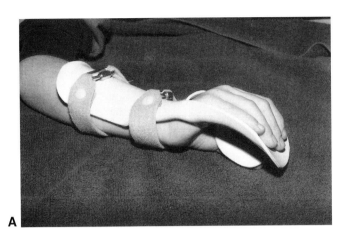

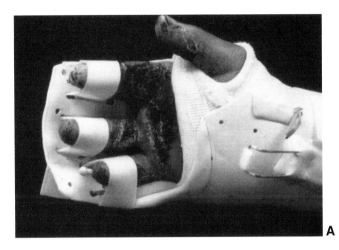

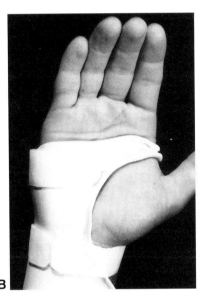

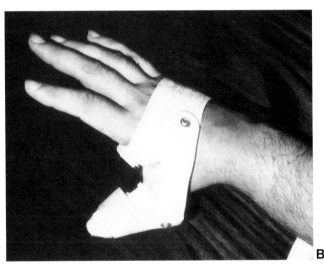

Fig. 10-5   A, Wrist extension, index–small finger flexion, thumb CMC palmar abduction and MP-IP extension mobilization splint, type 0 (16) B, Wrist neutral immobilization splint, type 0 (1) Flaring or rolling proximal and distal ends of a splint decreases edge pressure and eliminates the narrow sharp edge that is often present on precut, preformed, or custom-cut splinting material. [Courtesy **(A)** Joni Armstrong, OTR, CHT, Bemidji, Minn.]

Fig. 10-6   A, Index, ring, small finger extension, thumb CMC palmar abduction and MP flexion mobilization splint, type 1 (12); or index finger flexion, thumb CMC palmar abduction mobilization splint, type 1 (5) B, Thumb CMC radial abduction mobilization / MP-IP extension immobilization splint, type 0 (3) Splint edges that must be adjacent to areas of soft tissue of questionable viability should be contoured outward to decrease pressure. **A,** Splint also incorporates an outrigger for thumb and index finger mobilization (mobilization assist not attached) [Courtesy **(A)** Lin Beribak, OTR/L, CHT, Chicago, Ill.; **(B)** Joan Farrell, OTR, Miami, Fla.]

from the proximal nail bed (Fig. 10-10, *A,B*). This excess leverage could also cause damage to the nail itself. Patients with rheumatoid arthritis are particularly vulnerable to the nail bed becoming ischemic with pressure on the nail distally.

Proximal and distal straps should be attached as closely as possible to the respective ends of the splint. For optimum mechanical advantage, a strap that functions as the middle reciprocal force should be positioned over the joint on which it acts, provided it will not jeopardize tissue viability.

Leverage effects on finger cuffs may be diminished by placing the attachment site of the traction device

closer to the surface of the digit as advocated by Brand (Fig. 10-11, *A,B*).[1,2] This is especially helpful when dealing with insensitive hands. Dycem added to the cuffs also decreases slippage.

Patients should be instructed to remove their splints every 1 to 2 hours to check for areas of soft tissue embarrassment after the initial application of a splint. If cutaneous surfaces show no signs of distress, the frequency of checks may be decreased and splint-wearing time increased as needed.

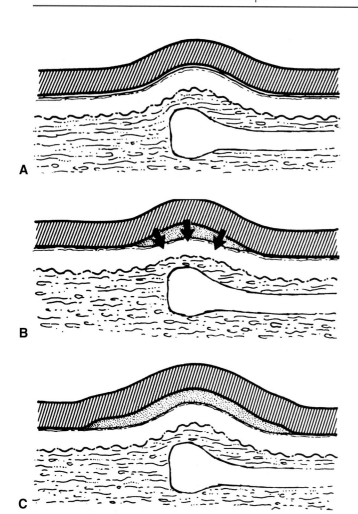

Fig. 10-7   **A,** The addition of padding must not compromise splint fit by diminishing contoured space. **B,** Incorrect. **C,** Correct.

Bone

Accommodate Bony Prominences

The bony prominences of the extremity must always be considered when fitting a splint. Subcutaneous soft tissue is at a minimum over these areas, rendering them more vulnerable to external pressure. Improper contouring of splint material may cause pressure ischemia, resulting in tissue necrosis.

In the hand, the most common problematic bony prominences include the ulnar styloid process, the pisiform, the radial styloid process, the heads of the metacarpals, and the base of the first metacarpal. The dorsal surface of the hand is particularly vulnerable in comparison to the palmar surface because of its relative lack of pressure-disseminating subcutaneous tissue. Moving proximally up the arm, the olecranon and lateral and medial epicondyles of the elbow, the shoulder glenohumeral joint, the spine of the scapula, and the clavicle all present potential problem areas

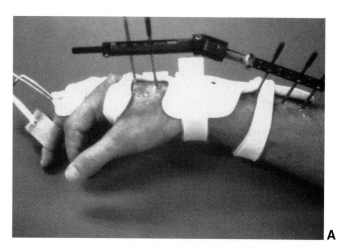

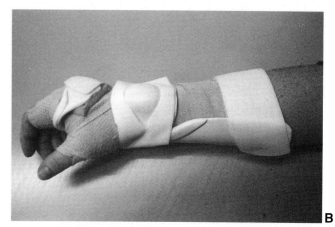

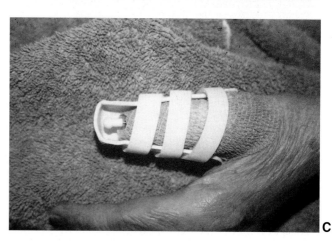

Fig. 10-8   **A,** Long finger PIP extension mobilization splint, type 2 (3) **B,** Wrist extension mobilization splint, type 0 (1) **C,** Thumb MP-IP extension immobilization splint, type 0 (2)
A, Careful splint fit is essential to minimize pressure around external fixators. Creating a domed area (**B**) or lengthening the end of the splint (**C**) protects protruding ends of external fixation pins. To avoid pressure on the pin, it is important that the pin not contact the splint material. [Courtesy (**A**) Robin Miller, OTR/L, CHT, Ft. Lauderdale, Fla.]

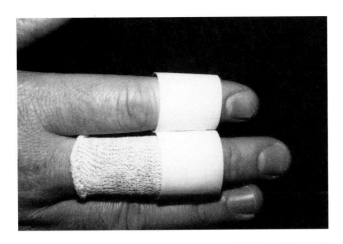

Fig. 10-9   Index finger MP-PIP extension and flexion torque transmission splint, type 2 (4)
Placement of stockinette or similar material between two adjacent cutaneous surfaces decreases friction. This splint allows an actively mobile digit to passively move an adjacent digit lacking full or partial active range of motion.

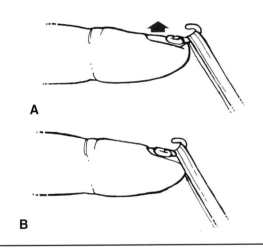

Fig. 10-10   Care should be taken to minimize the leverage effect of a fingernail attachment device on a fingernail bed by avoiding distal attachment. A, Incorrect. B, Correct.

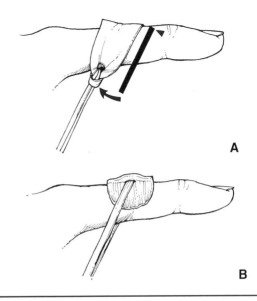

Fig. 10-11   A, Lack of 90° angle of pull produces edge pressure from this finger cuff with a long moment arm. B, By placing the attachment site of a mobilization assist closer to the finger, the leverage effect of the finger cuff is diminished and pressure is decreased even when pull is not at a 90° angle.

when fitting splints (Fig. 10-12, *A,B*). Caution must be employed when fitting parts of splints that come into contact with or are adjacent to bony prominences. Forearm or humeral bars/troughs, wrist or elbow bars, dorsal phalangeal bars, dorsal metacarpal bars, opponens bars, and other splint components specific to the larger elbow and shoulder joints such as special force or strapping systems, especially those with D-rings, all require careful fitting. Additionally, the iliac crest is often incorporated into shoulder splints for increased stability, requiring careful fitting of splint components over this wide, lower torso, bony prominence.

Reducing pressure by widening the area of force application is an important mechanical concept when dealing with bony prominences. If bony protuberances cannot be avoided, then decrease splint pressure over these protrusions by widening the area of force application through contiguous material contact or through the selective and judicious use of padding (Fig. 10-13, *A-C*).

Incorporate Dual Obliquity Concepts

Dual obliquity[9] is an important consideration in splint fitting that is determined by the skeletal configuration of the hand. Due to the hand's unique structural formation, two oblique lines may be drawn that particularly relate to splint design and fit. The first line, from a dorsal aspect, is created by the progressive metacarpal shortening (Fig. 10-14); the second line, from a distal transverse view, is the result of the progressive metacarpal descent from the radial to the ulnar side of the normal hand in a resting posture (Fig. 10-15). The anatomic foundations for dual obliquity include (1) the progressive decrease of length of the metacarpals from the radial to the ulnar aspect of the hand and (2) the immobility of the second and third metacarpals as compared to the mobile first, fourth, and fifth metacarpals.

Functionally, this anatomic arrangement means that, with the forearm fully supinated and resting on a table, a straight object gripped comfortably in the hand will not be parallel to the table but will be slightly higher on the radial side. When the wrist is held in a nondeviated posture, the object will also not be held

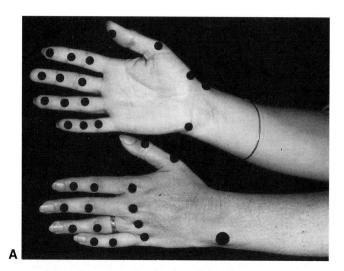

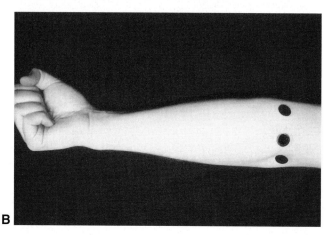

Fig. 10-12   Pressure over bony prominences may cause soft tissue damage.

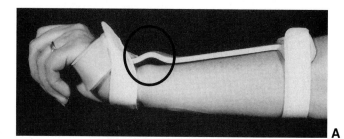

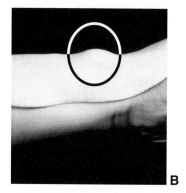

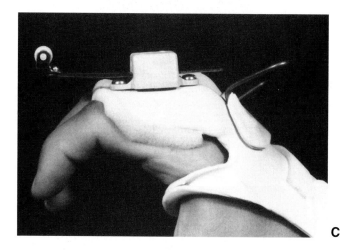

Fig. 10-13   A, Wrist extension immobilization splint, type 0 (1) Pressure over bony prominences may be decreased by avoidance (**A**), wider area of contact (**B**), or contoured padding (**C**).

perpendicular to the longitudinal axis of the forearm but will form an oblique angle with the more proximal portion of the angle occurring on the ulnar side of the hand and the distal portion on the radial aspect.

This concept of dual obliquity must then be translated to any splint part that supports or incorporates the second through fifth metacarpal bones. That is, a splint should be longer and higher on the radial side (Fig. 10-16, *A-C*) and at no time should it end or bend perpendicular to the longitudinal axis of the forearm when the wrist is not deviated to either side (Fig. 10-17).

Arches

Maintain Arches

The three skeletal arches of the hand (proximal transverse, distal transverse, and longitudinal) must be taken into consideration in attaining congruous splint fit. The distal transverse or metacarpal arch consists

of an immobile center post, the second and third metacarpal heads, around which the mobile first, fourth, and fifth metacarpals rotate (Fig. 10-18, *A,B*). The longitudinal arch (Fig. 10-19) on a sagittal plane embodies the carpals, metacarpals, and phalanges and allows approximately 280° of total active motion in each finger. The carpal or proximal transverse arch, although existent anatomically, is of secondary importance in splinting because the flexor tendons and palmar neurovascular structures that traverse through the arch obliterate its concavity exteriorly. These arches (Fig.10-20, *A,B*), which combine stability and flexibility, allow the normal hand to grasp an almost

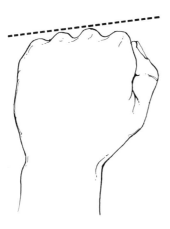

Fig. 10-14   Dorsally, the consecutive metacarpal heads create an oblique angle to the longitudinal axis of the forearm.

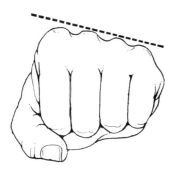

Fig. 10-15   Distally, the fisted hand exhibits an ulnar metacarpal descent that creates an oblique angle in the transverse plane of the forearm.

endless array of items of various sizes and shapes with a maximum or minimum of surface contact.

To maintain maximum potential mobility of the hand, the distal transverse and longitudinal arches must be preserved throughout the duration of treatment. The distal transverse arch should be apparent in any splint that incorporates the metacarpals (Fig. 10-21), provided significant dorsal and palmar swelling is not present. If this type of edema exists, care should be taken to adjust the parts of the splint that are responsible for supporting the arch as the edema subsides. Care should also be taken to continue the transverse arch configuration in splint parts that extend distal to the metacarpophalangeal joints, such as dorsal phalangeal bars or finger pans (Fig. 10-22, A,B).

Because of the mobility afforded by the longitudinal arch, splints that affect it are varied. Basically, any splint that incorporates the phalanges, either by immobilization, mobilization, restriction, or torque transmission, influences the state of this arch. The use of a finger pan, either in a "resting pan" splint or a

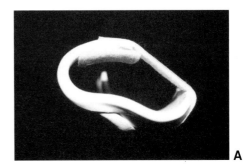

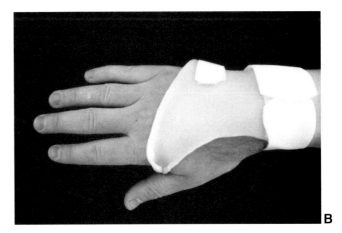

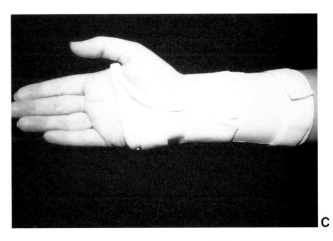

Fig. 10-16   **B,** Wrist neutral immobilization splint, type 0 (1) **C,** Wrist neutral immobilization splint, type 0 (1)
The concept of dual obliquity is reflected in the metacarpal bars of correctly fitted splints. **A,** A transverse angle mirrors the progressive reduction in radial to ulnar height of the metacarpals with the hand at rest. A dorsal **(B)** and volar oblique **(C)** angle follows the natural progressive radial to ulnar shortening of the lengths of metacarpals 2-5.

"safe position" splint, provides support for the entire length of the longitudinal arch. Extension or flexion outriggers, MP flexion cuffs, and elastic traction applied through the use of fingernail clips are examples of splint parts that are used to augment the passive range of motion of the longitudinal arch. When

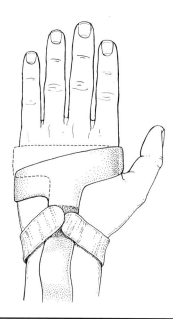

Fig. 10-17 **Wrist neutral immobilization splint, type 0 (1)**
The metacarpal bars should follow the oblique configuration of the
metacarpal heads. *Solid lines,* correct; *broken lines,* incorrect.

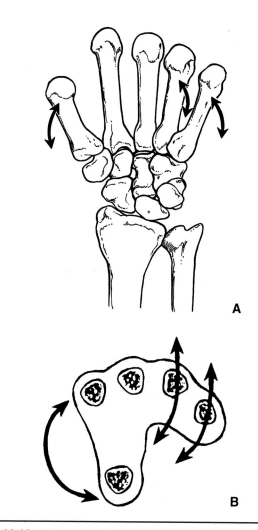

A

B

Fig. 10-18 The mobile first, fourth, and fifth metacarpals allow
the hand to assume an anteriorly concave configuration, which is
fundamental to coordinate grasp.

fitting splints that support only certain segments of
the longitudinal arch, care must be taken not to block
the motion of the remaining adjacent components
of the arch, either distally or proximally. This may
be done through careful attention to the dorsal and
palmar skin creases and their relationships to each
end of the splint (Fig. 10-23). Whenever support of
any part of the longitudinal arch is to be achieved, the
desired position of the involved MP and IP joints must
be predetermined before fitting may commence. This
determination of joint posture depends on the specific
purpose of the splint and the individual pathology with
which one is dealing.

Ligaments

Consider Ligamentous Stress

The preservation of ligamentous structures in correct
alignment and tension is another fundamental
anatomic principle of proper fitting of hand splints.
Because ligaments normally dictate joint stability and
direction, it is important that their biomechanical
functions be considered when attempting to augment
hand and/or upper extremity function with splinting
devices. The application of incorrect forces via an
improperly fitted splint may cause further damage to
an injured or diseased hand by erroneously stressing
periarticular structures, resulting in inflammation,
attenuation, and occasionally, disruption of ligamentous tissue.

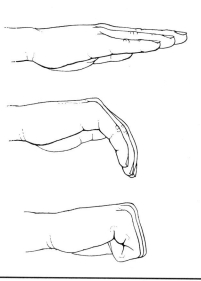

Fig. 10-19 In the sagittal plane the motion potential of the
segments comprising the longitudinal arch is approximately 280°.

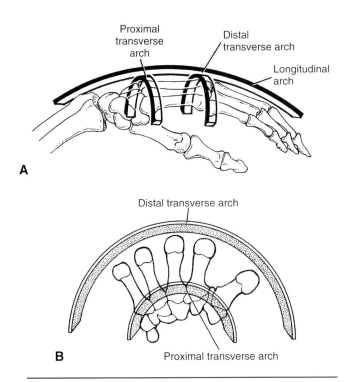

A

B

Fig. 10-20   **A,** The proximal transverse arch passes through the distal carpus; the distal transverse arch passes through the metacarpal heads. The longitudinal arch of the hand consists of the four digital rays and the carpus proximally. **B,** Proximal and distal transverse arches.

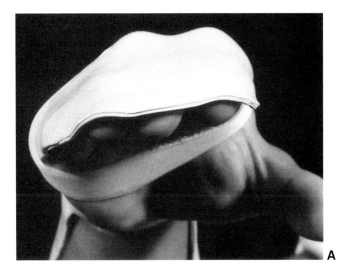

A

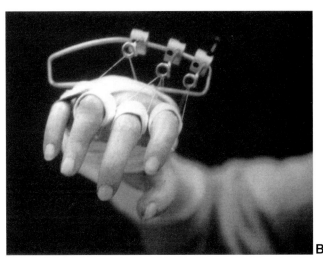

B

Fig. 10-22   **A,** Index–small finger extension restriction splint, type 1 (13) **B,** Index–small finger MP extension and radial deviation mobilization splint, type 1 (5)
The transverse metacarpal arch should be continued to splint parts that affect the fingers. [Courtesy **(B)** Lin Beribak, OTR/L, CHT, Chicago, Ill.]

From a simplistic point of view, each metacarpophalangeal and interphalangeal joint has three similar ligaments whose presence directly influences the construction of hand splints: two collateral ligaments and a palmar plate ligament. In hinged joints, such as digital interphalangeal joints, the collateral ligaments prevent joint mobility in the coronal plane, that is, ulnar and radial deviation.

Use Optimum Rotational Force. Because of this anatomic arrangement, splints designed to mobilize these joints must be constructed so that their line of pull or application of force is perpendicular to the joint axis (Fig. 10-24, *A-C*). It is important to monitor

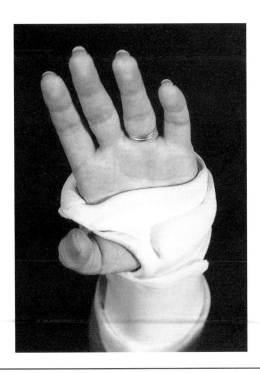

Fig. 10-21   **Wrist extension mobilization splint, type 0 (1)**
The metacarpal bar supports the transverse metacarpal arch.

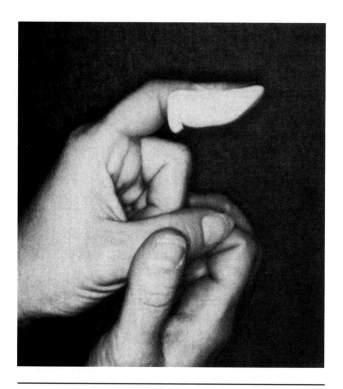

Fig. 10-23 Index finger DIP extension immobilization splint, type 0 (1)
Care should be taken not to impede motion of unsplinted segments of the longitudinal arch.

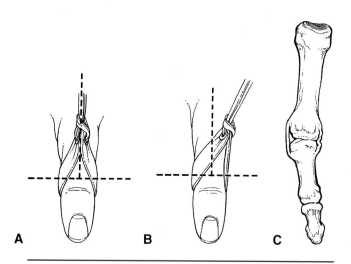

A   B   C

Fig. 10-24 A, Correct alignment. B, A nonperpendicular pull to the rotational axis of the joint, C, produces unequal stress on the collateral ligaments.

splints carefully as passive joint motion improves so that ligamentous structures are not overstretched. Immobilization splints should also be designed to protect this ligamentous support system to prevent instability. In general, after digital injury, which requires PIP joint immobilization, a splint that

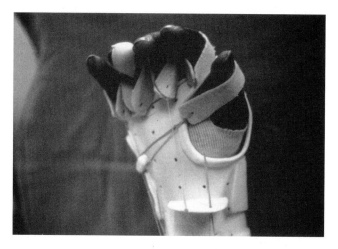

Fig. 10-25 Index–small finger MP flexion, thumb CMC palmar abduction and MP flexion mobilization splint, type 1 (7)
The finger metacarpophalangeal collateral ligaments become more taut as the mobilization assists pull the proximal phalanges into flexion. (Courtesy Lin Beribak, OTR/L, CHT, Chicago, Ill.)

maintains the joint in near-full extension will best preserve collateral ligament length and prevent flexion contracture.

Because of the cam-like structure of the metacarpals, the collateral ligaments of the metacarpophalangeal joints are not taut until the proximal phalanx is brought into near-full flexion, allowing finger abduction–adduction in extension and limited lateral motion when the fingers are flexed. This is an important concept to recognize when fitting splints that act on the MP joints (Figs. 10-25, 10-26). If the full length of the collateral ligaments of the MP joints is not maintained, a loss of flexion may occur, and the ensuing fixed contracture may be impossible to improve by conservative means. So-called "safe position" splints with finger MP flexion, IP extension, and thumb palmar or radial abduction positioning, such as the splints developed by the burn units at Brooke Army Hospital[3,4,10] and the University of Michigan Burn Center in Ann Arbor, Michigan (Fig. 10-27) embody this concept by positioning the metacarpophalangeal joints in flexion to maintain collateral ligament length. More difficult to envision, but equally important, is the action of a dorsal phalangeal bar (lumbrical bar) that determines the degree of extension allowed to the MP joints in some splint designs. If the potential for MP joint stiffness is present, the dorsal phalangeal bar should be adjusted to hold the proximal phalanges in near-full flexion (Fig. 10-28). The presence of dressings, extremity edema fluctuations, and other varying conditions necessitates careful monitoring and adaptation of splints to meet the specific physiologic and/or biomechanical changes presented.

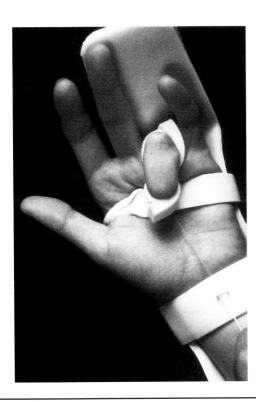

Fig. 10-26   **Long–small finger extension restriction / ring finger flexion mobilization splint, type 1 (10)**
When using a palmar pulley/fulcrum for a flexion assist, it is important to achieve a pull that equally stresses the collateral ligaments of the metacarpophalangeal joint. (Courtesy Stancie Trueman, OT, Missiauga, Ontario, Canada.)

A concept that is frequently misunderstood is the function of the finger MP collateral ligaments and the CMC ligaments of the fourth and fifth digits during simultaneous finger flexion. Bunnell,[5] in 1944, correctly noted that in the normal hand each finger points toward the scaphoid when flexed. However, over the years this observation created some confusion when some therapists applied it too literally to the fitting of hand splints designed to increase passive finger flexion. It is essential to understand the kinematic differences between digital alignment in single finger flexion and simultaneous multiple finger flexion. When the fingers are individually flexed, the tips of the digits touch the palm in a small area near the thenar crease. The distal transverse arch maintains a concave configuration, and the longitudinal axis of each digit aligns toward the scaphoid as Bunnell described. However, a study by Fess[6] demonstrates that when the fingers are flexed simultaneously, the distal transverse arch flattens and digital convergence points shift to the radial middle third of the forearm (Fig. 10-29). The dorsal rotation of the fourth and fifth metacarpals changes the alignment of the longitudinal axis of the ring and small fingers

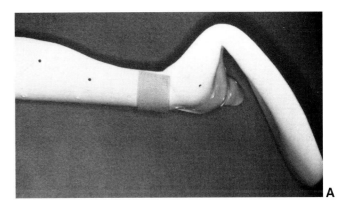

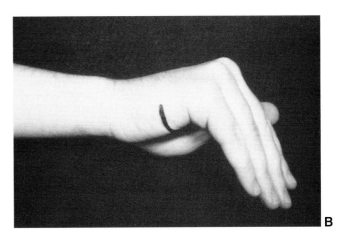

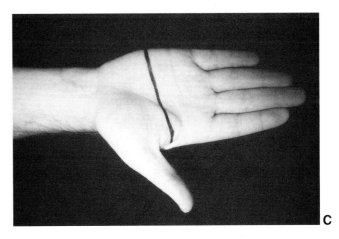

Fig. 10-27   **A, Index–small finger MP flexion and IP extension, thumb CMC radial abduction and MP-IP extension mobilization splint, type 1 (16)**
A, To preserve periarticular tissue length, this safe position splint maintains the metacarpophalangeal joints in flexion and the interphalangeal joints in extension. When fitting splints that position the MP joints in flexion, the flexion bend of the finger pan should occur approximately 2 centimeters proximal to the distal palmar crease, allowing space for swelling or bandages. B, Lateral view. C, Palmar view.

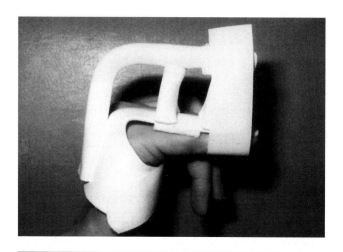

Fig. 10-28   Small finger IP extension mobilization splint, type 1 (6)
A dorsal phalangeal bar is used to position the metacarpophalangeal joints in near-full flexion to maintain the length of the collateral ligaments. (Courtesy Janet Bailey, OTR/L, CHT, Columbus, Ohio.)

away from the direction of the scaphoid toward a more ulnar orientation. Functionally this allows the hand to grasp objects without the fingers overlapping each other. It also permits optimal palmar surface contact of the hand on larger objects during palmar grip.

The lengths of the MP joint collateral ligaments and the ligaments of the fourth and fifth CMC joints are critical to digital spreading and mobility of the distal transverse arch. In splinting it is essential that the lengths of these ligaments be preserved. When flexion traction to more than one digit is required, the proximal ends of the traction devices at the wrist level should not be anchored at a single point, but should individually originate, allowing maintenance of the lengths of MP and CMC joint ligaments and permitting digital separation (Fig. 10-30). If, however, the traction anchor point is placed at a midforearm position, then a single attachment may be appropriate because the distally widening fan configuration of the mobilization assists results in separation of the traction forces at the wrist level (Fig. 10-31).

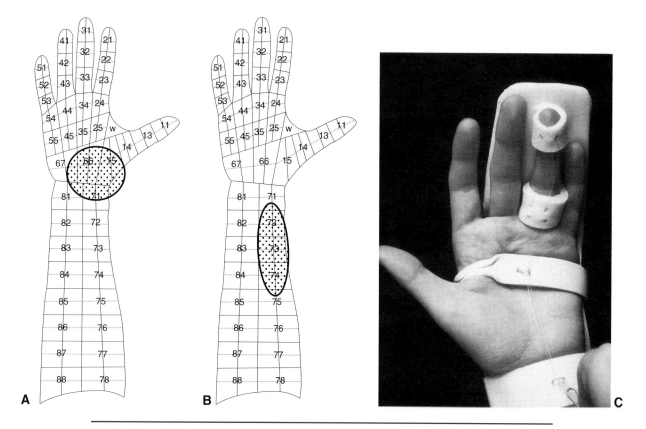

Fig. 10-29   C, Long–small finger extension restriction / ring finger flexion mobilization splint, type 1 (10)
A, When the fingers are flexed individually, their axes converge at the base of the thumb. B, When the fingers are flexed simultaneously, their extended longitudinal axes converge in an area on the middle third of the radial aspect of the forearm. C, The pulley/fulcrum located on the palmar strap assures a correct direction of pull of the finger flexion assist in this splint for a postoperative flexor tendon repair. (C Courtesy Stancie Trueman, OT, Missiauga, Ontario, Canada.)

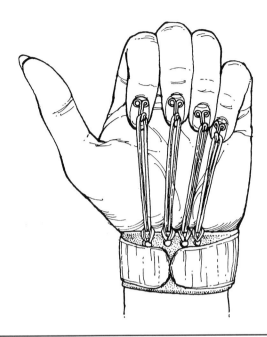

Fig. 10-30   Index–small finger flexion mobilization splint, type 0 (12)
To maintain the necessary ligament length at the 4-5 carpometacarpal and 2-5 metacarpophalangeal joints to allow simultaneous finger flexion, mobilization flexion assists should not overlap at the level of the wrist.

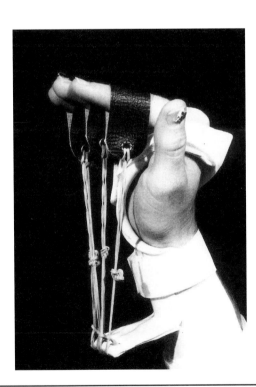

Fig. 10-31   Index–small finger MP flexion mobilization splint, type 1 (5)
Midforearm attachment of the mobilization assists allows a separation of forces at the wrist level when simultaneously mobilizing multiple digits into flexion. (Courtesy Roslyn Evans, OTR, CHT, Vero Beach, Fla.)

Because the rotation afforded by the ulnar two metacarpals varies from patient to patient, it is important that the angle of approach of the mobilizing force be evaluated carefully for each digit incorporated in the splint.

Palmar plate ligaments control the degree of hyperextension of the metacarpophalangeal and interphalangeal joints of the hand. Both finger MP hyperextension and thumb IP hyperextension are variable in normal individuals. Comparison with the uninvolved extremity is helpful when assessing baseline motion and subsequent follow-up measurements. When employing mobilizing splints to increase digital passive joint extension, such as outriggers, serial cylinder casts, or wire or spring three-point pressure splints, caution should be taken to prevent attenuation of palmar plate structures. This may be done by tension adjustment and by careful monitoring of the progress of the joint as it is brought to the neutral position (Fig. 10-32). X-rays with the splint in place may be helpful in attaining correct position in an immobilization, mobilization, restriction, or torque transmission splint (Fig. 10-33).

The thumb carpometacarpal joint is a saddle articulation that allows motion of the first metacarpal through all planes. There are five primary thumb carpometacarpal ligaments; when fitting thumb splints, one should give careful thought to the position in which the thumb is placed and the ultimate functional ramifications of this position.[2] Maintenance of the first web space is key to hand function, and for most supportive or positioning splints the thumb should be

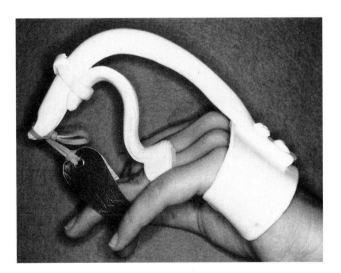

Fig. 10-32   Long finger PIP extension mobilization splint, type 1 (2)
Attenuation of the palmar plate with resultant hyperextension of the joint may occur with prolonged unsupervised extension traction.

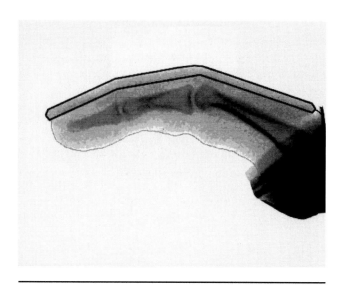

Fig. 10-33 Ring finger PIP extension restriction splint, type 1 (2)
After a PIP joint dorsal dislocation, the PIP joint is positioned in 30° of flexion to maintain joint reduction. An x-ray, taken with the splint in place, confirms the proper position of the joint. (Courtesy Maureen Stark, OTR, and James W. Strickland, MD, Indianapolis, Ind.)

held in wide palmar abduction. If a splint is required to increase passive range of motion of the thumb carpometacarpal joint, it must be fitted so that the mobilizing force is directed to the first metacarpal. Force applied incorrectly to the proximal phalanx creates undue stress on the ulnar collateral ligament of the metacarpophalangeal joint, potentially causing further damage by attenuating the ligament and creating an unstable joint (see Chapter 12). The posterior oblique ligament (POL) of the thumb may be thought of as an MP collateral ligament. The POL is tensed when the thumb is in both radial abduction and palmar abduction. When the thumb is in extension the POL is relaxed and can become contracted.

Palmar and dorsal ligament systems to the wrist include the dorsal and palmar radiocarpal, radioulnar articular capsule, radial and ulnar collateral, palmar ulnocarpal, dorsal and palmar intercarpal, pisohamate, pisometacarpal, and palmar and dorsal carpometacarpal ligaments. These ligaments assist in stabilizing the radiocarpal, distal radioulnar, intercarpal, and carpometacarpal joints of the wrist. Postinjury, a wrist immobilization splint may be required to correctly align and protect healing carpal ligaments. Also, depending on individual circumstances, the transverse carpal ligament may require splinting support to eliminate bowstringing in a postoperative carpal tunnel release.

The anterior, medial, and lateral aspects of the elbow joint are supported by the ulnar, radial collat-

eral, and annular ligaments. Repetitive overuse and loading of the joint are common etiologies that produce elbow ligament damage from strain, stress, or tear. Elbow immobilization or restriction splints provide rest and allow healing to the ligament system.

The shoulder ligamentous system provides stability to the acromioclavicular joint, sternoclavicular joint, and glenohumoral joint anterior and posterior capsule. Major ligamentous structures include coracoclavicular, coracohumeral, and glenohumeral ligaments. While these ligaments are a major focus for a vast array of therapeutic procedures, they are not generally the focus of splinting regimes, per se.

With the specificity of wrist, elbow, and shoulder pathology and the variability of subsequent treatments, close communication with referring physicians is essential. Therapy and splinting regimes may differ considerably, often depending on individual physician or therapist philosophies.

Joints

Align Splinting Forces According to Joint Rotational Axis and Bone Longitudinal Axis

Splinting of joints is dependent upon sound knowledge of ligamentous structures surrounding articular structures. Two mechanical principles prevail when fitting mobilization or restriction splints: (1) achievement of the correct alignment of the splint axis with the anatomic joint axis and (2) use of a 90° angle that is simultaneously perpendicular to the rotational axis of the joint.

Align Splint Axis with Anatomic Axis

Articulated splints (Fig. 10-34) must provide correct splint and joint alignment to allow achievement of full motion of the joint being splinted. If this is not accomplished, the splint may not only prove ineffective in increasing motion, but also may actually limit joint range and cause friction burns as splint components move independent of the joint. The approximate location of a specific anatomic joint axis may be found through observation of the joint as it moves in the plane in which it is to be splinted.

Use Optimum Rotational Force

When mobilization traction is used to increase the passive range of motion of a joint, the splint should be fitted to eliminate all translational forces and permit only rotational force in the desired plane. This is accomplished by positioning the distal end of the dorsal or palmar outrigger at a point that allows the mobilization assist, such as a rubber band, to pull at a 90° angle on the bone to be mobilized. This pull

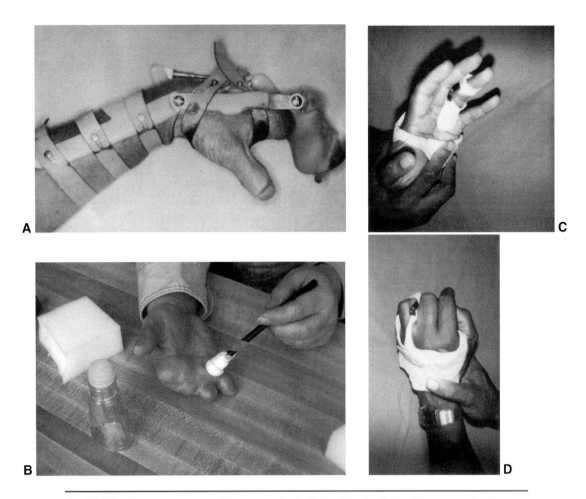

Fig. 10-34   A, Wrist extension [finger prosthesis flexion] / wrist flexion [finger prosthesis extension] torque transmission splint-prosthesis, type 0 (1) C,D, Ring finger PIP radial deviation mobilization splint, type 1 (2)
A, The rotational axis of a splint must be correctly aligned with the anatomic rotational axis of the joint to allow unhampered simultaneous movement of both joints. This partial hand prosthesis exhibits good alignment at the wrist joint. B, The hand without the partial prosthesis has limited function from lack of distal digital ray lengths. C,D, This splint allows full flexion and extension of the PIP joint while correcting an ulnar deviation deformity of the joint. [Courtesy (A) Lawrence Czap, OTR, orthotist, Columbus, Ohio; (C,D) Carol Hierman, OTR, CHT, Cedar Grove, N.C., Elisha Denny, PTA, OTA, Pittsboro, N.C. © UNC Hand Rehabilitation Center, Chapel Hill, N.C.]

should also be perpendicular to the rotational axis of the joint so that the supporting ligamentous structures are equally stressed. If a 90° angle of pull is not employed, and if the force is applied in the direction of the joint, significant pressure may be imparted to the cartilaginous surfaces of the joint as a result of compression of the two bones. If the force is directed away from the joint to be mobilized, the joint surfaces may be distracted, and the patient will have difficulty keeping the traction cuffs on the fingers. As the joint range of motion improves, the length of the outrigger must be changed to accommodate a continuous 90° angle of pull (Fig. 10-35, A-F).

As noted, two separate views of the hand must be analyzed simultaneously to determine correct rotational force. While the two 90° angles do not change in respect to the bone and joint upon which they act, their relative positions in space do change as the involved joint's range of motion changes. The Dual-Track-Along concept illustrated on the next few pages describes a simple method for defining splint outrigger length and position in space and the location of mobilization assists on an outrigger. Two 90° angles must be considered simultaneously: (1) the bone angle of rotation (BAR) and (2) the joint angle of rotation (JAR).

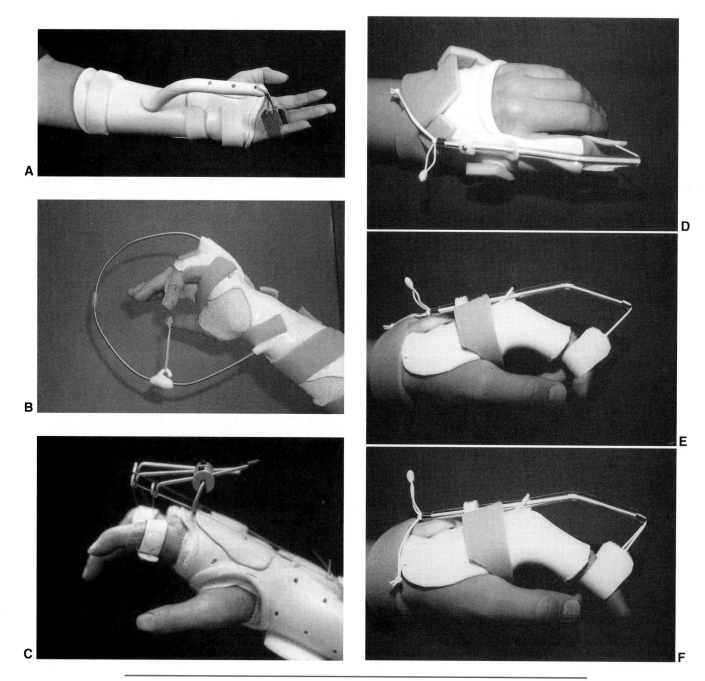

Fig. 10-35
For legend see opposite page.

The 90° BAR determines the length of an outrigger (Fig. 10-36, *A-E*). Generally speaking, the greater the angle formed by the involved bone segments, the longer the outrigger will need to be. As the contracture decreases, the length of the outrigger must also decrease to maintain a 90° mobilization assist BAR angle. Failure to correctly establish and maintain a 90° BAR as a patient progresses results in either a joint distraction force if the outrigger is too long or a joint compression force if the outrigger is too short. For splints designed to mobilize finger joints, complaints from patients are consistent and revealing. If the outrigger is too short, patients complain that the finger cuffs cut into their second, third, and/or fourth web spaces; if the outrigger is too long, they complain that the finger cuffs do not stay on their fingers.

Fig. 10-35   A, Ring–small finger MP flexion mobilization splint, type 1 (3) B, Small finger middle phalanx distraction, PIP distraction and extension or flexion mobilization splint, type 2 (3) C, Index–small finger MP extension and radial deviation mobilization splint, type 1 (5) D-F, Index finger PIP extension mobilization splint, type 1 (2)

A, As the finger position changes, the length of the outrigger must be altered to accommodate a 90° angle of the traction assist to the segment being mobilized. This palmar outrigger is designed to allow the patient to adjust the traction assist. **B,** The circular configuration of this outrigger allows distraction of the PIP joint via traction on the phalangeal pin as the finger is flexed or extended. It is especially important to correctly align this type of outrigger with the joint angle of rotation, allowing equal amounts of stress to be applied to the PIP joint collateral ligaments. **C,** A commercial outrigger system allows easy adjustment of individual outrigger lengths via adjustment screws in the individual metal housing disks on the transverse outrigger bar. **D,** This commercially available tube outrigger facilitates maintaining a 90° angle of pull to the proximal phalanx via adjustment of the screw in the plastic sleeve that holds the outrigger to the dorsal metacarpal bar. **E,** Note the relatively short outrigger length proximal to the setscrew when the outrigger length distally needs to be longer to accommodate the greater PIP flexion contracture. **F,** As the PIP joint flexion contracture becomes less, the outrigger is adjusted, by moving it proximally, to maintain a 90° angle of pull to the proximal phalanx. Note the longer length proximal to the setscrew. [Courtesy **(B)** Christopher Bochenek, OTR/L, CHT, Cincinnati, Ohio; **(C)** Lin Beribak, OTR/L, CHT, Chicago, Ill.; **(D-F)** Paul Van Lede, OT, MS, Orfit Industries, Wijnegem, Belgium.]

The 90° JAR determines outrigger and mobilization assist position in a plane parallel to the joint axis of rotation (Fig. 10-37, *A-E*). As a contracture decreases, the 90° JAR position of the outrigger and mobilization assist follow normal ray tracking, remaining, for the most part, unchanged as the length (BAR) of the outrigger changes. Failure to correctly establish and maintain a 90° JAR results in application of unequal force to collateral ligaments, eventually producing unwarranted attenuation of the greater-stressed ligament with concomitant joint instability.

Vascular and Neural Structures

Consider Vascular and Neural Status

Local vascular and/or neural structures are subjected to stress as splint mobilization forces are applied. Like other soft tissues, it is important that these structures are allowed to remodel through gradual application of low-load force. Too much splint force can cause lumen collapse of vascular structures, compression of nerves, and ultimately may cause tissue necrosis and/or nerve damage. If vessels or nerves have been repaired under tension, passive motion of associated joints must be carefully achieved through initial restriction of joint motion with gradual increases that allow remodeling over time (Fig. 10-38).

▥ KINESIOLOGIC CONSIDERATIONS

Kinesiologic considerations encompass two additional concepts pertaining to the actual shaping of a hand splint: kinematic principles and kinetic principles.

Kinematic principles deal with the differences between the hand at rest and the hand in motion, and kinetic principles address the mobilization force relationship between the hand and the splint. Both the design and form of a hand splint should reflect an understanding of these two major concepts.

Allow for Kinematic Changes

As the fingers and thumb move through an arc of motion from a fully extended position to an attitude of full flexion, basic external anatomic configurations change their relationships. In flexion, palmar skin creases approximate, arches deepen, dorsal bony prominences become more apparent, the dorsal surface area elongates, and the palmar length lessens. As the thenar and hypothenar masses move palmarly in opposition, the breadth of the hand changes to become convex dorsally and concave palmarly, resulting in the increase of dorsometacarpal surface area. A splint designed to allow motion must be fitted to accommodate anticipated relative changes in the arches and bony prominences. For example, finger extension cuffs must be cut to permit full proximal and distal phalangeal flexion (Fig. 10-39, *A-D*), whereas the entire width of flexion cuffs may be preserved to decrease pressure. Hypothenar bars should not inhibit motion of the first metacarpal, and phalangeal bars should allow unencumbered motion of the segments they do not support. If these types of adaptations are not executed, motion of the hand may be inhibited, pressure and friction/shear injury of the skin may occur, and the splint may be rendered ineffective.

Fig. 10-36   Bone Angle of Rotation (BAR)

EXAMPLE: METACARPOPHALANGEAL (MP) JOINT FLEXION CONTRACTURE

A, Normal MP joint.
B-E, Resolving MP joint flexion contracture.

* MP joint and proximal phalanx, lateral view

* MP in maximum comfortable extension

* Using the proximal phalanx (P_1) as a linear base, imagine/construct a perpendicular angle extending dorsally from the midpart of the proximal phalanx

    * This perpendicular angle to the bone = Bone Angle of Rotation (BAR)

    * The BAR = the angle of force application of the mobilizing assist = the angle of rubber band, spring, etc., to the proximal phalanx

* The outrigger must be long enough to reach the extended BAR

* As joint extension increases:

    * The BAR does not change its perpendicular angle to P_1

    * Because P_1 is moving into more extension, the BAR changes position in space

    * The outrigger length must change to maintain the BAR

Hint: Use an Allen wrench to help determine the Bone Angle of Rotation (BAR)

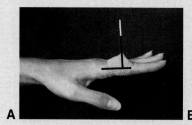
A
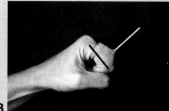
B
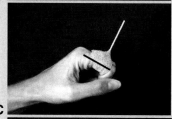
C
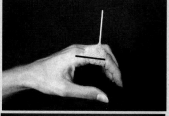
D
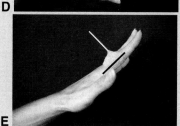
E

Employ Kinetic Concepts

The actual positioning of specific splint parts will augment or retard muscle action. An extension finger cuff placed on the proximal phalanx assists the long extensor tendons, while interossei and lumbrical forces are reinforced when the cuff is positioned at the middle phalanx. The fitting of a dorsal phalangeal bar to prevent metacarpal hyperextension augments extension of the fingers by maximizing the extrinsic extensor action at the IP joints (Fig. 10-40). Because of the relative lengths of the extrinsic digital flexors and extensors, a wrist bar fitted for extension transfers moment to finger flexors, and conversely a flexed wrist bar transfers moment to finger extensors. Knowledge of kinetic principles as they pertain to the hand and upper extremity is important in achieving the full potential of splints used to increase upper extremity function.

■ TECHNICAL CONSIDERATIONS

Numerous techniques of fitting hand splints are based on practical everyday experiences. These additional clinical considerations increase efficiency and make the fitting process run more smoothly.

Develop Patient Rapport

An explanation about the proposed splint—its functions, material, and method of forming—develops patient rapport and trust. Demonstration models of frequently used splints help patients visualize what splints are and how they work. A rehearsal of the desired position in which the splint will be fitted before the actual application of the material also expedites the fitting process. If thermal materials are used, the patient should be warned that the material will feel

Fig. 10-37 Joint Angle of Rotation (JAR)

EXAMPLE: METACARPOPHALANGEAL (MP) JOINT FLEXION CONTRACTURE

A, Normal MP joint.
B-E, Resolving MP joint flexion contracture.

- MP joint and proximal phalanx, transverse view

- MP in maximum comfortable extension

- Using the MP joint as a linear base, imagine/construct a perpendicular angle extending dorsally from the midpart of the joint

  - This is the perpendicular angle to the joint = Joint Angle of Rotation (JAR)

  - The JAR = the angle of force application of the mobilizing assist = the angle of the rubber band, spring, etc., to the joint axis

- The point of attachment of the mobilizing assist on the outrigger must be exactly in line with the JAR. It should not be positioned on either side of the JAR

- As joint extension increases:

  - The JAR does not change its perpendicular angle to the joint axis for the third and fourth digital rays. The second and fifth digits may abduct slightly to accommodate border digital spreading

  - If extension and radial deviation are needed, the angle of pull of the mobilizing assist will be slightly to the thumb (radial) side of the JAR

Hint: Use an Allen wrench to help determine the Joint Angle of Rotation (JAR)

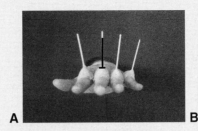
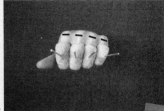
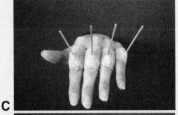
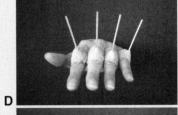
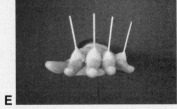

warm. Allowing a child to play with scraps of the material before fitting commences is ultimately well worth the extra time and effort!* When a splint is completed, specific instructions for its care, donning and doffing, wearing and exercise times, and precautions are given to the patient.** Both written and verbal instructions are essential to ensuring that the patient understands the splinting regimen. Quality patient education is as important as the designing, fabricating, and fitting of a splint. Without the cooperation of the patient, a splint, no matter how well conceived and executed, is useless.

Some patients may develop minor skin irritations from wearing their splints. Many clinics avoid this potential problem by routinely furnishing patients with a set of stockinette sleeves that provide a clean cotton interface between the extremity and the splint, and allow a practical wash/wear rotation where one sleeve is worn while the other is washed.

Consideration of the patient and attention to the small details that make the rehabilitation experience more pleasant is key to gaining patient rapport and trust. Taking extra time with patient education and providing "extras" like stockinette liners strengthen the therapeutic relationship that is so critical to a successful rehabilitative outcome.

Work Efficiently

The use of devices or methods that increase the efficiency of the molding time may also be of considerable benefit. Lightly wrapping a warmed, low-temperature, thermal material splint to the patient's hand and forearm with an elastic bandage allows the therapist's full attention to be directed to the positioning of the hand. Strategically applied tape holds

---

*See Chapter 18, Splinting the Pediatric Patient, for additional information.
**See Chapter 15, Exercise and Splinting for Specific Problems, for additional information.

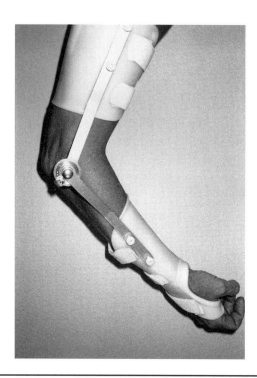

Fig. 10-38   Elbow extension restriction splint, type 2 (3)
The elbow-locking device restricts elbow joint extension, allowing remodeling of vascular and neural structures by gradually increasing the amount of elbow extension over time. (Courtesy Helen Marx, OTR, CHT, Wickenburg, Ariz.)

splint parts in position as they cool (Fig. 10-41) and an elevation board (Fig. 10-42) lessens patient muscle fatigue during the material cooling phase. Allowing gravitational forces to augment splint fabrication is another efficiency consideration of fit. Coated thermoplastics tend to slide off patients when working against gravity. Positioning the patient in a manner that allows the warmed splint material to be placed on top of the extremity allows normal gravitational pull to assist in formation of the splint. In general, a volar splint is fit with the hand in supination and a dorsal splint fit with the hand in pronation. Smooth strokes are used to shape splints. Rotate the hand into the desired position before the splint hardens completely. Unless otherwise indicated, splints that include the forearm should be formed with the hand in neutral or close to the patient's normal working position. Neutral position will best accommodate the changes in shape of the forearm as the wrist is rotated from pronation to supination. Exceptions may include specific jobs or sports where pronation or supination may be more appropriate. Splinting of larger joints such as the elbow or shoulder may require the assistance of another therapist or aide to efficiently manipulate the requisite greater amount of warmed splint material.

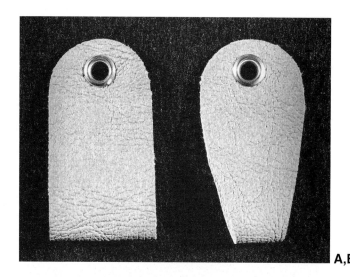

A,B

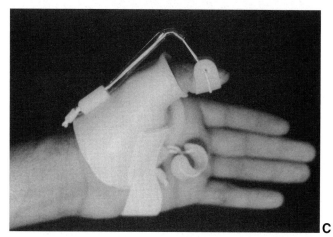

C

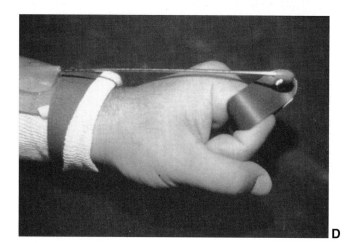

D

Fig. 10-39
For legend see opposite page.

Fig. 10-39   C, Thumb IP extension or flexion mobilization splint, type 2 (3) D, Wrist flexion: index–small finger MP extension / index–small finger MP flexion: wrist extension torque transmission splint, type 0 (5)
Depending on hand size, finger flexion cuffs (A) may be used without alteration, while extension finger cuffs (B) should be cut to allow finger flexion. C, In addition to having a wide area of force application, the mobilization assist attachments of this thumb IP extension cuff are separate, decreasing circumferential pressure on the distal thumb segment. D, This flexion cuff is contoured to allow unencumbered flexion of the MP and PIP joints. [Courtesy (C,D) Kathryn Schultz, OTR, CHT, Orlando, Fla.]

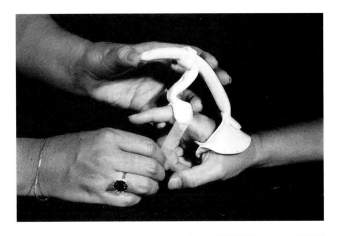

Fig. 10-41   Tape may be used to maintain splint position until plastic hardens.

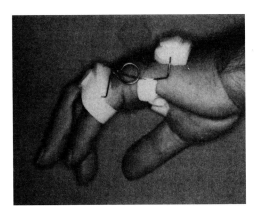

Fig. 10-40   Ring–small finger MP extension restriction / IP extension torque transmission splint, type 0 (6)
This dorsal phalangeal bar prevents metacarpophalangeal joint hyperextension and allows the excursion of extrinsic extensors to be focused on the interphalangeal joints.

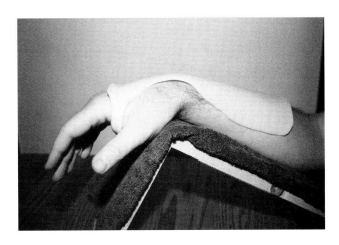

Fig. 10-42   Index–small finger extension torque transmission splint, type 1 (13)
A slant board assists arm positioning during the process of fitting a splint.

Some materials facilitate fitting against gravity. Original Aquaplast and Reveal Quick Bond's sticky surfaces hold splints in place, allowing splint fitting with the extremity in almost any position. The universal working time for $\frac{1}{8}$ inch thick material is approximately 3-6 minutes. Setting time may be abbreviated by cooling the material with cold packs or frozen exercise bands, or by removing the splint when it is partially set and holding it under cool water. Thermoplastic working time increases when fitting over dressings. Spot heating with a heat gun is useful for making smaller adjustments.

Change Method According to Properties of Materials Used

Different materials require the use of diverse approaches to the forming procedure (Fig. 10-43). For example, if a protective stockinette is used during the shaping of a splint constructed of high-temperature

material, or if removable spacers are used in thermoplastic materials, the resulting splint or splint component will be slightly large for the unprotected extremity, requiring further adjustment. Moisture should be eliminated from the surfaces of a material requiring wet heat before application to the patient, and the use of a separating substance such as petroleum jelly augments the removal of newly applied circumferential plaster splints. Depending on the material's propensity to collect dirt and grime with wear, external surfaces of finished splints may be protected with stockinette sleeves.

Adapt Prefabricated Splints when Appropriate

Over time, commercially available splints have improved in their abilities to meet requisite mechan-

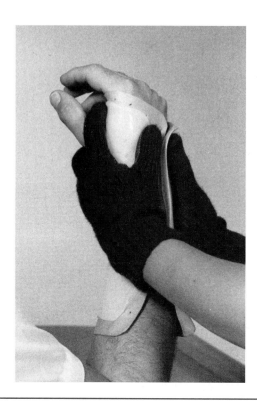

Fig. 10-43   Protective gloves are needed when working with high-temperature materials such as polyethylene. (Courtesy Theresa Bielawski, OT[C], Toronto, Ont., and Jane Bear-Lehman, PhD, OTR, New York, N.Y.)

ical, design, construction, and fit criteria. Use of prefabricated splints is contingent upon whether they meet the same basic criteria required of custom splints. If a prefabricated splint meets these requirements, then other decisive factors such as cost, time to fit, insurance restrictions, patient circumstances, and clinic situation may be evaluated in comparison to those of a same-purpose custom splint. Conversely, if a prefabricated splint fails to meet basic mechanical, design, construction, fit, and/or patient criteria, its use is automatically eliminated as an option. Ultimately placing a patient's rehabilitative potential in jeopardy, no justification is ever appropriate for applying a prefabricated splint that fails to achieve basic splinting purposes and principles.

When prefabricated splints are used, a trade-off is typically achieved between their higher initial cost and their lower construction/fit time as compared to same-purpose custom splints. Be certain that the initial saving in construction/fit time is not nullified by time-consuming adaptations, thus making the real cost of the splint prohibitive. A few prefabricated splints are so mass-produced that custom splints cannot equal their low cost. These inexpensive commercially available splints generally fall into a restric-

tion or "quasi-immobilization" category, allowing a wide fit range via soft material bases combined with easily adjustable straps or fasteners. If this type of splint is what the patient needs and it meets the technical criteria involving mechanical, design, construction, and fit standards, then its use benefits both patient, with its low cost, and therapist, by freeing him/her to treat more complicated upper extremity problems in the clinic. Unfortunately, these low-cost prefabricated splints frequently cannot provide the complicated splinting solutions required by patients with upper extremity dysfunction caused by injury or disease.

Assess Finished Splint

Although splints are continually assessed as they are fitted to patients, it is important to conduct a thorough assessment of the finished splint product. An exit checkout (see Chapter 5, Box 5-1) encompasses all of the phases of splint fabrication including design, construction, fit, mechanics, and client education. Mobilization splints need especially rigorous assessment because they employ active mobilization forces that influence tissue remodeling. In addition to addressing patient-specific diagnoses, splints must also be appropriate to socioeconomic, vocational, and avocational requisites of those for whom they were made.

■ SUMMARY

Those involved in the splinting process must arm themselves with knowledge of the anatomic, mechanical, kinesiologic, and technical principles that are an absolute prerequisite for proper fit. Failure to adhere to these principles often results in embarrassing pressure areas, splint disuse, and patient distrust, with the probable attendant decrease of extremity function.

The decision to use a splint on the hand/extremity of a particular patient is a serious consideration involving the physician and the therapist. A close communication between the two must exist so that the exact function expected from each splint may be realized. If the proper fit techniques are employed, the opportunity for maximum upper extremity function and patient satisfaction is provided.

REFERENCES

1. Brand PW: *Clinical mechanics of the hand,* Mosby, 1985, St. Louis.
2. Brand PW, Hollister A: *Clinical mechanics of the hand,* ed 2, Mosby, 1993, St. Louis.
3. Brook Army Medical Center B: *Finger nail hooks and their application,* Motion Picture Section, U.S. Army Surgical

Research Unit, Brooke Army Medical Center, 1968, Fort Sam Houston, TX.

4. Brooke Army Medical Center B: *Physical and occupational therapy for the burn patient*, Motion Picture Section, U. S. Army Surgical Research Unit, Brooke Army Medical Center, 1968, Fort Sam Houston, TX.

5. Bunnell S: *Surgery of the hand*, ed 1, JB Lippincott Company, 1944, Philadelphia.

6. Fess EE: Convergence points of normal fingers in individual and simultaneous flexion, *J Hand Ther* 2:12-9, 1989.

7. Malick M: *Manual on dynamic hand splinting with thermoplastic materials*, Harmarville Rehabilitation Center, 1974, Pittsburgh.

8. Malick M: *Manual on static hand splinting*, Rev ed, Harmarville Rehabilitation Center, 1972, Pittsburgh.

9. Mayerson E: *Splinting theory and fabrication*, Goodrich Printing and Lithographers, Inc., 1971, Clarence Center, NY.

10. Yeakel M, Gronley J, Tumbush W: Fiberglass positioning device for the burned hand, *J Trauma* 4:57-70, 1964.

PART FOUR

Anatomic Site

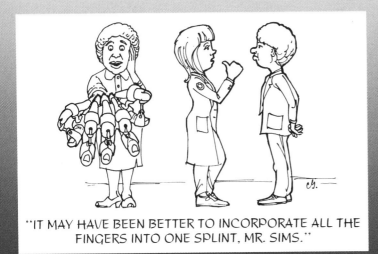

"IT MAY HAVE BEEN BETTER TO INCORPORATE ALL THE FINGERS INTO ONE SPLINT, MR. SIMS."

Splints Acting on the Fingers

Chapter Outline

T his chapter follows the expanded ASHT SCS format by first dividing splints into articular or nonarticular categories. In the articular category, splints are further grouped according to the primary joints they influence. Splints in the nonarticular category are defined by the anatomical segments upon which they are based.

Once articular splints are sorted according to their primary joints, they are divided according to one of four purposes: immobilization, mobilization, restriction, or torque transmission. Dual-purpose categories (e.g., mobilization / restriction or immobilization / mobilization) designate splints with more than one primary purpose. Each purpose category is then grouped according to direction of force application. In this chapter, force direction (e.g., abduction, extension, flexion, etc.) for finger splints is included as part of the purpose groupings. Purpose categories are further subdivided by *type*. *Type* identifies the number of secondary joint levels included in splints. Note: *Type* refers to the number of secondary joint levels, not to the total number of secondary joints in a splint. While not all categories and/or subcategories are represented in this chapter, the ESCS is sufficiently flexible to accommodate additional groupings as needed. For this chapter, sections describing splints that affect fingers precede sections about splints that include the fingers and thumb. The final section in this chapter discusses single-splint designs that combine more than one ESCS site or direction (e.g., MP-IP joint and IP joint torque transmission or finger extension and flexion mobilization).

It is important to remember that not all of the finger splints pictured in this book are illustrated in this designated chapter. To locate additional finger splints beyond those shown in this chapter, refer to the Splint Ranking Index©. The Index lists all splints in the book according to the expanded Splint Classification System, including page and figure number locations.

■ ARTICULAR SPLINTS

The purpose of this chapter is to review the concepts involved in splinting the fingers. Governed by anatomic, kinesiological, and mechanical variables, finger splints must also adhere to the principles of design, construction, fit, mechanics, and using outriggers and mobilization assists. The most common reasons for applying finger splints are protection of injured or repaired structures, correction or prevention of deformity, allowance of partial motion to specific joints, and transmission of torque to predetermined joints. Finger splinting may also be used to decrease pain, enhance grasp and release patterns, and provide stability to lax or unstable joints.

The functional capacity of the fingers depends on the integrated motion of its four proximally unified, distally independent articulated rays. These triarticular rays function as diverging open kinematic chains whose four segments provide a progressive summation of motion in the sagittal and coronal planes. The mobility afforded by the fourth and fifth CMC joints also provides an element of motion in the transverse plane to the ring and small fingers, allowing palmar and radial approximation of the ulnar border of the hand. The condylar metacarpophalangeal joints allow some rotation in addition to flexion, extension, abduction, and adduction of the fingers. Longitudinally each

successive joint adds an increment of sagittal mobility until at its greatest limit the cumulative palmar flexion possible per digit is approximately 280°.

The effect of restriction of a single joint or the loss of a distal segment on composite hand function is lessened when the rest of the hand has normal motion. However, as the number of stiffened joints or lost segments increases, the compensatory ability of the hand becomes progressively compromised.

In addition to supple joints, it is necessary to have muscles of adequate strength with adhesion-free tendon excursion to produce the highly integrated digital motion required for optimum hand function. In their normal state, the fingers represent a balance of intrinsic and extrinsic forces that, in conjunction with the thumb, are capable of functional patterns ranging from delicate prehension to powerful grasp.[11-15,26]

Because digital effectiveness depends on mobility, it is important to achieve and maintain adequate motion early in the rehabilitation process. Splinting and exercise programs should be designed to prevent the development of articular and musculotendinous limitations. In the presence of established deformity, emphasis should be placed on restoring lost motion. If muscle imbalance is present, splints that restrict motion or transfer active moments to other joints improve function and diminish potential for deformity.[3] Splinting and exercise programs should acknowledge the structural peculiarities at each joint level and be designed accordingly. The MP joints of the fingers have a propensity for becoming stiff in extension; the PIP joints more often become stiff in flexion.[10]

Sensibility also plays an important role in finger use. Impaired digital sensibility diminishes the ability of the hand to distinguish texture and pressure variables. This inability to adequately receive, relay, or interpret sensory impulses from the hand severely limits composite hand and upper extremity function. Splints whose designs are meant to encourage hand use should not encumber the palmar surfaces of the fingers, particularly at distal, more tactilely receptive areas.

Depending on individual patient needs, finger splints may be applied to immobilize, mobilize, or restrict finger motion. They may also be used to transmit mobilizing torque to joints within, distal to, or proximal to splint physical boundaries. Multipurpose splints tackle more complicated problems. For example, a splint may simultaneously immobilize a primary finger MP joint and restrict motion at the primary IP joints, protecting proximal healing structures while allowing predefined limited motion at the two more distal joints.

Immobilization splints prevent motion of the finger(s) or of selected segments within the finger rays to allow healing, control early postoperative motion, decrease pain, or enhance functional use. Inflammatory conditions and soft tissue injuries of finger structures often require splint immobilization. Postoperative immobilization between exercise periods effectively limits use while allowing early motion at uninvolved joints. Severe hand injuries, especially those with a component of crush or with median and/or ulnar nerve involvement, often produce insidious MP extension, IP flexion contractures, which, if permitted to persist, rapidly develop into rigid deformities that markedly limit finger function. It should be stressed that, for immobilization of finger joints which have not undergone surgical repair, the preferred or "safe" position for the metacarpophalangeal joints is usually considered to be 70-90° of flexion, and a 0-10° flexion posture is best for the IP joints.[9,10] These attitudes considerably decrease the potential for ligamentous contractures and the consequent limitation of articular motion.

Mobilization splints maintain or increase passive range of motion. For supple finger joints, in a paralyzed or partially paralyzed finger, mobilization splinting preserves passive range of motion and prevents deformity while permitting continued functional use. Since optimal effectiveness of the finger depends on mobility, when finger motion is tethered by scar and/or fibrosed soft tissues, restoration of motion of the finger joints is critical to the success of the rehabilitation process. Splinting and active range of motion exercises, combined with purposeful activity, are the cornerstones to mobilizing stiffened joints. Maximum passive range of motion of the involved joints must be acquired and maintained before a corresponding active range of motion may be achieved or before many surgical procedures may be attempted. Through application of prolonged gentle mobilization forces that cause soft tissue remodeling, splinting is the most effective means for improving finger passive range of motion.

Although finger mobilization splints assume a variety of configurations, all must meet certain criteria to be effective. To mobilize stiffened joints, understanding anatomy, kinesiology, surgical procedures, rehabilitation goals, mechanical concepts, properties of outriggers, mobilization assists, and the physiologic ramifications of applying a splint are equally important. A well-designed splint is rendered ineffective if not worn long enough to produce tissue growth; failure to combine splint and exercise regimens may result in good passive motion but poor active range; application of incorrect forces may actually cause further damage; and a beautifully executed surgical procedure may be jeopardized because of insufficient communication between the physician and the therapist during the postoperative phase. The patient's cooperation is also essential to achieving maximum rehabilitation potential. Too often the fitting of a splint is seen as an isolated experience. Nothing could be further from the truth! An appropriately used splint is but one of many tools an astute upper extremity specialist employs in close conjunction with other therapy techniques.

Mobilization splints may use elastic or inelastic traction to direct corrective forces. The angle of application of the mobilizing force directly influences the efficacy of the splint, in terms of efficiency in correcting deformity while providing optimum comfort. Elastic traction splints frequently require an outrigger component to serve as a base of attachment or as a fulcrum for mobilization assists. Aside from the obvious difference in mass, the height of an outrigger influences the number of times it must be adjusted as joint range of motion changes. High-profile outriggers maintain an angle of pull that is closer to 90° for a longer time and require fewer adjustments as change occurs than do low-profile configurations. Inelastic traction splints usually involve consecutive serial applications or depend on the patient to adjust the amount of force applied as joint motion improves. Selecting the type of traction and the configuration of specialized components depends on many factors. Each design option has distinct advantages and disadvantages. There are no universal answers. The more familiar upper extremity specialists become with the many choices available, the better prepared they are to best meet the needs of their individual patients.

Restriction splints limit specific joint motion to protect healing finger structures, influence reparative scar formation, decrease pain, or enhance functional use.

Torque transmission splints direct active mobilizing torque to selected joints that usually, but not always, lie outside the physical boundaries of splints to improve motion, to remodel soft tissue, and/or to increase functional capabilities of these selected joints.

To reduce potential error, careful deductive assessment of the extremity is imperative before final design decisions are reached. It is not unusual for a diseased or injured upper extremity to exhibit perplexing symptoms. An inaccurate assumption regarding etiology can lead an unwary person or novice to create a splint that may not only be ineffective but may actually cause further damage. For example, a rotational deformity of the metacarpal may be misinterpreted as pathology at the more distal MP or PIP joints. Lack of active motion at a joint may be the result of any number of problems, including shortening of periarticular structures, articular adhesions, intra-articular fracture, tendon rupture, tendon adhesions, or nerve disruption. A splint that is appropriate for one problem may actually be contraindicated for others. It is therefore critical that a complete and accurate concept of the pathology be determined before embarking on the design and fabrication of any splint.

Finger splints may involve one or more joints and may be fitted dorsally, palmarly, laterally, or circumferentially. Care should be taken to maintain correct ligamentous stress at each joint traversed, while allowing full motion of unsplinted joints. Because many finger splints have narrow configurations, contouring splinting material to half the segmental thickness provides splint strength. Splint components should be of sufficient length to fully control finger segment(s); and if the wrist is included secondarily or as a primary joint, the forearm trough should be at least two thirds the length of the forearm to achieve optimum mechanical performance. Straps placed at the level of the axis of joint rotation provide maximum mechanical purchase. Circumferentially designed finger splints eliminate the need for counterforce straps at joints by providing opposing forces along the entire length of the segment.

Finger splints may affect only articular motion or they may affect extrinsic musculotendinous units by including the wrist as a secondary joint. In the latter, wrist position increases or decreases the amount of tension on finger structures through modification of the tenodesis effect. A splint designed to affect both articular motion and extrinsic tendon problems must include the wrist.

Finger MP Splints

The metacarpophalangeal joints of the index, long, ring, and small fingers are condyloid with the rounded metacarpal head fitting into a small concavity at the base of the proximal phalanx. The ligamentous arrangement at each MP joint consists of two collateral ligaments and one palmar ligament that allow anteroposterior and mediolateral motion in addition to a slight amount of phalangeal rotation. Since the ligaments must extend around the cam-shaped palmar portion of the joint, the collateral ligaments are slack when the MP joint is in extension and taut when the joint is flexed. Pathologic conditions involving the metacarpophalangeal joints of the fingers frequently result in periarticular stiffness and eventually contracture in a position of extension or hyperextension. This deformity in a protracted state is extremely difficult to correct through conservative means. It is

important to anticipate this problem and make appropriate efforts to maintain adequate length of the metacarpophalangeal collateral ligaments through preventive antideformity flexion splinting and exercise programs that emphasize full metacarpophalangeal joint flexion.

In addition to the MP splints illustrated in this section, other chapters in this book include designated sections that describe splints that affect the MP joints. Refer to Chapter 16, Hand and Wrist Splinting for the Patient with Rheumatoid Arthritis, and Chapter 13, Splints Acting on the Wrist and Forearm.

Immobilization Splints

Finger MP immobilization splints may be used to promote healing, control early postoperative motion, or enhance functional use. These splints may involve one or more joints and, depending on the specific requirements, may be fitted dorsally, palmarly, or laterally. While some specialized postoperative splints immobilize the MPs in extension, it is far more common to immobilize the MP joints in flexion. The antideformity position for the MP joints is 70-90° of MP flexion, but other positions are used depending on patient-specific needs. For example, finger MP joint extension immobilization splints protect extensor digitorum communis repairs; and MP flexion immobilization splints prevent MP collateral ligament shortening. As noted above, the antideformity position holds MP joint collateral ligaments at full length, thereby preventing their recurrent predisposition to shorten when not under stress.[9,10,29]

Type 0. *Type 0 finger MP immobilization splints* incorporate only the MP joints as primary joints (Fig. 11-1, *A*). There are no secondary joints in *type 0 MP immobilization splints* and the wrist and finger interphalangeal joints are permitted full, unencumbered motion. The MP joints may be positioned in abduction, adduction, extension, flexion, radial deviation or ulnar deviation.

Type 1. In addition to incorporating the MP joints, *type 1 finger MP immobilization splints* incorporate one secondary joint either proximal or distal to the primary MP joints, depending on individual patient requisites.

Type 2. *Finger MP immobilization splints, type 2,* incorporate two secondary joints in addition to the primary MP joints. Secondary joints may lie proximal, distal (Fig. 11-1, *B*), or one proximal and one distal to the MP joints.

Mobilization Splints

Splinting for mobilization of a metacarpophalangeal joint should incorporate a 90° rotational force on the

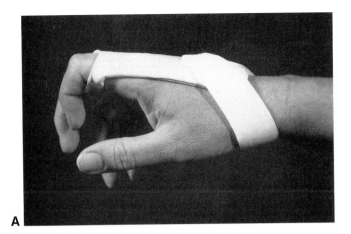

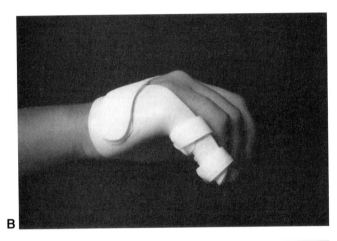

Fig. 11-1   A, Index finger MP extension immobilization splint, type 0 (1) B, Small finger MP flexion immobilization splint, type 2 (3)

A, Fitted dorsally, this immobilization splint prevents articular motion at the metacarpophalangeal joint. B, Incorporation of the lateral aspect of the fifth digit provides stability to this splint that maintains the metacarpophalangeal joint in flexion, allowing the radial collateral ligament to heal.

distal aspect of the proximal phalanx. This force must also be perpendicular to the axis of rotation in the mobilization plane of the involved joint. If a perpendicular pull is not achieved, unequal force will be applied to the periarticular ligaments, which may cause attenuation and result in harmful ulnar or radial deviation of the digit. To allow full flexion, the palmar metacarpal bar of an MP flexion splint should not extend beyond the distal palmar flexion crease. If distal migration of the splint limits metacarpophalangeal motion, an elbow cuff, triceps cuff, or diagonal splint straps may be added to further stabilize the splint on the extremity. A lining of nonskid material such as Dycem* may assist in limiting distal migration

*Dycem, P.O. Box 6920, 83 Gilbane St., Warwick, RI 02887

of the splint. The choice between a hand-based or forearm splint design depends on the presence or absence of extrinsic adhesions producing a tenodesis effect or on poor habitual posturing of the wrist. Mobilization assist design and material depend on the degree of contracture, length of time, and presence of end-range "give" of involved MP joints.

Type 0. *Finger MP mobilization splints* affect motion only at the primary MP joints. Secondary joint levels are not included in *type 0 MP mobilization splints*. These splints may be designed to improve MP abduction (Fig. 11-2, *A*), adduction, extension (Fig. 11-2, *B*), or flexion (Fig. 11-2, *C-E*).

Type 1. *Type 1 MP mobilization splints* incorporate one secondary joint, either proximally or distally to the primary focus MP joint(s). If the wrist is included as a secondary joint, extrinsic musculotendinous units are affected in addition to articular motion at the MP joint. *Type 1 MP mobilization splints* may be designed to improve finger MP abduction (Fig. 11-3, *A,B*), adduction, extension (Fig. 11-3, *C-E*), flexion (Fig. 11-3, *F-J*), supination, pronation, or circumduction.

Type 2. In addition to the primary MP joints, two secondary joints are included in *MP mobilization splints, type 2*. Secondary joints may be split with one proximal and one distal to the MP joints, or both secondary joints may be situated distal to the MPs. Two proximal secondary joints would include the elbow in addition to the wrist—an unlikely clinical scenario. *Type 2 MP mobilization splints* may be fitted to improve MP abduction, adduction, extension (Fig. 11-4, *A*), flexion (Fig. 11-4, *B,C*), supination, pronation, or circumduction.

Type 3 and More. *Type 3 MP mobilization splints* incorporate three secondary joints in addition to the primary MP joints. Usually, the secondary joints are split with one proximal (wrist) and two distal levels (PIP and DIP) (Fig. 11-5, *A,B*). *Type 5 MP mobilization splints* may exhibit idiosyncratic designs reflecting individual patient needs. For example, they may have unusual designs that include an innovative combination of same-level and distal secondary joints within two or more adjacent finger rays (Fig. 11-5, *C-E*).

Mobilization/Restriction Splints

Type 1. *Type 1* splints that both mobilize and restrict the MP joint have one secondary joint level, usually the wrist. *MP extension mobilization/flexion restriction splints, type 1*, typically are used to treat extensor tendon injuries in Zones V, VI, and VII (Fig. 11-6).

Text continued on p. 290

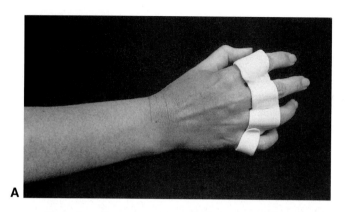

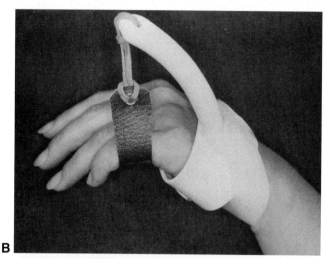

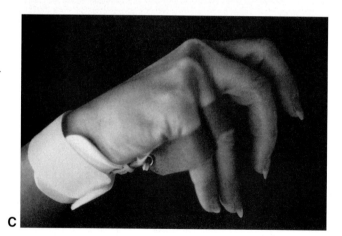

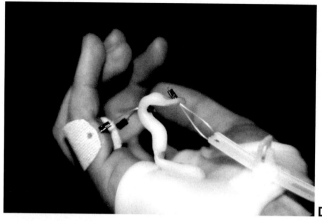

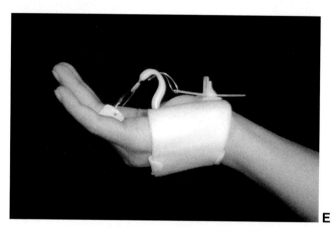

Fig. 11-2   A, Index, ring–small finger MP abduction mobilization splint, type 0 (4) B, Small finger MP extension mobilization splint, type 0 (1) C, Ring–small finger MP flexion mobilization splint, type 0 (2) D, Small finger MP flexion mobilization splint, type 0 (1) E, Ring finger MP flexion mobilization splint, type 0 (1)

Type 0 finger metacarpophalangeal mobilization splints may augment abduction (**A**), extension (**B**), or flexion (**C-E**). **A,** To improve finger MP abduction, the fingers are extended and mobilizing forces are directed toward the ulnar side of the index proximal phalanx, the radial sides of the ring, and small proximal phalanges, away from the stable long finger ray. **D-E,** This specialized outrigger maintains a 90° angle to the proximal phalanx as MP joint motion changes, and the unique inelastic mobilization assist facilitates tension adjustments. [Courtesy (**D,E**) Nelson Vazquez, OTR, CHT, Miami, Fla., and Damon Kirk, WFR Corporation, Wyckoff, N.J.]

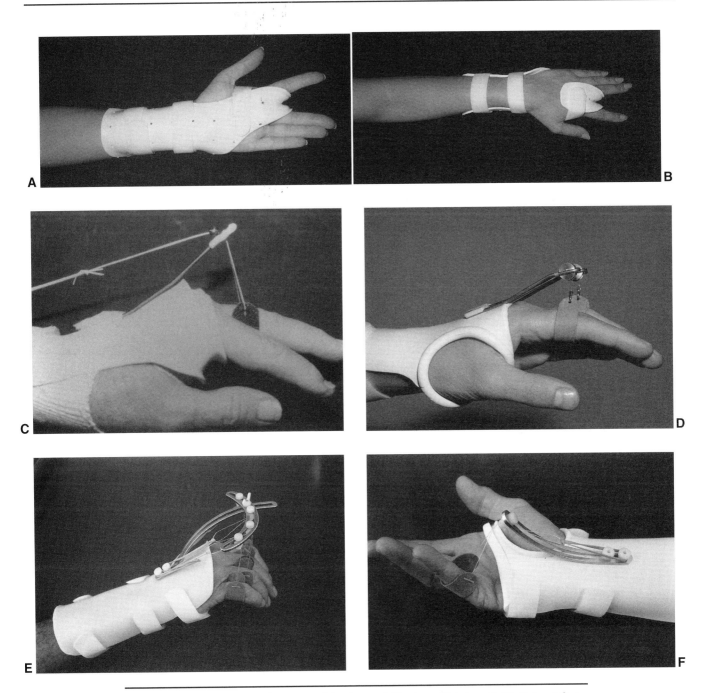

Fig. 11-3   A,B, Index–long finger MP abduction mobilization splint, type 1 (3) C, Long finger MP extension mobilization splint, type 1 (2) D, Index–long finger MP extension mobilization splint, type 1 (3) E, Index–small finger MP extension mobilization splint, type 1 (5) F, Small finger MP flexion mobilization splint, type 1 (2) G,H, Index–ring finger MP flexion mobilization splint, type 1 (4) I, Index–small finger MP flexion mobilization splint, type 1 (5) J, Index–small finger MP flexion mobilization splint, type 1 (5)

These *type 1 finger MP mobilization splints* are designed to increase abduction **(A,B)**, extension **(C-E)**, or flexion **(F-J)** of the MP joints. Despite different configurations and force directions, these splints function mechanically in a similar manner. **H,** Radial view of the splint shown in G. [Courtesy **(A,B)** Jerilyn Nolan, MA, OTR, CHT, Norwalk, Conn.; **(C)** Kathryn Schultz, OTR, CHT, Orlando, Fla.; **(D)** Esther May, PhD, OT, Adelaide, South Australia; **(E,F)** Helen Marx, OTR, CHT, Human Factors Engineering of Phoenix, Wickenburg, Ariz.; **(G,H)** Barbara Smith, OTR, Edmond, Okla.; **(J)** Rachel Dyrud Ferguson, OTR, CHT, Taos, N.M.; **(I)** Karen Schultz-Johnson, MS, OTR, FAOTA, CHT, UE-Tech, Edwards, Colo.]

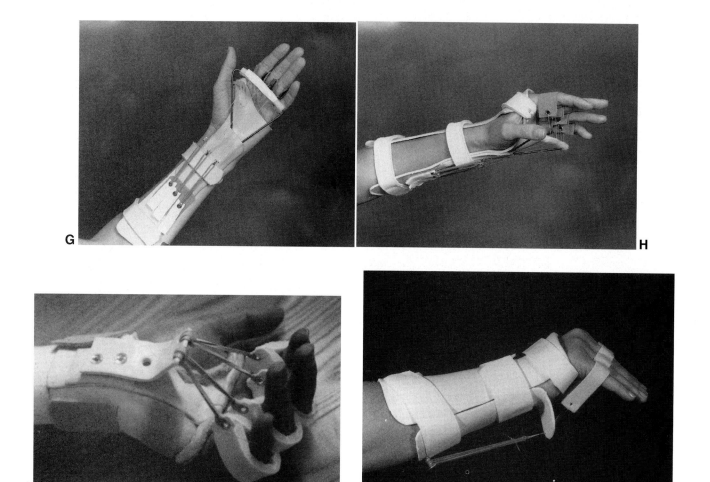

G

H

I

J

Fig. 11-3, cont'd
For legend see p. 287.

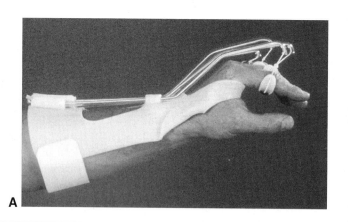

A

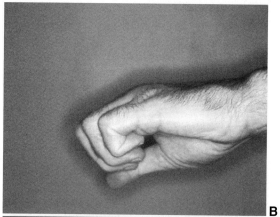

B

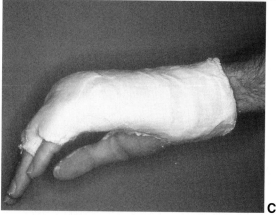

C

Fig. 11-4 A, Index–small finger MP extension mobilization splint, type 2 (9) C, Index small finger MP flexion mobilization splint, type 2 (9)

Incorporating two secondary joints, *type 2 mobilization splints* may use elastic (A) or inelastic (C) traction to remodel adherent soft tissues. (A) Rigid thermoplastic slings prevent full PIP joint motion, making this splint a *type 2*. Note the lack of MP flexion before splinting initiated (B) and after 2 weeks of serially applied MP flexion mobilization splints (C). [Courtesy (A) Paul Van Lede, OT, MS, Orfit Industries, Wijnegem, Belgium; (B,C) Christopher Bochenek, OTR/L, CHT, Cincinnati, Ohio.]

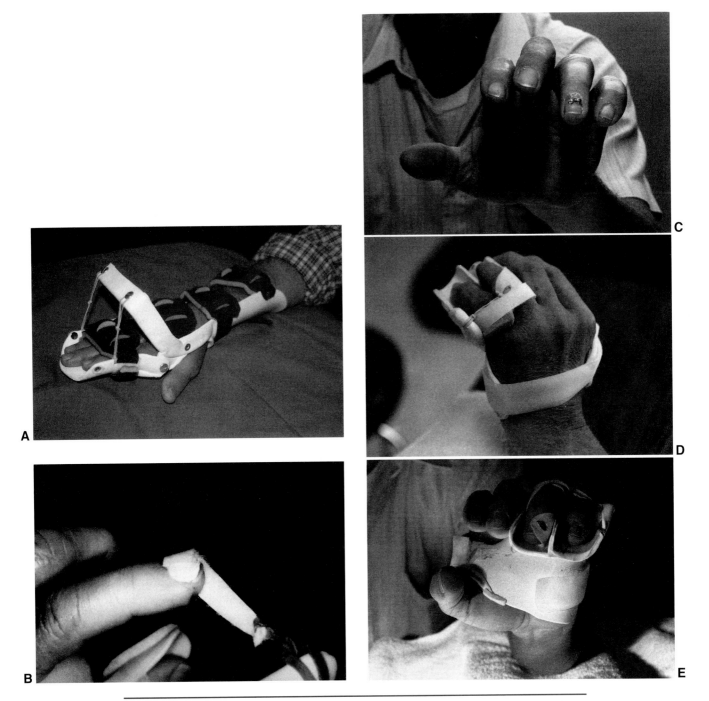

Fig. 11-5   A, Index–small finger MP extension mobilization splint, type 3 (13) B, Index finger MP supination mobilization splint, type 3 (4) D,E, Ring finger MP supination mobilization splint, type 5 (6)
A,B, *Type 3 MP mobilization splints* that incorporate two distal secondary joints utilize longer lever arms to affect MP joint motion. **C-E,** An innovative *type 5 MP supination mobilization splint* pairs the involved fourth finger with the normal fifth finger to achieve supination of the fourth MP joint, the only primary joint included in the splint. [Courtesy **(A)** Jason Willoughby, OTR, Richmond, Ky.; **(C-E)** Sandra Robinson, OTR, CHT, Elmira, N.Y., and Jill Townsend, PT, CHT, West Chester, Pa.]

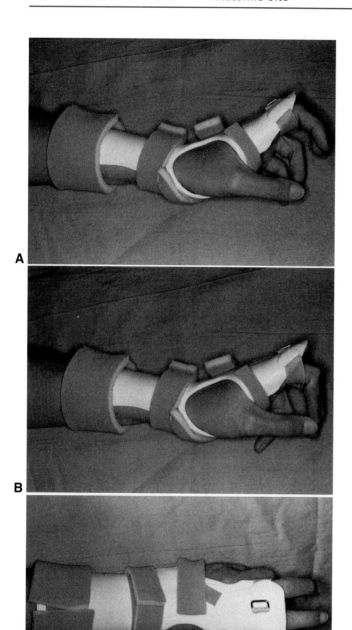

Fig. 11-6 A-C, Index–long finger MP extension mobilization / flexion restriction splint, type 1 (3)
With one secondary joint—the wrist—this splint (A) assists extension of the index and long finger MP joints and (B) restricts index and long finger MP flexion. C, Dorsal view. (Courtesy Lori Klerekoper DeMott, OTR, CHT, Columbus, Ohio.)

Restriction Splints

Splints designed to partially limit finger MP motion may affect motion in one or more planes and they may or may not incorporate secondary joints. Both articulated and nonarticulated MP restriction splints are used to control partial arcs of MP motion. Splint design and strap placement are predicated on specific criteria for fitting the splint and the need to obtain a firm purchase on the finger metacarpals and proximal phalanges while simultaneously allowing controlled motion of the primary MP joint(s).

Type 0. *Type 0 finger MP restriction splints* incorporate no secondary joints. They may be used to limit MP joint abduction, adduction, extension, flexion, supination, pronation, radial deviation (Fig. 11-7, *A*), ulnar deviation[23] (Fig. 11-7, *B-D*), or circumduction. The proximal aspects of *type 0 MP restriction splints* should not impede wrist motion, and to provide optimum mechanical advantage, phalangeal bars on these splints should extend as far distally on the proximal phalanx as possible without interfering with PIP joint motion. *Finger MP restriction splints, type 0,* allow healing of specific MP joint capsule structures while permitting motion that is not disruptive to the reparative process. They are also used to enhance finger function through improved MP joint positioning.

Type 1 and More. *Finger MP restriction splints* with one secondary joint level are classified as *type 1,* those with two secondary joint levels are *type 2,* and so on. Secondary joint levels lie proximal or distal to the primary focus MP joint(s) or they may be split with the primary MPs situated between the secondary joints.

Torque Transmission Splints

Finger MP torque transmission splints transfer moment to primary joints that are situated beyond the boundaries of the splint itself, or if primary joints are included within the splint, they are "driven" by harnessed secondary joints that are also included within the boundaries of the splint. Torque transmission splints may transfer moment longitudinally or transversely. Often referred to as "exercise" splints, these splints are used to remodel soft tissue structures and improve joint motion, and are often paired with specific exercises and with functional activities.

Type 1 and More. Torque transmission splints affecting finger MP joints may have one, two, or three secondary joint levels incorporated in these splints and are categorized as *type 1, type 2,* or *type 3,* respectively. Splints that function longitudinally to transmit torque to the MP joints limit motion of the IP joints distally so that extrinsic muscle power is focused on the MP joints. These splints also may be paired with MP torque transmission splints that limit secondary wrist motion proximally (Fig. 11-7, *E*).

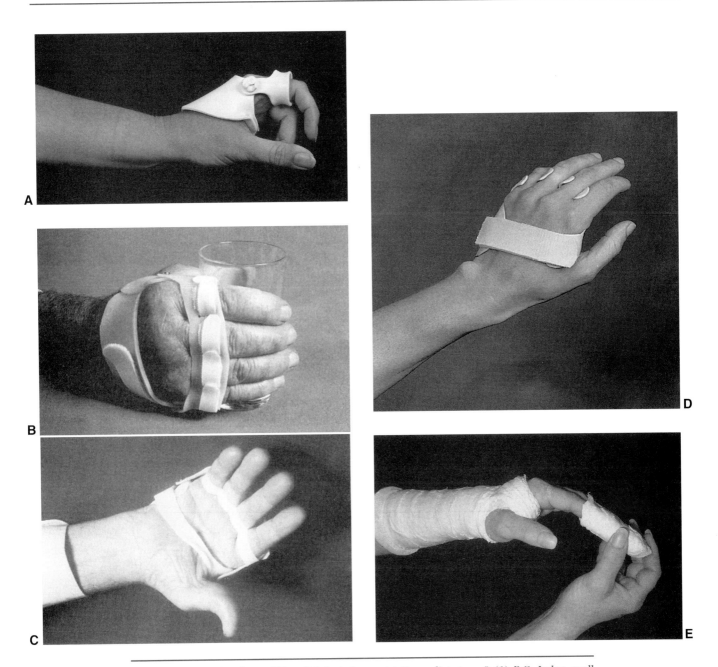

Fig. 11-7   A, Index finger MP radial deviation restriction splint, type 0 (1) B,C, Index–small finger MP ulnar deviation restriction splint, type 0 (4) D, Index–small finger MP extension, flexion, and ulnar deviation restriction splint, type 0 (4) E, Index–small finger MP extension and flexion torque transmission splint, type 2 (12) \\ Index–small finger MP extension and flexion torque transmission splint, type 1 (13)
Articulated **(A-C)** and nonarticulated **(D)** MP deviation restriction splints align MP joints to improve hand function. C, Palmar view of the splint shown in B. E, Torque transmission splints that affect the MP joints may control secondary IP joint levels, they may control the wrist secondarily, or the two splints may work together to transmit extrinsic muscle power to the MP joints. Note that the *type 2* splint includes the wrist and the *type 1* splint includes the fingers. [**(B,C)** from Rennie HJ: Evaluation of the effectiveness of a metacarpophalangeal ulnar deviation orthosis, *J Hand Ther* 9(4):371-7, 1996. Courtesy **(D)** Barbara Smith, OTR, Edmond, Okla.]

Finger MP, PIP Splints

Finger MP-PIP splints range from simple to complex designs depending on individual patient circumstances. Because MP joints are condyloid in nature and move in multiple planes, and PIP joints are hinge articulations with movement in one plane, proper alignment of these longitudinally situated joints is critical to successful splint application. Further, the combined length of proximal and middle phalanges in finger MP-PIP splints results in longer force arms and greater potential torque on respective MP joints, as compared to MP joint splints that incorporate only the proximal phalanges. If immobilization, mobilization, restriction, or torque transmission splints are incorrectly applied, MP, PIP, or MP-PIP joint instability may be produced through unequal collateral ligament remodeling. It is also important to remember that convergence points for single finger and simultaneous finger flexion[8] differ considerably, manifesting in unique normal extension-flexion arcs of motion for each finger. Joint axis of rotation, planes of motion, and arcs of motion alone and in the company of adjacent joints all must be considered when fabricating finger MP-PIP splints. Errors in joint alignment are magnified as successive longitudinal joints are incorporated in splints.

The interphalangeal joints of the fingers are true hinge, or ginglymoid, joints, allowing motion in only the sagittal plane. The ligamentous structure of these joints is similar to that of the metacarpophalangeal joints in that there are two collateral ligaments and one palmar plate ligament per joint. However, the interphalangeal joints differ from the metacarpophalangeal joints in that the articular surfaces of the interphalangeal joints travel in the same arc throughout their full range and produce an almost constant tension on the collateral ligaments regardless of joint position. The changes that do occur vary in the dorsal and palmar halves of the ligaments. When the proximal interphalangeal joint is in extension, the dorsal portion is slack and the palmar portion is taut. When the joint is flexed, the reverse is true. The interphalangeal joints, unlike the metacarpophalangeal joints, have a tendency to develop flexion contractures, although they may become contracted in extension as well.

Immobilization Splints

Splints that immobilize the finger MP and PIP joints follow the general concepts noted earlier. The antideformity position for the MP joints is 70-90° of MP flexion and the antideformity position for the PIP joint is 0-10°. The MP flexion and IP extension posture maintains optimal collateral ligament length at both joints, counteracting predictable deforming forces at these joints that occur after injury. Postoperative immobilization splinting is surgery-specific, requiring close communication between surgeon and therapist to ensure that splints meet highly specialized requisites of individualized operative procedures.

Mobilization Splints

Because two consecutive longitudinal joints are involved, splinting to increase motion simultaneously at the MP and PIP joints is more complicated than splinting to improve motion at either joint alone. The mobilizing angle of force application must be perpendicular to the rotational axes of both the MP and PIP joints and it must also be perpendicular to the proximal and middle phalanges. If only one mobilization force is employed on the middle phalanx, the combined lengths of the proximal and middle phalanges create a longer moment arm on the MP joint as compared to that of the single-segment length of the middle phalanx on the PIP joint. It is difficult to maintain appropriate levels of remodeling torque at both joints with just one mobilizing source. Splints using a one-force design must be carefully monitored to ensure that remodeling of joint structures progresses at an equal rate at both the MP and PIP joints. It is easy to create unequal changes between the two joints with the most common problem that of range of motion improvement at the MP joint but not at the PIP joint. The longer lever arm also increases the potential to apply too much torque to the MP joint, resulting in microscopic tearing of the tissue rather than the desired soft tissue remodeling.

Type 0. There are no secondary joints in *type 0 finger MP-PIP mobilization splints*. These splints are most often designed to improve extension or flexion of MP and PIP joints simultaneously and they may employ one or two mobilization forces (Fig. 11-8, *A*).

Type 1. *Type 1 finger MP-PIP mobilization splints* incorporate one secondary joint level, which may be positioned proximally or distally to the primary MP-PIP joints. Inclusion of the wrist as the secondary joint usually is indicative of extrinsic musculotendinous involvement, whereas if the DIP joint level is secondary, the problem is articular in nature (Fig. 11-8, *B-D*).

Type 2. Finger MP-PIP mobilization splints include two secondary joint levels, usually configured with one proximal to the primary MP-PIP joints and one distal. Splints are designed to improve either extension or flexion.

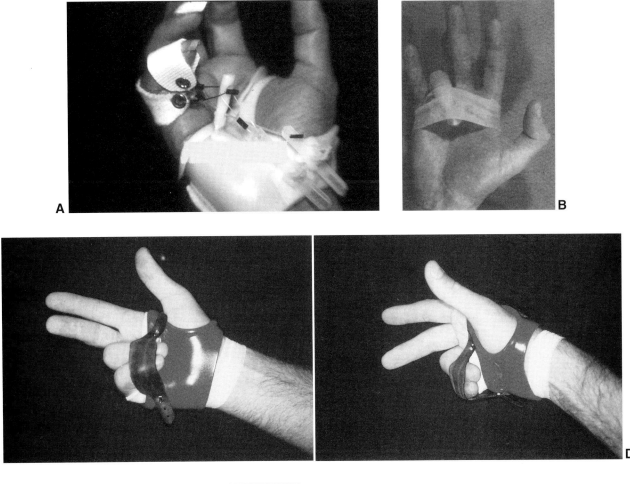

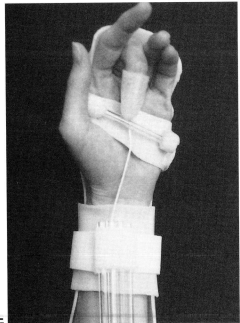

Fig. 11-8   **A, Small finger MP-PIP flexion mobilization splint, type 0 (2) B, Ring finger MP-PIP flexion mobilization splint, type 1 (3) C,D, Ring-small finger MP-PIP flexion mobilization splint, type 1 (6) E, Index–small finger MP extension restriction / long finger MP-PIP flexion mobilization splint, type 2 (7)**
A, Inelastic traction directed to each joint separately remodels soft tissue that restrains flexion motion of the fifth finger MP and PIP joints. **B-D,** These *type 1 MP-IP flexion mobilization splints* include the DIP joints as secondary joint levels. **D,** Another view of C. **E,** A palmar pulley controls MP joint rotation with long finger MP and PIP joint flexion in this *type 2* dual purpose restriction / mobilization splint. [Courtesy **(A)** Nelson Vazquez, OTR, CHT, Miami, Fla., and Damon Kirk, WFR Corporation, Wyckoff, N.J.; **(C,D)** Griet Van Veldhoven, OT, Orthop E., Heverlee, Belgium; **(E)** Paul Van Lede, OT, MS Hlth. Sc., Orfit Industries, Wijnegem, Belgium.]

Restriction/Mobilization Splints

MP-PIP restriction/mobilization splints have dual purposes. Occasionally used to treat patients with tendon repairs, these splints restrict motion of some MP or PIP primary joints while mobilizing other MP or PIP primary joints. Type ranges from 0 to 3. Exclusion of the DIP joints as primary joints renders these splints less efficient in their abilities to control and protect the entire lengths of the fingers (Fig. 11-8, *E*).

Torque Transmission Splints

Torque transmission splints are most often designed to transfer moments to joints external to the splints themselves, although there are instances when the recipient joints lie within the splint boundaries. The transfer of moment may be in a longitudinal or transverse direction to the secondary control joint(s). Single-purpose torque transmission splints have a minimum of one secondary joint level. These splints are often referred to as "exercise" splints because they are used to maintain or increase motion in conjunction with functional hand use.

Type 1. One secondary joint level is included in *type 1 finger MP-PIP torque transmission splints*. The secondary joint level may be proximal, as with the wrist, or distal, as with the DIP joint, to the primary MP-PIP joints. These splints control position of either the wrist or DIP joint in order to transfer moment to the MP and PIP joints to influence motion or remodeling of soft tissue periarticular structures.

Type 2. *Type 2 finger MP-PIP torque transmission splints* incorporate two secondary joint levels while affecting motion at the primary MP and PIP joints. When the transfer of moment is oriented transversely, the MP and PIP joints of an adjacent normal finger may act as secondary "drivers" for the problematic primary MP and PIP joints (Fig. 11-9, *A-C*).

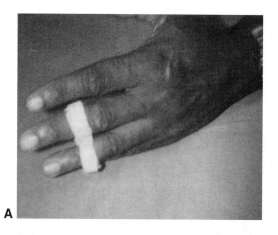

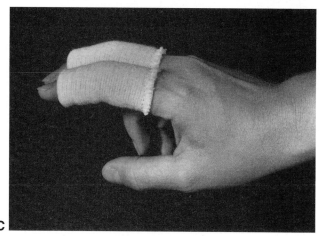

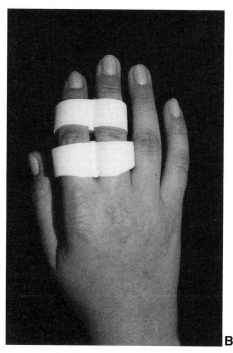

Fig. 11-9
For legend see opposite page.

Finger MP, PIP, DIP Splints

Splints that act on all three successive longitudinal joints of the fingers involve complex mechanical factors that, if not fully understood, may result in failure of splints to achieve their intended purposes. The respective axes of the MP, PIP, and DIP joints must be carefully aligned to apply equal force(s) to the collateral ligaments. Also, it is important to remember that alignment problems are magnified with the addition of each intercalated segment. Individual and simultaneous finger convergence points differ. The fingers, when flexed individually, converge most often at a point near the base of the thumb. In contrast, when the fingers are flexed simultaneously, the convergence point moves proximally to the radial aspect, middle third, of the forearm. Normal convergence points exhibit a fairly wide range of variations. It is critical that each patient be methodically assessed in this regard when splints affect motion at all three finger joints. Also, keep in mind that finger abduction is greater in extension than in flexion where the MP collateral ligaments are at their greatest tension. All of these concepts directly have bearing on splint design and fit, and on component shape and placement.

Immobilization Splints

Finger immobilization splints are applied to allow tissue healing or to provide optimal positioning of finger joints during times of rest. Splints whose primary purposes are to immobilize all three primary finger joints may or may not include the wrist as a secondary joint. When extrinsic tendons are not involved in the pathology, a hand-based splint may be fabricated to immobilize the MP, PIP, and DIP joints. If, however, wrist position negatively influences finger joint posture, stability, or physiologic homeostasis, the wrist, as secondary joint, must be included in the splint to control detrimental tenodesis effect or to prevent complications such as spread of infection.

Type 0. *Type 0 finger immobilization splints* have no secondary joint levels. The three most distal joints within the digital ray, the MP, PIP, and DIP joints are primary joints in these splints that are designed to immobilize a single finger (Fig. 11-10, *A*) or multiple fingers (Fig. 11-10, *B*). Care must be taken to ensure that these immobilization splints permit full active motion of the wrist joint. Finger joints may be positioned in abduction, extension, flexion, or a combination thereof. Straps should hold the fingers securely in the splint, disallowing finger joint motion; to increase splint mechanical advantage and durability, splint length should be as long as possible without limiting motion of proximal joints not included in the splint, and splint width should be one half the thickness of the segments being splinted.

Type 1. Incorporating the wrist as a secondary joint, *type 1 finger immobilization splints* control the effect of extrinsic tendons on the MP, PIP, and DIP joints of the finger(s). Allowing tension to be increased or decreased on the extrinsic tendons, the wrist may be positioned in neutral, extension, flexion, or deviation, depending on patient-specific requirements. As with type 0 finger immobilization splints, *type 1 finger immobilization splints* may be designed to include one or more fingers (Fig. 11-10, *C,D*).[21]

Mobilization Splints

Acting on the MP, PIP, and DIP joints simultaneously, finger mobilization splints are designed either to maintain or create joint motion of supple finger joints or to increase joint motion of stiffened finger joints through gradual soft tissue remodeling. Elastic or inelastic traction may be used in finger mobilization splints.

Type 0. *Type 0 finger mobilization splints* have no secondary joints; only the primary MP, PIP, and DIP joints are included. Full wrist motion is permitted in these hand-based splints. Single or multiple fingers may be incorporated (Fig. 11-11, *A*) and direction of the mobilizing force(s) must be perpendicular to the

Fig. 11-9   A, Long finger MP-PIP extension and flexion torque transmission splint, type 2 (4) B, Long finger MP-PIP extension and flexion torque transmission splint, type 2 (4) C, Long finger MP-PIP extension and flexion torque transmission splint, type 2 (4)
By harnessing adjacent digits together at the middle phalanx (**A**), at the middle and distal phalanges (**B**), or at the proximal and middle phalanges (**C**), torque transmission splints use active extension and flexion of the normal index finger to mobilize the MP and PIP joints of the adjacent long finger, which lacks full active range of motion. [Courtesy (**A**) Carol Hierman, OTR, CHT, Cedar Grove, N.C. and Elisha Denny, PTA, OTA, Pittsboro N.C.; © Hand Rehabilitation Center, UNC, Chapel Hill, N.C.; (**C**) Rachel Dyrud Ferguson, OTR, CHT, Taos, N.M.)

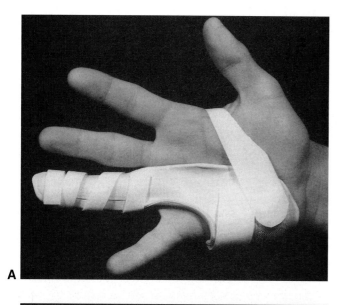

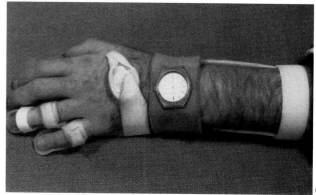

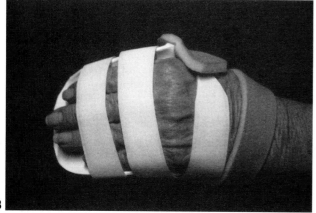

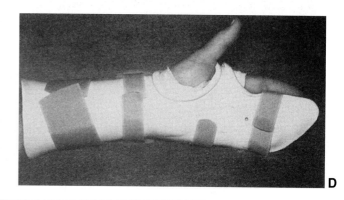

Fig. 11-10 **A,** Ring finger extension immobilization splint, type 0 (3) **B,** Index–small finger MP flexion and IP extension immobilization splint, type 0 (12) **C,** Ring–small finger extension immobilization splint, type 1 (7) **D,** Long–small finger extension immobilization splint, type 1 (10) **A,B,** *Type 0 finger immobilization splints* do not include the wrist as a secondary joint. **C,** Cleverly, this patient's watch has been included in the middle strap of his *type 1 finger immobilization splint!* Additions of jewelry, stickers, or artwork are but a few ways patients personalize their splints. **D,** Leaving the index finger and thumb unencumbered by this *type 1 finger immobilization splint* aids functional use of the extremity. [Courtesy **(C)** Brenda Hilfrank, PT, CHT, South Burlington, Vt.; **(D)** from Prosser R, Conolly WB: Complications following surgical treatment for Dupuytren's contracture, *J Hand Ther* 9(4):344-8, 1996.]

axis of each successive finger joint (Fig. 11-11, *B*). In addition, the mobilizing force(s) should be perpendicular to the three intercalated phalanges of the finger(s). Failure to achieve a 90° angle of force application may result in damaging collateral ligament attenuation. With a greater torque to the MP joint due to summation of phalangeal lengths, this is especially problematic when IPs joints are relatively stiffer than are their associated MP joint(s).

Type 1. The wrist, a secondary joint, is included in *type 1 finger mobilization splints*. One or multiple fingers may be included in these splints designed

to effect or increase motion of finger abduction, adduction, flexion (Fig. 11-11, *C-E*), or extension. In special circumstances when increased independent extrinsic tendon glide is needed, finger mobilization splints may be designed to increase simultaneous separate finger motion in opposite directions (Fig. 11-11, *F*).

Restriction/Mobilization Splints

Splints that restrict and mobilize MP, PIP, and DIP finger joints frequently are created to address specific postoperative needs, combining specialized compo-

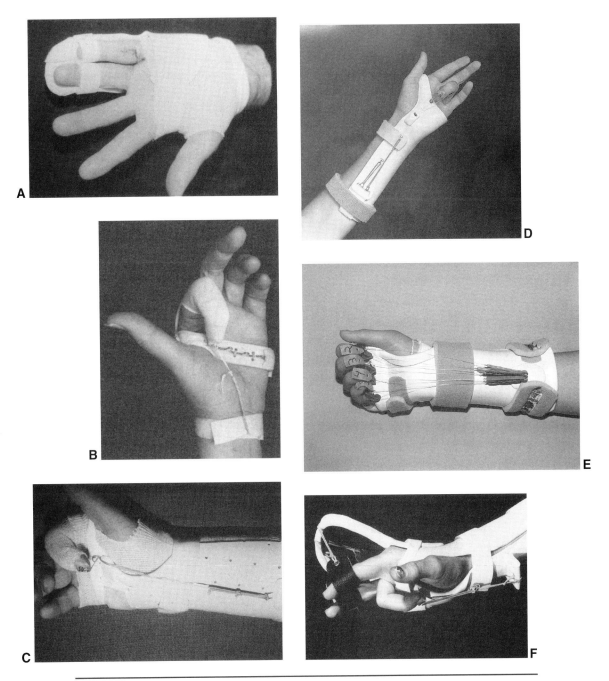

Fig. 11-11   **A,** Ring finger MP-PIP, small finger extension mobilization splint, type 0 (5) **B,** Index finger flexion mobilization splint, type 0 (3) **C,** Index finger flexion mobilization splint, type 1 (4) **D,** Ring finger flexion mobilization splint, type 1 (4) **E,** Index–small finger flexion mobilization splint, type 1 (13) **F,** Index, ring finger extension and long finger flexion mobilization splint, type 1 (10) or index–ring finger extension mobilization splint, type 1 (10) **A,** A *type 0 dorsal finger extension splint* allows the healing wound to be kept aerated and dry. **B,** This splint is constructed of materials other than low-temperature plastic. Work environments or patient allergies may dictate materials used in splint construction. **C-E,** Various and innovative methods for guiding and proximally attaching mobilization assists to their respective splints are demonstrated on these *type 1 finger flexion mobilization splints.* Velcro, thermoplastic material, and embedded paper clips are but a few of the many methods used to secure mobilization assists to splints. **F,** By controlling wrist position and applying a triad of alternate forces to adjacent fingers, final increments of tendon excursion are obtained. [Courtesy **(A)** Kathryn Schultz, OTR, CHT, Orlando, Fla.; **(B)** from Hollis LI: Innovative splinting ideas. In Hunter J, et al: *Rehabilitation of the hand,* ed 1, Mosby Company, 1978, St. Louis, Mo.; **(C)** Brenda Hilfrank, PT, CHT, South Burlington, Vt.; **(D)** Barbara Smith, OTR, Edmond, Okla.; **(E)** Joni Armstrong, OTR, CHT, Bemidji, Minn.; **(F)** Roslyn Evans, OTR, CHT, Vero Beach, Fla.]

nents into one combination splint. These innovative splints are often, but not always, associated with treatment of repaired flexor tendons in Zone II.

Type 1. *Type 1 finger restriction / mobilization splints* include the wrist as a secondary joint. Integration of a removable, semi-rigid palmar phalangeal bar in the splint design allows minute increments of DIP extension (Fig. 11-12, *A*). Mobilization assists passively flex the fingers (Fig. 11-12, *B*) and the dorsal finger pan restricts active finger extension from the flexed position (Fig. 11-12, *C*), generating an increment of extrinsic flexor tendon excursion to reduce and/or elongate tendon adhesions in the area of the Zone II flexor tendon repair. An adjustable wrist bar facilitates changes in wrist position as needed (Fig. 11-12, *D*).

Torque Transmission Splints

Torque transmission splints control one or more joints to transfer moment longitudinally or transversely to primary joints that frequently, but not always, are located outside the borders of the splints, effecting active motion of supple joints or soft tissue remodeling of shortened soft tissue structures. Due to the obligatory presence of at least one secondary joint, the type category in single-purpose torque transmission splints is always greater than zero.

Type 1. *Type 1 finger torque transmission splints* incorporate the wrist proximally as a secondary joint, allowing longitudinal transference of moment to the MP, PIP, and DIP joints (Fig. 11-13). The wrist may be positioned in neutral, flexion, or extension depending on patient-specific requisites. Neutral wrist posi-

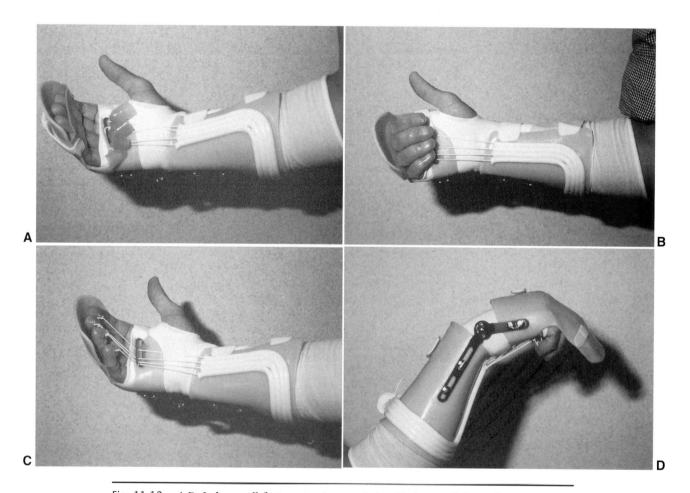

Fig. 11-12   A-D, Index–small finger extension restriction / index–small finger flexion mobilization splint, type 1 (13)
An intelligently creative design allows finger mobilization and restriction purposes in one splint. Used for treating flexor tendon repairs in Zone II, many concepts incorporated in this splint may be adapted to other situations. Multipurpose splints simplify patient wearing schedules by decreasing time spent changing splints; and for tendon repair patients, multipurpose splints are safer, in that there is no time when healing extremities are left unprotected during splint donning and doffing. (Courtesy Griet Van Veldhoven, OT, Orthop. E., Heverlee, Belgium.)

tion balances finger extension and flexion torque transmission; wrist flexion facilitates finger extension torque transmission; and wrist extension assists finger flexion torque transmission.

Type 3. When moment is shifted transversely in finger torque transmission splints, an adjacent normal finger is harnessed as the "drive" finger. The normal finger's three joints are secondary joints to the corresponding three primary joints of the involved finger. A *type 3 finger torque transmission splint* incorporates the distal phalanges of at least two adjacent fingers.

Finger PIP Splints

Anatomy of the proximal interphalangeal joint is complex; it is important that all those involved in treating PIP joint pathology understand normal and abnormal biomechanics of this joint before embarking on any type of treatment intervention. Although approximately 6° of supination occurs with joint flexion,[2] the PIP joint is a hinge joint that allows motion in one plane, extension-flexion. Radial and ulnar collateral ligaments and the palmar plate combine to provide strong articular stability. The central extensor tendon, lateral bands, transverse retinacular ligament, and the oblique retinacular ligament further reinforce PIP joint stability. Generally, the position of antideformity of the PIP joint is 0-10°, although injury-specific positions may differ. To avoid asymmetrical healing or remodeling of collateral ligaments, splints should be designed and fitted so that they apply equal amounts of force to the two respective PIP joint collateral ligaments. The serious consequence of attenuation of a PIP collateral ligament from unbalanced splinting forces is lateral joint instability. While the palmar plate is very strong, it too may be attenuated with incorrectly applied splinting forces.

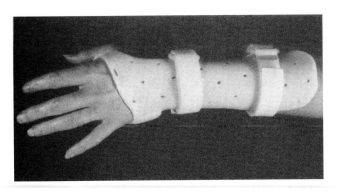

Fig. 11-13 Index–small finger extension and flexion torque transmission splint, type 1 (13)
Secondary wrist immobilization facilitates active finger motion in this *type 1 torque transmission splint*. (Courtesy Sharon Flinn, MEd, OTR/L, CHT, Cleveland, Ohio.)

Communication with the referring physician is fundamental to achieving optimal rehabilitative potential of a proximal interphalangeal joint.

Immobilization Splints

Immobilization splints usually are applied to the proximal interphalangeal joint to prevent injury, to allow healing of injured or repaired tissues, or to externally reinforce various types of surgical hardware used in internal fixation. Tape, rather than straps, is often used to provide accurate and secure splint application, especially in early postoperative cases.

Type 0. *Type 0 PIP immobilization splints* have no secondary joint levels. Only the primary PIP joint is included in these splints (Fig. 11-14, *A*). The PIP joint is most often immobilized in extension but splints may be fitted to immobilize the PIP in degrees of flexion depending on particular patient requisites.

Type 1. One secondary joint level is incorporated in *type 1 PIP immobilization splints*. The secondary joint may be situated proximal or distal (Fig. 11-14, *B,C*) to the primary PIP joint.

Mobilization Splints

Splinting for PIP joint mobilization requires that the angle of approach of the applied rotational force be 90° to the middle phalanx. This force should also be perpendicular to the axis of joint rotation to create equal stress on the collateral ligaments (Fig. 11-15). Because the proximal interphalangeal joint is the intermediate joint of the three digital articulations, splints that influence it often must affect the joints proximal and/or distal to it. If all the joints within the ray possess similar degrees of mobility, and if wrist position does not affect digital motion, a hand-based splint design that applies a single mobilizing force to all three longitudinally oriented joints in the ray may be chosen. However, if discrepancies exist in the relative mobility of the successive joints within the digital ray, measures must be taken to control the more mobile joint(s) and allow traction to be concentrated on the stiffer PIP joint. Splint designs may provide concomitant secondary stabilization of a segment and primary mobilization of another within the same longitudinal ray. When wrist patterns are poor, or when decreased extrinsic musculotendinous amplitude creates a tenodesis effect on finger joints, secondary wrist immobilization is required. When multiple joints of a digital ray are incorporated within a splint, little room for error exists because the multiple lever arms involved tend to accentuate deformity. It is important that mobilizing forces are correctly applied to all joints they influence. Alignment of a small finger in a PIP mobilization splint can be challenging, requiring extra attention due to the lack of an ulnar supporting border digit and the inherent mobility of the fifth CMC joint.

The PIP joint is by far the most frequently splinted joint in the hand, with mobilization splinting of the PIP joint representing slightly more than 12% of the total number of splints illustrated in this book.

By necessity, the format of this section of the chapter is altered, allowing PIP mobilization splints to be grouped according to direction (e.g., PIP extension splints are presented together, PIP flexion splints are together, etc.).

Extension. Generally speaking, a PIP joint whose fixed flexion deformity is greater than 35° responds more readily to custom-made *PIP extension mobilization splints* using elastic traction or inelastic traction depending on the acuteness of the joint injury.[5] Experience has also shown that for extremely stiff PIP joints, splinting with inelastic traction results in better passive motion than that achieved with elastic traction.

Type 0. *Type 0 PIP extension mobilization splints* employ inelastic (Fig. 11-16, *A,B*) or elastic[20] traction (Fig. 11-16, *C,D*) to remodel capsular and pericapsular soft tissue structures, improving PIP joint motion in extension. Only the primary PIP joints are splinted in these type 0 extension splints. No secondary joints are included. Full motion of the MP and DIP joints is permitted. The decision whether to use elastic or inelastic traction usually depends on the acuteness of the PIP flexion contracture. Requiring careful monitoring, some spring-coil and spring-wire splints have the potential to apply too much rotational force to joints.[7] Correction of long-standing, chronic PIP flexion deformities almost always requires application of inelastic traction in the form of serial splints or serial adjustment to mobilization assists. In contrast, acute PIP flexion deformities, in which the inflammatory process continues, respond well to application of either elastic or inelastic traction.

Type 1. One secondary joint level is incorporated into *type 1 PIP extension mobilization splints*. The secondary joint level may be proximal or distal to the PIP joint. All of the illustrated type 1 PIP extension mobilization splints in this section are three-point reciprocal pressure splints regardless of whether inelas-

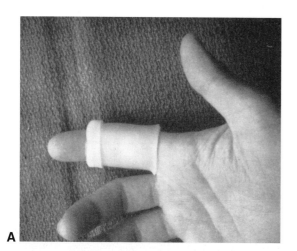

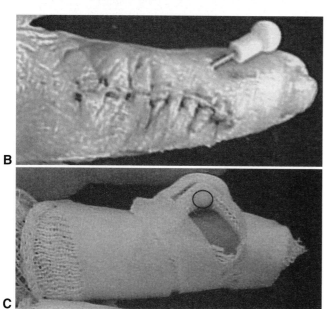

Fig. 11-14   A, Index finger PIP extension immobilization splint, type 0 (1) C, Long finger PIP extension immobilization splint, type 1 (2)
A, Although moment is transferred to the DIP joint, this splint's SCS technical name indicates that its primary purpose is PIP joint immobilization, not torque transmission. **B,** A fixation pin is protected and reinforced by (**C**) a *PIP extension immobilization splint*. [Courtesy (**A**) Brenda Hilfrank, PT, CHT, South Burlington, Vt.]

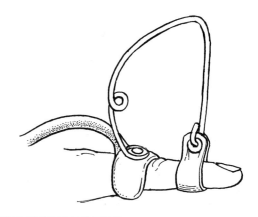

Fig. 11-15   For maximum benefit of traction, the angle of approach should be 90° to the proximal phalanx and perpendicular to the axis of rotation of the PIP joint.

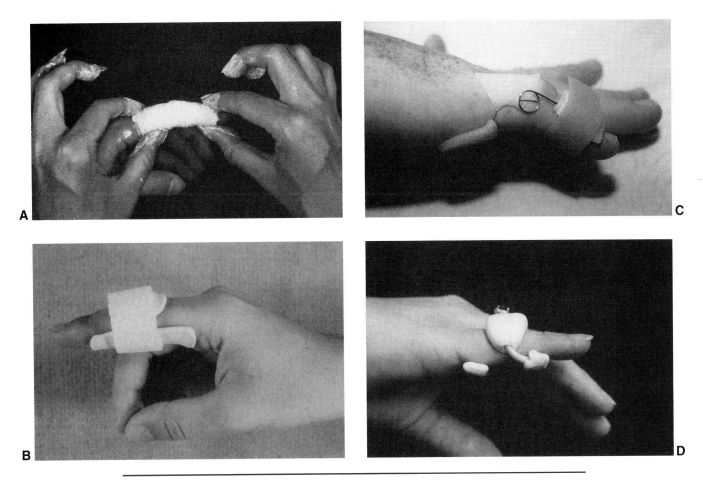

Fig. 11-16 **A,** Index finger PIP extension mobilization splint, type 0 (1) **B,** Index finger PIP extension mobilization splint, type 0 (1) **C,** Small finger PIP extension mobilization splint, type 0 (1) **D,** Small finger PIP extension mobilization splint, type 0 (1)
Type 0 mobilization splints for PIP extension have numerous design options. Splints may employ **(A,B)** inelastic or elastic traction **(C,D).** It is important to monitor spring wire and spring coil splints to ensure that they do not exceed the recommended 100-300 grams of applied mobilizing force. **(A)** Distal edges of this splint will be folded back to allow full DIP motion. [Courtesy **(B)** Jill White, MA, OTR, New York, N.Y.; **(C)** Rosemary Prosser, BApSc, CHT, Sydney, Australia.]

tic[24] (Fig. 11-17, *A-D*) or elastic[27] traction (11-17, *E-K*) is applied. While inclusion of the DIP joint as the secondary joint level mechanically lengthens the mobilizing lever arm to the full length of the middle phalanx, care must be taken during fitting to ensure that the distal reciprocal force is directed to the distal aspect of the middle phalanx and not to the distal phalanx, diminishing rotational force at the PIP joint and causing potentially damaging DIP joint extension/hyperextension. Experience and analysis of mechanical factors find that commercial three-point pressure inelastic traction digital splints, including the "safety pin" and "joint jack," are more effective at correcting flexion deformities that measure approximately 35° or less (see Chapter 6: Mechanical Principles) than they are at correcting flexion contractures greater than 35°.

If MP joints are included as secondary joints, the dorsal phalangeal bar must have a 90° angle of force application to the dorsum of the proximal phalanges to eliminate shear; it must also achieve full-width, contiguous contact with the dorsal aspect of the proximal phalanges to reduce the pressure at this site of middle reciprocal force application (Fig. 11-17, *E*). For acute flexion deformities with end-range "give," palmar phalangeal bars may not be required to prevent MP joint subluxation that can occur as an opposite reaction to the extension forces applied to the middle phalanges. An important concept to remember is that the more flexed the MP joints, the less potential for MP subluxation to occur because the MP collateral ligaments become progressively more taut with increased MP flexion. However, when splinting to correct fixed PIP flexion contractures with little

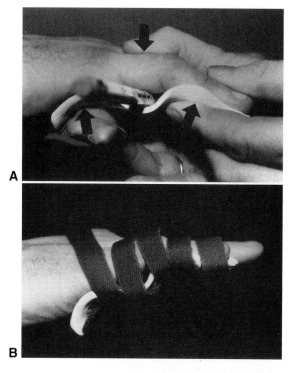

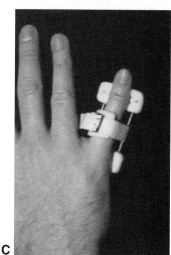

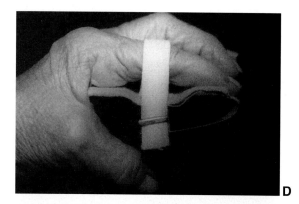

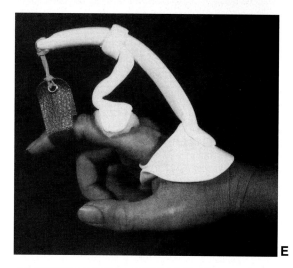

Fig. 11-17 **A-B,** Small finger PIP extension mobilization splint, type 1 (2) **C,** Small finger PIP extension mobilization splint, type 1 (2) **D,** Index finger PIP extension mobilization splint, type 1 (2) **E,** Index finger PIP extension mobilization splint, type 1 (2) **F,G,** Index finger PIP extension mobilization splint, type 1 (2) **H,** Index finger PIP extension mobilization splint, type 1 (2) **I,** Index–long finger PIP extension mobilization splint, type 1 (4) **J,** Index–ring finger PIP extension mobilization splint, type 1 (6) **K,** Index–small finger PIP extension mobilization splint, type 1 (8)

Despite considerable differences in their external configurations, all of these *type 1 PIP extension splints* function similarly through application of three reciprocal mobilizing forces. During fit stage **(A)** a gap is created to provide three-point purchase *(arrows)* **(B)** of the inelastic traction on the joint. **(B-D)** Mechanical advantage for inelastic traction three-point pressure splints is greater for improving proximal interphalangeal joint contractures of 35° or less. **(E-K)** Clinician experience with the many types of dynamic assists, pulleys, and anchors available is important to maintaining clinical competency and expanding options for splint design. Design choice is determined by many factors, including the patient's availability to return for therapy, the acuteness of the deformity, and/or required construction and fitting time. [Courtesy **(A,B)** Elaine LaCroix, MHSM, OTR, CHT, Stoneham, Mass.; **(F,G)** Peggy McLaughlin, OTR, CHT, San Bernadino, Calif.; **(H,J)** Paul Van Lede, OT, MS, Wijnegem, Belgium; **(I)** Theresa Wollenschlaeger, OTR, Ocala, Fla.; **(K)** Barbara Boling, OSSY, North Coast Medical, Inc., Morgan Hill, Calif., and from Srinivasan MS, Knowles D, Wood J: The OSSY splint, a new design of dynamic extension splint, *Br J Hand Ther* 5(3):72-4, 2000.]

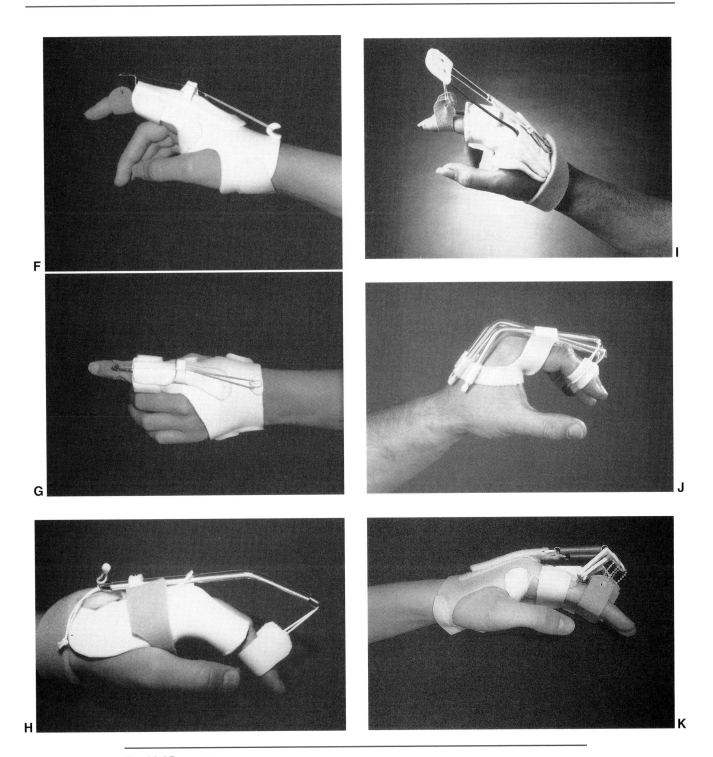

Fig. 11-17, cont'd
For legend see opposite page.

to no end-range "give," addition of palmar phalangeal bar components to protect reaction forces from causing adverse MP subluxation or MP collateral ligament remodeling is requisite to achieving successful results (Fig. 11-17, *F-K*).

Type 2. *Type 2 PIP extension mobilization splints* include two secondary joint levels in addition to the primary PIP joints. The secondary joints may be split proximally and distally on the same finger with the PIP joint between (Fig. 11-18, *A-E*), one secondary joint may be proximal or distal to the PIP joint while the other secondary joint is situated on a different digit altogether, for example, a thumb CMC joint (Fig. 11-18, *F*), or both secondary joints may lie proximal to the PIP joint (Fig. 11-18, *G-J*). The mechanical concepts discussed above for *type 1 PIP extension mobilization splints* also are applicable to *type 2 PIP extension mobilization splints*. Individual finger PIP torque transmission splints may be used concurrently with a *type 2 PIP extension mobilization splint* to

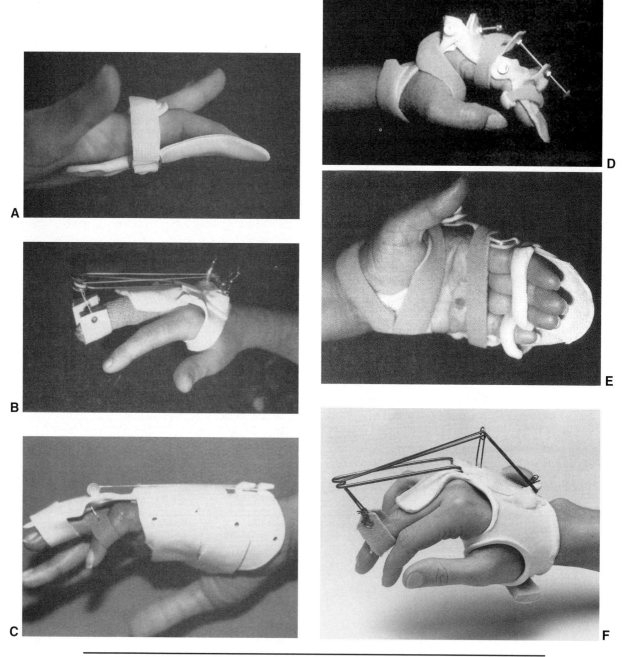

Fig. 11-18
For legend see opposite page.

further focus mobilizing forces on the PIP joints (Fig. 11-18, *J*). Splinting to correct extrinsic flexor tightness may require this two-splint approach where joints proximal and distal to the PIP joints are splinted to affect the multijoint extrinsic digital flexor tendons.

If the *DIP torque transmission splints* are omitted and only the *type 2 extension mobilization splint* is used, adherent flexor digitorum profundi tendons passively flex the DIP joints, abating the effects of the *type 2 splint.*

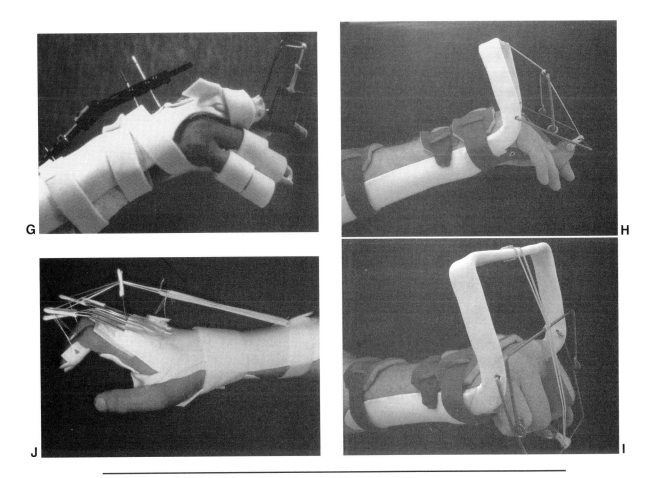

Fig. 11-18   **A,** Index finger PIP extension mobilization splint, type 2 (3) **B,** Long–ring finger PIP extension mobilization splint, type 2 (6) **C,** Ring–small finger PIP extension mobilization splint, type 2 (6) **D,E,** Index–small finger PIP extension or flexion mobilization splint, type 2 (12) **F,** Long finger PIP extension mobilization splint, type 2 (3) **G,** Long finger PIP extension mobilization splint, type 2 (3) \\ Ring finger IP extension immobilization splint, type 0 (2) \\ Small finger IP extension immobilization splint, type 0 (2) **H,I,** Long finger PIP extension mobilization splint, type 2 (3) **J,** Index–small finger PIP extension mobilization splint, type 2 (9) \\ Finger PIP extension torque transmission splint, type 1 (2); 4 splints @ finger separate

A, For mild PIP joint contractures, an extension splint including the MP and DIP joints provides greater mechanical advantage. Use of a D-ring permits greater ease of adjustment. **B,** Considered a *type 2 splint* (the DIP and MP are secondary joints), this splint incorporates the MERIT ™ SPS Component for easy adjustment of the nonelastic mobilization assist tension. Inclusion of the DIP joint increases mechanical advantage of the splint on the PIP joint. **C,** This splint incorporates two forms of mobilization assists: inelastic (ring finger strap) and elastic (small finger). **D,E,** Originally described for active exercise of DIP joints, this splint may also be used to increase extension and/or flexion of stiff PIP joints. **F,** The thumb CMC and long finger MP joints are secondary joint levels in this *type 2 PIP extension mobilization splint.* **G,** Accommodating an external fixation device, the first splint mobilizes the long finger PIP joint. In the second and third splints, ring and small finger IP joints are immobilized in extension. **H,I,** A Crane outrigger maintains a 90° angle as the long finger PIP joint moves through its arc of motion. **J,** Individual *finger PIP extension torque transmission splints* add to mobilizing forces generated by this *type 2 PIP extension mobilization splint.* [Courtesy **(B)** Kathryn Schultz, OTR, CHT, Orlando, Fla.; **(C)** Lin Beribak, OTR/L, CHT, Chicago, Ill.; **(D,E)** From Rose H:MP/PIP adjustable digit blocking splint, *J Hand Ther* 9(3): 247–248, 1996; **(F)** Barbara Allen, OTR, Oklahoma City, Okla.; **(G)** Robin Miller, OTR, CHT, Ft. Lauderdale, Fla.; **(H,I)** Jason Willoughby, OTR, Richmond, Ky.; **(J)** Jill Francisco, OTR, CHT, Cicero, Ind.]

Type 3. In addition to the primary PIP joint(s), three secondary joint levels are included in *type 3 PIP extension mobilization splints*. At least one, and often two, of the secondary joints are situated on the same ray as the problematic PIP joint; the wrist may be included as a secondary joint and, occasionally, a secondary joint may be found on an entirely different digital ray as when the thumb CMC joint is included secondarily to help secure a splint on the hand (Fig. 11-19, *A*). Finger cuffs may control secondary DIP joint posture if the cuffs are sufficiently wide, are made of a semirigid material, and are positioned such that their distal borders extend beyond the DIP joint flexion crease (Fig. 11-19, *B*).[18]

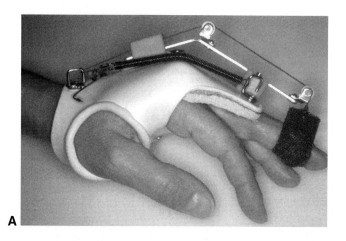

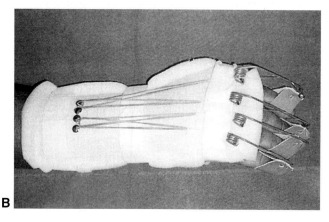

Fig. 11-19   A, Long finger PIP extension mobilization splint, type 3 (4) B, Index–small finger PIP extension mobilization splint, type 3 (13)

A, On a hand-based splint, the mobilization assist is routed through a D-ring to preserve its length. Outrigger adjustments are quick and easy via a setscrew in the plastic block on the dorsal aspect of the splint. B, Finger cuffs hold DIP joints in extension, increasing the rotational moment arm on the PIP joints. [Courtesy (A) Jean Claude Rouzaud, Montpellier, France; (B) from Mazon C, Ulson HJ, Davitt M, et al: The use of synthetic plaster casting tape for hand and wrist splints, *J Hand Ther* 9(4):391-3, 1996.]

Extension, Distraction. Historically associated with poor results, splints that simultaneously place distraction forces on fractures and mobilize and distract associated primary joints are increasingly more accepted as yet another means to provide early motion to capsular and pericapsular soft tissue structures with concomitant phalangeal fractures. A long way from the old "banjo" splint that produced so many problems in the 1940s, these new splints are custom fitted and they reflect more sophisticated understanding of the complex biomechanical concepts involved. Close communication with referring surgeons is an absolute requisite. Previously discussed concepts regarding 90° angle of force application to the axis of joint rotation become even more important with splints that mobilize as they distract fractures and associated articular surfaces. The smallest error in splint alignment may produce misalignment or nonunion of the fracture, or unequal remodeling of soft tissues surrounding primary joints. Careful limitation and monitoring of mobilizing/distracting force magnitude is also critical to ensure that injurious microscopic tissue tearing does not occur instead of tissue growth or remodeling. Because these splints seem to effect soft tissue changes more rapidly than conventional splints, mobilization/distraction splints must be conscientiously monitored once they are applied. The consequences of inattention are poor fracture healing, joint instability, pain, and diminished function.

Type 1. One secondary joint level is incorporated in *type 1 PIP extension and distraction mobilization splints*. The DIP joint is almost always included as the secondary joint in these splints (Fig. 11-20, *A*).

Type 3. *Type 3 PIP extension and distraction mobilization splints* include three secondary joint levels: the wrist, MP joints, and DIP joints (Fig. 11-20, *B,C*).

Flexion. Splints designed to mobilize primary PIP joints into flexion must neutralize or control the more proximally situated MP joints in order to prevent flexion mobilizing forces from being dissipated at the supple MP joints. Depending on splint design and relative acuteness of the extension deformity, control of secondary MP joints may be achieved through dorsal or palmar phalangeal bar components that are continuations of corresponding dorsal or palmar metacarpal bar components.

Type 1. Incorporating one secondary joint, *type 1 PIP flexion mobilization splints* exhibit a variety of configurations, although nearly all of these splints have the commonality of including MP joints secondarily. Both dorsal- and palmar-based designs may be found. Some designs include an articulated outrigger that maintains 90° force application

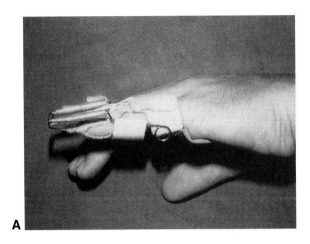

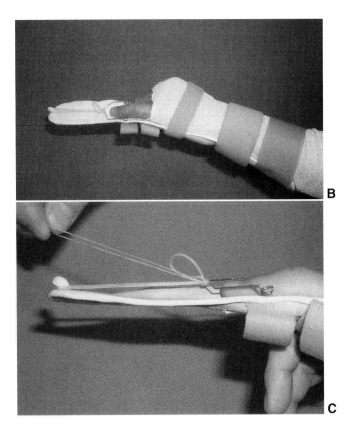

Fig. 11-20   A, Small finger middle phalanx distraction, PIP extension and distraction mobilization splint, type 1 (2) B-C, Small finger middle phalanx distraction, PIP extension and distraction mobilization splint, type 3 (4)
Longitudinal splint extensions or outriggers form platforms to which mobilization assists are attached distally on splints that distract and extend the PIP joint. C, Lateral view of the splint shown in B. [Courtesy (A) Carol Hierman, OTR, CHT, Cedar Grove, N.C., and Elisha Denny, PTA, OTA, Pittsboro N.C.; © Hand Rehabilitation Center, UNC, Chapel Hill, N.C.; (B,C) Christopher Bochenek, OTR/L, CHT, Cincinnati, Ohio.]

(Fig. 11-21, A-G),[28] while others achieve the requisite 90° pull through site-specific attachments of elastic traction material (Fig. 11-21, H,I) or the use of palmar pulleys embedded in the splint (Fig. 11-21, J).

Type 2. Two secondary joint levels are incorporated into *type 2 PIP flexion mobilization splints.* The MP joint level is almost universally included in these splints with the second secondary joint being either the DIP joint or the wrist, depending on patient-specific needs. *PIP flexion mobilization splints, type 2* may be based dorsally[16] (Fig. 11-22, A) or palmarly (Fig. 11-22, B,C) on the hand and forearm.

Ulnar deviation, extension

Type 0. *Type 0 PIP ulnar deviation mobilization splints* have no secondary joints. Only the primary PIP joint is included. These splints are fitted to correct radial deviation deformity at the PIP joint caused by attenuation or disruption of the PIP joint ulnar collateral ligament (Fig. 11-23, A). Splints apply radial directed force to the radial aspect of the proximal phalanx and ulnar-corrective force to the ulnar side of the middle phalanx with a strap that secures the finger into the ulnar aspect of the splint (Fig. 11-23, B).

Type 1. Providing additional mechanical advantage through a longer distal lever arm, one secondary joint, the DIP, is included in a *type 1 PIP ulnar deviation mobilization* splint (Fig. 11-23, C). Because PIP joints have a tendency to become swollen with injury, splints should be closely monitored and adjusted as edema subsides. Fit tolerances on these lateral force application splints are close and if adjustments are not made as finger size decreases, healing in an angulated position may occur.

Restriction Splints

Used to protect healing structures or to improve function by preventing extremes of motion, PIP restriction splints limit primary PIP joint motion in extension, flexion, extension and flexion, radial and/or ulnar deviation.

Extension

Type 0. No secondary joint levels are included in *type 0 PIP extension restriction splints.* Only the primary PIP joints are included and full flexion of the PIP joint is permitted. *PIP extension restriction splints, type 0,* are often used with rheumatoid arthritis patients to counteract existing PIP swan neck deformities. Athletes and musicians also find these splints helpful for maintaining better joint posture and for protecting against recurring injuries. Easily fabricated from thermoplastic materials (Fig. 11-24, A-D) or available commercially (Fig. 11-24, B-D), these splints are also useful for preoperative assessment of potential surgical procedures to correct PIP hyperextension problems.

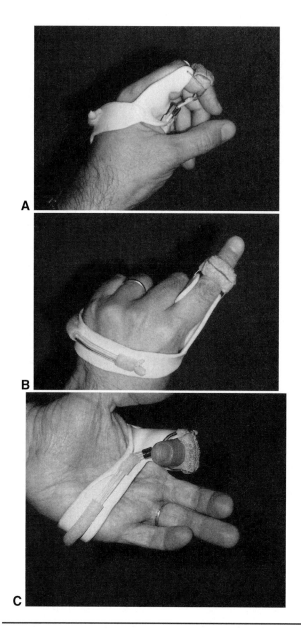

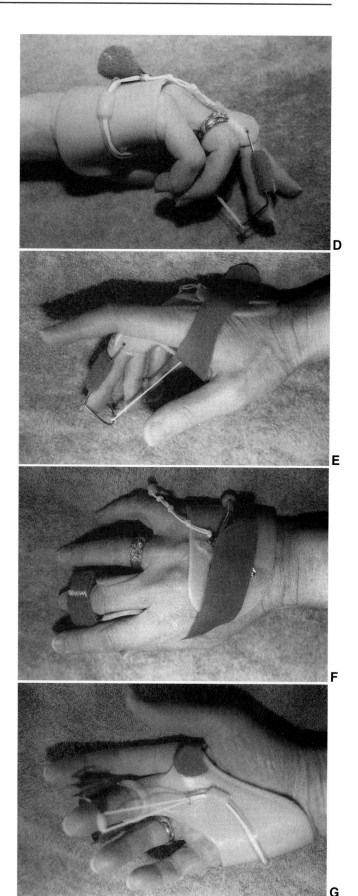

Fig. 11-21   A-C, Index finger PIP flexion mobilization splint, type 1 (2) D-G, Long finger PIP flexion mobilization splint, type 1 (2) H,I, Small finger PIP flexion mobilization splint, type 1 (2) J, Index–long finger IP, small finger PIP flexion mobilization splint, type 1 (9)

These four splints are *type 1 PIP flexion mobilization splints* or have *type 1 PIP flexion mobilization components*, in addition to other elements. Articulated outriggers maintain 90° angles of approach to the index (A-C) and long finger middle phalanges (D-G). In this innovative *type 1 PIP flexion mobilization splint* (H,I), an elastic strap serves as a mobilization assist. J, An outrigger and embedded pulleys direct mobilization assists to multiply involved digits. [Courtesy (A-C) Jean-Christophe Arias, Saint-Etienne, France; (D-G) Griet Van Veldhoven, Heverlee, Belgium; (H,I) Lin Beribak, OTR/L, CHT, Chicago, Ill.; (J) Shelli Dellinger, OTR, CHT, San Diego, Calif.]

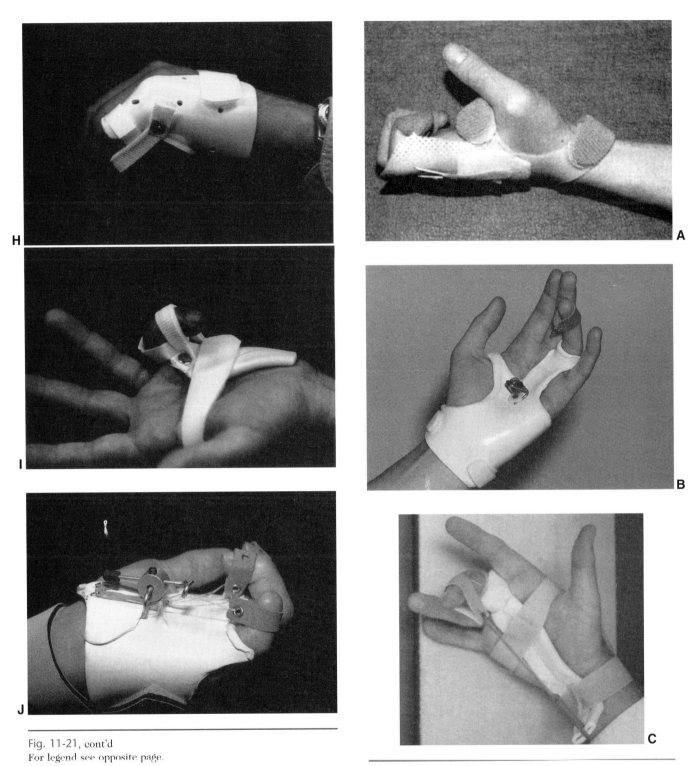

Fig. 11-21, cont'd
For legend see opposite page.

Fig. 11-22   A, Index–small finger PIP flexion mobilization splint, type 2 (8) B, Ring finger PIP flexion mobilization splint, type 2 (3) C, Long finger PIP flexion mobilization splint, type 2 (3)

Ranging from full extension to approximately 60° flexion, the positions of secondary MP joints differ as do their surfaces of application in these three *type 2 PIP flexion mobilization splints*. [(**A**) from Lei B, Lei E: Hand-based PIP flexion assist splint, *J Hand Ther* 6(4):339-40, 1993; Courtesy (**B**) Esther May, PhD, OT, Adelaide, South Australia; (**C**) Linda Shuttleton, OTR, Long Beach, Calif.]

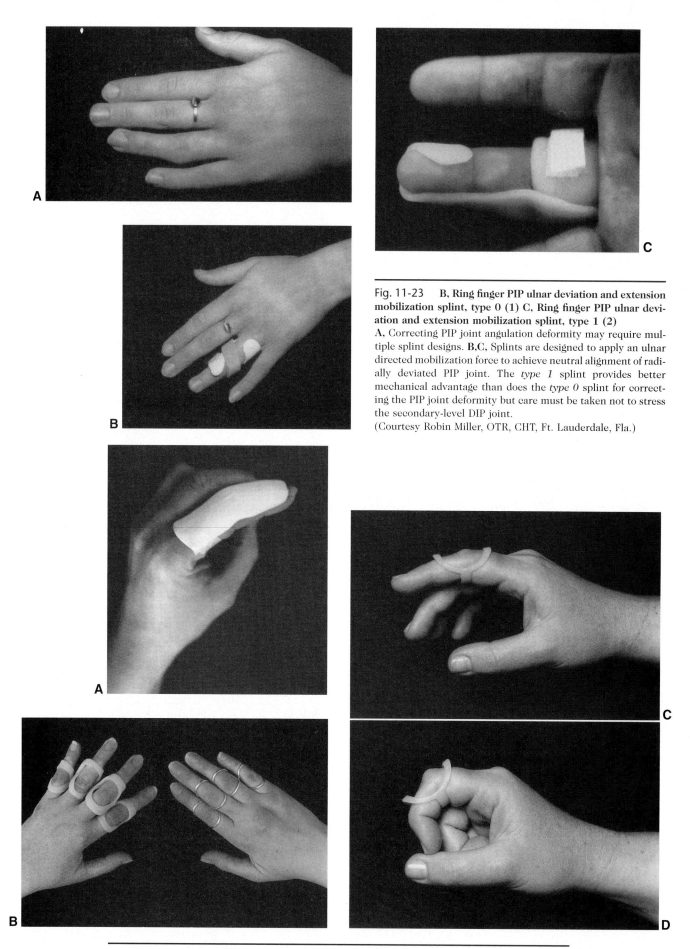

Fig. 11-23   B, Ring finger PIP ulnar deviation and extension mobilization splint, type 0 (1) C, Ring finger PIP ulnar deviation and extension mobilization splint, type 1 (2)
A, Correcting PIP joint angulation deformity may require multiple splint designs. B,C, Splints are designed to apply an ulnar directed mobilization force to achieve neutral alignment of radially deviated PIP joint. The *type 1* splint provides better mechanical advantage than does the *type 0* splint for correcting the PIP joint deformity but care must be taken not to stress the secondary-level DIP joint.
(Courtesy Robin Miller, OTR, CHT, Ft. Lauderdale, Fla.)

Fig. 11-24
For legend see opposite page.

Extension, flexion

Type 0. *PIP extension and flexion restriction splints, type 0,* limit both PIP joint extension and PIP joint flexion. *Type 0* splints affect motion only at the PIP joints and they have no secondary joints. Originally developed for volleyball players,[1] they are also used in other sports to protect PIP joints. These splints allow defined PIP arcs of motion and protect the joint from extremes of motion (Fig. 11-25, *A,B*).

Extension, deviation

Type 1. Restricting both PIP joint extension and PIP joint radial (Fig. 11-25, *C*) or ulnar deviation, *type 1 PIP extension and deviation restriction splints* incorporate one secondary joint. The secondary joint may be situated proximal or distal to the primary PIP joint.

Deviation

Type 1 and Type 2. *Type 1* and *type 2 PIP deviation restriction splints* are critical to attaining and maintaining PIP joint stability when injury or the disease process cause PIP joint collateral ligament partial tears or complete ruptures or when PIP arthroplasties are done. Restricting PIP joint radial or ulnar deviation, or both, PIP deviation restriction splints may include one or two secondary joints (Fig. 11-26, *A-C*) in addition to the primary PIP joint. These splints allow full PIP joint extension and flexion.

Restriction/Mobilization Splints

Extension, distraction

Type 3. Designed to treat stable or unstable intra-articular PIP fractures,[4,6,25] *type 3 PIP extension restriction/distraction mobilization splints* include three secondary joint levels: the wrist, MP joint, and DIP joint (Fig. 11-27, *A,B*). Requiring close communication between surgeon, therapist, and patient, these splints allow early motion of the PIP joint to prevent adhesions of ligaments and capsular structures.

Torque Transmission Splints

Transferring moment longitudinally or transversely, PIP torque transmission splints control one or more

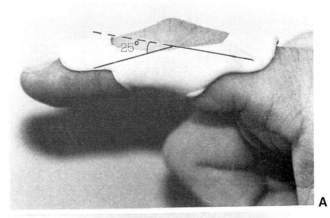

A

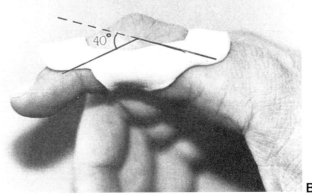

B

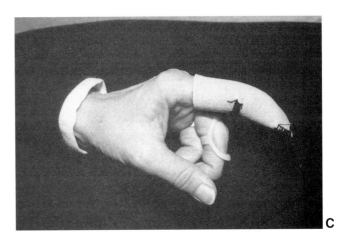

C

Fig. 11-25   A,B, Index finger PIP extension and flexion restriction splint, type 0 (1) C, Index finger PIP extension and radial deviation restriction splint, type 1 (2) \\ Long finger PIP extension restriction splint, type 0 (1)

A,B, This modified *type 0 PIP restriction splint* is designed to limit extension to 25° and flexion to 40°. C, A circumferential neoprene finger "sleeve" provides lateral PIP joint support, inhibiting radial deviation; and incorporation of a tuck sewn volarly PIP restricts PIP joint extension. [(A) from Benaglia P, Sartorio F, Ingenito R: Evaluation of a thermoplastic splint to prevent the proximal interphalangeal joints of volleyball players, *J Hand Ther* 9(1):52-6, 1996; Courtesy (C) Joni Armstrong, OTR, CHT, Bemidji, Minn.]

Fig. 11-24   A, Index finger PIP extension restriction splint, type 0 (1) B, Finger separate PIP extension restriction splint, type 0 (1); 4 splints @ finger \\ Finger PIP extension restriction splint, type 0 (1); 4 splints @ finger separate C,D, Index finger PIP extension restriction splint, type 0 (1)

With several design options, *type 0 PIP extension restriction splints* may be custom fabricated or they may be purchased commercially [B(right), C-D]. These splints prevent full extension of the PIP joint while allowing full active PIP joint flexion. [Courtesy (B) Cindy Garris, OTR, Silver Ring Splint Company, Charlottesville, Va.; (C,D) Julie Belkin, OTR, CO, MBA, 3-Point Products, Annapolis, Md.]

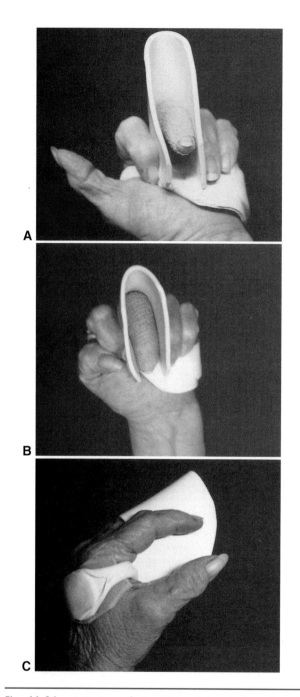

Fig. 11-26 **A-C, Long finger PIP radial and ulnar deviation restriction splint, type 2 (3)**
Preventing radial and ulnar deviation of the long finger PIP joint, this postoperative replacement arthroplasty splint allows PIP joint extension and flexion.

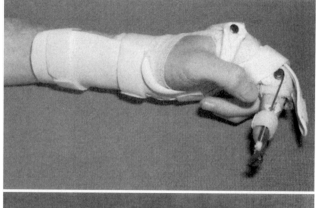

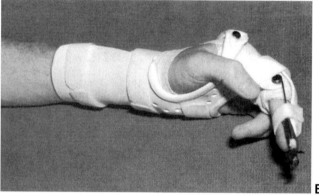

Fig. 11-27 **A,B, Index finger PIP extension restriction / distraction mobilization splint, type 3 (4)**
An articulated outrigger applies traction throughout PIP joint active range of motion with full extension restricted. (From Byrne A, Yau T: A modified dynamic traction splint for unstable intra-articular fractures of the proximal interphalangeal joint, *J Hand Ther* 8(3):216, 1995.)

joints to affect motion at primary PIP joints outside the borders of the splints. These torque transmission splints promote active motion of supple PIP joints or soft tissue remodeling of shortened soft tissue PIP joint periarticular structures. The type category in single-purpose torque transmission splints is always greater than zero, due to the obligatory presence of at least one secondary joint.

Type 1. *Type 1 PIP extension torque transmission splints* incorporate one secondary joint in addition to the primary PIP joint. The secondary joint may be proximal or distal to the PIP joint. *PIP extension torque transmission splints, type 1,* with distally situated secondary joints may be used alone or with other PIP extension mobilization splints (Fig. 11-18, *J*) to increase PIP joint extension.

The review of PIP splints using modified text format concludes here. Regular text format is used for the remainder of this chapter.

Finger PIP, DIP Splints

Immobilization Splints

Interphalangeal joint immobilization splints allow healing of injured or repaired tissues or they externally reinforce various types of surgical hardware used in internal fixation of fractures. They may be fitted dorsally, palmarly, laterally, or circumferentially, depending on patient-specific requirements and materials used. As with other digital immobilization splints, paper tape, rather than straps, provides a more stable and accurate method of securing IP immobilization splints to fingers.

Type 0. With no secondary joints, *type 0 IP immobilization splints* prevent motion at the PIP and DIP joints (Fig. 11-18, *G*, ring and small fingers). Straps or tape placed over the axes of the two joints helps keep these splints in proper position. Because these splints commonly are worn for several weeks as tissue healing progresses, skin maceration and/or pin track infections may occur if patients are not taught proper hygiene and skin care.

Type 1 and More. *Type 1 IP immobilization splints* incorporate the MPs as one secondary joint level; *type 2* includes the MP joint level and the wrist for two secondary joint levels. Often used to immobilize IP joints during the acute phase of wound healing, these splints are injury-specific and surgery-specific regarding joint positioning.

Mobilization Splints

Increasing range of motion of the two finger interphalangeal joints simultaneously requires thoughtful ingenuity. Splint design is influenced by the amount of motion present at the PIP and DIP joints. In general, when flexion is needed, the more IP joint flexion present, the less complicated is the splint design. The same is true for extension, in that splint designs become simpler with increasing presence of IP joint extension. A 90° angle of approach to the rotational axes of the PIP and DIP joints is fundamental to applying equal amounts of corrective force to the collateral ligaments of the two joints. Mobilizing forces should also be 90° to longitudinal axes of the middle and distal phalanges. As with all mobilizing splints, magnitude of the force applied should not exceed 100-300 grams.

Type 0. *Type 0 finger IP mobilization splints* include no secondary joint levels. Only the primary PIP and DIP joints are incorporated in these splints that may be designed to improve either extension or flexion (Fig. 11-28, *A-D*). It is important to remember that *type 0 IP mobilization splints* commonly produce a certain amount of translational force due to lack of true 90° force application. These splints must be carefully assessed to ensure that rotational (corrective) force is in fact greater than translational force (joint compression or distraction). Two-stage serial plaster casting is an excellent technique for increasing PIP extension and DIP flexion simultaneously (Fig. 11-28, *E-G*) and joint compression problems from too much translational force are almost nonexistent when this two-stage technique is applied properly.

Type 1. One secondary joint level, the MP joint, is included in *type 1 finger IP mobilization splints*. For PIP-DIP mobilization splints, complete immobilization of a secondary metacarpophalangeal joint with concomitant mobilization force to the two primary interphalangeal joints may be one of the most difficult tasks in splint fabrication. For IP flexion mobilization splints, because the primary intent of the splint is to produce a flexion force, one's initial impulse is to design a palmar-based splint. This design, however, can result in frustration and mechanical failure when the distal mobilizing flexion force overpowers the more proximal secondary immobilizing extension force. Upon reassessment, it becomes apparent that the proximal extension force must be equal to or greater than the distal flexion torque to produce complete immobilization of the metacarpophalangeal joint. Therefore a dorsally based splint or a palmar-based splint with a dorsal or circumferential proximal phalanx component generates better mechanical advantage for immobilizing a secondary metacarpophalangeal joint against a distal flexion force to the IP joints (Fig. 11-29, *A-D*). Inclusion of MP joints as a secondary joint level when mobilizing IP joints into flexion is an effective method for splinting intrinsic tightness.

Type 1 IP extension mobilization splints have the same mechanical challenges except that the requisite of dorsal proximal phalanx components is reversed to palmar proximal phalangeal components in order to fully stabilize the secondary MP joints.

Type 2. *Type 2 finger IP mobilization splints* have two secondary joint levels in addition to the two primary IP joints. One of the secondary joint levels is at the MP joint while the second secondary joint may be the thumb CMC joint (Fig. 11-30, *A*) or the wrist joint, depending on individual patient needs. Finger IP mobilization splints may be fitted to increase extension (Fig. 11-30, *B*) or flexion of the IP joints (Fig. 11-30, *C-E*). As described above for *type 1 IP extension mobilization splints*, palmar proximal phalangeal components are requisite in order to fully control position of the secondary MP joint in *type 2 IP extension mobilization splints*. The reverse, dorsal proximal phalangeal components, are needed for *type 2 IP flexion mobilization splints*. Fingernail clips or Velcro buttons facilitate attachment of mobilization assists to the fingers and increase mechanical advantage by allowing the full length of the distal phalanx to be used.

Mobilization/Restriction/Torque Transmission Splints

With seemingly simple configurations, finger IP mobilization/restriction/torque transmission splints involve very sophisticated biomechanical concepts. These splints are often employed to treat resistant PIP

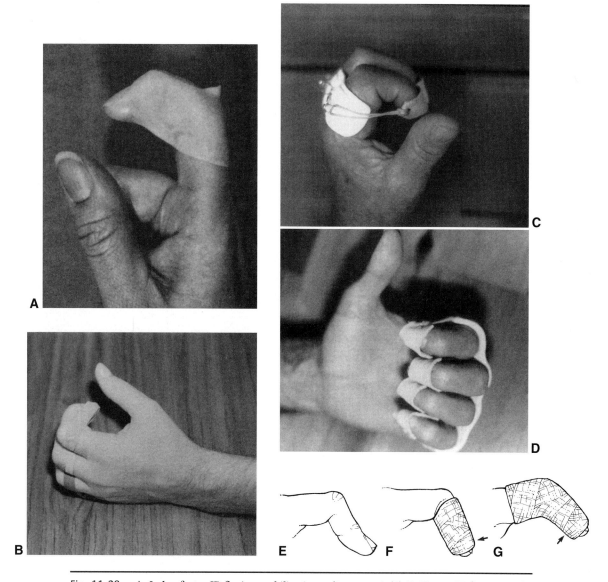

Fig. 11-28   A, Index finger IP flexion mobilization splint, type 0 (2) B, Finger IP flexion mobilization splint, type 0 (2); 4 splints @ finger separate C,D, Index–small finger IP flexion mobilization splint, type 0 (8) F, Finger DIP flexion mobilization splint, type 0 (1) G, Finger PIP extension, DIP flexion mobilization splint, type 0 (2)

A, Simple yet effective *type 0 IP flexion mobilization splints* may be made by cutting transverse bands from fingers of unused surgical gloves or **(B)** applying wide short rubber bands that may be found in the vegetable departments of grocery stores. While these simple elastic bands may seem innocuous, they must be monitored carefully to ensure that they do not apply too much mobilizing force to the IP joints. **C,D,** A thermoplastic band distributes pressure in this type 0 IP flexion mobilization splint. **E-G,** Two-stage plaster serial casting is an excellent method to correct long-standing IP extension contractures. Inelastic mobilization forces produce soft tissue remodeling (i.e., tissue growth), increasing IP joint motion. [Courtesy **(B)** Darcelle Decker, OTR, CHT, Danville, Pa.; **(C,D)** Kathryn Schultz, OTR, CHT, Orlando, Fla.; **(E-G)** Judith Bell-Krotoski, OTR, FAOTA, CHT, Baton Rouge, La.]

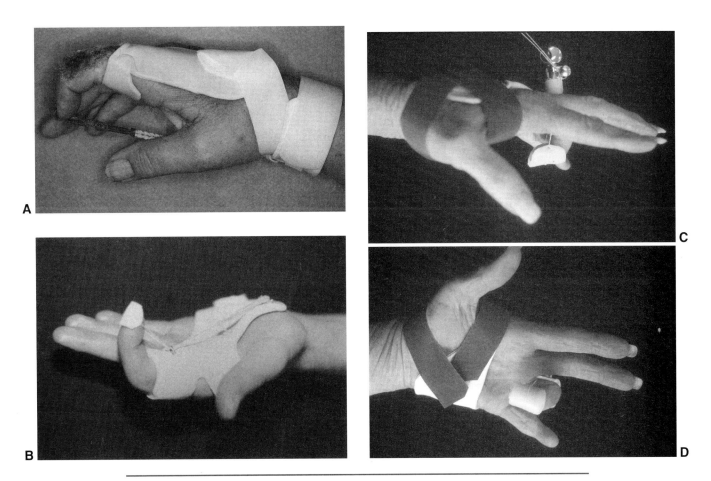

Fig. 11-29   A, Index finger IP flexion mobilization splint, type 1 (3) B, Index finger IP flexion mobilization splint, type 1 (3) C,D, Ring finger IP flexion mobilization splint, type 1 (3)
A-D, Splint designs that incorporate dorsal phalangeal or dorsal phalangeal-metacarpal components provide better control of secondary MP joint position and stronger counter to mobilizing forces to the IP joints. Elastic or inelastic traction is gently applied to remodel shortened periarticular soft tissues. **C,D,** To alleviate potential finger "crowding" from a volarly fitted splint as IP joint flexion nears normal range, the "power generator" (MERIT™ SPS Component) for this splint is situated dorsally to allow unrestricted mobilization of IP joints into maximum flexion. [Courtesy **(B)** Kathryn Schultz, OTR, CHT, Orlando, Fla.; **(C,D)** Karen Schultz-Johnson, MS, OTR, FAOTA, CHT, UE-Tech, Edwards, Colo.]

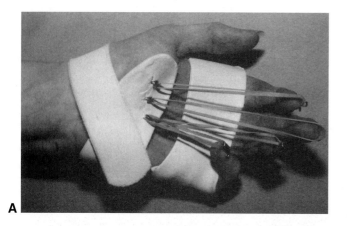

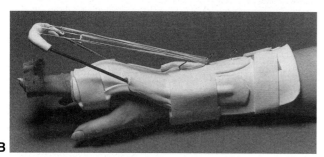

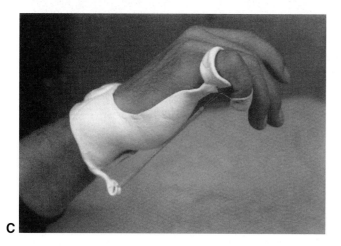

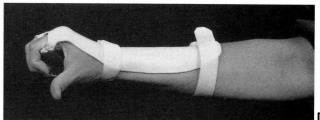

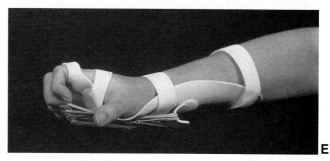

Fig. 11-30   **A,** Index–small finger IP flexion mobilization splint, type 2 (13) **B,** Index–ring finger IP extension mobilization splint, type 2 (10) **C,** Small finger IP flexion mobilization splint, type 2 (4) **D,** Index–small finger IP flexion mobilization splint, type 2 (13) **E,** Index–small finger IP flexion mobilization splint, type 2 (13)
The thumb CMC joint **(A)** and wrist **(B-E)** are secondary joints in these *type 2 IP flexion mobilization splints*. **A,C-E,** Dorsal phalangeal components are important to controlling position of secondary MP joints in *type 2 IP flexion splints* and **(B)** palmar phalangeal components are critical to preventing MP joint subluxation in *type 2 IP extension splints*. [Courtesy **(A)** Donna Reist-Kolumbus, OTR, CHT, Jacksonville, Fla.; **(B)** Lisa Dennys, BSc, OT, London, Ont.; **(C)** Carolina deLeeuw, MA, OTR, Tacoma, Wash.]

flexion contractures that are accompanied by DIP extension stiffness. When, due to injury or disease process, the PIP lateral bands move volar to the PIP joint axis of rotation causing PIP joint flexion, resultant tension on the oblique retinacular ligaments creates an extension force at the DIP joint. If the lateral band volar subluxation is not corrected, over time, insidious PIP flexion and DIP joint extension contractures develop.

Type 0. No secondary joints are included in *type 0 finger PIP extension mobilization / DIP extension restriction / DIP flexion torque transmission splints* (Fig. 11-31, *A-D*). These splints are designed to remodel and lengthen PIP joint soft tissue structures to increase

joint extension while simultaneously remodeling and lengthening the oblique retinacular ligaments through transferred flexion moment to the DIP joint. Because of the biomechanical complexity of this two-joint zigzag deformity, application of inelastic traction through serial plaster mobilization splints is more effective in remodeling shortened soft tissue structures than are splint designs relying on elastic traction.

Restriction Splints

Type 0. *Type 0 IP restriction splints* include no secondary joints. Only the primary PIP and DIP joints are included in these splints that may be designed to restrict IP joint extension, flexion, or a combination

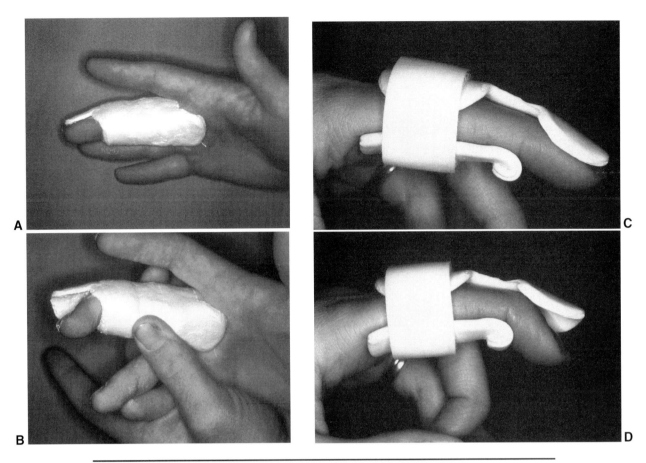

Fig. 11-31 **A,B, Long finger PIP extension mobilization / DIP extension restriction / DIP flexion torque transmission splint, type 0 (2) C,D, Index finger PIP extension mobilization / DIP extension restriction / DIP flexion torque transmission splint, type 0 (2)**
Constructed from different materials, these two splints involve sophisticated understanding of PIP and DIP joint biomechanics. Both splints use torque transmission to actively move the DIP joint and over time to remodel shortened oblique retinacular ligaments. Concomitantly, through serial adjustments, both splints use inelastic traction to remodel PIP soft tissues and increase PIP joint extension. [Courtesy **(A,B)** Christopher Bochenek, OTR/L, CHT, Cincinnati, Ohio; **(C,D)** Diane Collins, MEd, PT, CHT, New Canaan, Conn.]

of extension and flexion. Limiting extremes of IP extension and flexion, *IP restriction splints, type 0*, made of neoprene rest tender arthritic joints while providing neutral warming to the finger (Fig. 11-32).

Restriction/Immobilization Splints

Designed to allow restricted PIP joint mobility and DIP joint stability, these injury-specific splints allow motion and protect healing tissue in the postoperative phase of rehabilitation.

Type 0. With two different purposes, this classification of splints restricts motion at the PIP joint while immobilizing the DIP joint. No secondary joints are incorporated in *type 0 PIP extension restriction / DIP extension immobilization splints.* One innovative design securely fixes the splint distally on the finger and leaves the proximal PIP extension restric-

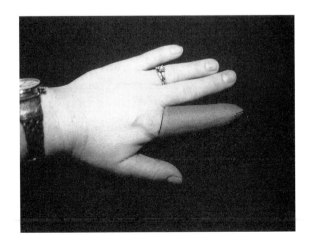

Fig. 11-32 **Index finger IP flexion restriction splint, type 0 (2)**
Neoprene finger "sleeve" restricts IP flexion and provides an increment of neutral warmth.

tion component of the splint free, allowing full PIP joint flexion (Fig. 11-33, *A,B*).[30]

Finger DIP Splints

Because the DIP joints are also hinge articulations with collateral ligaments and palmar plate stabilization, mechanical principles similar to those of the proximal interphalangeal joints are applicable. From a practical point of view, however, the small area of purchase provided by the distal phalanx makes elaborate mobilization traction techniques less successful in correcting stiffness at this joint. Three-point pressure splints that utilize inelastic traction sometimes prove more effective in correcting flexion deformities,

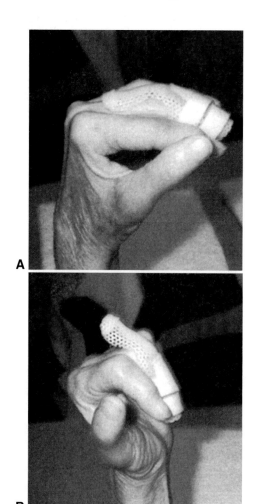

Fig. 11-33   A,B, Long finger PIP extension restriction / long finger DIP extension immobilization splint, type 0 (2)
The proximal end of this splint moves up and away from the dorsum of the proximal phalanx as the PIP joint flexes, allowing full PIP flexion. As the PIP joint extends, the splint is reseated on the phalanx, restricting full PIP extension. Distally, the DIP joint is immobilized by the splint. (From Wong S: Combination splint for distal interphalangeal joint stability and protected proximal interphalangeal joint mobility, *J Hand Ther* 8(4):269, 1995.)

and simple straps or rubber bands may best overcome extension stiffness.

Immobilization Splints

Immobilization splints prevent motion of the DIP joints to allow healing of injured or repaired structures, protect sensitive fingertips, and reinforce surgical hardware such as internal or external fixation devices for fractures.

Type 0. *Type 0 DIP extension immobilization splints* incorporate no secondary joints; only the primary DIP joints are included. These *type 0* splints may be designed simply to immobilize the DIP joint or they may cover the entire fingertip to protect healing tissue from unintentional bumping and to decrease noxious sensory stimulation as the hand is used (Fig. 11-34, *A*). Fitted dorsally, palmarly (Fig. 11-34, *B,C*), or circumferentially (Fig. 11-34, *D*), *DIP extension immobilization splints, type 0*, are frequently used to treat terminal extensor tendon ruptures or lacerations in Zones I and II. The DIP joint is immobilized in 0° extension to slight hyperextension. Studies indicate that immobilizing the DIP joint in too much hyperextension diminishes blood supply to dorsal skin.[17,22] Because of this potential complication, DIP joint immobilization beyond 50% of its normal hyperextension should be avoided.[22] Careful monitoring of the involved fingertip for color changes and for increased swelling is important. Because these splints typically are worn for 6-10 weeks depending on patient-specific circumstances, patient education regarding wearing regimen and skin hygiene is an important factor to achieving successful outcomes.

Mobilization Splints

DIP mobilization splints present varied configurations but all have the same purpose, to improve motion of the DIP joint through gentle application of inelastic or elastic traction. A 90° angle of approach to the rotational axes of the DIP joint allows equal amounts of corrective force to be applied to the DIP joint collateral ligaments. Mobilizing forces should also be 90° to the longitudinal axes of the distal phalanges. As with all digital mobilizing splints, magnitude of the force applied should not exceed 100-300 grams. DIP mobilization splints pose a special problem in securing the splints to the finger. Splint mechanical advantage and purchase progressively improve, as secondary joints are included in splint designs. Identifying the etiology of DIP joint stiffness is critical to splint design. For example, DIP extension deformities are often associated with lateral band subluxation at the PIP joint, requiring splints that affect both the PIP and DIP joints, not just the DIP joint.

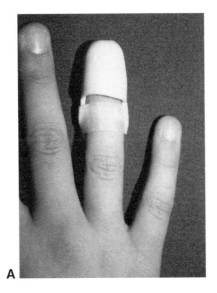

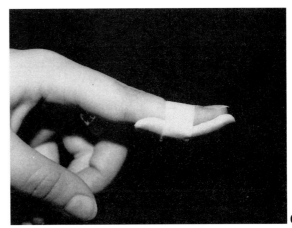

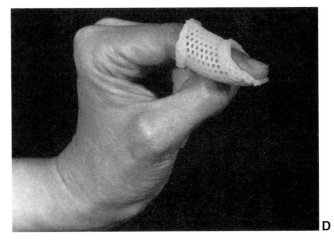

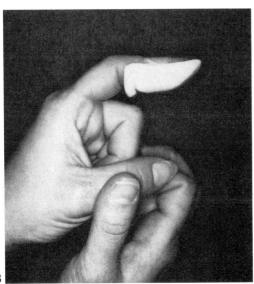

Fig. 11-34   A, Ring finger DIP extension immobilization splint, type 0 (1) B, Index finger DIP extension immobilization splint, type 0 (1) C, Index finger DIP hyperextension immobilization splint, type 0 (1) D, Index finger DIP extension immobilization splint, type 0 (1)
DIP immobilization splints **(A)** protect sensitive fingertips and **(B-D)** healing tendon/soft tissue structures about the DIP joint. **A,** Additional material covering dorsal distal phalanx area may be used to protect nail bed injuries/repairs. [Courtesy **(D)** Rachel Dyrud Ferguson, OTR, CHT, Taos, N.M.]

Type 0. Only the primary DIP joint is included in *type 0 DIP mobilization splints*. Secondary joint levels are absent in this splint classification. Designed to increase extension (Fig. 11-35) or flexion of the DIP joint, *type 0 DIP mobilization splints* may be fabricated in a variety of splint materials. Inelastic (Fig. 11-28, *F*) or elastic traction applies gentle mobilizing force to capsular and pericapsular soft tissue to affect tissue remodeling.

Type 1. *Type 1 DIP mobilization splints* incorporate one secondary joint level, the PIP joint, in addition to the primary DIP joint. Providing increased mechanical advantage and purchase area, *type 1 DIP mobilization splints* are designed to increase extension (Fig. 11-36, *A,B*) or flexion (Fig. 11-36, *C*) range

of motion of finger DIP joints through soft tissue remodeling.

Type 2. Incorporating secondary MP and PIP joint levels, *type 2 DIP mobilization splints* increase extension (Fig. 11-37, *A*) or flexion (Fig. 11-37, *B-D*) at primary DIP joints.

Finger, Thumb CMC Splints
Immobilization Splints

Finger, thumb CMC immobilization splints prevent motion of the finger MP, PIP, DIP joints and the thumb CMC joint to rest or to allow healing of soft tissue. The decision of whether to immobilize in an antideformity position or a functional position is key, especially

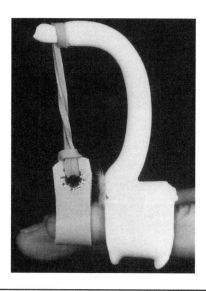

Fig. 11-35   **Small finger DIP extension mobilization splint, type 0 (1)**
To avoid causing injury from shear, splints designed to mobilize the DIP joint must be well stabilized on the finger. Elastic mobilization forces produce soft tissue remodeling (i.e., tissue growth), increasing DIP joint motion. (Courtesy Norma Arras, MA, OTR, CHT, Springfield, Ill.)

when treating acute hand cases involving soft tissue trauma, including burn or crush injuries. An antideformity position splint holds the MP joints in flexion and the IP joints in extension, thereby maintaining collateral ligament length. In contrast, a functional position splint allows the MP collateral ligaments to slacken and over time, shorten, and its obligatory IP flexion attitude predisposes flexion deformities of interphalangeal joints. Since the early 1970s, use of functional positional splints has gradually lost favor as increased awareness of the important role antideformity splints play in maintaining the intricate biomechanical balance of the hand. Once almost universally prescribed, functional position immobilization splints are now relegated to treatment of hands afflicted by rheumatoid arthritis and other diagnoses where the potential for reduced collateral ligament tension is diminished.

Type 0. *Type 0 finger, thumb CMC immobilization splints* have no secondary joints. Only the primary finger MP, PIP, DIP joints and the thumb CMC joint are included in these immobilization splints. These hand-based splints that leave the thumb MP and IP joints free are infrequently used because they do not control the effect of extrinsic tendons crossing the wrist joint; nor are they as comfortable as *type 1* splints that further disperse pressure through greater mechanical advantage afforded by the presence of forearm troughs.

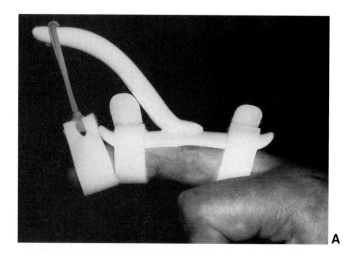

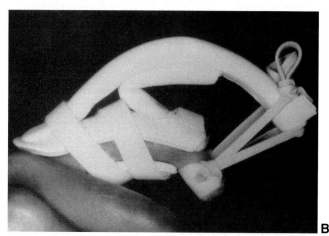

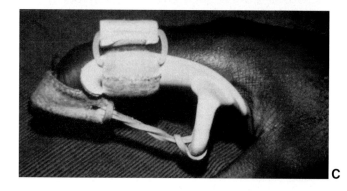

Fig. 11-36   **A, Long finger DIP extension mobilization splint, type 1 (2) B, Long finger DIP extension mobilization splint, type 1 (2) C, Index finger DIP flexion mobilization splint, type 1 (2)**
With incorporation of the secondary PIP joint, *type 1 DIP mobilization splints* have improved mechanical advantage over *type 0* splints. These splints may be fitted to increase DIP extension (**A,B**) or flexion (**C**). [Courtesy (**B**) Jill Francisco, OTR, CHT, Cicero, Ind.; (**C**) Kathryn Schultz, OTR, CHT, Orlando, Fla.]

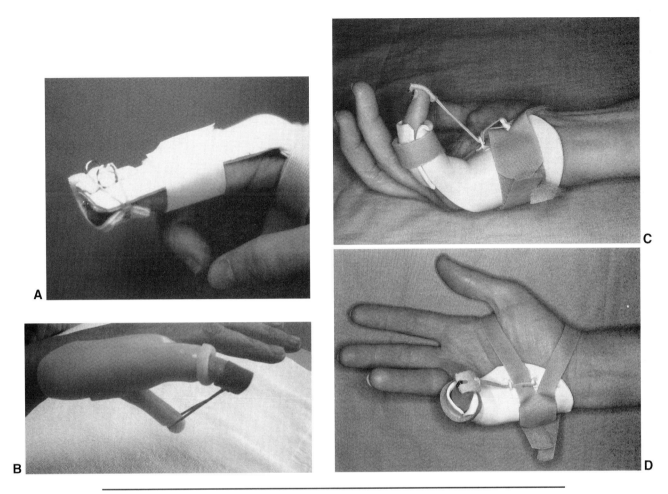

Fig. 11-37   **A, Index finger DIP extension mobilization splint, type 2 (3) B, Small finger DIP flexion mobilization splint, type 2 (3) C,D, Small finger DIP flexion mobilization splint, type 2 (3)** *Type 2 DIP mobilization splints* include the MP and PIP joints as secondary levels. These splints have the advantage of being hand-based rather than finger-based and tend to be more stable on the extremity. They may be fitted to improve DIP extension **(A)** or flexion **(B-D)**. **D,** Palmar view of the splint shown in C. [Courtesy **(A)** Robin Miller, OTR, CHT, Ft. Lauderdale, Fla.; **(B)** Jason Willoughby, OTR, Richmond, Ky.; **(C,D)** Lori Klerekoper DeMott, OTR, CHT, and Janet Bailey, OTR, CHT, Columbus, Ohio.]

Type 1. Immobilizing all three joints of the fingers and the thumb CMC joint, *type 1 finger, thumb CMC immobilizing splints* incorporate one secondary joint—usually, but not always—the wrist. Although it is possible that the thumb MP joint, instead of the wrist, may be included as the sole secondary joint level, it is not very probable clinically. *Finger, thumb CMC immobilization splints, type 1*, typically hold the hand and thumb CMC in an antideformity, "safe," position or in a functional position (Fig. 11-38, *A,B*). Often recommended for rheumatoid arthritic patients as resting or night splints, *type 1 finger, thumb CMC immobilization splints* are used with a variety of diagnoses. Leaving thumb MP and IP joints free in these splints permits limited thumb use, an especially helpful factor for individuals wearing bilateral splints.

Regardless of whether these splints are antideformity position or functional position, custom fabricated or purchased through commercial sources, good splint fit and mechanics are imperative.

Mobilization Splints

Design, construction, and fitting become more challenging when mobilization of the thumb CMC joint must proceed simultaneously with mobilization of the finger joints. Concurrent coordination of joint alignment variables, including 90° angle of force application to rotational joint axes and to longitudinal phalangeal axes, with other factors such as digital convergence points for both the fingers and the thumb requires a thorough understanding of anatomy, biomechanics, and the mechanical principles of splinting.

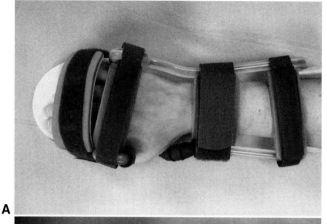

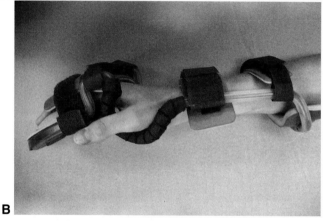

Fig. 11-38 A,B, Index–small finger MP flexion and IP extension, thumb CMC palmar abduction immobilization splint, type 1 (13)

Designed for warm climates and commercially available in bright primary colors, this inventive TUBOform *finger, thumb CMC immobilization* splint is easily adjustable via its plastic tubing lateral supports. (Courtesy Expansao, Sao Paulo, Brazil.)

Type 0. Only the primary joints—finger MP, PIP, DIP, and thumb CMC—are included in *type 0 finger, thumb CMC mobilization splints*. There are no secondary joints in these splints. Absence of the wrist as a secondary joint results in no ability to control extrinsic tenodesis effect and the obligatory hand-based design does not disperse pressure as efficiently as do *type 1* designs.

Type 1. *Type 1 finger, thumb CMC mobilization splints* incorporate the wrist as a secondary joint. *Finger, thumb CMC mobilization splints, type 1*, may be fitted to improve finger abduction, extension, or flexion, and thumb CMC radial or palmar abduction. Because thumb position can impede finger flexion mobilization, splints designed to increase finger flexion, while at the same time increasing thumb CMC palmar abduction or opposition, are especially difficult. Separate flexion outriggers for fingers and thumb are invaluable in this situation. (Also see combination splint section of this chapter.)

Finger, Thumb Splints

Finger, thumb splints include the finger MP, PIP, and DIP joints and the thumb CMC, MP, and IP joints as primary joints. The only difference between the splints described in this section and the splints described in the immediately preceding section is the addition of the thumb MP and IP joints to the splints included in this category. All of the concepts discussed above are applicable to splints in this section. Further, splint complexity increases from a minimum total of 13 joints included for finger, thumb CMC splints to a minimum total of 15 joints included in this group of finger, thumb splints.

Immobilization Splints

Again, the key factor for *finger, thumb immobilization splints* is joint position. With the cam-like configuration of the heads of the metacarpal bones, MP joint collateral ligament length is best maintained with the MP joints in 70-90° of flexion; the IP joints, with their predisposition to flexion contractures, are best splinted in full extension to very slight, 10°, flexion.[9,10] Providing no other superseding condition exists (e.g., tendon repair, unstable fracture, etc.) and the splinting goal is full hand immobilization, the anti-deformity position for the fingers and thumb CMC joint are the postures of choice for immobilizing hands with local or more proximal forearm or upper extremity injuries. In the presence of upper extremity trauma, *finger, thumb immobilization splints* that maintain hands in functional positions do little to counteract the insidious deforming forces of MP extension/hyperextension and IP flexion. In contrast, functional position *finger, thumb immobilization splints* are used as resting or night splints for rheumatoid arthritic patients.

If patients wearing *finger, thumb immobilization splints* habitually rest their palmarly abducted splinted thumbs on mattresses, chair arms, lapboards, etc., thumb or splint post components must be added to prevent thumb ulceration from prolonged pressure and shear forces from theses semirigid/rigid surfaces. This is especially problematic for patients with no or poor cognition, and those who lack thumb protective sensation.

Type 0. *Type 0 finger, thumb immobilization splints* contain no secondary joint levels. Only the primary finger MP, PIP, and DIP and thumb CMC, MP, and IP joints are included in these hand-based splints. Because the wrist is not incorporated in these *type 0 splints*, the extrinsic tenodesis effect is uncontrolled.

Type 1. The wrist is included as a secondary joint level in *finger, thumb immobilization splints, type 1*. Finger MP, PIP, and DIP joints and thumb CMC, MP, IP joints are considered primary joints in these

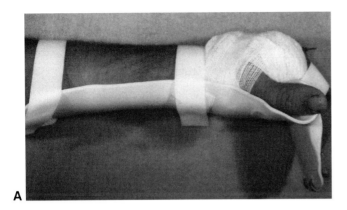

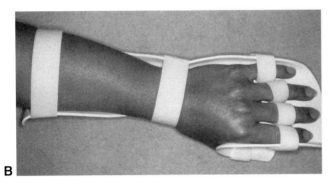

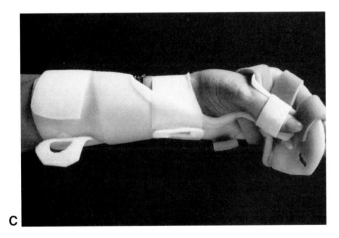

Fig. 11-39   A, Index–small finger MP flexion and IP extension, thumb CMC radial abduction and MP-IP extension immobilization splint, type 1 (16) B, Index–small finger MP flexion and IP extension, thumb CMC palmar abduction and MP-IP extension immobilization splint, type 1 (16) C, Index–small finger flexion, thumb CMC palmar abduction and MP-IP flexion immobilization splint, type 1 (16)

Immobilization of the hand is a serious undertaking determined by patient-specific diagnosis and/or surgical procedure, coupled with objective assessment data. Finger, thumb immobilization splints typically maintain the hand in an antideformity position (**A**) or a functional position (**B**) depending on patient-specific requirements. **C**, "Catch-holes" in the ends of straps ease splint doffing and donning.

splints. *Type 1 finger, thumb immobilization splints* typically, but not always, maintain the hand in an antideformity position (Fig. 11-39, *A*) or a functional position (Fig. 11-39, *B,C*). Other etiology-specific finger or thumb articular postures may be appropriate, depending on individual patient requirements.

Mobilization Splints

Type 0. *Type 0 finger, thumb mobilization splints* do not include the wrist as a secondary joint. These hand-based splints are designed to increase both finger and thumb motion simultaneously through application of gentle remodeling forces from inelastic (Fig. 11-40, *A,B*) or elastic traction. Finger, thumb mobilization splints may be fitted dorsally or palmarly, depending on patient requisites and optimum splint

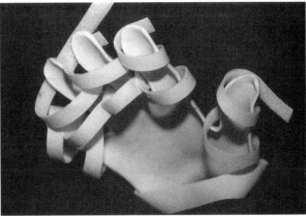

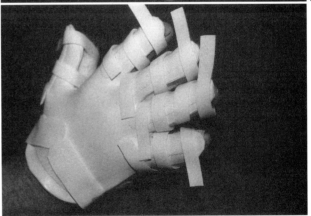

Fig. 11-40   A,B, Index–small finger extension, thumb CMC radial abduction, and MP-IP extension mobilization splint, type 0 (15)

Exceptional draping capacity of some thermoplastic splinting materials allows excellent contiguous fit for dorsal *finger, thumb mobilization splints*. Spirally wrapped long straps increase strap durability and ease of closure. The dorsal design leaves palmar wounds free of splint pressure. **B**, Dorsal view of the splint shown in **A**. (Courtesy Elizabeth Spencer Steffa, OTR/L, CHT, Seattle, Wash.)

mechanical advantage. Angle of force application must be 90° to all mobilized joint rotational axes and to the longitudinal axes of mobilized digital segments to prevent corrective forces from applying damaging, disproportionate forces to articular surfaces and supporting structures.

Type 1. Including the wrist as a secondary joint, *finger, thumb mobilization splints* affect articular motion of finger MP, PIP, and DIP and thumb CMC, MP, and IP joints. Inelastic traction *finger, thumb mobilization splints, type 1,* often are used to main-

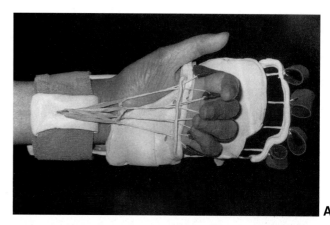

A

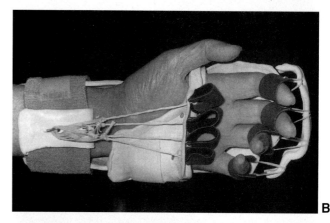

B

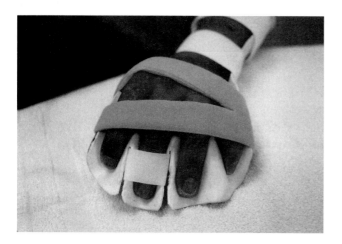

Fig. 11-41   Index, ring–small finger MP abduction, index–small finger extension, thumb CMC palmar abduction and MP-IP extension mobilization splint, type 1 (16)
Individual troughs increase finger extension and abduction, and thumb palmar abduction, in this *type 1 finger, thumb mobilization splint.* Incorporation of the wrist as a secondary joint controls extrinsic finger and thumb tenodesis effect. (Courtesy Joni Armstrong, OTR, CHT, Bemidji, Minn.)

Fig. 11-42   A, Index–small finger MP flexion mobilization splint, type 1 (5) or index–small finger PIP extension mobilization splint, type 2 (9) B, Index–small finger PIP extension mobilization splint, type 2 (9) or index–small finger MP flexion mobilization splint, type 1 (5) C, Index–small finger flexion, thumb MP extension mobilization splint, type 2 (16) or index–small finger extension, thumb MP flexion mobilization splint, type 2 (16) D, Index finger flexion, thumb CMC palmar abduction mobilization splint, type 1 (5); or Index, ring, small finger extension, thumb CMC palmar abduction and MP flexion mobilization splint, type 1 (12)
A,B, Incorporating multiple splint functions into the design of a single splint improves patient compliance by omitting extraneous steps. This combination splint permits alternating use of PIP extension mobilization and MP flexion mobilization options. **C, D,** Elastic and inelastic mobilization assists increased finger flexion and extension respectively, while the thumb is maintained in a functional position. Achieving digital motion at the expense of the thumb, even if it is uninjured, may result in a hand that cannot pick up objects or hold a pen, although the fingers regain full range of motion. [Courtesy **(A,B)** Diana Williams, MBA, OTR, CHT, Macon, Ga.; **(C,D)** Lin Beribak, OTR/L, CHT, Chicago, Ill.]

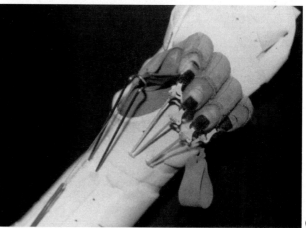

C

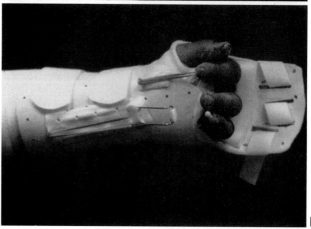

D

tain range of motion gained during the day through exercises and other kinds of mobilization splinting (Fig. 11-41). These splints are serially adjusted to keep pace with progressive joint changes. Elastic traction *finger, thumb mobilization splints, type 1,* are unusual in that it is difficult mechanically to direct corrective forces to all fifteen digital joints simultaneously.

Combination Splints

As experienced hand rehabilitation specialists know, hand problems seldom seem to present themselves in simple textbook formats. Requiring considerable creativity and ingenuity, splints often must be designed to meet multiple rehabilitative goals. For example, the integration of several splints into one eases the changing process from flexion splinting to extension splinting (Fig. 11-42, *A-D*), specialized, removable splint components allow the focus of torque transmission splints to be redirected without changing splints (Fig. 11-43, *A,B*), and the commercial availability of articulated splint components considerably simplifies crucial alterations in wrist position on a splint whose primary focus is enhancing digital motion (Fig. 11-44). The concept that each splint must be created "from the inside out" to meet individual needs cannot be overemphasized. Attempts at rigid, predetermined assignation or matching of given splint configurations to specific diagnoses might be not only ineffective, but also may be harmful to patients.

■ NONARTICULAR SPLINTS

Nonarticular splints do not affect joint motion. Applied to support or reinforce healing or repaired tissue, and employing two-point coaptation forces, many of these splints fit around the circumference of a digital segment or, in the case of metacarpal fracture braces, around the second through fifth metacarpals. Nonarticular splints also may protect healing finger or thumb tips from inadvertent bumping or from dysesthesias and noxious sensory stimuli as the hand is used.

Finger Proximal Phalanx Splints

Nonarticular finger proximal phalanx splints may be fitted to reinforce healing soft tissue structures such as repaired tendon pulleys (Fig. 11-45, *A*) or to immobilize fractures, as with metacarpal or phalangeal fractures (Fig. 11-45, *B*).[19] Because these splints fit circumferentially, it is important to ensure that they do not constrict blood supply or impede venous drainage

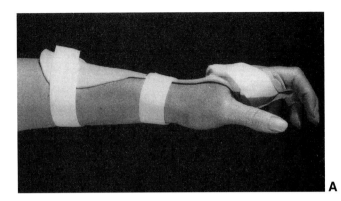
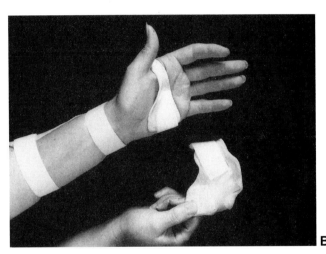

Fig. 11-43   A, Index–small finger IP extension and flexion torque transmission splint, type 2 (13) B, Index–small finger extension and flexion torque transmission splint, type 1 (13) A removable palmar proximal interphalangeal bar allows easy changeover from a *type 2 IP torque transmission splint* to a *type 1 finger torque transmission splint*. (Courtesy Sharon Flinn, MEd, OTR/L, CHT, Cleveland, Ohio.)

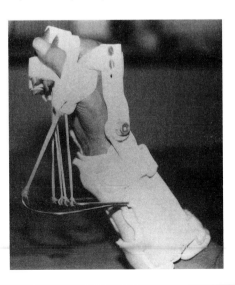

Fig. 11-44   Index–small finger flexion, thumb CMC palmar abduction mobilization splint, type 1 (13) Adjustable wrist unit facilitates tension changes to extrinsic musculotendinous units. (Courtesy Kathryn Schultz, OTR, CHT, Orlando, Fla.)

at or distal to the site of splint application. Nonarticular proximal phalanx splints allow full motion of the adjacent MP and PIP joints. Patient education programs are fundamental to successful outcomes using these splints.

Finger Middle Phalanx Splints

Protecting healing structures of finger amputations, *nonarticular finger middle phalanx splints* (Fig. 11-46) allow early use of remaining finger segments.

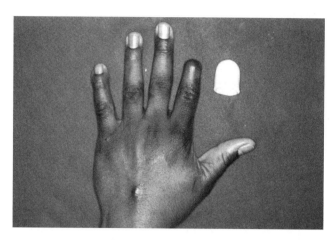

Fig. 11-46   Nonarticular index finger middle phalanx splint
Allowing full PIP joint motion, a middle phalanx splint protects a sensitive amputation stump. Protective splints must be revised as the stump changes shape and becomes less edematous. Through desensitization programs, patients gradually discontinue stump protection splints.

Full articular motion of the MP and PIP joints is permitted.

Finger Distal Phalanx Splints

Nonarticular finger distal phalanx splints protect sensitive digital tips, provide pressure to healing nail beds, or reinforce distal phalangeal internal fixation hardware. These splints do not impede DIP joint motion.

■ SUMMARY

Pericapsular fibrosis resulting in stiffening of the metacarpophalangeal or interphalangeal joints of the fingers represents the most common disabling problem following hand injury, disease, or surgery. Preventive splints that immobilize or restrict joints in positions least likely to cause stiffness, or mobilizing or torque transmission splints designed to overcome existing contracture are important tools to those involved in the hand rehabilitative process. A sound knowledge of normal anatomy and those factors contributing to the pathologic condition at a given joint is required to make decisions about the design of finger splints. As in any treatment method, the purpose and expected goals of a splint must be well planned and carefully explained to the patient. Once the splint has been applied, it is important to closely monitor progress and to make appropriate alterations in the splint, the wearing schedule, and/or the exercise routine as changes occur throughout the rehabilitation period.

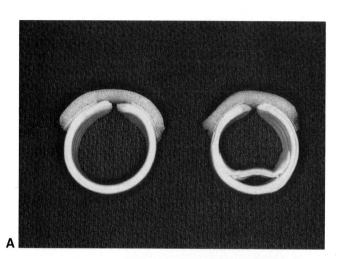

A

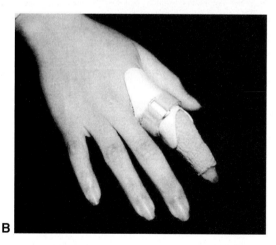

B

Fig. 11-45   A, Nonarticular finger proximal phalanx splint. B, Nonarticular index finger proximal phalanx splint
A, Two different designs of nonarticular finger proximal phalanx splints protect digital pulley injuries/repairs. The splint on the left provides a uniform circumferential pressure around the proximal phalanx, while the splint on the right is designed to minimize the outward force placed on the pulley during active finger flexion through the added palmar pressure bar. **B,** A fracture brace stabilizes the proximal phalanx while allowing PIP motion. [Courtesy **(A)** Diane Collins, MEd, PT, CHT, New Canaan, Conn.; **(B)** from Oxford K, Hildreth D: Fracture bracing for proximal phalanx fractures, *J Hand Ther* 9(4):404, 1996.]

REFERENCES

1. Benaglia PG, Sartorio F, Ingenito R: Evaluation of a thermoplastic splint to protect the proximal interphalangeal joints of volleyball players, *J Hand Ther* 9(1):52-6, 1996.
2. Bowers W: *The interphalangeal joints*, Churchill Livingstone, 1987, Edinburgh.
3. Brand PW, Hollister A: *Clinical mechanics of the hand*, ed 2, Mosby, 1993, St. Louis.
4. Byrne A, Yau T: A modified dynamic traction splint for unstable intra-articular fractures of the proximal interphalangeal joint, *J Hand Ther* 8(3):216-8, 1995.
5. Colditz JC: Low profile dynamic splinting of the injured hand, *Am J Occup Ther* 37(3):182-8, 1983.
6. Dennys L, Hurst L, Cox J: Management of proximal interphalaneal joint fractures using a new dynamic traction splint and early active motion, *J Hand Ther* 5(1):16-24, 1992.
7. Fess EE: Force magnitude of commercial spring-coil and spring-wire splints designed to extend the proximal interphalangeal joint, *J Hand Ther* 2:86-90, 1988.
8. Fess EE: Convergence points of normal fingers in individual and simultaneous flexion, *J Hand Ther* 2(1):12-9, 1989.
9. James JIP: Fractures of the proximal and middle phalanges of the fingers, *Acta Orthop Scand* 32:401-12, 1962.
10. James JIP: Common, simple errors in the management of hand injuries. In *Royal Society of Medicine*, Royal Society of Medicine, 1970, London.
11. Landsmeer JM: Observations on the joints of the human finger, *Ann Rheum Dis* 28(5 Suppl):11-4, 1969.
12. Landsmeer JM: Cross-section analysis of the human finger, *J Anat* 111(3):474-5, 1972.
13. Landsmeer JM: The interphalangeal joints in man, *Acta Morphol Neerl Scand* 13(3):240-1, 1975.
14. Landsmeer JM: The proximal interphalangeal joint, *Hand* 7(1):30, 1975.
15. Landsmeer JM, Long C: The mechanism of finger control, based on electromyograms and location analysis, *Acta Anat* (Basel), 60(3):330-47, 1965.
16. Lei B, Lei E: Hand-based PIP flexion assist splint, *J Hand Ther* 6(4):339-40, 1993.
17. Macht S, Watson S: The Moberg volar advancement flap for digital reconstruction, *J Hand Surg* 5(4):372-6, 1980.
18. Mazon C, Ulson HJ, Davitt M, et al: The use of synthetic plaster casting tape for hand and wrist splints, *J Hand Ther* 9(4):391-3, 1996.
19. Oxford K, Hildreth D: Fracture bracing for proximal phalanx fractures, *J Hand Ther* 9(4):404-5, 1996.
20. Prosser R: Splinting in the management of proximal interphalangeal joint flexion contracture, *J Hand Ther* 9(4):378-86, 1996.
21. Prosser R, Conolly WB: Complications following surgical treatment for Dupuytren's contracture, *J Hand Ther* 9(4):344-8, 1996.
22. Rayan GM, Mullins P: Skin necrosis complicating mallet finger splinting and vascularity of the distal interphalangeal joint overlying skin, *J Hand Surg* 12(4):548-52, 1987.
23. Rennie HJ: Evaluation of the effectiveness of a metacarpophalangeal ulnar deviation orthosis, *J Hand Ther* 9(4):371-7, 1996.
24. Rose II: MP/PIP adjustable digit blocking splint, *J Hand Ther* 9(3):247-8, 1996.
25. Schenck RR: Dynamic traction and early passive movement for fractures of the proximal interphalangeal joint, *J Hand Surg* [Am] 11(6):850-8, 1986.
26. Spoor CW, Landsmeer JM: Analysis of the zigzag movement of the human finger under influence of the extensor digitorum tendon and the deep flexor tendon, *J Biomech* 9(9):561-6, 1976.
27. Srinivasan MS, Knowles D, Wood J: The OSSY splint, a new design of dynamic extension splint, *Br J Hand Ther* 5(3):72-4, 2000.
28. van Veldhoven G: Proximal interphalangeal joint swing traction splint, *J Hand Ther* 8(4):265-8, 1995.
29. Von Prince K, Yeakel M: *The splinting of burn patients*, Charles C. Thomas, 1974, Springfield, IL.
30. Wong S: Combination splint for distal interphalangeal joint stability and protected proximal interphalangeal joint mobility, *J Hand Ther* 8(4):269, 1995.

SUGGESTED READING

Brand PW, Hollister A: *Clinical mechanics of the hand*, ed 3, Mosby, 1999, St. Louis.
Green DP, Hotchkiss R, Pederson W: *Operative hand surgery*, ed 4, Churchill Livingstone, 1998, London.
Mackin EJ, Callahan AD, Osterman AL, et al: *Hunter, Mackin & Callahan's rehabilitation of the hand and upper extremity*, ed 5, Mosby, 2002, St. Louis.
Van Lede P, van Veldhoven G: *Therapeutic hand splints: a rational approach*, Vol 1, Provan, 1998, Antwerp, Belgium.

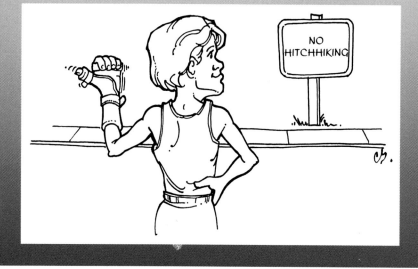

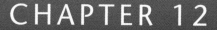

CHAPTER 12

Splints Acting on the Thumb

Chapter Outline

This chapter follows the expanded ASHT Splint Classification System format by first dividing splints into articular or nonarticular categories. In the articular category, splints are next grouped according to the primary joint or joints they influence. Splints in the nonarticular category are defined by the anatomical segments upon which they are based.

Once articular splints are grouped according to their primary joints, they are further defined by direction of force application and then divided according to one of four purposes: immobilization, mobilization, restriction, or torque transmission. Splints with more than one primary purpose are designated by dual-purpose categories (e.g., mobilization/restriction or immobilization/mobilization). In this chapter, force direction (e.g., palmar abduction, radial abduction, flexion, extension, etc.) for thumb splints is included in the purpose groupings. Purpose categories are further subdivided by *type*. *Type* identifies the number of secondary joint levels included in splints. Note: *Type* refers to the number of secondary joint levels, not the total number of secondary joints in a splint. While not all categories and/or subcategories are represented in this chapter, the ESCS is sufficiently flexible to accommodate additional groupings as needed.

The importance of the thumb in almost all aspects of hand function cannot be overstated. The presence of an opposable thumb gives the human species a manual dexterity that is unparalleled in lower animal forms. Insurance companies assess a 40% functional loss to a hand that is missing the thumb; the real loss may be substantially greater. Because of the tremendous disability resulting from thumb loss, hand surgeons have long striven to develop techniques to salvage or restore thumb function. Loss may result from congenital absence, traumatic amputation, disease, or injury.

The functional requirements of the thumb differ substantially from those of the other four digits. Thumb stability, for example, is much more important than mobility, and a thumb unit with basilar joint motion alone permits adequate function despite fused distal joints. Even a completely immobile first metacarpal may serve as a stable post for prehension with the mobile adjacent digits if it is in the correct position. In addition to stability, it is important that the thumb unit retains sufficient length for pinch and grasp functions and sensibility of at least a protective grade without pain and hypersensitivity. The maintenance of proper thumb position, therefore, is extremely important. Splints that correct thumb deformities, establish and maintain an adequate first web space, help mobilize stiffened thumb joints, and/or transmit torque to improve motion and function are among the most important discussed in this book.

Consisting of three joints, the thumb ray is a multiarticular, open kinematic chain that moves through three planes and combinations thereof. The distal segment of the chain is allowed a high degree of freedom of movement as the result of the sum of the participating joints (Fig. 12-1). This arrangement helps minimize the disabling effect of the restriction or loss of motion at any of the individual joints as the result of trauma or disease. Circumduction and opposition motions allowed by the CMC joint are critical to positioning the thumb for pinch and grasp tasks.[1] Flexion, extension, and slight rotation of the MP joint facilitate grasp and release of a wide range of objects of differing sizes. Adding the final increment of refinement, the thumb IP joint plays an important role in very fine, precision activities.

Depending on individual patient needs, thumb splints may be applied to immobilize, mobilize, restrict, or transmit torque. Multipurpose splints tackle more complicated problems. For example, a splint may simultaneously immobilize the thumb CMC joint and restrict motion at the MP and IP joints, protecting proximal healing structures while allowing predefined limited motion at the two more distal joints.

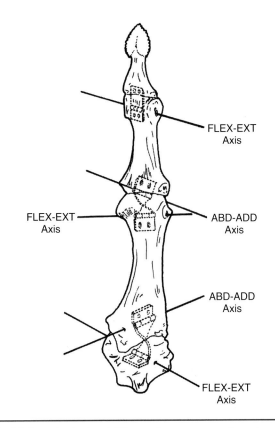

Fig. 12-1   The CMC and MP joints have two axes of rotation while the IP joint has one, allowing multiplanar motion at the CMC and, to a much lesser degree, at the MP joints and single plane motion at the IP joint. (From Brand PW, Hollister A: *Clinical mechanics of the hand*, ed 3, Mosby, 1999, St Louis.)

Immobilization splints prevent motion of the entire thumb or of selected segments within the thumb ray to allow healing, control early postoperative motion, decrease pain, or enhance functional use. Inflammatory conditions and soft tissue injuries of thumb structures often require splint immobilization. Postoperative immobilization between exercise periods effectively limits use while allowing early motion. *Mobilization* splints maintain or increase passive range of motion. For supple thumb joints, in a paralyzed or partially paralyzed thumb, mobilization splinting preserves passive range of motion and prevents deformity while permitting continued functional use. Since optimal effectiveness of the thumb depends on combined mobility and stability, when thumb motion is limited by tethering scar and fibrosed soft tissues, restoration of motion of the three thumb joints is an important part of the rehabilitation process. Splinting and active range of motion exercises, combined with purposeful activity, are the cornerstones of mobilizing stiffened joints. Maximum passive range of motion of the involved joints must be accomplished and maintained before a corresponding active range of motion may be achieved or before surgical procedures may be attempted. Through application of prolonged gentle mobilization forces that cause soft tissue remodeling, splinting is the most effective means for improving thumb passive range of motion. *Restriction* splints limit specific joint motion to protect healing thumb structures, influence reparative scar formation, decrease pain, or enhance functional use. Thumb *torque transmission* splints transfer moment to joints beyond the physical boundaries of splints to increase motion of supple joints or to remodel stiff joints.

Thumb splints involve one or more joints and may be fitted dorsally, palmarly, laterally, or circumferentially. Care should be taken to maintain correct ligamentous stress at each joint traversed, while allowing full motion of unsplinted joints. Because many thumb splints have narrow configurations, contouring splinting material to half the segmental thickness provides splint strength. C-bar and/or thumb post components should be of sufficient length to fully control thumb segment(s); if the wrist is included, the forearm trough should be at least two thirds the length of the forearm to achieve optimum mechanical performance. Straps placed at the level of the axis of joint rotation provide maximum mechanical purchase. Circumferentially designed thumb splints eliminate the need for counterforce straps at joints by providing opposing forces along the entire length of the segment.

Severe hand injuries, particularly if a component of crush is involved, often produce an insidious contracture of the first web space, which, if permitted to persist, rapidly develops into a rigid adduction deformity that will markedly limit thumb function. Wrist position increases or decreases the amount of tension on thumb structures through alteration of the tenodesis effect. When extrinsic thumb musculotendinous units are involved, the wrist must be included in the splint as a secondary joint.

Regardless of the intent of splint application, the basic principles of mechanics, outriggers and mobilization assists, design, construction, and fit must be implemented to create splints that meet the requirements of presenting situations. The purpose of this chapter is to discuss splinting techniques as they relate to the thumb.

■ ARTICULAR THUMB SPLINTS
Thumb CMC Splints

The carpometacarpal joint of the thumb is a triaxial saddle articulation that allows movement through multiple planes. CMC joint ligaments provide first metacarpal stability in palmar abduction and allow

metacarpal rotation in neutral. Palmar ligaments include the anterior intermetacarpal ligament, the anterior oblique carpometacarpal ligament, and the radial carpometacarpal ligament. Dorsal ligaments are the posterior oblique carpometacarpal and the posterior intermetacarpal ligaments. The larger posterior ligament is similar to the collateral ligament at the finger MP joints with relaxation in extension and tension in flexion and opposition. To maintain or gain CMC joint ligament length, the splinted position of the first metacarpal should be alternated from full radial abduction to full palmar abduction to minimize the possibility of shortening of the five carpometacarpal articular ligaments as described by Haines[5] and Napier.[8] This may be accomplished through use of two splints with differing directional forces, one toward full palmar abduction and the other toward full radial abduction, and through a carefully supervised exercise routine. Some clinicians opt for a middle-of-the-road approach by positioning the first metacarpal midway between palmar and radial abduction. However, this requires vigilant monitoring of CMC joint motion to ensure that full palmar and radial abduction motion is not compromised inadvertently.

Immobilization Splints

Preventing motion at the most proximal thumb joint, *CMC immobilization splints* may include the CMC joint alone or they may incorporate one or more secondary joints sited distal or proximal to the thumb CMC joint. To achieve complete immobilization of the CMC joint, it is important that at least one proximal joint and one, preferably two, distal joints are included as secondary joint levels. *Thumb CMC immobilization splints* frequently position the thumb in palmar abduction but also may be used for thumb radial abduction, depending on patient-specific requisites.

Patients with CMC arthritis find a *thumb carpometacarpal palmar abduction immobilization splint* decreases pain with prehension activities by alleviating stress on the thumb joint. These splints are fabricated in many designs, furnishing multiple options for adaptation according to each patient's lifestyle.

Type 0. *Type 0 immobilization splints* include only the primary thumb CMC joint. No secondary joints are integrated in *type 0 thumb CMC immobilization splints* (Fig. 12-2, A-C). Because purchase on the first metacarpal is difficult to achieve, exacting fit of the splinting material to the contours of the thenar eminence, first web space, and palmar arch is critical in order to immobilize the CMC joint in a *type 0* splint. Even with good fit, increments of

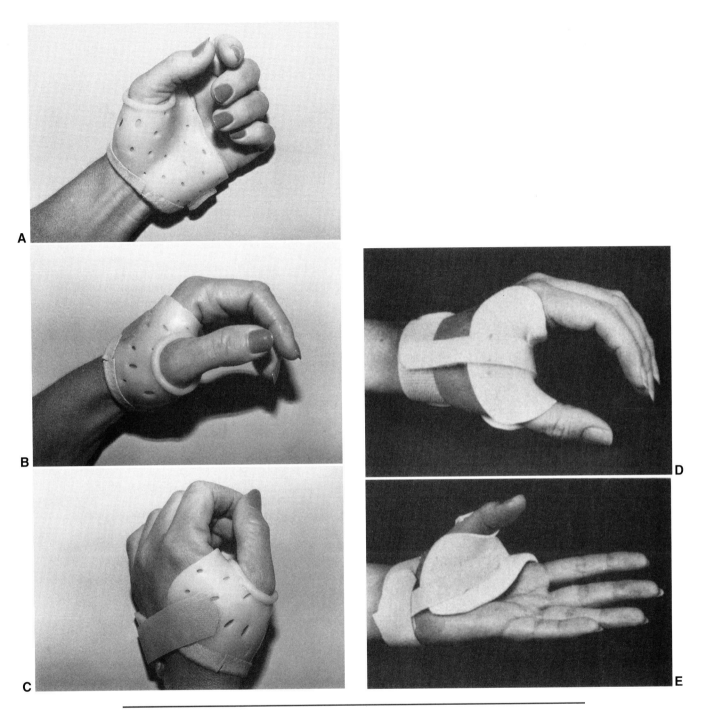

Fig. 12-2   **A-C, Thumb CMC palmar abduction immobilization splint, type 0 (1) D,E, Thumb CMC palmar abduction immobilization splint, type 1 (2) F,G, Thumb CMC palmar abduction immobilization splint, type 1 (2) H, Thumb CMC palmar abduction immobilization splint, type 2 (3) I, Thumb CMC radial abduction immobilization splint, type 3 (4)**

A-C, A type 0 immobilization splint is commonly used to decrease pain associated with overuse of the CMC joint. This splint nicely incorporates a rolled edge to allow unencumbered use of the MP joint and a padded proximal edge for comfort during wrist motion. **D-G,** A carpometacarpal immobilization splint, type 1 allows full range of motion of adjacent finger metacarpophalangeal joints while holding the first metacarpal stationary. **D,E,** Straps are designed to prevent distal migration of the splint. **H,** Mechanically, a type 2 CMC immobilization splint that incorporates both a proximal and a distal secondary joint provides excellent immobilization control of the thumb CMC joint. **I,** This CMC radial abduction splint protects the fracture supported by the external fixation device. The splint does not interfere with the orthopaedic appliance but immobilizes all segments distal to the injury and the index metacarpophalangeal joint for increased stability. [Courtesy **(A-C)** Rebecca Duncan, PT, Lynchburg, Va.; **(F,G)** Barbara Smith, OTR, Edmond, Okla.; **(I)** Brenda Hilfrank, PT, CHT, South Burlington, Vt.]

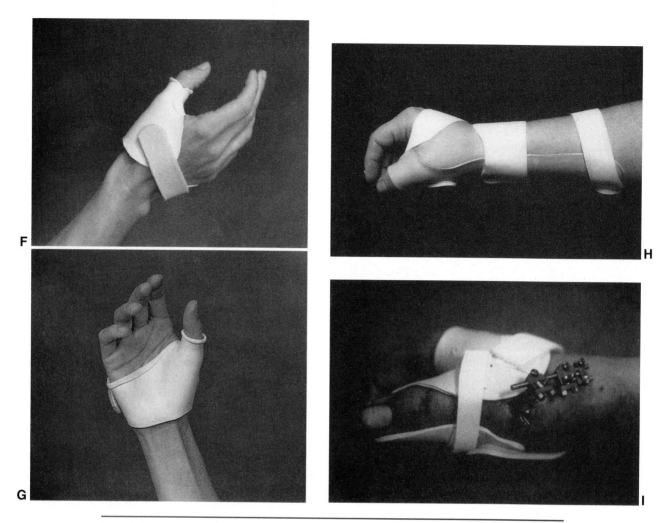

Fig. 12-2, cont'd
For legend see p. 331.

motion may occur at the CMC joint in splints in this classification.

Type 1 and Up. *Type 1* and higher *thumb CMC immobilization splints* include one or more normal secondary joints. Distally sited secondary joints in *thumb CMC immobilization splints* may include the thumb MP (*type 1*), thumb MP and IP (*type 2*), the thumb MP, IP, and index MP (*type 3*), and so on. In contrast, proximally sited secondary joints are usually limited to the wrist (*type 1*) or occasionally the wrist and forearm (*type 2*). If both proximal and distal secondary joints are included, the type count may range from *type 2* upward, depending on how many secondary joint levels are involved. For example, if thumb MP and IP and index finger MP joints are distal secondary joints and the wrist and forearm also are included proximally as secondary joints, the resulting splint is defined as a *thumb CMC immobilization splint, type 5 (6).*

Incorporation of one secondary joint, either the thumb MP or the wrist, increases splint mechanical advantage on the CMC joint, providing more secure immobilization control of the thumb CMC joint than a *type 0* splint (Fig. 12-2, *D-G*). A *type 1* CMC splint that immobilizes the wrist as a proximal secondary joint instead of the distal MP joint permits full motion of both thumb MP and IP joints. CMC immobilization splints that include two secondary joint levels are designated *type 2* and may incorporate the thumb MP and IP joints, the wrist and forearm joints, or the wrist and thumb MP as secondary joints. A *type 2* or *type 3* splint that incorporates both a proximal and a distal secondary joint mechanically provides superior immobilization control of the thumb CMC joint than do splints that include two or more proximal or two or more distal secondary joints (Fig. 12-2, *H*). Hand-based splint designs that include, as secondary joints, the index finger MP in addition to the thumb

MP and IP joints to better stabilize the CMC joint are examples of *type 3 CMC immobilization splints* (Fig. 12-2, *I*). Despite inclusion of three or more distally situated secondary joints, these splints are not as efficient at immobilizing the thumb CMC joint as are splints that include a combination of both proximal and distal secondary joints.

Immobilization splinting of the CMC joint in arthritis patients has been shown to be an effective method of treatment that diminishes but does not eliminate symptoms of basilar joint disease.[16,17] Clinically, patients with CMC joint disease seem to prefer *type 1 CMC immobilization splints* that leave the wrist free, although a study by Weiss, LaStayo, et al. found that splinting does not increase pinch strength or alter pain associated with pinch strength assessment.[16]

Mobilization Splints

Pathologic conditions at the carpometacarpal joint level will often result in limited motion of the first metacarpal with concomitant narrowing of the first web space. Any splint designed to maintain or increase passive range of thumb carpometacarpal motion must have its site of force application on the first metacarpal. Practically speaking, however, this is difficult because of the intervening soft tissue of the first web space. Many ill-conceived splints fitted with the intent of increasing CMC motion actually apply most of the rotational force to the proximal phalanx, resulting in attenuation of the ulnar collateral ligament of the metacarpophalangeal joint, radial deviation of the proximal phalanx, pressure over the radiometacarpal condyle, and instability of the thumb. Care must be taken to ensure that as much of the distal aspect of the first metacarpal is included in the splint as possible and that the primary site of the rotational force is directed toward the metacarpal (Fig. 12-3, *A,B*). To decrease the amount of pressure on the first metacarpal, the area of force application may be widened to include the proximal phalanx as a secondary joint. This addition, however, must not jeopardize the stability of the metacarpophalangeal joint by exerting a stretching force on the ulnar collateral ligament. In most instances the splint need not be extended distally beyond the interphalangeal flexion crease, thus allowing full motion of the distal phalanx. The splint should also be fitted proximal to the distal palmar flexion crease, permitting full metacarpophalangeal flexion of the adjacent fingers.[10] When fingers and thumb both are involved, the thumb CMC joint should be positioned carefully. Radial abduction of the thumb to permit full digital flexion may compromise CMC joint motion by allowing unwarranted ligament shortening. Mobilization of the

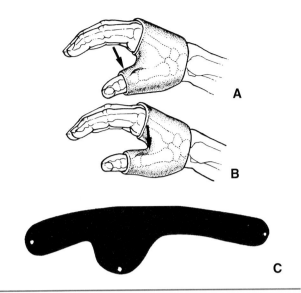

Fig. 12-3   A,B, Thumb CMC palmar abduction mobilization splint, type 1 (2)
To avoid damage to the metacarpophalangeal ulnar collateral ligament when mobilizing a thumb carpometacarpal joint, force should be directed toward the head of the first metacarpal instead of the proximal phalanx. **A,** Incorrect. **B,** Correct. **C,** When using elastic traction to mobilize the thumb carpometacarpal joint, this modified Phelps/Weeks thumb sling fits on the first metacarpal and provides two-directional force application to the first metacarpal. [**(A,B)** from Fess EE: Splinting for mobilization of the thumb. In Hunter JM, et al: *Rehabilitation of the hand,* ed 2, Mosby, 1984, St. Louis; **(C)** Karen Priest Barrett, OTR, Atlanta, Ga.]

thumb carpometacarpal joint in palmar abduction is critical to attaining a functional hand. A thumb held in adduction cannot be used in opposition. Radial abduction is also important to hand function, allowing wider grasp span and open hand contact for push movements.

Type 0. *Type 0 CMC mobilization splints* affect motion at the CMC joint without incorporating secondary joints. Depending on CMC joint mobility, these splints may be fabricated from various materials whose properties range from flexible to rigid. If a CMC joint is supple or near supple, maintenance of joint motion may be accomplished with simple splint designs in soft or semirigid materials (Fig. 12-4, *A,B*). If full passive range of motion is not present at the carpometacarpal joint, slow, progressive, inelastic mobilization traction may be applied through the use of serial *CMC abduction mobilization splints* (Fig. 12-4, *C*) that are adjusted to increase palmar or radial abduction every 2 or 3 days. Progressive splinting of the thumb is continued until the passive measurements of abduction duplicate those of the normal thumb or until the passive motion remains unchanged for three or four consecutive splint adjustments. In

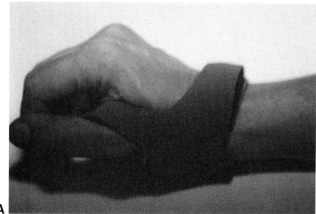

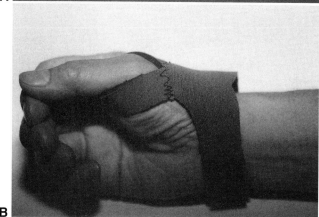

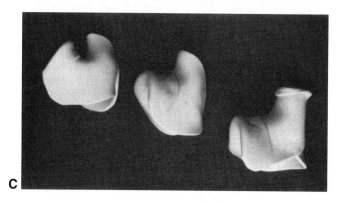

Fig. 12-4   A,B, Thumb CMC radial abduction mobilization splint, type 0 (1) C, Thumb CMC palmar abduction mobilization splint, type 1 (2)

A,B, A splint fabricated in neoprene is comfortable, lightweight, and easy to apply and remove. The thumb strap component mobilizes the CMC into radial abduction. C, Serial CMC mobilization splints are widened every 2 or 3 days. [Courtesy **(A,B)** Elizabeth Spencer Steffa, OTR/L, CHT, Seattle, Wash.; **(C)** from Fess EE: Splinting for mobilization of the thumb. In Hunter JM, et al: *Rehabilitation of the hand,* ed 2, Mosby, 1984, St. Louis, Mo.]

most instances, inelastic serial carpometacarpal mobilization splints are more effective than elastic traction splinting for increasing the passive range of motion of the thumb carpometacarpal joint. This, of course, depends on the patient's ability to return for frequent splint changes.

Type 1 and Up. *Type 1 CMC mobilization splints* incorporate one normal secondary joint, sited either proximally or distally, to improve splint control and enhance mechanical effect. These splints often include the thumb MP as a distal secondary joint to achieve better purchase on the first metacarpal (Fig. 12-2, *D-G*). As noted above, corrective forces must be applied to the first metacarpal, *not* to the proximal phalanx.

CMC mobilization splints that include more than one secondary joint are classified according to the number of secondary joint levels incorporated in each splint. As with *CMC immobilization splints, type 3* mobilization splints often include the index finger MP joint in addition to the thumb MP and IP joints to disperse pressure and increase mechanical advantage (Fig. 12-5, *A,B*). If thumb extrinsic tendons are tethered by scar, incorporation of the wrist as a secondary joint is necessary to remodel restraining scar tissue (Fig. 12-5, *C*).

Restriction Splints

Fitted to protect healing tissues, decrease pain, or increase function, thumb CMC restriction splints limit one or more selected motions of the CMC joint. Secondary joints may or may not be included in these splints, depending on individual patient needs. Generally speaking, unidirectional splints that restrict motion in one plane frequently are based on a single layer "wrapped strap" design while circumduction restriction splints tend to be more circumferential in design or they incorporate multiple layers of "strapping."

Type 0. Only CMC joint motion is affected with *type 1 thumb CMC restriction splints.* These "strap" splint designs may be constructed in soft materials when splinting smaller hands or when minimal to moderate control is required. For example, functional hand use may improve with a neoprene *type 0 thumb CMC radial adduction restriction splint* that blocks the final 10-20° thumb adduction arc of motion. These simple splints bring the thumb out of the palm while allowing other CMC joint motions for patients with upper motor neuron dysfunction (Fig. 12-6, *A,B*).

Type 1. A *thumb CMC restriction splint, type 1 (2)* includes one secondary joint, usually the thumb MP. As with *type 0* splints, restricted motion may involve one (Fig. 12-6, *C,D*) or multiple planes (Fig. 12-6, *E-H*) as dictated by patient requirements.

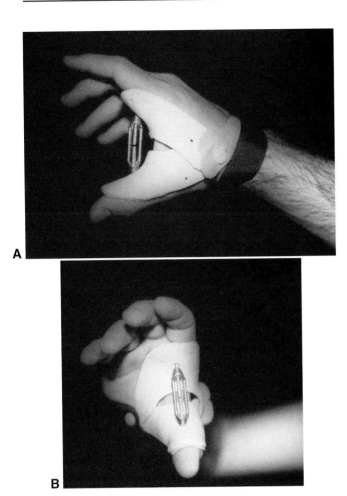

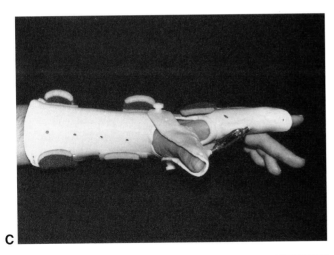

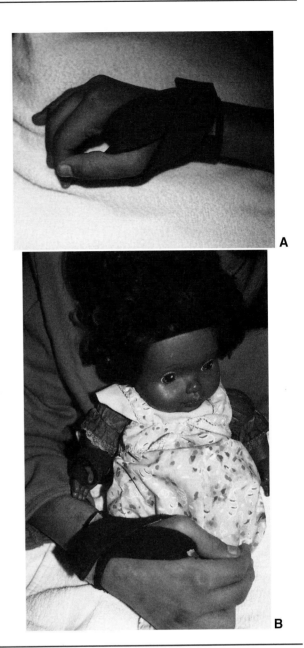

Fig. 12-5   **A,B, Thumb CMC palmar abduction mobilization splint, type 3 (4) C, Thumb CMC radial abduction mobilization splint, type 5 (6)**
A,B, This two-piece jointed splint mobilizes the thumb CMC by serially adjusting the first metacarpal into palmar abduction. **C,** To increase lever arms for CMC radial abduction, five secondary joints are included in the splint's design. (Courtesy Daniel Lupo, OTR, CHT, Ventura, Calif.)

Fig. 12-6   **A,B, Thumb CMC adduction restriction splint, type 0 (1) C,D, Thumb CMC adduction restriction splint, type 1 (2) E,F, Thumb CMC circumduction restriction splint, type 1 (2) G,H, Thumb CMC circumduction restriction splint, type 1 (2) I, Thumb CMC circumduction restriction splint, type 2 (3) J,K, Thumb CMC circumduction torque transmission splint, type 2 (3) L, Thumb CMC circumduction torque transmission splint, type 3 (4)**
A,B, A neoprene splint restricting the final degrees of thumb CMC adduction allows functional activities to be achieved through lateral prehension of the thumb and index finger. **C,D,** Strap direction of pull on this circumferentially fitting neoprene splint limits CMC adduction. **E-H,** By altering the placement and configuration of wrapping, soft splinting materials restrict thumb CMC joint motion. **I,** This commercially available soft splint restricts the extremes of thumb CMC joint motion. **J,K,** These type 2 and **(L)** type 3 torque transmission splints focus transferred active thumb motion to the thumb CMC. [Courtesy **(A,B)** Joni Armstrong, OTR, CHT, Bemidji, Minn.; **(C,D)** Shelli Dellinger, OTR, CHT, San Diego, Calif.; **(E-H)** Bobbie-Ann Neel, OTR, Opelika, Ala. (Splint, patent pending.)]

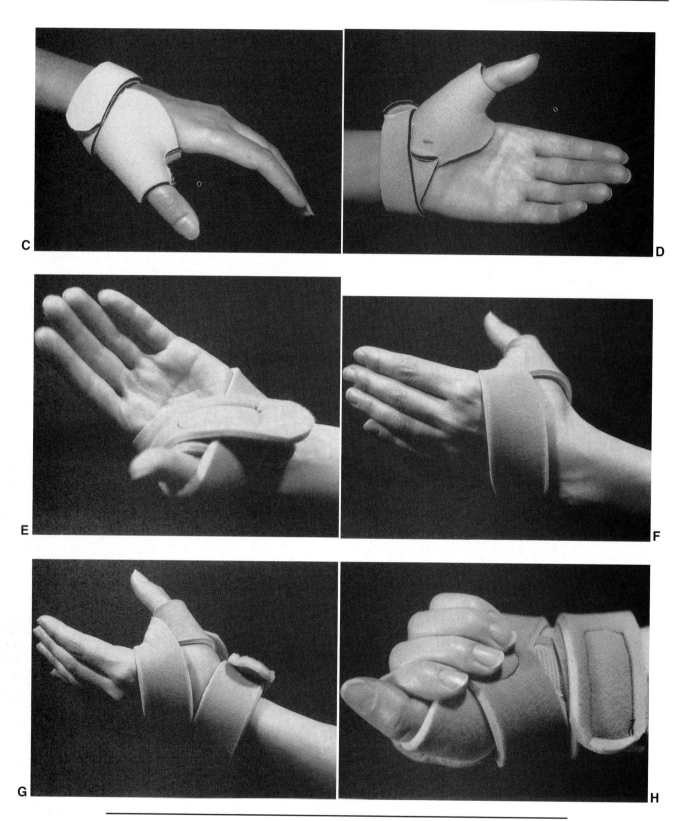

Fig. 12-6, cont'd
For legend see p. 335.

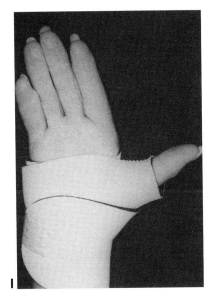

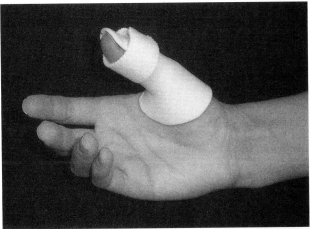

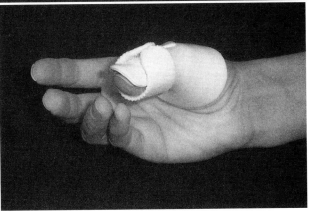

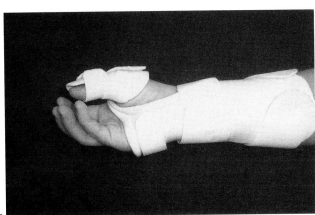

Fig. 12-6, cont'd
For legend see p. 335.

Type 2. With two secondary joints, the wrist and thumb MP, more stability is provided to the CMC joint while allowing motion in all planes with extremes of motion restricted (Fig. 12-6, *I*).

Torque Transmission Splints

Torque transmission splints may be used to transfer moment to the thumb CMC joint, to mobilize the CMC joint if it is supple, or to remodel it if passive range of motion is limited.

Type 2. *Type 2 CMC torque transmission splints* include two secondary joints in addition to the primary thumb CMC joint. The two secondary joints are almost always situated distal to the CMC joint (Fig. 12-6, *J,K*).

Type 3. The wrist, thumb MP, and IP joint levels are incorporated secondarily in *type 3 thumb CMC*

torque transmission splints (Fig. 12-6, *L*). Specific thumb CMC joint motions may be facilitated by positioning the wrist in attitudes that either encourage or discourage thumb extrinsic tendon excursion.

Thumb CMC, MP Splints

Incorporating two primary thumb joints, these splints immobilize, mobilize, restrict motion, or transmit torque at/to the thumb CMC and MP joints. Proximal and/or distal secondary joints may or may not be included in thumb CMC, MP splints. Although similar in configuration to earlier described CMC *type 1* splints that include a normal thumb MP as a secondary joint in order to enhance inherent splint mechanical action, these splints differ in that both CMC and MP joints are primary joints, indicating that pathology exists at the MP as well as the CMC joint.

Immobilization Splints

Thumb CMC, MP immobilization splints halt passive and active motion at both the thumb CMC and MP joints. Secondary joints may or may not be included in these splints.

Type 0. Stopping motion at the thumb's two most proximal joints, *type 0 CMC, MP immobilization splints* usually hold the CMC joint in either palmar abduction or radial abduction and the MP joint in extension to allow healing of injured or surgically repaired thumb structures (Fig. 12-7, *A,B*). *Type 0 CMC, MP splints* do not include adjacent proximal or distal normal articulations as secondary joints.

Mobilization Splints

Corrective forces are focused on both the thumb CMC and MP joints in thumb CMC, MP mobilization splints. These splints may or may not include secondary joints to improve mechanical application.

Type 0. Because both thumb CMC and MP joints are mobilized in *type 0 CMC, MP mobilization splints*, it is critical that the force line of application be carefully analyzed and directed. The force line of application must be perpendicular to the rotational axis of the MP joint. If it is not perpendicular, unequal mobilization forces will be directed to thumb MP joint radial and ulnar collateral ligaments, causing differential remodeling of the ligaments and eventual joint instability. Thumb CMC joint articular structures remodel in line with the mobilization forces directed to the MP joint, meaning that full CMC joint motion may not be attained if limitations exist in extreme radial or palmar abduction. Progress of passive CMC joint motion must be monitored carefully to ensure that desired motion is accomplished in all planes. There are no secondary joints in *type 0 thumb CMC, MP mobilization splints* (Fig. 12-8, *A-C*).

Mobilization/Immobilization Splints

In *thumb CMC mobilization / MP immobilization splints*, remodeling forces are applied to the CMC joint and stabilizing forces are applied to the MP joint simultaneously, allowing healing of MP periarticular structures and corrective remodeling of problematic CMC structures. Normal adjacent joints may or may not be included as secondary joints.

Type 0. Mobilization forces to the thumb CMC joint may include elastic traction mobilization assists (Fig. 12-9, *A*) or inelastic traction in the form of sequential serial adjustments (Fig. 12-9, *B*). The MP joint may be immobilized in full extension or in designated increments of flexion, depending on the specific rationale for splint application. No secondary joints are included in *type 0 CMC mobilization/MP*

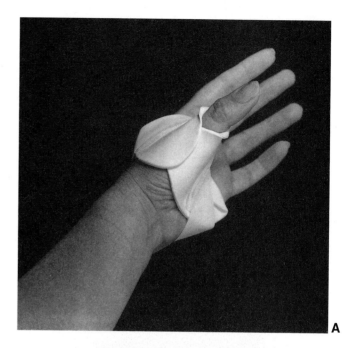

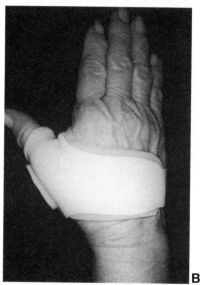

Fig. 12-7   A, Thumb CMC palmar abduction and MP extension immobilization splint, type 0 (2) B, Thumb CMC palmar abduction and MP flexion immobilization splint, type 0 (2) Three-point pressure forces are dispersed along the length of the splinted thumb first metacarpal, MP joint, and proximal phalanx in these circumferential design splints that immobilize the CMC and MP joints.

immobilization splints. Both the CMC and MP joints are primary joints.

Thumb CMC, MP, IP Splints

All three thumb joints are included as primary joints in thumb CMC, MP, IP splints. These splints may be single purpose to immobilize, mobilize, or restrict thumb joint motion or they may be multipurpose with combined objectives, e.g., simultaneous mobilization of two thumb joints with restriction of motion at the third joint. Adjacent joints may or may not be included as secondary joints.

Immobilization Splints

Halting motion at all three thumb joints, thumb CMC, MP, IP immobilization splints allow healing of injured or surgically repaired thumb structures. Secondary joints may or may not be included depending on specific patient requirements.

Type 1. *Type 1 thumb[1] (CMC, MP, IP) immobilization splints* incorporate the wrist as a secondary joint. These splints frequently are employed to manage thumb extrinsic tendon inflammation problems, tendon repairs, some fractures, and selected reconstructive procedures (Fig. 12-10, *A,B*). Wrist and thumb positions are critical and diagnosis specific. Close communication between referring surgeons and those clinicians responsible for designing and fabricating splints is important to ensure that all involved, including patients, understand the rationale for splint application.

Mobilization Splints

Traction forces are simultaneously directed to all three thumb articulations in thumb mobilization splints. Incorporation of secondary joints may or may not be present.

Type 0. A *type 0 thumb (CMC, MP, IP) mobilization splint* uses a unidirectional corrective force to mobilize all three joints of the thumb simultaneously. The mobilizing force must be applied perpendicular to the rotational axes of the thumb MP and IP joints to avoid unequal force application on the respective MP and IP joint collateral ligaments (Fig. 12-11, *A,B*). Collateral ligament attenuation and ensuing joint instability of the MP, IP, or of both joints may result if application of the mobilizing force is not perpendicular. Because the resultant mobilizing force to the CMC joint follows the direction of force application at the MP and IP joints, full passive CMC joint motion may not be realized in all CMC motion planes. Careful monitoring of CMC joint passive motion is requisite to achieving multiplanar CMC joint passive motion.

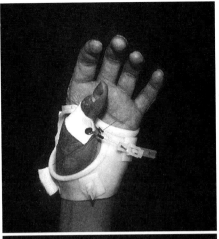
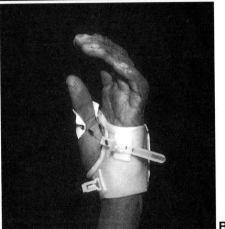
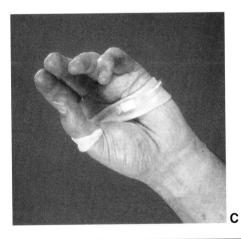

Fig. 12-8   A,B, Thumb CMC palmar abduction and MP flexion mobilization splint, type 0 (2) C, Thumb CMC palmar abduction and MP flexion mobilization splint, type 0 (2)

A,B, Incremental adjustments of the mobilization assist are facilitated with this innovative commercially available mobilization assist. **C,** Applying elastic traction, this splint is simple in design and aesthetically pleasing. [Courtesy **(A,B)** Nelson Vazquez, OTR, CHT, Miami, Fla.; **(C)** Provan, Knokke, Belgium.]

---

[1]When all joints of a digital ray are designated primary joints, the ESCS location is identified by the name of the digital ray, e.g., thumb, index finger, etc.

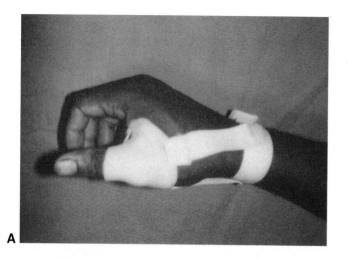

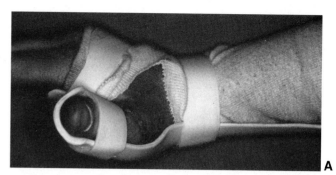

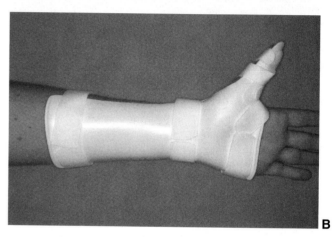

A

B

Fig. 12-10 A, Thumb CMC radial abduction and MP-IP extension immobilization splint, type 1 (4) B, Thumb CMC radial
abduction and MP-IP extension immobilization splint, type 1 (4)
The wrist is included as a secondary joint in these type 1 immobilization splints.

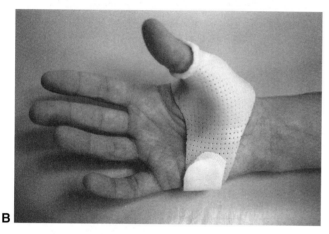

Fig. 12-9 A, Thumb CMC radial abduction mobilization /
thumb MP flexion immobilization splint, type 0 (2) B, Thumb
CMC palmar abduction mobilization / thumb MP flexion immobilization splint, type 0 (2)
Different in their designs, both these splints have dual purposes: to
mobilize and to immobilize simultaneously. While both immobilize
the thumb MP joint in slight flexion, the CMC joint is mobilized into
radial abduction using elastic traction in splint (A) and into palmar
abduction using inelastic traction through sequential serial adjustments in splint (B). [Courtesy (A) Carol Hierman, OTR, CHT, Cedar
Grove, N.C., and Elisha Denny, PTA, OTA, Pittsboro, N.C., © UNC
Hand Rehabilitation Center, Chapel Hill, N.C.]

Restriction/Mobilization Splints

With all thumb joints involved, specified joint motion
is restricted while the remaining joint or joints are
mobilized in *thumb restriction / mobilization* splints.
Secondary joints may or may not be included to
enhance mechanical effect.

Type 1. *Type 1 thumb restriction / mobilization
splints* usually restrict specific motion at the thumb
CMC joint and, at the same time, act to increase
motion at all three joints or only at the thumb MP and
IP joints. One secondary joint, the wrist, is included

in *type 1 thumb restriction / mobilization splints* (Fig.
12-12, A,B).

Thumb CMC, IP Splints

Reflecting unique patient requirements, thumb CMC,
IP splints incorporate the MP joint as a secondary
joint. These splints may immobilize, mobilize,
restrict, or transmit torque to the thumb CMC and IP
primary joints.

Mobilization Splints

Type 1. A *type 1 thumb CMC, IP mobilization
splint* focuses traction forces on the thumb CMC and
IP joints to increase motion at these two joints. The
thumb MP joint is included in the splint as a secondary
joint (Fig. 12-13). Mobilization forces may be elastic,
inelastic, or a combination of the two. In designing
and fitting this splint, it is important that the splinting material fully extends around the proximal
phalanx of the thumb, thus rendering the metacarpophalangeal joint immobile and diminishing the

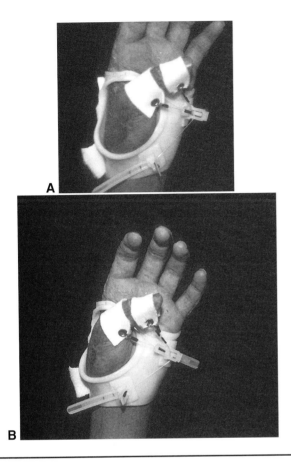

Fig. 12-11   A,B Thumb CMC palmar abduction and MP-IP flexion mobilization splint, type 0 (3)

All three joints of the thumb are mobilized in this splint using two assists to apply individual mobilizing forces perpendicular to the MP and IP joint rotational axes. (Courtesy Nelson Vazquez, OTR, CHT, Miami, Fla.)

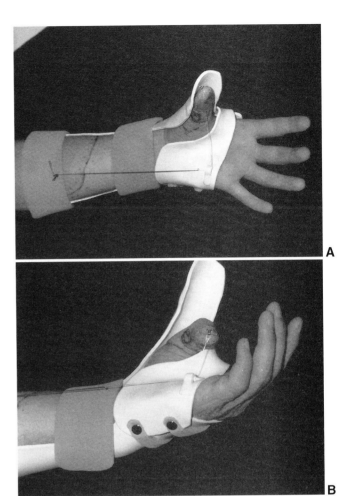

Fig. 12-12   A,B Thumb CMC radial abduction and MP-IP extension restriction / thumb CMC palmar abduction and MP-IP flexion mobilization splint, type 1 (4)

Used in treatment of flexor tendon repairs, the dorsal portion of this splint restricts full active radial abduction and extension of the thumb while the volar splint passively mobilizes the thumb into CMC palmar abduction and MP-IP flexion during exercise. (Courtesy Peggy McLaughlin, OTR, CHT, San Bernardino, Calif.)

pressure on the palmar aspect of the phalanx. Once again, the angle of approach of the rubber band should be at a 90° angle to the distal phalanx and perpendicular to the center of the axis of rotation of the interphalangeal joint. The metacarpophalangeal joints of the fingers should also be permitted a full range of motion into flexion.

Thumb MP Splints

The middle joint in the important thumb intercalated chain is the metacarpophalangeal joint. At this level, stability is a more important consideration than mobility. A wide discrepancy exists in the amount of thumb metacarpophalangeal motion found in the general population, with flexion ranging from only a few degrees to 90°. It is apparent that the functional sequela of limited or absent metacarpophalangeal motion is negligible if the joint is positioned properly

and is stable and pain free. According to some authors, the metacarpophalangeal joint of the thumb, unlike those of the fingers, tends to be more nearly of the ginglymoid, or hinge, type. In mobilizing this joint, care should be taken to apply a rotational force perpendicular to the center of the axis of rotation of the metacarpophalangeal joint. If this concept is disregarded, attenuation of either the ulnar or radial collateral ligament may occur with resulting deviation of the proximal phalanx and metacarpophalangeal joint instability. The angle of the mobilizing force should also be 90° to the proximal phalanx. Splints acting on the MP joint may immobilize, mobilize, restrict, or transmit torque. Secondary joints may or may not be included in these splints.

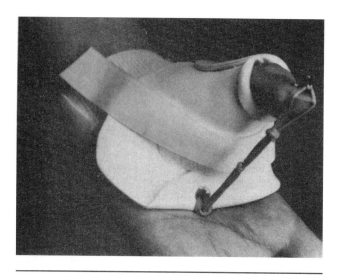

Fig. 12-13 Thumb CMC palmar abduction and IP flexion mobilization splint, type 1 (3)
The combination of inelastic mobilization traction at the CMC joint and elastic mobilization assist consisting of a fingernail clip and rubber band permits simultaneous mobilization of carpometacarpal and interphalangeal joints, respectively.

Immobilization Splints

Thumb MP immobilization splints halt motion at the thumb MP joint and may or may not include adjacent normal joints secondarily. Immobilization splints allow healing of thumb MP articular and/or periarticular structures and also are used to decrease pain.

Type 0. Stopping motion at the middle thumb articulation, *type 0 thumb MP immobilization splints* use three-point force application to limit MP joint motion. Although these splints may be fitted dorsally or palmarly, partial circumferential or circumferential splint designs provide more secure immobilization to the thumb MP joint (Fig. 12-14, *A,B*). Splints usually immobilize the MP joint in extension or slight flexion.

Type 1. A *type 1 thumb MP immobilization splint* incorporates one secondary joint, either proximally or distally, in addition to the primary MP joint where motion is stopped. In a better position to oppose the fingers, the IP joint is frequently left free. Arthritic patients with MP hyperextension deformities find these splints improve hand function because position of the thumb is improved when MP joint subluxation is eliminated (Fig. 12-14, *C*).[2,4] *Type 1 thumb MP immobilization splints* are also used as conservative treatment for ulnar collateral ligament injuries (Fig. 12-14, *D,E*).[3,6,11,13]

Type 2. Two secondary joints are included in *type 2 thumb immobilization splints*. Secondary joints may be the thumb IP and CMC joints for proximal and distal stabilization, or they may include the CMC and wrist joints for proximal control. Ulnar collateral ligament injuries are also treated in *type 2 MP immobilization splints* that include the CMC and wrist joints secondarily to further extend proximal splint control.

Mobilization Splints

Splints designed to maintain or increase thumb MP passive motion often incorporate the CMC joint as a secondary joint to improve mechanical effect on the MP joint. As with metacarpophalangeal joint mobilization in the fingers, the most carefully designed and constructed splints may totally fail to overcome MP joint contracture (usually extension) despite the most vigorous efforts of both therapist and patient. It must be realized at the onset that in many instances this type of fixed deformity has such rigid underlying fibrosis and ligamentous pathologic conditions that no amount of splinting, however well conceived, may be expected to succeed. To avoid frustration, a realistic understanding by all those involved of the possibility of failure is essential when the splinting program is initiated.

Type 0. A *type 0 metacarpophalangeal mobilization splint* in the form of a wristband with an elastic mobilization assist is one of the least complicated means of facilitating thumb metacarpophalangeal flexion. However, it must be remembered that this splint affects motion along the entire thumb ray, including the thumb CMC, MP, and, if a nail hook is used, IP joints, and therefore may be ineffective in cases where only one joint in the thumb ray is passively limited. Further, an incorrect force angle may cause medial or lateral rotation of the first metacarpal with stretching of the carpometacarpal ligaments and intra-articular pressure, as well as undue stressing of the metacarpophalangeal collateral ligaments and joint surfaces (Fig. 12-15, *A*). This kind of MP mobilization splint is rarely effective.

Type 1. *Type 1 thumb MP mobilization splints* include the thumb CMC as a secondary joint in order to better direct mobilization forces to the thumb MP joint. Although traction is usually elastic, inelastic mobilization may be applied through sequential serial adjustments. *Type 1 MP mobilization splints* are designed to increase either MP extension or MP flexion. The direction of force application must be perpendicular to MP joint axis of rotation and perpendicular to the proximal phalanx to avoid unequal stress to the MP collateral ligaments (Fig. 12-15, *B,C*).

Type 2. *Type 2 thumb metacarpophalangeal mobilization splints* allow the application of the full magnitude of the mobilizing force on the metacar-

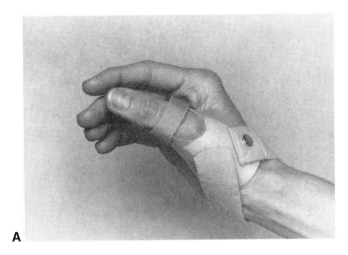

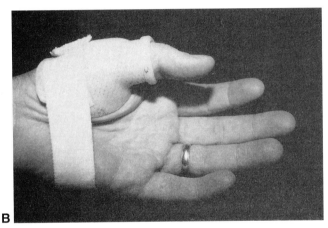

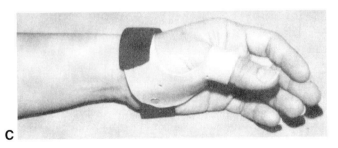

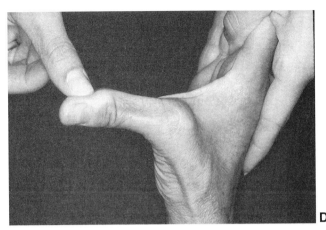

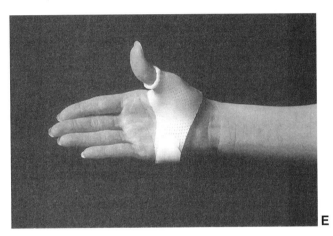

Fig. 12-14   A, Thumb MP flexion immobilization splint, type 0 (1) B, Thumb MP flexion immobilization splint, type 0 (1) C, Thumb MP flexion immobilization splint, type 1 (2) E, Thumb MP flexion immobilization splint, type 1 (2)

Type 0 thumb MP immobilization splints may be used in the treatment of thumb MP collateral ligament injuries (A) and osteoarthritis of the MP joint (B). The design of these splints along with the use of an elastic strap securing the splint to the hand permits CMC motion. C, The thumb CMC joint is a secondary joint in this type 1 MP immobilization splint. D, Disruption or attenuation of the ulnar collateral ligament of the MP joint creates painful instability of the thumb. E, This splint immobilizes the thumb MP joint while including the CMC joint as a secondary joint level. The IP joint is free. [Courtesy (A) Julie Belkin, OTR, CO, MBA, 3-Point Products, Annapolis, Md; (C) from Galindo A, Suet L: A metacarpophalangeal joint stabilization splint, *J Hand Ther* 15(1):83-4, 2002.]

pophalangeal joint by stabilizing both the thumb carpometacarpal joint and the wrist as secondary joints. In special situations, these splints may also be used to direct longitudinal mobilization forces to distract a fractured first metacarpal (Fig. 12-15, *D-F*). For thumb MP joint flexion or extension mobilization, the force angle of approach must be directed 90° to the prox-

imal phalanx and perpendicular to the center of the axis for rotation of the metacarpophalangeal joint. Wrist position through tenodesis effect influences tension on the extrinsic thumb musculotendinous units. *Type 2 thumb MP mobilization splints* may be fitted dorsally, palmarly, radially, or circumferentially.

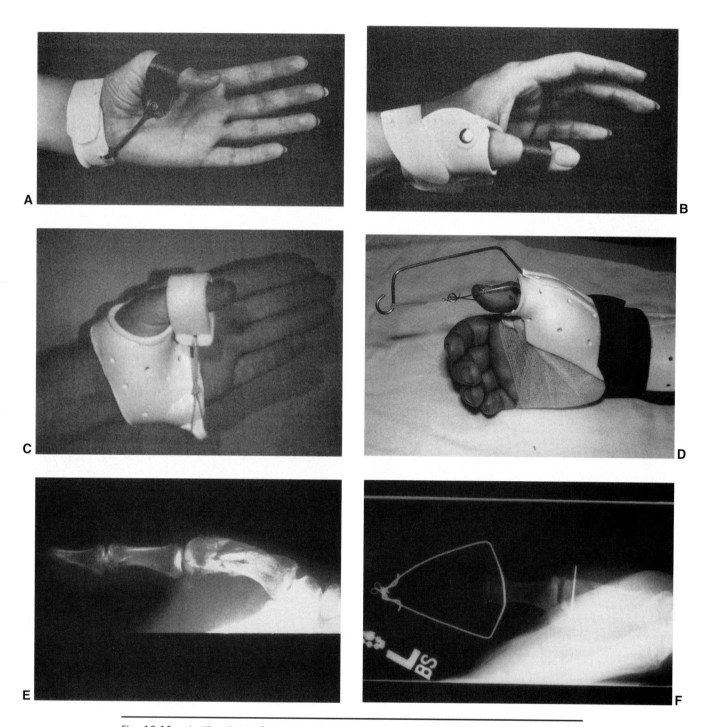

Fig. 12-15   A, Thumb MP flexion mobilization splint, type 1 (2) B, Thumb MP flexion mobilization splint, type 1 (2) C, Thumb MP flexion mobilization splint, type 1 (2) D, First metacarpal distraction, thumb MP distraction mobilization splint, type 2 (3)
A, Mobilization forces intended for the MP joint are dissipated at the normal CMC joint. This attempt at improving MP joint passive motion would be more effective if the CMC joint were immobilized secondarily. B,C, Secondary immobilization of the CMC joint allows mobilization forces to be fully directed to the MP joint. Through application of a longitudinally directed force (D), this splint assists in the alignment and healing process of a comminuted intra-articular metacarpal fracture. F, Note the use of a clip attaching the splint's mobilization assist to the intraosseous distraction wire as seen in this radiograph. [(B) from Fess EE: Splinting for mobilization of the thumb. In Hunter JM, et al: *Rehabilitation of the hand*, ed 2, Mosby, 1984, St. Louis, Mo.; Courtesy (C) Susan Emerson, MEd, OTR, CHT, York, Maine; (D-F) Suzanne Brand, OTR, CHT, Needham, Mass.]

Restriction Splints

Limiting active and passive motion, thumb MP restriction splints control the amount of motion allowed in a normally occurring arc of MP extension or flexion motion or they restrict undesired motion, such as MP radial or ulnar deviation, to allow healing of MP periarticular soft tissue structures and to decrease pain. If the wrist is included as a secondary joint, variations of these splints maybe used in specific extrinsic tendon early motion protocols.

Type 1. *Type 1 thumb MP restriction splints* incorporate one secondary joint, either proximally or distally, to maximize splint mechanical effectiveness on the MP joint. When included as the secondary joint, the CMC joint may be immobilized or it may have near full motion, depending on the specific design of the splint (Fig. 12-16, A-C).[2,12,14] Frequently applied to reduce stress to injured MP ulnar collateral ligaments, these splints are fabricated in many designs. A comfortable and very effective design uses radial and ulnar deviation bars at the thumb IP joint level to restrict thumb MP ulnar deviation. In this splint, the unencumbered area over the dorsal MP joint, proximal phalanx, IP joint, and distal phalanx allows free IP extension and flexion in addition to increments of MP flexion and full MP extension (Fig. 12-16, D,E).

Thumb MP, IP Splints

Splints in this ESCS category focus on both the thumb MP and IP joints as primary joints. Immobilizing, mobilizing, restricting motion at, or transmitting torque to the MP and IP joints, these splints may or may not include secondary joints to improve their mechanical function.

Immobilization Splints

Type 0. *Type 0 MP-IP immobilization splints* stop motion at both the MP and IP joints of the thumb (Fig. 12-17, A). There are no secondary joints included in this splint classification.

Type 1. Incorporating the thumb CMC joint as a secondary joint, *type 1 thumb MP-IP immobilization splints* stop motion at the thumb MP and IP joints to allow healing of injured thumb structures. Although many different designs have been advocated, splints with a contoured thumb post (Fig. 12-17, B) and those with circumferential designs provide better immobilization to the MP and IP joints than do those with flatter designs. Whenever a circumferential design is used care must be taken to ensure that the thumb is not constricted if edema increases. Also, if the splint is too light or flimsy, it may cause an increase in edema due to inconstant application of pressure.

Immobilization/Restriction Splints

Type 1. A *type 1 thumb MP immobilization / IP restriction splint* permits limited motion at the distal thumb joint while simultaneously stopping motion at the middle thumb articulation, the MP joint.[7] The thumb CMC is included in the splint as a secondary joint to improve purchase on the first metacarpal (Fig. 12-17, C,D).

Restriction/Torque Transmission Splints

Type 2. Incorporating the wrist and thumb CMC joints secondarily, *type 2 thumb MP restriction / MP-IP torque transmission splints* transfer moment to the MP and IP joints to promote active motion of supple joints or to remodel stiff MP and IP joints. The transmitted motion is restricted at the MP joint by these splints (Fig. 12-17, E).

Thumb IP Splints

Although strong interphalangeal joint motion is valuable to thumb performance, its absence is not critical. In most cases thumb functions are possible if there is a good carpometacarpal joint and perhaps some metacarpophalangeal joint motion. Thumb IP splints are applied to immobilize, mobilize, restrict, or transmit torque to the IP joint. Secondary joints are often incorporated in these splints but are not mandatory.

Immobilization Splints

Type 0. Only the distal thumb joint is immobilized in a *type 0 thumb IP immobilization splint*. These splints are used to treat a variety of injuries to the distal thumb including selected mallet thumb problems (Fig. 12-18, A,B).[9]

Type 1. *Type 1 thumb immobilization splints* include the thumb MP joint as a secondary joint to improve immobilization leverage on the IP joint. These splints may be applied dorsally, volarly, or circumferentially to permit healing of distally sited thumb structures.

Mobilization Splints

Since the interphalangeal joint of the thumb is a true uniaxial hinge articulation, the mechanical principles previously mentioned regarding mobilization of the thumb metacarpophalangeal joint are applicable to the mobilization of the thumb interphalangeal joint. For optimum results, the angle of approach should be 90° to the distal phalanx of the thumb and perpendicular to the center of the axis of rotation of the interphalangeal joint.

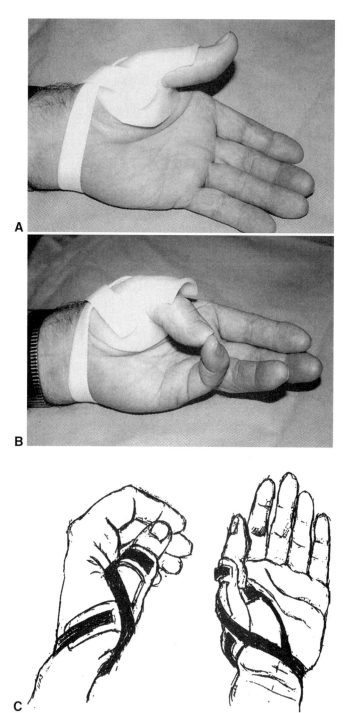

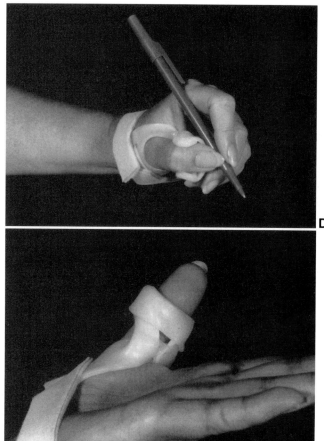

Fig. 12-16   A,B, Thumb MP extension restriction splint, type 1
(2) C, Thumb MP extension restriction splint, type 1 (2) D,E,
Thumb MP radial and ulnar deviation restriction splint, type 1 (2)
A,B, A *type 1 MP extension restriction splint* blocks MP extension
at 30° to unload the thumb basal joint. C, This "strap splint" positions the thumb MP in an antideformity posture for better function.
D,E, This innovative design restricts MP joint deviation while allowing easy thumb use. [(A,B) from Poole JU, Pellegrini VD: Arthritis
of the thumb basal joint complex, *J Hand Ther* 13(2):91-107, 2000;
(C) from Wajon A: Clinical splinting successes: the thumb "strap
splint" for dynamic instability of the trapeziometacarpal joint, *J
Hand Ther* 13(3):236, 2000; courtesy (D,E) Donna Breger Stanton,
MA, OTR, CHT, Kensington, Calif.]

Type 2. Incorporating the thumb CMC and MP
joints as secondary joints to better direct mobilization
forces to the IP joint, *type 2 thumb IP mobilization
splints* increase passive flexion or extension motion
at the thumb IP joint (Fig. 12-19, A-C). The mobilization assist is attached to the thumb via a sling or a
finger-nail attachment (clip or Velcro). To decrease
the amount of pressure incurred by inhibiting motion

at the carpometacarpal and metacarpophalangeal
joints, a *type 2 thumb IP mobilization splint* should
be extended as far distally as possible along the proximal phalanx without interfering with full interphalangeal flexion. Room for complete flexion of the
adjacent digital metacarpophalangeal joints and
support of the transverse metacarpal arch should
also be provided. Some innovative designs include

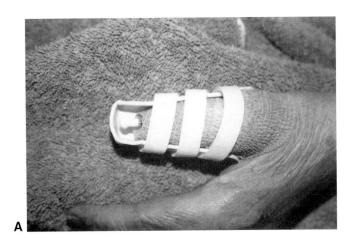

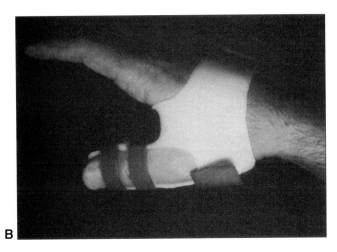

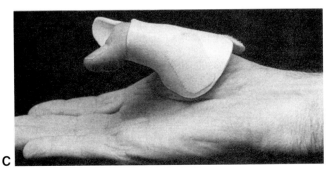

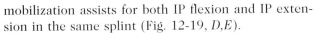

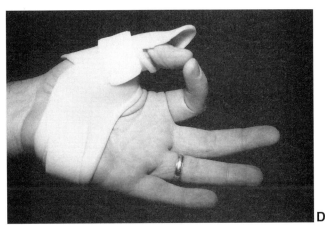

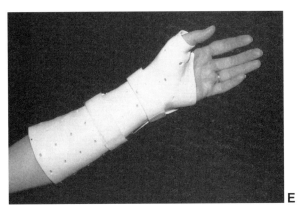

Fig. 12-17   A, Thumb MP-IP extension immobilization splint, type 0 (2) B, Thumb MP-IP extension immobilization splint, type 1 (3) C, Thumb MP extension immobilization / IP ulnar deviation restriction splint, type 1 (2) D, Thumb MP flexion immobilization / thumb IP extension restriction splint, type 1 (3) E, Thumb MP flexion restriction / MP-IP extension and flexion torque transmission splint, type 2 (4)
A, Immobilization splints are often used to protect the thumb MP and IP joints postoperatively. B, To increase material strength, narrow components such as this thumb post should be contoured to half the thickness of the segment being immobilized. C,D, These two type 1 MP immobilization / IP restriction splints restrict IP motion in different planes. E, The wrist and thumb CMC joints are considered secondary joints in this splint that transfers moment to the thumb MP and IP joints while restricting full flexion of the MP joint. [Courtesy (B) Elaine LaCroix, MHSM, OTR, CHT, Stoneham, Mass.; (C) from Moore JW, Braverman: Splinting for radial instability of the thumb MCP joint: a case report and description, *J Hand Ther* 3(4):202, 1990.]

mobilization assists for both IP flexion and IP extension in the same splint (Fig. 12-19, *D,E*).

Type 3. When thumb extrinsic tendons are tethered by scar tissue, the wrist must be included secondarily to control tenodesis effect. A *type 3 thumb IP mobilization splint* has three secondary joints, the wrist, CMC, and MP joints, and one primary joint, the IP joint (Fig. 12-19, *F,G*).

Torque Transmission Splints

Type 3. Transferring moment to the thumb IP joint to actively move a supple joint or to remodel a stiff IP joint, *type 3 thumb IP torque transmission splints* include the wrist, thumb CMC and MP joints as secondary joint levels (Fig. 12-20). These splints may be used to maximize the effect of the extrinsic tendons that influence motion at the thumb IP joint.

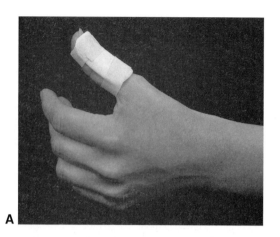

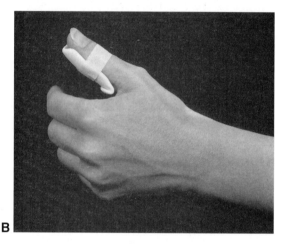

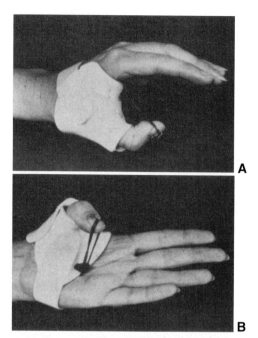

Fig. 12-18   A, Thumb IP extension immobilization splint, type 0 (1) B, Thumb IP extension immobilization splint, type 0 (1) Although the placement of straps differs between dorsal (A) and palmar (B) thumb immobilization splints, the mechanical function of both splints is identical. Proximal and distal pressure is applied palmarly and the opposing middle force is applied dorsally.

■ NONARTICULAR THUMB SPLINTS

Nonarticular thumb splints traverse no thumb joints and do not affect articular motion. Fitted to protect healing structures or influence soft tissue remodeling, these splints are applied to the segments of the thumb ray, e.g., the first metacarpal, or proximal or distal phalanx, rather than the thumb joints. Commonly used to support healing tendon pulleys, or to shape injured/repaired thumb nail beds, thumb nonarticular splints may fit circumferentially or they may contour to fit dorsally or volarly, according to patient requisites. Nonarticular thumb splints are classified according to the segment of application.

Thumb Distal Phalanx Splints

Thumb nail bed splints and splints that protect the tip of the thumb without incorporating thumb joints are

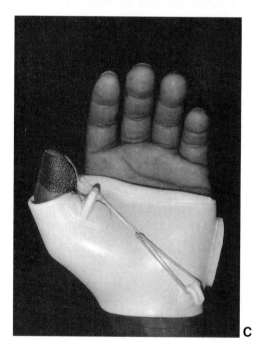

Fig. 12-19   A,B, Thumb IP flexion mobilization splint, type 2 (3) C, Thumb IP flexion mobilization splint, type 2 (3) D,E, Thumb IP extension or flexion mobilization splint, type 2 (3) F, Thumb IP extension mobilization splint, type 3 (4) G, Thumb IP extension mobilization splint, type 3 (4)
A-C, Using a variety of mobilization assists and outriggers, these type 2 IP flexion splints allow the application of elastic traction to affect only the distal thumb joint. The clip, a dressmaker's no. 2 hook, is attached with ethyl cyanoacrylate glue. D,E, This type 2 IP mobilization splint has a dual-purpose design with outriggers positioned for increasing either flexion or extension. F,G, Designed to increase passive thumb interphalangeal joint extension, these splints use elastic traction with different height outriggers. [(A,B) from Fess EE: Splinting for mobilization of the thumb. In Hunter JM, et al: *Rehabilitation of the hand*, ed 2, Mosby, 1984, St. Louis; Courtesy (C) Peggy McLaughlin, OTR, CHT, San Bernardino, Calif.; (D,E,F) Kathryn Schultz, OTR, CHT, Altamonte Springs, Fla.; (G) Kenneth Flowers, PT, CHT, San Francisco, Calif.]

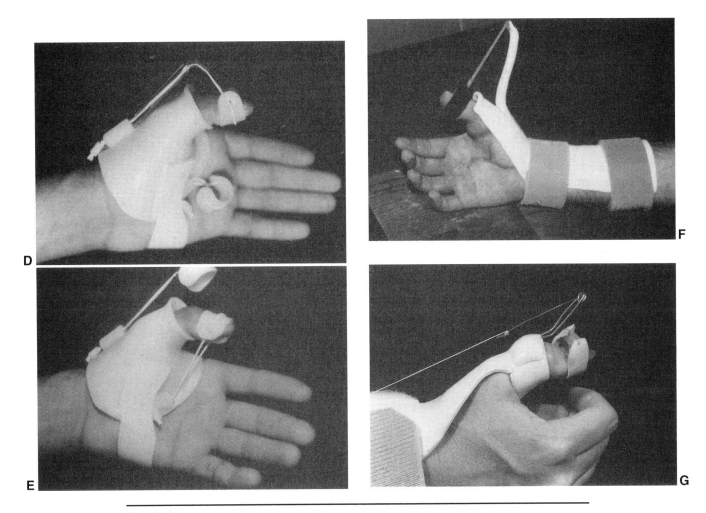

Fig. 12-19, cont'd
For legend see opposite page.

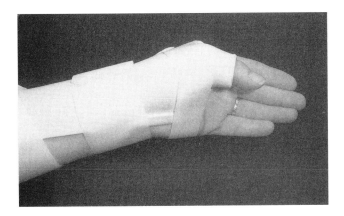

Fig. 12-20   Thumb IP extension and flexion torque transmission splint, type 3 (4)
Secondary control of the wrist, and thumb CMC and MP joints in this splint allows transmission of torque to the thumb IP joint, producing active extension and flexion of the IP joint.

classified as *nonarticular distal phalanx splints* (Fig. 12-21). These splints are often taped on the phalanx instead of strapped to ensure that they remain in place without slippage.

■ SUMMARY

It is of utmost importance that thumb splints be created to provide functional position, stability, and at least basilar joint mobility. Although careful adherence to the basic design, mechanics, use of outriggers and mobilization assists, construction and fit principles remains important, the thumb must be considered as a separate, unique unit. Splints should be used to carefully provide a maximum return of thumb participation in the important pinching and grasping activities of the hand. If done properly, the combination of splinting, exercise, and purposeful activity may help minimize the disabling effect of disease and

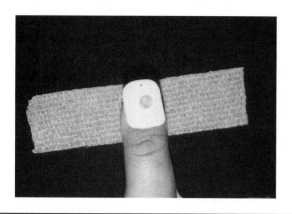

Fig. 12-21   Nonarticular thumb distal phalanx splint
This thumb nail bed splint helps remodel and shape the nail bed as it heals.

trauma to the thumb and enhance the results of surgery.

REFERENCES

1. Brand PW, Hollister A: *Clinical mechanics of the hand*, ed 3, Mosby, 1999, St. Louis.
2. Diaz J: Three-point static splint for chronic volar subluxation of the thumb metacarpophalangeal joint, *J Hand Ther* 7(3):195-7, 1994.
3. Fricker R, Hintermann B: Skier's thumb. Treatment, prevention and recommendations, *Sports Med* 19(1):73-9, 1995.
4. Galindo A, Suet L: A metacarpophalangeal joint stabilization splint, *J Hand Ther* 15(1):83-4, 2002.
5. Haines R: The mechanism of rotation at the first carpometacarpal joint, *J Anat* 78:44-6, 1944.
6. Landsman JC, et al: Splint immobilization of gamekeeper's thumb, *Orthopedics* 18(12):1161-5, 1995.
7. Moore JW, Braverman S: Splinting for radial instability of the thumb MCP joint: a case report and description, *J Hand Ther* 3(4):202, 1990.
8. Napier J: The form and function of the carpometacarpal joint of the thumb, *J Anat* 89:362, 1955.
9. Patel MR, Lipson LB, Desai SS: Conservative treatment of mallet thumb, *J Hand Surg [Am]* 11(1):45-7, 1986.
10. Phelps PE, Weeks PM: Management of the thumb–index web space contracture, *Am J Occup Ther* 30(9):543-50, 1976.
11. Pichora DR, McMurtry RY, Bell MJ: Gamekeeper's thumb: a prospective study of functional bracing, *J Hand Surg [Am]* 14(3):567-73, 1989.
12. Poole JU, Pellegrini VD: Arthritis of the thumb basal joint complex, *J Hand Ther* 13(2):91-107, 2000.
13. Sollerman C, Abrahamsson SO, Lundborg G, et al: Functional splinting versus plaster cast for ruptures of the ulnar collateral ligament of the thumb. A prospective randomized study of 63 cases, *Acta Orthop Scand* 62(6):524-6, 1991.
14. Wajon A: Clinical splinting successes: the thumb "strap splint" for dynamic instability of the trapeziometacarpal joint, *J Hand Ther* 13(3):236-7, 2000.
15. Weiss AP, Hastings H: Distal unicondylar fractures of the proximal phalanx, *J Hand Surg [Am]* 18(4):594-9, 1993.
16. Weiss S, LaStayo P, et al: Prospective analysis at splinting the first carpometacarpal joint: an objective, subjective, and radiographic assessment, *J Hand Ther* 13(3):218-26, 2000.
17. Wolock BS, Moore JR, Weiland AJ: Arthritis of the basal joint of the thumb. A critical analysis of treatment options, *J Arthroplasty* 4(1):65-78, 1989.

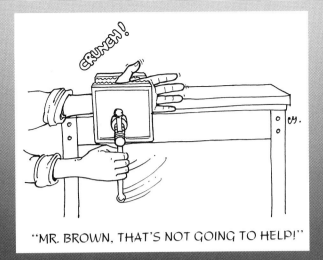

"MR. BROWN, THAT'S NOT GOING TO HELP!"

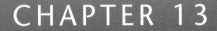

CHAPTER 13

Splints Acting on the Wrist and Forearm

Chapter Outline

T his chapter follows the expanded ASHT ESCS format by first dividing splints into articular or nonarticular categories. In the articular category, splints are next grouped according to the primary joint or joints they influence. Splints in the nonarticular category are defined by the anatomical segments upon which they are based.

Once articular splints are grouped according to their primary joints, they are further defined by direction of force application and then divided according to one of four purposes: immobilization, mobilization, restriction, or torque transmission. Splints with more than one primary purpose are designated by dual-purpose categories (e.g., mobilization/restriction or immobilization/mobilization). In this chapter, force direction (e.g., flexion, extension, supination, etc.) for wrist and forearm splints is included in the purpose

groupings. Purpose categories are further subdivided by *type*. *Type* identifies the number of secondary joint levels included in splints. Note: *Type* refers to the number of secondary joint levels, not the total number of secondary joints in a splint. While not all categories and/or subcategories are represented in this chapter, the expanded SCS is sufficiently flexible to accommodate additional groupings as needed.

Wrist and forearm articulations are key elements to upper extremity function in that they fine-tune positioning of the distally sited hand, providing proficiency in self-care, work, and leisure activities. Essential to normal hand function, the wrist and forearm refine motion of more proximal upper extremity joints through progressive, proximal-to-distal summation of intercalated joint motion. When integrated with selective joint stabilization, this cumulative joint motion allows the hand to be positioned in a seemingly infinite number of attitudes, further maximizing its capacity for interaction within the environment. With powerful extrinsic tendon systems traversing the wrist and inserting in the hand and digits, hand strength, digital posture, and fine finger/thumb motions are dependent on the integrity and positioning of wrist and forearm joints.

The ulna and radius, connected by a fibrous interosseous membrane, create two articulations: the proximal radioulnar joint (PRUJ) and the distal radioulnar joint (DRUJ). Together the proximal and distal radioulnar joints form a bicondylar joint with the radial head rotating axially and the distal ulna head fixed regarding rotation.[7-9,17] These integrated osseous and ligamentous forearm components provide critical rotational movement to the entire distal portion of the upper extremity open kinematic chain. With an axis of motion that travels proximally through the head of the radius and distally through the head of the ulna, the radius rotates in relation to the ulna. The two bones are positioned parallel to each other in supination, and the radius crosses over the ulna in pronation. One may consider the forearm as a two-part unit with the hand and radius being the mobile unit and the ulna and humerus as the fixed unit about which the radius-hand unit rotates. As the radius rotates, the ulna moves volarly in supination and dorsally in pronation. The ulna head glides in the sigmoid notch of the radius from the dorsal pronation position to the volar supination position. The interosseous membrane, although not considered an anatomical joint of the forearm, is an important structure in that it binds the radius and ulna together and limits extremes of forearm rotation.

Following the arc of the radius, the hand may be rotated approximately 180°. Combined, the radioulnar joints allow a single arc of transverse rotational motion—pronation-supination—and form a uniaxial joint with 1° of freedom of movement. Coalescence of forearm and wrist motion results in hand positioning in the sagittal, coronal, and transverse planes. Normally, axial load is shared between the radius and ulna with the radius accepting 82% of the workload and the ulna 18%, with the triangular fibrocartilage complex (TFCC) stabilizing the distal RU joint.[17] Disruption of the PRUJ, DRUJ, and/or interosseous membrane may compromise forearm rotation, causing substitution patterns of shoulder internal or external rotation to compensate for limited forearm pronation or supination.

The osseous anatomy of the wrist consists of the distal radius and ulna and eight carpal bones. The wrist is classified as a condylar diarthrosis with a wide range of motion resulting from its many small internal joints. Intrinsic stability is provided by a complex ligamentous arrangement. As the most proximal segment in the intercalated chain of hand joints, the wrist is the key to function at the more distal joint levels. The wrist is vulnerable to a wide assortment of injuries and diseases, thus making it subject to acute or secondary patterns of deformity, instability, or collapse that may significantly interfere with hand performance.

The collective carpal bones form the anteriorly concave proximal transverse arch, whose functional position directly influences the kinetic interaction of structures composing the longitudinal arch. It appears that the once widely held concept of the wrist carpus as two transverse four-bone rows is a substantial oversimplification of its complex dynamic motion patterns. Taleisnik,[18,20] in refining the work of Navarro, defines the carpal scaphoid as the lateral or mobile column of the wrist, with the triquetrum serving as the medial or rotation column and the remaining six bones comprising the central or flexion-extension column. Taleisnik notes that the anatomic positioning of the wrist ligaments, particularly on the palmar side, permits these intricate columnar movements and provides a sound rationale for understanding the dynamic anatomy of the wrist, its function, and its behavior during injury. Garcia-Elias and Dobyns[5] describe six compartment articulations with interdependent kinematic behaviors. These include distal radioulnar joint, radiocarpal joint, midcarpal joint, pisotriquetral joint, trapeziometacarpal joint, and common CMC joint. These joints provide stability of grip and a wide range of motion for fine prehension.

Direct or adjacent trauma, particularly when accompanied by crushing or prolonged edema, may result in fibrotic changes in the tightly articulated wrist joints, resulting in limited range of motion. The obligatory immobilization of fracture, tendon, or ligament injuries in this area increases the possibility of motion loss. Conversely, ligamentous rupture or attenuation secondary to inflammatory disease processes may result in wrist instability and collapse patterns that can compromise digital performance to an even greater extent than that produced by wrist stiffening. Surgical intervention may include partial wrist fusions to decrease pain and increase wrist stability. Injuries commonly referred to therapists for splinting include diagnoses ranging from repetitive strain injuries to scaphoid and lunate fractures. Close communication between referring surgeons and therapists is critical because wrist pathology and surgical intervention is often esoteric and highly individualized. Knowledge of anatomic idiosyncrasies is also important. For example, the poor blood supply to carpal bones such as the scaphoid and lunate may delay healing and necessitate splinting to stabilize the wrist and prevent movement.

The wrist serves as the key joint to distal hand function and influences both digital strength and dexterity. It is therefore important to give very careful consideration to proper joint positioning and protection, as well as the restoration and preservation of a satisfactory range of motion. A program that integrates splinting and exercise often provides the essential elements to maintain wrist function.

It is also important that the effect of wrist position be thoroughly considered in the preparation of any hand splint. Wrist dorsiflexion tightens extrinsic flexor tendons and permits the synergistic wrist extension–strong finger flexion function employed in power grasp. Wrist palmar flexion tightens the long extrinsic extensor tendons, allowing the hand to open automatically, while greatly reducing digit flexion efficiency. Splints designed either to relax or protect extensor tendons or to promote active digital flexion should support the wrist in an appropriate degree of dorsiflexion as determined by the presenting pathology. Conversely, splinting the wrist in a flexed attitude enhances active digital extension or allows protection for flexor tendon healing. One must take care, however, to avoid positioning the wrist in either excessive palmar flexion or dorsiflexion, which could lead to attenuation of delicate soft tissue structures or cause pressure on the median nerve as it passes through the carpal canal. Understanding and careful application of these kinetic mechanisms will aid healing and motion programs in the hand.

The purpose of this chapter is to discuss splinting of the wrist and forearm with regard to anatomic, kinesiologic, and mechanical factors. It is much more common to use wrist and forearm splints for immobilization purposes. With the limited exception of splints designed to correct deformation, the majority of splints in the preceding list require immobilization techniques.

◼ ARTICULAR WRIST AND FOREARM SPLINTS

Wrist Splints

When used to control articular motion, wrist splints affect motion of the multiple carpal joints in a similar manner. They may be used to immobilize, mobilize, restrict motion, or transmit torque. It is important to understand that in order to control digital extrinsic muscle/tendon glide, the wrist must be included in the splint. Recommendations and designs for wrist splints are numerous. Much of this is due to the proliferation of upper extremity cumulative trauma cases over the past few decades. Currently, no specific splint

design has been proven to prevent the occurrence of cumulative trauma, but splints seem to be effective at decreasing or eliminating symptoms on a case-by-case basis. With all wrist splints, whether designed to immobilize, mobilize, restrict motion, or transmit torque, care must be taken to diminish pressure over bony prominences such as the ulnar styloid process, the first metacarpal, and the head of the radius, and to avoid pressure over the superficial branch of the radial nerve.

Wrist splints are constructed in a variety of materials, including thermoplastics, leather, vinyl, cloth, and athletic tape, with popular designs including volar, dorsal, circumferential, bivalve, radial, or ulnar bases. When choosing the best design and material for a wrist splint, it is important to assess the occupational performance demands of the patient. Splints may be custom made or prefabricated. If a prefabricated splint is used, it must meet the same principles of mechanics, using outriggers and mobilization assists, design, construction, and fit criteria as custom splints. In an age of easy accessibility of a wide range of splinting materials, there is no excuse for application of an ill-fitting prefabricated splint.

In the following review, wrist splints are grouped according to their expanded SCS designations. Remember, according to the expanded SCS nomenclature, primary joints are specifically identified and their purpose(s) and direction(s) are explicitly defined, type notes secondary joint levels, and the number in parentheses is the total number of joints included in the splint.

Immobilization Splints

Wrist immobilization splints allow healing of inflamed or injured structures of the distal forearm and wrist. Depending on the purpose of application, these splints may be fitted to affect motion in either or both the sagittal and coronal planes. Wrist immobilization splints are, for many therapists, the most frequently made splints. Proper fit is essential to healing and achievement of functional results. Generally, for optimum mechanical advantage, the forearm trough of a wrist splint should be two-thirds the length of the forearm and half its thickness.[15,16] The metacarpal bar should allow full MP flexion and extension, support the distal transverse arch, and reflect dual obliquity configuration (Fig. 13-1). Straps should be placed at the far distal and proximal ends of the splint and, if possible, directly over the wrist axis of rotation.

Type 0. The primary joint of a *type 0 wrist immobilization splint* is the wrist itself. There are no secondary joints included in a *type 0* wrist splint. While there are many approaches to immobilizing a wrist, without doubt the most commonly used splint is the

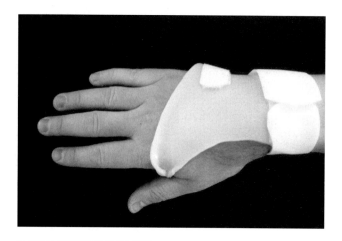

Fig. 13-1 **Wrist neutral immobilization splint, type 0 (1)** Anatomical and kinesiological factors form the foundation for well-fitting wrist splints.

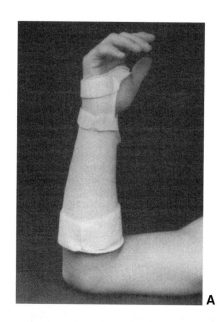

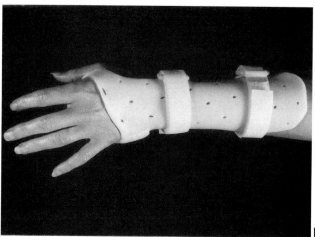

Fig. 13-2 **A, Wrist extension immobilization splint, type 0 (1) B, Wrist neutral immobilization splint, type 0 (1) C, Wrist neutral immobilization splint, type 0 (1) D, Wrist extension immobilization splint, type 0 (1) E, Wrist flexion immobilization splint, type 0 (1)** Type 0 wrist immobilization splints may be designed to fit volarly (**A**), dorsally (**B,E**), or circumferentially (**C,D**). [Courtesy (**B**) Sharon Flinn, MEd, OTR, CHT, Cuyahoga Heights, Ohio; (**C**) Lin Beribak, OTR/L, CHT, Chicago, Ill.; (**D**) Paul Van Lede, OT, MS, Orfit Industries, Wijnegem, Belgium.]

wrist extension immobilization splint, type 0 (1), which, in most cases, positions the wrist in approximately 10-30° of extension to allow maximum composite hand function (Fig. 13-2, *A*). Neutral wrist position is also used frequently and, in this instance, the splint is called a *wrist neutral immobilization splint, type 0 (1)* (Fig. 13-2, *B,C*). Radial and ulnar deviation bars may be necessary to prevent coronal movement of the hand. Deviation bars have the additional effect of reinforcing potentially weak areas of the splint. Circumferential designs provide the greatest amount of wrist immobilization (Fig. 13-2, *D*).[11] The wrist may also be positioned in flexion with a *type 0 wrist flexion splint* (Fig. 13-2, *E*). If a wrist splint is to be worn while the patient is working at a computer, the flare on the proximal end may be eliminated for comfort.

Type 1. A *type 1 wrist immobilization splint* indicates the presence of one secondary joint level included in the splint in addition to the primary joint, the wrist. The secondary joint most often included in a *wrist immobilization splint, type 1 (2)* is the thumb CMC joint, which is held motionless by a carefully fitted first metacarpal bar component. *Type 1 wrist immobilization splints* that include the thumb CMC may be used to help control and/or decrease wrist pain (Fig. 13-3). Because mechanical purchase on the first metacarpal is challenging, complete immobilization of the CMC joint is difficult to achieve with a *type 1 wrist immobilization splint.*

Type 2. *Type 2 wrist immobilization splints* incorporate two secondary joint levels in addition to the wrist, the primary joint. Secondary joint(s) may be situated either proximal or distal to the wrist depending on the specific purpose of the splint. For example, splints may include both the thumb CMC and MP as distally located secondary joint levels (Fig. 13-4, *A-D*) or they may include the forearm and elbow as proximal secondary level joints (Fig. 13-4, *E*). *Type 2 wrist immobilization splints* that incorporate the thumb are sometimes used to provide additional stabilization for partial fusions or fractures on the radial side of the wrist including scaphoid fractures, or radial wrist ligament injuries where thumb IP joint motion is permitted.

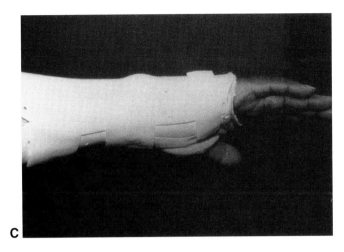

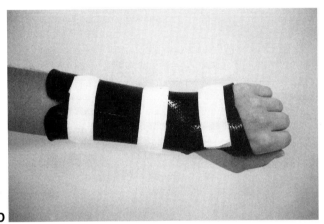

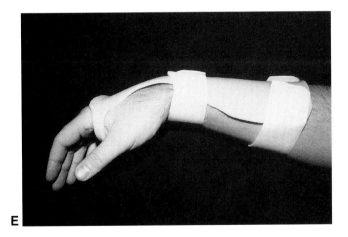

Fig. 13-2, cont'd
For legend see opposite page.

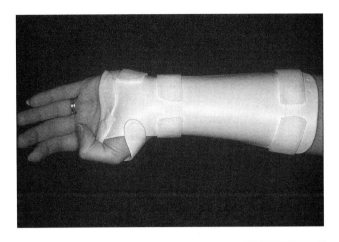

Fig. 13-3   Wrist extension immobilization splint, type 1 (2)
The thumb CMC joint is included in this wrist immobilization splint as a secondary joint.

Mobilization Splints

Wrist mobilization splinting focuses on two main problem areas: (1) supple wrists that lack active motion, and (2) stiff wrists with limited passive range of motion. For the most part, flaccid or paralyzed wrists lacking full or partial active motion require simple mobilization splints that facilitate and improve hand function. Occasionally, more complicated splinting utilizing torque transmission may be required to substitute for absent movement in supple wrists. In contrast, mobilizing the stiffened wrist through splinting is a more difficult assignment. Certainly no externally applied splinting device may selectively differentiate its force application to the radiocarpal or midcarpal joints. When columnar or compartmental wrist motion patterns are considered, the problem of mobilizing specifically targeted fibrosed wrist articulations becomes even more difficult. Nonetheless, carefully prepared splints that attempt to gently mobilize immobile carpal articulations without damaging uninjured ligamentous structures often prove beneficial. This chapter does not differentiate between wrist mobilization splints applied to supple joints and those applied to stiff joints because they represent opposite extremes of the same continuum. Splinting characteristics exist that are common to both problem areas. Assessment of progress is essential in determining effectiveness of a wrist splint, especially one applied to improve motion of fibrosed carpal articulations. Because increasing passive range of motion of a stiff wrist, even with splinting, may be a daunting task, if no measurable change in passive wrist motion occurs over a 10- to 14-day period of continuous wear, the patient should be reevaluated by the referring physician.

Type 0. *Type 0 wrist mobilization splints* have no secondary joints and may be fitted to produce wrist flexion, extension, deviation, or a combination of these motions. Wrist mobilization splints may be adjusted serially (Fig. 13-5, *A-C*), or they may be constructed as a single unit, or as two pieces connected

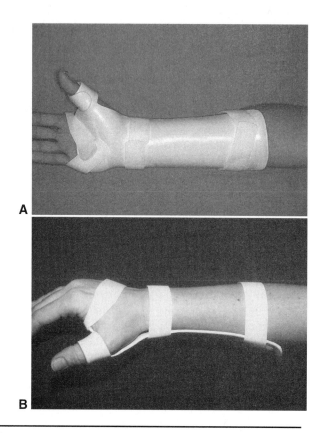

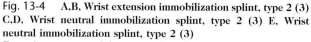

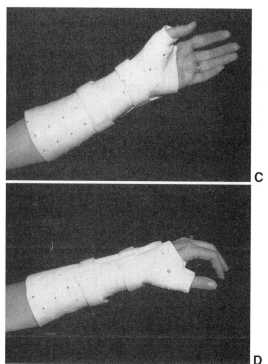

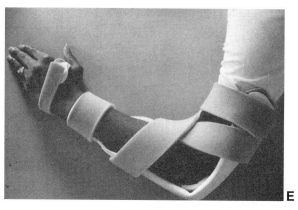

Fig. 13-4   A,B, Wrist extension immobilization splint, type 2 (3) C,D, Wrist neutral immobilization splint, type 2 (3) E, Wrist neutral immobilization splint, type 2 (3)
Type 2 wrist immobilization splint designs vary according to whether secondary joints are distal **(A-D)** or proximal and distal **(E)** to the wrist. [Courtesy **(C,D)** Shelli Dellinger, OTR, CHT, San Diego, Calif.]

by a traction device or by an articulated joint(s) (Fig. 13-6, *A-J*). Both one- and two-piece splint designs should provide continuous 90° angle of pull to the metacarpals through the use of appropriate length outriggers (Fig. 13-7, *A,B*).

Some highly specialized splints direct mobilization forces to specific anatomical parts of the wrist. For example, a midcarpal instability splint mobilizes the pisiform bone dorsally and the proximal carpal row into extension, reducing the ulnar sag of the wrist and the volar flexed position of the proximal carpal row (Fig. 13-7, *C-F*). A splint for midcarpal instability is designed to correct ulnar wrist sag using a diagonal adjustable tension strap that provides an extension-oriented distal ulnar to proximal radial pull to the ulnar aspect of the wrist (Fig. 13-7, *G*). This splint encourages functional use of the wrist.

If the wrist is passively mobile, an outrigger may not be required for splints that substitute for lost motion (Figs. 13-5, 13-6, *G*, 13-8). In these splints, the wrist bar may be absent or hinged (Fig. 13-9, *A,B*). To reduce pressure, the longitudinal length of the metacarpal bar should be as long as possible without inhibiting wrist motion proximally and MP joint motion distally. It should also maintain the distal transverse metacarpal arch. Thumb motion should be preserved and, as with wrist immobilization splints, the forearm trough should be two-thirds the length of the forearm and, if using low-temperature plastic, half its thickness. An elbow cuff, triceps cuff or strap, or Dycem inside of the splint may be necessary to prevent distal migration of the forearm trough on the forearm (Fig. 13-10, *A,B*). Because of the magnitude of the forces involved in mobilizing a wrist, careful attention

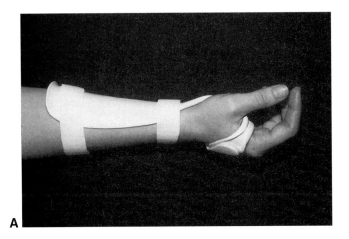

A

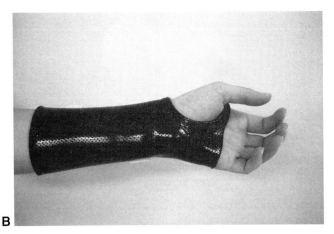

B

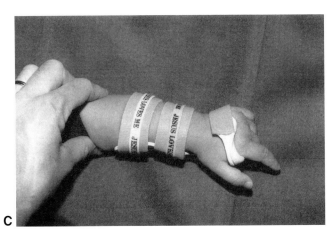

C

Fig. 13-5   A, Wrist extension mobilization splint, type 0 (1) B, Wrist extension mobilization splint, type 0 (1) C, Wrist extension mobilization splint, type 0 (1)

Type 0 wrist mobilization splints may be fitted to provide mobilization forces to stiff, weakened, or paralytic joints. When used to increase passive joint range of motion, they may be serially adjusted allowing continuous application of mobilization forces until the desired goal is achieved. [Courtesy (C) Joni Armstrong, OTR, CHT, Bemidji, Minn.]

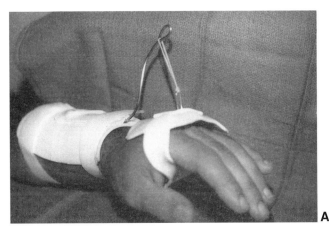

A

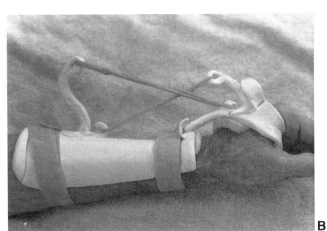

B

Fig. 13-6   A, Wrist extension mobilization splint, type 0 (1) B, Wrist extension mobilization splint, type 0 (1) C, Wrist extension mobilization splint, type 0 (1) D, Wrist extension mobilization splint, type 0 (1) E, Wrist extension mobilization splint, type 0 (1) F, Wrist flexion mobilization splint, type 0 (1) G, Wrist extension mobilization splint, type 0 (1) H, Wrist extension mobilization splint, type 0 (1) I, Wrist extension mobilization splint, type 0 (1) J, Wrist extension mobilization splint, type 0 (1)

Type 0 wrist mobilization splints present a variety of designs and methods of force application, including elastic (A,B,E-J) and inelastic (C,D) mobilization assists. These splints may be constructed as single units (C-E,G-J) or two-piece units (A,B,F). (F) Designed at the Hand Rehabilitation Center of Indiana, Indianapolis, Ind. [Courtesy (A) Cynthia Philips, MA, OTR, CHT, Boston, Mass.; (B) Carolina deLeeuw, MA, OTR, Tacoma, Wash.; (C,D) Shelli Dellinger, OTR, CHT, San Diego, Calif.; (E) Carol Hierman, OTR, CHT, Cedar Grove, N.C., and Elisha Denny, PTA, OTA, Pittsboro, N.C., © UNC Hand Rehabilitation Center, Chapel Hill, N.C.; (G) Paul Van Lede, OT, MS, Orfit Industries, Wijnegem, Belgium; (H) DeRoyal/LMB, Powell, Tenn.; (I) Ultraflex Systems, Inc., Dowingtown, Pa.; (J) G. Roger Williams, OTR, Midwest City, Okla., and North Coast Medical, Inc. Morgan Hill, Calif.]

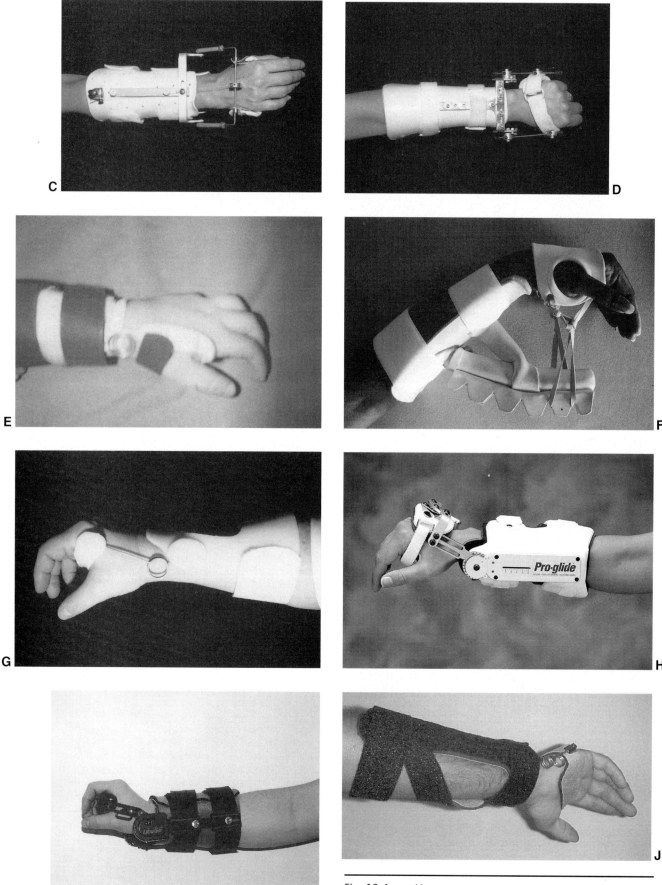

Fig. 13-6, cont'd
For legend see p. 357.

should be directed to underlying cutaneous surfaces. Splints should be removed for skin inspection a minimum of every hour during initial wearing phases. Padding may be necessary at the proximal and distal end of the forearm trough and/or along the length of the metacarpal bar. It is not unusual for a wrist mobilization splint to produce transient median nerve compression with paresthesia in the distribution of the

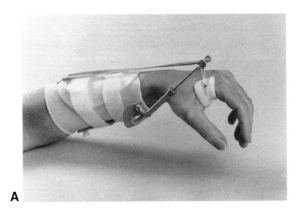

A

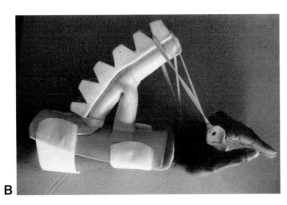

B

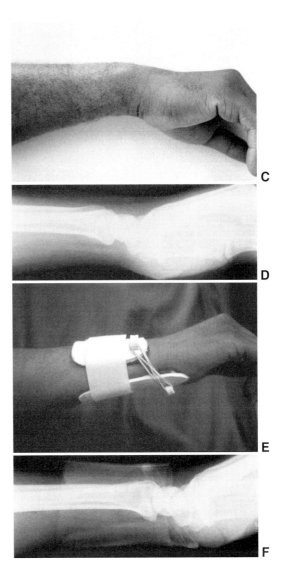

C

D

E

F

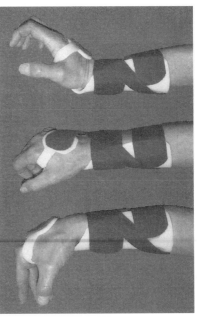

G

Fig. 13-7   A, Wrist extension mobilization splint, type 0 (1) B, Wrist extension mobilization splint, type 0 (1) E,F, Pisiform dorsal, proximal carpal row extension mobilization splint, type 0 (1) G, Wrist radial extension mobilization splint, type 0 (1)
A,B, As wrist motion changes, the outrigger must be adjusted to maintain a 90° angle of force application of the mobilization assist to the metacarpals. Additionally, the angle of pull must be perpendicular to the joint axis of rotation and, as adjustments are made, the mobilization assist should track according to the normal anatomic arc of motion of the joint. Note that the base and outrigger design shown in splint **B**, a.k.a. "the dinosaur," and in Figs. 13-6F, 13-13B, and 13-13E is interchangeable for flexion or extension with dorsally or volarly fitted metacarpal bars. **C-F,** This innovative and highly sophisticated splint corrects palmar translation of the distal carpal row and the volar flexed orientation of the proximal carpal row by applying a dorsal mobilization force to the pisiform and an extension force to the proximal carpal row. **G,** This splint is designed to correct midcarpal instability ulnar wrist sag while encouraging functional use of the wrist. (B) Designed at the Hand Rehabilitation Center of Indiana, Indianapolis, Ind. [Courtesy (A) Helen Marx, OTR, CHT, Human Factors Engineering of Phoenix, Wickenburg, Ariz.; (C-F) Terri Skirven, OTR, CHT, King of Prussia, Penn.; (G) Roger Williams, OTR, Midwest City, Okla.]

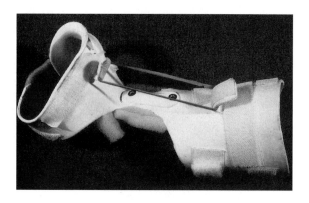

Fig. 13-8   Wrist extension mobilization splint, type 0 (1)
When the wrist is passively supple and the splint is applied to
substitute for absent active motion, extended outriggers and a 90°
angle of pull are not required.

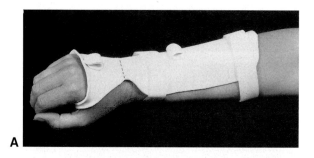

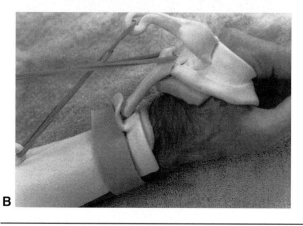

Fig. 13-9   A, Wrist extension mobilization splint, type 0 (1)
B, Wrist extension mobilization splint, type 0 (1)
Whether one or two pieces, a hinged wrist bar must be aligned
(A. *broken line*) with corresponding wrist creases to permit unin-
hibited motion. [Courtesy (B) Carolina deLeeuw, MA, OTR,
Tacoma, Wash.]

nerve. If a patient complains of numbness or tingling
in the fingers from wearing a wrist mobilization splint,
remove and adjust the splint and revise the wearing
schedule. If the numbness returns when the adjusted
splint is reapplied, the splint must be discontinued.

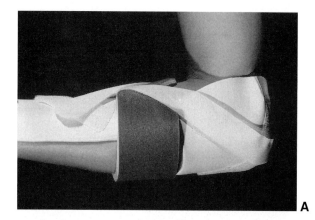

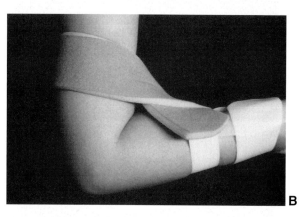

Fig. 13-10   Distal migration of a forearm trough may be controlled with an elbow cuff (A) or triceps strap (B). An elbow
cuff must be fitted with considerable care to avoid damaging pressure on elbow bony prominences and/or the ulnar nerve. Wider
triceps straps disperse pressure on the posterior upper arm, diminishing chances for inadvertent irritation of the ulnar and/or radial
nerves.

For wrist radial or ulnar deviation mobilization
splints, correct alignment is determined by the second
or fifth metacarpal, respectively (Fig. 13-11, *A,B*).
Thumb position is not involved in identifying
the correct line of force application for *type 0 wrist
deviation splints*.

Type 1. One secondary joint level is included in a
type 1 wrist mobilization splint. As with *type 1 wrist
immobilization splints*, the thumb CMC joint is the
most common secondary joint to be included in *type
1 wrist mobilization splints*. Inclusion of the first
metacarpal in a wrist mobilization splint may better
focus corrective forces on stiffened articulations, or it
may improve stabilization of the splint on the hand,
or both (Fig. 13-12, *A-C*).

Type 3. Despite passively supple joints, extrinsic
tendon adhesions may inhibit simultaneous passive
flexion or extension of both the wrist and digital joints
secondary to a tenodesis phenomenon. To increase

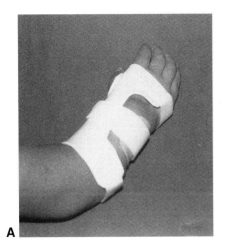

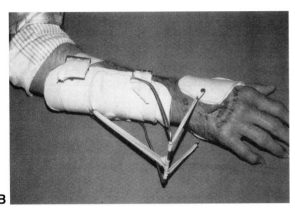

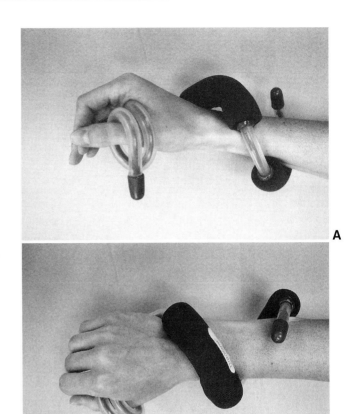

Fig. 13-11   A, Wrist ulnar deviation mobilization splint, type 0 (1) B, Wrist ulnar deviation mobilization splint, type 0 (1)
Although methods of mobilizing differ, these type 0 wrist ulnar deviation mobilization splints are designed to apply an ulnarly directed force to achieve neutral wrist alignment. **A,** When treating radial club hand deformities, splint serial changes improve wrist position through gradual tissue remodeling. [Courtesy **(A)** Karen Mathewson, OTR/L, CHT, Cranston, R.I.; **(B)** Carol Hierman, OTR, CHT, Cedar Grove, N.C., Elisha Denny, PTA, OTA, Pittsboro, N.C., © UNC Hand Rehabilitation Center, Chapel Hill, N.C.]

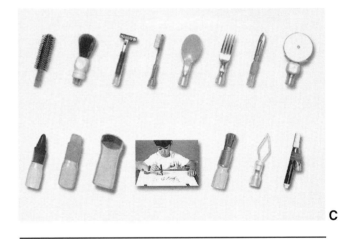

Fig. 13-12   A,B, Wrist extension mobilization splint, type 1 (2)
A,B, An adjustable TUBOform type 1 wrist extension mobilization splint positions a weak or paralytic wrist in a more functional posture. The moldable wire frame wraps around the base of the first metacarpal to provide splint stability by including the thumb CMC joint as a secondary joint, hence the type 1 classification. The distal end of the wire thumb post serves as an attachment point for a variety of Spander™ accessories **(C)** used to increase independence in activities of daily living. (Courtesy Expansao, Sao Paulo, Brazil, expansao@expansao.com.)

tendon excursion and convert the tenodesis effect, a splint must be designed either to immobilize the wrist and mobilize the fingers or mobilize the wrist and immobilize the fingers. Care must be taken to avoid tendon attenuation when splinting to mobilize scar-bound tendons. This is especially true of adhered extensor tendons following tendon repairs. With their flatter, ribbon-like configurations, scar-bound extensor tendons may require staged splinting programs to prevent tendon attenuation, including isolated tenodesis splinting followed by composite mobilization assists. Both staged and nonstaged splinting techniques enhance the mechanical focus of mobilization forces.

In a *type 3 wrist mobilization splint,* the posture of the wrist and the direction of the traction are dictated by whether flexor or extensor tendon excursion is limited. When flexor tendon adhesions are present, a volar or dorsal finger pan may be used to immobilize the fingers in extension, while extension mobilization traction is applied to the wrist (Fig. 13-13, A-D). If extrinsic extensor adhesions limit simultaneous wrist and finger flexion, the fingers may be immobilized in a flexed attitude and gentle flexion traction applied to the wrist (Fig. 13-13, E). To provide optimum rotational effect, the traction assist for either extension or flexion splints should pull at a 90° angle to the metacarpals and should also be perpendicular to the center of the sagittal axis of rotation of the wrist. The metacarpal bar should support the distal transverse metacarpal arch and, in the case of a *type 3 wrist flexion mobilization splint,* should allow full MP flexion. The forearm trough should be of sufficient length and width to provide good mechanical advantage, reduction of pressure, and splint durability. Application of *type 3 wrist mobilization splints* in the form of serial plaster casts is one of the most effective methods for increasing wrist passive range of motion when scar-bound extrinsic tendons are present. Serial casting may be applied to increase either flexion or extension motion using this method. If thumb extrinsic tendons are involved instead of finger extrinsic tendons, the three joints of the thumb may be immobilized as the wrist is mobilized into extension or flexion either through serial adjustments (inelastic traction) or through elastic traction (Fig. 13-13, F).

Type 6. A *type 6 wrist mobilization splint* is effective for decreasing wrist ligament and capsular tightness. This splint includes finger and thumb joints as secondary joints. Remember, only the joint level is counted when describing *type,* not the number of individual joints themselves. In the splint illustrated in Fig. 13-14, the thumb CMC, MP, and IP joints are added as the 4th, 5th, and 6th type levels. The finger MP and IP secondary joints represent levels 1, 2, and 3.

Note: As previously mentioned, efforts to mobilize digital joints may be compromised by the position the wrist is allowed to assume. The tenodesis effect of wrist extensors on extrinsic digital flexors is an important consideration in the design of *type 1* finger and *type 1* thumb splints where the wrist is immobilized as a secondary joint. Although the wrist is included as a secondary joint, the primary purpose of *type 1* digital immobilization, mobilization, restriction, or torque transmission splints is directed toward influencing digital motion, not wrist motion. See Chapter 11, Splints Acting on the Fingers, and Chapter 12, Splints

Acting on the Thumb, for further information on digital splints.

Mobilization/Restriction Splints

Type 0. Some wrist mobilization splints allow motion in one plane but inhibit motion in another, usually through the use of sequential changes (Fig. 13-15, A,B) or articulated hand and forearm pieces (Fig. 13-15, C). When fitting this style of splint, it is imperative to match the rotational axis of the splint with the anatomic joint axis. Improper alignment of the two joints produces deforming forces across the wrist joint, which could lead to further damage, including inhibition of motion, and shear or friction damage to underlying skin and subcutaneous structures. Articulated splints are often used with post wrist arthroplasty patients when medial and lateral hinges are needed to provide stability and eliminate radial and ulnar deviation while allowing wrist extension and flexion motion as healing occurs.

Restriction Splints

Restriction splints are used in situations when expressly identified motions are prohibited or where defined arcs of active wrist motion are required. Limitation of specific wrist motion may be controlled completely through the use of inflexible materials (e.g., thermoplastic, metal, etc.) or motion may be controlled in gradations by using less rigid materials like neoprene, leather, vinyl, tape, or other similar flexible materials.

Type 0. *Type 0 wrist restriction splints* control motion at one primary joint, the wrist. There are no secondary joints included in *type 0 restriction splints.* Restriction splints may be designed and fit to allow full or limited wrist extension/flexion while preventing radial and ulnar deviation or vice versa, or they may simply limit motion in one direction while allowing increments of motion in other directions (Fig. 13-16, A,B). Wrist circumduction restriction splints allow varying degrees of overall wrist mobility while providing external support for sports, work, and/or avocational activities. These splints are constructed in softer materials including tape[10] (Fig. 13-16, C), neoprene (Fig. 13-16, D), or fabric (Fig. 13-16, E).

Type 2. *Type 2 wrist restriction splints* limit gradations of wrist motion and are used with a variety of diagnoses. They are often worn during sports or work activities. Generally, these splints allow normal motion while limiting extreme motion in extension and/or flexion, or in radial and/or ulnar deviation. One of the most commonly used *type 2 wrist restriction splints* includes the thumb CMC and MP as secondary joints (Fig. 13-16, F).

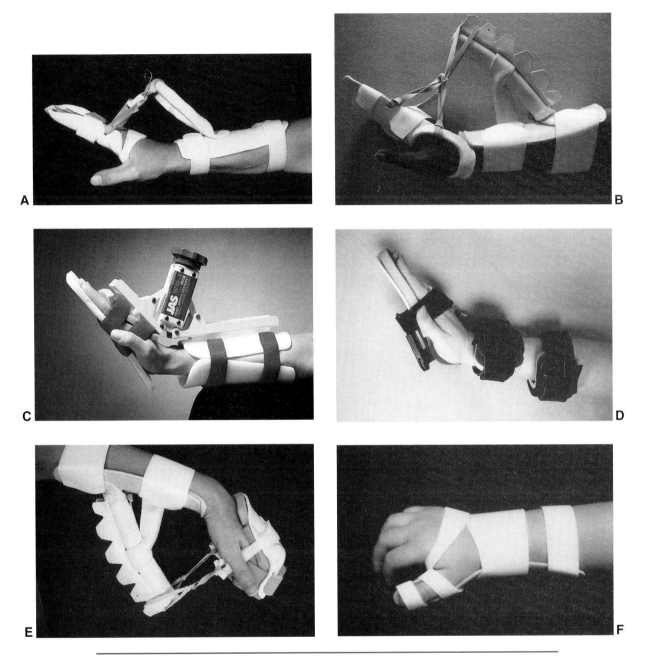

Fig. 13-13   A, Wrist extension mobilization splint, type 3 (13) B, Wrist extension mobilization splint, type 3 (13) C, Wrist extension mobilization splint, type 3 (14) D, Wrist extension mobilization splint, type 3 (14) E, Wrist flexion mobilization splint, type 3 (13) F, Wrist extension mobilization splint, type 3 (4)

Type 3 wrist mobilization splints may be used to treat extrinsic flexor tightness (A-D,F) or extrinsic extensor tightness (E). Due to the multijoint nature of the extrinsic digital extensors and flexors, it is necessary to provide secondary control to joints distal to the wrist in order to effectively mobilize scar-bound extrinsic tendons. All of the splints illustrated are type 3 wrist mobilization splints because they incorporate three secondary joint planes, at the finger MP, PIP, and DIP levels (A-E) or at the thumb CMC, MP, IP levels (F). (E) Designed at the Hand Rehabilitation Center of Indiana, Indianapolis, Ind. [Courtesy (C) Joint Active Systems, Inc. Effingham, Ill.; (D) EMPI, St. Paul, Minn.]

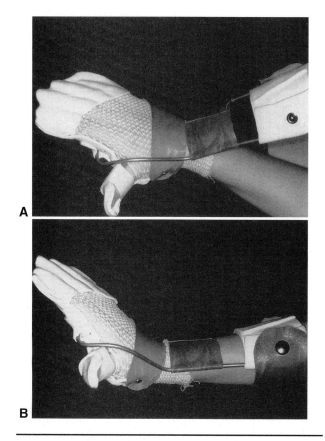

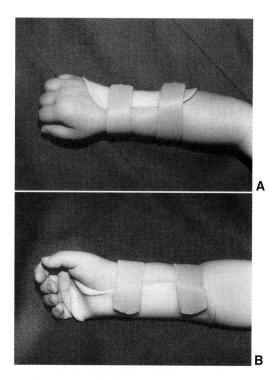

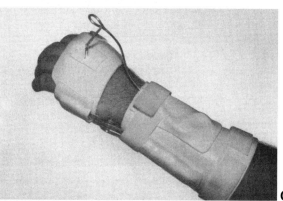

Fig. 13-14   **A,B, Wrist extension mobilization splint, type 6 (16)**
Incorporating the thumb and fingers as secondary joints in addition to the primary wrist joint, this type 6 wrist splint focuses mobilization forces to the wrist while the digital joints are held in extension. **A,** Donning this splint incorporates leverage of the dorsal forearm trough to bring the wrist and digits into extension. **B,** Splint applied. Malleable wire allows predetermined adjustment of the wrist angle. (Courtesy Dominique Thomas, RPT, MCMK, Saint Martin Duriage, France.)

Fig. 13-15   **A,B, Wrist extension mobilization / ulnar deviation restriction splint, type 0 (1) C, Wrist extension mobilization / radial and ulnar deviation restriction splint, type 0 (1)**
A,B, An ulnarly based splint design simultaneously restricts wrist ulnar deviation and moves the wrist into extension to improve hand use. **C,** Articulated wrist hinges restrict wrist radial/ulnar deviation as an outrigger and mobilization assist focus extension directed forces to the wrist. [Courtesy **(A,B)** Joni Armstrong, OTR, CHT, Bemidji, Minn.; **(C)** Cynthia Philips, MA, OTR, CHT, Boston, Mass.]

Torque Transmission Splints

Wrist torque transmission splints transfer moment to primary joints that are situated beyond the boundaries of the splint itself, or if primary joints are included within the splint, they are "driven" by harnessed secondary joints that are also included within the boundaries of the splint. Wrist torque transmission splints transfer moment longitudinally. Often referred to as "exercise" splints, these splints are used with specific exercises and with functional activities.

Types 3 and 4. Torque transmission splints affecting the wrist joint may have three or four secondary joint levels incorporated, and are categorized as *type 3* or *type 4*, respectively. These splints function longitudinally by controlling finger joint motion to transmit torque to the wrist joint proximally so that extrinsic muscle power is focused exclusively on the wrist joint (Fig. 13-17, *A-D*).

Wrist, Finger Splints

Some splints include both wrist and digital joints as primary joints. These dual primary purpose splints involve immobilization, mobilization, restriction, or torque transmission of primary proximal joints of the fingers and/or thumb in addition to the primary focus wrist joint. Because the expanded SCS groups splints

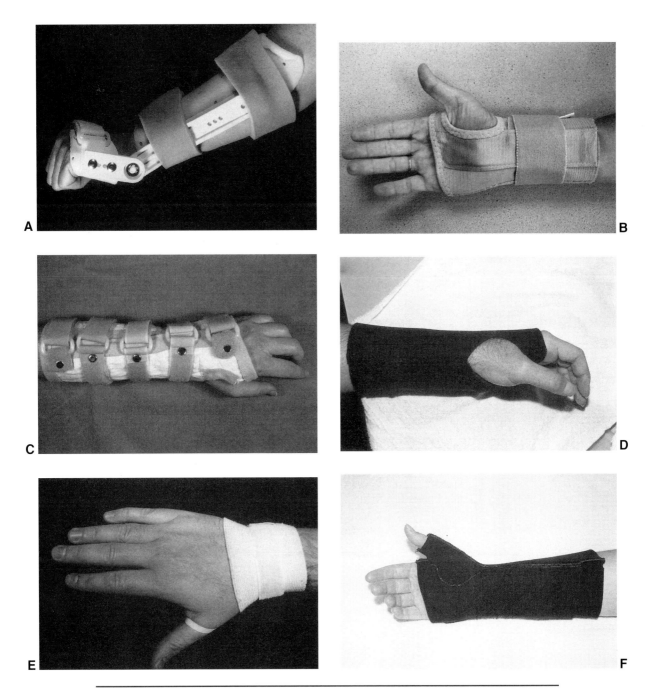

Fig. 13-16   A, Wrist ulnar deviation restriction splint, type 0 (1) B, Wrist flexion restriction splint, type 0 (1) C, Wrist circumduction restriction splint, type 0 (1) D, Wrist circumduction restriction splint, type 0 (1) E, Wrist circumduction restriction splint, type 0 (1) F, Wrist flexion restriction splint, type 2 (3)

A-E, Incorporating no secondary joints, type 0 wrist restriction splints may limit one or more specific wrist motions or they may restrict wrist motion in all planes. Restriction splints are constructed from a variety of materials with varying degrees of inherent resistance, resulting in gradations of restricted motion. F, A type 2 wrist flexion restriction splint usually includes the thumb CMC and MP as secondary joints. [Courtesy **(A)** Sharon Flinn, MEd, OTR, CHT, Cuyahoga Heights, Ohio; **(C)** Jennifer L. Henshaw, OTR; **(D,F)** Joni Armstrong, OTR, CHT, Bemidji, Minn.]

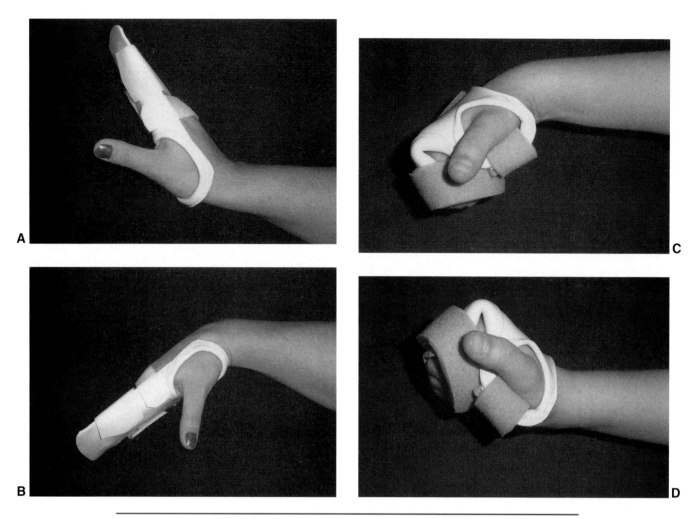

Fig. 13-17   A,B, Wrist extension and flexion torque transmission splint, type 3 (13) C,D, Wrist extension and flexion torque transmission, type 4 (14)
A-D, These designs of wrist torque transmission splints may be used for specific isolation of the wrist extensor or flexor musculature when patients incorrectly utilize digital extrinsics to move the wrist. An alternative to C and D is composite digital taping in lieu of low-temperature thermoplastic material.

according to the most proximal primary joint(s), these splints are classified as wrist splints even though the splints affect both carpal and digital articulations. In contrast, when the wrist is considered a *secondary* joint and digital joints are primary joints, the splint is classified as a finger or thumb splint accordingly. With the exception of the torque transmission splints that fit in this general category, primary wrist and digital splints tend to be highly individualized, one-of-a-kind designs allowing personalized solutions to uniquely differing pathology.

Mobilization Splints

Type 0. *Type 0 wrist finger splints* do not include secondary joints. Splints in this category are designed to increase motion at the wrist and finger or thumb joints simultaneously. Direction of mobilizing forces may be identical for the wrist and digital joints or they may differ for wrist and digital joints. For example, the wrist may be moved into extension while finger MPs are moved into flexion, or vice versa (Fig. 13-18).

Wrist, Thumb Splints

Restriction/Immobilization Splints

Type 1. Splints in this category are highly individualized and may be created to protect healing structures while allowing limited motion. *Type 1 wrist, thumb restriction / immobilization splints* incorporate one secondary joint along with the wrist and

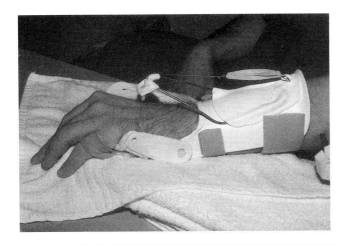

Fig. 13-18   Wrist extension, small finger MP flexion mobilization splint, type 0 (2)
Splints may be designed to apply separately directed mobilization forces to different primary joints. For example, this splint simultaneously mobilizes the wrist into extension and the small finger MP joint into flexion. (Courtesy Joni Armstrong, OTR, CHT, Bemidji, Minn.)

thumb CMC joint. This innovative splint design is advocated for treating various wrist problems (Fig. 13-19, A-C).[2] The secondary joint level for this splint is the thumb MP.

Wrist: Finger Splints
Torque Transmission Splints

Type 0. In the ESCS, use of a colon punctuation mark (:) in a splint's technical name indicates a torque transmission splint in which the joint immediately preceding the colon is the driver or power joint. For example, a *wrist extension: index–small finger MP flexion torque transmission splint, type 0 (5)* uses active wrist extension to produce passive finger MP joint flexion. Splints in this group may be single-joint power-driven as noted in the example or, as is often the case, they may be reciprocal alternating multijoint powered with active wrist flexion producing MP extension and active MP flexion producing wrist extension (Fig. 13-20, A,B). The latter are sometimes used to improve hand function in radial nerve injuries. There are no secondary joints in a *type 0 wrist: finger torque transmission splint.*

Wrist: Finger, Thumb Splints
Torque Transmission/Immobilization Splints

Type 2. As noted earlier, the presence of a colon punctuation mark (:) in a splint's technical name indicates the splint transfers active motion at one or more joints to create passive joint motion at another joint

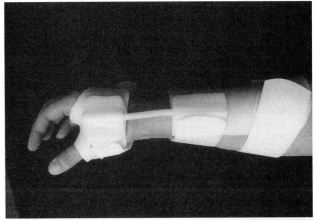
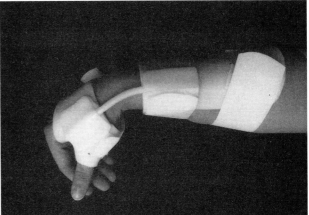
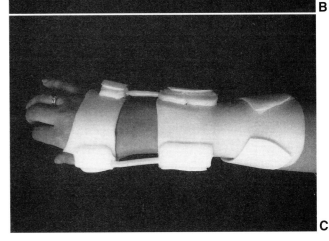

Fig. 13-19   A-C, Wrist radial and ulnar deviation restriction / Thumb CMC palmar abduction immobilization splint, type 1 (3) This splint incorporates flexible thermoplastic tubes to restrict wrist deviation and allow active wrist extension, while the thumb components immobilize the thumb CMC and MP joints. (Courtesy Terri Skirven, OTR, CHT, King of Prussia, Penn.)

or joints. Wrist: finger, thumb splints use wrist torque transmission to power finger and thumb joints and are frequently used to increase hand function for patients that have good wrist extension but poor digital grasp, as with C7 spinal cord injuries. A *type 2 wrist:*

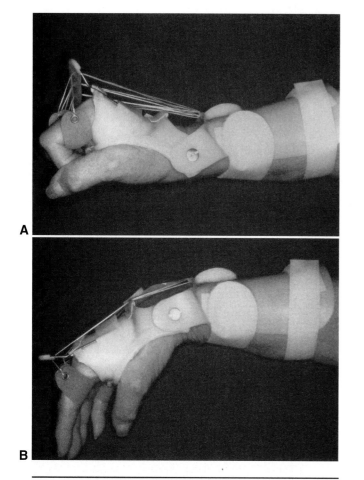

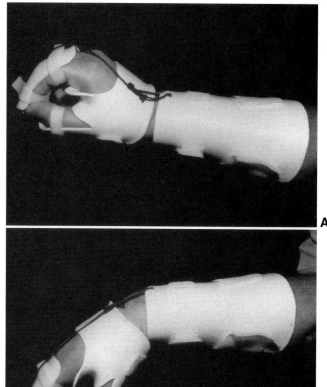

Fig. 13-20   A,B, Wrist flexion: index–small finger MP extension / index–small finger MP flexion: wrist extension torque transmission splint, type 0 (5)
A type 0 wrist: finger driven tenodesis splint creates reciprocal passive finger motion through torque transmission of active wrist motion and vice versa. **A,** Active wrist flexion creates tension on the inelastic mobilization assists resulting in passive finger MP joint extension. **B,** Conversely, active MP joint flexion tenses the inelastic mobilization assists to produce passive wrist extension. There are no secondary joints in a type 0 wrist: finger driven torque transmission splint. (Courtesy Jill Francisco, OTR, CHT Cicero, Ind.)

Fig. 13-21   A,B, Wrist extension: index–long finger flexion torque transmission / Wrist flexion: index–long finger extension torque transmission / Thumb CMC palmar abduction and thumb MP-IP extension immobilization, type 2 (10)
A type 2 wrist driven tenodesis torque transmission splint includes two secondary joint levels, usually the finger IPs, to improve passive finger prehension. **A,** Active wrist extension allows the natural tenodesis action of the hand to bring the index and long fingertips into contact with the tip of the thumb. A volar inelastic mobilization assist increases prehension strength as tension is applied through transmitted active wrist extension. Wrist flexion, assisted by gravity, creates tension on the dorsal inelastic mobilization assist resulting in transmitted extension of the index and long fingers and "opening" of the hand. (Courtesy Cheryl Kunkle, OTR, CHT, Allentown, Pa.)

finger, thumb splint controls two secondary joint levels, usually finger PIPs and DIPs, to further enhance tenodesis prehension (Fig. 13-21).

Forearm Splints

Splints may be applied to immobilize, mobilize, restrict, or transmit torque to radioulnar joint motion. Because of the orientation of the rotational axis of the forearm and the problems presented in obtaining a secure mechanical hold from which to base splinting forces, designing and fitting splints to limit or increase supination or pronation range of motion may be a very

difficult task. Understanding that the combined rotational axis of the radioulnar joints almost parallels the lengths of the ulna and radius (Fig. 13-22) is essential in dealing successfully with radioulnar problems requiring splinting. Also, when fitting forearm splints that incorporate the elbow as a secondary joint, considerable care must be taken to avoid excess pressure on the lateral and medial epicondyles, the olecranon, and the ulnar and radial nerves. The combined length and weight of the forearm and hand have the potential of becoming a formable moment arm for applying

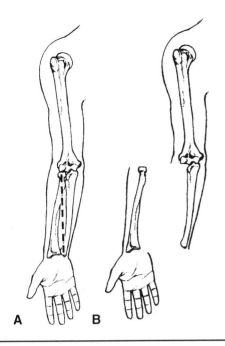

Fig. 13-22   **A,** Rotational axis of the forearm runs almost parallel to the lengths of the ulna and radius. **B,** The hand and radius act as a single unit rotating around a fixed ulna.

harmful pressure to the posterior and lateral aspects of the distal upper arm.

Immobilization Splints

Pain or discomfort associated with forearm rotation may necessitate immobilization for healing or protection. Splints may be used to immobilize the forearm in supination, pronation, or in neutral position, depending on the individual patient requirements. To completely immobilize the radioulnar joint, splints must incorporate both the wrist and elbow as secondary joints. Inclusion of either the elbow or wrist as a single secondary joint allows an increment of forearm motion at the joint left free.

Type 1. *Type 1 forearm immobilization splints* incorporate either the wrist or the elbow as a secondary joint in addition to the forearm, which is the single primary joint. A common error may occur when attempting to fabricate what is sometimes referred to as a "Munster" splint. In this epicondylar-bearing splint, the wrist is included as a secondary joint and two proximal extensions of the forearm trough clasp the lateral and medial epicondyles to limit radioulnar rotation. Unfortunately, when the proximal extensions of this splint are constructed in low-temperature plastic, they seldom provide the requisite proximal forearm rotational control due to lack of sufficient material strength, hence the *type 1* classification (Fig. 13-23, *A,B*). If rotational control were truly afforded

to the proximal forearm, the splint would be defined as a *type 2 forearm immobilization splint* and would be included in the next classification group. *Type 1 forearm immobilization splints* that include the elbow as the secondary joint leave the wrist free.

Type 2. *Type 2 forearm immobilization splints* incorporate two secondary joint levels in addition to the primary radioulnar joint. Secondary joint levels may include the wrist and thumb CMC joint for distal control or the wrist and elbow joints for optimum proximal and distal control of the forearm (Fig. 13-23, *C-F*).[4]

Mobilization Splints

To be effective, mobilizing forces must have a 90° angle of approach to the axis of joint rotation. Therefore, mobilization traction that is intended to increase supination or pronation should be applied at an angle perpendicular to the length of the forearm. When attempting to increase forearm rotation, a tight interosseous membrane can alter the focus of mobilization forces. Other structures may also be involved in stiffness, including, but not limited to, the palmar leaf of the distal radioulnar joint, which is implicated in problems achieving full supination.[12] It is important to avoid inadvertently applying mobilization forces to joints of lesser resistance, such as those of the wrist and hand, when attempting to improve passive motion of a resistive radioulnar joint. Additionally, congruous fit is very important in radioulnar mobilization splints. If this is not obtained, friction/shear injury to the underlying cutaneous surface can occur. As with wrist mobilization splints, if the patient complains of numbness or tingling in the digits, the splint should be removed immediately.

Type 0. A *forearm coaptation mobilization splint, type 0 (1)* may be applied to increase stability to the distal ulna joint and decrease pain following surgical procedures that alter the anatomical configuration of the distal radioulnar joint as with Darrach and Suave Kapinjii procedures. This simple cuff gently pulls the distal radius and ulna together to provide an increment of support and to decrease movement of the two bones away from each other during postoperative healing (Fig. 13-24). *Type 0 forearm mobilization splints* do not include secondary joints.

Type 2. Requiring considerable ingenuity, radioulnar mobilization splint designs assume unusual configurations. To obtain maximal purchase on the extremity, the wrist and elbow are included as secondary joints and the length of the forearm trough should be at least two-thirds the length of the forearm. Outriggers may run perpendicular (Fig. 13-25, *A-C*) or parallel (Fig. 13-26, *A,B*) to the axis of rotation. A two-piece splint, without outriggers, that incorporates the

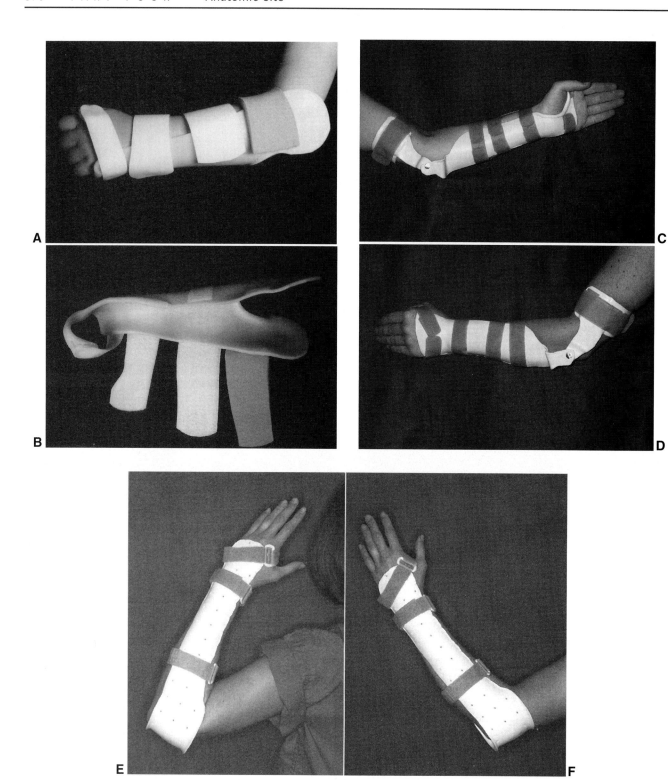

Fig. 13-23   A,B, Forearm neutral immobilization splint, type 1 (2) C,D, Forearm neutral immobilization splint, type 2 (3) E,F, Forearm neutral immobilization splint, type 2 (3)
Splints designed to immobilize forearm motion include the wrist or elbow, or both, as secondary joints. Type 1 forearm immobilization splints that incorporate one secondary joint (A,B), either the elbow or wrist, generally fail to achieve total forearm immobilization because the remaining free joint allows an increment of forearm rotation. In contrast, type 2 forearm immobilization splints incorporate both the wrist and elbow to better limit forearm rotation. C,D, Active elbow motion is permitted via an articulated joint or the elbow may be immobilized (E,F), or as shown in Fig. 13-4E. (Note: The expanded SCS technical name for the splint shown in E changes if its primary purpose is immobilization of the forearm instead of the wrist.) [Courtesy (C,D) Rebecca Banks, OTR, CHT, MHS, Blackburn, Australia; (E,F) from Contesti L: The radioulnar joints and forearm axis: therapist's commentary, *J Hand Ther* 12(2):86, 1999.]

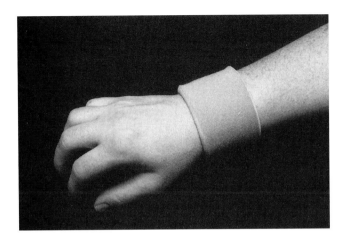

Fig. 13-24   **Forearm coaptation mobilization splint, type 0 (1)** Fabricated from a 2-inch wide soft strap with a D-ring for ease of donning, this axial mobilization splint applies multiple inwardly directed 2-point pressure forces to support the distal radioulnar joint.

elbow and wrist as secondary joints may be serially adjusted into pronation or supination (Fig. 13-27, *A-E*). The simplicity of this design allows more efficient construction and fit and, therefore, may be more cost effective despite its use of more material when compared with other smaller, but more complicated, forearm mobilization splints.

Supination or pronation mobilization splints incorporating long serpentine mobilization assists that diagonally cross the longitudinal axis of the forearm simultaneously create joint compression forces as well as desired rotational force to the radioulnar joint. Because of this, it is important to understand that serpentine designs inherently lose some of their rotational forces to translational compressive forces. Attempts to compensate for diminished rotational forces by increasing tension on the mobilization assist create greater compressive forces, often resulting in a splint that is not well tolerated by patients. Serpentine design splints are useful so long as their inherent mechanical confines are fully understood and patient selection is well thought out. Components in these serpentine splints usually do not follow the two-thirds forearm length requisite. Generally, forearm mobilization splints are better suited to patients whose stiffness is not long-standing (Fig. 13-28, *A-E*).

Commercially available forearm mobilization splints may decrease construction time, providing extensive modification is not required and cost is not prohibitive (Fig. 13-29, *A,B*). Because some commercial splints may not achieve a completely congruous fit on the extremity, it is prudent to check frequently during early wearing periods for pressure areas on

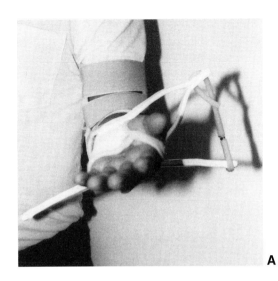

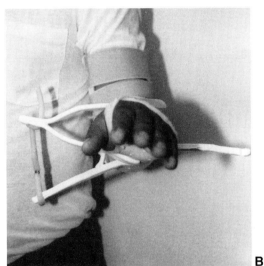

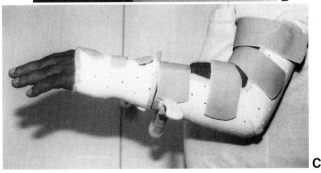

Fig. 13-25   **A, Forearm supination mobilization splint, type 2 (3) B,C, Forearm pronation mobilization splint, type 2 (3)** Designed to increase supination (**A**) and pronation (**B,C**), this splint uses mobilization forces perpendicular to the axis of rotation of the combined radioulnar joints. (Courtesy Janet Kinnunen Lopez, OTR, CHT, San Antonio, Texas.)

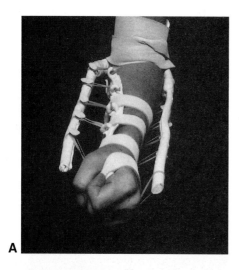

A

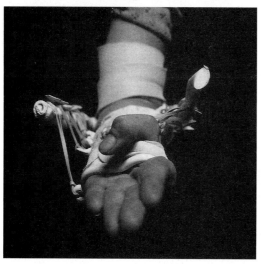

B

Fig. 13-26 A, Forearm pronation mobilization splint, type 2 (3) B, Forearm supination mobilization splint, type 2 (3) Dual outriggers that run parallel to the forearm provide multiple attachment sites for mobilization forces (rubber bands) that pull perpendicular to the rotational axis of the forearm, enhancing pronation (A) and supination (B). (Courtesy Kay Colello-Abraham, OTR, CHT, Orange, Calif.)

underlying cutaneous surfaces. Most problems with both custom and commercial forearm mobilization splints, however, arise from overenthusiastic application of mobilization forces rather than from lack of appropriate fit.

Forearm, Finger Splints
Mobilization/Restriction Splints

Type 1. *Type 1 forearm mobilization, finger restriction splints* are usually one-of-a-kind splints that reflect unique needs specific to individual patients. These splints incorporate the distal forearm

and some or all finger joints as primary joints and the wrist is included as a secondary joint (Fig. 13-30).

Forearm, Wrist, Thumb Splints
Mobilization Splints

Type 0. A *type 0 forearm, wrist, thumb splint* will include as primary joints the forearm, wrist, and thumb. Patients note improved function with the thumb positioned in palmar abduction, wrist in extension, and forearm in supination. The splint is typically fabricated for children with mild hypertonia (Fig. 13-31).

■ NONARTICULAR FOREARM SPLINTS

Nonarticular forearm splints use coaptational forces to support, restrict, or facilitate underlying soft tissues and/or osseous structures. Allowing graded force application to meet individual patient requirements, splints in this classification may be fabricated from a wide selection of materials ranging from rigid to flexible or combinations thereof (Fig. 13-32).

■ SUMMARY

The integrity of the wrist joint with its complex anatomic and motion architecture has been established as the key to hand function. It is uniquely vulnerable to a variety of injury and disease processes that may result in pain, stiffness, or instability, which may interfere with normal upper extremity function at all levels. The management of these wrist maladies may be substantially enhanced by proper splinting with objectives ranging from pain relief and protection to prevention and correction of deformity. In addition, wrist splinting may be used to negate or augment long extrinsic tenodesis functions in the management of digital pathologic conditions. Postoperative splinting protects healing structures while allowing predefined motion to involved and noninvolved joints. Therefore, it is imperative that careful consideration be directed toward the anatomic, kinesiologic, and functional effects of any splint created to traverse this important joint.

The radioulnar joints provide the distal extremity with the very important increment of transverse rotation, allowing the hand to be positioned in a multitude of functional attitudes. In addition to a thorough knowledge of forearm anatomy, the key to splinting these joints lies in understanding their cooperative kinesiologic role.

Close communication between therapist, surgeon, and patient is crucial to attaining optimum patient

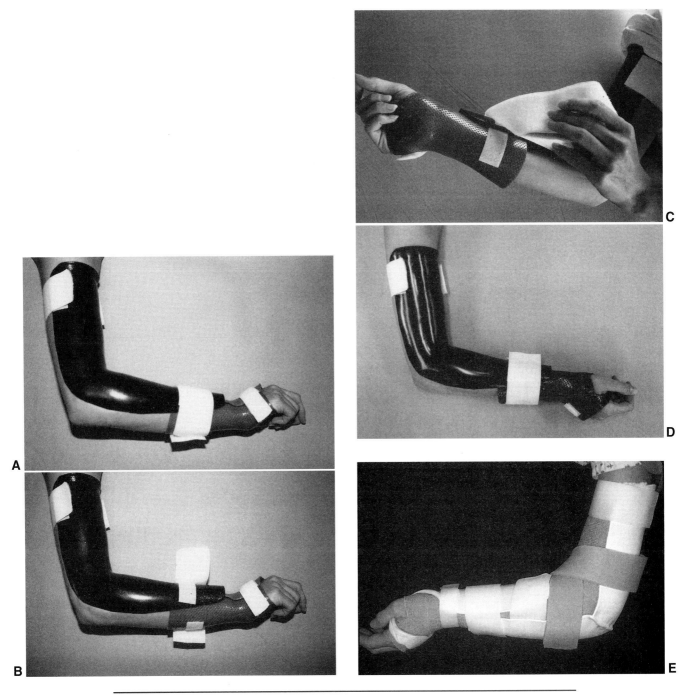

Fig. 13-27   A,B, Forearm pronation mobilization splint, type 2 (3) C,D, Forearm supination mobilization splint, type 2 (3) E, Forearm supination mobilization splint, type 2 (3)
This two-piece combination elbow and wrist splint for forearm mobilization in pronation (A,B) and supination (C-E) is simple in design and efficient in fabrication time. The two-piece design permits serial adjustments through an adjustable strap that firmly attaches the two splints together. [Courtesy (A-D) Paul Van Lede, OT, MS, Orfit Industries, Wijnegem, Belgium.]

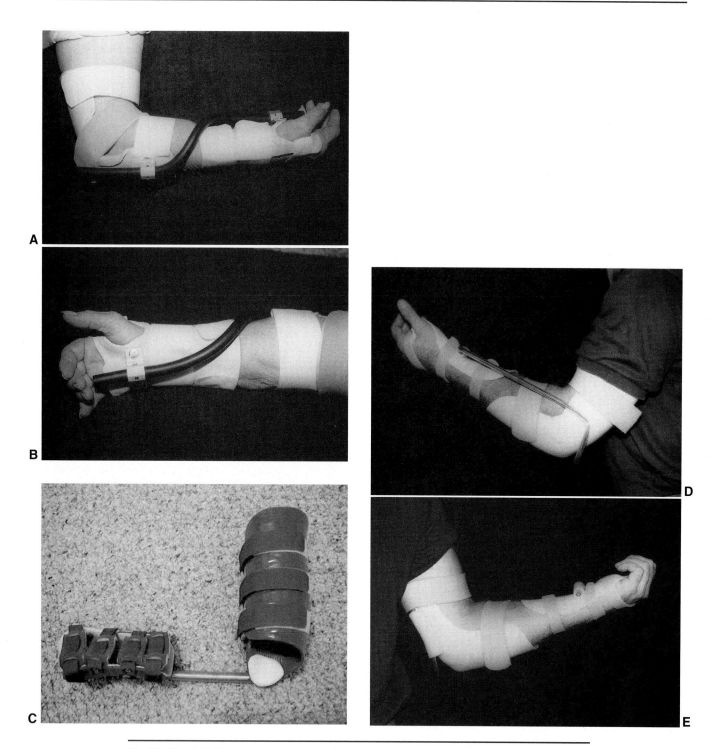

Fig. 13-28   A,B, Forearm supination mobilization splint, type 2 (3) C, Forearm supination mobilization splint, type 2 (3) D,E, Forearm supination mobilization splint, type 2 (3)
Forearm mobilization splints vary in design and materials. The elbow and wrist are secondary joints (A-E). [Courtesy (C) Jason Willoughby, OTR, Richmond, Ky.; (D,E) Connor McCullough, OTR, Canoga Park, Calif.]

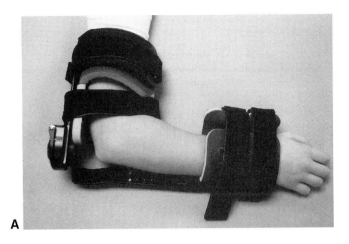

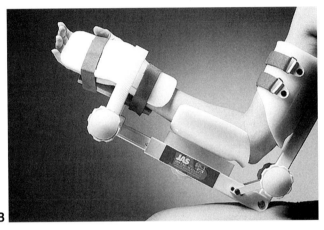

Fig. 13-29   **A, Forearm supination mobilization splint, type 2 (3) B, Forearm pronation mobilization splint, type 4 (8)**
Forearm mobilization splints are available commercially in various prefabricated forms (not all inclusive of the many splints available). [Courtesy **(A)** EMPI, St. Paul, Minn.; **(B)** Joint Active Systems, Inc., Effingham, Ill.]

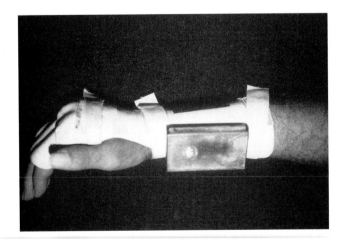

Fig. 13-30   **Forearm pronation mobilization / Index–small finger MP extension restriction splint, type 1 (6)**
This innovative splint design uses a radially mounted weight as a mobilization assist to increase forearm pronation while restricting extension of the finger MP joints. (Courtesy Robin Miller, OTR/L, CHT, Ft. Lauderdale, Fla.)

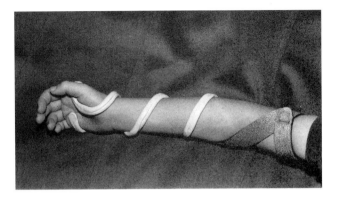

Fig. 13-31   **Forearm supination, wrist extension, thumb CMC palmar abduction mobilization splint, type 0 (3)**
This type 0 splint assists supination, wrist extension, and thumb palmar abduction by facilitating functional use of the extremity without inhibiting sensory input. (Courtesy Joni Armstrong, OTR, CHT, Bemidji, Minn.)

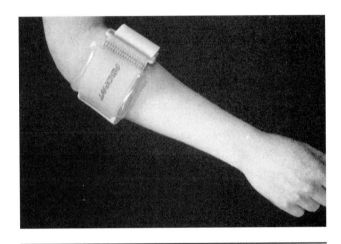

Fig. 13-32   **Nonarticular proximal forearm splint**
This Aircast Armband is but one of many splints commercially available that may be used for treating lateral epicondylitis.

rehabilitation potential. Assessment and adaptation of patients' work, home, and/or avocational environments also may be necessary to allow independent return to normal activities.

REFERENCES

1. Alexander CE, Lichtman DM: Ulnar carpal instabilities, *Orthop Clin North Am* 15(2):307-20, 1984.
2. Bora FW Jr, Culp RW, Osterman AL, et al: A flexible wrist splint, *J Hand Surg* [Am] 14(3):574-5, 1989.
3. Brown DE, Lichtman DM: Midcarpal instability, *Hand Clin* 3(1):135-40, 1987.
4. Contesti LA: The radioulnar joints and forearm axis: therapist's commentary, *J Hand Ther* 12(2):85-91, 1999.
5. Garcia-Elias M, Dobyns J: Bones and joints. In Cooney W, Linscheid RL, Dobyns J: *The wrist: diagnosis and operative treatment*, Mosby, 1998, St. Louis.
6. Green DP: Carpal dislocations and instabilities. In Green DP: *Operative hand surgery*, Churchill Livingstone, 1994, London.

7. Hagert CG: Distal radius fracture and the distal radioulnar joint—anatomical considerations, *Handchir Mikrochir Plast Chir* 26(1):22-6, 1994.

8. Hagert CG: The distal radioulnar joint, *Hand Clin* 3(1):41-50, 1987.

9. Hagert CG: The distal radioulnar joint in relation to the whole forearm, *Clin Orthop* (275):56-64, 1992.

10. Henshaw J, Satren J, Wrightsman J: Semi-flexible support: an alternative for the hand-injured worker, *J Hand Ther* 2(1):35, 1989.

11. Jansen C, Olson S, Hasson S: The effectiveness of use of a wrist orthosis during functional activities on surface electromyography of the wrist extensors in normal subjects, *J Hand Ther* 10(4):283-9, 1997.

12. Kleinman W: DRUJ contracture release, *Tech Hand Upper Extremity Surg* 3(1):13-22, 1999.

13. Lichtman DM, Galenslen E, Pollock G: Midcarpal and proximal carpal instabilities. In Lichtman DM: *The wrist and its disorders*, Saunders, 1977, Philadelphia.

14. Lichtman DM, Bruckner JD, Culp RW, et al: Palmar midcarpal instability: results of surgical reconstruction, *J Hand Surg* [Am] 18(2):307-15, 1993.

15. Malick M: *Manual on static hand splinting*, vol 1, Rev ed, Harmarville Rehabilitation Center, 1972, Pittsburgh.

16. Malick M: *Manual on dynamic hand splinting with thermoplastic materials*, Harmarville Rehabilitation Center, 1974, Pittsburgh.

17. Palmer A, Werner F: Biomechanics of the distal radioulnar joint, *Clin Orthop* 187:26-35, 1984.

18. Taleisnik J: Carpal kinematics. In Taleisnick J: *The wrist*, Churchill Livingstone, 1985, London.

19. Taleisnick J: *The wrist*, Churchill Livingstone, 1985, London.

20. Taleisnik J: *Wrist: anatomy, function and injury, American Academy of Orthopaedic Surgeons' Instructional Course Lectures* 27:61, 1978.

21. Taleisnik J, Watson HK: Midcarpal instability caused by malunited fractures of the distal radius, *J Hand Surg* [Am] 9(3):350-7, 1984.

22. Wright TW, Dobyns J: Carpal instability non-dissociative. In Cooney W, Linsheid R, Dobyns J: *The wrist: diagnosis and operative treatment*, Mosby, 1998, St. Louis.

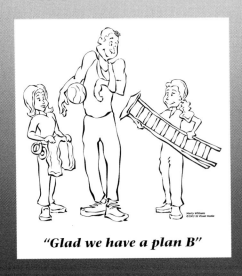

"Glad we have a plan B"

CHAPTER 14

Splints Acting on the Elbow and Shoulder

Chapter Outline

The format of this chapter follows the expanded ASHT Splint Classification System[2] hierarchy in that elbow and shoulder splints respectively are first divided into articular or nonarticular categories with articular splints described and illustrated before the nonarticular classification splints. Within the articular category, splints are grouped according to the primary joint or joints they influence. Splints in the nonarticular category are defined according to the anatomical segments upon which they are based.

Once the elbow or shoulder articular splints are grouped according to their primary joints, they are further defined by direction of force application and then divided according to one of four purposes: immobilization, mobilization, restriction, or torque transmission. Splints with more than one primary purpose are designated by dual-purpose categories (e.g., mobilization/restriction or immobilization/mobilization). In this chapter, the force direction (e.g., extension, flexion, rotation) is

included with the purpose groupings rather than as a free-standing subcategory. Purpose categories are further subdivided by *type*. *Type* identifies the number of secondary joint levels included in splints. Note: *Type* refers to the number of secondary joint levels, *not* the total number of secondary joints in a splint. While not all categories and/or subcategories are represented in this chapter, the ESCS is sufficiently flexible to accommodate additional groupings as needed.

Splinting the elbow and shoulder presents unique challenges for physicians and therapists. A team approach is important to successful patient outcomes. Conferring with referring physicians is crucial to gathering pertinent patient data. Diagnosis, prognosis, precautions, and the purpose of splints must be clearly defined before splint designs are begun. It is not unusual for referring physicians to define very specific elbow or shoulder joint postures and angles that splints must accomplish, especially for splints used postoperatively. The principles of splinting mechanics, outriggers and mobilization assists, design, construction, and fit previously outlined for forearm, wrist, and digits also are applicable to the larger elbow and shoulder joints. Both the elbow and shoulder have joint-specific splinting requirements. Injuries to these joints often involve multiple structures, including soft tissue, nerve, and bone.

ARTICULAR ELBOW, ELBOW-FOREARM, AND SHOULDER SPLINTS

Elbow splints

The elbow joint is critical to upper extremity function. Considered a trochoginglymoid joint, the elbow has two articulations, the ulnohumeral joint, a hinge joint, and the radiohumeral and proximal radioulnar joint, an axial rotation joint.[26] These two articulations combine to permit two degrees of freedom of motion, flexion–extension and supination–pronation. Without sufficient elbow flexion, the ability to get one's hand to the face and mouth is significantly compromised; lack of elbow extension makes reaching objects in the environment and performing some personal care activities difficult or impossible. Several authors report that good upper extremity function is possible with elbow motion of −30° extension to 130° flexion.[13,24,27] Successful treatment is predicated on thorough evaluations and close monitoring to allow timely intervention of exercise and splinting programs. Even experienced clinicians find that elbows are often difficult to rehabilitate. It is important to keep in mind that elbows do not respond well to aggressive or forceful therapy.[28] "Because of the tight congruity of the elbow joint, the closely applied and vulnerable soft tissues, and the proximity of the muscles that move the elbow, stiffness is extremely difficult to overcome . . . Further, excessive passive stretch of the joint is to be assiduously avoided."[28] "A slow continuous force that stretches the damaged contracted tissue must be distinguished from the sudden, quick maneuver (manipulation) that tears tissue and may evoke a response that results in further contracture."[28] Prolonged gentle splinting improves elbow range of motion through remodeling of contracted soft tissue structures.

When splinting elbow injuries, it is important to avoid pressure over the ulnar nerve. This nerve may be injured at the time of the original trauma. Therefore, prior to splinting, it is essential to evaluate the neurovascular status of the extremity to provide a baseline for follow-up assessments. Further, it is important to remember that nerve involvement may not appear immediately and may be a late sequela of a fracture. Patients should be instructed to contact their

therapists immediately if changes in neurovascular status occur, allowing timely adjustment of splints and notification of referring physicians.

Immobilization Splints

Elbow immobilization splints promote tissue healing, control early postoperative motion, and/or rest joints that are debilitated from overuse. These splints may be applied to the anterior, posterior, lateral, or medial aspect of the elbow and they may include one or more secondary joints in addition to the primary elbow joint. Conditions commonly requiring immobilization of the elbow include arthritis, cubital tunnel syndrome, ligamentous injuries, dislocations, fractures, bicep tendon repairs, ulnar nerve transpositions, or total elbow arthroplasties.[7]

Depending upon the kind and severity of the injury, elbow fractures may be treated with either closed reduction or open reduction and internal fixation. When treating elbow fractures, it is important that all those involved in the rehabilitation process be aware of concomitant soft tissue injuries and/or repairs because associated ligament or nerve injuries are often present. Upper extremity sensory and motor evaluations should be routinely performed to allow early detection of changes in sensibility or muscle strength. Elbow immobilization splint designs that provide protection during bone healing may or may not include the forearm and wrist as secondary joints. Wearing schedules vary and usually are diagnosis-specific. For example, an *elbow immobilization splint* that postoperatively protects a biceps tendon repair is usually worn full time except during prescribed exercise sessions and showering. Immobilization splints facilitate early and frequent exercise sessions to uninvolved joints. *Elbow immobilization splints* almost always immobilize the elbow in some degree of flexion, depending on diagnosis.

Type 1. *Type 1 elbow immobilization splints* include one primary joint, the elbow, and one secondary joint, which usually is the forearm. These splints are used to hold the elbow in a position of extension or flexion. *Type 1 splints* are commonly used in acute overuse injuries to the elbow (Fig. 14-1).

Type 2. *Type 2 elbow immobilization splints* incorporate two secondary joints, both of which almost always are situated distal to the primary elbow joint. Inclusion of these secondary joints increases splint stabilization and improves elbow immobilization by stabilizing the forearm and wrist (Fig. 14-2).

Mobilization Splints

Elbow mobilization splints maintain or increase passive range of motion in either elbow extension or

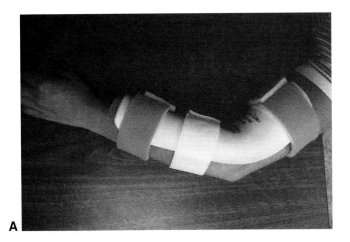

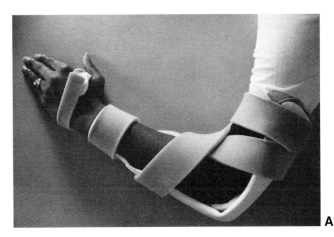

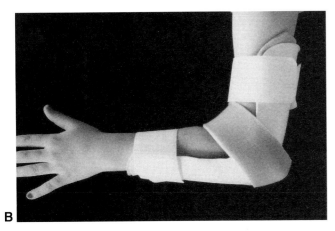

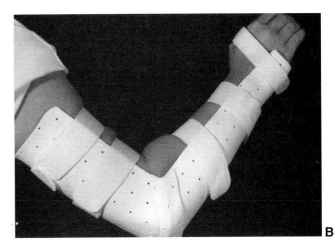

Fig. 14-1   A, Elbow flexion immobilization splint, type 1 (2) B, Elbow flexion immobilization splint, type 1 (2)
Elbow splints may be designed to fit anteriorly (A) or posteriorly (B). Most elbow immobilization splints position the elbow in some degree of flexion. An anterior design splint may be used to limit elbow flexion and rest an irritated ulnar nerve in a patient with cubital tunnel syndrome.

Fig. 14-2   A, Elbow flexion immobilization splint, type 2 (3) B, Elbow flexion immobilization splint, type 2 (3)
To more completely immobilize the elbow, two secondary joints are incorporated in the splint, increasing both splint stability and patient comfort. The two joints most often included are the forearm and wrist. [Courtesy (B) Rachel Dyrud Ferguson, OTR, CHT, Taos, N.M.]

flexion.[14,15,20,23] These splints provide low-load prolonged mobilization forces through elastic or inelastic traction to resolve elbow flexion or extension contractures. Subsequent to injury, elbow contractures may be manifested in thickening and shortening of the anterior and posterior capsules, with increasing contracture of the collateral ligaments and muscles surrounding the elbow as time progresses.[13] Other causes of elbow stiffness may include fracture/dislocations of the elbow, burns, or heterotopic bone formation most commonly seen after head injuries.[13] Clinically, restoration of passive elbow extension may be more difficult to achieve than is passive elbow flexion. Elbow mobilization is frequently a goal following injury to the elbow and various design options are needed to fit the specific patient requirements. Mobilization splinting using inelastic traction is especially

helpful in restoring functional extension to the elbow.[5,13,16]

The forearm is considered a secondary joint in most elbow mobilization splints. In order to obtain sufficient splint mechanical advantage on the elbow joint, the forearm must be included in the splint, resulting in impedance of forearm pronation/supination ranging from minuscule to near total immobilization. Distinguishing between *type 0* and borderline *type 1 elbow* mobilization splints can be difficult and is dependent on the length and contiguousness of fit of the forearm component. Strapping also plays an important role in that strapping with an increment of elasticity allows more forearm rotation than does strapping with no stretch properties. "Full supination and pronation can be achieved only when both the proximal and distal radioulnar joints are

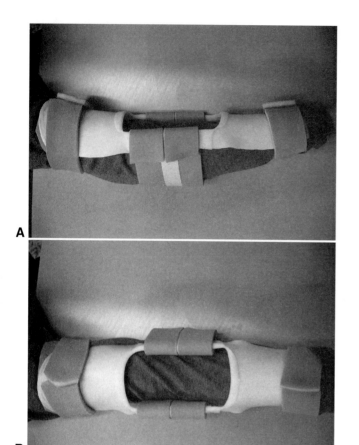

A

B

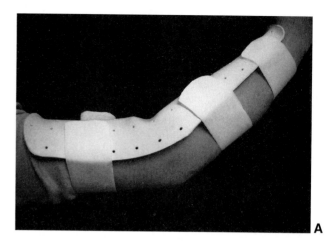

A

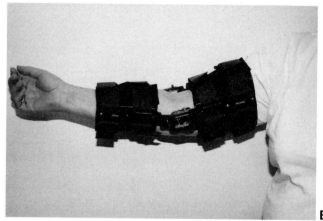

B

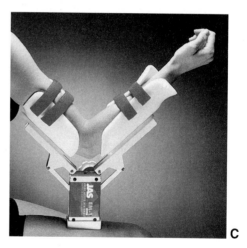

C

Fig. 14-3 A,B, Elbow extension mobilization splint, type 0 (1) This custom-fabricated splint is more appropriate for an elbow contracture with less severe angulation. It uses adjustable inelastic traction strapping that is pulled through the splint window located directly over the elbow joint. This particular splint is classified as type 0 because of its relatively short forearm component and the presence of a distal soft strap. For most contractures, supplemental night splinting is essential to maintain gains made during exercise, functional use, and mobilization splinting during the day.

Fig. 14-4 A, Elbow extension mobilization splint, type 1 (2) B, Elbow extension mobilization splint, type 1 (2) C, Elbow extension mobilization splint, type 1 (2)
Type 1 elbow extension splints may be custom fitted (A) or they may be obtained through commercial sources (B,C). [Courtesy (B) Ultraflex Systems, Inc., Downington, Pa.; (C) Joint Active Systems, Inc., Effingham, Ill.]

normal in their relationship, the relative length of the radius and ulna is anatomic, and the interosseous membrane is unaltered."[30]

Type 0. *Type 0 elbow mobilization splints* affect only the primary elbow joint. No secondary joints are incorporated into these splints. Mobilization forces may improve either elbow extension (Fig. 14-3) or flexion range of motion. Splints may be applied to the anterior, posterior, medial, or lateral aspect of the elbow, depending on the specific diagnosis of the patient and the presence or absence of associated injuries.

Type 1. One secondary joint, usually the forearm, is included in an *elbow mobilization splint, type 1.* These splints may be fitted to increase elbow extension (Fig. 14-4) or flexion (Fig. 14-5). If needed, extension and flexion splints may be alternated. To obtain

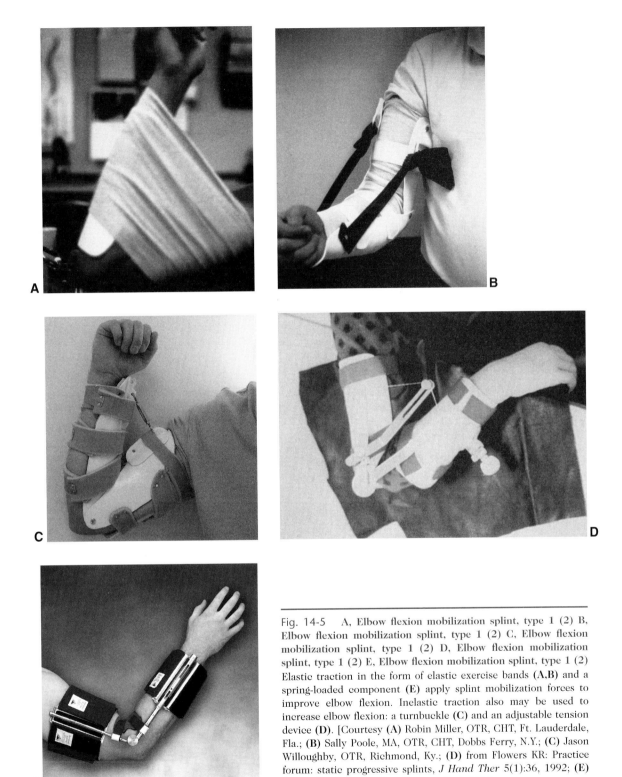

Fig. 14-5   A, Elbow flexion mobilization splint, type 1 (2) B, Elbow flexion mobilization splint, type 1 (2) C, Elbow flexion mobilization splint, type 1 (2) D, Elbow flexion mobilization splint, type 1 (2) E, Elbow flexion mobilization splint, type 1 (2) Elastic traction in the form of elastic exercise bands (**A,B**) and a spring-loaded component (**E**) apply splint mobilization forces to improve elbow flexion. Inelastic traction also may be used to increase elbow flexion: a turnbuckle (**C**) and an adjustable tension device (**D**). [Courtesy (**A**) Robin Miller, OTR, CHT, Ft. Lauderdale, Fla.; (**B**) Sally Poole, MA, OTR, CHT, Dobbs Ferry, N.Y.; (**C**) Jason Willoughby, OTR, Richmond, Ky.; (**D**) from Flowers KR: Practice forum: static progressive splints, *J Hand Ther* 5(1):36, 1992; (**E**) Dynasplint Systems, Inc., Severna Park, Md.]

sufficient purchase and to distribute pressure, the majority of elbow mobilization splints controls secondarily some increment of forearm rotation. Including the forearm also directs mobilization forces to the elbow by excluding some or all forearm rotation.

Type 2. The forearm and wrist, secondary joints, are included in an *elbow mobilization splint, type 2.* Incorporating the forearm and wrist directs mobilization forces to the elbow by excluding forearm rotation (Fig. 14-6, *A-E*).

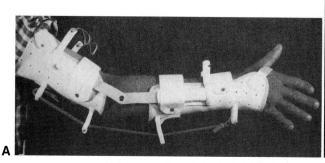

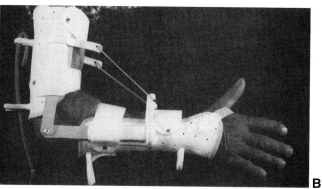

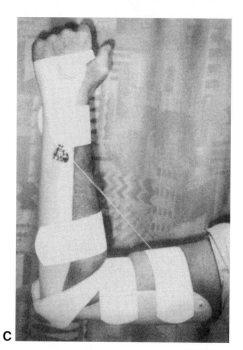

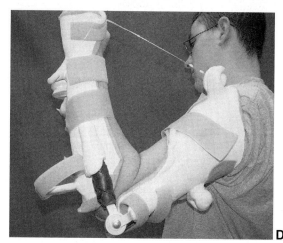

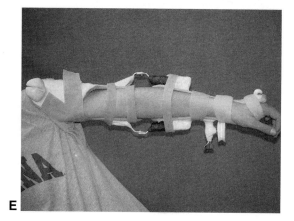

Fig. 14-6   A, Elbow extension mobilization splint, type 2 (3) B, Elbow flexion mobilization splint, type 2 (3) C, Elbow flexion mobilization splint, type 2 (3) D, Elbow flexion or extension mobilization splint, type 2 (3) E, Elbow extension or flexion mobilization splint, type 2 (3)

A-C, These elbow mobilization splints direct force to the elbow by completely eliminating forearm rotation through inclusion of the forearm and wrist as secondary joints. D,E, This elbow splint is designed to provide elbow flexion (D) or elbow extension (E) mobilization forces. D, Note the unlinked extension outriggers on the proximal and distal forearm trough. Mechanical advantage is also excellent in this splint. Both the humeral and forearm-wrist components are long and wide, increasing splint strength and comfort. [(A,B) from Nirschl RP, Morrey BF: Rehabilitation. In Morrey BF: *The elbow and its disorders*, ed 3, WB Saunders, 2000, Philadelphia; (C) from Bash D, Spur M: An alternative to turnbuckle splinting for elbow flexion, *J Hand Ther* 13(3):239, 2000; (D,E) Christopher Bochenek, OTR, CHT, Cincinnati, Ohio.]

Restriction Splints

With numerous design options, *elbow restriction splints* limit the elbow's normal arc of motion to promote healing or to decrease pain. Fitted for a wide variety of elbow problems, these splints may affect motion in one or more planes and their design options are diagnostic-specific. For example, an elbow fracture that is unstable within a particular arc of motion requires stabilization that may be provided by an articulated elbow joint component with adjustable stops, which is incorporated in an *elbow restriction splint,* allowing protected movement within a safe range of motion as determined by the physician. As healing progresses, the adjustable hinge may be incrementally reset to allow increasing range of motion over a specified period of time. Another example, a tendon transfer for elbow flexion, requires an elbow splint that may be adjusted into gradual extension per the physician's orders and the patient's progress. A final example, an anterior *elbow flexion restriction splint* is often helpful in relieving cubital tunnel symptoms. The splint is worn when sleeping to prevent elbow flexion. During the day, an elbow pad is worn to protect the posterior elbow. In addition to elbow restriction splints that allow precise restriction of motion through adjustable elbow hinges or dial-like devices, more simple elbow restriction splints may be fabricated in neoprene to provide only a minimal amount of restriction especially at the end ranges of motion.

Type 0. Affecting only the primary elbow joint, *type 0 elbow restriction splints* incorporate no secondary joints. These splints may limit elbow extension, flexion, or deviation. Prevention of extremes of normally occurring arcs of elbow motion helps protect healing structures (Fig. 14-7).

Type 1. *Type 1 elbow restriction splints* incorporate one secondary joint, the forearm, while restricting elbow extension (Fig. 14-8), flexion (Fig. 14-9), both extension and flexion (Fig. 14-10), or deviation (Fig. 14-11). These splints may be custom fitted with or without commercial components, or they may be obtained through commercial sources, depending on individual patient requirements.

Torque Transmission Splints

Elbow torque transmission splints are designed to transfer moment to joints external to the splints themselves. These splints transfer moment longitudinally by controlling secondary joint(s). Single purpose torque transmission splints have a minimum of one secondary joint level. These splints are often referred to as "exercise" splints because they are used to maintain or increase motion in conjunction with functional

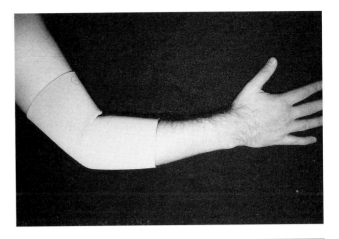

Fig. 14-7   Elbow extension and flexion restriction splint, type 0 (1)
A neoprene sleeve frequently is used following discontinuation of more rigid splinting to provide a lighter form of restriction. This soft splint also has high patient compliance when it is used to treat arthritic conditions of the elbow. Patients report that it provides support and warmth to the elbow and helps reduce pain and increases overall function of the arm. Some patients with epicondylitis find these splints beneficial as well.

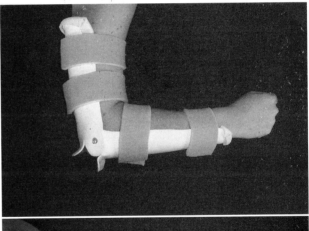

A

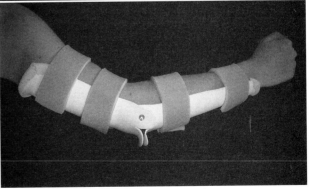

B

Fig. 14-8   A,B, Elbow extension restriction splint, type 1 (2)
Inclusion of the forearm as a secondary joint in an elbow restriction splint limits a portion of forearm rotation secondarily, depending on the length of the forearm component. This custom splint incorporates an innovative blocking mechanism to restrict elbow extension. It also includes almost the entire length of the forearm secondarily, dispersing splint pressure and increasing patient comfort.

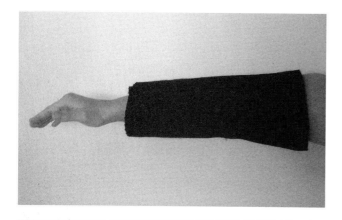

Fig. 14-9   Elbow flexion restriction splint, type 0 (1)
Type 1 elbow flexion restriction splints may be used to reduce ulnar nerve compression at the cubital tunnel by preventing full elbow flexion.

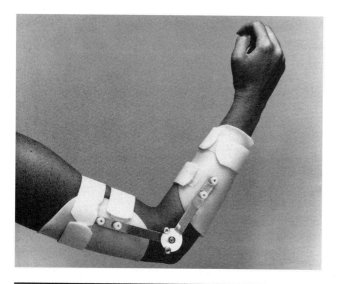

Fig. 14-10   Elbow extension and flexion restriction splint, type 1 (2)
An articulated *elbow restriction splint, type 1* limits both elbow extension and flexion via adjustable "stops" in the elbow joint of this restriction splint. (Courtesy Helen Marx, OTR, CHT, Human Factors Engineering of Phoenix, Wickenburg, Ariz.)

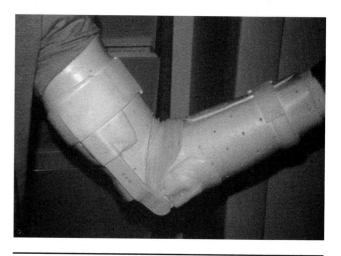

Fig. 14-11   Elbow lateral and medial deviation restriction splint, type 1 (2)
A hinged elbow restriction splint, type 1 prevents medial and lateral deviation of the elbow while including the forearm as a secondary joint. (Courtesy Sally Poole, MA, OTR, CHT, Dobbs Ferry, N.Y.)

activities, an *elbow extension and flexion torque transmission splint, type 1 (2)* may be considered to eliminate undesirable shoulder substitution patterns. More realistic is the concept of incorporating the wrist secondarily to transfer moment to the elbow to improve motion or to remodel elbow soft tissue. For example, if active elbow flexion is limited and a patient tends to compensate by flexing his wrist during exercise and functional activities designed to increase elbow flexion, an *elbow extension and flexion torque transmission splint, type 1 (2)* that controls the wrist secondarily may be fitted to eliminate wrist motion and to increase active elbow motion.

Elbow, Forearm Splints
Mobilization Splints

Splints that mobilize both the elbow and forearm joints typically are diagnosis-specific in design. These splints may be used preoperatively to substitute for lost active motion, or they may maintain or improve passive joint motion. Postoperatively they protect healing structures and improve joint motion.

Type 1. With the elbow and forearm designated as primary joints, *type 1 elbow, forearm mobilization splints* incorporate either the wrist distally or the shoulder proximally as secondary joints (Fig. 14-12).

Restriction/Immobilization Splints

Splints that restrict and immobilize the elbow and forearm restrict elbow motion within a protected arc while simultaneously immobilizing an additional primary joint, the forearm.

upper extremity use. Of the hundreds of photographs submitted for inclusion in the third edition of this book, no elbow torque transmission splints were included.

Type 1. *Type 1 elbow torque transmission splints* incorporate one secondary joint in addition to the primary elbow joint. Although in theory the secondary joint may be situated proximal or distal to the elbow, the practicality of including the shoulder joint secondarily to improve elbow motion is arguable. However, if a patient persists in substituting shoulder motion when performing elbow flexion exercises or functional

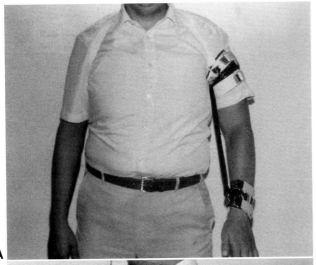

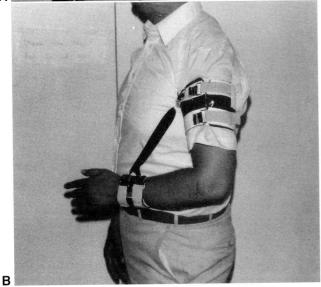

Fig. 14-12   **A,B, Elbow flexion, forearm neutral mobilization splint, type 1 (3)**
Substituting for lost active motion, this splint uses an elastic band to substitute for a nonfunctioning brachioradialis muscle. The shoulder harness makes this a type 1 ESCS classification. (Courtesy Carol Hierman, OTR, CHT, Cedar Grove, N.C., and Elisha Denny, PTA, OTA, Pittsboro, N.C.; © UNC Hand Rehabilitation Center, Chapel Hill, N.C.)

Type 1. *Type 1 elbow restriction / forearm immobilization splints* restrict elbow motion while the forearm is immobilized in neutral, supination, or pronation. For these splints, both the elbow and forearm are considered primary joints and the wrist is a secondary joint. The splint further isolates restricted elbow motion by immobilizing the forearm primarily and wrist secondarily (Fig. 14-13).

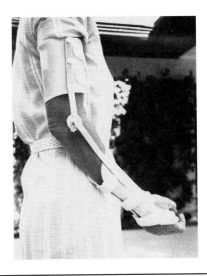

Fig. 14-13   **Elbow extension restriction / Forearm supination immobilization splint, type 1 (3)**
An adjustable "stop" at the elbow joint limits elbow extension as the forearm is immobilized in supination. (Courtesy Helen Marx, OTR, CHT, Human Factors Engineering of Phoenix, Wickenburg, Ariz.)

Shoulder Splints

Because of its inherent complexity and size, splinting the shoulder is one of the more challenging splinting endeavors clinicians may encounter. The shoulder is a composite of four articulations that work together in a complex symphony to provide three degrees of freedom of motion in multiple planes. The four joints of the shoulder include the glenohumeral joint, the sternoclavicular joint, the acromioclavicular joint, and the scapulothoracic joint.[24] Positioning of the shoulder following injury or surgery depends on the injury, the reparative procedure performed, and surgeon preference.

Clinicians have a wide range of shoulder splint design options from which to choose, ranging from custom-fabricated splints to commercially available splints. Deciding whether to make a shoulder splint or to apply a prefabricated splint involves careful consideration of numerous factors including patient, staff, and third-party reimbursement variables. Unfortunately, some custom-designed shoulder splints are time-consuming to fabricate and they often require the assistance of a second person to obtain a proper fit. In today's therapy world, not only is this not practical, but it often is not possible in some clinics! With an increasing number of commercial shoulder splints on the market, some clinicians seem to be gradually moving away from making custom-fitted shoulder splints. Interestingly, a defining element of this trend involves purpose of splint application, in that most shoulder immobilization splints continue to be custom fabricated to exactingly meet individual patient needs. In contrast, lack of an easily constructed and adjusted shoulder mobilization splint design may be intimidating to some clinicians, insidiously shrinking acceptance criteria in favor of less efficacious but quicker and easier shoulder mobilization splinting solutions. This unfortunate situation, however, is rectified with a simple, adjustable shoulder mobilization splint devised by McClure and Flowers[25] (see section on shoulder mobilization splints).

Sometimes a prefabricated shoulder splint may be the splint of choice. If a commercially manufactured splint is used, it must satisfy all of the principles (mechanics, outriggers and mobilization assists, design, construction, and fit) discussed earlier in this book. There is never any excuse for an improperly fitting or poorly functioning splint, whether custom or commercially made.

When fitting shoulder splints, care should be taken to avoid overstretching of the brachial plexus and to avoid pressure over the radial nerve. Wounds involving both bone and soft tissue require innovative splinting solutions. For example, humeral fractures are commonly associated with radial nerve injuries.* In complex cases such as these, splinting must satisfy multiple purposes including immobilizing the humeral fracture and providing splintage for the associated radial nerve palsy.

A clinical hint that is applicable to fitting most shoulder splints is as follows: To prevent a patient from assuming an adverse scoliotic spinal posture from supporting the weight of his arm in a shoulder splint, design the splint so that its inferior-lateral border includes the upper portion of the patient's iliac crest. This stabilizes the splint on the hip, allowing an upright and comfortable posture. Poor spinal posture is not a problem with bilateral shoulder splints because arm weight is balanced evenly. Other clinical hints for fitting shoulder splints include putting the patient in a side lying or supine position to make efficient use of gravitational forces as the splint material is applied, and using elastic wraps to secure the distal portion of the splint to free the therapist's hands for fitting more proximal portions of the shoulder splint.

Immobilization Splints

Shoulder immobilization splints prevent movement of the shoulder in predefined planes of motion according to injury-specific and/or surgery-specific requisites. Many shoulder immobilization splints include

*References 1, 3, 4, 6, 12, 18, 22.

multiple secondary joint levels, allowing arm weight to be dispersed over a larger area, thus providing greater comfort than would splints that incorporate only the shoulder and humerus. The majority of these splints incorporate the elbow, forearm, and wrist as secondary joints to improve splint mechanics. For example, if the elbow is not included in a shoulder splint, control of shoulder external and internal rotation is difficult if not impossible, and destructive pressure on the distal portion of the humerus occurs as the forearm and hand are allowed to assume a dangerous, edema producing, dependent position at rest. As each successive, more distal joint is incorporated into the design of a shoulder splint, control of shoulder joint position and splint comfort increase. While finger and thumb joints frequently are free of splint material, inclusion of the wrist as a secondary joint is an important consideration in shoulder splint design. Leaving the wrist free allows better hand function but the trade-off that must seriously be considered is the potentially injurious dependent position of the hand at rest that is allowed. As a solution, a removable wrist immobilization splint may be used—removed to allow for hand use and donned for comfort and protection.

Incorporating the shoulder and elbow as primary joints, *shoulder, elbow immobilization splints* may be used postoperatively to protect healing tissues after procedures such as arthroplasty, acromioplasty, Bankart repair, rotator cuff repair, and tendon transfers.[7] For postoperative rotator cuff repairs, shoulder position is dependent on the specific repair and surgeon preference. The shoulder may be positioned in abduction for a period of time to protect the repair or the arm may be positioned at the patient's side in a sling or shoulder immobilization splint.[8,31] Debate continues regarding optimum postoperative treatment for rotator cuff repairs. For example, in a study by Watson, it was found that the results of splinting the shoulder in abduction did not enhance the outcome of rotator cuff repairs and that after 5 weeks splinted shoulders were often stiff with winging scapulas.[31]

Close communication with referring physicians is mandatory when working with postoperative shoulder repairs. Cookbook approaches to splinting protocols are inappropriate in this arena. Various positioning splint designs are available to clinicians and many factors must be considered to appropriately correlate splint design with individual patient needs. Determining variables include, but are not limited to, injury and amount of damage, surgical procedures, physician preferences, patient requirements, and third-party payer criteria.

Type 1. *Type 1 shoulder immobilization splints* include the elbow as a secondary joint in addition to the primary shoulder joint (Fig. 14-14, *A*). These splints may be used to immobilize the shoulder in abduction or adduction and/or shoulder external or internal rotation. Inclusion of the elbow in a flexed posture allows control of shoulder rotation positioning.

Type 3. *Type 3 shoulder immobilization splints* incorporate one primary joint, the shoulder, and three secondary joint levels, the elbow, forearm, and wrist (Figs. 14-14, *B*, 14-15). The shoulder may be positioned in abduction or adduction, and in external or internal rotation, or combinations thereof, depending on patient-specific requirements. These splints are used to immobilize shoulders in precisely defined attitudes. Inclusion of the elbow, forearm, and wrist as secondary joint levels reinforces shoulder immobilization forces.

Mobilization Splints

Mobilization of a passively supple shoulder requires, at a minimum, force sufficient to abduct, extend, flex, or rotate this proximal upper extremity joint that is both complex in structure and large in size. No other upper extremity joint requires force levels of this magnitude to simply move the joint through its normal passive range of motion. Splinting the complex glenohumeral, sternoclavicular, acromioclavicular and scapulothoracic joint composite requires incorporation of more secondary joints than are typically employed in splints designed to mobilize more distal, smaller, upper extremity joints. Inclusion of these secondary joints allows improved purchase, stabilization, and torque to be applied to achieve specific shoulder positions. Mobilization splints may be used in the conservative treatment of stiff or frozen shoulders, or for postoperative shoulder procedures such as manipulation or capsulectomies. These mobilization splints maintain or increase shoulder passive range of motion through application of low-load prolonged tension on associated soft tissues.[19,25] While most shoulder mobilization splints mechanically function using three-point pressure systems, some specialized mobilization splints work through two-point systems, applying coaptation forces. Examples of two-point pressure splints may be found in some of the splints that minimize or passively correct shoulder subluxation. Classified as articular *shoulder coaptation mobilization splints*, these splints apply opposing, longitudinally directed forces that approximate the humerus and glenoid fossa.

Type 1. *Shoulder mobilization splints, type 1* include one secondary joint, the elbow, in addition to the primary shoulder joint (Fig. 14-16).

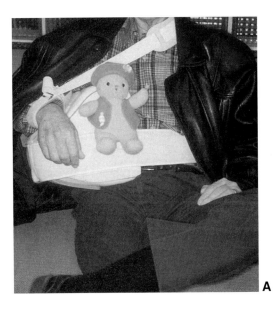

A

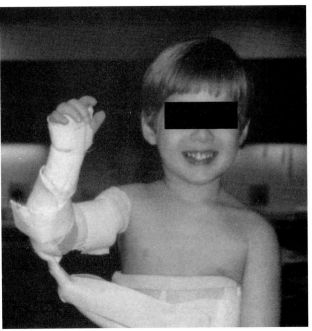

B

Fig. 14-14   A, Shoulder abduction and neutral rotation immobilization splint, type 1 (2) B, Shoulder abduction and external rotation immobilization splint, type 3 (4)

A, A foam pillow with straps immobilizes the shoulder in abduction and neutral rotation. **B,** Colloquially known as the "airplane" or "Statue of Liberty" splint, this shoulder abduction and external rotation immobilization splint is used during the initial period of rest following tendon transfer surgery to restore shoulder abduction and/or external rotation. With the initiation of exercises, the splint's purpose changes and it is serially adjusted to allow gradual mobilization of the shoulder into adduction and internal rotation while active abduction and external rotation exercises are performed within the limit of the splint. With the change in purpose, the splint is renamed a shoulder adduction and internal rotation mobilization / restriction splint, type 3 (4).

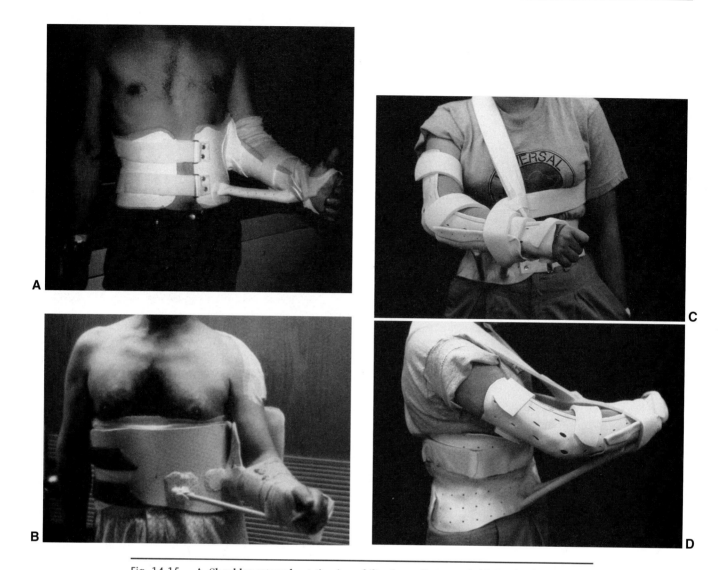

Fig. 14-15   A, Shoulder external rotation immobilization splint, type 3 (4) B, Shoulder external rotation immobilization splint, type 3 (4) C,D, Shoulder flexion and internal rotation immobilization splint, type 3 (4)
Colloquially labeled "gunslinger" splints, these shoulder splints incorporate the elbow, forearm, and wrist as secondary joints. Attaining correct shoulder position is more easily accomplished when these three distal joints are included in shoulder splints. The wide torso portion of the splint improves patient comfort. A dual-purpose connector bar spans the distance between the torso base and the distal splint, providing the support needed to immobilize the entire extremity and controlling shoulder and forearm positions. Strapping placed anteriorly (A) and laterally (B-D) allows removal of the torso splint sections. [Courtesy (A,B) Sally Poole, MA, OTR, CHT, Dobbs Ferry, N.Y.; (C,D) Lin Beribak, OTR/L, CHT, Chicago, Ill.]

Type 3. In addition to the primary shoulder joint, three secondary joints—elbow, forearm, and wrist—are included in *shoulder mobilization splints, type 3.* Incorporating three secondary joint levels increases mechanical advantage, improving shoulder positioning, splint stability, and patient comfort. *Type 3 shoulder mobilization splints* may be fitted to improve shoulder abduction or adduction and/or shoulder external or internal rotation.

As noted earlier in this chapter, mobilization splints are used with much greater frequency to treat joints distal to the shoulder. Custom-fabricated shoulder mobilization splints are less accepted by clinicians due to the perceived and actual degree of difficulty of fabricating these splints. Rectifying this unfortunate situation, McClure and Flowers advocate the use of a simply constructed, easy-to-adjust splint capable of effectively mobilizing the shoulder into whatever of connector bar. Serial adjustments of this splint are accomplished by simply changing the length and/or position of the connector dowel rod (Fig. 14-17, *B*). Once the beauty of this minimalistic design is fully understood and appreciated, all sorts of adaptations come to mind. For example, incorporation of specialized thermoplastic "change-out cups" that hold the ends of the dowel rod make alterations even easier. Trustworthy patients who are unable to return to the clinic for frequent adjustments may be given a series of different-length dowels and taught to change the dowel connector bar as shoulder range of motion improves. Further, by cutting the dowel in half and inserting an appropriate-size spring between the two cut ends of the dowel, elastic traction rather than inelastic traction may be applied to the shoulder. Application of a thermoplastic collar around the dowel-spring-dowel unit stabilizes and reinforces the connector bar, creating a spring-loaded dowel. Wound care and axilla hygiene are also easy with this remarkable splint design. Flowers notes that compliance may be a problem with this splint due to its inherent bulk, but when compared to other *type 3 splints*, this design is streamlined.

The application of splinting low-load, prolonged gentle tension to remodel contracted soft tissues is a fundamental concept to hand/upper extremity specialists but, for various reasons, in clinical practice these concepts have not been applied in their entirety to the shoulder. Lack of an efficacious splint design and the fact that shoulder treatment has been almost exclusively "manual therapy, electrotherapy, active exercises, and various forms of passive stretching"[25] have delayed clinical acceptance of splinting to remodel stiffened or frozen shoulders. With a simple shoulder mobilization splint design, there no longer is an excuse for therapists to avoid making custom shoulder mobilization splints. Easier shoulder splint fabrication also means that research studies may be initiated to identify the most efficacious methods for mobilizing stiff shoulder joints. Just as forceful manual manipulation of digital joints is now considered harmful and passé, so too may these nonsplinting shoulder mobilization techniques become in the future! Further, questions regarding duration of shoulder splint wearing times may be put to rest through research studies that compare continuous, or nearly continuous, splint wear to short duration, 2-3 times a day, wear.

More complicated *type 3* shoulder mobilization splint designs are available, providing a range of options from which clinicians may coordinate appropriate shoulder mobilization splints with patients' individual needs (Fig. 14-17, *C-E*).

Type 7. *Type 7 shoulder mobilization splints* include the primary shoulder joint and seven

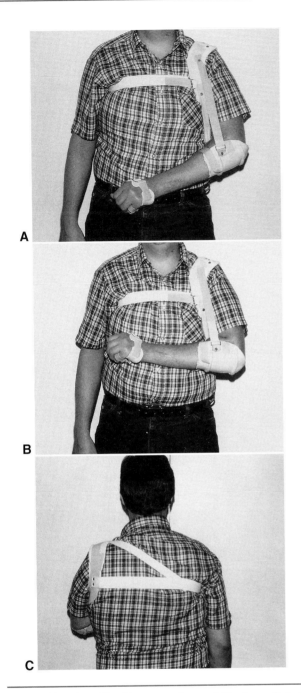

Fig. 14-16   A-C, Shoulder coaptation mobilization splint, type 1 (2) \\ Small finger MP flexion mobilization splint, type 0 (1) A-C, An articular coaptation mobilization splint is used with a brachial plexus injury to minimize subluxation of the humerus while permitting function. A,B, A hand-based MP flexion mobilization splint increases small finger MP flexion motion. C, Posterior view of harness design. (Courtesy Carol Hierman, OTR, CHT, Cedar Grove, N.C., and Elisha Denny, PTA, OTA, Pittsboro, N.C. © UNC Hand Rehabilitation Center, Chapel Hill, N.C.)

altitude is required (Fig. 14-17, *A*).[25] With a design predicated on efficiency, the McClure-Flowers splint essentially is a wrist immobilization splint attached to a torso-base component via a dowel rod or other kind

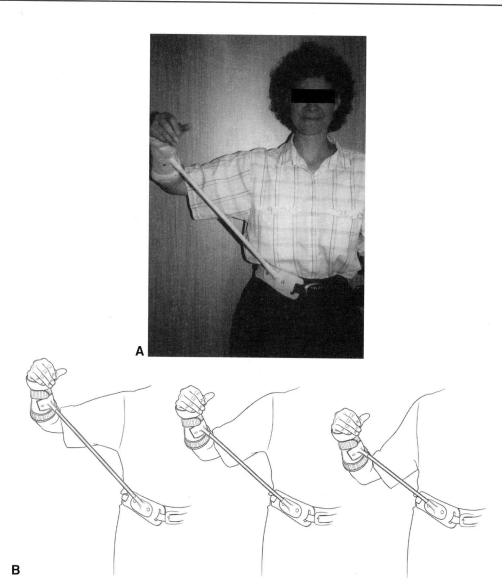

Fig. 14-17 A, Shoulder abduction and external rotation mobilization splint, type 3 (4) B, Shoulder abduction and external rotation mobilization splint, type 3 (4) C, Shoulder abduction and neutral rotation mobilization splint, type 3 (4); right \\ Shoulder abduction and neutral rotation mobilization splint, type 3 (4); left D, Shoulder abduction and external rotation mobilization splint, type 3 (4) E, Shoulder flexion mobilization splint, type 3 (4)

Custom (A-C) and prefabricated (D,E) *type 3* splint designs for shoulder mobilization. A,B, Shoulder abduction and external rotation may be increased through lengthening of the connector bar in a custom-fabricated splint based on the design by McClure and Flowers. C, Bilateral "airplane" splints are worn for scar remodeling after burn injury. D,E, Prefabricated splints require the patient to be supine during the application of a low-load tension to the shoulder. [Courtesy (C) Indiana University School of Health and Rehabilitation Sciences Department of Occupational Therapy, Indianapolis, Ind.; (D,E) Dynasplint Systems, Inc., Severna Park, Md.]

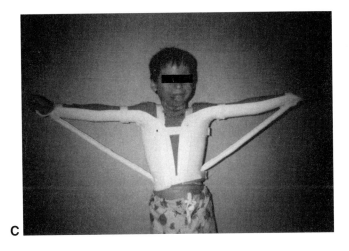

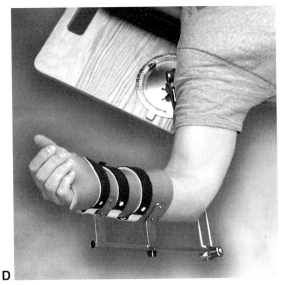

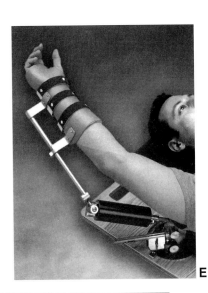

Fig. 14-17, cont'd
For legend see opposite page.

secondary joint levels including elbow, forearm, wrist, finger MP-PIP, and thumb CMC-MP joints. *Type 7* splints may be custom fitted or they may be obtained through commercial sources (Fig. 14-18). Inclusion of digital joints to enhance splint comfort may be optional in some commercial *type 7* splints.

Mobilization/Restriction Splints

Shoulder mobilization / restriction splints are designed to limit a specific range of shoulder motion to protect healing tissue structures while simultaneously mobilizing other shoulder motions. These splints are often used to rehabilitate postoperative tendon transfers done to provide shoulder external rotation and abduction. Tendon transfer procedures usually require that postoperative exercises be performed within a specific range while shoulder range of motion

is gradually increased.[7,17] To accomplish this, an adjustable shoulder mobilization/restriction splint allows incremental increases in adduction and internal rotation. Adjustable, prefabricated shoulder restriction splints are commercially available in adult sizes; however, children may require custom-fabricated splints in order to achieve a proper fit.[7] When designing a shoulder mobilization/restriction splint that will be periodically adjusted to change the angle of motion restriction, use of screw rivets rather than bonding of adjacent surfaces to join the humeral portion of the splint to the torso-base portion of the splint will save therapist time and effort during the adjustment process. If this is not done, frequent adjustments of solid splint bonds may result in a stretched-out and weakened splint that may require replacement.

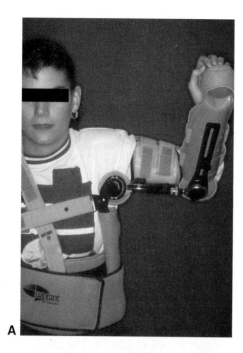

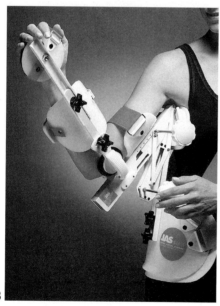

Fig. 14-18   A, Shoulder abduction and external rotation mobilization splint, type 7 (14) **B,** Shoulder abduction and external rotation mobilization splint, type 7 (14)
These prefabricated splint designs allow adjustments to be made in varying degrees of shoulder abduction and external rotation. Inclusion of hand joints is for patient comfort. Commercial splints may provide the heavy durability needed to mobilize the large and complex shoulder composite joint. [Courtesy **(A)** DJ Orthopedics Inc., Vista, Calif.; **(B)** Joint Active Systems, Inc., Effingham, Ill.]

Type 3. *Shoulder mobilization / restriction splints* include three secondary joint levels; the elbow, forearm, and wrist improve splint stability and positioning of the shoulder.

Torque Transmission Splints

Shoulder torque transmission splints are designed to transfer moment to joints external to the splints themselves. These splints transfer moment longitudinally and proximally to the shoulder joint through control of one or more distal secondary joint(s). Single-purpose torque transmission splints have a minimum of one secondary joint level. These splints are often referred to as "exercise" splints because they are used to maintain or increase motion in conjunction with functional upper extremity use.

Type 1. *Type 1 shoulder torque transmission splints* incorporate one distal secondary joint, the elbow, in addition to the primary joint, the shoulder. By controlling the elbow secondarily, unwanted elbow substitution patterns that incorrectly compensate for shoulder motion may be eliminated. Further, specific shoulder motions including but not limited to internal and/or external rotation may be encouraged by controlling the elbow to transmit active moment to the shoulder joint to improve shoulder motion or to remodel soft tissue. Although many *shoulder torque transmission splints, type 1 (2)* are used as exercise splints, these splints may also be used over time to remodel soft tissues about the shoulder joint. A word of caution: Care must be taken to ensure that elbow joint motion is not compromised through the requisite secondary immobilization or restriction of the elbow.

■ NONARTICULAR HUMERUS SPLINTS

Nonarticular splints do not cross joints or affect joint motion. They often are used to protect healing fractures as in the case of humeral fractures. Circumferential or bivalve designed *nonarticular humerus splints* employ two-point coaptation forces to support humeral fractures. Constriction of blood or venous flow at the distal edge of the *nonarticular humerus splint* should be monitored due to its circumferential nature.

Humerus Splints

Functional splinting of the humerus following a humerus diaphysis fracture has been an accepted form of treatment for a number of years. While exact percentages vary with individual studies, this technique is associated with a high rate of fracture

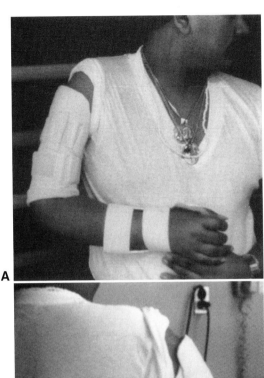

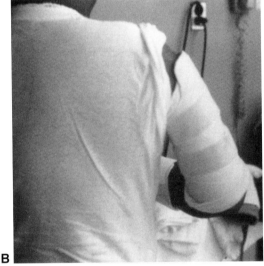

Fig. 14-19   **A, Nonarticular humerus splint \\ Wrist extension mobilization splint, type 0 (1) B, Nonarticular humerus splint**
Through its circumferential application, a nonarticular humerus splint provides a coaptation force for support of a humerus fracture. This patient also had concomitant radial nerve palsy secondary to the humeral fracture and wears a splint for wrist extension mobilization. (Courtesy Sally Poole, MA, OTR, CHT, Dobbs Ferry, N.Y.)

healing.[11,21,29] Depending upon therapist skill and preference, custom or prefabricated *nonarticular humerus splints* are used.[9] This splint is fit circumferentially or in a bivalve design around the humerus and secured with strapping.[10] By providing compression of the soft tissues surrounding the humerus, a *nonarticular humerus splint* (Fig. 14-19) protects the fracture site during the healing phase while allowing shoulder and elbow motion. The period of immobilization and the exercise program is determined by the patient's physician according to the specific needs of the patient.

SUMMARY

Splinting the elbow and shoulder provides a number of challenges. The therapist's understanding of the patient's condition, good communication with the referring physician, and the knowledge of splinting principles and design options will optimize the chance for a positive outcome for the patient.

REFERENCES

1. Alnot J, Osman N, Masmejean E, et al: Lesions of the radial nerve in fractures of the humeral diaphysis. Apropos of 62 cases, *Rev Chir Orthop Reparatrice Appar Mot* 86(2):143-50, 2000.
2. ASHT: *American Society of Hand Therapists Splint Classification System*, ed 1, The American Society of Hand Therapists, 1992, Chicago.
3. Bodner G, Huber B, Schwabegger A, et al: Sonographic detection of radial nerve entrapment within a humerus fracture, *J Ultrasound Med* 18(10):703-6, 1999.
4. Bodner G, Buchberger W, Schocke M, et al: Radial nerve palsy associated with humeral shaft fracture: evaluation with US—initial experience, *Radiology* 219(3):811-6, 2001.
5. Bonutti PM, Windau JE, Ables BA, et al: Static progressive stretch to reestablish elbow range of motion, *Clin Orthop* Jun(303):128-34, 1994.
6. Bostman O, Bakalim G, Vainionpaa S, et al: Radial palsy in shaft fracture of the humerus, *Acta Orthop Scand* 57(4):316-9, 1986.
7. Cannon N, et al: *Diagnosis and treatment manual for physicians and therapists*, ed 4, The Hand Rehabilitation Center of Indiana, 2001, Indianapolis.
8. Chase JM, Friedman BG, Fenlin JM: Diagnosis and management of common shoulder problems. In Mackin EJ, Callahan AD, Osterman AL, et al: *Hunter, Mackin, & Callahan's rehabilitation of the hand and upper extremity*, ed 5, Mosby, 2002, St. Louis.
9. Colditz J: Functional fracture bracing. In Mackin EJ, Callahan AD, Osterman AL, et al: *Hunter, Mackin, & Callahan's rehabilitation of the hand and upper extremity*, ed 5, Mosby, 2002, St. Louis.
10. Davila S: Humeral fracture brace, *J Hand Ther* 5(3):157-8, 1992.
11. Fjalestad T, Stromsoe K, Salvesen P, et al: Functional results of braced humeral diaphyseal fractures: why do 38% lose external rotation of the shoulder? *Arch Orthop Trauma Surg* 120(5-6):281-5, 2000.
12. Foster RJ, Swiontkowski MF, Bach AW, et al: Radial nerve palsy caused by open humeral shaft fractures, *J Hand Surg* [Am] 18(1):121-4, 1993.
13. Gelinas JJ, Faber KJ, Patterson SD, et al: The effectiveness of turnbuckle splinting for elbow contractures, *J Bone Joint Surg Br* 82(1):74-8, 2000.
14. Griffith A: Therapists' management of the stiff elbow. In Mackin EJ, Callahan AD, Osterman AL, et al: *Hunter, Mackin, & Callahan's rehabilitation of the hand and upper extremity*, ed 5, Mosby, 2002, St. Louis.
15. Hepburn G: Case studies: contracture and stiff joint management with Dynasplint, *J Orthop Sports Phys Ther* 8(10):498-504, 1987.
16. King GJ, Faber KJ: Posttraumatic elbow stiffness, *Orthop Clin North Am* 31(1):129-43, 2000.
17. Kozin S, Ciocco R, Speakman T: Tendon transfers for brachial plexus palsy. In Mackin EJ, Callahan AD, Osterman AL, et al:

Hunter, Mackin, & Callahan's rehabilitation of the hand and upper extremity, ed 5, Mosby, 2002, St. Louis.

18. Larsen LB, Barfred T: Radial nerve palsy after simple fracture of the humerus, *Scand J Plast Reconstr Surg Hand Surg* 34(4):363-6, 2000.

19. LaStayo P, Jaffe R: Assessment and management of shoulder stiffness: a biomechanical approach, *J Hand Ther* 7(2):122-30, 1994.

20. LaStayo P, Cass R: Continuous passive motion for the upper extremity: why, when, and how. In Mackin EJ, Callahan AD, Osterman AL, et al: *Hunter, Mackin, & Callahan's rehabilitation of the hand and upper extremity*, ed 5, Mosby, 2002, St. Louis.

21. Latta LL, Sarmiento A, Tarr RR: The rationale of functional bracing of fractures, *Clin Orthop* Jan-Feb(146):28-36, 1980.

22. Levitskii VB, Kvasha VP, Shramko VI: The diagnosis and combined treatment of humeral fractures complicated by involvement of the radial nerve, *Lik Sprava* 2(3):138-41, 1993.

23. MacKay-Lyons M: Low-load, prolonged stretch in treatment of elbow flexion contractures secondary to head trauma: a case report, *Phys Ther* 69(4):292-6, 1989.

24. Magee DJ: *Orthopedic clinical assessment*, ed 2, WB Saunders, 1992, Philadelphia.

25. McClure P, Flowers K: Treatment of limited shoulder motion: a case study based on biomechanical considerations, *Phys Ther* 72(12):929-36, 1992.

26. Morrey BF: Anatomy of the elbow joint. In Morrey BF: *The elbow and its disorders*, ed 3, WB Saunders, 2000, Philadelphia.

27. Morrey BF, Askew LJ, Chao EY: A biomechanical study of normal functional elbow motion, *J Bone Joint Surg Am* 63(6):872-7, 1981.

28. Nirschl RP, Morrey BF: Rehabilitation. In Morrey BF: *The elbow and its disorders*, ed 3, WB Saunders, 2000, Philadelphia.

29. Sarmiento A, Zagorski JB, Zych GA, et al: Functional bracing for the treatment of fractures of the humeral diaphysis, *J Bone Joint Surg Am* 82(4):478-86, 2000.

30. Volz R, Morrey BF: The physical examination of the elbow. In Morrey BF: *The elbow and its disorders*, ed 3, WB Saunders, 2000, Philadelphia.

31. Watson M: Major ruptures of the rotator cuff. The results of surgical repair in 89 patients, *J Bone Joint Surg Br* 67(4):618-24, 1985.

Special Situations

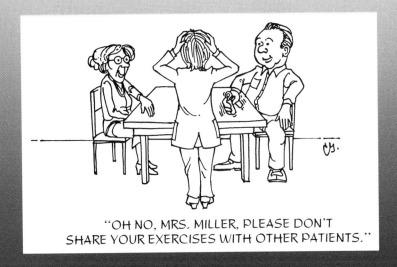

CHAPTER 15

Exercise and Splinting for Specific Upper Extremity Problems

Chapter Outline

Encompassing a number of frequently encountered clinical upper extremity conditions, this chapter suggests appropriate splinting approaches to each problem. Although there may be considerable variation in the individual presentation of a particular upper extremity problem, certain common features must be dealt with in each situation. The underlying pathologic condition of each of these problems is reviewed, as well as an integrated program with emphasis on splinting to help restore the afflicted extremity to its best functional level.

While specific splint designs illustrate this chapter, it should be noted that these do not represent the only solutions for the problems described. The important concept is to understand how a splint functions in relation to the pathologic condition presented. As

397

has been emphasized throughout this book, there are often several different splint configurations, all of which function in a similar manner, that may be used to treat a given upper extremity problem. It is up to the specialist to decide which design is most applicable for an individual, on a patient-by-patient basis.

Additionally, it should be clearly understood that in most cases it is necessary to use splinting as a part of a more comprehensive rehabilitation program directed by a knowledgeable physician-therapist team. It is therefore appropriate to include general exercise concepts in this chapter.

■ EXERCISE

To produce optimum results during rehabilitation programs, splinting and exercise must be carefully integrated. All too often splinting is erroneously viewed as an isolated treatment technique. Splints are used to immobilize, mobilize, restrict, and/or transmit torque. Infrequently they are even designed to provide resistance to weakened muscles. However, the application of an external device such as a hand splint will do little to enhance the critically important active range of motion that must be provided by voluntary use of strong muscles whose tendinous extensions have adhesion-free excursion and smooth gliding beds. Active motion through exercise and purposeful activity is the true key to establishing and maintaining the functional capacity of an upper extremity (Fig. 15-1).

The maximum passive range of motion of a joint must be realized before a corresponding range of active motion may be achieved. In other words, AROM of a joint cannot exceed its PROM! Splinting, therefore, is frequently employed as one of the initial treatment modalities when exercise alone is insufficient to attain an acceptable level of motion. A combination of appropriate splinting augmented with a structured and individualized exercise program best provides for the restoration of the maximum functional potential in a given upper extremity problem.

Since entire books are available that deal solely with the subject of exercise, the purpose of this chapter is not to compete with these works, but rather to review the fundamental concepts of exercise to produce a common framework of terminology and theory that may then be related to the clinical use of splinting of the upper extremity.

Basically, there are three types of exercise: (1) passive exercise, in which a joint is moved through an arc of motion by an external force without the assis-

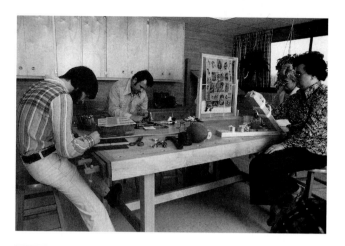

Fig. 15-1   Group interaction helps maintain enthusiasm and interest during the rehabilitation process. Patients are encouraged to use their afflicted hands in functional activities as soon as it is medically feasible.

tance of active muscle contraction; (2) active exercise, in which joint movement is the result of physiologic muscle contraction; and (3) resistive exercise, in which an external opposing force is applied against the mobile segment of the joint as active motion is attempted. The focus of each type of exercise is centered on different anatomic structures, and the respective objectives and methods of implementation of each are significantly different.[12,45]

Passive Exercise

Passive exercise produces gliding of the articular surfaces and excursion of tendons and capsular structures through the use of externally applied forces such as manipulation techniques or traction devices. Splinting is an effective conservative means of attaining passive mobility and, when used appropriately, produces a gradual remodeling of the pericapsular structures and an elongation of adhesions through directed gentle traction. The small joints of the hand, with their delicate pericapsular ligamentous arrangement, are uniquely susceptible to stiffening and deformity resulting from direct trauma or chronic edema. Overzealous attempts to improve passive range of motion of a joint by too much splinting traction or poorly applied manual techniques (Fig. 15-2) may not only fail to improve motion, but may actually create further tissue damage and edema. Any passive method of joint mobilization should be carefully monitored with specific attention to patient discomfort, edema, skin temperature, and changes in range of motion. On occasion, automated splints in the form of controlled passive motion units (CPM) for digits,

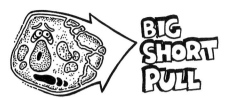

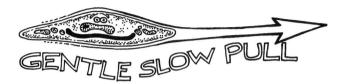

Fig. 15-2   Forceful passive range of motion may tear delicate structures, resulting in increased inflammatory response and additional scar formation.

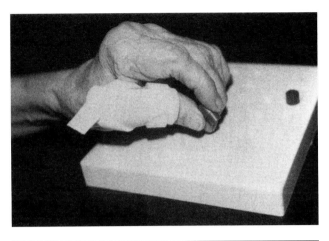

Fig. 15-3   **Thumb MP flexion immobilization splint, type 0 (1)** Support to the MP joint decreases pain and increases thumb stability, allowing active exercise to the CMC and IP joints through functional activities.

wrist, forearm, elbow, or shoulder may be indicated for postoperative passive exercise to allow continual joint motion.

Active Exercise

Active exercise through purposeful activity such as self-care, leisure, work, or sports and individualized exercise routines produces joint motion affected by muscle contraction and resultant tendon excursion. Achievement of a functional level of active motion depends on the presence of adequate muscle strength and passively supple joints (Fig. 15-3). Active range of motion is benefited by correctly implemented passive motion and splinting techniques that are designed to mobilize arthrofibrosed joints and adherent tendons or lengthen myostatically shortened muscles or tight pericapsular structures. For joints whose diminished range of motion is secondary to an extrinsic tenodesis effect from tendon adhesion or muscle shortening rather than a pericapsular pathologic condition, the active improvement from mobilization or transmission of torque splinting may be substantial. Since the application of traction has little effect on motion at the musculotendinous level once the full passive mobility of a joint is established and the tenodesis effect minimized, splinting should not be used exclusively to increase active motion. However, an appropriately applied splint designed specifically to supplement prescribed exercises may augment an active exercise or ADL program (Fig. 15-4). Allowing greater function than would otherwise take place, this kind of splint often supports weaker muscles, stabilizes adjacent (usually proximal) joints, particularly the wrist, maximizes tendon amplitude at a given joint, or uses or negates a tenodesis effect (Fig. 15-5).

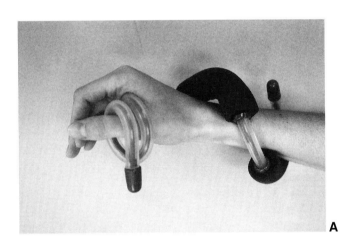

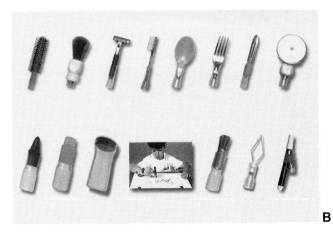

Fig. 15-4   **A, Wrist extension, thumb CMC palmar abduction and MP extension mobilization splint, type 0 (3)**
A, Splints provide a base for attaching items that allow patients to live independently. B, Items that may be attached to the TUBOform splint. [B Courtesy Gisleine Martin Philot (Occupational Therapist) and George Guarany Philot (Designer)—inventors—www.tuboform .com.br<http://www.tuboform.com.br>.]

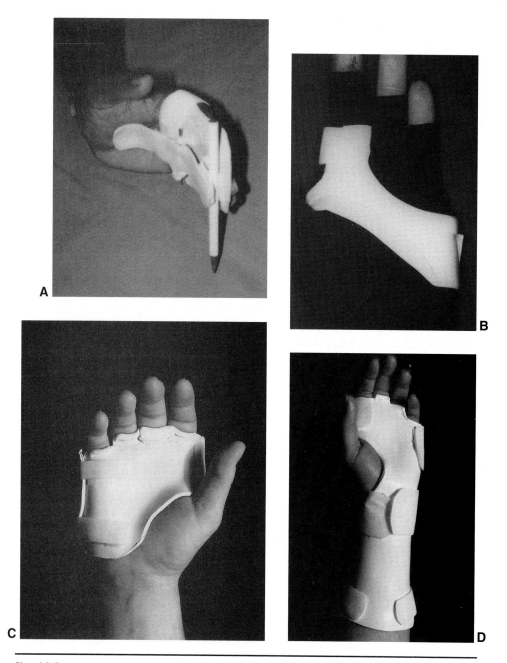

Fig. 15-5   **A,** Index–small finger MP extension and flexion torque transmission / MP flexion restriction splint, type 2 (12) **B,** Long finger IP extension and flexion torque transmission splint, type 1 (3) **C,** Index–small finger IP extension and flexion torque transmission splint, type 1 (12) **D,** Index–small finger IP extension and flexion torque transmission splint, type 2 (13)

A, This exercise splint effectively isolates MP motion. **B-D,** Blocking exercise increases flexor digitorum superficialis tendon excursion. Some patients may not be able to accomplish this critical exercise due to inability to understand how to perform the exercise, poor coordination, or bilateral injury. Torque transmission splints assist in accomplishing the exercise successfully. [Courtesy **(A)** Carol Hierman, OTR, CHT, Cedar Grove, N.C., and Elisha Denny, PTA, OTA, Pittsboro, N.C.; © UNC Hand Rehabilitation Center, Chapel Hill, N.C.]

Repetitive active motion in the form of specific structured exercises and the use of the extremity in functional adapted and graded activities are the most productive means for increasing and maintaining strength and amplitude at the musculotendinous level. Generally, specific exercises are to be performed slowly, smoothly, and in accordance with precise program parameters as directed by a therapist.

Resistive Exercise

The purpose of resistive exercise is to produce sufficient muscle strength to allow maximum tendon excursion, full joint motion, and the execution of normal daily activities. This may be accomplished through purposeful graded activities and progressive resistive exercises. Strengthening is traditionally divided into isometric, eccentric, and concentric exercises. Emphasis includes improving endurance and/or strengthening. Caution is needed in adapting strengthening programs for patients with repetitive strain disorders, especially if pain is experienced for 1 to 2 hours after exercise. An external splinting force applied to a wrist or hand joint has little appreciable effect on improving muscle strength, since strengthening requires voluntary effort of muscles to enhance power. In addition to strengthening muscles, resistive exercises may be used to provide a form of biofeedback to the patient, allowing increased awareness of the position and function of key muscle groups (Fig. 15-6). Resistive exercises may be used at many stages of rehabilitation but should not be relied on solely to increase passive range of motion of stiffened joints. Mechanically, because of the angle of approach of a tendon to a given joint, the inherent strength of a muscle is often lost in translational force when attempting active mobilization of a stiff joint. From a physiologic viewpoint, the musculotendinous unit cannot provide the long-term tension on the joint needed to cause pericapsular remodeling. Splinting produces a more advantageous and sustained angle of pull because of its external position, producing better results with less force (Fig. 15-7).

Basic exercises may be effectively merged to meet the needs of the individual situation. For example, active assistive exercise is a combination of active and passive exercises in which the involved joint is moved actively as far as possible with passive completion of the remaining arc of motion.

A sequential program employing these basic kinds of exercises in a logical order eliminates many hours of nonproductive exercise for the patient. Achievement of passively supple joints is a prerequisite to the establishment of active range of motion and resistive exercises. It must be recognized that the active

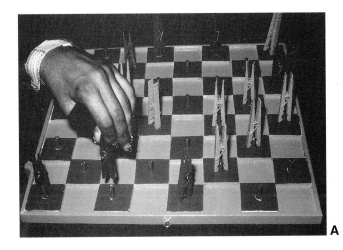

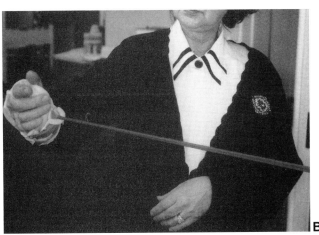

Fig. 15-6   **A,** Specific graded activities are often coupled with projects that encourage gross and fine motion of the extremity. **B,** A thermoplastic hook attached to the splint allows the patient to perform shoulder strengthening exercises while protecting healing structures. Adding resistance to splints enhances patient endurance and strength. This technique is effective when treatment goals include strengthening while simultaneously protecting an injured adjacent joint or healing structure. (Courtesy **(A)** Joan Farrell, OTR, Miami, Fla.)

motion of a joint cannot be greater than its existing passive range of motion, and, regardless of the strength or amplitude of the involved musculotendinous unit, absence of satisfactory passive joint motion will negate its functional effect. Adequate active joint motion depends on a minimum of fair grade muscle strength. In the presence of resistance-producing tendon adhesions, the involved musculature should be functioning on a good or normal level to effect excursion change.

Muscle atrophy, with or without myostatic contracture, will have a profound effect on the ultimate performance of a joint after it has been successfully mobilized. Therefore, it is essential to initiate and

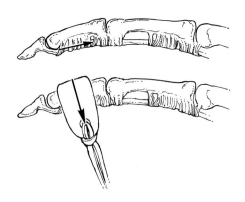

Fig. 15-7 Because extrinsic digital tendons normally run parallel to the phalanges, their force angle of approach to the joints they cross is not as mechanically advantageous as that which may be achieved by an externally positioned splint.

maintain muscle-strengthening exercises early in the rehabilitation process, often well in advance of the ability of the muscle to effect appreciable motion at the joints it crosses. It is also important that these strengthening exercises be carried out in all extremity muscle groups, not only in those whose weakness or atrophy is obvious.

▇ TORQUE TRANSMISSION SPLINTS

A special group of splints transmit internal torque to joints that are situated, for the most part, outside the physical boundaries of the splint. Often dubbed "exercise splints" or "substitution splints," these sophisticated splints were only recently recognized by the authors as a uniquely different group of splints that encompass a fourth purpose classification to the expanded SCS. Proper use of these splints requires a thorough knowledge of normal anatomy and kinesiology, a comprehensive understanding of upper extremity pathology and its effect on functional patterns, and an in-depth proficiency in splinting. In hindsight, it is ironic that what is in all probability the most advanced of the splint purpose groups was not given due respect because of the simple external appearance of many of these splints. They often lack more complicated components like mobilization assists, outriggers, etc. Torque transmission splints position or control selected joints within a digital ray to allow predetermined internal muscle tendon units to create articular motion at joints lying distal or proximal to the controlled joint(s). Direction of the transmitted torque may be longitudinal or it may be transverse (Fig. 15-8). While all splints transmit torque to unsplinted joints, the differential factor between torque transmission splints and other splints that immobilize, mobilize, or restrict joint motion is that

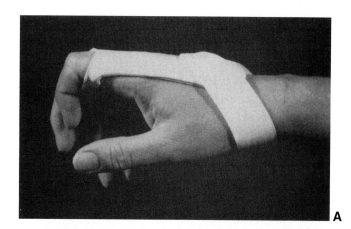

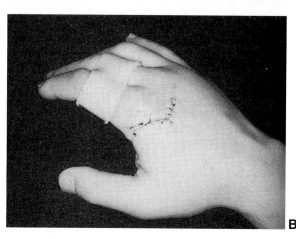

Fig. 15-8 **A,** Index finger IP extension and flexion torque transmission splint, type 1 (3) **B,** Long finger MP extension and flexion torque transmission splint, type 1 (2)
Torque transmission splints generate motion at selected longitudinally (**A**) or transversely (**B**) oriented joints outside the physical borders of splints. [(**B**) from Thomas D, Moutet F, Guinard D: Postoperative management of extensor tendon repairs in Zones V, VI, and VII, *J Hand Ther* 9(4):309-14, 1996.]

the primary purpose of torque transmission splints is to internally conduct muscle-tendon moment to predetermined joints to bring about active motion at these joints. Because they often lack external mobilization components, these splints are the ultimate in "low-profile" splint designs.

Torque transmission splints are used to transmit internal forces to supple joints to produce motion or to contracted joints to affect soft tissue remodeling. Splint configuration is the same for both purposes; only the condition of the target joint(s) differs.

From experience in casting Hansen's disease patients' hands, Brand noted that prolonged use of torque transmission splints can result in gradual correction of contractures through soft tissue remodeling.[6-10] This technique differs from serial casting to correct joint contracture in that the plaster cast is not changed sequentially. Instead, the plaster splint is worn for a long duration, holding key joints in predefined postures, allowing extrinsic tendons to affect motion at contracted joints outside the splint itself. With functional use and over time, the pericapsular structures around these external-to-the-splint joints remodel, and range of motion improves. Described by Brand* in the 1950s, and routinely used by many clinicians, Colditz has further popularized this technique the past few years.[24]

Historically, torque transmission splints are not new. They have been used for centuries to improve function. The only difference is that these splints have not previously been classified as a separate group. Torque transmission splints are included in the exercise section of this chapter because they frequently are used to maximize active tendon excursion and articular motion. (For other torque transmission splints in this chapter, see Figures 15-5, *A-D*; 15-8, *A,B*; 15-14, *B-I*; 15-15, *A, C-G*; 15-16, *A-C*; 15-18, *B-D*; 15-19, *F-J*; 15-22, *A*; 15-24, *B*; 15-31, *H*.)

TIMING AND TYPE OF EXERCISE

Exercise, like splinting, should be adapted to correspond to the physiologic stages of wound healing. Knowledge of the inflammatory process and the reparative schedule of the various tissue types found in the hand are paramount to successful therapeutic intervention. Individual factors such as anatomic structures involved, etiology, surgical procedures, concomitant patient risk factors, medications, age, intelligence, motivation, and prognosis all influence the timing and form of exercise used. For example, although tension may be applied to some cutaneous and soft tissue repairs within a few hours postoperatively, the use of full-range active exercise may be contraindicated for tendon or ligament repairs. Resistive exercises are frequently delayed until tissue tensile strength is sufficient. Some exercise routines, such as early passive or active mobilization of tendon repairs, are used for adults, but they are inappropriate for young children or those whose motivation or abilities are limited. And, although full active motion may be attained quickly, unrestricted use of the hand may not be permitted at 12 weeks in a flexor tenolysis patient who has a history of previous rupture.

Throughout the rehabilitative period care should be taken to ensure that the implemented splinting and exercise program is truly effective. Range of motion measurements provide numeric verification of the progress being made and assessment of volume; skin color and skin temperature ensure that detrimental ramifications such as local inflammation or increased edema are prevented.

COORDINATION OF EXERCISES AND SPLINTING SCHEDULES

The coordination of exercise and splinting schedules is dictated by individual patient requirements. Although general guidelines based on diagnosis must be followed, the rigid adherence to a predetermined routine without consideration of specific patient factors produces less than desired results. It is important to remember that, although they may have similar diagnoses, no two patients respond to therapeutic intervention exactly alike. The astute upper extremity specialist has an overall concept of the course of treatment to pursue, but this is guided, refined, and adapted to meet the unique needs of the patient.

Before a schedule is devised, splinting and exercise parameters must first be defined with measurements obtained from precise and accurate assessment instruments. Some schedules are straightforward and fairly routine; many others require experience and open-minded creativity on the part of the upper extremity specialist. For example, if three weeks after PIP joint capsulectomy, a patient has greater limitation in active and passive extension than in flexion, then, to focus on the extension problem, the patient may be instructed to wear his extension splint twice as long as he wears his flexion splint while at the same time continuing his active flexion and extension exercises on an hourly basis (Fig. 15-9, *A*). If, after a week, routine goniometric measurements indicate that passive and active flexion has improved considerably but passive extension has plateaued, the patient is instructed to further increase the amount of time in the extension splint, and the flexion splint time and frequency of active exercise are relatively decreased. Splint care and wearing instructions help ensure that patients understand proper care and use of the splint (Fig. 15-9, *B*). If the patient does not progress as expected, the use of additional treatment techniques or modalities may be considered, providing no contraindications are present (Fig. 15-10).

Assessment data provide guideposts for coordinating splinting and exercise programs. Without evaluation, splinting and exercise programs are directionless and limited in their effectiveness. Each tied to the other, assessment, splinting, and exercise play unique and critical roles in the rehabilitation process of a diseased or injured upper extremity.

*See Chapters 1 and 3.

SPLINT-EXERCISE SCHEDULE

Wear *EXTENSION* splint *0* hour, *50* minutes.

Exercise *10* minutes.

Wear *EXTENSION* splint *0* hour, *50* minutes.

Exercise *10* minutes.

Wear *FLEXION* splint *0* hour, *50* minutes.

Exercise *10* minutes.

Repeat schedule throughout day. Sleep in *NIGHT* splint.

Call Hand Rehabilitation Center if you have questions.

A

SPLINT-EXERCISE SCHEDULE

Wear *EXTENSION* splint *1* hour, *50* minutes.

Exercise *12* minutes.

Wear *EXTENSION* splint *1* hour, *50* minutes.

Exercise *10* minutes.

Wear *FLEXION* splint *0* hour, *50* minutes.

Exercise *10* minutes.

Repeat schedule throughout day. Sleep in *NIGHT* splint.

Call Hand Rehabilitation Center if you have questions.

B

SPLINT INSTRUCTIONS

Patient _____ Date _____

A _____ splint has been made for you. The purpose of the splint is to
_____
_____

You are to wear the splint _____.

Other instructions for you to follow are: _____
_____
_____
_____
_____

Precautions:

1. Note any areas of redness, pressure, or rash on your skin or any pain or numbness. If any of these problems develop *notify therapist* to have necessary adjustments made.
2. Keep splint away from heat such as a stove or heating unit. Do not leave your splint in the car in the hot weather. The heat will soften the splint and change its shape.
3. The splint may be cleaned with mild soap and cool water. The inside of the splint may be cleaned with rubbing alcohol. The pieces of stockinette given to you with your splint should be worn under the splint and should be kept clean.

If you have any further questions or if any problems develop with the splint contact your therapist.

Therapist: _____

Phone: _____

C

Courtesy Cynthia Philips, M.A., O.T.R., C.H.T.

Fig. 15-9 A-C, Examples of splint care and wear instruction forms. **A,B,** By increasing the periods of extension splinting while decreasing flexion splinting and exercise times, passive joint extension is emphasized.

◼ SPECIAL PROBLEMS ACCORDING TO ANATOMICAL STRUCTURE

Bone

Fractures

Occurring at all ages, trauma resulting in upper extremity fractures is prevalent. Fracture of the small bones of the hand is one of the most commonly encountered injuries of the upper extremity.[28] Fractures of the distal phalanx occur most frequently, followed by metacarpal, proximal phalangeal, and finally, middle phalangeal fractures.[27] The potential functional loss from this kind of injury may be underestimated. Even if fracture healing occurs uneventfully, residual joint stiffness may become a serious factor that limits composite hand function.

Strickland et al.[94] reported that fracture immobilization beyond 4 weeks has a dramatically unfavorable effect on digital performance, although no clear-cut evidence is available to indicate that mobilization before the third week has any profound effect on the final range of motion. Fracture comminution

and, perhaps most important, associated tendon injuries also have a strongly detrimental effect on the final outcome of digital motion following fracture.

In the presence of a fracture, it is important to maintain the mobility of adjacent joints and digits to prevent magnification of the original injury through the development of secondary periarticular pathology (Fig. 15-11). Internal or external fixation of fractures with Kirshner wires, small compression plates, or external fixation devices usually eliminates the need to immobilize uninvolved joints and allows early mobilization of the hand, which is the key to preventing residual joint stiffness.

Splints should be designated to forestall the insidious development of deformity caused by edema and accompanying arthrofibrosis. Because the mechanical and physiologic repercussions of a fracture differ according to the severity of the injury, site of the fracture, quality of reduction, and method of immobilization used,[47] each patient must be objectively evaluated and splint and exercise programs created to meet patient-specific needs.[74] Splint(s) should also be

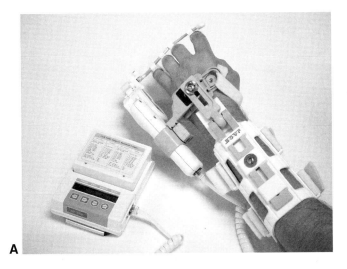

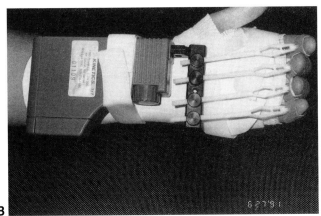

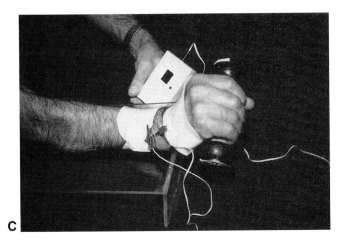

Fig. 15-10   A, Index–small finger extension and flexion mobilization splint, type 1 (13) B, Index–small finger IP extension and flexion mobilization splint, type 2 (13)
A,B, CPM or (C) biofeedback or other modalities may augment splinting programs. [Courtesy (A) JACE Systems, Cherry Hill, N.J; (B) Laura McCarrick, OTR, Manchester, Conn.; (C) Helen Marx, OTR, CHT, Human Factors Engineering of Phoenix, Wickenburg, Ariz.]

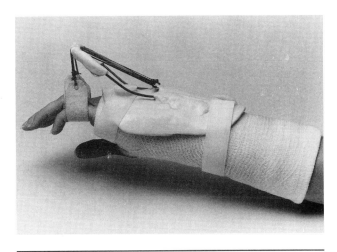

Fig. 15-11   Index–small finger MP extension mobilization splint, type 1 (5)
A detachable outrigger allows this patient with a forearm cast to begin early motion of distal finger joints. Because the cast is rigid and distributes pressure evenly, the need for a longer base of attachment of the outrigger is negated. (Courtesy Barbara Allen Smith, OTR., Oklahoma City, Okla.)

adapted to support the fractured segment and avoid protruding fixation pins. Pressure on pins may lead to pin-site irritation or possible infection. Splints with secondary level wrist immobilization usually are not required in treating stable phalangeal fractures but may be of use with metacarpal fractures or unstable finger fractures where wrist control may lessen deforming tendon forces. It is not uncommon to splint for both flexion and extension of adjacent joints of a segment that has sustained a fracture.

Tendon injuries associated with phalangeal fractures have a particularly prejudicial effect because of the tendency for the tendon to become strongly adherent to the site of fracture healing. This obligatory loss of tendon amplitude, most often involving the extensor mechanism or flexor digitorum superficialis over the proximal phalanx or profundus over the middle phalanx, severely limits distal joint excursion by virtue of its checkrein effect. In these instances it is extremely dangerous to rely on strong manipulative or mobilization traction techniques to improve digital joint motion because the restrictive adhesions may be so strong that tendon rupture or attenuation occur, resulting in irreparable consequences. More gentle range of motion techniques and careful gentle splinting are indicated with consideration for early surgical tenolysis with or without capsulectomy when a strong tendon-bone bond is apparent.

The presence of associated ligament or neurovascular injury considerably alters the mode of conservative treatment. Consultation among members of the rehabilitation team is of paramount importance to establish goals and guidelines for post reduction management.

See Chapter 17, Splinting for Work, Sports, and the Performing Arts, for further information on other upper extremity fractures.

Joint

Capsulotomy/Capsulectomy

Capsulectomy involves the surgical division (capsulotomy) or excision (capsulectomy) of a portion of the collateral ligaments of a digital joint with normal articular surfaces but limited passive motion due to contracted periarticular ligamentous structures. Although a substantial improvement of motion may be reliably anticipated at the MP level, the results of a capsulectomy procedure at the PIP joint are less predictable.[14,44,85,100,109] Mobilization efforts are usually initiated within 1 to 7 days postoperatively. These efforts routinely involve assertive and focused splinting and exercise programs, which are vigilantly monitored.

Preoperative splinting and exercises are designed to attain as much passive joint motion as possible, enhancing the postoperative arc of motion and assuring adhesion-free tendon excursion essential to the active maintenance of passively improved postoperative motion. Splints are adapted to meet individual patient variations. The decision as to the type of splint to be applied depends on the presence or absence of wrist-produced tenodesis effect. If the limitation is purely articular, a hand-based splint will suffice (Fig. 15-12, A,B). Splints with secondary level wrist immobilization are required to control the effects of wrist position on distal joints in the presence of extrinsic tendon adhesions or poor postural habits that unfavorably affect digital joint mechanics (Fig. 15-12, C).

Splinting of a joint that has undergone a capsulectomy procedure maintains the motion gained from the combined preoperative and operative efforts. Because of potential recurrence of extension contractures, the MP joints are usually splinted to encourage joint flexion. In contrast, extension is often more difficult to regain than is flexion in the capsulectomized PIP joint. For this reason extension splinting, which is interspersed with frequent exercise periods, and limited flexion splinting may need to be prolonged to prevent recurrence of deformity. It is important that postcapsulectomy splinting and exercise programs are frequently reevaluated by members of the rehabilitation team during the first 2 or 3 postoperative months, and appropriate changes be instigated to ensure optimum results. One should emphasize to the

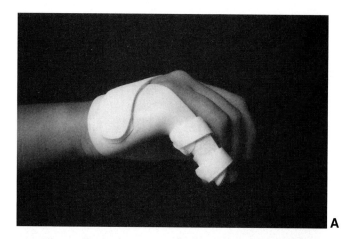

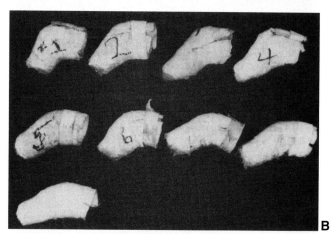

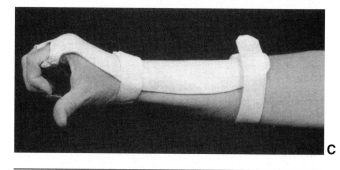

Fig. 15-12   A, Small finger MP flexion immobilization splint, type 2 (3) B, Finger PIP extension mobilization splint, type 1 (2) C, Index–small finger IP flexion mobilization splint, type 2 (13) A, Immobilization of the small finger MP joint allows collateral ligament healing. B, Serial cylinder casts, which are changed every 2 or 3 days, may be used to enhance passive PIP joint motion before a capsulotomy/capsulectomy procedure is undertaken. Cylinder casts are also effective in maintaining postoperative motion once the initial edema subsides and the incision is healed. C, Splint designs that incorporate the wrist eliminate compensatory tenodesis effect as traction is applied to more distal joints.

patient undergoing these difficult joint mobilization procedures that the tendency for recurrent stiffening of the involved joints is great and that splinting may be necessary for many months.[21]

Neurovascular

Peripheral Nerve Injuries

The potential for the restoration of optimum hand function after peripheral nerve injuries of the upper extremity depends on the preservation of good passive joint motion. It is also necessary to protect periarticular structures and denervated musculature by avoiding improper positioning of the partially paralyzed extremity.[39,42] In the presence of existing deformity, splints may be designed to restore passive mobility to upper extremity joints. Adapted to the individual requirements of the patient, these splints range from uncomplicated rubber bands to complex multifunction splints. Once free gliding of articular surfaces has been established, maintenance and positioning splints may be used until reinnervation occurs or until tendon transfer procedures are carried out to restore balance to the hand. These positioning splints should be used in conjunction with a high-quality exercise program. Splints serve to prevent deformity that results from the unopposed antagonists of the paralyzed muscles as well as to position the hand for use while awaiting nerve regeneration. These splints often assume predictable design configurations based on the nerve(s) involved[69] and they must be light, without excessive components, and easily applied or they will not be worn.

In the supple hand, the need for protective splinting varies according to the type of lesion and the inherent laxity of the ligamentous structure of the individual hand.[5] For example, not all patients who have sustained ulnar nerve injuries proceed to develop the classic claw hand posture of hyperextension of the fourth and fifth MP joints and concomitant IP flexion. Some have unusually firm palmar plate restraint at the MP joints and are not predisposed to hyperextension deformities, despite the lack of intrinsic opposition to the long extensor muscles. It is important, however, that these patients be monitored throughout rehabilitation to ensure that late-blooming deformity does not occur. In contrast, all patients with total loss of radial nerve innervations to the wrist and digital extensors develop wrist drop, requiring external support to properly position the hand, both to avoid deformity and to allow function.

Median Nerve. The median nerve provides the critical sensory perception to the palmar surface of the hand with the exception of the small finger and ulnar half of the ring finger. This nerve is also respon-

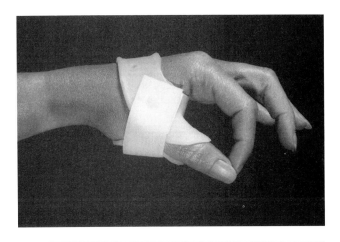

Fig. 15-13   Thumb CMC palmar abduction mobilization splint, type 1 (2)
This splint prevents first web space contracture in a median nerve injury. (Courtesy Sharon Flinn, MEd, OTR/L, Cleveland, Ohio.)

sible for innervations of the pronator teres and pronator quadratis, the flexor carpi radialis, the flexor digitorum superficialis, flexor digitorum profundus of the index and long fingers, and the flexor pollicis longus of the thumb. At a more distal level, the median nerve innervates the intrinsic thenar muscles, whose function is abduction and opposition. High median nerve lesions, therefore, are more disabling than is interruption at the wrist level, with the former affecting extrinsic as well as intrinsic digital function. However, a main functional disability with a median nerve lesion is loss of sensibility.

Splinting median nerve injuries depends on the level of lesion and the etiology.[83,110] Emphasis is placed on maintenance of passive mobility of the involved joints and enhancement of function. High, proximal interruption may require splints that assist finger flexion as well as opposition of the thumb.[30] Emphasis may be reduced to the prevention of thumb web contractures after more distal loss (Fig. 15-13). Splinting is frequently used in treating nerve entrapment problems such as carpal tunnel syndrome.* An understanding of each patient's functional capacity and substitution patterns is important before a splint design is initiated. For example, many patients whose long thumb flexor or short abductor and opponens action has been lost achieve adequate thumb use through substitution of the abductor pollicis longus, flexor pollicis brevis (deep head), and adductor pollicis

---

*References 15, 61, 66, 83, 104, 107, 110, 111.

Radial Nerve. A high-level radial nerve injury results in loss of active wrist, thumb, and finger extension and a weakening of supination and thumb radial abduction. Because the wrist provides the key to hand function at the digital level, the loss of the ability to properly position the hand in extension markedly weakens grasp and diminishes coordination. The coexisting deficit of metacarpophalangeal extension presents a less significant problem because the intrinsic muscles provide active extension of the interphalangeal joints.

The most important objective in splinting a high radial nerve injury is to support the wrist in extension, enhancing hand function and preventing overstretching of the extensor muscle groups. For most patients the use of a *wrist extension splint* is sufficient to allow satisfactory hand use (Fig. 15-14, *A*). Extension outrigger attachments are sometimes considered excessive and should be used in situations in which full digital extension is required for successful accomplishment of given tasks.[23,39,48,69,102] Since these are substitution rather than correction splints, low-profile outrigger configurations are preferable. Several different splint designs improve hand function for radial nerve patients (Fig. 15-14, *B-M*).

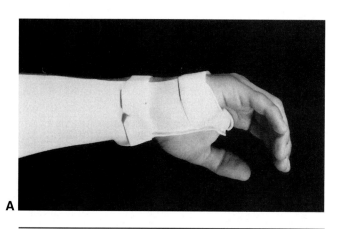

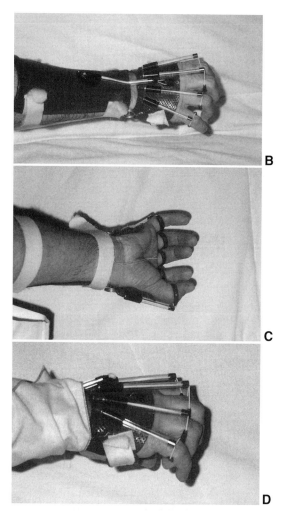

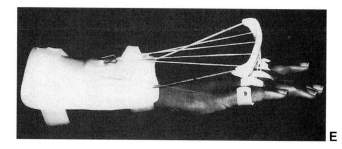

Fig. 15-14 A, Wrist extension mobilization splint, type 0 (1) B-D, Wrist flexion: index–small finger MP extension / index–small finger MP flexion: wrist extension torque transmission / thumb CMC radial abduction and MP extension mobilization splint, type 0 (7) E, Wrist flexion: index–small finger MP extension / index–small finger MP flexion: wrist extension torque transmission splint, type 0 (5) F, Wrist flexion: index–small finger MP extension / index–small finger MP flexion: wrist extension torque transmission splint, type 0 (5) G-I, Wrist flexion: index–small finger MP extension / index–small finger MP flexion: wrist extension torque transmission splint, type 0 (5) J, Index–small finger MP extension, thumb CMC radial abduction and MP extension mobilization splint, type 1(7) K-M, Index–small finger MP extension, thumb CMC radial abduction and MP extension mobilization splint, type 1 (7)
A, Stabilization of the wrist allows functional use of the hand in radial nerve palsy. **B-D,** This splint mobilizes the wrist and digits in extension, encouraging hand use. **E-I,** Other splints for radial nerve palsy make use of torque transmitted to the wrist or MP joints to produce synergistic tenodesis extension or flexion. Splints **J-M,** demonstrate a fourth design option that mobilizes the primary finger MP and thumb CMC and MP joints while the wrist is immobilized secondarily. [Courtesy **(B-D)** Jean-Christophe Arias, Saint-Etienne, France; **(E)** from Colditz JC: Splinting for radial nerve palsy, *J Hand Ther* 1(1):18-23, 1987; **(F)** Paul Van Lede, OT, MS, Orfit Industries, Wijnegem, Belgium; **(G-I)** Lori Klerekoper DeMott, OTR, CHT, Columbus, OH; **(J)** Christine Heaney, BSc, OT, Ottawa, Ontario; **(K-M)** Dominique Thomas, RPT, MCMK, Saint Martin Duriage, France.]

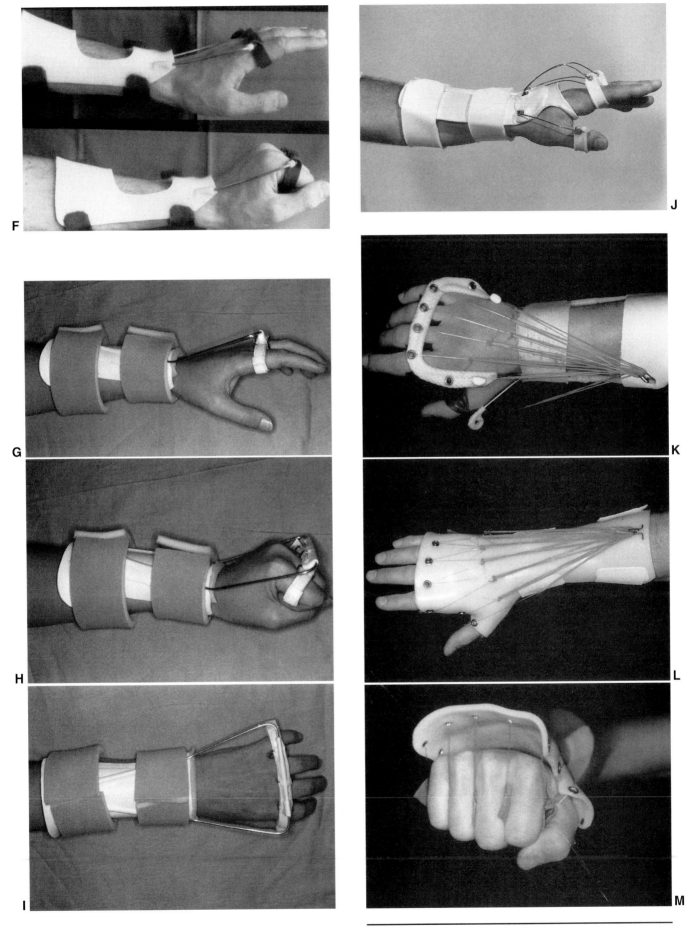

Fig. 15-14, cont'd
For legend see opposite page.

Ulnar Nerve. The ulnar nerve, with its important intrinsic innervation, is largely responsible for delicate coordinated movements of the hand. In addition, it also influences flexion of the ring and small fingers and ulnar deviation and flexion of the wrist.[49,79] Disruption of the ulnar nerve may result in the development of a claw deformity with metacarpophalangeal joint hyperextension and interphalangeal joint flexion of the fourth and fifth digits. Loss of small finger abduction and opposition and adduction of the thumb with the resultant weakness of pinch also accompanies ulnar paralysis.

The goals of splinting a hand that has sustained an ulnar nerve lesion are directed toward the attainment and maintenance of full passive motion and the improvement of hand function.[72] Existing joint limitations, often at the PIP joint of the ring or small finger, must be corrected before maintenance or substitution-splinting programs may be initiated. Splints designed to correct deformity should be specifically created to meet individual needs and should be changed to maintain optimum mechanical purchase as joint motion improves. When full passive motion has been established, or if the hand is supple at the time of initial examination, preventive splinting may commence.

Positioning the fourth and fifth MP joints in slight flexion allows the amplitude of the extrinsic digital extensor muscles to act effectively on the IP joints. Numerous splint designs accomplish this objective. One of the most acceptable is a three-point piano wire splint described by Wynn Parry.[75,76] Adaptation of this splint to the use of low-temperature materials for the dorsal and palmar metacarpal bars and dorsal phalangeal bar makes construction and fitting easier (Fig. 15-15, *A*). Splinting, using a selection of suitable designs until nerve regeneration is complete or until tendon transfer procedures are done, is a critical element in successful management of nerve injuries. (Fig. 15-15, *B-G*).

Combined Nerve Injuries. Damage to multiple nerves of the upper extremity is not uncommon, and the resulting potential for the development of deformity is, of course, magnified. Splinting programs should continue to incorporate the concepts previously mentioned for each individual injury, with even more care taken to monitor progress and make necessary adaptations as changes occur. Designs for the combined median and ulnar nerve injury resemble single-nerve ulnar or median nerve splints but multinerve splints encompass all digits (Fig. 15-16).

Splinting patients with peripheral nerve injuries must be augmented with individually designed exercise programs that promote the maintenance of active and passive motion and enhance hand dexterity.

Although the goals of exercise and splinting programs are almost identical, each brings a unique contribution to minimizing the resultant disability, and in conjunction with one another they provide an integrated and practical approach to rehabilitation. Each splint and exercise routine should also be interspersed with periodic objective reevaluation sessions, which allow program modification and continued patient progress.

See Chapter 17, Splinting for Work, Sports and the Performing Arts, for further information on peripheral nerve compression.

Spinal Cord Nerve Injury: Tetraplegia

Splinting of the quadriplegic upper extremity depends on the level of the spinal cord lesion.[26,41,60,65] Extremities that lack innervation above the seventh cervical nerve (C7) level often require the development of a passive or active tenodesis function for grasp, whereas those at C7 have active gross grasp and release through innervated extrinsic flexors and extensors. The intrinsic muscles of the hand are usually innervated at the first thoracic nerve level, allowing normal hand function.

Fifth Cervical Nerve. Patients with lesions at this level usually have active elbow flexion and deltoid shoulder movements, allowing gross positioning of the forearm and hand. Paralyzed wrist and hand musculature necessitates external wrist support in the form of a wrist immobilization splint to provide distal stability of the extremity. Accommodation of the splint to serve as the basis of attachment for adapted equipment is important to establishing independence in activities of daily living. Thumb CMC position and passive motion may be maintained through alternately positioning the thumb in palmar and radial abduction. Wrist and thumb splints are usually combined into one (Fig. 15-17).

If the patient is a candidate for an externally powered splint, development of a passive tenodesis hand may be considered (see next section). Most externally powered splints create a gross grasp or pinch by providing a power source to drive a conventional wrist-operated tenodesis splint. Power sources vary, as do triggering mechanisms (Fig. 15-18, *A*).

Sixth Cervical Nerve. In spinal cord lesions at this level, shoulder and elbow motions are stronger, resulting in more coordinated extremity positioning, but active elbow extension is absent. The important wrist extensors are spared, permitting a tenodesis hand in which grasp is achieved through an active wrist extension–passive finger flexion pattern. Tenodesis hands can be maximally developed through carefully supervised exercise and splinting programs (Fig. 15-18, *B-D*).[73] Exercises are oriented toward allowing

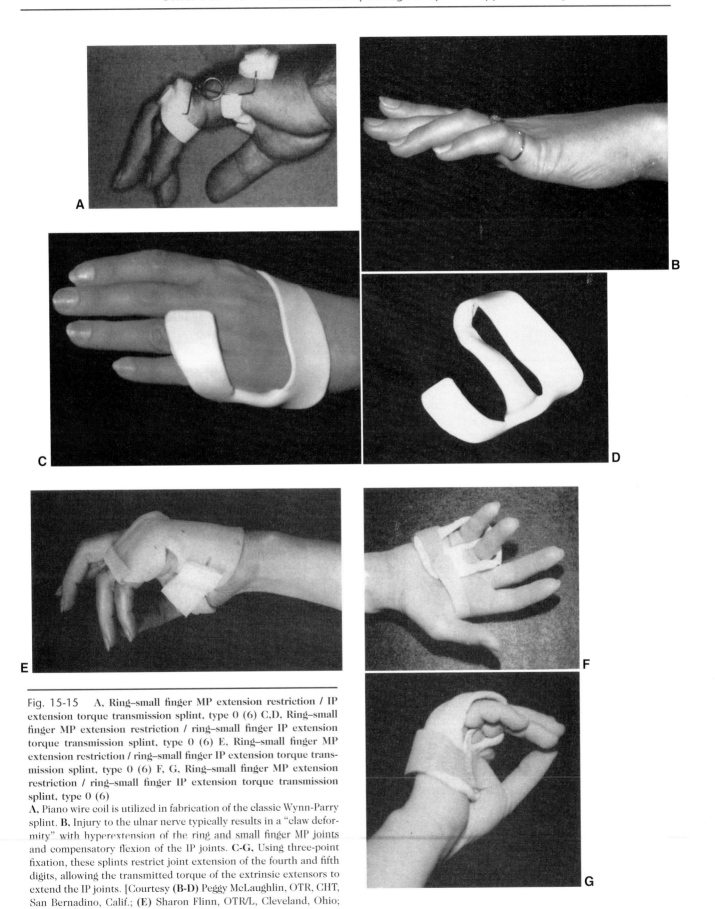

Fig. 15-15   A, Ring–small finger MP extension restriction / IP extension torque transmission splint, type 0 (6) C,D, Ring–small finger MP extension restriction / ring–small finger IP extension torque transmission splint, type 0 (6) E, Ring–small finger MP extension restriction / ring–small finger IP extension torque transmission splint, type 0 (6) F, G, Ring–small finger MP extension restriction / ring–small finger IP extension torque transmission splint, type 0 (6)
A, Piano wire coil is utilized in fabrication of the classic Wynn-Parry splint. B, Injury to the ulnar nerve typically results in a "claw deformity" with hyperextension of the ring and small finger MP joints and compensatory flexion of the IP joints. C-G, Using three-point fixation, these splints restrict joint extension of the fourth and fifth digits, allowing the transmitted torque of the extrinsic extensors to extend the IP joints. [Courtesy (B-D) Peggy McLaughlin, OTR, CHT, San Bernadino, Calif.; (E) Sharon Flinn, OTR/L, Cleveland, Ohio; (F,G) Sandra Artzberger, MS, OTR, Milwaukee, Wis., and Bonnie Fehring, LPT, Fond du Lac, Wis.]

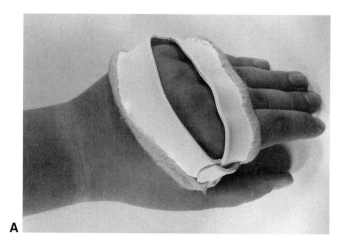

A

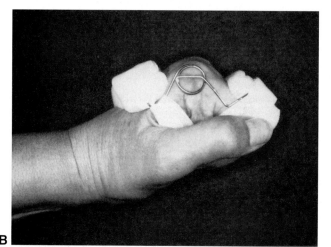

B

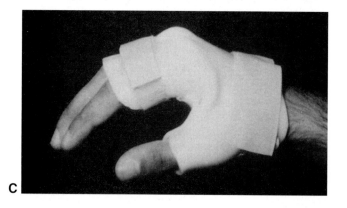

C

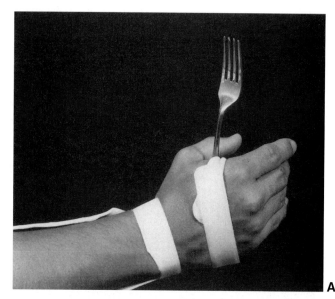

A

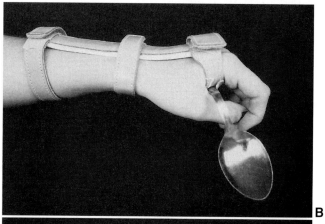

B

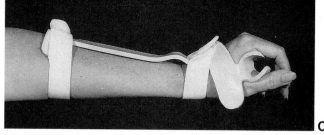

C

Fig. 15-16   A, Index–small finger MP extension restriction / IP extension torque transmission splint, type 0 (12) B, Index–small finger MP extension restriction / IP extension torque transmission splint, type 0 (12) C, Index–small finger MP extension restriction / index–small IP extension torque transmission / thumb CMC palmar abduction and MP extension mobilization splint, type 0 (14)
These splints prevent hyperextension of the second through fifth MP joints while allowing partial to full digital flexion. They may be used for treating combined ulnar and median nerve lesions. Extrinsic extensor torque transmission to the IPs for extension is accomplished by preventing hyperextension of the MPs. [Courtesy (A) Ruth Coopee, OTR, CHT, Athol, Mass.; (C) Gretchen Maurer, OTR, CHT, Norfolk, Va.]

Fig. 15-17   A, Wrist extension mobilization splint, type 0 (1); with grasp assist B, Wrist extension mobilization splint, type 0 (1); with grasp assist C, Wrist extension, thumb CMC palmar abduction mobilization splint, type 0 (2)
A, To help patient independence, splints may be designed to hold ADL, homemaking, or work-related equipment. B,C, Several splint designs may be used to stabilize the wrist and accomplish independent function. D, This wrist and thumb CMC/MP positioning splint also stabilizes the wrist and maintains the first web space of a C5 spinal cord lesion patient. [Courtesy (B) Allyssa Wagner, MS, OTR, Indianapolis, Ind.]

controlled extrinsic flexor tightness to occur while maintaining passive range of motion of the wrist and digits. Finger extension exercises are performed with the wrist in flexion, and finger flexion exercises are carried out with the wrist in extension. Splints designed to augment these patterns are used to reinforce the tenodesis motion in functional activities. As habit patterns become established, gradual weaning from the splint is encouraged, allowing increasingly independent tenodesis hand use.

Moberg[70] describes a surgical procedure for using the wrist extensors to enhance flexor hinge key grip of the thumb. Splinting for this procedure involves maintaining passive motion of the thumb carpometacarpal and metacarpophalangeal joints preoperatively and protecting splinting of the transfer during the early postoperative mobilization phase. A thumb abduction splint may occasionally be required to maintain carpometacarpal joint motion as postoperative time increases.

Seventh Cervical Nerve. Patients with lesions at the C6 level usually have gross active finger flexion and extension but lack the intrinsic musculature that allows fine hand coordination and dexterity. Splinting and exercise programs are directed toward maintenance of passive joint range of motion with emphasis on thumb CMC joint mobility and prevention of extension deformities at the MP joints. Splinting to position the thumb in opposition enhances prehension of small objects.

As a result of severe muscle imbalance and limited active motion, many tetraplegic hands have a tendency to become slightly edematous and to assume a resting posture of MP joint extension, PIP joint flexion, and thumb adduction. These factors may lead insidiously to stiffness and eventually to severe joint contractures, which are correctable only through surgical

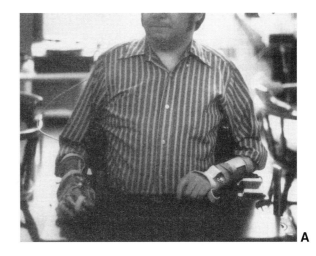

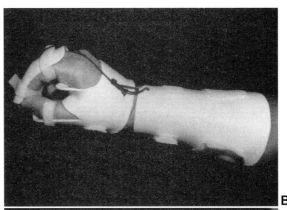

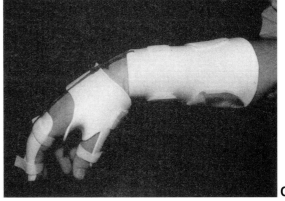

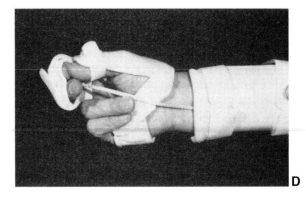

Fig. 15-18 A, Index–long finger extension and flexion, thumb CMC palmar abduction and MP-IP extension mobilization splint, type 1 (7); left. \\ Wrist extension mobilization splint, type 0 (1); with prop; right B,C, Wrist extension: index–long finger flexion / wrist flexion: index–long finger extension torque transmission / thumb CMC palmar abduction and thumb MP-IP extension immobilization splint, type 2 (10) D, Wrist extension: index–long finger flexion / wrist flexion: index–long finger extension torque transmission / thumb CMC palmar abduction and MP-IP extension immobilization splint, type 2 (10)

A, A battery-powered external orthosis allows this C5 quadriplegic patient to grasp and release objects. The orthosis is triggered when the patient touches his watchband to the copper plate mounted on his lapboard. (United States patent No. 3967321: Ryan, Fess, Babcock et al.). B-D, These tenodesis splints produce passive approximation of the index and long fingers to the thumb through active wrist extension. [Courtesy **(B,C)** Cheryl Kunkle, OTR, CHT, Allentown, Pa.]

intervention. In anticipation of these problems, preventive measures should be initiated within the first week after injury, since joint stiffness and contractures severely limit rehabilitative potential. As with direct injury to the hand, it is important to position the resting tetraplegic hand in a posture of antideformity to prevent shortening of digital ligaments. So-called functional position splints do not provide sufficient MP joint flexion and PIP joint extension to prevent collateral ligament shortening. With the wrist in neutral position, the MP joints should be splinted in 70-90° of flexion, the IP joints in 0-10° of flexion, and the thumb CMC joint in palmar or radial abduction (safe position). Although a vigil for early deforming forces must always be maintained, the need for safe position splinting during periods of rest diminishes as the patient increases the use of his hands in functional compensatory patterns and the potential for edema subsides.

Muscle–Tendon

Tendon

Extensor Tendon Repair. Traditionally, extensor tendon repairs have been treated by immobilizing the wrist and digital joints in extension.[81] Problems of adhesions between the repair site and the gliding bed are not as limiting to extensor tendons as they are to flexor tendons because of the relatively long fibroosseous canals through which the flexor tendons course. However, with severe extensor tendon injuries in which periosteum, retinaculum, or soft tissues are involved, adhesions can significantly restrict active motion and limit the patient's potential for rehabilitation.

Based on physiologic concepts similar to those used with early mobilization of flexor tendon repairs, Evans and Burkhalter[37] reported an average total active motion of 210.4° using a method of early mobilization of extensor tendon repairs, which they devised.[34,36] Incorporating the wrist in approximately 45° extension and allowing 5 mm extensor tendon glide, a *finger extension mobilization / finger flexion restriction splint* is fitted 2 to 5 days after repair. On a predetermined daily protocol, the patient is instructed to flex the MP joints until the fingers touch the flexion restriction portion of the splint, and to allow the mobilization assists to passively return the digits to 0°. Prescribed passive IP joint exercises are done with the wrist and MP joints in extension to avoid stress to the repair. The authors emphasize the need to calculate extensor tendon excursion in relation to MP joint motion to obtain the appropriate motion allowed by the splint. The extension finger cuff is wider than normal, encompassing both the PIP and DIP joints, allowing only MP motion. Twice a day the patient exercises in a torque transmission splint fit in 30° wrist extension and 0-10° MP extension for the purpose of exercising the IP joints. At night an extension immobilization splint is worn. The level of repair and the adjunct injuries will determine extensor tendon repair splint design (Fig. 15-19, A-D). Other programs for mobilizing repaired extensor tendons employ different splint designs (Fig. 15-19, E-J).*

See Chapter 17, Splinting for Work, Sports, and the Performing Arts, for further information on mallet and boutonniere injuries.

---

*References 3, 4, 13, 18, 19, 35, 38, 91, 97, 101.

Fig. 15-19   A,B, Index–small finger MP-PIP extension mobilization / index–small finger flexion restriction splint, type 1 (13) C,D, Index–small finger MP extension mobilization / index–small finger flexion restriction splint, type 1 (13) E, Index–small finger flexion restriction splint, type 1 (13) F, Index–small finger MP flexion restriction / index–small finger IP extension-flexion torque transmission splint, type 1 (13) G,H, Long finger MP extension and flexion torque transmission / long finger MP flexion restriction splint, type 1 (4) \\ Wrist extension immobilization splint, type 0 (1) I,J, Index finger IP extension mobilization / PIP flexion restriction / DIP flexion torque transmission splint, type 2 (4). A-D, Allowing passive finger extension and limited active finger flexion, these splints were designed for use with early passive mobilization of complex extensor tendon injuries. E,F, While protecting extensor tendon repairs by positioning the wrist and MP joints in extension, the distal portion of this splint can be removed to permit IP joint exercises. G,H, Splinting post zone III extensor laceration of the long finger utilizes restriction of flexion and allows IP motion through torque transmission. Note: wrist splint. I,J, Dorsal and lateral views of an IP extension mobilization splint that uses a simple "safety pin" for the dynamic assist and an added Velcro strap while DIP exercises are done. [Courtesy (A,B,E,F) Roslyn Evans, OTR, CHT, Vero Beach, Fla.; (C,D) Barbara Smith, OTR, Edmond, Okla.; (G,H) from Merritt WH: Written on behalf of the stiff finger, *J Hand Ther* 11(2):74-9, 1998; (I,J) from Schreuders T, et al: Dynamic extension splint: Rotterdam design, *J Hand Ther* 10(3):240-1, 1997.]

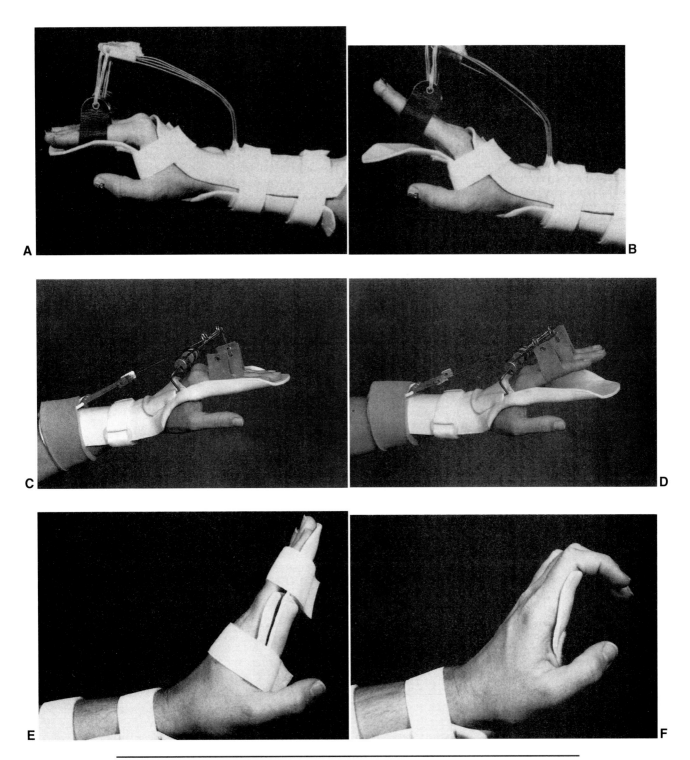

Fig. 15-19
For legend see p. 414.

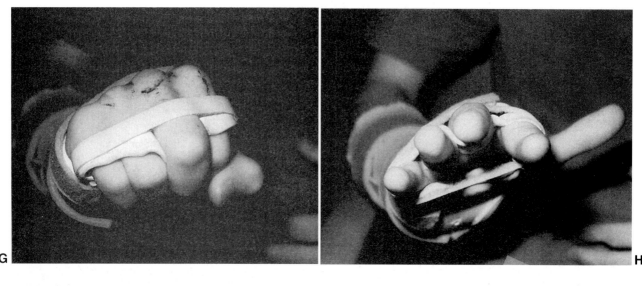

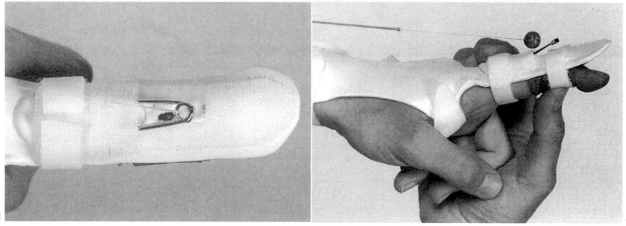

Fig. 15-19, cont'd
For legend see p. 414.

Flexor Tendon Repairs. Splinting involved in flexor tendon repairs falls into three categories: splints used with (1) early passive or active mobilization techniques for flexor tendon repairs, and those used (2) to protect or (3) to enhance motion once active motion of the repair has been initiated.

Historically, tendon repairs were immobilized from 3 to 5 weeks before motion was permitted. However, it has been well demonstrated by Mason that there is little or no tensile strength at a flexor tendon repair site until it is subjected to stress.[67] Kleinert and associates[57,58] and Duran[31,32] developed methods for early passive mobilization of repaired flexor tendons in "no-man's land" that seems to lessen the effect of amplitude-limiting adhesions on the repaired tendon. The method of Kleinert and colleagues is based on use of antagonistic active extension, whereas Duran advocates passive motion at the interphalangeal joints.

Both methods require careful adherence to specific splinting and exercise routines, and neither should be undertaken without a thorough understanding of the concepts involved. Early active flexor tendon programs require a stronger repair that allows protected active motion. Although splints developed to be used with these early mobilization techniques differ in configuration, similarities exist.[40] Each requires a posture of wrist flexion to decrease tension on the repair and some method of eliminating/restricting active digital flexion and passive digital extension while permitting periods of limited passive or active excursion of the flexor tendon repair (Table 15-1) (Fig. 15-20).*

*References 22, 25, 38, 46, 55, 57, 58, 68, 77, 86, 88, 89, 93, 95, 96, 99.

Text continued on p. 421

TABLE 15-1 Published Zone II Flexor Tendon Splints: ESCS Classifications and Splint Sequenced Ranking Index© Order

Primary Joint(s)	Purpose	Direction	Type	Total Joints	Digits	Articular/Nonarticular SCS Name	Author
						Articular	
Wrist, finger MP, PIP, DIP	Restriction / Mobilization	Extension: flexion	0	(07)	Index	Wrist extension: index-small finger MP extension restriction and index finger flexion mobilization / wrist flexion: index-small finger MP extension restriction and index finger IP extension mobilization splint, type 0 (7)	Cooney[2]
		Extension: flexion	0	(13)	Index–Small	Wrist extension restriction: index-small finger flexion mobilization / index–small finger extension restriction / wrist flexion: index-small finger extension restriction splint, type 0 (13)	Strickland[8]
Finger MP, PIP, DIP	Restriction	Extension	1	(13)	Index–Small	Index-small finger extension restriction splint, type 1 (13)	Gratton[5]
	Restriction / Mobilization	Extension, flexion	1	(07)	Index, Long	Index-long finger extension restriction / index finger flexion mobilization splint, type 1 (7)	Kleinert[6]
		Extension, flexion	1	(07)	Small	Index-small finger MP extension restriction / small finger flexion mobilization splint, type 1 (7)	Duran[3]
		Extension, flexion	1	(07)	Ring–Small	Ring-small finger MP extension restriction / ring-small finger flexion mobilization splint, type 1 (7)	Silfverskiold[7]
		Extension, flexion	1	(10)	Long	Long-small finger extension restriction / long finger flexion mobilization splint, type 1 (10)	Werntz[10]
		Extension, flexion	1	(13)	Index–Small	Index-small finger extension restriction / index-small finger flexion mobilization splint, type 1 (13)	Evans[4]
		Extension, flexion	1	(13)	Index	Index-small finger extension restriction / index finger flexion mobilization splint, type 1 (13)	Chow[1]
		Extension, flexion	1	(13)	Index–Small	Index-small finger extension restriction / ring finger flexion mobilization splint, type 1 (13)	Trueman[9]

Total number of splints classified: 10
*The SCS and ESCS group splints according to Primary Joints.
Type = number of secondary joint level(s).
Total joints = count of all joints in splint ( ).
References:
1. Chow JA, Thomes LJ, Dovelle S, et al: A combined regimen of controlled motion following flexor tendon repair in "no man's land," Plast Reconstr Surg 79(3):447-55, 1987.
2. Cooney W, Lin G, An KN: Improved tendon excursion following flexor tendon repair, J Hand Ther 2(2):102-6, 1989.
3. Duran R, et al: Management of flexor tendon lacerations in Zone 2 using controlled passive motion postoperatively. In Hunter J, Schneider L, Mackin E: Tendon surgery in the hand, Mosby, 1987, St. Louis.
4. Evans R, Thompson D: Immediate active short arc motion following tendon repair. In Hunter J, Schneider L, Mackin E: Tendon and nerve surgery in the hand, a third decade, Mosby, 1997, St. Louis.
5. Gratton P: Early active mobilization after flexor tendon repairs, J Hand Ther 6(4):285-9, 1993.
6. Kleinert HE, Kutz J, Cohen M: Primary repair of zone 2 flexor tendon lacerations. In Hunter J, Schneider L: American Academy of Orthopaedic Surgeons symposium on tendon surgery in the hand, Mosby, 1975, St. Louis.
7. Silfverskiold KL, May EJ: Flexor tendon repair in zone II with a new suture technique and an early mobilization program combining passive and active flexion, J Hand Surg [Am] 19(1):53-60, 1994.
8. Strickland JW, Gettle K: Flexor tendon repair: the Indianapolis method. In Hunter J, Schneider L, Mackin E: Tendon and nerve surgery in the hand, a third decade, Mosby, 1997, St. Louis.
9. Trueman S, Bio-dynamic finger component, J Hand Ther 11(3):209-11, 1998.
10. Werntz JR, Chesher SP, Breidenbach WC, et al: A new dynamic splint for postoperative treatment of flexor tendon injury, J Hand Surg [Am] 14(3):559-66, 1989.

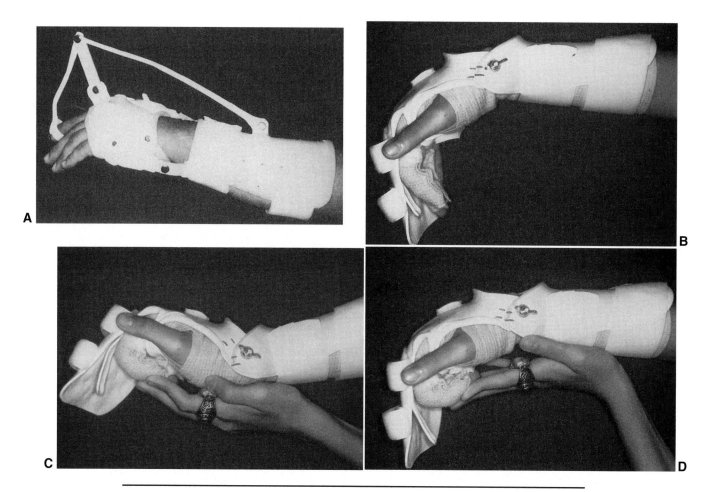

Fig. 15-20 **A,** Wrist extension: index–small finger MP extension restriction and index finger flexion mobilization / wrist flexion: index–small finger MP extension restriction and index finger IP extension mobilization splint, type 0 (7) **B-D,** Wrist extension restriction: index–small finger flexion mobilization / index–small finger extension restriction / wrist flexion index–small finger extension restriction splint, type 0 (13) **E,** Wrist extension restriction: index–small finger flexion mobilization / index–small finger extension restriction / wrist flexion: index–small finger extension restriction splint, type 0 (13) **F,G,** Index–small finger extension restriction splint, type 1 (13) **H,** Long–small finger extension restriction / long finger flexion mobilization splint, type 1 (10) **I-L,** Long–small finger extension restriction / ring finger flexion mobilization splint, type 1 (10) **M,N,** Index–small finger MP extension restriction / index–small finger flexion mobilization splint, type 1 (13) **O,P,** Index–long finger extension restriction / index–long flexion mobilization / ring–small MP flexion IP extension immobilization splint, type 1 (13) **Q,R,** Thumb CMC radial abduction and MP-IP extension restriction / thumb CMC palmar abduction and MP-IP flexion mobilization splint, type 1 (4)

A, Cooney's prototype for flexor tendon repairs uses wrist motion to mobilize the index finger IP joints through the dorsal outrigger. **B-E,** Strickland's early active program for zone II tendon repairs employs a splint that allows wrist flexion with IP extension and a place-hold exercise with restricted wrist extension and finger flexion. **F,G,** Passive flexion and extension are performed with the Duran early passive motion technique for zone II flexor tendon repairs. **H-R,** Varied splint designs are available for treating flexor tendon repairs. [Courtesy **(A)** from Cooney W, Lin G, An KN: Improved tendon excursion following flexor tendon repair, *J Hand Ther* 2(2):102-6, 1989; **(B-E)** Jill Francisco, OTR, CHT, Cicero, Ind.; **(H)** from Werntz JR, et al: A new dynamic splint for postoperative treatment of flexor tendon injury, *J Hand Surg* [Am] 14(3):559-66, 1989; **(I-L)** Stancie Trueman, Missiauga, Ontario, Canada; **(M,N)** from Evans R, Thompson D: Immediate active short arc motion following tendon repair. In Hunter J, Schneider L, Mackin E: *Tendon and nerve surgery in the hand, a third decade*, Mosby, 1997, St. Louis; **(O,P)** Joanne Kassimir, OTR, photography by Owen Kassimir; **(Q,R)** Peggy McLaughlin, OTR, CHT, San Bernardino, Calif.]

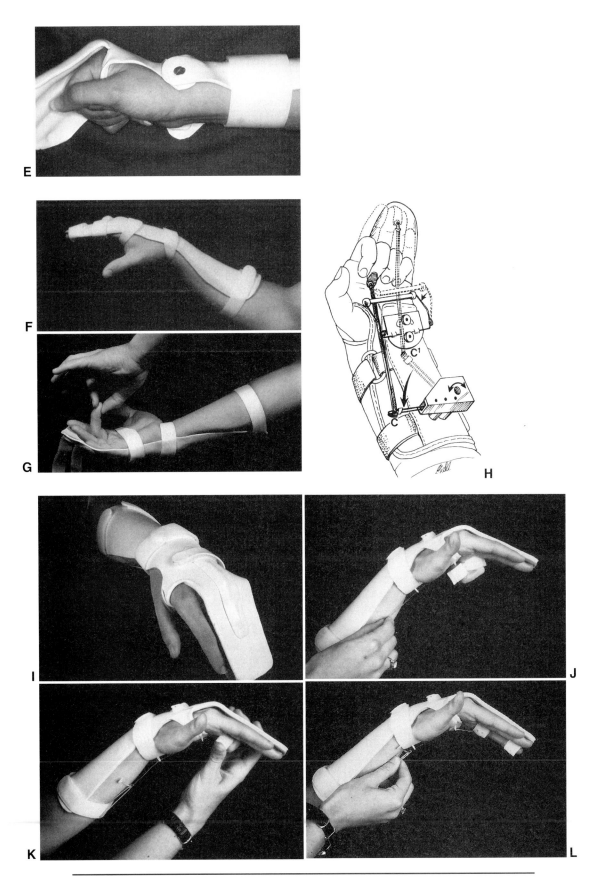

Fig. 15-20, cont'd
For legend see opposite page.

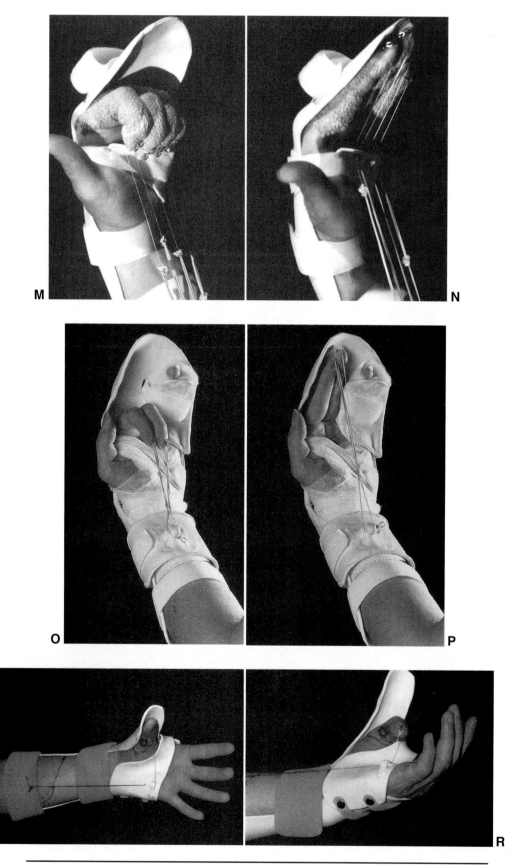

Fig. 15-20, cont'd
For legend see p. 418.

When designing a splint for flexor tendon repairs, one should consider the effect of integrated motion of the flexor tendons, which to some degree limits independent digital action. Because the index finger and the thumb are considered the only truly independent digits, repair of the long, ring, or small flexor tendons necessitates inclusion of all three digits in the splint.

Early passive and active mobilization concepts may be used for repairs of tendons other than those in zones I and II (Fig. 15-21). Again, it is important that all members of the rehabilitation team are included during the initial planning stages, for poor communication or misunderstandings may seriously jeopardize the patient's ability to reach his full rehabilitative potential.

Repaired flexor or extensor tendons that have been treated with initial immobilization may require a period of protective splinting to prevent undue accidental stress to the repair site between controlled exercise periods. Flexion of the wrist and digital joints decreases tension on flexor repairs; conversely, extensor repairs are protected with extension positioning. It should be remembered, however, that these positions require greater active excursion of the tendon to effect joint motion, and active exercises done in these splints may be less effective than with reverse positioning to increase tension. The patient should thoroughly understand the exercise and splinting programs before being allowed to proceed with an unsupervised course of self-therapy. As tensile strength increases, the protective positioning is gradually changed and ultimately discarded. If joints that have become stiffened during the period of immobilization do not respond to exercises, mobilization splinting in the direction of the repair that does not impart stress to the tendon repair may be required. Gentle mobilization splinting in a direction that stresses the tendon repair site may be applied concomitant with the initiation of light resistive exercises about 6 to 12 weeks after surgery.

Secondary Procedures Post Tendon Repair

Tendon Grafts. Tendon grafting involves the bridging of a gap in a tendon with an autogenous donor tendon from the same or a separate extremity. Commonly used donor tendons include the palmaris longus, the plantaris, and, on occasion, a toe extensor. One of the most important criteria for a successful tendon graft procedure is the establishment and maintenance of good passive motion of the involved segment and adjacent rays. Splinting may be effectively employed for creating and preserving supple digits, both preoperatively and during the postoperative course.

Postoperative splinting should be designed to meet the individual problems presented. If wrist position

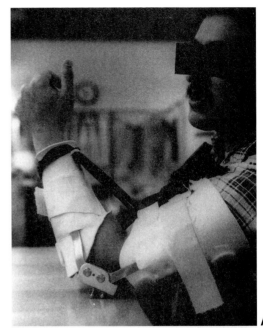

A

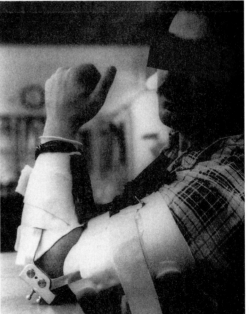

B

Fig. 15-21   **A,B, Elbow extension restriction / elbow flexion mobilization / forearm neutral immobilization splint, type 0 (2)** Designed for modified early passive mobilization of a biceps tendon repair, this splint allows active elbow extension **(A)** with passive flexion **(B)** provided by a mobilization assist of elastic tubing. The amount of elbow extension is controlled by an adjustable hinge component that may be changed to allow greater motion as healing permits. If forearm position cannot be maintained in neutral, the wrist must also be included in this splint design. (Courtesy Linda Tresley, OTR/L, and Barbara Sopp, OTR/L, Chicago, Ill.)

does not influence passive motion, splints such as a *finger PIP extension splint, finger flexion splint,* or *thumb CMC palmar abduction splint* are usually efficient devices for maximizing passive joint motion.[20,59] If, however, significant wrist-produced tenodesing of the extrinsic flexor or extensor tendons is present, the wrist must be incorporated into the splint to control its influence at digital levels. Once passive motion is reestablished, the splinting program is directed at maintaining joint status. This often involves uncomplicated night splinting and a routine exercise program during the day (Fig. 15-22).

The philosophy of postoperative management to which one subscribes dictates the kind of splinting program employed after surgical attachment of the tendon graft. Some authors advocate immobilization for 3 weeks to promote tendon healing before initiating splinting and conservative therapy, whereas others begin early controlled passive motion in hopes of diminishing scar formation between the sutured graft and its gliding bed. It appears, however, that many of the adhesion-modifying benefits of early controlled motion after primary flexor tendon repair are not as applicable to tendon grafting, and results following the application of these techniques to grafts have been disappointing. Because splinting programs differ considerably, the postoperative management of tendon grafts should not be undertaken without a thorough knowledge of the surgical and rehabilitation plans for each patient. A comprehensive understanding of the concepts involved is the key to attaining patient rehabilitation potential. (See also the section in this chapter on postoperative splinting of tendon repairs.)

Staged Flexor Tendon Grafts. The general concepts employed in the management of single-stage tendon grafts may be applied to the treatment of two-stage flexor tendon grafting procedures, except that the pregraft time period is expanded to allow the development of a pseudosheath around a flexible tendon implant, which is removed at the time of grafting. As with the one-stage grafts, a supple hand is a prerequisite to surgical procedures. Once this is established, a flexible tendon implant is inserted with its distal end anchored to the tendon stub or to bone. Postoperatively, the hand and wrist are immobilized in flexion posture for approximately 3 weeks, during which time the pseudosheath forms, providing a smooth gliding bed for the second-stage autogenous graft. Early splinting may be required to reestablish preoperative passive motion levels. Finger taping, frequent conscientious exercise periods, and individualized splinting such as extension immobilization to prevent flexion contractures or torque transmission splinting in the form of "buddy taping" to assist passive motion are the

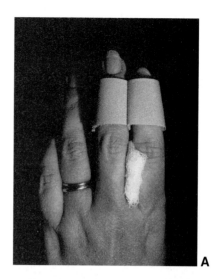

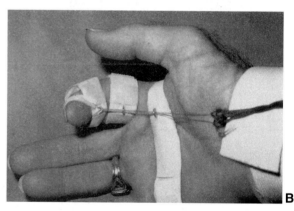

Fig. 15-22   A, Index finger MP-PIP extension and flexion torque transmission splint, type 2 (4) B, Index finger flexion mobilization splint, type 1 (4)

The use of a torque transmission splint (**A**) or a finger flexion mobilization splint (**B**) facilitates the maintenance of passive motion during the preoperative phase of a tendon graft procedure. [Courtesy (**B**) Carol Hierman, OTR, CHT, Cedar Grove, N.C., and Elisha Denny, PTA, OTA, Pittsboro, N.C.; © UNC Hand Rehabilitation Center, Chapel Hill, N.C.]

keys to maintaining good passive motion during the first stage of the postoperative phase.

Once the implant is removed and the tendon graft connected, the two-stage procedure is treated similarly to the single-stage tendon graft.

Active Tendon Implant. The active tendon implant designed by Hunter et al.[52] allows controlled active motion during stage one postoperative phase. With a preoperative stage similar to those for tendon grafting and the two-stage tendon implant, stage one postoperative management of the active tendon follows a regime similar to that of early passive mobilization of a tendon graft with some modifications. While in the dorsal restriction splint with elastic flexion mobilization traction, "passive hold" exercises are begun in addition to the active extension–passive flexion with elastic band exercises. At 6 to 8 weeks the dorsal splint is replaced with a wristband with elastic flexion traction for continued protection. Active exercises are begun at 8 to 10 weeks and, at 10 to 11 weeks, postoperatively graded resistive exercises may be initiated. As with the passive two-stage implant, the active implant is removed and replaced with a tendon graft at stage two surgery. Because this is an unusual technique, before embarking on a treatment regime for an active tendon implant, it is recommended that those involved in the rehabilitation process familiarize themselves with the specific protocols outlined by the Hand Rehabilitation Center, Philadelphia, Pa.

Tenolysis. Tenolysis involves the surgical freeing of adhesions around a tendon to improve tendon gliding and excursion. Active range of motion exercises and splinting are usually initiated within 24 hours after surgery.

A tenolysis program employs splinting to achieve and maintain passive motion preoperatively and to maintain passive range of motion postoperatively.[16,19,85] Preoperative splints are designed to correct specific joint limitations and may be used at night to sustain passive motion once it has been achieved. Alteration of both flexion and extension splints may be required and, despite the involvement of extrinsic tendons, the need to immobilize the wrist is unusual. However, if the patient consistently assumes a protective wrist posture that is unfavorable to attainment of maximum tendon amplitude, a splint that favorably positions the wrist secondarily to digital mobilization should be applied. For instance, after flexor tenolysis, if the patient uses an inefficient wrist

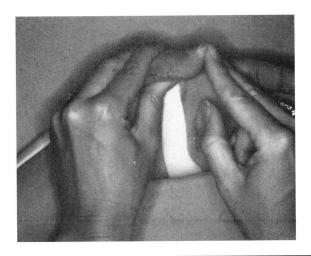

Fig. 15-23   Manual application of mild resistance to a segment as it is volitionally moved through its arc of motion may be used as a form of biofeedback.

flexion posture when flexing the digits, immobilizing the wrist in extension encourages flexor tendon excursion.

Because active motion is paramount after a tenolysis procedure, splint-wearing times must be interspersed with frequent exercise periods. Depending on individual circumstances, patients are often instructed to exercise 15 minutes of every hour and to alternate extension and flexion splints every 1 to 2 hours during the day (Fig. 15-23). In addition, patients are usually instructed to sleep in the splint that either mobilizes or positions to counteract problem motion.

Often delayed for 6–12 weeks, resistive exercises should be initiated only after consultation with the surgeon. Since tenolysis causes interruption in the blood supply, resistance applied too early may lead to tendon rupture. This is especially true if previous surgical procedures have been done on the tendon. To decrease the chance of rupture, it is important for the surgeon to inform those who are responsible for postoperative management about the condition of the tendon at the time of the tenolysis.

Exercise and splinting programs must be continuously reevaluated and adapted as changes in motion status occur. As active motion improves, the splinting program is gradually curtailed to permit progressively longer durations of unassisted functional hand use. Night splinting is continued until the patient is able to consistently maintain active and passive motion through exercise alone.

Digital extensor/flexor tenolysis is more common than at other levels of the upper extremity due to the complicated and interrelated anatomic structures involved. Preoperatively, an extensor lag is generally present, and postoperatively the extensor lag is unchanged or decreased by 5-10° with an increase in flexion. If extensor adherence is secondary to a diagnosis other than tendon laceration, resistance can be initiated at 4-6 weeks when flexion is limited. Extension splinting is necessary to minimize extensor lag combined with tendon glide when active flexion is performed after positioning in extension. Preoperatively, a flexor adherence will have decreased active extension and limited flexion while after surgery full motion can be expected.

Tendon Transfers

In developing a rehabilitation program for the patient with a partially paralyzed hand who is a candidate for the transference of muscle power, it is imperative that the therapist work closely with the physician to understand the exact deficit and the specific plans for surgical restoration. Postoperatively, it is equally important to gain a comprehensive appreciation of the transfers used, their course, and realistic functional goals. Without this understanding the patient may be subjected to ineffective and unwarranted exercise and splinting programs that often diminish the benefit of the tendon transfers.

The splint and exercise program used with tendon transfers is divided into three chronological subcategories: (1) preoperative phase, (2) early postoperative phase, and (3) late postoperative phase. Each phase is characterized by distinctly different purposes for exercise and splinting.

It is important that exercise programs be implemented at an early stage in the management of the patient who has developed paralysis secondary to the interruption or disease of a major peripheral nerve. When tendon transfers are anticipated, the strengthening of donor muscles is helpful, particularly if testing indicates that weakness has developed secondary to disuse. Predictable patterns of paralysis are seen after nerve loss, and consultation with the upper extremity reconstructive surgeon provides valuable information regarding anticipated functional return, potential tendon transfers, and the therapeutic needs of a specific patient.*

To obtain maximum benefit from tendon transfer procedures, the joints affected by the transfer must be supple. During the preoperative phase, emphasis is placed on attaining and maintaining maximum passive range of motion of all the joints crossed by the intended tendon transfer, including wrist and digital joints. If joints exhibit restricted passive motion, mobilization splints must be designed and fitted to correct the specific joint limitations. However, when full passive motion is present and maintenance of this mobility is the indication for splint application, splints that substitute for lost active motion may be considered. Manual muscle test data and active range of motion measurements govern the designing of a splint used to prevent the development of joint stiffness while allowing improved functional use of the partially paralyzed extremity. Splints employed to prevent deformity from occurring in some of the more common types of peripheral upper extremity paralyses are described in the section of this chapter on peripheral nerve injury.

Early postoperative splinting encompasses three facets: (1) protection of the transfer after dressing removal, (2) correction of stiffness secondary to the immobilization necessitated by surgery, and (3) controlled increase of tension on the transferred musculotendinous unit(s).

Splinting may be used to protect tendon transfers during the earliest stages of mobilization. These splints are designed to decrease tension on the transfer and are used before and during exercise periods and at night (Fig. 15-24, A).

Because a period of immobilization is required to promote healing after surgical intervention, adjacent uninvolved joints may become stiff. In some cases splinting is required to regain diminished passive motion. Joints whose stiffness originates from this relatively brief period of immobilization usually respond quickly to splinting efforts and require little more than exercise to maintain motion once it has been regained.

The third reason for employing splinting in the early postoperative phase is to gradually increase the tension on transferred tendons to help lengthen any adhesion that may have formed and to allow for the initiation of mechanically advantageous active motion. Careful control of splint mobilization traction during this phase can allow the splinted joints to regain the desired range of motion without the unfavorable reverse deformity that sometimes accompanies tight transfers. Because some lengthening may occur as function returns, care must be taken not to place too much tension on a transfer, or muscle imbalance may recur. Timing of this kind of splinting

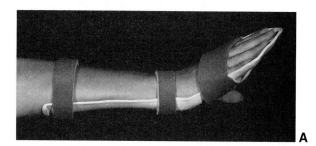

A

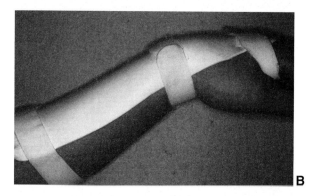

B

Fig. 15-24   **A,** Index–small finger flexion restriction splint, type 1 (13) **B,** Index–small finger extension and flexion torque transmission splint, type 1 (13)
A, This type 1 finger restriction splint eliminates tension on an extrinsic transfer that runs dorsal to the wrist axis of rotation. **B,** Wrist flexion increases the tension on a dorsally placed extrinsic donor tendon and mechanically facilitates active digital extension.

*References 10, 11, 42, 43, 63, 70, 92.

usually corresponds with the initiation of light resistive exercises and activities. This is the most challenging aspect of tendon transfers. Too aggressive mobilization of a tendon transfer can stretch out the transfer and compromise function.

Altering the position of joints crossed by the specific musculotendinous combination of a given transfer permits an increase or decrease in the tension stress on the tendon. Immobilizing the wrist in a direction opposite to the side in which the tendon transfer was routed effectively tightens the transfer and maximizes its function. An example of this tenodesis effect may be seen in the tension imparted to a donor motor tendon that passes volarly to the wrist axis by placing the wrist in extension. Similarly, a posture of wrist flexion will intensify the pull on a dorsally placed extrinsic donor (Fig. 15-24, B). In cases of tendon transfers designed to function across multiple digital joints, the splint may be extended distally to position consecutive joints in attitudes that will effectively control tension. As the amplitude and tensile strength increase and active motion of the involved joints improves, the use of splints may be gradually eliminated to permit unassisted use of the transfer.

Splinting in the late postoperative phase involves the conversion of learned substitution patterns by gradually eliminating the mechanically advantageous use of wrist tenodesis and requiring greater excursion of the donor musculotendinous unit(s). The wrist may now be gradually positioned in an attitude opposite to that used in the early postoperative phase with active contraction of the motor tendon replacing the tension created by the splint. The concept now is to decrease the postural tension on the donor musculotendinous unit and force greater tendon excursion to accomplish segmental motion.

It is important to note that the requirement for splinting during the postoperative phase of tendon transfers is variable, depending substantially on the specific transfer procedure used, the expertise of the surgeon, and the inherent adaptability of the patient. Many patients require only initial instruction at the time of dressing removal, readily accommodating to the altered kinetic and kinematic effects of the transfer procedure. This is particularly true in patients whose tendon transfers have been synergistic with wrist flexors used for finger extension and wrist extensors for finger flexion. Others, often with "out-of-phase" transfers, require considerable assistance in the form of splinting, exercise, and guidance to attain acceptable tendon transfer performance. Synergy, however, is not considered to be a major factor in choosing a muscle for transfer; the direction of pull of the transfer is far more important.

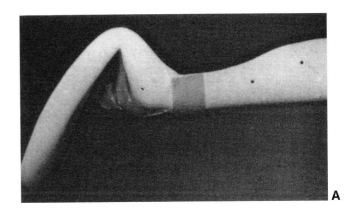

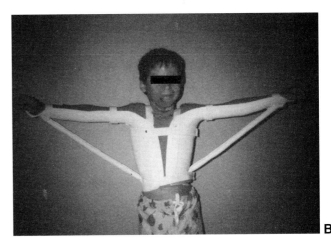

Fig. 15-25   A, Index–small finger MP flexion and IP extension, thumb CMC radial abduction and MP-IP extension mobilization splint, type 1 (16) B, Shoulder abduction and neutral rotation mobilization splint, type 3 (4); right \\ Shoulder abduction and neutral rotation mobilization splint, type 3 (4); left
A, MP flexion, IP extension of the digits, with thumb radial abduction and extension mobilization splints are frequently used during the early stages of burn, crush, or frostbite injuries. Splinting is critical to prevent unwanted deformity. B, Bilateral shoulder abduction and neutral rotation splints are fitted on this burn patient. [Courtesy (B) Indiana University School of Health and Rehabilitation Sciences, Department of Occupational Therapy, Indianapolis, Ind.]

Soft Tissue

Crush, Burn, and Cold Injuries

Although of dissimilar etiologies, extensive soft tissue damage resulting in crush, burn, and frostbite injuries often requires similar conservative treatment. Splinting requirements after these injuries depend on the site and extent of tissue damage. When a major portion of the hand is involved, early use of an anti-deformity or "safe position" splint (*finger MP flexion, IP extension immobilization splint*) alternated with exercise facilitates preservation of collateral ligament length by maintaining joint postures that place these ligaments at near-maximum tension (Fig. 15-25, A).*

---

*References 29, 53, 54, 98, 105, 106, 112.

Philosophies regarding optimum thumb position in a "safe position" splint differ. Full CMC thumb palmar abduction is advocated by some, whereas others prefer radial abduction. The key concept involved, however, is to maintain maximum passive range of motion at the first CMC joint and to adapt the splint to meet the individual requirements of the patient. To prevent the occurrence of additional arthrofibrotic changes in a hand already predisposed to swelling and stiffness, an immobilization splint must be accompanied by frequent periods of passive and active exercises to the wrist and digital joints. Shoulder, elbow, and forearm motion are also critical. The extent to which range of motion of these more proximal joints is emphasized depends on their direct and indirect involvement in the injury (Fig. 15-25, *B*). It is important to remember that more proximal normal joints can become stiff secondarily to more distal injuries. As the extent of the injury becomes more apparent and additional splinting is required to maintain passive motion of specific joints, an antideformity splint may be alternated with mobilization splints or used only at night in deference to daytime exercise and mobility splinting.

Splints fitted on extremities with soft tissue loss or damage must be altered at the design stage to adapt for the presence of surface defects, skin grafts, and draining areas. Underlying fractures are often present in this form of injury and protruding internal fixation wires may require adjustments in the basic splint design. To enhance cleanliness and decrease the chance of tissue maceration from the presence of excessive moisture, splints are fitted over several layers of light bandage. To ensure consistent and contiguous splint application, care must be taken to keep these dressings to a minimum. Padding is usually considered inappropriate in splints used on extremities that have sustained extensive soft tissue damage because it tends to become contaminated with tissue exudates. The use of wide straps or overlapping rolled gauze or elastic wrap diminishes the possibility of circumferential constriction with the resultant propagation of increased edema. Once healing has occurred, patients sometimes compain of cold intolerance or sensory dysesthesia. Soft splints and sensory reeducation programs may be beneficial in treating these patients (Fig. 15-26).

Dupuytren's

Preoperative splinting of Dupytren's contractures is generally considered to be ineffective and can on occasion, increase local inflammatory response.[1,87] In contrast, postoperative splinting is almost always recommended.* An active and passive exercise program

---

*References 33, 56, 64, 71, 78, 80.

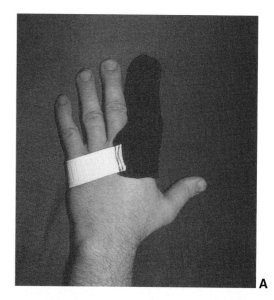
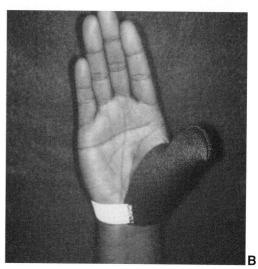

Fig. 15-26   A,B, Neoprene provides warmth and, therefore, comfort from the cold. Neoprene garments and splints may be custom fabricated using a sewing machine or, alternatively, using neoprene glue and iron on Velcro. A sewing machine may be helpful to further customize the neoprene garment. Because these neoprene sleeves are applied for warmth, they do not have expanded SCS classifications. (Courtesy Joni Armstrong, OTR, CHT, Bemidji, Minn.)

with extension immobilization splinting usually is initiated 24-72 hours after a subtotal palmar fasciotomy. Immobilization splinting is employed at this time due to the flexibility of the recently released palmar structures. Postoperative splints may be hand-based or they may include the wrist, depending on severity of involvement. Extension and/or flexion mobilization splinting may be initiated as needed to increase passive range of motion. Dupuytren's flare can occur between 4-6 weeks postoperatively. When this occurs,

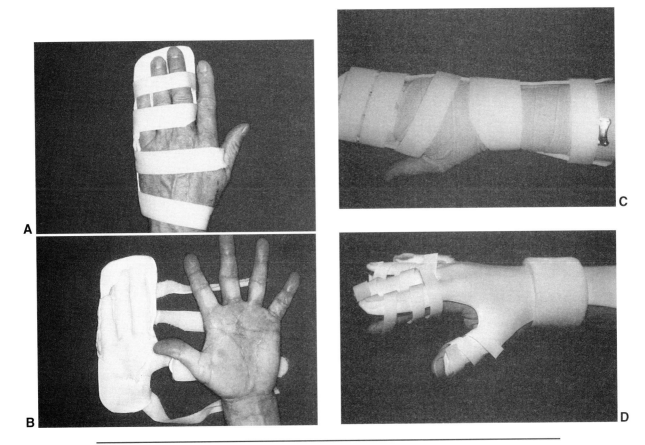

Fig. 15-27   A,B, Long–small finger extension mobilization splint, type 0 (9) C, Long–small finger extension mobilization splint, type 1 (10) D, Index–small finger extension, thumb CMC radial abduction and MP-IP extension mobilization splint, type 1 (16)
A, Post Dupuytren's release, an extension mobilization splint may include a Silastic insert (**B**) to minimize scarring. **C,** If full finger extension is difficult a design that includes the wrist increases the mechanical advantage of the splint. **D,** A dorsal extension mobilization splint provides an effective design for patients with sensitive or open palmar wounds. [Courtesy (**D**) Elizabeth Spencer Steffa, OTR/L, CHT, Seattle, Wash.]

the therapy program may need to be augmented and the surgeon may implement steroidal therapy. Careful documentation of range of motion and an emphasis on active motion are important elements toward identifying and preventing postoperative loss of active and/or passive joint motion. The program for the open palm technique differs only from the closed techniques with the addition of wound management until closure. Inelastic extension mobilization splinting is continued as needed during the healing phase between exercises and/or at night to maintain full digital extension (Fig. 15-27).

Nail Bed Repair

Nail bed injuries are among the most frequent hand injuries and often occur in conjunction with distal phalangeal fractures.[62,114-116] Initial treatment generally consists of protecting the fingertip with a *DIP extension immobilization splint, type 0 (1)* (Fig. 15-28, *A*). Once the nail bed wound is healed, a dorsally applied *nonarticular distal phalanx splint* may be applied at night to apply gentle pressure to aid in the flattening/remodeling nail bed scar tissue to minimize deformities of the fingernail as it regrows (Fig. 15-28, *B*). Periodic splint adjustments are necessary to accommodate changes in the developing nail.[17]

See Chapter 17, Splinting for Work, Sports, and the Performing Arts, for further information on splinting soft tissue sprains, strains, tears, and joint subluxations and dislocations. See Chapter 1, History of Splinting, for historical information about splinting thermal injuries.

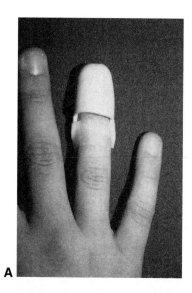

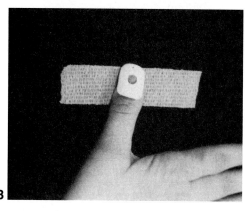

Fig. 15-28 **A, Ring finger DIP extension immobilization splint, type 0 (1) B, Nonarticular thumb distal phalanx splint**
A, Commonly referred to as a "tip protector," this splint shields the fingertip. **B,** Nail bed splints are used to influence tissue remodeling of the digital nail beds. These splints may be fabricated from thermoplastic or Silastic material and are secured with an elastic wrap or tape. The hole in the center of the splint anchors elastomer to the nail bed side of the splint.

Extensive Injuries to Multiple Structures
Ray Resection

Splinting post third or fourth digital ray resection without ray transposition is designed to protect the surgical reapproximation of the transverse intermetacarpal ligament of the digits adjacent to the excised metacarpal. Splint buttressing of this ligament reapproximation is accomplished by fitting a *nonarticular metacarpal splint* (Fig. 15-29) over the site of the ligament and around the remaining metacarpals. Resection of the second or fifth rays generally does not require protective splinting. Ray resection with accompanying metacarpal transposition requires protection of the osseous fixation site in addition to protection of the reapproximated transverse inter-

metacarpal ligament.[108] Splinting following this procedure is essentially similar to treating an openly reduced and fixated proximal metacarpal fracture with additional attention to the reapproximated transverse intermetacarpal ligament.[17]

Replantation/Free Tissue Transfer/Transplantation

Splinting programs employed with patients who have undergone replantation, free tissue transfer, or transplantation procedures emphasizes attainment and maintenance of motion in adjacent uninvolved joints and in the replanted segment.* Because of the obligatory immobilization of repaired structures to promote healing, the interval between the initiations of each type of splinting is often several weeks.

Depending on the level of severance, viability status of the replant or transplant, and size of the postoperative dressing, splinting and exercises may be carried out on joints not included in the dressing within the first postoperative week, provided that the mobilization does not stress repaired structures. Initiation of exercises to the replanted/transferred/transplanted part is determined by the particular operative procedures performed and the patient's status as he advances through the requisite physiologic stages of wound healing. It is imperative that splints and exercises appropriately correspond with the healing stages through which the patient progresses (e.g., early active or passive vs. active or passive). Close coordination between surgeon, therapist, and patient is essential, first toward preserving viability of the reattached/attached part and later toward achieving maximum patient rehabilitative potential.

With immobilization splints providing external support to internally fixated fractures and healing soft tissue structures, gentle mobilization traction designed according to individual requirements may be initiated. Because of lack of sensation and the potential damaging effect of edema, careful attention must be directed to obtaining a congruous splint fit that does not produce pressure, obstruct venous return, or impair arterial flow. Straps and splint components may be widened to alleviate undue pressure on underlying soft tissue (Fig. 15-30). Splints that apply small areas of three-point pressure or are circumferential in design are contraindicated during the early mobilization of a replanted segment. Careful monitoring of the replant is essential after splint application. An alteration of digital color or increase in edema of the replanted segment necessitates immediate removal of the splint. As the vascular status becomes less tenuous, its sensitivity to pressure decreases, allowing the use of more conventional splint designs.

*References 51, 56, 82, 84, 90, 113.

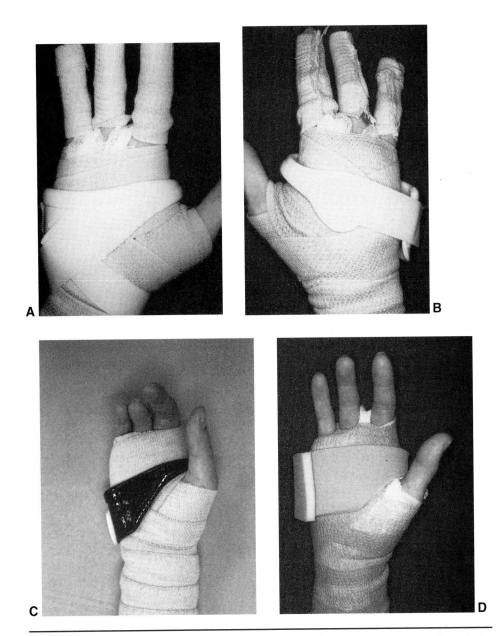

Fig. 15-29   A, Nonarticular metacarpal splint B, Nonarticular metacarpal splint C, Nonarticular metacarpal splint D, Nonarticular metacarpal splint

A, Along with a well-formed palmar bar supporting the transverse metacarpal arch, the radial and ulnar bars of this splint apply a gentle medially directed force to protect the healing transverse intermetacarpal ligament. **B,** As postoperative edema decreases the splint becomes loose and nonsupportive, necessitating periodic adjustments. **C,** Fabricating the splint in a thin, flexible thermoplastic material, rather than the standard $\frac{1}{8}$-inch rigid material, allows the patient to tighten the splint as needed in response to its loosening as edema decreases. **D,** Another splinting option includes use of a strap or an elastic wrap to provide support to the healing transverse intermetacarpal ligament. This option allows simple yet effective adjustments as edema decreases. Careful attention to fit is necessary to ensure that the transverse metacarpal arch is not flattened or exaggerated once the strap or elastic wrap is secured in place. Since the splint fits circumferentially, it is important to make certain that vascular structures are not compromised.

Amputation

Unfortunately, amputation of portions of a digit or hand may occur after severe injury. From both a psychological and functional standpoint, it is important that all efforts be devoted to rapidly restoring the amputation victim to a productive status.

Splinting a hand that has undergone amputation of a part may be directed toward (1) the maintenance of motion of uninvolved joints, (2) protective splinting to the area of amputation, and (3) functional splinting to improve prehensive patterns.[2,103,108] Emphasis is placed on prevention of adhesions and the return of

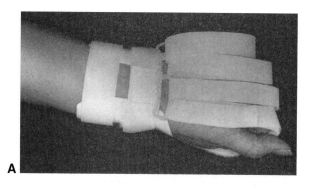

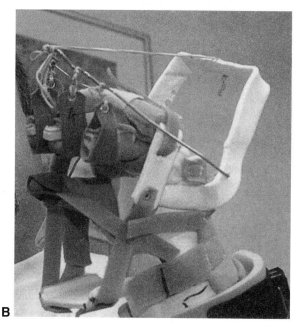

Fig. 15-30   A, Index–small finger flexion mobilization splint, type 1 (13) B, Wrist neutral immobilization / index–small finger MP extension restriction / index–small finger PIP extension, thumb CMC palmar abduction and MP-IP flexion mobilization splint, type 0 (16) \\ Finger DIP extension immobilization splint, type 0 (1); 4 splints @ finger separate

A, The wristband of this finger flexion splint has been widened to decrease pressure from the splint on the distal forearm. B, Used with the nation's first upper extremity transplant patient, this splint was designed to increase finger IP extension, and thumb palmar abduction and MP-IP flexion. The index–small finger DIPs are immobilized in extension with individual extension immobilization splints. [Courtesy (B) Jewish Hospital, Louisville, Ky.]

maximum function commensurate with the particular loss. The unnecessary stiffening of unaffected joints after amputation usually reflects a failure to establish motion programs at an early stage. The patient with an amputation is often reluctant to remove bandages and resume motion because of self-consciousness and fear of pain. The upper extremity specialist must be especially supportive, while reinforcing constantly the need to use the extremity and to resume social contacts.

Fingertip amputations are generally the most common kind of amputation seen in the therapy clinic. A tip protector may be needed along with wound management, exercises, and edema control (see Fig. 15-28, A). Stump wrapping to the digit and Silastic molds can improve the final cosmetic appearance and decrease stump hypersensitivity.

Amputation often results in generalized edema of the extremity, increasing the risk of stiffness in the remaining adjacent joints. Splinting therefore may be required to augment exercise programs. In the early postamputation phase, joints in adjacent digits readily respond to uncomplicated traction devices, such as wide rubber bands and glove rubber bands for flexion and three-point fixation splints for extension. Joints proximal to the site of amputation may be more resistant to the establishment and maintenance of good passive and active range of motion, requiring more complicated splints to attain an acceptable level of motion. To encourage early use of the hand in purposeful activity, a temporary splint may be designed to fit over the distal aspect of the remaining digit (Fig. 15-31, A-C). This prevents unintentional bumping of the tender stump and allows more uninhibited use of the hand as healing progresses. These splints are frequently fitted over dressings and should be removed during inactive periods for cleaning and to allow ventilation. Care should be taken to prevent wound maceration from an improper splint-wearing schedule and poor skin hygiene.

The potential for dependence on a protective splint should be acknowledged, and measures taken to gradually wean the patient from the splint as self-confidence increases and area sensitivity decreases. The initiation of a desensitization program is often instrumental in hastening unprotected hand use. Persistent hypersensitivity at the healed site of amputation may indicate unresolved problems such as retained terminal neuromas, and evaluation by a physician should be requested.

Functional splinting of a partially amputated hand permits accomplishment of special occupational tasks (Fig. 15-31). Splint design ranges from relatively simple to extremely complicated, depending on specific anatomic loss and patient requirements. Durability of the splint is often a key factor and may necessitate collaboration with an orthotist.

Individualized, beautifully made cosmetic prostheses are available for cosmetic coverage of digital, hand, and forearm amputations. Above-elbow and below-elbow amputees require evaluation and training with conventional functional body-powered or electric-powered prostheses.

It is important that an excellent rapport is established with the amputation patient. Initial education

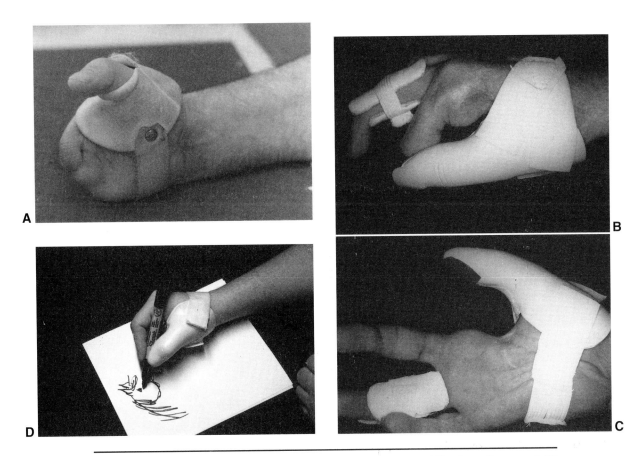

Fig. 15-31   A, Thumb CMC palmar abduction and MP extension mobilization splint, type 0 (2) B, Thumb MP-IP splint-prosthesis \\ Long finger PIP extension immobilization splint, type 0 (1) C, Thumb CMC circumduction / [thumb MP-IP flexion fixed] torque transmission splint-prosthesis, type 0 (1) D, Thumb CMC circumduction / [thumb MP-IP flexion fixed] torque transmission splint-prosthesis, type 0 (0) E, [Thumb CMC radial abduction, MP-IP flexion fixed] splint-prosthesis, type 0 (0) F, G, Index finger MP flexion immobilization / [index finger IP flexion, long–small finger flexion fixed] splint-prosthesis, type 0 (1) H, Wrist extension: [finger prosthesis flexion] / wrist flexion: [finger prosthesis extension] torque transmission splint-prosthesis, type 0 (1)

A, This thumb CMC mobilization splint helps prevent joint contracture and loss of thumb motion in a hand that has sustained a partial amputation. B,C, A nonskid thumb pad and simulated thumbnail increase functional prehension for this patient using his prototype thumb splint-prosthesis. Prototypes for prostheses may be fabricated in thermoplastic materials, allowing identification of optimal functional designs. D, This splint-prosthesis simulated a final prosthetic device and allowed the patient to perform daily tasks ensuring the final design would meet the patient's needs. E, Prosthetic thumb post provides a stable surface against which normal fingers can oppose for pinch and grasp activities. F,G, Provision of an adapted gripping surface against which the thumb may oppose allowed this patient to grasp and use a hammer. H, Because this man required splint durability that could not be attained with routine splinting materials, he was referred to an orthotist who specializes in metal hand braces. [Courtesy (A,E) Jolene Eastburn, OTR, Scranton, Pa.; (B-D) J. Robin Janson, MS, OTR, CHT, Indianapolis, Ind.; (F,G) Joan Farrell, OTR, Miami, Fla. (H) Lawrence Czap, OTR, Columbus, Ohio;]

for phantom sensation and nightmares is essential for every patient post-amputation. The loss of a body part is a severe psychological blow, regardless of the level, and the patient must be gently brought to understand the importance of accepting the loss and devoting efforts toward maintaining and restoring maximum function in the remaining hand. See Chapter 23, Splint Prostheses, for additional information.

USE OF PREFABRICATED COMMERCIAL SPLINTS

The same principles of mechanics, outriggers and mobilization assists, design, construction and fit that define custom-made splints must also be used to analyze prefabricated splints. Application of these principles is unconditionally fundamental to ensuring

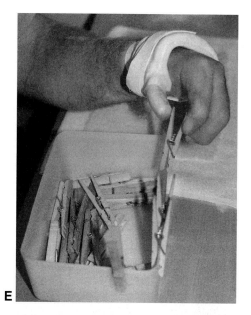

E

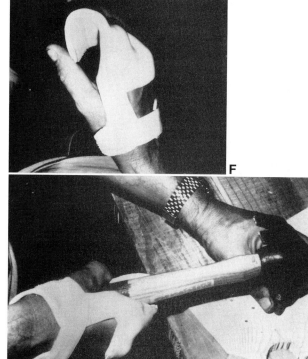

F

G

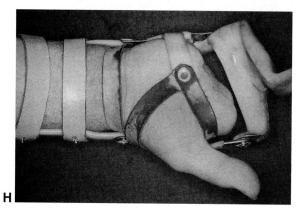

H

Fig. 15-31, cont'd
For legend see p. 431.

the effectiveness and safety of prefabricated splints as treatment modalities. Inattention to these time-honored splinting principles when applying any splint, whether custom or prefabricated, has considerable potential to cause patient harm.

Typically purchased through commercial vendors, prefabricated splints are premolded to "fit" various upper extremity sections/parts. These splints are available in a multiplicity of designs, according to mass-production standard sizes, in a variety of materials including low- and high-temperature thermoplastics, leather, vinyl, fabric, and neoprene. Prefabricated splints may be a splinting source for clinicians who are not proficient at custom splint fabrication and for experienced splint makers; in special circumstances, they may be more cost efficient than custom-fabricated splints. Because of these perceived advantages, prefabricated splints have found widespread use in clinical settings.

Some prefabricated splints permit minor adjustments to achieve better fit. For example, material may

be trimmed to clear flexion creases so long as splint fit and structural stability are not sacrificed. Metal stays in many prefabricated wrist immobilization splints do not fit the normal contour of the volar wrist and proximal palm and stays may not bend at the proper angle required for the diagnosis for which the splints are issued. To correct these problems, metal stays may be reformed or replaced with custom-fabricated low-temperature thermoplastic stays to achieve greater contiguous fit and proper wrist angle.

Appropriate selection between a custom and prefabricated splint is predicated on the complexity of patient-specific requirements. For example, prefabricated splints, when properly fitted, may be adequate for the conservative treatment of carpal tunnel syndrome. In contrast, custom-fitted splints are indicated for postoperative splinting of flexor tendon repairs where well-fitting splints that accurately position joints at precise angles are required. When choosing between a custom or prefabricated splint for a shoulder condition, after an analysis of the cost, time, and feasibility of fabrication, a properly fitted prefabricated shoulder splint may be the splint of choice simply because of the large physical mass and inherent strength requisites associated with an adult-size shoulder splint. However, if optimum fit and mechanics cannot be achieved with a prefabricated splint, its use is contraindicated. See Chapter 14, Splints Acting on the Elbow and Shoulder, for further information.

As emphasized in the introduction of this chapter, various splint configurations and designs may be appropriate for any given upper extremity condition. Once a splint's purpose and basic design have been determined, the next sequential phase is splint construction. It is at the construction stage that the pros and cons of custom-fabricated splints versus prefabricated splints may be analyzed as they relate to the patient-specific situation at hand. This is a critical decision as it entails profound consequences that will significantly influence the efficacy of the patient's rehabilitative course.

Deciding whether or not to use a prefabricated splint is dependent on fundamental questions that must be addressed with candor and unbiased analysis: (1) Does a prefabricated splint achieve the same purpose as a custom splint? (2) Does it meet the same standards of mechanics, outriggers and mobilization assists, design, and fit as a custom splint? (3) Will its produced outcome be as clinically effective as that of a custom splint? (4) Does it meet individual patient needs as well as a custom splint? (5) Is it as adjustable as is a custom splint, if adjustments are required? (6) In the long run, will it be as cost-effective as a custom splint? The ability of the patient to achieve maximum rehabilitation potential is always paramount. If the answer is "no" to any of the above questions, then use of a prefabricated splint is inappropriate.

The judicious use of prefabricated splints requires time to study the splints available on the market and to stay current with changing products.[50] Preliminary trial fittings with careful attention to detail help separate potentially useful splints from useless contraptions and cost analysis is a must. Prefabs are not indicated for every splinting situation, but they do provide additional choices when they fit properly. Remember, it may take longer to adjust a preformed splint properly than it would take to make and fit a custom splint from scratch, thus negating anticipated cost and time efficacy.

While many prefabricated splints can be stocked in the clinic in various sizes, other prefabricated commercial splints must be rented or purchased through medical supply companies that take care of paperwork (billing, etc.) and send a representative to fit the

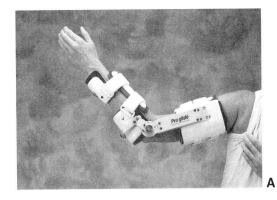

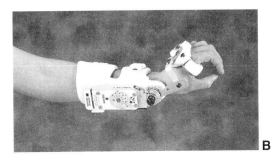

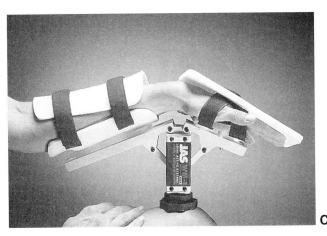

Fig. 15-32   A, Elbow extension mobilization splint, type 1 (2) B, Wrist extension mobilization splint, type 0 (1) C, Wrist flexion mobilization splint, type 5 (14)
Not limited to the illustrated examples, prefabricated wrist and elbow splints are available commercially in many designs. Special care is required to achieve correct alignment of joints and proper splint positioning. Splinting principles must be followed in fitting all prefabricated splints. [Courtesy (**A,B**) DeRoyal/LMB, Powell, Tenn.; (C) Joint Active Systems, Effingham, Ill.]

splints. These splints are typically more expensive, including CPMs and complicated mechanized wrist, elbow, and shoulder splints. The bottom line, however, is that patient care is the responsibility of the clinician, not the company representative. When a company representative fits a splint on your patient, it is essential that you, the therapist, evaluate and approve the fit (Fig. 15-32).

As noted above, a prefabricated splint, as with a custom splint, must meet exacting patient requisites according to the specific diagnosis for which it is applied. If a prefabricated splint fails to achieve required parameters, it is not a suitable treatment option regardless of how cost-effective or time saving it may be.

■ SUMMARY

One can see that special problems relating to upper extremity injury and disease and the appropriate surgical management of these conditions present somewhat predictable splinting requirements. Although broad generalization with regard to the splinting of these problems may be offered, it is obvious that wide variations occur in the clinical presentation of each problem and its therapeutic approach. Armed with an appreciation of the potential peculiarities of each of these general categories, one must become familiar with the individual circumstances and subsequently initiate the most applicable splinting and exercise program.

REFERENCES

1. Abbott K, Burke FD, McGrouther DA: A review of attitudes to splintage in Dupuytren's contracture, *J Hand Surg* [Br] 12(3):326-8, 1987.
2. Bennett JE: Skin and soft tissue injuries of the hand in children, *Pediatr Clin North Am* 22(2):443-9, 1975.
3. Blair WF, Steyers CM: Extensor tendon injuries, *Orthop Clin North Am* 23(1):141-8, 1992.
4. Blue AI, Spira M, Hardy SB: Repair of extensor tendon injuries of the hand, *Am J Surg* 132(1):128-32, 1976.
5. Bracker MD, Ralph LP: The numb arm and hand, *Am Fam Physician* 51(1):103-16, 1995.
6. Brand PW: The reconstruction of the hand in leprosy, *Ann Royal College of Surg* 11:350, 1952.
7. Brand PW: Rehabilitation of the hand with motor and sensory impairment, *Orthop Clin North Am* 4:1135-9, 1973.
8. Brand PW: *Clinical mechanics of the hand*, Mosby, 1985, St. Louis.
9. Brand PW, Hollister A: *Clinical mechanics of the hand*, ed 2, Mosby, 1993, St. Louis.
10. Brand PW, Hollister A: *Clinical mechanics of the hand*, ed 3, Mosby, 1999, St. Louis.
11. Brand PW, Hollister A: Operations to restore muscle balance to the hand. In Brand PW, Hollister A: *Clinical mechanics of the hand*, ed 3, Mosby, 1999, St. Louis.
12. Brooks G: *Exercise physiology: human bioenergetics and its applications*, ed 3, Mayfield Publishing, 2000, Mountain View, CA.
13. Browne EZ, Ribik CA: Early dynamic splinting for extensor tendon injuries, *J Hand Surg* [Am] 14(1):72-6, 1989.
14. Buch VI: Clinical and functional assessment of the hand after metacarpophalangeal capsulotomy, *Plast Reconstr Surg* 53(4):452-7, 1974.
15. Burke DT, Burke MA, Bell R, et al: Subjective swelling: a new sign for carpal tunnel syndrome, *Am J Phys Med Rehabil* 78(6):504-8, 1999.
16. Cannon N: Enhancing flexor tendon glide through tenolysis . . . and hand therapy, *J Hand Ther* 2(2):122-38, 1989.
17. Cannon N, et al: *Diagnosis and treatment manual for physicians and therapists*, ed 4, Hand Rehabilitation Center of Indiana, 2001, Indianapolis.
18. Chester DL, Beale S, Beveridge L, et al: A prospective, controlled, randomized trial comparing early active extension with passive extension using a dynamic splint in the rehabilitation of repaired extensor tendons, *J Hand Surg* [Br] 27(3):283-8, 2002.
19. Chow JA, Dovelle S, Thomes LJ, et al: A comparison of results of extensor tendon repair followed by early controlled mobilisation versus static immobilisation, *J Hand Surg* [Br] 14(1):18-20, 1989.
20. Chow JA, Thomes LJ, Dovelle S, et al: Controlled motion rehabilitation after flexor tendon repair and grafting. A multicentre study, *J Bone Joint Surg Br* 70(4):591-5, 1988.
21. Chowdhury SR, Chowdhury AK: Management of long standing post burn deformities of hand, *J Indian Med Assoc* 87(11):251-3, 1989.
22. Citron ND, Forster A: Dynamic splinting following flexor tendon repair, *J Hand Surg* [Br] 12(1):96-100, 1987.
23. Colditz JC: Splinting for radial nerve palsy, *J Hand Ther* 1(1):18-23, 1987.
24. Colditz JC: Preliminary report on a new technique for casting motion to mobilize stiffness in the hand. In Proceedings, American Society of Hand Therapists 22nd annual meeting, *J Hand Ther* 13(1):72-73, 2000.
25. Cooney W, Lin G, An KN: Improved tendon excursion following flexor tendon repair, *J Hand Ther* 2(2):102-6, 1989.
26. Curtin M: Development of a tetraplegic hand assessment and splinting protocol, *Paraplegia* 32(3):159-69, 1994.
27. de Jonge JJ, et al: Phalangeal fractures of the hand. An analysis of gender and age-related incidence and aetiology, *J Hand Surg* [Br] 19(2):168-70, 1994.
28. de Jonge JJ, Kingma J, van der Lei B, et al: Fractures of the metacarpals. A retrospective analysis of incidence and aetiology and a review of the English-language literature, *Injury* 25(6):365-9, 1994.
29. deLeeuw C: Personal communication from Carolina deLeeuw: fingernail hooks for positioning burned hands, E.E. Fess, Editor. 1963, deLeeuw, C.: Tacoma, WA.
30. Dillingham T, et al: Orthosis for the complete median and radial nerve-injured war casualty, *J Hand Ther* 5(4):212-5, 1992.
31. Duran R, Houser R: Controlled passive motion following flexor tendon repair in zones 2 and 3. In Hunter J, Schneider L: *American Academy of Orthopaedic Surgeons symposium on tendon surgery in the hand*, Mosby, 1975, St. Louis.
32. Duran R, et al: Management of flexor tendon lacerations in Zone 2 using controlled passive motion postoperatively. In Hunter J, Schneider L, Mackin E: *Tendon surgery in the hand*, Mosby, 1987, St. Louis.
33. Ebskov LB, et al: Results after surgery for severe Dupuytren's contracture: does a dynamic extension splint influence outcome? *Scand J Plast Reconstr Surg Hand Surg* 34(2):155-60, 2000.
34. Evans R: An analysis of factors that support the early active short arc motion of the repaired central slip, *J Hand Ther* 5(4):187-201, 1992.
35. Evans RB: Clinical application of controlled stress to the healing extensor tendon: a review of 112 cases, *Phys Ther* 69(12):1041-9, 1989.
36. Evans RB: Immediate active short arc motion following extensor tendon repair, *Hand Clin* 11(3):483-512, 1995.

37. Evans RB, Burkhalter WE: A study of the dynamic anatomy of extensor tendons and implications for treatment, *J Hand Surg* [Am] 11(5):774-9, 1986.
38. Evans RB, Thompson DE: The application of force to the healing tendon, *J Hand Ther* 6(4):266-84, 1993.
39. Eversmann WW: Compression and entrapment neuropathies of the upper extremity, *J Hand Surg* [Am] 8(5 Pt 2):759-66, 1983.
40. Fess EE: Splinting flexor tendon injuries, *Hand Surg* 7(1):101-8, 2002.
41. Formal CS, Cawley MF, Stiens SA: Spinal cord injury rehabilitation. 3. Functional outcomes, *Arch Phys Med Rehabil* 78(3 Suppl):S59-64, 1997.
42. Frykman GK, Waylett J: Rehabilitation of peripheral nerve injuries, *Orthop Clin North Am* 12(2):361-79, 1981.
43. Goloborod'ko S: Training splint for EIP to EPL transfer, *J Hand Ther* 10(1):48, 1997.
44. Gould JS, Nicholson BG: Capsulectomy of the metacarpophalangeal and proximal interphalangeal joints, *J Hand Surg* [Am] 4(5):482-6, 1979.
45. Gowitzke B, Milner M: *Understanding the scientific basis of human movement*, ed 2, Williams & Wilkins, 1984, Baltimore.
46. Gratton P: Early active mobilization after flexor tendon repairs, *J Hand Ther* 6(4):285-9, 1993.
47. Gustilo RB, Simpson L, Nixon R, et al: Analysis of 511 open fractures, *Clin Orthop* 66:148-54, 1969.
48. Hannah S, Hudak P: Splinting and radial nerve palsy: a single-subject design, *J Hand Ther* 14(3):216-8, 2001.
49. Harper B: The drop-out splint: an alternative to the conservative management of ulnar nerve intrapment at the elbow, *J Hand Ther* 3(4):199, 1990.
50. Harrell P: Splinting of the hand. In Robbins L, et al: *Clinical care in the rheumatic diseases*, American College of Rheumatology, 2001, Atlanta.
51. Hodges A, Chesher S, Feranda S: Hand transplantation: rehabilitation—a case report, *Microsurgery* 20:389-92, 2000.
52. Hunter JM, Singer DI, Jaeger SH, et al: Active tendon implants in flexor tendon reconstruction, *J Hand Surg* [Am] 13(6):849-59, 1988.
53. James JIP: Fractures of the proximal and middle phalanges of the fingers, *Acta Orthop Scand* 32:401-12, 1962.
54. James JIP: Common, simple errors in the management of hand injuries. In *Royal Society of Medicine*, Royal Society of Medicine, 1970.
55. Jansen C, Minerbo G: Comparison between early dynamically controlled mobilization and immobilization after flexor tendon repair in zone 2 of the hand, *J Hand Ther* 3(1):20-5, 1990.
56. Kasabian A, McCarthy J, Karp N: Use of a multiplanar distracter for the correction of a proximal interphalangeal joint contracture, *Ann Plast Surg* 40(4):378-81, 1998.
57. Kleinert HE, Kutz J, Cohen M: Primary repair of zone 2 flexor tendon lacerations. In Hunter J, Schneider L: *American Academy of Orthopaedic Surgeons symposium on tendon surgery in the hand*, Mosby, 1975, St. Louis.
58. Kleinert HE, et al: Primary repair of flexor tendons in no-man's land, *J Bone Joint Surg* 49A:577, 1967.
59. Konirova M, Sinkorova B: Early rehabilitation of the hands after the suture of flexors and after tendon grafts with the use of dynamic splints, *Acta Chir Plast* 37(2):58-9, 1995.
60. Krajnik SR, Bridle MJ: Hand splinting in quadriplegia: current practice, *Am J Occup Ther* 46(2):149-56, 1992.
61. Kruger VL, Kraft GH, Deitz JC, et al: Carpal tunnel syndrome: objective measures and splint use, *Arch Phys Med Rehabil* 72(7):517-20, 1991.
62. Lille S, Brown RE, Zook EE, et al: Free nonvascularized composite nail grafts: an institutional experience, *Plast Reconstr Surg* 105(7):2412-5, 2000.
63. Littler JW: Tendon transfers and arthrodesis in combined median and ulnar nerve paralysis, *J Bone Joint Surg* 31A:225-34, 1949.
64. Mackin EJ: Prevention of complications in hand therapy, *Hand Clin* 2(2):429-47, 1986.
65. Malick M, Meyer C: *Manual on management of the quadriplegic upper extremity*, Harmarville Rehabilitation Center, 1978, Pittsburgh.
66. Manente G, Torrieri F, Di Blasio F, et al: An innovative hand brace for carpal tunnel syndrome: a randomized controlled trial, *Muscle Nerve* 24(8):1020-5, 2001.
67. Mason ML: Injuries to nerves and tendons of the hand, *JAMA* 116(13):1375-97, 1941.
68. May EJ, Silfverskiold KL, Sollerman CJ: Controlled mobilization after flexor tendon repair in zone II: a prospective comparison of three methods, *J Hand Surg* [Am] 17(5):942-52, 1992.
69. Messer RS, Bankers RM: Evaluating and treating common upper extremity nerve compression and tendonitis syndromes...without becoming cumulatively traumatized, *Nurse Pract Forum* 6(3):152-66, 1995.
70. Moberg E: Surgical treatment for absent single-hand grip and elbow extension in quadriplegia. Principles and preliminary experience, *J Bone Joint Surg Am* 57(2):196-206, 1975.
71. Mullins PA: Postsurgical rehabilitation of Dupuytren's disease, *Hand Clin* 15(1):167-74, 1999.
72. Neviaser J: Splint for correction of claw hand, *J Bone Joint Surg* 12:440-3, 1930.
73. Nichols PJ, Peach SL, Haworth RJ, et al: The value of flexor hinge hand splints, *Prosthet Orthot Int* 2(2):86-94, 1978.
74. Opgrande JD, Westphal SA: Fractures of the hand, *Orthop Clin North Am* 14(4):779-92, 1983.
75. Parry W: *Rehabilitation of the hand*, ed 3, Butterworth, 1973, London.
76. Parry W: *Rehabilitation of the hand*, ed 4, Butterworth, 1981, London.
77. Peck F, et al: An audit of flexor tendon injuries in Zone II and its influence on management, *J Hand Ther* 9(4):306-8, 1996.
78. Peterson-Bethea D: Static progressive splint for Dupuytren's release, *J Hand Ther* 10(4):312, 1997.
79. Posner MA: Compressive neuropathies of the ulnar nerve at the elbow and wrist, *Instr Course Lect* 49:305-17, 2000.
80. Prosser R, Conolly WB: Complications following surgical treatment for Dupuytren's contracture, *J Hand Ther* 9(4):344-8, 1996.
81. Purcell T, Eadie PA, Murugan S, et al: Static splinting of extensor tendon repairs, *J Hand Surg* [Br] 25(2):180-2, 2000.
82. Robbins F, Reece T: Hand rehabilitation after great toe transfer for thumb reconstruction, *Arch Phys Med Rehabil* 66(2):109-12, 1985.
83. Sato Y, Kaji M, Tsuru T, et al: Carpal tunnel syndrome involving unaffected limbs of stroke patients, *Stroke* 30(2):414-8, 1999.
84. Scheker LR, Chesher SP, Netscher DT, et al: Functional results of dynamic splinting after transmetacarpal, wrist, and distal forearm replantation, *J Hand Surg* [Br] 20(5):584-90, 1995.
85. Schneider LH: Tenolysis and capsulectomy after hand fractures, *Clin Orthop* (327):72-8, 1996.
86. Schneider LH, McEntee P: Flexor tendon injuries. Treatment of the acute problem, *Hand Clin* 2(1):119-31, 1986.
87. Schultz-Johnson K: Static progressive splinting, *J Hand Ther* 15(2):163-78, 2002.

88. Silfverskiold KL, May EJ: Flexor tendon repair in zone II with a new suture technique and an early mobilization program combining passive and active flexion, *J Hand Surg* [Am] 19(1):53-60, 1994.

89. Silfverskiold KL, May EJ, Tornvall AH: Tendon excursions after flexor tendon repair in zone. II: Results with a new controlled-motion program, *J Hand Surg* [Am] 18(3):403-10, 1993.

90. Silverman P, Willett-Green V, Petrilli J: Early protective motion in digital revascularization and replantation, *J Hand Ther* 2(2):84-101, 1989.

91. Slater RR, Bynum DK: Simplified functional splinting after extensor tenorrhaphy, *J Hand Surg* [Am] 22(3):445-51, 1997.

92. Smith RJ: *Tendon transfers of the hand and forearm*, Little, Brown, 1987, New York.

93. Strickland JW: Biologic rationale, clinical application, and results of early motion following flexor tendon repair, *J Hand Ther* 2(2):71-83, 1989.

94. Strickland JW, et al: *Factors influencing digital performance following phalangeal fractures*, Presented at American Society for Surgery of the Hand, Annual Symposium 1979, San Francisco.

95. Strickland JW, Glogovac SV: Digital function following flexor tendon repair in Zone II: A comparison of immobilization and controlled passive motion techniques, *J Hand Surg* [Am] 5(6):537-43, 1980.

96. Strickland JW, Gettle K: Flexor tendon repair: the Indianapolis method. In Hunter J, Schneider L, Mackin E: *Tendon and nerve surgery in the hand: a third decade*, Mosby, 1997, St. Louis.

97. Stuart D, Zambia L: Duration of splinting after repair of extensor tendons in the hand, *J Bone Joint Surg* 47B:72-9, 1965.

98. Taams KO, Ash GJ, Johannes S: Maintaining the safe position in a palmar splint. The "double-T" plaster splint, *J Hand Surg* [Br] 21(3):396-9, 1996.

99. Tajima T: Indication and techniques for early postoperative motion after repair of digital flexor tendon pratically in zone II. In Hunter J, Schneider L, Mackin E: *Tendon and nerve surgery in the hand: a third decade*, Mosby, 1997, St. Louis.

100. Talbot JD, Villemure JG, Bushnell MC, et al: Evaluation of pain perception after anterior capsulotomy: a case report, *Somatosens Mot Res* 12(2):115-26, 1995.

101. Thomas D, Moutet F, Guinard D: Postoperative management of extensor tendon repairs in Zones V, VI, and VII, *J Hand Ther* 9(4):309-14, 1996.

102. Thomas FB: A splint for radial (musculospiral) nerve palsy, *J Bone Joint Surg* 26(July):602-5, 1944.

103. Upton J, Littler JW, Eaton RG: Primary care of the injured hand, part 1, *Postgrad Med* 66(2):115-22, 1979.

104. Verdugo RJ, et al: Surgical versus non-surgical treatment for carpal tunnel syndrome, *Cochrane Database Syst Rev* (2):CD001552, 2002.

105. Von Prince K, Yeakel M: *The splinting of burn patients*, Charles C. Thomas, 1974, Springfield, Ill.

106. Von Prince KM, Curreri PW, Pruitt BA: Application of fingernail hooks in splinting of burned hands, *Am J Occup Ther* 24(8):556-9, 1970.

107. Walker WC, Metzler M, Cifu DX, et al: Neutral wrist splinting in carpal tunnel syndrome: a comparison of night-only versus full-time wear instructions, *Arch Phys Med Rehabil* 81(4):424-9, 2000.

108. Ware LC: Digital amputation and ray resection. In *Hand rehabilitation: a practical guide*, Churchill Livingstone, 1998, London.

109. Weeks PM: Volar approach for metacarpophalangeal joint capsulotomy, *Plast Reconstr Surg* 46(5):473-6, 1970.

110. Weimer LH, et al: Serial studies of carpal tunnel syndrome during and after pregnancy, *Muscle Nerve* 25(6):914-7, 2002.

111. Whitley JM, McDonnell DE: Carpal tunnel syndrome. A guide to prompt intervention, *Postgrad Med* 97(1):89-92, 95-6, 1995.

112. Willis B: The use of orthoplast isoprene splints in the treatment of the acutely burned child: preliminary report, *AJOT* 23(1):57-61, 1969.

113. Wilson CS, Alpert BS, Buncke HJ, et al: Replantation of the upper extremity, *Clin Plast Surg* 10(1):85-101, 1983.

114. Zook EG: Nail bed injuries, *Hand Clin* 1(4):701-16, 1985.

115. Zook EG, Russell RC: Reconstruction of a functional and esthetic nail, *Hand Clin* 6(1):59-68, 1990.

116. Zook EG, Guy RJ, Russell RC: A study of nail bed injuries: causes, treatment, and prognosis, *J Hand Surg* [Am] 9(2):247-52, 1984.

SUGGESTED READING

Brand PW, Hollister A: *Clinical mechanics of the hand*, Mosby, ed 3, 1999, St. Louis.

Green DP, Hotchkiss R, Pederson W: *Operative hand surgery*, ed 4, London, 1998, Churchill Livingstone.

Mackin EJ, Callahan AD, Osterman AL, et al: *Hunter, Mackin & Callahan's rehabilitation of the hand and upper extremity*, ed 5, Mosby, 2002, St. Louis.

Omer G, Spinner M, Van Beek A: *Management of peripheral nerve problems*, ed 2, W. B. Saunders, 1998, Philadelphia.

Strickland JW, ed. *The hand*, Lippincott-Raven 1998, Philadelphia.

"MRS. GRAHAM, I THINK YOU'RE EXPECTING TOO MUCH FROM YOUR NEW JOINTS."

CHAPTER 16

Splinting for Patients with Rheumatoid Arthritis of the Hands and Wrists

GENERAL SPLINTING CONCEPTS

Pathomechanics

Before undertaking a splinting program with a patient with rheumatoid arthritis, the therapist must understand the pathomechanics of the disease process.

Rheumatoid arthritis is a chronic autoimmune disease that causes inflammation primarily in synovial tissue, often leading to tendon, ligament, and bone involvement.[2] The disease is usually polyarthritic, in that it affects multiple joints, and may have systemic manifestations. The course of the disease is unpredictable, but it is usually one of exacerbations and remissions. The small joints of the hands and feet are most commonly affected, often in a symmetrical pattern. Predominant signs and symptoms include joint swelling, inflammation, and stiffness. "The inflammatory sites are characterized by infiltration of activated lymphocytes and macrophages into the synovial membrane, and the proliferation of synovial cells. The local production of a number of cytokines by proliferative synovial cells as well as by infiltrating cells appears to account for many of the pathological and clinical manifestations in rheumatoid arthritis."[33] Associated systemic signs such as generalized malaise, fever, chills, fatigue, and anorexia may also be present. In severe cases there can be lung, heart, or vascular involvement.

Early involvement of the hands may show dorsal tenosynovitis of the wrist. The extensor tendons glide in synovial sheaths that extend approximately 1 cm above and 1 cm below the extensor retinaculum. Since rheumatoid arthritis involves synovial tissue, dorsal tenosynovitis follows this anatomic pattern.

In contrast, the flexor tendons glide in synovial sheaths at the wrist, palm, and digits and therefore may be affected in any of those areas. Volarly, tenosynovitis at the wrist may compress the median nerve, leading to carpal tunnel syndrome. When the palm and digits are involved, limited active motion or digital triggering or locking may result.

Swelling of the metacarpophalangeal joints is also a sign of early hand involvement. The proximal interphalangeal joints are characterized by fusiform swelling, pain, and limited motion. The distal interphalangeal joints are often not affected to the same extent as are the other joints of the hand, but frequently are involved secondary to musculotendinous imbalance, as seen in swan neck and boutonniere deformities.

In the normal hand there is a fine balance between the bony architecture, the capsuloligamentous system, and the muscle and tendon system. In rheumatoid arthritis both internal and external forces disrupt this intricate relationship. It should be remembered that all rheumatoid deformities originate either primarily or secondarily from the synovial hypertrophy that occurs within the joint. This synovitis may stretch out the capsuloligamentous system and invade the tendons that glide in synovial sheaths. This then leads to a compromise in the normal biomechanics of the hand and wrist. A musculotendinous imbalance occurs, as does a disruption of the normal bony archi-

tecture, due to stretching of the supporting soft tissue structures. Later erosive bone changes may occur. This leads to the deformities that are frequently seen in a patient with rheumatoid arthritis (Fig. 16-1, A,B).[28]

Deformities at the MP joints are usually manifested by palmar subluxation and increasing ulnar deviation (Fig. 16-1, C).[30] The metacarpophalangeal joints allow a wide range of motion and are subjected to greater stresses during functional activities. The extensor tendons are vulnerable to disruption and often sublux ulnarly into the valleys between the metacarpal heads. Forces generated by the flexor tendons during grip and pinch may cause stretching of the collateral ligaments and lead to an ulnar displacement of the flexor tendons. As the normal restraining mechanisms of the MP joints become attenuated, the intrinsic muscles are placed at a greater mechanical advantage and may become a deforming factor themselves. Normally when a fist is made, the metacarpal heads slope in an ulnar direction. As palmar subluxation and ulnar drift occur, use of the hand in daily activities continues to aggravate this situation. Other factors,

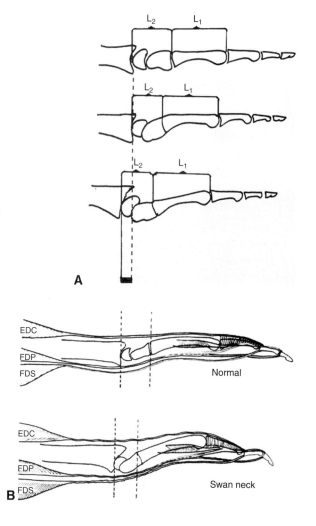

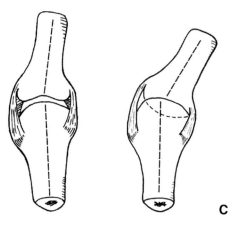

Fig. 16-1   A,B, Ligamentous attenuation from synovial inflammation compounded by contributions of cartilage thinning, carpal row positioning, and erosion alters the carpal/metacarpal ratio.[34] This causes volar, sagittal plane, subluxation of the wrist, which contributes to the deforming forces at the finger joints that result in a sagittal plane "zigzag" pattern of deformity. C, The MP joint normally exhibits a slight resting tendency toward ulnar deviation in the coronal plane (right MP joint, dorsal view). In the rheumatoid arthritic hand, the motion planes of MP volar subluxation and ulnar deviation become more pronounced, forming the wrist radial deviation and finger MP joint ulnar deviation "zigzag" pattern of deformity commonly exhibited in rheumatoid arthritic hands and wrists. [(A,B) from Shapiro JS: The wrist in rheumatoid arthritis, *Hand Clin* 12(3):480, 483, 1996; (C) from Stirrat CR: Metacarpophalangeal joints in rheumatoid arthritis of the hand, *Hand Clin* 12(3):516, 1996.]

including the condition of the wrist, may also affect ulnar deviation at the metacarpophalangeal joints. As the wrist shifts radially, associated metacarpophalangeal joint ulnar deviation occurs, resulting in the characteristic zigzag deformity. The distal radioulnar joint and the middle scaphoid are early sites for synovial involvement.

At the proximal interphalangeal joint level, synovitis of the joint leads to shortening of the collateral ligaments and stretching of the joint capsule and the central slip. This results in palmar displacement of the lateral bands and eventually leads to a boutonniere deformity, with flexion of the proximal interphalangeal joint and hypertension of the distal interphalangeal joint.

Swan neck deformity, which is characterized by hyperextension of the proximal interphalangeal joint and flexion of the distal interphalangeal joint, may have its origin at any of the three digital levels. It may begin when the metacarpophalangeal joints become involved and tight intrinsic muscles develop, leading to a musculotendinous imbalance. Swan neck deformity may also develop when the proximal interphalangeal joint becomes involved, stretching out the volar plate or causing the lateral bands to become stuck dorsally. Another cause of this deformity is a ruptured superficialis tendon. At the distal interphalangeal joint a mallet deformity may lead to an imbalance resulting in a swan neck deformity.

Wrist involvement in rheumatoid arthritis has a significant effect on overall hand and upper extremity function. Involvement is often seen early in the course of the disease and affects the radiocarpal, intercarpal, distal radioulnar, or any combination of these joints.

Indications for Splinting

The patient with rheumatoid arthritis presents numerous treatment challenges to the rehabilitation team.[3,23] Whether or not to splint is a major decision. A rheumatoid arthritic hand may be splinted for the following reasons: (1) to help decrease inflammation, (2) to rest and support weakened joint structures, (3) to properly position joints, (4) to help minimize joint contractures, or (5) to help improve function through better positioning of the joints.

Controversy, however, still surrounds this subject.[6,19] Most agree that splinting has a place, especially in the acute stage, in a total rehabilitation program for the person with rheumatoid arthritis. However, there are few documented or well-established indications for splinting the rheumatoid hand. Therefore, before any splinting program is undertaken for a patient with rheumatoid arthritis, a careful evaluation must be done to determine the feasibility and appropriate-

ness of splinting. This helps insure that each splint fabricated will then fit the individual needs of the patient. Patients with longstanding rheumatoid arthritis and those taking certain medications, such as corticosteroids, may have thin, delicate skin that bruises easily. In these cases special precautions need to be taken to prevent skin breakdown, and more frequent checks of the splint are necessary.

Alexander,[1] Feinberg,[9,10] Gault,[16] Mills,[24] Partridge,[26] Rotstein,[27] and Souter[29] have advocated a combination of hand splints and rest when the joints are inflamed. During periods of inflammation, the joints are more vulnerable to damage from both internal and external forces. Splinting has been noted to reduce pain and decrease inflammation and muscle spasm, thus reducing stress to the joints and allowing increased motion and function. A study by Zoeckler and Nicholas[36] showed that 63% of the patients who responded to their questionnaire found moderate or great relief from pain and morning stiffness by using splints.

Immobilization Splints

Immobilization splints, either for the whole hand or for the wrist, are often recommended for use during acute periods of inflammation. It is suggested that the splints be worn full time except for brief periods of gentle range of motion exercises and to perform necessary self-care tasks. As inflammation subsides, the splints are worn intermittently. The splints should be worn at night for several weeks after resolution of acute inflammation. If bilateral splints are necessary, alternating the use of each splint often seems more reasonable to the patient and leads to better acceptance and compliance. The patient's activities may be gradually increased as tolerated, and joint protection may be taught at this time. In cases where the metacarpophalangeal joints are involved, but the interphalangeal joints are not, a resting splint may be fabricated to include the MP joints while leaving the IP joints free (Fig. 16-2, A). This kind of splint may also be used as an exercise (torque transmission) splint for intrinsic lengthening. For this situation, the metacarpophalangeal joints are held in full extension to remodel intrinsics. The patient then puts the splint on for short periods of exercise several times during the day.

When positioning an arthritic hand in a wrist and hand immobilization splint, one should keep in mind the pathomechanics of the disease. The tendency, as previously mentioned, is for the metacarpophalangeal joints to sublux palmarly. Therefore the metacarpophalangeal joints should be held in about 25-30° of flexion to provide palmar support to those joints and surrounding soft tissue (Fig. 16-2, B,C). The proximal interphalangeal joints are then held in approximately

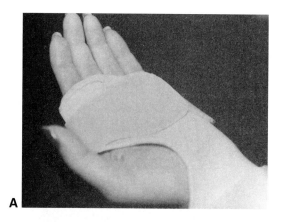

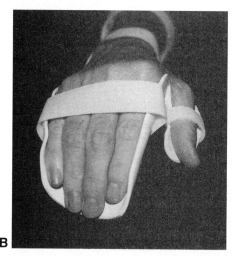

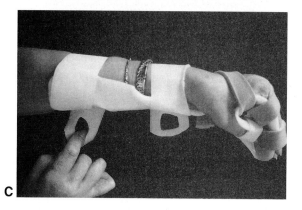

Fig. 16-2   A, Wrist neutral, index–small finger MP extension immobilization splint, type 0 (5) B, Wrist extension, index–small finger flexion, thumb CMC radial abduction and MP flexion, IP extension immobilization splint, type 0 (16) C, Wrist neutral, index–small finger flexion, thumb CMC palmar abduction and MP-IP flexion splint, type 0 (16)

A, A resting splint for the wrist and metacarpophalangeal joints. This splint may also be used as an exercise splint for the proximal interphalangeal joints. When used to increase range of motion at the IP joints, the purpose of this splint changes to an index-small finger IP extension and flexion torque transmission splint, type 2 (13). B, An immobilization splint positions wrist and hand during a period of acute inflammation. C, Adapted straps allow easy doffing and donning of immobilization splints.

30° of flexion. The wrist should, if possible, be positioned in neutral to 10° of dorsiflexion. Too much dorsiflexion increases pressure in the carpal tunnel and may lead to median nerve symptoms. This is especially significant if there is evidence of flexor tenosynovitis at the wrist, a frequent cause of median nerve compression in rheumatoid arthritis. When the thumb is included in the splint, it should be positioned in palmar abduction or slight radial abduction depending on individual circumstances.

The position for resting a rheumatoid hand is different from the "safe" or "antideformity" position for splinting an injured hand. After injury, the metacarpophalangeal joints are held in 70-90° of flexion with the interphalangeal joints in full extension to protect the collateral ligaments. A rheumatoid hand held in the "antideformity position" could increase palmar subluxation of the MP joints and stiffness of the PIP joints. Metacarpophalangeal and interphalangeal joints should be held in only slight flexion in the rheumatoid hand.

Mobilization Splints

Mobilization splints using elastic traction are used to minimize joint contractures, to position joints, or to aid in postoperative positioning. A study of elastic mobilization splinting in 51 nonsurgical rheumatoid arthritic patients done by Convery et al.[7,8] and Li-Tsang et al.[21] suggested that hand function was not improved and the progression of deformity was not uniformly prevented. They also found that correction of preexisting deformity was not achieved. The authors felt that there was a greater loss of motion than would have been expected if splints had not been used. Others, however, such as Granger,[17] Young,[35] and Swanson,[31] report that a well-designed and properly fitted mobilization splint may help in both preoperative and postoperative management. None suggests that an established deformity may be corrected by splinting. Flatt[15] stresses the necessity for gentle continuous pull and avoidance of sudden violent force on a joint when any mobilization splinting is used. Forceful manipulation may cause permanent damage to the joints and supporting structures already under stress from the disease process.

Postoperative Splinting

Another important use of splinting is in postoperative management where immobilization, mobilization, restriction, or torque transmission splints, or a combination thereof, may be used. For example, an immobilization splint to position the hand at night may supplement gains made with mobilization splinting. The type of splint design and its accompanying exercise program (Fig. 16-3) are determined by the

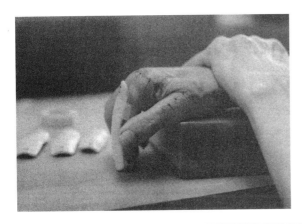

Fig. 16-3 Index finger MP extension and flexion torque transmission splint, type 2 (3)

Postoperative exercise programs are important for attaining active range of motion. Secondary immobilization of the index finger IP joints in slight flexion allows the effects of active extrinsic tendon glide to be concentrated on mobilizing the MP joint. (Courtesy Jolene Eastburn, OTR, Scranton, Pa.)

surgery performed and the status of the patient's soft tissue. Therefore good communication between the therapist and the physician is necessary to design the most effective splint.

Arthroplasty. In the postoperative management of metacarpophalangeal joint replacement arthroplasty, the purposes of elastic traction mobilization splinting are to maintain alignment of the joints and allow guarded motion while the new capsuloligamentous system is forming (Fig. 16-4, A-M).[20,22] Outrigger design in postoperative MP arthroplasty splints must be chosen with a thorough understanding of inherent mechanical effect. Because high-profile outriggers require patients to have less volitional strength to flex actively against extension mobilization assists than do low-profile outriggers, patients with weak finger flexion are able to more easily achieve desired active MP flexion range if they are placed in high-profile outrigger splints.[4,11-14,18] If finger flexion strength is not an issue, either high- or low-profile outrigger designs are appropriate so long as obligatory extension-radial deviation mobilizing forces are fully achieved. When using low-profile commercial outriggers, be certain that the angle of approach of the extension–radial deviation pull on the index MP joint is fully attained. Many prefabricated outriggers must be reshaped on the radial side to provide the correct angle of force application to the index MP joint. When success of arthroplasty procedures is defined by programmed joint encapsulation, no excuse exists for accepting less than the requisite angle of pull from an outrigger.

Postoperative MP arthroplasty splinting using a regimen that alternates two splints to mobilize the MP

joints first into extension and then into flexion is also becoming more widely practiced. Although these splints possess no moving parts, they are classified as mobilization splints because their purposes are to move the MP joints into extension and flexion.[5]

Index finger supination mobilization assists may be applied according to one of two general formats. As with outrigger design, choice of a supinator component for the index finger depends on mechanical concepts. A mobilization assist that attaches to the index fingernail and wraps around the distal phalanx to pull the finger into supination affects capsule remodeling while the index finger is in extension. Because this type of "passive" supinator relies on a small moment arm to effect proximal phalanx rotation, the mobilization assist is often inelastic, and is unhooked for exercise sessions (Fig. 16-4, N-O). In contrast, an "active" supinator requires flexion of the index PIP joint to achieve supination of the index finger. With this supinator design, as active PIP flexion increases to 90°, the rotational moment arm on the proximal phalanx lengthens, providing strong rotational torque to the index MP joint. Characterized by a shorter radial outrigger that ends at the level of the PIP joint, an "active" supinator requires very minimal mobilization assist tension because of the long moment arm created upon active PIP flexion (Fig. 16-4, P). If mobilization assist force of an "active" supinator is too aggressive, damaging torque may be applied to the MP joint, resulting in unwarranted attenuation of healing ulnar capsular structures.

When a wrist arthroplasty is done, the goals of the surgery are to provide a stable, pain-free wrist with about a 50° arc of motion. Therefore the wrist is placed in an immobilization splint for 4 to 6 weeks. In some cases a controlled *mobilization / restriction splint* is used after the removal of the immobilization splint (Fig. 16-5). It is recommended that the patient always wear a wrist immobilization splint for protection when performing heavier tasks.

Tendon reconstruction. Following surgery for correction of a boutonniere deformity, immobilization splinting is used. The length of immobilization depends on the exact nature of the surgery performed. When motion is started, the immobilization splint is usually worn between exercise sessions for a period of time until the soft tissue has stabilized. Mobilization splinting may be introduced as an adjunct to immobilization splinting. The patient may then progress to daytime intermittent mobilization splinting and night immobilization splinting. A long-term splinting and exercise program may be necessary to prevent recurrent deformity.

Tendon ruptures are a frequent complication of rheumatoid disease. Extensor tendons rupture more

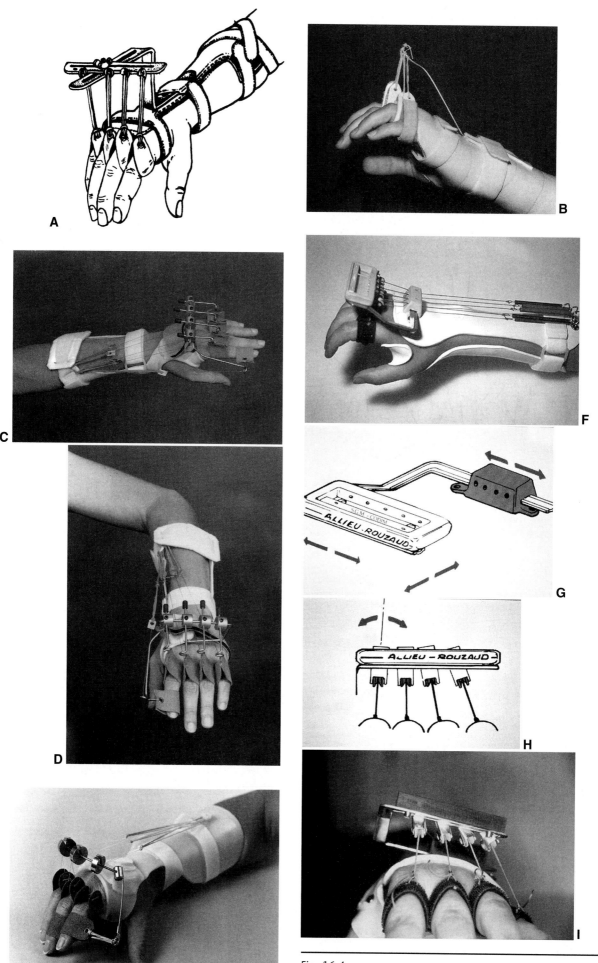

Fig. 16-4
For legend see p. 443.

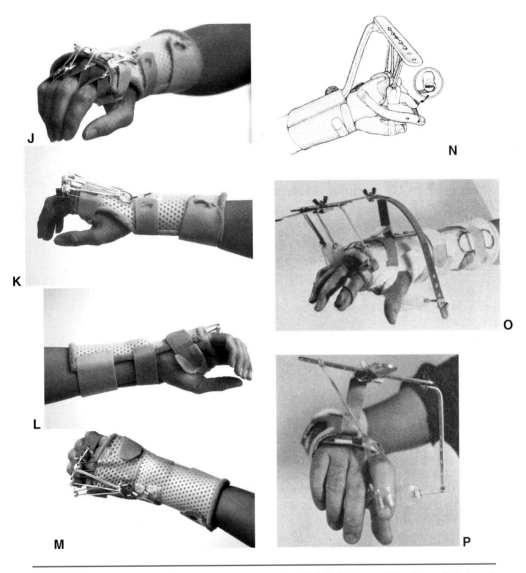

Fig. 16-4   A, Index–small finger MP extension and radial deviation mobilization splint, type 1 (5) B, Index–small finger MP extension and radial deviation mobilization splint, type 1 (5) C,D, Index–small finger MP extension and radial deviation, index finger MP supination mobilization splint, type 3 (7) E, Index–ring finger MP extension and radial deviation, index–long finger MP supination mobilization splint, type 3 (8) F, Index–small finger MP extension and radial deviation mobilization splint, type 3 (7) I, Index–small finger MP extension and radial deviation mobilization splint, type 1 (5) J-M, Index–small finger MP extension and radial deviation mobilization splint, type 1 (5) N, Index–small finger MP extension and radial deviation, index finger MP supination mobilization / thumb CMC radial abduction and MP–IP flexion immobilization splint, type 3 (10) O, Index–small finger MP extension and radial deviation, index finger MP supination, thumb CMC radial abduction and MP extension mobilization splint, type 3 (9) P, Index finger MP supination mobilization splint, type 3 (4)

Postoperative mobilization splints for MP joint replacement arthroplasties vary in design. These splints maintain proper alignment of the MP joints and allow guarded motion while a new capsuloligamentous system is forming. Various outrigger designs permit individual positioning of MP joints into required increments of extension and radial deviation. A, Mobilization assist radial extension may be accomplished through progressively longer rubber bands attached to a stationary radially placed extension outrigger (B) or through adjustable outriggers (C-O). Depending on the extent of surgical repair, flexion mobilization assists may also be directed radially to further reinforce development of a tight radial joint capsule (not shown). A supination outrigger with a Velcro fingernail attachment device, (N) a serpentine supination splint (O), or a two-sling force couple (P) protects the surgical repair to the index or other fingers to minimize pronation deformity. [Courtesy (A,O,P) from Swanson AB, Swanson GG, Leonard J: Postoperative rehabilitation program in flexible implant arthroplasty of the digits. In Hunter JM, et al: *Rehabilitation of the hand*, ed 2, Mosby, 1984, St. Louis; (C,D) Barbara (Allen) Smith, OTR, Edmond, Okla.; (E) Helen Marx, OTR, CHT, Human Factors Engineering of Phoenix, Wickenburg, Ariz.; (F-I) Jean Claude Rouzaud, Montpellier, France; (J-M) Margareta Persson, PT, Uppsala, Sweden.]

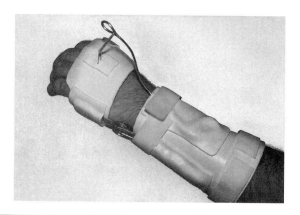

Fig. 16-5 **Wrist extension mobilization / wrist radial and ulnar deviation restriction splint, type 0 (1)**
A controlled wrist mobilization / restriction splint is used to allow protected wrist motion following removal of the immobilization splints when a wrist arthroplasty has been performed.

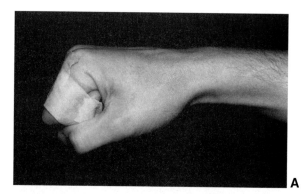

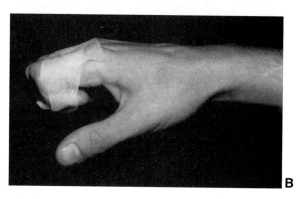

Fig. 16-6 Taping exercise has been found helpful after tendon transfer to transmit torque by isolating the long extensors. **A,** In flexion. **B,** In extension.

frequently than do the flexor tendons. Tendons rupture through attrition caused by the tendon rubbing on a bony spur, through direct synovial invasion into the tendon, and through pressure of the hypertrophied synovium on the tendons. It is often not possible to do an end-to-end repair of the tendons, since patients often do not seek immediate medical attention after tendon rupture. Also, the condition of soft tissue may be poor. Therefore tendon transfer is frequently undertaken to restore function.

When tendon transfers have been performed for extensor tendon ruptures, immobilization splinting with the metacarpophalangeal joints in extension is used for the first 3 weeks to support the wrist and MP joints while the transfer heals. Later in the rehabilitation program a mobilization splint for extension may be used if the patient cannot obtain adequate extension. A helpful exercise in rehabilitating a patient who has undergone tendon transfer is to tape the interphalangeal joints into a claw-like position to transmit torque to the MP joints by isolating the long extensors. The patient then flexes and extends the MP joints with the fingers held in this position (Fig. 16-6). Practice is important, and the patient needs to be aware that several months of rehabilitation may be required to optimize a functional recovery. The number of tendon ruptures and the condition of the soft tissue determine the outcome of tendon transfers.

Splinting to Enhance Function

Functional splints for the person with rheumatoid arthritis help a patient who is having difficulty with daily tasks perform with more ease and safety. From time to time functional splints are used instead of surgery for patients who, for one reason or another, are not surgical candidates. When assessing a patient

for a functional splint, it is important to remember that the degree of deformity does not always correlate with loss of function.

Wrist. The wrist is often a source of pain that interferes with a person's functioning. This is usually manifested in decreased grip strength and inability to perform many routine activities. A *wrist immobilization splint* supports the wrist, often increases grip strength, and allows an improvement in activities of daily living by relieving wrist pain (Fig. 16-7).

Fingers. A common problem seen in rheumatoid arthritis is ulnar deviation of the metacarpophalangeal joints. This may not necessarily cause functional loss and does not routinely require splinting. In some cases, though, a patient may express a need to have a splint to continue with certain activities. Some patients lose dexterity due to inability to effectively position thumb, index, and midfingers for pinch. In these cases, either an immobilization, mobilization, restriction, or torque transmission splint to help position the MP joints may benefit the patient (Fig. 16-8, *A-G*). The design should fulfill individual patient requirements. The splint should provide palmar support to the metacarpophalangeal joints, since palmar subluxation is often a component of ulnar drift (Fig. 16-8, *C,D*). Commercial splints are also available

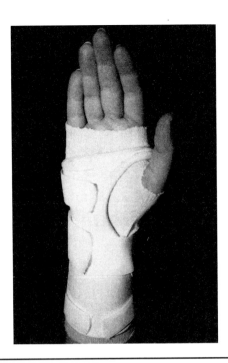

Fig. 16-7   **Wrist extension immobilization splint, type 0 (1)**
A wrist immobilization splint is used to aid function and protect the wrist.

in various designs (Fig. 16-8, *E-G*). It is unrealistic, however, to expect these splints to correct ulnar deviation of the MP joints. This needs to be explained to the patient before the splint is made.

Immobilization, mobilization, restriction, or torque transmission splints that control unwanted motion at the PIP joints may increase hand function by positioning fingers in more advantageous postures that facilitate hand dexterity and coordination. Although not appropriate for correcting fixed PIP joint deformities, many of these splints are designed to correct PIP joint swan neck or boutonniere deformities that are passively supple (Fig. 16-9, *A,D*).

It is important to remember that deformities resulting from rheumatoid arthritis are usually insidious in onset, allowing gradual patient adaptation and retention of surprisingly good levels of functional capacity. When corrective splints are applied, they may actually impair hand dexterity rather than improve it due to the sudden postural change of the digits. Both therapist and patient must understand that, if good splint-wearing compliance is to be achieved, a splint must provide bona fide functional improvement, not just cosmetic realignment of joints. A quick functional dexterity test such as the Jebsen Hand Dexterity Test, the Flinn Performance Screening Test, or the Minnesota Rate of Manipulation Test given pre- and post-splint application provides valuable insight into the true usefulness of splints designed to increase function by improving passive joint alignment at the MP and/or PIP joints.

Thumb. When the thumb becomes involved in the rheumatoid process, the function of the hand is often significantly compromised.[32] This is especially true with activities requiring fine manipulation. Thumb deformities in rheumatoid arthritis have been classified by Nalebuff.*[25]

Type I deformity has its origin at the metacarpophalangeal joint and is characterized by MP joint flexion and IP joint hyperextension. This deformity is further accentuated by normal pinch forces in daily activities. This deformity may be referred to as an extrinsic minus deformity, since there is a loss of extrinsic extensor power at the metacarpophalangeal joint level.

Type II deformity has its origin at the carpometacarpal joint and is characterized by the flexion at the MP joint and hyperextension at the IP joint. It looks similar to the type I deformity except that adduction of the metacarpophalangeal joint occurs due to contracture of the adductor pollicis.

Type III deformity follows the same pattern as type II except that it is characterized by hyperextension of the MP joint and flexion of the IP joint. This deformity also has metacarpophalangeal joint adduction.

Type IV deformity is the result of stretching or rupture of the ulnar collateral ligament. The proximal phalanx deviates laterally at the MP joint with the

---

*Nalebuff's thumb deformity classifications are *not* related to the expanded Splint Classification System's "type" nomenclature.

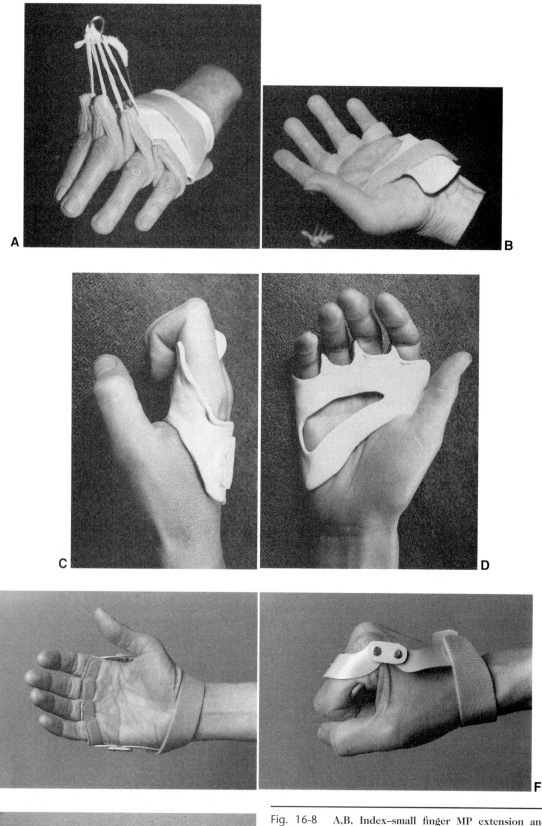

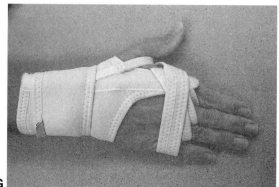

Fig. 16-8   A,B, Index–small finger MP extension and radial deviation mobilization splint, type 0 (1) C,D, Index–small finger MP flexion and ulnar deviation restriction splint, type 0 (4) E,F, Index–small finger MP ulnar deviation restriction splint, type 0 (4) G, Index–small finger MP ulnar deviation restriction splint, type 1 (5)

A small hand-based MP extension radial deviation splint is helpful in increasing function when ulnar deviation is present. A, Dorsal aspect of splint. B, Volar aspect of splint. C,D, This MP ulnar deviation restriction splint also limits MP flexion. E,F, The innovative hinge on this MP restriction splint allows MP flexion and extension while preventing ulnar deviation. G, This commercially available splint provides MP ulnar deviation restriction. [Courtesy (C,D) KP MacBain, OTR, Vancouver, BC; (E,F) Julie Belkin, OTR, CO, MBA, 3-Point Products, Annapolis, Md.]

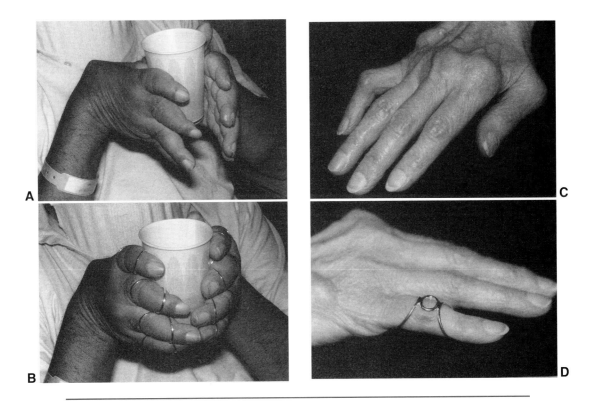

Fig. 16-9   B, Finger PIP extension restriction splint, type 0 (1); 4 splints @ finger separate; left \\ Finger PIP extension restriction splint, type 0 (1); 4 splints @ finger separate; right D, Small finger PIP extension mobilization splint, type 0 (1)
A,B, Enhancing functional hand use, these splints prevent PIP hyperextension, swan neck deformity at the PIP joints. C,D, A passively supple boutonniere deformity is corrected with this simple, commercially available splint. [Courtesy (A-D) Cindy Garris, OTR, Silver Ring Splint Company, Charlottesville, Va.]

first metacarpal secondarily assuming an adducted position.

In type V deformity, the major deforming factor is an attenuated palmar plate of the metacarpophalangeal joint. The metacarpophalangeal joint becomes hyperextended and the distal joint assumes a flexed position. Unlike the type III deformity, the metacarpal does not become adducted.

Type VI deformity is distinguished by collapse and loss of bone. Patients with this deformity demonstrate thumbs that are short and often unstable. Although this deformity is specific to the thumb, it is most often associated with similar problems of the other digits.

As in all rheumatoid deformities, these thumb deformities are the results of muscle and tendon imbalance occurring between the joints of the thumb ray. In each case the alteration of posture at one joint influences the posture at adjacent joints.

Splinting may have particular value for the thumb, both for function, by stabilizing the joints, and in postoperative care. In the postoperative phase of thumb reconstruction, extended periods of splinting are necessary to ensure stability for effective pinch.

When the carpometacarpal joint becomes involved, the synovitis stretches out the joint capsule, leading to joint subluxation or dislocation. The metacarpal often assumes an adducted position. Rehabilitation goals at this point are to prevent an adduction contracture and to maintain a functional range of motion. A *type 2 thumb CMC immobilization splint* may be fabricated to protect and stabilize the CMC joint and maintain the first web space (Fig. 16-10). The thumb MP and wrist are included in this splint as secondary joints. The splint should extend two-thirds up the forearm and distally to the interphalangeal joint crease. The IP joint should be left free to move. A *type 1 thumb CMC immobilization splint*, where the MP joint is the sole secondary joint, is sometimes made for this problem, but in many cases this proves ineffective. The *type 1* splint often does not provide the needed support when the carpometacarpal joint is involved. A *type 2* splint that includes the wrist and MP as secondary joints ensures good CMC joint protection while helping to maintain the thumb metacarpal in the corrected position. Patients generally wear this splint during the day when performing functional activities and at night for

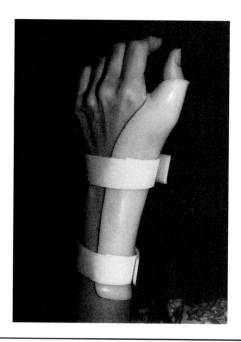

Fig. 16-10 **Thumb CMC palmar abduction immobilization splint, type 2 (3)**
This thumb splint protects the carpometacarpal joint, relieves pain, and improves thumb function.

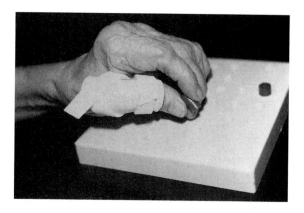

Fig. 16-11 **Thumb MP flexion immobilization splint, type 0 (1)**
Designed to support the metacarpophalangeal joint of the thumb, this splint enhances functional use of the thumb.

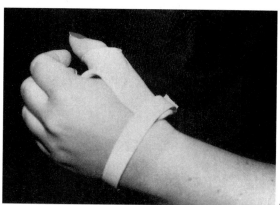

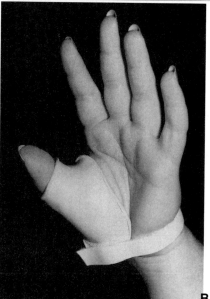

Fig. 16-12 **A,B, humb MP extension immobilization splint, type 1 (2)**
The metacarpophalangeal joint of the thumb is protected in this immobilization splint. **A,** Dorsal aspect of splint. **B,** Volar aspect of splint.

positioning. Patients should be instructed to remove the splint several times a day to perform light range of motion exercises.

When the thumb metacarpophalangeal joint is involved, the goals are to prevent the deformity from becoming fixed, to improve function, and to help protect the joint from external forces that could produce further joint damage and deformity. One way to accomplish this is to use a small splint that will protect the metacarpal joint. In this case, neither the carpometacarpal nor the interphalangeal joints need to be immobilized. The exception to this is if there is also deformity or involvement at the adjacent joints. The MP joint may be immobilized with a small aluminum and foam splint or a splint made from thermoplastic (Figs. 16-11, 16-12). Immobilizing the metacarpophalangeal joint often improves function by providing a more stable base for pinching, and protecting the joint from external forces. The interphalangeal joint also may be controlled with the use of a *type 1 thumb immobilization splint* of aluminum and foam (Fig. 16-13, *A*) or thermoplastic, providing both stability and protection of this joint. If IP joint hyperextension is problematic, a *type 1 thumb IP extension restriction splint* may suffice (Fig. 16-13, *B*). Continued pinching activities may lead to stretching of the supporting soft tissue, leaving the joint unstable and pinching difficult. If the joint becomes unstable, splinting may improve the patient's functional level.

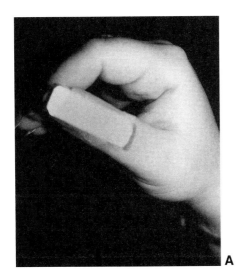

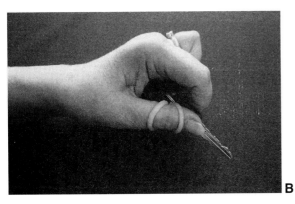

Fig. 16-13   A, Thumb IP extension immobilization splint, type 0 (1) B, Thumb IP extension restriction splint, type 0 (1)
Both these splints provide extension stability to the thumb IP joint through either immobilization (**A**) or restriction (**B**) of IP joint motion.

Postoperative immobilization of the thumb is maintained for approximately 4 to 6 weeks to ensure good capsular healing and joint stability. During the immobilization period, the patient should be encouraged to perform range of motion of the fingers several times a day to prevent stiffness. After discontinuation of splinting, therapy is directed toward functional use of the thumb. The goal of the therapy program is to obtain a stable, pain-free, functional pinch.

Once a splint has been made, it is necessary to monitor the patient periodically for proper fit and any change in status. When embarking on a functional splinting program for a patient with rheumatoid arthritis, it is important to remember that splinting one area places more stress on adjacent areas. Therefore the patient should be monitored for signs of inflammation in surrounding joints. Because the patient does have a chronic disease, splints are used

for a long time and will need adjustments or replacement from time to time. Because the disease is unpredictable, the patient's needs often change and should be reassessed. Splinting should be only a part of a well-coordinated rehabilitation program.

CASE STUDY*

The subject is a 62-year-old female who developed rheumatoid arthritis (RA) at the age of 27. Pain and progressive digital instability compelled her to give up her practice as a dental hygienist and begin teaching as a university professor. Over the years, progressive bilateral hand involvement forced the subject to relinquish activities such as playing the piano, typing fluently on a keyboard, manipulating small objects (e.g., jewelry), and grasping large objects unilaterally (e.g., drinking glasses). The subject consulted an experienced hand surgeon, and bilateral reconstructive surgery was recommended to improve hand function and decrease pain. She opted to have the nondominant, left hand reconstructed first (Fig. 16-14).

Prior to surgery, two different splints were fitted to the subject's left thumb to determine which positional splint was most functional (Fig. 16-15, *A-D*).

Multiple complex deformities of the left thumb and fingers (Table 16-1) required careful preoperative planning to provide the best potential for postoperative hand function (Fig. 16-16, *A,B*). Surgical procedures to the left digits included arthrodeses, replacement MP arthroplasties, extensor revision and tenotomy, and a capsulodesis (Table 16-2).

TABLE 16-1	Indications for Surgical Reconstruction, Nondominant Left Hand
Thumb	MP and IP joint instability
	IP joint hyperextension deformity
Index finger	MP joint subluxation and destruction
Long finger	MP joint subluxation and destruction
	PIP joint extension lag
Ring finger	MP joint subluxation and destruction
	PIP joint fixed flexion deformity, joint destruction
	DIP joint hyperextension deformity, joint destruction
Small finger	MP joint subluxation and destruction
	PIP joint fixed flexion deformity, joint destruction
	DIP joint hyperextension deformity, joint destruction

*The authors express their gratitude to James W. Strickland, MD, and K. E. Gable, EdD, for their invaluable and generous assistance in preparing this case study.

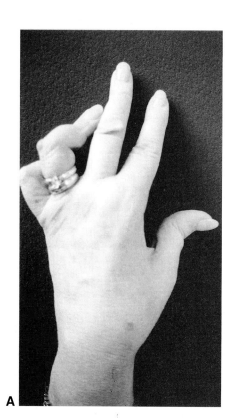

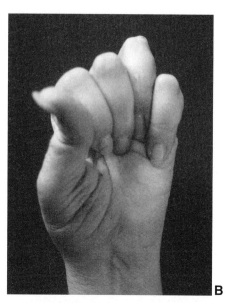

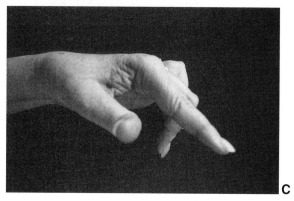

Fig. 16-14   Preoperative thumb and finger deformities resulting from rheumatoid arthritis. A, Left hand. B, Preoperative flexion and C, Preoperative extension of fingers.

TABLE 16-2	Surgical Reconstruction Procedures, Nondominant Left Hand
Thumb	MP arthrodesis
	IP flexion capsulodesis
Index finger	MP replacement arthroplasty
Long finger	MP replacement arthroplasty
	Extensor tendon revision of PIP with tenotomy of terminal extensor tendon
Ring finger	MP replacement arthroplasty
	PIP arthrodesis
	DIP arthrodesis
Small finger	MP replacement arthroplasty
	PIP arthrodesis
	DIP arthrodesis

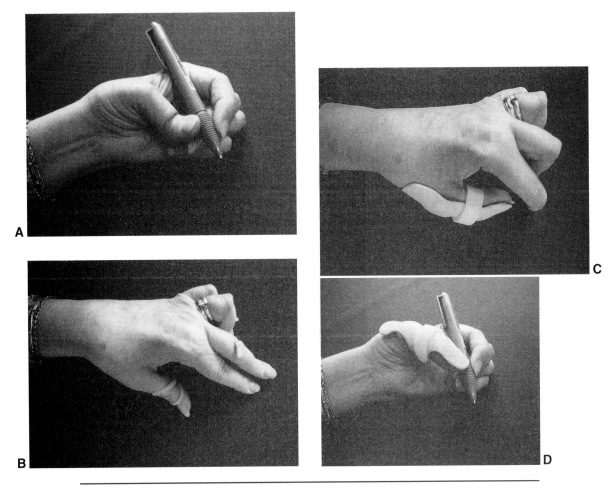

Fig. 16-15   B, Thumb IP extension restriction splint, type 0 (1) C,D, Thumb IP extension restriction splint, type 1 (2)

B,C, Trials using two separate splint designs, with different type classifications, to restrict IP extension were carried out to determine which design afforded the best function. **A,** Without splinting, the thumb collapsed into MP flexion and IP hyperextension during pinch, resulting in poor prehension. Subject preferred the *type 1* splint design due to the added stabilization **(C)** and positioning **(D)** of the thumb MP joint, which allowed the pulp of the thumb to contact objects rather than the ulnar aspect of the thumb IP joint and distal phalanx provided by the *type 0* splint design **(B).**

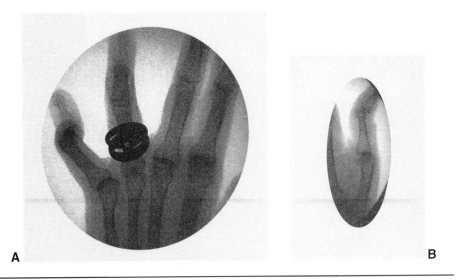

Fig. 16-16   Preoperative fluoroscans of left fingers (A) and thumb (B).

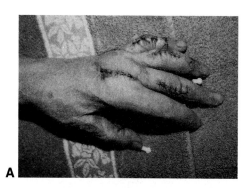

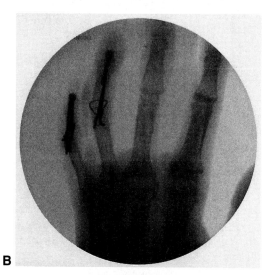

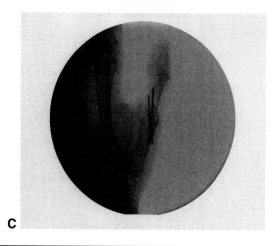

Fig. 16-17   A, Appearance of left hand following removal of bulky dressing. B, Postoperative fluoroscans of fingers with MP replacement arthroplasties and arthrodesis hardware in ring and small fingers (**B**) and thumb (**C**).

Therapy was initiated on the 12th postoperative day following removal of the bulky dressing (Fig. 16-17, A-C). In addition to exercise, edema control, and implementation of one-handed ADL and vocational compensatory strategies, splinting was an integral part

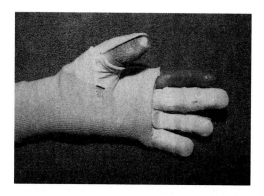

Fig. 16-18   Thumb MP flexion immobilization / IP extension restriction splint, type 0 (2) \\ Long finger PIP extension immobilization splint, type 1 (2) \\ Ring finger IP flexion immobilization splint, type 0 (2) \\ Small finger IP flexion immobilization splint, type 0 (2)
(Radial to ulnar), the thumb splint protects MP arthrodesis and prevents IP extension, to avoid stretching of volar IP capsulodesis, while allowing active and passive IP flexion. Long finger splint prevents PIP motion to allow healing of PIP extensor tendon centralization, with the DIP included as a secondary joint. Ring and small finger splints provide external support at the respective PIP and DIP joints to protect arthrodeses at these joints.

of the rehabilitation program.* Upon pin and suture removal, and application of edema control digital "socks," *finger and thumb immobilization splints* were fitted for continuous wear (Fig. 16-18). Once these digital splints were applied, an *index–small finger MP extension and radial deviation, index–ring finger MP supination mobilization splint, type 3 (11)* was fitted to influence/control MP joint capsular remodeling (Fig. 16-19, A,B). An additional splint was fabricated for night and as-needed day wear (Fig. 16-20).

Active range of motion was initiated for the long finger PIP joint on the 6th postoperative week. Day and night extension splinting to the long finger continued between exercise sessions to minimize potential development of an extensor lag.

With fluoroscopic confirmation of bone healing, all digital immobilization splints protecting arthrodeses were discontinued at the 8th postoperative week. The *index–small finger MP extension and radial deviation, index–ring finger MP supination mobilization splint, type 3 (11)* was discontinued at 10 weeks postoperatively. Night splinting and as-needed day splinting, during moderate to heavy hand use, was continued with an *index–small finger MP extension mobilization and ulnar deviation restriction splint, type 1 (5)* for support and protection of the finger MP joints (Fig. 16-21). Joint protection concepts and techniques were also reviewed with the subject.

*Detailed description of therapy procedures other than the splinting program is not within the scope of this case study.

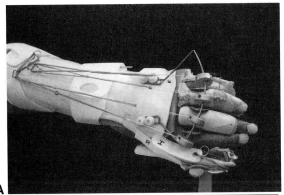

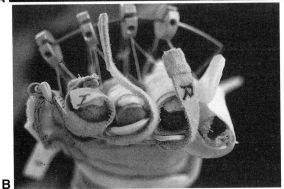

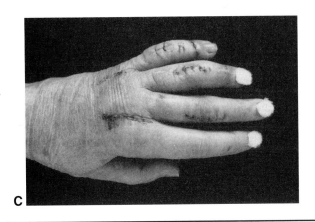

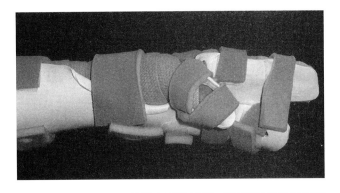

Fig. 16-20   Index–small finger MP extension, long finger PIP extension, ring–small finger IP flexion, thumb MP-IP flexion immobilization splint, type 4 (16)
Night and as-needed day immobilization splint protects healing structures and maintains neutral alignment of MP joints. For positioning and stabilization, the wrist, index finger IP joints, long finger DIP joint, and thumb CMC joint are included as secondary joints.

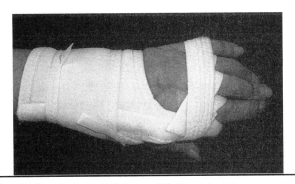

Fig. 16-21   Index–small finger MP ulnar deviation restriction splint, type 1 (5)
This splint supports the MP joints during functional use.

Fig. 16-19   A,B, Index–small finger MP extension and radial deviation, index–ring finger MP supination mobilization splint, type 3 (11) \\ Thumb MP flexion immobilization / IP extension restriction splint, type 0 (2) \\ Long finger PIP extension immobilization splint, type 1 (2) \\ Ring finger IP flexion immobilization splint, type 0 (2) \\ Small finger IP flexion immobilization splint, type 0 (2)
A, Mobilization assists pull the finger MP joints into extension and radial deviation to control remodeling of MP joint capsules with radial tightening. B, MP supination mobilization assists counteract pronation tendencies of the index, long, and ring fingers following surgery. C, Appearance of hand at 2 1/2 weeks postoperatively. The Velcro loop "buttons" are adhered with cyanoacrylate glue to the fingernails. These allow attachment of the MP supination mobilization assists.

At the 6th postoperative month, both function and cosmesis were improved considerably (Fig. 16-22, A-D) and the subject reported high outcome satisfaction (Fig. 16-23, A-C) and a desire for surgical reconstruction of her dominant, right hand to be done as soon as possible! Reconstructive surgery of the subject's right hand was accomplished with similar results.

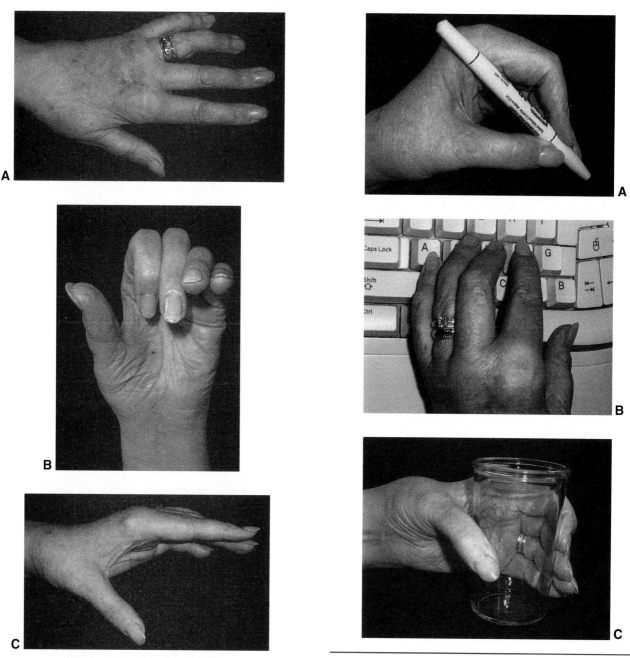

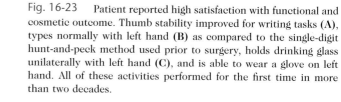

Fig. 16-23   Patient reported high satisfaction with functional and cosmetic outcome. Thumb stability improved for writing tasks (**A**), types normally with left hand (**B**) as compared to the single-digit hunt-and-peck method used prior to surgery, holds drinking glass unilaterally with left hand (**C**), and is able to wear a glove on left hand. All of these activities performed for the first time in more than two decades.

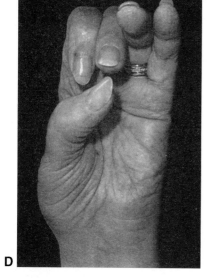

Fig. 16-22   **A,** Reconstructed left hand at 6th postoperative month with pleasing cosmesis, active finger flexion (**B**), active finger extension (**C**), and active thumb flexion (**D**). (Compare to Fig. 16-14.)

SUMMARY

Splinting the rheumatoid hand is controversial but may often be beneficial in both medical and surgical management along with a well-planned rehabilitation program. Knowledge of the biomechanics of the disease process, good communication with the physician and other team members, and careful assessment of the patient's individual situation and functional status all help the patient to derive maximum benefit from the splinting program.

REFERENCES

1. Alexander G, Hortas C, Bacon P: Bed rest, activity and the inflammation of rheumatoid arthritis, *Br J Rheumatol* 22(3):134-40, 1983.
2. Alter S, Feldon P, Terrono A: Pathomechanics of deformities in the arthritic hand and wrist. In Mackin E, et al: *Hunter, Mackin, & Callahan's rehabilitation of the hand and upper extremity*, ed 5, Mosby, 2002, St. Louis.
3. Biese J: Therapist's evaluation and conservative management of rheumatoid arthritis in the hand and wrist. In Mackin E, et al: *Hunter, Mackin, & Callahan's rehabilitation of the hand and upper extremity*, ed 5, Mosby, 2002, St. Louis.
4. Boozer JA, Sanson MS, Soutas-Little RW, et al: Comparison of the biomedical motions and forces involved in high-profile versus low-profile dynamic splinting, *J Hand Ther* 7(3):171-82, 1994.
5. Burr N, Pratt AL, Smith PJ: An alternative splinting and rehabilitation protocol for metacarpophalangeal joint arthroplasty in patients with rheumatoid arthritis, *J Hand Ther* 15(1):41-7, 2002.
6. Callinan NJ, Mathiowetz V: Soft versus hard resting hand splints in rheumatoid arthritis: pain relief, preference, and compliance, *Am J Occup Ther* 50(5):347-53, 1996.
7. Convery FR, Minteer MA: The use of orthoses in the management of rheumatoid arthritis, *Clin Orthop* 0(102):118-25, 1974.
8. Convery FR, Conaty J, Nickel V: Dynamic splinting of the rheumatoid hand, *Orth Pros* 22:41-5, 1968.
9. Feinberg J: Effect of the arthritis health professional on compliance with use of resting hand splints by patients with rheumatoid arthritis, *Arthritis Care Res* 5(1):17-23, 1992.
10. Feinberg J, Brandt KD: Use of resting splints by patients with rheumatoid arthritis, *Am J Occup Ther* 35(3):173-8, 1981.
11. Fess EE, Philips C: *Hand splinting principles and methods*, ed 2, Mosby, 1987, St. Louis.
12. Fess EE: Principles and methods of dynamic splinting. In Hunter J, et al: *Rehabilitation of the hand*, ed 2, Mosby, 1984, St. Louis.
13. Fess EE: Principles and methods of splinting for mobilization. In Hunter J, et al: *Rehabilitation of the hand*, ed 3, Mosby, 1989, St. Louis.
14. Fess EE: Splints: mechanics versus convention, *J Hand Ther* 8(2):124-30, 1995.
15. Flatt A: *Care of the arthritic hand*, ed 4, Mosby, 1983, St. Louis.
16. Gault S, Spyker M: Beneficial effect of immobilization of joints in rheumatoid and related arthritides: a splint study using sequential analysis, *Arthritis Rheum* 12(1):34-44, 1969.
17. Granger C, et al: Laminated plaster-plastic bandage splints, *Arch Phys Med* 46:585-9, 1965.
18. Gyovai J, Howell J: Validation of spring forces applied in dynamic outrigger splinting, *J Hand Ther* 5(1):8-15, 1992.
19. Hanten D: The splinting controversy in rheumatoid arthritis. In *AOTA Physical disabilities special interest section newsletter*, 1982.
20. Kozin SH: Arthroplasty of the hand and wrist: surgeon's perspective, *J Hand Ther* 12(2):123-32, 1999.
21. Li-Tsang C, Hung LK, Mak AF: The effect of corrective splinting on the flexion contracture of rheumatoid fingers, *J Hand Ther* 15(2):185-91, 2002.
22. Luban J, Wolfe T: Joint replacement in the rheumatoid hand: surgery and therapy. In Mackin E, et al: *Hunter, Mackin, & Callahan's rehabilitation of the hand and upper extremity*, ed 5, Mosby, 2002, St. Louis.
23. Melvin J: *Rheumatic diseases in the adult and child: occupational therapy and rehabilitation*, ed 3, Davis, 1989, Philadelphia.
24. Mills J, et al: Value of bed rest in patients with rheumatoid arthritis, *N Eng J Med* 284:453-8, 1978.
25. Nalebuff EA: Diagnosis, classification and management of rheumatoid thumb deformities, *Bull Hosp Joint Dis* pp. 119-137, 1968.
26. Partridge R, Duthie J: Control trial of the effects of complete immobilization of the joints in rheumatoid arthritis, *Ann Rheum Dis* 22:91-9, 1963.
27. Rotstein J: Use of splints in conservative management of acutely inflamed joints in rheumatoid arthritis, *Arch Phys Med Rehabil* 46:198-9, 1965.
28. Shapiro JS: The wrist in rheumatoid arthritis, *Hand Clin* 12(3):477-98, 1996.
29. Souter W: Splintage in the rheumatoid hand, *Hand* 3:144-51, 1971.
30. Stirrat CR: Metacarpophalangeal joints in rheumatoid arthritis of the hand, *Hand Clin* 12(3):515-29, 1996.
31. Swanson AB, Coleman JD: Corrective bracing needs of the rheumatoid arthritic wrist, *Am J Occup Ther* 20(1):38-40, 1966.
32. Terrono A, Nalebuff E, Philips C: The rheumatoid thumb. In Hunter J, Mackin E, Callahan A: *Rehabilitation of the hand: surgery and therapy*, ed. 4, Mosby, 1995, St. Louis.
33. Tucci MA, Baker R, Mohamed A, et al: Synovial tissues collected from rheumatoid patients undergoing total joint arthroplasty express markers for acute inflammation, *Biomed Sci Instrum* 34:169-74, 1997.
34. Youm Y, McCurthy RY, Flatt AE, et al: Kinematics of the wrist I. An experimental study of radial-ulnar deviation and flexion-extension, *J Bone Joint Surg [Am]* 60(4):423-31, 1978.
35. Young P: Use of splintage in the rheumatoid hand after surgery, *Physiotherapy* 66:371-4, 1980.
36. Zoeckler A, Nicholas J: Prenyl hand splint for rheumatoid arthritis, *Phys Ther* 49:377-9, 1969.

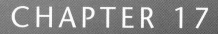

"Did that 'Flight of the bumble bee' sound slow?!"

Marty Williams
©2003 IU Visual Media

CHAPTER 17

Splinting for Work, Sports, and the Performing Arts

Chapter Outline

CASE EXAMPLES
Musician
Worker
Athlete
COMMON HAND INJURIES/CONDITIONS
Mallet Finger
Boutonniere
Metacarpal Fractures
Silicone Rubber Playing Casts
Proximal Phalanx Fracture
Trigger Finger (Stenosing Tenosynovitis)
Thumb MP Ulnar Collateral Ligament Tear or Rupture
COMMON WRIST INJURIES/CONDITIONS
Carpal Tunnel Syndrome
deQuervain's Disease
Dorsal Carpal Ganglion (DCG)
Scaphoid Fractures

COMMON FOREARM AND ELBOW
 INJURIES/CONDITIONS
Cubital Tunnel Syndrome
Lateral Epicondylitis
Medial Epicondylitis
Elbow Dislocations/Fractures
COMMON SHOULDER INJURIES/CONDITIONS
Humeral Fracture
Shoulder Subluxation/Dislocation
Posterior Subluxation/Dislocation
Anterior Subluxation/Dislocation
INSTRUCTIONS FOR SILICONE RUBBER PLAYING CAST
 FABRICATION
Materials
Fabrication
SUMMARY

The upper extremity is vulnerable to injury and overuse especially among workers involved in physically demanding jobs, professional and nonprofessional athletes, and all classes of musicians.[25,27] A distinctive patient population, workers, athletes, and musicians have unique but related physical demands that make them susceptible to injury, including repetitive stress problems. With livelihoods and futures dependent on their abilities to work and/or to compete, these individuals, particularly athletes and musicians, are highly motivated to return to their activities as quickly as possible, often to the very behavior patterns that caused them injury initially.

Splinting programs for these individuals must be tailored to perform within the demands of the respective specialized professions. This is a true challenge to clinicians' creativity! Clinicians responsible for designing and fabricating splints for workers, athletes, or musicians must first understand the details of their patients' vocational and/or avocational activities. This requires learning and analyzing postures used for playing musical instruments, work tasks implemented on the job, and actions performed in specific sports.

Guided by individual diagnoses, each patient's activity and particular job, sport, or performing art must be thoroughly analyzed in order that appropriate splints may be designed that allow expedient return to work, practice, or competition. The most frequent indications for splinting workers, athletes, or musicians include, but are not limited to, (1) restriction of unwanted motion during specific activities, (2) protection from further injury as healing progresses, and (3) following postoperative procedures. Generally, diagnosis-specific postoperative care for this population parallels traditional guidelines used for conservative and surgical intervention for the general population. However, more restrictive splints that afford better protection to healing structures are required when activities involve potential for recurring injury.

■ CASE EXAMPLES

To illustrate the unique approaches needed in treating workers, athletes, and musicians, the following three scenarios are presented.

Musician

A professional musician, who sustained an index finger distal phalanx amputation, wants to return to playing the violin in an orchestra, a job he held prior to the injury. Traditionally, a finger prosthesis would be the treatment of choice, providing cosmetic coverage, patient acceptance, and some functional use. However, finger sensation is required to precisely place the fingertips on the strings of a violin as it is played and, because of this, the patient rejected the prosthesis. Analysis of the remaining length of the amputated digit found that splinting and adapting the violin would accommodate the slight decrease in finger length. This solution required a concentrated team effort that included the musician, violin teacher, violin maker, therapist, and physician to evaluate and successfully integrate the instrument, playing technique, and physical capacity of the patient.

General treatment goals for musicians include delaying return to performances until the appropriate time, accommodating to alterations in anatomy and/or soft tissue status, and adapting daily practice schedules. Pain levels document problems and progress and define timing of treatment reevaluations.[18] While the therapist's role is valuable, input from the music professional is equally critical and must not be ignored. Dividing splints into three categories, protective, assistive, and limiting, Johnson[14] designates splints worn during playing of musical instruments as "playing splints." Protective splints allow early return to practice as they protect healing structures, assistive splints decrease stress over painful areas, and limiting splints protect from inflammation or are used

as training splints to avoid injurious playing techniques.[14] For the violin player described above, a combination of splinting and adaptations to the instrument itself allowed his quick return to playing the violin.

Worker

A worker experiences repetitive trauma to his right thenar eminence as he works on a factory assembly line. After analyzing the situation, a therapist recommends that the equipment with which the employee works be adapted with an antivibratory material such as Sorbothane. It is also recommended that the worker change specific motions he uses as he works, decreasing further repetitive trauma to his thumb.

Splinting and postural or usage changes are effective approaches toward alleviating potential injurious work situations. Judiciously planned work rotation schedules also help decrease repetitiveness of workers' activities. Analyzing workers at their specific jobs is fundamental to defining and initiating the most efficacious treatment possible. Further, recommendations for adapting job situations may prevent other employees from being injured. Employers want job-injured workers to return to a working situation as early as possible and splinting plays an important role toward accomplishment of this goal.

"Soft splints," e.g., antivibration gloves with Viscolas, or neoprene splints, are used to absorb repetitive shear to working hands and digits. These splints may be molded as workers grip their specific work-related tools or equipment; they may be fitted over or into work gloves, depending on individual needs. Splints worn over work gloves must be fitted with the donned gloves in place and as tools or equipment are gripped until thermoplastic materials cool. For the worker described above, an adapted splint protected his thumb as he worked at his assembly line job, allowing him to continue to be productive without incurring further injury.

Athlete

Football, baseball, basketball, and other sports are national passions and players often are obsessed with playing regardless of whether they are grade schoolers or professionals! The third example, a professional football player with a stable long finger metacarpal fracture, wants to return to playing football as soon as possible. The splinting goal for this football player is to maintain the hand in a position that facilitates safe healing of his metacarpal fracture. The referring physician deems the fracture stable and recommends a protective playing cast. The therapist fabricates an adapted fiberglass cast for the patient to wear during practice and games, allowing quick return to competition for this professional athlete.

Before incurring cost to patients, it is prudent to identify the kinds of splints approved by the sanctioning body of the specific sports involved. Rules and regulations vary from sport to sport and between different levels of a given sport. Remember, officials at the game make the final decisions on allowing devices to be worn. Sanctioned materials may include thermoplastics, silicone, foam, padding, and tape. If plaster or fiberglass splints are allowed, they are padded externally to protect other players. Tape or elastic wrap may be used to secure splints during practices and competition events. Alternate low-temperature thermoplastic splints frequently are fitted for off-field wear.

With their high motivation for successful results, workers, athletes, and musicians are truly an exceptional group of patients to splint and treat, presenting many opportunities for therapists to exercise their creative talents. It is important to remember that diagnoses are not the sole determinants of splint design; instead, patients' special interests and requirements, in addition to their specific diagnoses, determine successful splint designs. In contrast to other splinting venues, splinting materials that are soft and supportive are more frequently used to treat workers, athletes, and musicians. These materials require very different fabrication skills, often challenging even adroit splint fabricators.

■ COMMON HAND INJURIES/CONDITIONS

This section reviews typical upper extremity diagnoses that workers, athletes, and musicians may encounter. Good communication with referring physicians is absolutely imperative when treating the injuries described in this chapter. Knowing general treatment protocols is entry-level expertise that is, for the most part, incompatible with successful treatment of these high-functioning individuals. Astute upper extremity clinical specialists are aware of the multiplicity of variables that may, and frequently do, occur and they integrate physician preference, individual patient factors, and in-depth understanding of anatomy, biomechanics, and timing of wound healing, with splinting principles and exercise concepts to devise effective treatment programs that allow patients to achieve their optimum rehabilitative potentials. There is no place in this arena for therapists with "nine-to-five" attitudes who rigidly treat according to rote protocols, without communicating with physicians and other relevant professionals. A team approach that involves patient, therapist, physi-

cian, and associated occupation-specific professionals is necessary to produce high-level functional outcomes for this special group of patients.

The following describe standard, not all, splinting approaches used in treating injuries that frequently involve workers, athletes, and musicians. Splints illustrated in this chapter are described according to expanded Splint Classification System terminology. The ESCS identifies splints according to function rather than form or configuration. It is not unusual for splints that look alike to have dissimilar technical names because their purposes are different for differing situations. In some instances, colloquial splint names are included along with ESCS terminology. It is not within the scope of this chapter to address associated surgical procedures, therapy techniques, or complicating circumstances. Readers are encouraged to pursue independent study of the many excellent references cited throughout this book.

Mallet Finger

"Mallet finger," "baseball finger," and "drop finger" are interchangeable colloquial terminology for the most common closed tendon injury in the athletic patient population.[1,2,34,35,48] Disruption of the terminal extensor tendon at its insertion may occur when catching a ball (baseball finger) or whenever an excessive external flexion force is applied to the distal interphalangeal joint (DIP) while the joint is extended (mallet finger). This injury is frequently seen in athletes who catch or hit balls as in baseball, football, basketball, and volleyball, and the history usually involves a ball hitting a straightened finger, forcing DIP flexion.[34,35] The terminal extensor tendon may be avulsed with or without a bone fragment, or it may be ruptured or stretched. These injuries are frequently treated conservatively with DIP joint immobilization.

Clinically the patient presents with a DIP joint flexion deformity and pain over the dorsal aspect of the distal digit.[23,24] Joint flexion is caused by an unopposed flexor digitorum profundus. Providing no extenuating circumstances exist, a *finger DIP hyperextension immobilization splint, type 0 (1)* is applied to immobilize the DIP joint in 5-10° hyperextension. The splint, fitted dorsally, palmarly, or circumferentially, is secured to the finger with paper tape, prohibiting splint migration (Fig. 17-1). Hyperextension greater than half the DIP joint's normal hyperextension range must be avoided to maintain adequate vascularity to local soft tissues.[36] Duration of splinting is usually 6 weeks for acute injuries and 8 weeks for chronic conditions, depending on patient-specific variables. Patient instructions include removal of the splint for periodic cleaning. It is critical that the patient understand that the DIP joint must be held in

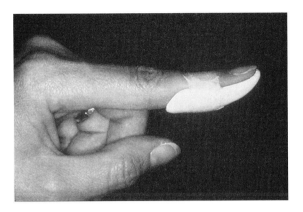

Fig. 17-1   Index finger DIP hyperextension immobilization splint, type 0 (1)
Worn continuously except for removal for hygiene, this splint, for "mallet finger," is fit in full extension or slight hyperextension to avoid an extension lag when exercises are initiated.

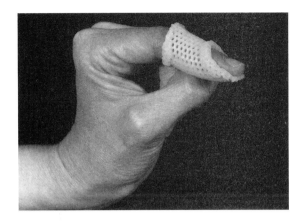

Fig. 17-2   Index finger DIP hyperextension immobilization splint, type 0 (1)
A perforated low-temperature thermoplastic material decreases potential for skin maceration with splints that are worn for long periods of time. Splints made of perforated materials must have contiguous fit, and smooth internal and external surfaces and edges to ensure that pressure areas do not develop. Using powder between the digit and splint or changing to a dry splint as needed during the day diminishes problems from moist skin. (Courtesy Rachel Dyrud Ferguson, OTR, CHT, Taos, N.M.)

continuous hyperextension whenever the splint is removed. If the patient is unable to carry out the splinting program independently, a family member or friend must be enlisted to help.

Dorsal splinting is preferable for workers, athletes, and musicians who require input from fingertip tactile sensation. A combination of volar and dorsal splints or a circumferential splint may be utilized for heavy-duty activities or if the injury causes hypersensitivity and the fingertip needs extra protection. *Type 1 finger DIP hyperextension immobilization splints* may be padded if worn during contact sports. Multiple splints that allow a rotational wearing schedule or splints made of perforated materials are often necessary to allow skin aeration and to avoid maceration (Fig. 17-2). Typically, patients are unable to perform fine dexterous activities but are able to return to normal activities so long as they wear their splints continuously. When active DIP motion is initiated, splint wear is continued at night. Additional wearing of splints during the day is dependent on maintenance of full DIP extension.

Boutonniere

Dubbed "boutonniere" or "buttonhole deformity," injury to the extensor tendon central slip is the second most frequently occurring closed tendon injury in athletes. Etiology of this injury involves trauma to the central slip or a sudden forced flexion of the PIP joint, as with a blow to the dorsal middle phalanx that forces PIP flexion as the digit is extended. Boutonniere injuries are more frequently associated with contact sports such as football,[34,35] but also occur in nonsports situations. Often these injuries go unrecognized as with the basketball player who experiences a PIP joint

palmar lateral dislocation that was "pulled" back into place and forgotten. Other scenarios include the worker who reports a fall on a digit or being trapped in a machine or a musician who experiences a fall or direct blow to the PIP joint. Initially no deformity may be observed, but as the lateral bands move volar to the axis of joint rotation, a PIP flexion deformity becomes apparent, followed later in time by an associated DIP hyperextension deformity. Symptoms usually include local edema and pain, decreased active extension of the PIP joint, and diminished active and passive flexion of the DIP joint with the MP joint held in flexion.

If the injury is acute and full passive PIP extension is present, a *finger PIP extension immobilization splint* is applied and worn continuously for 6 weeks. A volar *finger PIP extension immobilization splint, type 0 (1)* of thermoplastic material may be used if edema is present, but if edema is not a concern, a cylinder cast provides excellent immobilization. It is important to understand that both these splints are *finger PIP extension immobilization splint, type 0 (1)*; only the material and surfaces of application differ. If the amount of extension provided by either of these splints is in doubt, a lateral radiograph should be taken to ensure that the PIP joint is in full extension. Generally a cast or circumferential splint gives greater security for the duration of treatment and allows early return to activities, including contact sports. Because circumferential casts help reduce edema, they must be monitored to ensure that these splints continue to provide correct extension positioning to injured joints or fingers. It is not unusual to replace a cast that initially fit but fails to maintain desired PIP extension as edema subsides. These *type 0 finger PIP extension immobilization splints* should allow DIP joint passive and active flexion, which maintains and/or remodels oblique retinacular ligament length.

Chronic boutonniere injuries often present with stiff or fixed PIP joint flexion contractures, requiring *finger PIP extension mobilization splints* to correct these deficits. Splint design is determined by the angle-degree of the contracture, its "end-range feel," and the time interval since initial injury. If the PIP joint flexion deformity is less than 30°, a *finger PIP extension mobilization splint, type 1 (2)* in the form of a commercially available Bunnell "safety pin" splint or serial *finger PIP extension mobilization splint, type 0 (1)* casts that employ inelastic traction are effective. However, a *finger PIP extension mobilization splint, type 1 (2)* using elastic or inelastic traction may be useful if the deformity is greater than 30° and if noticeable give to extension "end-range feel" is present, indicating that the deformity is not fixed.[46] In contrast, if the deformity is long-standing, greater than 30°, and no extension end-range give is felt, elastic traction splints are relatively worthless. Inelastic traction mobilization splints, in the form of serial casts or splints with mobilization assists that allow incremental adjustments of inelastic traction, are the most efficient method to improve fixed PIP flexion deformities. Associated DIP extension or hyperextension stiffness may be treated with active and passive flexion exercises or two-stage serial casting, or with *finger PIP extension mobilization / DIP flexion torque transmission splints,* (Fig. 17-3) depending on the extent of involvement of the DIP joint.

All of the splints described above for improving PIP joint flexion deformities are hand-based and are

classified as either *type 0* or *type 1 finger PIP extension mobilization splints*. Only individual design options differ between these splints whose purposes are identical. Different design options allow these *finger PIP extension mobilization splints* to be correlated appropriately with individual patient variables.

Once full passive PIP joint extension is attained, a program of extension immobilization splinting is initiated and the passively supple PIP joint is immobilized in an appropriately designed and fitted *finger PIP extension immobilization splint* for 8 weeks of uninterrupted wear. At about 8 weeks when active range of motion is initiated, immobilization splinting is continued and time in the immobilization splint is gradually decreased. Program aggressiveness and scheduling of both AROM exercises and immobilization splinting are altered as PIP extension is maintained and flexion increases. For example, if PIP joint extension is 0°, then PIP flexion exercises or splinting may be more aggressive in frequency and duration. It is important to monitor PIP joint extension carefully. If an extension lag occurs, the program must be adjusted to decrease flexion exercises and/or flexion mobilization splinting and increase extension immobilization splinting. An astutely balanced splinting and exercise program that is studiously monitored and adjusted to reflect individual patient factors is the key to a successful result.

Metacarpal Fractures

Various etiologies lead to metacarpal fractures, including direct or indirect blows to metacarpal shafts or jolts that apply indirect compression torsion to the metacarpal bones.[34,35] Associated with work injuries, metacarpal fractures may also occur when a crushing force over the dorsum of the hand forcefully drives the hand into a solid surface or sandwiches it between two hard objects. Fractures of the neck of the fifth metacarpal are common and are often caused by a clenched fist impacting a hard object such as a wall. Fractures to the base of the metacarpal more often are the result of a direct blow, with clenched fist, to the distal end of the metacarpal, transmitting force down the shaft. Symptoms include pain and tenderness over the site of the break.[30] A cast or a splint may be used to position a closed, stable metacarpal fracture providing alignment is satisfactory without rotatory displacement. For metacarpal shaft, head, neck, or unstable base fractures, a *wrist extension, finger MP flexion immobilization splint, type 1 (3)* or cast may be used to immobilize the wrist in 15-20° extension and the MP joints of the fractured digit and an adjacent stabilizing digit in 65-70° of flexion.[44] Positioning the MP joints in flexion prevents shortening of the collat-

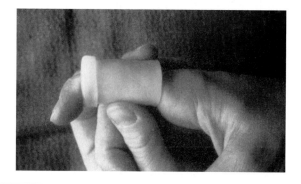

Fig. 17-3 Index finger PIP extension mobilization / DIP flexion torque transmission splint, type 0 (2)
With the PIP held in full extension the DIP is actively exercised, allowing remodeling to lengthen the oblique retinacular ligament. (Courtesy Brenda Hilfrank, PT, CHT, South Burlington, Vt.)

eral ligaments. Splinting a metacarpal fracture requires contiguous conforming fit that supports the fracture and surrounding soft tissue, including the normal architecture of the transverse and longitudinal arches. As an alternate option, a stable metacarpal fracture may be treated with a *nonarticular metacarpal splint* ("fracture brace"). A *wrist extension immobilization splint, type 0 (1)* may be fitted to protect a stable metacarpal base or proximal shaft fracture.

The inherent length of a digital ray amplifies metacarpal fracture rotational problems. For each degree of malrotation present at a metacarpal fracture site, as much as 5° of associated rotation occurs at the distal tip of the digit.[31,34,35] A *torque transmission splint,* such as a "buddy tape," may harness the injured digit to its normal adjacent digit to help control a rotational problem, but this should be done only with the consent of the referring physician.

With radiographic confirmation that the fracture has healed and the referring physician's approval, at about 3 weeks post injury, active range of motion may be initiated with continuation of protective splinting between exercise sessions. As the patient returns to work or to the sports arena, splint protection of the fracture is frequently required. In the case of an athlete returning to practice and/or competitive sports, the trainer, therapist, and patient work together to create an appropriate splint design that is within acceptable limits of the sanctioning body of the sport. For contact sports, splints may include rigid supports and protective dorsal padding. Splint design options are dependent on specific fracture sites. A *wrist extension immobilization splint, type 0 (1)* for base fractures, a *nonarticular metacarpal splint* for shaft fractures, and a *finger MP flexion immobilization splint, type 0 (2)* for distal fractures may be used to protect healing or recently healed metacarpal fractures (Fig. 17-4). Another option, a room temperature vulcanizing silicone rubber wrist splint or wrist and finger and/or thumb splint may be appropriate for practice and contact sports.

Silicone Rubber Playing Casts

General diagnoses for athletes include sprains, dislocations, and fractures.[40-42,49] Players want to return to their sports immediately but must be released by the physician to do so. While low-temperature thermoplastic splints may be worn off the playing field, more protective sport-specific splints are required for practice and game situations. Splints must be lightweight and they must absorb external stress if used in contact sports. "No-heat" or layered materials such as room temperature vulcanizing silicone rubber are practical for practice and contact sports providing injuries are stable. A silicone rubber playing cast has both elas-

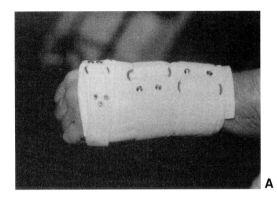

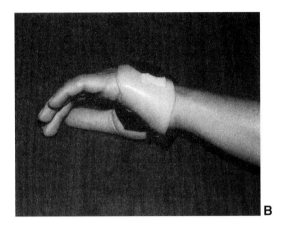

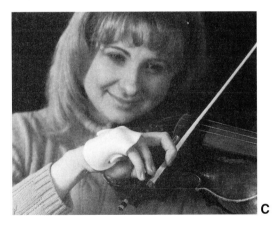

Fig. 17-4   A, Wrist extension immobilization splint, type 0 (1) B, Nonarticular index–small metacarpal splint C, Ring–small finger MP flexion immobilization splint, type 0 (2)
The metacarpal fracture site determines the splint design used. A, A wrist extension immobilization splint protects a base fracture. B, A nonarticular splint for a stable metacarpal shaft fracture supports the healing fracture. C, A hand-based MP flexion splint immobilizes a distal metacarpal fracture. [Courtesy (A) Lin Beribak, OTR/L, CHT, Chicago, Ill.; (B) Suzanne Brand, OTR, CHT, Needham, Mass.; (C) Rick Beets Photographic, Indianapolis, Ind.]

ticity and strength properties that serve to protect both the patient-player and others who may come in contact with the cast as play progresses. Because silicone rubber is a closed cell material, it should not be worn longer than 3 or 4 hours at a time.

As noted previously, it is important to verify with the regulatory board of the sport in question the rules regarding materials permissible during play. The newsletter of the National Association of Sports Officials provides resources for rule interpretation.[12] Also, financial obligations may necessitate clarification. For example, will the school or team compensate for the playing cast or is the patient responsible for its cost? Insurance companies generally do not reimburse for casts or splints to play sports. Soft protective playing casts are advocated in the literature* and their fabrication is detailed by several authors.[6,10,15,20,25]

Instructions for fabrication of playing casts are included at the end of this chapter.

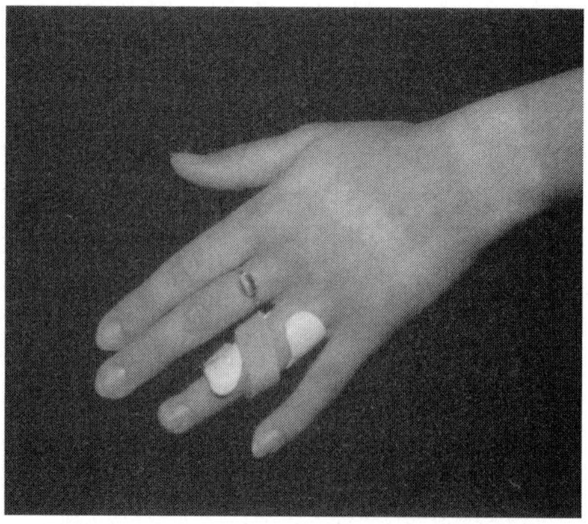

Proximal Phalanx Fracture

Proximal phalangeal fractures are also commonly encountered sports and work injuries. These fractures may have complicated medical courses because of the intricate balance of extrinsic and intrinsic muscle tendon units, extensor mechanism, and ligamentous structures that may be involved. The proximal phalanx is more commonly fractured than the distal or middle phalanx because under certain circumstances the length of the finger imparts a mechanical leverage on the proximal phalanx.[30] Suddenly catching an extended finger between two opposing solid objects or surfaces may produce a proximal phalangeal fracture. For example, trapping a finger between a playing surface and a shoe cleat, or a tool or object falling on an extended finger, may cause a proximal phalanx to break. Forceful hyperextension of the finger produces shaft or base fractures of a proximal phalanx. This is similar to the kind of force that leads to proximal interphalangeal joint or metacarpophalangeal joint dislocations. In contrast, a fracture of the distal end of a proximal phalanx usually occurs with the finger flexed, a force similar to that causing a metacarpal neck fracture.[30] Symptoms may present with edema, pain, and tenderness over the fracture site. Site of injury determines the kind of immobilization for stable fractures. Proximal phalangeal head and neck fractures are fit with a *finger PIP extension immobilization splint, type 0 (1)* (Fig. 17-5). When edema is not a concern, a *finger PIP extension immobilization splint, type 0 (1)* "cylinder cast" in full extension may replace the *finger IP extension immobilization splint, type 0 (2)*. A proximal phalanx base or shaft fracture typically is immobilized in the intrinsic plus or antideformity position using a *wrist extension, finger MP flexion and IP extension immobilization splint* that holds the wrist in 15-25° exten-

---

*References 4, 10, 11, 15, 20, 24.

Fig. 17-5   **Ring finger PIP extension immobilization splint, type 0 (1)**
This splint design provides a buffer for dorsal sensitivity from a proximal phalangeal fracture. (Courtesy Robin Miller, OTR, CHT, Ft. Lauderdale, Fla.)

sion, the MPs in 65-70° flexion, and the IPs in extension.[44] Immobilization splints are worn continuously for 3 weeks or until bone healing is confirmed by radiograph and the referring physician determines active range of motion may be initiated along with protective splint wearing between exercises and at night.

For athletes with proximal phalangeal fractures, stable protective splinting is mandatory for practice and game situations. *Finger PIP extension immobilization splint, type 0 (1)* in the form of "cylinder casts" or "gutter" splints are used frequently as protection splints for proximal phalanx fractures. However, proximal phalangeal base fractures require splints that also include the MP joints. *Torque transmission splints* that harness the injured digit to its neighboring adjacent uninjured digit (e.g., "buddy tapes") may be considered to prevent sudden application of torque to the involved digit but it is important to remember that these splints are made of soft materials (Fig. 17-6) that afford only limited protection.

If a contracture of the PIP joint develops, a *finger PIP extension mobilization splint* may be initiated pending approval of the referring physician (Fig. 17-7).[44] See the previous section on splinting boutonniere deformities for details.

Trigger Finger (Stenosing Tenosynovitis)

Repetitive trauma to the area of the A-1 digital pulley is seen in baseball catchers, gymnasts, weightlifters, workers who employ handled gripping tools such as pliers, and musicians who encounter persistent pressure from holding an instrument.[20] Direct pressure from a hard surface applied to the flexor tendon at the

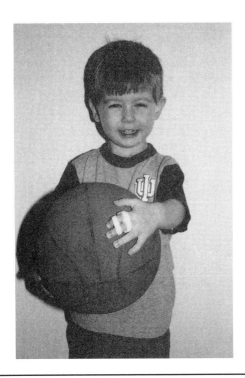

Fig. 17-6   **Long finger PIP extension and flexion torque transmission splint, type 2 (4)**
A noninjured digit protects an adjacent digit with a newly healed stable fracture from further injury in this nonarticular splint.

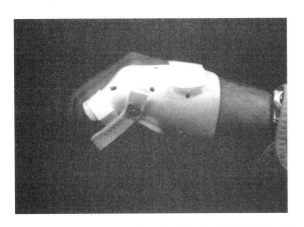

Fig. 17-7   **Small finger PIP flexion mobilization splint, type 1 (2)**
Support and protection to the proximal phalanx allows mobilization of the proximal interphalangeal joint. (Courtesy Lin Beribak, OTR/L, CHT, Chicago, Ill.)

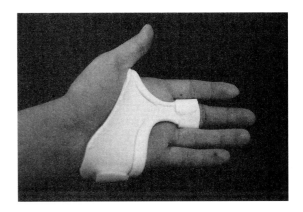

Fig. 17-8   **Long finger MP flexion restriction splint, type 0 (1)**
Repetitive trauma to the A-1 pulley is reduced by restricting flexor tendon glide at the metacarpophalangeal joint.

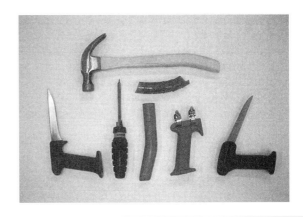

Fig. 17-9   Shock-absorbing material applied to tools, equipment, or instruments decreases pressure on an irritated A-1 pulley.

distal metacarpal may precipitate symptoms, including point tenderness, and catching or triggering of the thumb or finger. Musicians often notice these symptoms upon rising in the morning or during and after practice sessions.[7]

An increasingly recognized program of conservative management to decrease triggering is described by Evans et al.[8] A hand-based, *finger MP flexion restriction splint, type 0 (1)* that holds involved finger MP joints in 0° extension is fitted and worn for 6 weeks, restricting tendon glide distally and decreasing irritation (Fig. 17-8). Night splinting is indicated for musicians only in cases where pain is extreme. Padded or antivibration gloves* may be fitted and worn during tool, equipment, or instrument use. Made of leather with Viscolas in the palmar area, these gloves are available commercially in various styles. An alternative to gloves, tools, equipment, or instruments may be adapted with shock-absorbing materials to shield the A-1 pulley area and the palmar area (Fig. 17-9). Multiple-area contusions including, but not limited to, the thenar eminence frequently evidence repetitive trauma. The addition of a Silastic interface to a glove, splint, or directly to the area of injury helps protect these areas from further damage.

*Steel Grip Inc., 700 Garfield St., Danville, IL 61832; www.steelgripinc.com.

Thumb MP Ulnar Collateral Ligament Tear or Rupture

The metacarpophalangeal joint of the thumb is vulnerable when the thumb is abducted because, in abduction, the MP joint is locked, allowing forces to the distal thumb to be transmitted to the MP joint. Lateral stress with the thumb in abduction stresses the ulnar collateral ligament (UCL).[30] Commonly referred to as "gamekeeper's thumb" or "skier's thumb," injuries to the ulnar collateral ligament of the thumb MP joint precipitate MP joint instability. Causative factors include falling with the thumb entangled in a ski pole strap, creating torque, and forceful abduction of the thumb.[26] It is estimated that 15-25% of all skiing injuries involve the thumb.[34,35] Ski poles without grip restraints, which in a fall are discarded cleanly, seem to be the safest for avoiding thumb MP joint UCL injuries. Other sports where this injury occurs include basketball, gymnastics, rugby, volleyball, and hockey. Football-related UCL injuries are also reported when players' abducted thumbs strike other players' helmets. Additionally, stress to UCLs occurs from repetitive trauma in working situations or from continual stress from inappropriate positioning on playing instruments resulting in ligamentous deterioration and instability of the MP joint. A UCL injury negates thumb-index pinch, which is vital for most activities.[23,24]

Symptoms of a UCL injury include weakness, instability, edema, and pain with palpation or stress, indicating a need for immobilization. A *thumb MP radial and ulnar deviation restriction splint, type 1 (2)* holds the thumb CMC joint in approximately 40° palmar abduction and the MP joint in slight flexion. Worn until pain decreases, generally 4-6 weeks,[44] this splint combines stability and freedom of movement during most activities (Fig. 17-10). A less confining restriction splint may be considered as healing progresses (Fig. 17-11). If more protection and stability are needed, a *type 2, thumb MP radial and ulnar deviation restriction splint* that includes the wrist and thumb CMC joints proximally may be fitted. When less protection is needed, a *type 0, thumb MP flexion immobilization splint* may suffice to limit radial or ulnar stress until pain abates and joint stability improves. For athletes with UCL injuries, a silicone rubber playing cast with the thumb fully adducted may be required for practice and games. A simple neoprene thumb sleeve may be used for restricting work or performing arts activities. Taping techniques provide a continuum of thumb postures for protection to healing UCL injuries. For example, taping may prohibit thumb abduction while allowing full thumb adduction or the thumb may be positioned in slight abduction with extremes of motion prevented.

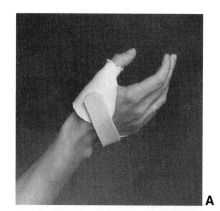
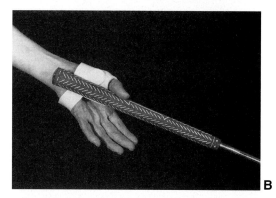
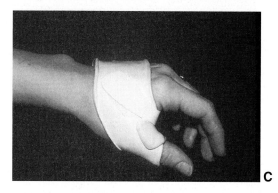

Fig. 17-10   **A,** Thumb MP radial and ulnar deviation restriction splint, type 1 (2) **B,** Thumb MP radial and ulnar deviation restriction splint, type 1 (2) **C,** Thumb MP radial and ulnar deviation restriction splint, type 1 (2)
Multiple designs provide individual options for this basic splint that protects the thumb MP collateral ligaments and allows continuation of sport, work, or playing an instrument. [Courtesy **(A)** Barbara Smith, OTR, Edmond, Okla.; **(B)** Rachel Dyrud Ferguson, OTR, CHT, Taos, N.M.]

■ COMMON WRIST INJURIES/CONDITIONS

Common wrist injuries/conditions include carpal tunnel syndrome (CTS), deQuervain's disease, dorsal carpal ganglion cysts (DCG), and scaphoid fractures.

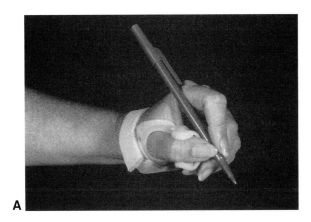

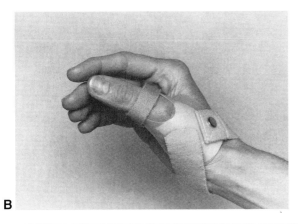

Fig. 17-11   A, Thumb MP radial and ulnar deviation restriction splint, type 1 (2) B, Thumb MP radial and ulnar deviation restriction splint, type 0 (1)

As stability of the thumb MP collateral ligament increases **(A)**, the CMC is unsplinted while protection from lateral or medial stress is continued to the metacarpophalangeal joint **(B)**. [Courtesy **(A)** Donna Breger Stanton, MA, OTR, CHT, Kensington, Calif.; **(B)** Julie Belkin, OTR, CO, MBA, 3-Point Products, Annapolis, Md.]

Carpal Tunnel Syndrome

To upper extremity clinicians, carpal tunnel syndrome (CTS) seems as though it is the nerve compression that won't go away! By far the most common neuropathy in the upper extremity, high incidence of CTS is found in workers, athletes, and performing artists.[55] The large variety of commercially available splints and "soft splints" attests to the fact that commonly employed treatment approaches have not completely alleviated patients' symptoms. CTS is caused by compression of the median nerve at the level of the carpal tunnel. Accompanied by eight finger flexor tendons and the flexor pollicis longus, the median nerve is vulnerable to compression injury as it traverses, along with the nine flexor tendons, through the confined space of the carpal tunnel.[30] With direct implications for splinting, Weiss et al. found that the lowest carpal tunnel pressure occurs with the

wrist in 2° extension (+/−9°) and 2° ulnar deviation (+/− 6°).[54]

CTS symptoms include pain, numbness, or dysesthesia, or a combination thereof, occurring distal to the carpal tunnel and following the median nerve distribution. Nocturnal intensification of symptoms may be present and symptoms may progress to include muscle weakness and sensory changes. Precipitating factors often involve a fall on an outstretched hand, repetitive use of the wrist, or static wrist flexion and vibration. High incidence is reported in workers in the aircraft and electronic industries and in automobile assembly. CTS is also prevalent in string instrumentalists who relax in a wrist flexion posture. Some of the most publicized reports of CTS involve computer keyboard users.

Conservative management may involve 6 weeks of continual wearing of a *type 0, wrist immobilization splint* that maintains the wrist in −7° to 9° extension or dorsiflexion and −4° to 8° ulnar deviation (Fig. 17-12).[54] Based on literature review and a cadaver study, Apfel et al. recommend, for night wear, a splint that holds the wrist in neutral and restricts finger flexion beyond 75% of a full fist to prevent incursion of proximal lumbrical muscles into the distal carpal canal.[3a] Accompanying exercise regimes vary considerably but most include periodic removal of the splint to allow specific exercises designed for treatment of CTS, including tendon-gliding exercises and active range of motion. Modalities may or may not be included.

Upper extremity clinicians analyze probable occupational or avocational sources for symptoms and recommend ergonomic changes, which may incorporate use of improved body mechanics during symptom-producing activities, avoidance of vibration stimuli, modification of workplace design, introduction of job rotations and rest periods, and adaptation of tools, musical instruments, or athletic equipment. Reduction of playing time and alteration of technique or practice patterns are essential considerations for performing artists with CTS. Having patients document in journals times and duration of their practice sessions, and incidence and intensity of their pain, is especially valuable for better understanding nerve compressions and/or tendonitis problems incurred from overuse activities. Logs often reveal specific activities preceding pain. For musicians, early goals are to rest but avoid the effects of immobilization, and to decrease pain.[18] Musicians' playing splints should minimally limit motion, be lightweight, have little to no strapping, conform closely, and have no unnecessary parts (Fig. 17-13).[14] For workers, antivibratory gloves offer an inner lining of Viscolas to absorb shock and protect the hand from vibration or repetitive trauma (Fig. 17-14). These gloves are available in

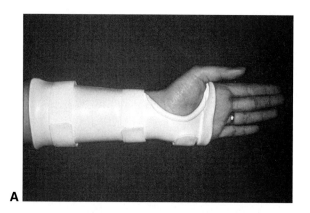

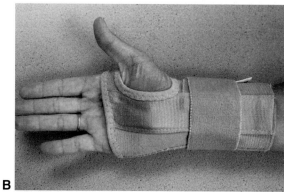

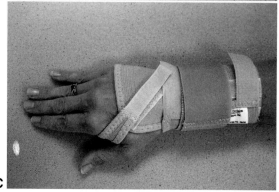

Fig. 17-12   A, Wrist extension immobilization splint, type 0 (1) B,C, Wrist extension immobilization splint, type 0 (1) Immobilization is accomplished with a low-temperature thermoplastic splint (**A**) or with an elastic fabric splint with a volar metal bar insert (**B,C**). The kind of insert will determine low, medium, or high stability. These splints are but two of many designs of wrist splints currently available.

various sizes and styles. Antivibratory material such as Viscolas* or Sorbothane† may be applied to tools and equipment for protection or used as liners or inserts in splints or gloves. For example, baseball bats or hammer handles may be adapted to better absorb

*Viscolas, Inc., 8801 Consolidated Drive, Soddy Daisy, TN 37379; www.viscolas.com.
†Sorbothane, Inc., 2144 State Route 59, Kent, OH; www.sorbothane.com.

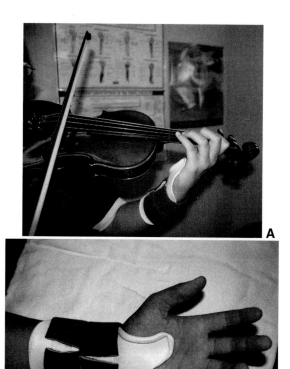

Fig. 17-13   A,B, Wrist flexion restriction splint, type 0 (1) Repetitive wrist flexion, which may be a precipitator of carpal tunnel syndrome, is restricted in this training splint. The splint reinforces learning ergonomically correct positioning and technique. (Courtesy Joni Armstrong, OTR, CHT, Bemidji, Minn.)

shock and shear forces.[5] To decrease repetitive wrist motion or extremes of wrist extension/flexion, "soft splints" may be worn throughout activities (Fig. 17-15). Articulated, semirigid, and soft splints are popular with workers and athletes requiring wrist protection while simultaneously allowing ranges of wrist motion depending on patient-specific requisites (Fig. 17-16).

deQuervain's Disease

deQuervain's disease is a stenosing tenosynovitis of the extensor pollicis brevis and abductor pollicis longus in the first dorsal compartment. Inflammation of the peritenons of the EPB and APL can be quite debilitating because of their role in thumb function.[7] Workers, athletes, and musicians may complain of pain occurring with thumb flexion when the wrist is ulnarly deviated and palmarly flexed. Common examples of sports that involve repetitive hand and wrist motion are bowling and golfing; professional golfers are especially susceptible to deQuervain's problems.[22] Higher incidences are also reported for occupations requiring fine manipulation actions in conjunction with postures of

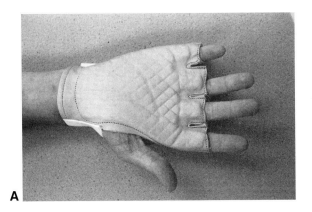

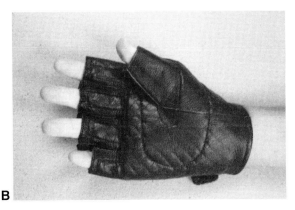

Fig. 17-14   **A,B,** A shock-absorbing material inserted in the glove reduces vibration and trauma to the hand during use. The gloves come in a variety of styles and sizes without a thumb **(A)** and with a thumb **(B).** The therapist may also make or buy a glove and add a shock-absorbing material insert.

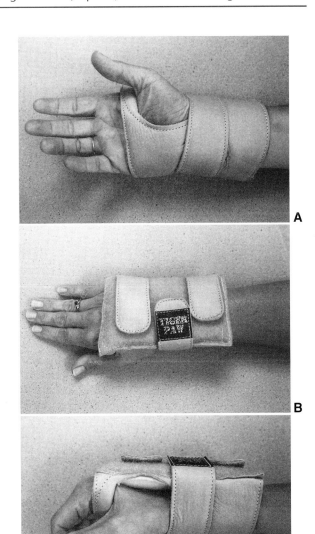

Fig. 17-15   A-C, Wrist extension and flexion restriction splint, type 0 (1)
A variety of inserts can be placed in the dorsal pocket to provide more or less restriction. Options may include no insert for less restriction, or one or more foam inserts for greater restriction. Multiple views of the same splint are shown.

wrist flexion and ulnar deviation. Symptoms include wrist pain with use and localized edema. Definitive testing for deQuervain's involves elicitation of a positive pain response when the thumb is passively held in flexion and the wrist is adducted (Finkelstein's test). To decrease tendon glide of the EPB and APL, a *wrist extension, thumb CMC palmar abduction and MP flexion immobilization splint, type 0 (3)* is fitted to immobilize the wrist and thumb in a position of rest. The wrist is positioned in approximately 15° extension or dorsiflexion, the thumb CMC joint in 40° palmar abduction, and the thumb MP joint in 10° flexion (Fig. 17-17). The thumb IP joint is not incorporated in the splint since neither the EPB nor APL traverses this joint. Accompanying exercise regimes and modality use are dependent on individual therapist and physician preferences. Throughout the immobilization phase, it is important that therapist and patient work together to analyze and modify the patient-specific causative factors of the stenosing tenosynovitis. *Wrist, thumb restriction splints* fabricated in soft materials may be fitted to limit overuse and impede extremes of wrist and thumb motion as patients return work, practice, or competition (Fig. 17-18).

Dorsal Carpal Ganglion (DCG)

The most common soft tissue tumors of the wrist are ganglions that originate from the dorsal scapholunate ligament.[3,45,50] Minor sprains to dorsal wrist capsules or repeated manipulations with the wrists in extension may, in time, cause dorsal ganglions to develop. Gymnasts report wrist ganglia associated with other wrist complaints to be major problems.[53] Ganglions may originate either extra-articularly or intra-articularly and the cysts generally involve adjacent tendon sheaths and joint capsules. DCGs are commonly found over scapholunate ligaments with symptoms including

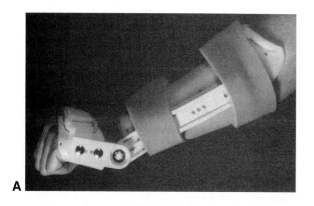

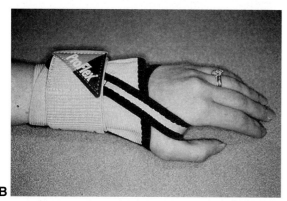

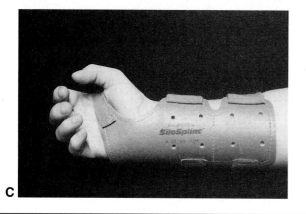

Fig. 17-16   A, Wrist extension restriction splint, type 0 (1) B, Wrist circumduction restriction splint, type 0 (1) C, Wrist circumduction restriction splint, type 0 (1)

These splints have variable degrees of restriction as determined by material and by the length of the forearm component. As the length decreases, so does the amount of restriction. It is not feasible for a clinic to carry numerous kinds of commercially available wrist restriction splints. Evaluate various designs and use those that most suit your patient population.

wrist pain and tenderness, especially with palmar flexion, which may decrease grip strength and range of motion.[45] A *wrist extension immobilization splint, type 0 (1)* is fabricated to reduce local area stress. A Silastic cover over the ganglion is secured with elastic wrap, allowing use for sports while protecting the DCG. If relief is not achieved with these conservative

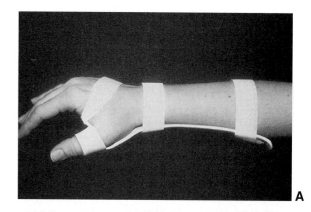

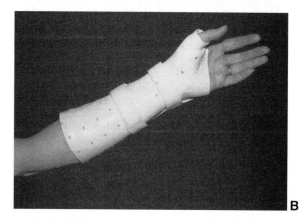

Fig. 17-17   A, Wrist extension, thumb CMC palmar abduction and MP flexion immobilization splint, type 0 (3) B, Wrist extension, thumb CMC palmar abduction immobilization / MP flexion restriction splint, type 0 (3)

deQuervain's may be treated by resting the EPB and APL tendons in a splint that positions the wrist in extension, the thumb CMC in palmar abduction, and the MP in slight flexion. [Courtesy **(B)** Shelli Dellinger, OTR, CHT, San Diego, Calif.]

methods, and the sport season is not yet concluded, a *wrist circumduction restriction splint, type 0 (1)* in a soft material helps limit extremes in wrist range of motion, which tend to compress the ganglion and elicit pain. Splints that immobilize or restrict wrist motion may help extend athletes' participation in their chosen sports, allowing completion of seasonal competition before surgical removals of DCGs are undertaken (Fig. 17-19). Postoperatively, a compressive dressing over the wrist may lessen local tenderness, as may a Silastic cover positioned with an elastic wrap.

Scaphoid Fractures

Biomechanical action and anatomical structure combine to predispose scaphoid bones to fractures. Because the scaphoid bridges the intercarpal joint, it is impinged upon the radius with wrist extension/dorsiflexion and radial deviation. Further, the scaphoid bone's narrow waist makes it vulnerable to

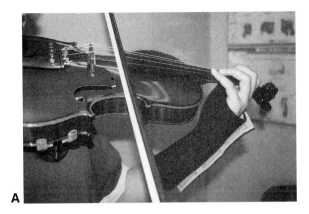

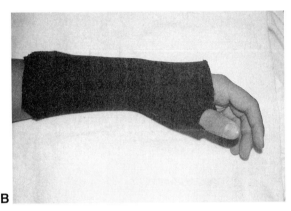

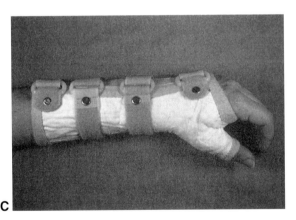

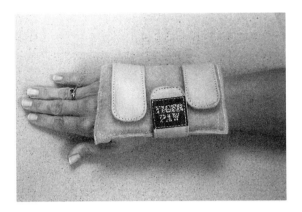

Fig. 17-19   **Wrist circumduction restriction splint, type 0 (1)**
Dorsal splint coverage may decrease pain through disseminated gentle pressure on the dorsal carpal ganglion. The soft splint restricts extremes of motion, which allows practice and competition to be better tolerated.

Fig. 17-18   **A,** Wrist circumduction, thumb CMC circumduction and MP flexion restriction splint, type 0 (3) **B,** Wrist circumduction, thumb CMC circumduction and MP flexion restriction splint, type 0 (3) **C,** Wrist circumduction, thumb CMC circumduction and MP flexion restriction splint, type 0 (3)
Allowing wrist motion, splints provide gentle support. Neoprene **(A,B)** and tape **(C)** splints. **A,B,** Neoprene also provides mild warmth for a patient's extremity. [Courtesy **(A)** Joni Armstrong, OTR, CHT, Bemidji, Minn.; **(B)** Jennifer L. Henshaw, OTR, Santa Rosa, Calif.]

fractures[30] and its large intraosseous areas are supplied by only one blood vessel, making the scaphoid susceptible to avascular necrosis.[32,56] With a prevalence of nonunion and avascular necrosis problems, scaphoid fractures are treated with caution. The

mechanism of injury is often a fall onto outstretched palms with the wrist dorsiflexed.[40] Scaphoid fracture symptoms include tenderness in the anatomic snuffbox and local edema. Undisplaced fractures usually respond to early continuous immobilization.

It is important that the worker, athlete, or musician with a scaphoid fracture understand that immobilization is mandatory and that the duration of immobilization is determined by fracture stability and method of internal fixation used. Immobilization in a long or short arm wrist and thumb cast or splint may indeed require months before fracture healing is achieved. Stable nondisplaced fractures may be immobilized with the wrist in slight volar flexion and radial deviation.[40,52] The decision as to whether a cast or splint is applied is the responsibility of the physician. If a transition splint is needed from cast to unrestricted motion, a splint with both dorsal and volar hand/forearm components increases splint stability and immobilizing capacity, as complete wrist immobilization is the predominant requisite (Fig. 17-20). These splints must be remolded or replaced every few weeks to keep pace with receding edema and changes in forearm and hand size. If casting is used to immobilize a scaphoid fracture and healing progresses on schedule and the fracture is stable, the physician may decide to replace the long or short arm-thumb spica cast with a volarly fitted *wrist neutral, thumb CMC palmar abduction and MP flexion immobilization splint, type 0 (3)* that is worn between exercises with the wrist positioned at neutral and the thumb CMC in palmar abduction and MP in 0-10° flexion. For noncontact competition events, addition of a dorsal component to this splint adds stability and further prevents extension/dorsiflexion of the wrist. Responsibility for deciding when it is appropriate to return to

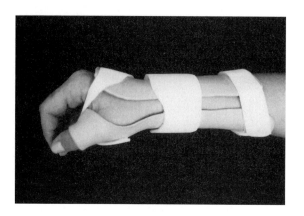

Fig. 17-20 Wrist extension, thumb CMC palmar abduction and MP flexion immobilization splint, type 0 (3) \\ Wrist extension immobilization splint, type 0 (1)
A combination volar and dorsal splint increases stability of the immobilized joints, decreases pain, and also allows adjustment for edema; used during the transition period between cast and unrestricted use.

work or competition rests solely with the referring physician. When an athlete is released to return to competition, a wrist and thumb silicone rubber playing cast for sports is usually necessary to further protect the newly healed scaphoid with its narrow waist configuration and its inherently tenuous blood supply.

■ COMMON FOREARM AND ELBOW INJURIES/CONDITIONS

Common forearm and elbow injuries/conditions include cubital tunnel syndrome, lateral epicondylitis, medial epicondylitis, and elbow dislocations/fractures.

Cubital Tunnel Syndrome

The ulnar nerve is vulnerable to injury at the elbow as it courses under fascia at the medial epicondyle and is tethered by the flexor carpi ulnaris.[55] Cubital tunnel syndrome may result from direct trauma, as in being hit on the elbow by a batted ball, or from sustained elbow flexion that compresses the ulnar nerve, as in playing a musical instrument that requires prolonged elbow flexion postures. For musicians, nerve compressions and tendonitis necessitate evaluation of postures, changes in technique (often correlates with changes in teachers), increases in playing times, and inefficient movement patterns. Cubital tunnel syndrome also is associated with athletes who play sports that increase tension and compression forces at the elbow, including baseball, tennis, racquetball, and javelin throwing. Workers whose jobs involve sustained elbow flexion are more prone to cubital tunnel syndrome problems.

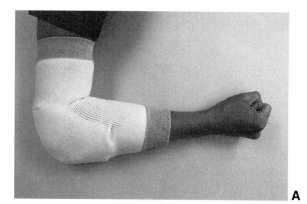

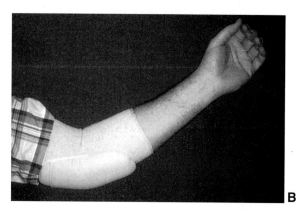

Fig. 17-21 A,B, An elbow pad or knee pad gives protection to the ulnar nerve at the elbow. An elbow pad may be custom made from foam and elastic stockinette.

Acute symptoms include pain, tingling, or numbness of the ring and small finger that may, over time, progress to weakness of the ulnar nerve innervated intrinsic muscles of the hand. Treatment goals include patient education and limiting elbow motion. Symptom-producing activities are identified and adapted with the intent of decreasing elbow flexion during instrument playing, sports, or work and eliminating prolonged elbow flexion during sleep. Simple padding solutions often suffice. A posterior elbow pad may be worn to protect the ulnar nerve from external compression (Fig. 17-21); worn on the anterior medial aspect of the elbow, a padded spandex kneepad protects the nerve by restricting elbow flexion. Pads are fitted loosely and must never escalate existing compression problems. Immobilization of the elbow is sometimes needed to avoid elbow flexion postures during the day and at night when patients are less aware of their elbow postures. To avoid further nerve compression, elbow immobilization splints are fitted anteriorly in approximately 45° of elbow flexion (Fig. 17-22). Posterior elbow pads may be added for additional elbow protection. If the ulnar nerve is hypermobile, subluxes anteriorly, and becomes inflamed as it shifts with elbow motion, the nerve requires immobilization in its posterior position,

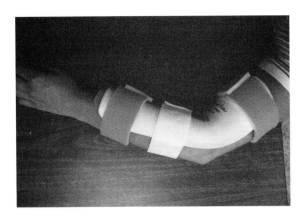

Fig. 17-22   Elbow flexion restriction splint, type 0 (1)
An elbow splint is worn during the day to avoid repetitive flexion and/or at night to avoid extreme flexion that increases ulnar nerve symptoms. At night, if symptoms are mild, a pillow or elbow pad may be secured to the anterior elbow instead of a splint to avoid extreme elbow flexion.

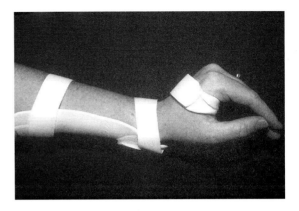

Fig. 17-23   Wrist extension immobilization splint, type 0 (1)
The wrist splint is positioned in extension to reduce strain at the common extensor origin.

which may correlate with almost full elbow extension.[7] Ergonomic changes must be included in daily routines to prevent further trauma to the ulnar nerve and patient education emphasizes avoidance of activities that (1) combine elbow flexion and pronation, (2) cause pressure to the nerve (e.g., resting elbows on arm rests or tables), and (3) require prolonged static elbow flexion. As pain is eliminated and positive behavioral changes are incorporated into patients' routines, elbow pads may be helpful not only for elbow protection but also as reminders to patients to monitor their elbow postures.

Lateral Epicondylitis

Frequently referred to as "tennis elbow," "rug beater's elbow," or "jailer's elbow," lateral epicondylitis is a common condition found in athletes, workers, and musicians. Arising from the humeral lateral epicondyle, the extensor-supinator muscles may be strained or contused through repetitive shear activities that cause microscopic tearing and inflammation at the origin of the common extensor tendon. Gripping an instrument, a piece of sporting equipment, or a tool further aggravates the injury. The exact etiology of lateral epicondylitis continues to be debated with mechanical, metabolic, and occupational theories cited. Riek et al. attribute lateral epicondylitis to the eccentric contraction at near maximum length of the extensor carpi radialis brevis,[43] and Lieber et al point to the ECRB's biphasic sarcomere length as the elbow moves from full extension to full flexion, resulting in eccentric muscle contraction.[17] Poor conditioning and/or poor technique may result in stress and inflammation of the extensor supinator muscle group, as with a racquet player who repetitively leads with the elbow on a back-

hand shot.[34] Symptoms of lateral epicondylitis include pain localized to the lateral epicondyle or lateral aspect of the elbow. A common history includes exertion involving grip and deviation of the wrist. Baseball pitchers may not be able to grip a ball and throw with elbow extension, while carpenters overuse their arms with hammering, and politicians describe symptoms secondary to shaking countless hands. Instrument players, especially violin and keyboard players, who use excessive twisting motions and/or poor coordination patterns have increased propensity for developing lateral epicondylitis.[18,19]

As with other overuse injuries, early treatment goals include reducing stress to the involved muscle groups, identification and adaptation of damaging use patterns, and patient education. Two separate randomized controlled trials (RCT) document wrist immobilization as a statistically significant, effective method for treating lateral epicondylitis. One RCT study found no significant difference between patient groups receiving wrist immobilization splinting and corticosteroid injections,[13] and another RTC study found no statistically significant difference between immobilization casting of the wrist and taking a recognized nonsteroidal anti-inflammatory.[16] Both studies recommended splinting/casting over injection or pharmacological intervention because splinting/casting lacks adverse side effects associated with drug-administered therapy.

For acute problems, a *type 0, wrist extension immobilization splint* immobilizes the wrist in dorsiflexion, decreasing tension on the ECRB and other muscles in the extensor-supinator group (Fig. 17-23). In severe cases an *elbow flexion, forearm neutral, wrist extension immobilization splint, type 0 (3)* may be used to immobilize the wrist in dorsiflexion, forearm in neutral, and elbow in 90° flexion. Designed to reduce irritation and control abusive force over-

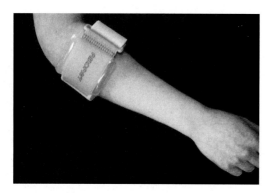

Fig. 17-24 Nonarticular proximal forearm splint
This nonarticular forearm splint design may reduce pain during activities that induce lateral epicondylitis. A variety of nonarticular forearm splint design options are available. (Courtesy Aircast, Summit, N.J.)

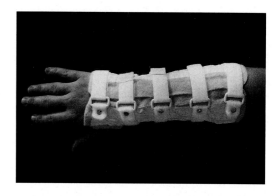

Fig. 17-25 Wrist neutral immobilization splint, type 0 (1)
Conservative management of medial epicondylitis may include 6-8 weeks of splinting the wrist at neutral or slight flexion to decrease activity level.

loads, *nonarticular forearm splints*, such as the Aircast* pneumatic armband, are also options (Fig. 17-24).[28,29] Nonarticular forearm splints are not positioned directly over the lateral epicondyle but over the tender area of the forearm, which is easily identified with resistive wrist extension. Splinting is augmented with exercise and patient education programs. Accompanying exercise regimes and modality use differ considerably from clinic to clinic. While many devices and techniques are touted for treating lateral epicondylitis, none provides relief to all individuals. Patients must be treated on a case-by-case basis to find the best possible solution for each person.

As pain diminishes, the rehabilitative program increasingly focuses on identifying, analyzing, and changing detrimental use patterns. It is important to identify the aggravating activity so that further injury is avoided upon return to work, sport, or playing a musical instrument. Reconditioning and balanced muscle strengthening combined with adaptation of the job situation, playing techniques, and/or equipment used are key elements to preventing recurrence of symptoms. Activities that repeatedly combine wrist extension and supination with resistance must be identified as well as grasp patterns used with tools and sports equipment. For musicians, decreasing the relative weight of instruments through use of a tripod stand or a harness often helps. Splints should not obstruct instruments' sound capacity or the motions required in playing.[14] For tennis players, this means defining and altering improper stroke mechanics, assessing the racquet and experimenting with different sized racquet grips, heads, and string tensions. Mea-

surement of the ring finger along the radial border from the proximal palmar crease to the tip of the ring is a good technique for determining handle size.[4a,28,29]

Medial Epicondylitis

Medial epicondylitis is similar to lateral epicondylitis but involves the muscles originating on the medial epicondyle of the humerus. Repetitive pronation with wrist flexion often leads to medial epicondylitis. Stress and microtearing to the pronator teres, flexor carpi radialis, flexor digitorum sublimus, and flexor carpi ulnaris occur in pitchers in the acceleration phase of throwing, during tennis serves, hitting a forehand shot, and with golf swings. Gymnasts place stress traction on the medial collateral ligament and epicondyle by using the upper extremity as a weight-bearing surface as when working on a vaulting horse.[53] "Golfer elbow," another term for medial epicondylitis, may be caused by not pulling the club through with the left side using the legs, back, and shoulder.[22] Symptoms include medial epicondyle tenderness upon palpation and pain on the medial aspect of the elbow with resistive wrist flexion or with passive wrist extension with the elbow extended. Conservative care may include a *type 0, wrist neutral immobilization splint* that holds the wrist in neutral to slight flexion for 6-8 weeks (Fig. 17-25). If discomfort continues and greater immobilization is indicated, an *elbow flexion, forearm neutral immobilization splint, type 0 (2)* that holds the elbow at 90° and the forearm in neutral may be added to the *wrist immobilization splint*. As pain decreases and immobilization splinting is no longer needed, progression to a *nonarticular forearm splint* adds extra support for the common flexor origin.[28]

---

*Aircast Corporation, Box T, Summit, NJ 07901; www.aircast.com.

Placement of *a nonarticular forearm splint* is distal to the medial epicondyle and, as with lateral epicondylitis, reconditioning and strengthening along with adaptation of the job and/or performance activity are implemented when appropriate diminished pain levels are achieved.

Elbow Dislocations/Fractures

Hyperextension is the most common reason for elbow dislocations. The coronoid process and the medial and lateral collateral ligaments provide stability for anterior/posterior movement while the biceps and brachialis supply negligible support in a hyperextension injury.[51] If the injury is of greater magnitude, an associated coronoid, epicondylar, or radial head fracture may occur along with ligament damage requiring surgical repair. These injuries are commonly seen in contact sports, gymnastics, or traumatic injuries on the job and many will require surgical repair. It is not within the scope of this discussion to review surgical intervention or postoperative care for elbow injuries. Only nonoperative elbow problems will be discussed in this section.

When treating acute elbow injuries, it is important not to force passive elbow extension, which may cause further injury or delay healing. Adjustable splints that control extension and flexion may be used to limit end range motion that may aggravate symptoms. Used with a dislocation or hyperextension sprain, a double hinged *elbow lateral and medial restriction splint, type 2 (3)* provides elbow stability while allowing motion. Adjustment options may include permitting full flexion and limiting extension, or allowing elbow full extension and limiting flexion (Fig. 17-26). An elbow sports splint may incorporate medial and lateral hinges but the medial hinge is detachable and is taped on for added stability for practice or competition. Padding is added to protect other athletes from the hinges. Elbow pads and neoprene sleeves are useful for protecting dislocations or fractures when sports or work are resumed. Useful for protecting the proximal ulna and olecranon bursa, these "soft splints" are elastic and foam combinations that vary in density from light open and closed cell foam, to Sorbothane, a dense viscoelastic polymer.[37,39] If an elbow flexion contracture occurs, an *elbow mobilization splint* is needed to increase passive elbow range of motion.

■ COMMON SHOULDER INJURIES/CONDITIONS

Common shoulder injuries/conditions include humeral fractures and anterior/posterior subluxation/dislocation.

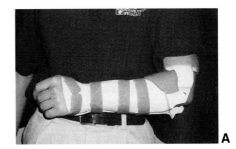
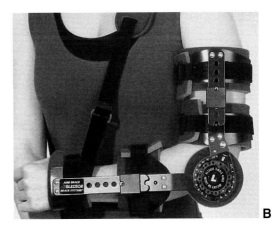

Fig. 17-26   A, Elbow lateral and medial restriction splint, type 2 (3) B, Elbow extension and flexion restriction splint, type 2 (3) A, Elbow stability is provided while flexion and extension are permitted in this splint. B, A commercially available splint limits varying degrees of extension and flexion. [Courtesy (A) Rebecca Banks, OTR, CHT, MHS, Blackburn, Australia; (B) Bledsoe Brace Systems, Grand Prairie, Texas]

Humeral Fracture

Trauma or a blow to the humeral region, as in direct impact or repeated blows by a ball, helmet, or striking by an opposing blocker, may cause a humeral fracture; a fall on the outstretched arm of a gymnast, worker, bicycler, or skier may also fracture the humerus. Rotational forces when the forearm is used as a lever can fracture the humerus as well, as in wrestling or shotput. Treatment involves protecting the area from additional trauma and avoiding circumstances that would interfere with fracture healing. Initial protection and external stabilization for reduced or minimally displaced fractures may be provided by a *nonarticular humeral splint* or a humeral "fracture brace" (Fig. 17-27); a posterior *elbow flexion immobilization splint, type 2 (3)* that maintains the elbow at 90°, forearm in neutral, and wrist in slight extension (Fig. 17-28); or a sling with the arm at the side. When return to sports, work, or activities is permitted, a neoprene sleeve or a padded sleeve constructed from cloth or foam and tape is often used as transitional protection.

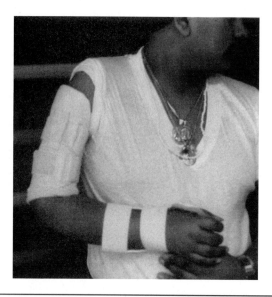

Fig. 17-27   **Nonarticular humerus splint \\ Wrist extension mobilization splint, type 0 (1)**
First splint: A nonarticular humerus splint protects a reduced or minimally displaced fracture from additional trauma. Second splint: Focusing on an associated radial nerve injury, a wrist mobilization splint maintains the wrist in slight extension, improving hand function. (Courtesy Sally Poole, MA, OTR, CHT, Dobbs Ferry, N.Y.)

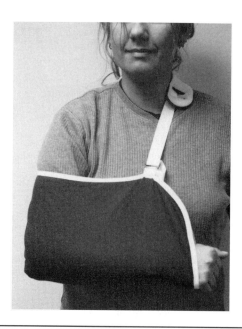

Fig. 17-29   During the healing and rest phase, a sling helps immobilize the shoulder following a posterior subluxation/dislocation.

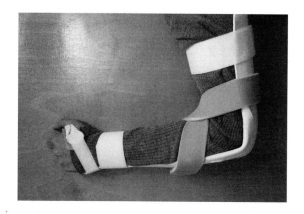

Fig. 17-28   **Elbow flexion immobilization splint, type 2 (3)**
Immobilization of the elbow, forearm, and wrist reduces stress and torque on a humeral fracture. The soft figure-eight strap provides secure placement of the elbow.

Shoulder Subluxation/Dislocation

Complete separation of the articular surfaces by a direct or indirect force results in a dislocation of the glenohumeral joint.[47] Dislocation includes a disruption of the ligaments of the joint, while a partial dislocation involves a subluxation of the shoulder joint, the sequela of a sprain. A dislocation may self-reduce, or be reduced by a teammate, coach, trainer, or physi-

cian. A minimum of 6 weeks is considered necessary for ligaments to mend, with protection that limits shoulder motion, obligatory for healing to take place. Shoulder instability is classified as anterior, posterior, superior, inferior, or multidirectional and may be congenital, acute, chronic, or recurrent.

Posterior Subluxation/Dislocation

A posterior shoulder dislocation may result from direct posterior force to the humerus or a fall on an outstretched hand, a direct blow to the anterior shoulder, or an indirect force of flexion, adduction, and internal rotation. Other etiology may also cause posterior dislocation of the shoulder, such as a worker who sustains an electric shock to the shoulder region.[47] Interestingly, an increment of posterior shoulder instability is sometimes desirable in swimming, volleyball, pitchers, and weightlifters. Symptoms include posterior shoulder pain with internal rotation, or flexing the arm to mimic strain or partial avulsion of the external rotator muscles.[30] The patient is unable to fully supinate the forearm and hand with the arm in forward flexion.[47] Treatment involves sling or splint immobilization with the arm adducted to the side and internally rotated, and the forearm positioned across the chest, providing this posture is not painful (Fig. 17-29). If internal rotation is painful, a cast is used to hold the shoulder in anatomic position, the elbow at 90° and the forearm forward (shoulder neutral rotation).[30] Splinting protection of the shoulder usually lasts for 3-6 weeks.

Anterior Subluxation/Dislocation

Anterior-inferior subluxation is the most frequent kind of athletic injury to the shoulder.[30] A force applied with the upper extremity in abduction, external rotation, and extension may cause attenuation of the anterior stabilizers of the joint.[47] Symptoms include pain anteriorly, muscle spasm, and a sensation the shoulder is "slipping out." External rotation and abduction are not permissible during healing, with immobilization of the shoulder varying from 1 to 6 weeks depending on the patient's age, the specific injury, and the sport in which the patient is involved. Consider occupation, dominant side, and general health in determining a conservative program. A sling is used to immobilize the arm at the side with a circumferential swathe to prevent external rotation-abduction between specific exercises for increasing the strength of muscles that stabilize the shoulder. Generally, older patients require a shorter immobilization to avoid shoulder stiffness and younger patients a longer phase to avoid shoulder joint laxity. Active use of the hand is permitted in the sling. A commercial shoulder harness is available to control shoulder instability by avoiding abduction and external rotation with lacing connecting the chest vest to the biceps cuff restraining abduction in varying degrees. One commercially available harness is the C.D. Denison-Duke Wyres shoulder vest.[38] Accurate application of a sling will permit the unaffected shoulder to support the affected upper extremity owing to the posterior diagonal strap and the hand, wrist, and forearm rest in the sling trough in a nondependent position.[20,21] After the immobilization period is completed and full ROM is achieved, a strengthening program is initiated.

▇ INSTRUCTIONS FOR SILICONE RUBBER PLAYING CAST FABRICATION

Materials

- Disposable towel or barrier to drape area of application
- Nonsterile surgical gloves
- 3-4 rolls 2-inch gauze wrap
- Prewrap, cotton stockinette, or petroleum jelly
- Emesis basin or similar container
- Tongue depressor
- 1-pound can RTV11* silicone rubber and catalyst
- Blunt-ended scissors
- Adhesive or nonadhesive open cell foam padding, $\frac{3}{8}$-inch thickness (1-2 sheets, 16 inches by 24 inches)

- Moleskin (1-2 sheets, 16 inches by 24 inches, needed if foam padding is adhesive)
- 2-inch or 3-inch elastic wrap or self-adherent, non-adhesive elastic wrap

Fabrication

- Cover working area with disposable drape.
- Apply a nonsterile surgical glove to the patient's injured hand. Proximal to the glove apply petroleum jelly to prevent adherence of RTV11 silicone rubber to skin and hair followed by prewrap or cotton stockinette (Fig. 17-30).
- If the foam padding has an adhesive side, remove paper backing. Moleskin is applied to the sticky side of the padding. The adhesive foam padding side will be against the skin and the moleskin side is exposed. The foam-padding seam is opposite the injury site. If moleskin is not applied, the sticky side of the adhesive foam padding faces the skin. A word of caution: This sticky surface does not embed well into the curing silicone rubber.
- Wrap the involved digits, hand, wrist, and $\frac{2}{3}$ the length of the forearm with 2-inch gauze wrap, overlapping $\frac{1}{2}$ the width of each wrap (Fig. 17-31).
- Trace the RTV11 cast pattern onto the foam padding.
- Don nonsterile surgical gloves.
- Open 1-pound can of RTV11 silicone rubber and add catalyst, avoiding skin contact with the raw catalyst. Thoroughly stir with a tongue depressor and pour in emesis basin. If less than 1 pound is required use 20 drops of the catalyst to 4 ounces RTV11. (Note: Prior to opening RTV11, store in cool location to maximize shelf life.) (Fig. 17-32)
- A thin layer of RTV11 silicone rubber is spread over the gauze wrap with a tongue depressor. This layer is thin but should be sufficient to saturate the gauze. (Remember that two additional, thicker layers will be applied when judging the amount used on the first layer.) (Fig. 17-33)
- Position the extremity as needed for the injury and participation in the specific sport.
- Gently wrap and overlap gauze over the first layer of RTV11 silicone rubber.
- Apply a second layer of RTV11 silicone rubber over the gauze. This layer will be thicker than the first (Fig. 17-34).
- Gently wrap and overlap a third layer of gauze over the RTV11 silicone rubber.
- Apply the third layer of RTV11 silicone rubber over the gauze. This layer should be heavily applied.

---

*General Electric Co., Silicone Rubber Products Division, 260 Hudson River Road, Waterford, NY 12188; www.gesilicones.com.

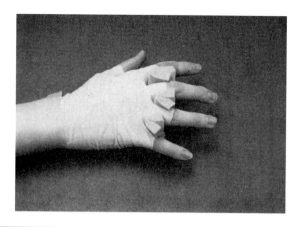

Fig. 17-30 Place a surgical glove on the patient's hand and use prewrap to cover the portion of the forearm exposed above the glove. Place small foam pads between the fingers to maintain the hand in a functional position. (Courtesy Cheri Alexy, CHT, OTR, Methodist Sports Medicine Center, Indianapolis, Ind.)

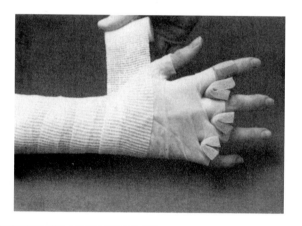

Fig. 17-31 Wrap the glove and prewrap with one layer of gauze. (Courtesy Cheri Alexy, CHT, OTR, Methodist Sports Medicine Center, Indianapolis, Ind.)

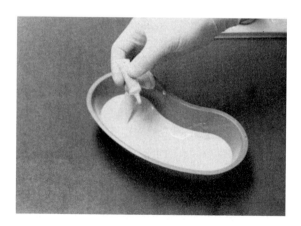

Fig. 17-32 While wearing surgical gloves, pour approximately half the RTV11 silicone rubber into the disposable bowl. Add about half the catalyst and mix thoroughly with a tongue depressor. (Courtesy Cheri Alexy, CHT, OTR, Methodist Sports Medicine Center, Indianapolis, Ind.)

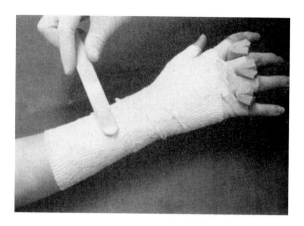

Fig. 17-33 Spread the RTV11 silicone rubber onto the prepared surface using a tongue depressor. Apply generously, covering the gauze completely without contacting the patient's skin. (Courtesy Cheri Alexy, CHT, OTR, Methodist Sports Medicine Center, Indianapolis, Ind.)

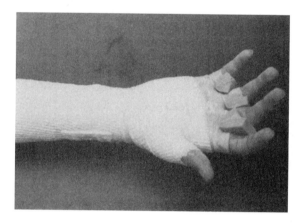

Fig. 17-34 Repeat steps shown in Figs. 17-31 and 17-32 two to four times, depending on the severity of the injury and the desired thickness of the cast. The outer layer at this stage will be silicone rubber rather than gauze. (Courtesy Cheri Alexy, CHT, OTR, Methodist Sports Medicine Center, Indianapolis, Ind.)

- Immediately apply the nonadhesive side of the foam padding over the layers of gauze and RTV11 silicone rubber with the seam of the foam padding opposite to the side of the injury. The foam will become embedded in the uncured RTV11 silicone rubber, adhering the foam to the layers of silicone rubber coated gauze (Fig. 17-35).
- Secure the playing cast with an outer elastic wrap (Fig. 17-36). If the patient needs to hold an object such as handlebars or a steering wheel, position the arm as needed. The fingertips of the surgical glove may be removed on the uninjured digits.
- Allow 3-4 hours for the RTV11 silicone rubber to cure before removal.* Cut the cast with blunt scissors on the opposite side of the injury, along the foam-padding seam (Fig. 17-37). After removal

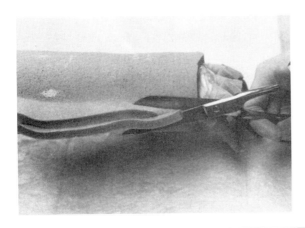

Fig. 17-35   Wrap the adhesive foam padding carefully around the cast, forming a seam on the side opposite to the injury and trim excess. (Courtesy Cheri Alexy, CHT, OTR, Methodist Sports Medicine Center, Indianapolis, Ind.)

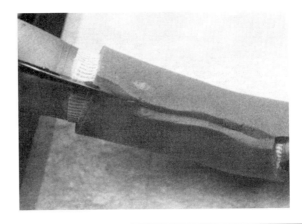

Fig. 17-37   Instruct the patient to cut the cast off using blunt scissors at home after 3-4 hours. The cut, which is made on the side opposite the injury along the seam of the pad, will cause the patient little discomfort. (Courtesy Cheri Alexy, CHT, OTR, Methodist Sports Medicine Center, Indianapolis, Ind.)

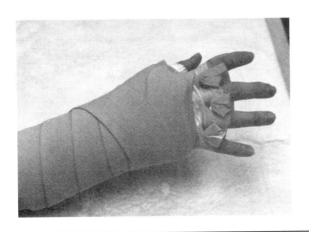

Fig. 17-36   Wrap the entire cast using the 2-inch or 3-inch elastic bandage. (Courtesy Cheri Alexy, CHT, OTR, Methodist Sports Medicine Center, Indianapolis, Ind.)

of the surgical glove, the protective inner layer of prewrap or stockinette may be discarded; remove the petroleum jelly from the patient's arm. Wash arm with soap and water.

- Always check for skin reaction to the cast materials both during fabrication and wearing of a cast. If a reaction is noted, fabrication and use of the silicone rubber playing cast should be discontinued immediately.
- The playing cast is secured with tape or elastic wrap during practice or competition. The patient's hand and forearm may be dusted with powder or covered with a stockinette to absorb moisture before application of the cast to protect the skin.

*See Canelon MF, Karus AJ: A room temperature silicone rubber sport splint, *AM J Occup Ther*: 49(3):244-49, 1995, for alternative techniques.

SUMMARY

Overall considerations for splinting workers, athletes, and musicians are as follows:

- Consider splint design as a means of early return to the job, sport, or play.
- Incorporate the tool, equipment, or musical instrument in splint fit if appropriate.
- Ensure the splint does not create a fulcrum for a new injury.
- Tape and elastic wrap, which are more secure than Velcro straps, have excellent conforming abilities for holding splints on extremities during work, sports, or play.
- Padding the outside of a splint protects other players who may come in contact with the splint from being injured.

REFERENCES

1. Abouna J: Splint for mallet finger, *Br Med J* 54:432-44, 1965.
2. Abouna JM, Brown H: The treatment of mallet finger, *Br J Surg* 55:653, 1968.
3. Angelides AC, Wallace PF: The dorsal ganglion of the wrist: its pathogenesis, gross and microscopic anatomy, and surgical treatment, *J Hand Surg* 1(3):228-35, 1976.
3a. Apfel E, Johnson M, Abrams R: Comparison of range of motion constraints provided by prefabricated splints used in the treatment of carpal tunnel syndrome: A pilot study, *J Hand Ther* 15(3):226-33, 2002.
4. Bergfeld JA, Welker GG, Andrish JT, et al: Soft playing splints for protection of significant hand and wrist injuries in sports, *Am J Sports Med* 10(5):293-6, 1982.
4a. Borkholder CD, Hill VA, Fess EE: The efficacy of splinting for lateral epicondylitis: A systematic review, *J Hand Ther* 17(2) (in press).

5. Brown AP: The effects of anti-vibration gloves on vibration-induced disorders: a case study, *J Hand Ther* 3(2):94-100, 1990.

6. Canelon MF: Material properties: a factor in the selection and application of splinting materials for athletic wrist and hand injuries, *J Orthop Sports Phys Ther* 22(4):164-72, 1995.

7. Eaton RG: Entrapment syndromes in musicians, *J Hand Ther* 5(2):91-6, 1992.

8. Evans R, Hunter J, Burkhalter W: Conservative management of the trigger finger: a new approach, J Hand Ther 1(2):59-68, 1988.

9. Evans RB, Burkhalter WE: A study of the dynamic anatomy of extensor tendons and implications for treatment, *J Hand Surg* [Am] 11(5):774-9, 1986.

10. Gieck JH, Mayer V: Protective splinting for the hand and wrist, *Am J Sports Med* 7:275-86, 1986.

11. Hankin FM, Peel SM: Sports-related fractures and dislocations in the hand, *Hand Clinics* 6:429-53, 1990.

12. Hillfrank B: Protecting the injured hand for sports, *J Hand Ther* 4(2):51-6, 1991.

13. Jensen B, Bliddal H, Danneskiold-Samsoe B: [Comparison of two different treatments of lateral humeral epicondylitis—"tennis elbow." A randomized controlled trial], *Ugeskr Laeger* 163(10):1427-31, 2001.

14. Johnson CD: Splinting the injured musician, *J Hand Ther* 5(2):107-10, 1992.

15. Kuland DN: *The injured athlete*, J.B. Lippincott, 1982, Philadelphia.

16. Labelle H, Guibert R: Efficacy of diclofenac in lateral epicondylitis of the elbow also treated with immobilization. The University of Montreal Orthopaedic Research Group, *Arch Fam Med* 6(3):257-62, 1997.

17. Lieber RL, Ljung BO, Friden J: Sarcomere length in wrist extensor muscles. Changes may provide insights into the etiology of chronic lateral epicondylitis, *Acta Orthop Scand* 68(3):249-54, 1997.

18. Lowe C: Treatment of tendinitis, tenosynovitis, and other cumulative trauma disorders of musicians' forearms, wrists, and hands: restoring function with hand therapy, *J Hand Ther* 5(2):84-90, 1992.

19. Markison RE: Tendinitis and related inflammatory conditions seen in musicians, *J Hand Ther* 5(2):80-3, 1992.

20. Mayer V, Gieck J: Protection of athletic injuries of the hand and wrist. Hand and wrist injuries and treatment, *Sports Injury Management* 2:72-90, 1989.

21. Mayer VA et al: Rehabilitation and protection of the hand and wrist. In Nicholas JA, Elliott MD, Hershman B, Posner MA: *The upper extremity in sports medicine*, Mosby, 1990, St. Louis.

22. McCarroll JR: Evaluation, treatment, and prevention of upper extremity injuries in golfers. In Nicholas JA, Elliott MD, Hershman B, Posner MA: *The upper extremity in sports medicine*, Mosby, 1990, St. Louis.

23. McCue FC, Cabrera JM: Common athletic digital joint injuries of the hand. In Strickland JW, Rettig AC: *Hand injuries in athletes*, W.B. Saunders, 1992, Philadelphia.

24. McCue FC, Garroway RY: Sports injuries to the hand and wrist. In Schneider RC, Kennedy JC, Plant ML: *Sports injuries: mechanisms, prevention and treatment*, Williams & Wilkins, 1985, Baltimore.

25. Mendoza FX, Nicholas JA, et al: The upper extremity in sports medicine. In Nicholas JA, Elliott MD, Hershman B, Posner MA: *The upper extremity in sports medicine*, Mosby, 1990, St. Louis.

26. Neviaser RJ: Collateral ligament injuries of the thumb metacarpophalangeal joint. In Strickland JW, Rettig AC: *Hand injuries in athletes*, W.B. Saunders, 1992, Philadelphia.

27. Nicholas JA, Elliott MD, Hershman B, Posner MA: *The upper extremity in sports medicine*, Mosby, 1990, St. Louis.

28. Nirschl RP: Tennis injuries. In Nicholas JA, Elliott MD, Hershman B, Posner MA: *The upper extremity in sports medicine*, Mosby, 1990, St. Louis.

29. Nirschl RP, Sabol J: *Tennis elbow: prevention and treatment*, Medical Sports Publishing 1989, Arlington.

30. O'Donoghue DH: *Treatment of injuries to athletes*, W.B. Saunders, 1984, Philadelphia.

31. Opgrande JD, Westphal SA: Fractures of the hand, *Orthop Clin North Am* 14(4):779-92, 1983.

32. Panagis JS, Gelberman RH, et al, The arterial anatomy of the human carpus II, the intraosseous vascularity, *J Hand Surg* 8:375, 1983.

33. Parks BJ, Barrett KP, Voss K: The use of Hexcelite in splinting the thumb, *Am J Occup Ther* 37(4):266-7, 1983.

34. Posner MA: Injuries to the hand and wrist in athletes, *Ortho Clinics N Am* 8:593, 1977.

35. Posner MA: Hand injuries. In Nicholas JA, Elliott MD, Hershman B, Posner MA: *The upper extremity in sports medicine*, Mosby, 1990, St. Louis.

36. Rayan GM, Mullins PT: Skin necrosis complicating mallet finger splinting and vascularity of the distal interphalangeal joint overlying skin, *J Hand Surg* 12(4):548-52, 1987.

37. Reese PC, Burruss TP, et al: Athletic taping and protective equipment. In Nicholas JA, Elliott MD, Hershman B, Posner MA: *The upper extremity in sports medicine*, Mosby, 1990, St. Louis.

38. Reese RC, Burruss TP, et al: Shoulder equipment. In Nicholas JA, Elliott MD, Hershman B, Posner MA: *The upper extremity in sports medicine*, Mosby, 1990, St. Louis.

39. Reese RC, Burruss TP, et al: Athletic training and protective equipment. In Nicholas JA, Elliott MD, Hershman B, Posner MA: *The upper extremity in sports medicine*, Mosby, 1990, St. Louis.

40. Rettig AC: Current concepts in management of football injuries of the hand and wrist, *J Hand Ther* 4(2), 1991.

41. Rettig AC: Closed tendon injuries of the hand and wrist in the athlete, *Clin Sports Med* 11(1):77-99, 1992.

42. Rettig AC, Ryan RO, et al: Epidemiology of hand injuries in sports. In Strickland JW, Rettig AC: *Hand injuries in athletes*, W.B. Saunders, 1992, Philadelphia.

43. Riek S, Chapman AE, Milner T: A simulation of muscle force and internal kinematics of extensor carpi radialis brevis during backhand tennis stroke: implications for injury, *Clin Biomech* (Bristol, Avon) 14(7):477-83, 1999.

44. Sadler JA, Koepfer JM: Rehabilitation and splinting of the injured hand. In Strickland JW, Rettig AC: *Hand injuries in athletes*, W.B. Saunders, 1992, Philadelphia.

45. Saunders WF: The occult dorsal carpal ganglion, *J Hand Surg* 10(2):257-60, 1985.

46. Schultz-Johnson K: Static progressive splinting, *J Hand Ther* 15(2):163-78, 2002.

47. Skybar MJW, et al: Instability of the shoulder. In Nicholas JA, Elliott MD, Hershman B, Posner MA: *The upper extremity in sports medicine*, Mosby, 1990, St. Louis.

48. Stamos BD, Leddy JP: Closed flexor tendon disruption in athletes, *Hand Clin* 16(3):359-65, 2000.

49. Strickland JW, Rettig AC: *Hand injuries in athletes*, W.B. Saunders, 1992, Philadelphia.

50. Taleisnik J: Soft tissue injuries of the wrist. In Strickland JW, Rettig AC: *Hand injuries in athletes*, W.B. Saunders, 1992, Philadelphia.

51. Tullos HS, Bennett J: Acute injuries to the elbow. In Nicholas JA, Elliott MD, Hershman B, Posner MA: *The upper extremity in sports medicine*, Mosby, 1990, St. Louis.

52. Webber RE, Chao EY: An experimental approach to the mechanism of scaphoid wrist fractures, *J Hand Surg* 3:142-8, 1978.

53. Weiker GG: Upper extremity gymnastic injuries. In Nicholas JA, Elliott MD, Hershman B, Posner MA: *The upper extremity in sports medicine*, Mosby, 1990, St. Louis.

54. Weiss ND, Gordon L, Bloom T, et al: Position of the wrist associated with the lowest carpal-tunnel pressure: implications for splint design, *J Bone Joint Surg Am* 77(11):1695-9, 1995.

55. Whitaker JH, Richardson GA: Compressive neuropathies. In Strickland JW, Rettig AC: *Hand injuries in athletes*, W.B. Saunders, 1992, Philadelphia.

56. Zemel NP: Carpal fractures. In Strickland JW, Rettig AC: *Hand injuries in athletes*, W.B. Saunders, 1992, Philadelphia.

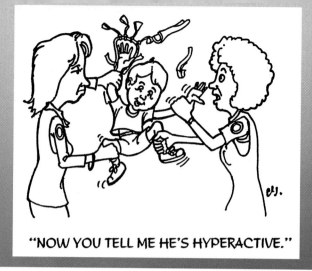

"NOW YOU TELL ME HE'S HYPERACTIVE."

CHAPTER 18

Splinting the Pediatric Patient

Joni Armstrong, OTR, CHT*

Chapter Outline

Splinting in the pediatric population can occur as early as the neonatal intensive care unit and may persist into adulthood for those who continue to be challenged by abnormal tone. Review of the literature finds very little objective research in the area of pediatric splinting.[1] This is probably due to difficulty finding a sufficient number of children in a given area who have a similar diagnosis with a comparable clinical picture on which to do a comparative study. Because of this and the resulting unfamiliarity of pediatric therapists with splinting options available, splinting is perhaps an underused form of treatment in the field of pediatrics. Although not a replacement for other forms of therapy, it can be a valuable adjunct to other therapeutic techniques.

This chapter focuses primarily on splinting for children who have developmental disabilities with subsequent difficulties in hand function. Although the splints discussed in this chapter have been observed to be clinically effective, lack of conclusive research and the variety of opinions specifically regarding splinting of the spastic hand mean that splint appropriateness must be evaluated on an individual basis and carefully monitored for effectiveness.

The overall goal of splinting in the pediatric population is to maximize hand function. This can be achieved through splint use with the following goals: (1) provide protection and support to weak muscles and joints, (2) provide proximal support and stability for improved distal function, (3) normalize muscle tone, (4) provide positioning of a joint, which then allows overall limb use and improved body movement and function, (5) compensate for muscle imbalance, (6) substitute for muscles that are not functional, (7) increase joint range of motion, (8) improve joint alignment, (9) decrease edema, (10) prevent or correct deformities, (11) make skin care and hygiene tasks easier, and (12) assist in task performance.

When selecting a splint for a pediatric patient, consider not only the problems associated with the upper extremity but also the strengths. Make certain that

---

*All figures in this chapter courtesy Joni Armstrong, OTR, CHT, Bemidji, Minn.

strengths are not eliminated with the problem's solution. Because most children with developmental disabilities have experienced the problems since birth, they have learned compensation techniques that allow them to use their hand quite functionally. Unless function is evaluated through observation, it can be easy to eliminate this functional use by splinting to fix another problem. Examples of this might be splinting the thumb in a position of palmar abduction and therefore preventing the functional use of the lateral pinch; or splinting a child's hand in functional position to prevent contracture formation, but using a splint that is too heavy for the child to wave his hand in greeting.

Problem areas seldom occur in isolation with the pediatric hand. Typically, several problems occur simultaneously. In splint selection, one needs to prioritize the problems, and then decide if all of these can be addressed at the same time in the same splint or if focus on one problem should be delayed in favor of initially focusing on another. Often a variety of splints with varying wearing schedules are an option to address more than one goal. Consideration of splints that are designed to increase function for performance of a specific task may also be warranted and these splints would only be worn during that task performance time.

As with adult hand splinting, there are many pediatric splinting options available to address the specific goals. A table of common pediatric problem areas describes splinting options presented in this chapter (Table 18-1). Selection varies with each patient's needs, caregiver compliance and preference, and therapist familiarity.

Compliance with the basic splinting principles described in this book for fabrication and fit of an adult splint is also recommended when fabricating pediatric splints; however, additional points also need to be considered for pediatric splinting success. Skin integrity of a child is often less than in an adult, so precautions need to be taken during the fabrication process and in monitoring to avoid burns and skin breakdown. This is particularly true for children who are underweight with little subcutaneous fat tissue. Splint monitoring by a responsible adult is very important as children often don't or can't complain of pain or discomfort. This is especially important if there is an accompanying sensory deficit. Children characteristically grow at a very rapid rate, so splints need to be monitored for appropriate fit and may frequently need replacing as they are outgrown. With the hopefully active lifestyle of children, splints may tend to wear out rapidly and this may necessitate replacement more often than with adults. Due to a high activity level and lack of mature judgment, damage to pediatric splints is not infrequent. Excuses given are

similar to those for the question, "What happened to your homework?" such as "My dog ate it," and "It fell out the bus window." As many children realize the importance of a splint, sometimes a reluctance to report damage that might "be their fault" is seen. This can result in not wearing the splint, improper application, or pressure areas.

In pediatrics, abnormal muscle tone is commonly the problem that therapists try to address. As a positioning change is made in one joint with abnormal tone or decreased range of motion, that change will most likely affect an adjacent joint as a way of compensation. An example of this would be as wrist extension is increased, increased finger flexion is also observed. Therefore, it may be necessary to compromise the ideal position of the splint (splint at less than maximum range) of one joint in order to avoid increased stresses on adjacent joints resulting in decreased function. Make certain that a splint does not prevent hand use that was previously achieved. Is an important action being taken away to gain something else? Which is more important?

IDEAS TO AID IN SPLINT CONSTRUCTION

Pediatric splinting can be fun but also really quite challenging, due to a number of factors including increased muscle tone, presence of primitive reflexes, splint size, short attention span, and lack of ability or desire to cooperate.

If the child being splinted has a significant amount of hypertonicity or behaviors that make splint fabrication difficult, it is recommended that another person be available to assist, not with the actual splint fabrication, but with positioning and distracting of the child. It is not recommended that a parent, teacher, or caregiver assist in the actual fabrication because their focus tends to be on control of the child with resulting fingerprints and pressure in the portion of the splint being held rather than the desired contour. However, their assistance in holding, positioning, and comforting the child can be of great value. Although a toy may be nice to occupy the child during the splinting process, it is not recommended that the child hold articles in the opposite hand due to the frequent overflow of tone to the hand being splinted which may make positioning difficult. Wrapping the forearm piece with elastic wrap or exercise band cooled in a refrigerator or freezer is also an option when an extra hand is needed. Quick cooling with cold spray is often helpful if positioning is difficult to hold due to behavior or spasticity. When another experienced therapist or aide is available to assist in fabrication, this situation is ideal.

TABLE 18-1   Common Pediatric Problems and Associated Splinting Options

Elbow Splints
Problem: Elbow Flexion

ESCS	Common Name
Elbow extension mobilization splint, type 0 (1)	*Elbow extension (volar) Elbow extension (circumferential) Elbow extension (bivalve) Air splint Turnbuckle elbow extension
Elbow extension mobilization splint, type 0 (1)	*Orthokinetic cuff

Forearm Splints
Problem: Limited Supination

ESCS	Common Name
Forearm supination, wrist extension, thumb CMC palmar abduction mobilization splint, type 0 (3)	*Long serpentine (proximal neoprene strap)
Forearm supination, wrist extension, thumb CMC radial abduction and MP extension mobilization splint, type 0 (4)	*Long neoprene thumb abduction with serpentine strap
Elbow flexion, forearm supination, wrist extension mobilization splint, type 0 (3)	Long arm (positioned in elbow flexion and forearm supination)

Wrist Splints
Problem: Wrist Flexion

ESCS	Common Name
Wrist extension, index–small finger extension, thumb CMC palmar abduction and MP-IP extension mobilization splint, type 0 (16)	*Resting hand (used serially if contractures have formed)
Wrist extension mobilization splint, type 0 (1)	*Radial bar wrist cock-up (volar) Radial bar wrist cock-up (dorsal) Wrist cock-up (thumb hole) Wrist cock-up (palmar support only) Wrist cock-up (circumferential thumb hole) Long neoprene (volar or dorsal stay)
Wrist extension, thumb CMC radial abduction and MP extension mobilization splint, type 0 (3)	*Long neoprene thumb abduction (volar or dorsal stay)
Forearm supination, wrist extension, thumb CMC palmar abduction mobilization splint, type 0 (3)	Long serpentine (for mild hypertonicity)
Wrist extension, index, ring–small finger MP abduction, index–small finger extension, thumb CMC palmar abduction and MP-IP extension mobilization splint, type 0 (16)	Antispasticity
Wrist extension mobilization splint, type 0 (1)	*Orthokinetic cuff

Problem: Wrist Ulnar Deviation

ESCS	Common Name
Wrist extension mobilization / wrist ulnar deviation restriction splint, type 0 (1)	Ulnar gutter Wrist cock-up with ulnar support
Wrist extension, thumb CMC radial abduction and MP extension mobilization / wrist ulnar deviation restriction splint, type 0 (3)	Long neoprene thumb abduction with ulnar gutter insert

Problem: Wrist Radial Deviation

ESCS	Common Name
Wrist extension, thumb CMC palmar abduction and MP extension / wrist radial deviation restriction splint, type 0 (3)	Long thumb spica Long thumb opponens
Wrist extension, thumb CMC palmar abduction mobilization / wrist radial deviation restriction splint, type 0 (2)	Dorsal radial bar wrist cock-up with thumb C-bar

TABLE 18-1   Common Pediatric Problems and Associated Splinting Options—cont'd

Hand Splints
Problem: Thumb-in-Palm Positioning

ESCS	Common Name
Thumb CMC radial abduction and MP extension mobilization splint, type 0 (2)	*Neoprene thumb abduction Short thumb opponens Short thumb spica
Thumb CMC radial abduction mobilization splint, type 0 (1)	*Thumb loop
Wrist extension, thumb CMC radial abduction and MP extension mobilization splint, type 0 (3)	Long thumb opponens Long thumb spica Wrist cock-up with thumb loop
Wrist extension, thumb CMC palmar abduction mobilization splint, type 0 (2)	Serpentine (short)
Thumb CMC palmar abduction mobilization splint, type 0 (1)	Thumb c-bar
Forearm supination, wrist extension, thumb CMC palmar abduction mobilization splint, type 0 (3)	Serpentine
Forearm supination, wrist extension, thumb CMC palmar abduction and MP-IP extension mobilization splint, type 0 (5)	Serpentine with thumb piece

Problem: Hand Fisting

ESCS	Common Name
Wrist extension, index, ring–small finger MP abduction, index–small finger extension, thumb CMC radial abduction and MP-IP extension mobilization splint, type 0 (16)	Antispasticity ball Antispasticity (dorsal) with finger pan (volar) *Resting hand (can add finger spacers)
Wrist extension, index–small finger MP extension mobilization splint, type 0 (5)	MacKinnon
Index–small finger extension, thumb CMC radial abduction and MP-IP extension mobilization splint, type 0 (15)	Cone

Problem: Difficulty Weight Bearing

ESCS	Common Name
Wrist extension, index–small finger MP extension and IP flexion, thumb CMC radial abduction and MP-IP extension mobilization splint, type 0 (16)	*Weight bearing
Elbow extension mobilization splint, type 0 (1)	Elbow extension *Elbow air (water wings)

Problem: Inability to Maintain Grasp

ESCS	Common Name
Wrist extension mobilization splint, type 0 (1)	*Wrist cock-up
	*Neoprene grasp assist
Thumb CMC radial abduction and MP extension mobilization splint, type 0 (2)	*Thumb abduction with sewn neoprene grasp assist Neoprene thumb abduction with sewn elastic pocket

Problem: Difficulty with Finger Isolation for Task Performance

ESCS	Common Name
Wrist extension, index finger MP flexion and IP extension, thumb CMC radial abduction and MP extension mobilization splint, type 0 (6)	*Long thumb opponens with index finger extension *Long or short neoprene thumb abduction with index finger included

*Indicates this author's favorites.

If hypertonicity is one of the challenges, it may be beneficial to decrease the tone through gentle passive range of motion exercises, massage, or neutral warmth application prior to splint fabrication. These techniques may also be helpful for use prior to splint application.

Awareness of the presence of primitive reflexes is important because they may be elicited by a change in body position. Positioning to elicit or inhibit the reflex assists in splint fabrication. For example, a child who exhibits a strong asymmetrical tonic neck reflex will exhibit extension in the upper extremity with his head turned to that side, decreasing the flexor tone in that extremity. If the head is turned to the opposite side, strong flexion can be seen in the extremity, making splint fabrication difficult.

When a child is frightened or uncertain about allowing a splint to be fabricated on his hand, allowing that child to play with scraps of the splinting material so he can see how it feels will often make him feel more at ease. Another technique is to have the child assist while making a splint on her doll or stuffed toy. A doll or toy that the therapist has wearing splints may also be helpful (Fig. 18-1).

■ MATERIALS SELECTION

A variety of materials are available for use in pediatric splinting. Some of the most commonly used and those recommended in this text include low-temperature thermoplastics, neoprene, elastomers, elastic wraps,

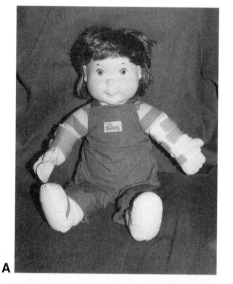

A

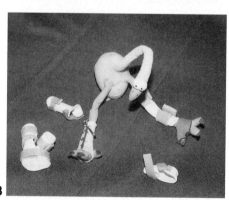

B

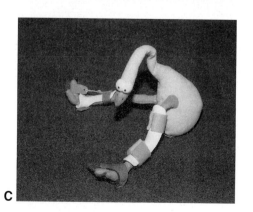

C

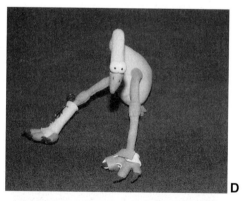

D

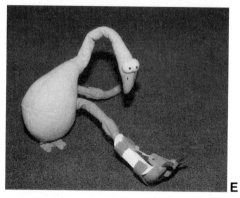

E

Fig. 18-1   A-E, Demonstrating and playing with dolls or toys that have been fit with splints will instill a positive introduction to children before application of splints to the actual pediatric arm.

and a variety of strapping materials. Selection of thermoplastics varies with each therapist and each child splinted. A variety of thermoplastics are available with pros and cons for the use of each.

Rubber-based thermoplastics work well with the pediatric population because they allow a great deal of control. They can be worked aggressively and have a high resistance to fingerprinting and stretch. Memory is fairly good if reforming or serial splinting is necessary. This material does need to be worked somewhat and held in place to maintain conformability. It is not as durable as some of the other splinting materials, so it may need reinforcement to prevent stress fractures. Rubber-based thermoplastics are a good choice for children who have a great deal of spasticity or who demonstrate behaviors that are not conducive to splinting. It is also a good choice for larger splints. Rubber-based thermoplastics are probably the easiest material to work with for beginning splinters.

Plastic-based thermoplastics are good material choices if a great deal of conformability is desired, especially for very small splints. It stretches easily and is not resistant to fingerprints. This material has very little memory, so it is not a good choice for serial splinting. Working time is short, which may or may not be an advantage. It is quite rigid when hard. Due to the high degree of stretch, the tendency to stick to itself, and little resistance to fingerprinting, it is difficult to use with children who have a high degree of spasticity or behaviors that are not conducive to splinting. It is typically a difficult material for beginning splinters.

Elastic-based thermoplastics are excellent choices for serial splinting due to their high degree of memory. Conformability is similar to that of rubber-based and is resistant to stretch and fingerprinting. Although rigidity is not high, this material is durable and will typically hold up to hard use. Working time is long, which may or may not be an advantage. It is not recommended to cool this material with cold spray because the top layer cools more quickly than the bottom, resulting in a twisting of the material. It can also lose some contour if removed from the hand and cooled quickly under cold water or if removed before cooling is complete.

Rubber-plastic-based thermoplastics are splinting materials that balance control and conformability. They self-edge nicely with some resistance to stretch and fingerprinting. These are a good choice for settings that see a variety of patient types, but only carry one type of splinting material. These materials may not have the desired control for children with a high degree of spasticity.

In the ideal situation, it is nice to carry an example of each of the four types of thermoplastics described above and use them to best meet patient needs. However, in many settings (particularly school-based therapists), the budget will allow purchase of only one type of thermoplastic. In this situation, the author recommends a thermoplastic that is primarily rubber-based because it will allow for the control needed when working with hands that have a high degree of spasticity, a shorter working time for impatient patients, and the memory that would allow for reforming or serial splinting situations. Opinions may vary among therapists and their respective experience. Using the material with which the therapist is the most comfortable is often best.

Neoprene is a fabric-covered synthetic rubber sheet, which provides a semidynamic stretch and good conformability in splint fabrication. It is available in Lycra or rubber-backed and some are available in a loop surface that is sensitive to Velcro hooks. It can be found in a variety of color choices depending on the source. A variety of thicknesses are also available. One may choose a thicker neoprene if more assistance or support is desired. A thicker neoprene sometimes works well in providing just enough resistance in a circumferential elbow splint to prevent self-abusive behavior. The Lycra-backed type will make splint application easier and may be more comfortable for wear, while the rubber-backed type prevents slipping and can be used to stabilize objects or a part of the hand. In addition to its other qualities, neoprene also maintains hand warmth, which can assist in decreasing spasticity, and is useful for splinting hands that have a cold hypersensitivity.

Elastomer is a silicone-based putty that conforms exceptionally well. They are used in pediatric splinting for thumb positioning or finger spacers. They also work well for scar softening and help to decrease scar hypersensitivity. Many types are available through splinting product catalogs. The putty types with a gel catalyst or the 50/50 mix are probably the easiest to work with because they can be mixed in the hand and varied in stiffness by adding more or less catalyst.

Because of the need for frequent small splint sizes, additional but inexpensive tools are sometimes valuable to have. After a splint has been fabricated, one is often hesitant to use a large heat gun to soften and smooth a small area because there is risk with such tiny splints of losing the entire contour and form. A smaller heat gun, such as the Ultratorch, works nicely to touch up small areas, but if one is not available, a turkey baster or eyedropper can be used to apply hot water directly to hard to reach places (Fig. 18-2, A). A pen, pencil, small dowel, or chopstick (the author's favorite is a laminated chopstick) is sometimes a helpful tool to use in smoothing out tiny areas that are smaller than the end of the therapist's finger (Fig.

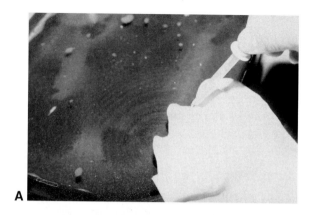

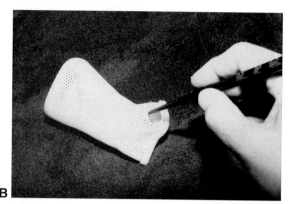

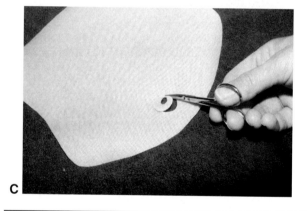

Fig. 18-2   **A,** A turkey baster, eye dropper, or Ultratorch are tools applicable to spot heating a small area on a pediatric splint. **B,** This chopstick can be maneuvered to smooth out hard to access areas. **C,** Tiny curves can be cut with small manicure scissors.

18-2, *B*). Small, curved fingernail scissors can be used to cut tiny curves (Fig. 18-2, *C*).

Because many children tend to have very active lifestyles, pediatric splints may require reinforcement to prevent early stress fractures in thermoplastics. Particularly, splints on hands with a great deal of spasticity may require reinforcement. Any technique that increases contour increases material strength. Contoured reinforcing bars or posts can be easily added to increase the strength of a splint. The thermoplas-

tic can also be doubled; however, this is often not recommended because it significantly increases the weight of the splint.

HOW TO IMPROVE THE LIKELIHOOD THAT A SPLINT WILL BE WORN

Whenever possible, ask the parent, caregiver, and teaching staff for their assistance in planning the wearing schedule. It is important to try to make the wearing schedule compatible with the child's typical routine and the caregiver's schedule. This consultation allows caregivers to know that the therapist has respect for their opinions and time, allows the therapist an opportunity to stress the reason and importance of splint use, and helps the therapist plan a wearing schedule that is appropriate for the child, as well as being possible for caregiver compliance.

In an alternate-care or school setting, plan where the splint may be kept during nonuse times to ensure compliance with the wearing schedule and prevent splint loss (e.g., in a backpack or wheelchair bag in school or in a bag that attaches with Velcro to the bed, crib, or isolette at home or in a hospital or institutional setting). Mark all splints with the child's name and the hand to which it is applied to assist in proper application and decrease the chance of its being lost. Sometimes including the wearing schedule or the therapist's phone number is also helpful.

The hand therapist's version of Murphy's Law is, "If a splint can be applied incorrectly, it will be." Anything that gives added information about splint application improves the likelihood that the splint will be applied correctly. A photograph of the splint on the hand along with the application instructions is helpful especially if there will be a variety of people applying the splint. If splint parts or straps are removable, the part or strap and the spot to which it is applied can be numbered or marked with a picture to ensure proper application following removal.

IDEAS TO AID IN SPLINT DESIGN

The more input the patient has into the planning and design of a splint, the more likely that he or she will comply with splint use. With that in mind, it is desirable to ask a patient's opinion about design choices that do not alter the basic goal and purpose of the splint.

Allow the child a choice of thermoplastic, neoprene, or Velcro color if this is available in your facility. This is the ideal, although highly unlikely, pediatric splinting situation. Most facilities will not have the budget for all these options so the following ideas using a neutral-colored thermoplastic might be considered. Apply decorative ribbon available in many designs at fabric stores to the straps. This ribbon is easily stitched on with a sewing machine (Fig. 18-3, *A*). Pictures can be drawn on the splint either before or after fabrication with permanent markers. The therapist or patient can do this. It can be done on the thermoplastic as a fine motor therapy activity prior to making the splint with resulting enthusiasm for fabrication and subsequent use. "Strap Pals" can be made out of thermoplastic by coloring a picture onto a scrap with permanent markers, cutting it out, then attaching it to the strap with self-adhesive Velcro hook. Designs can be traced with carbon paper onto the thermoplastic from a coloring book or children's book.

A variety of other items can be used for splint decoration. Take caution that the child will not remove and accidentally swallow these. Baby barrettes can be applied to the strap. Fabric paints can be used by the therapist or the patient to draw pictures or write a name on the straps. Material designs can be appliquéd onto the straps or orthokinetic cuffs with an iron-on adhesive. They can be finished by sewing with a close zigzag stitch or edged with fabric paints. Shoelaces are available in a variety of colors and designs and can be used to secure a splint. "Bow Biters" or shoelace charms can also be added for decoration. Stickers applied to the splint are an easy option that most

STRAP CRITTER PATTERNS

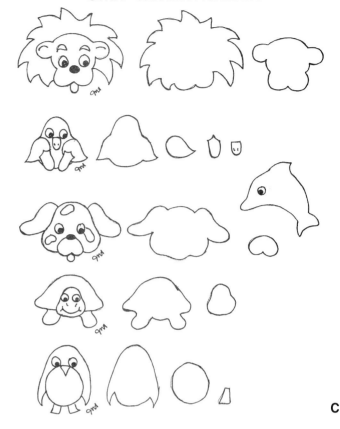

C

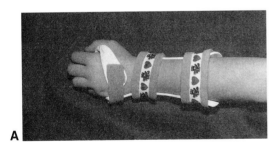

A

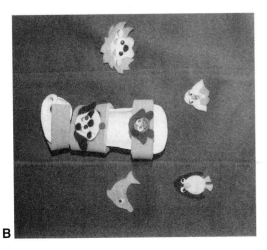

B

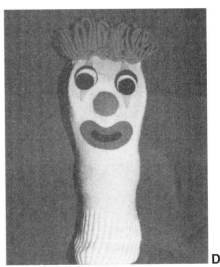

D

Fig. 18-3   **A, Wrist extension mobilization splint, type 0 (1). B, Wrist extension mobilization splint, type 0 (1)**

A, Decorative ribbon added to straps, drawings, or **(B,C)** strap critters with movable eyes enhancing the appearance of splints will increase the child's acceptance to their new splint. **D,** Covering the splint with a sock puppet can be a great fun project for the child and will have the added benefit of warmth.

children enjoy. "Strap Critters" can be made out of felt; add movable eyes and Velcro hook, and attach them to the splint straps (Fig. 18-3, *B,C*). These can also easily be used as a reward for doing well in therapy and provide a small change that can encourage continued splint use. For older individuals, decorative lapel pins can be used on the strap as long as they are attached only through the first layer of the velfoam strapping or the back is covered with moleskin to prevent pressure. Sock puppets can be made out of tube socks for a fun splint covering and are great to use when mittens don't fit over the splint (Fig. 18-3, *D*). Splint covers may also be sewn out of polar fleece with Velcro closure, for use when splints do not fit under mittens.

Sometimes just the way a splint is described can encourage wearing compliance. For example, describing a neoprene splint as a "scuba diver's glove" or "the kind of glove Batman wears" can make a child feel like this splint is something that's "really cool" and fun to wear.

To facilitate independence in splint application and removal, especially for patients who are bilaterally involved, simple strapping adaptations can be made. Lengthening the ends of the straps, allowing them to overlap where there is no Velcro, makes them easier to grasp. Adding a thumb loop or cutting a hole in the strap so that the thumb can be inserted and used to pull the strap is helpful when functional pinch is not present. Consider the line of pull of the strap. Is it easier to apply and remove from one direction than the other? Using their teeth instead of hand grasp for applying and removing straps is frequently a good option for patients (often the one chosen or discovered by patients).

■ IDEAS TO PREVENT UNWANTED SPLINT REMOVAL

Each therapist has treated those "little Houdinis" who are able to get out of any splint applied; they are the ultimate challenge to one's problem-solving skills. Since splints are not effective if not worn, adaptations to the conventional strapping techniques may need to be made. Reinforcing a Velfoam strap with Velcro loop makes it harder to remove and also increases the strap life. Riveting straps makes removal more difficult and ensures that straps will not be lost or applied incorrectly. A D-ring strap that wraps over the top of itself is more difficult to remove than the standard Velcro strap. Shoelaces for attachment rather than Velcro straps are often more challenging for removal. The shoelace can also be sewn onto the end of the strap and brought through the D-ring for added reinforcement or sewn onto the strap and then tied after the

Velcro has been fastened. "Bow Biters," little plastic critters that tie on the lace and then clamp down on the bow after it is tied, can also be used to secure the lace, therefore making removal more difficult (Fig. 18-4, *A,B*). Luggage locks work as fasteners even if they are not locked; it is difficult for little hands to push down the button and pull it out at the same time with one hand. Decorative "Friendship Bracelets" that have a push down/pull out type of fastener can be sewn onto the strap and hooked after the Velcro has been fastened, adding decoration and making the strap difficult to remove (Fig. 18-4, *C,D*). Swivel snaps and rings (available on key chains or at hardware stores) are nearly impossible to remove with one hand and secure the splint nicely. Metal C-rings with screw closures, available at hardware stores, take more time to apply but are very difficult for little hands to remove. Placing an elasticized stockinette or the cuff of a decorative sock over the splint or splint strap also makes removal more difficult. A strip of Dycem or rubber-backed neoprene placed inside the splint can prevent distal migration or help to keep a thumb in place.

In one case study, a female patient at an institution for severely and profoundly handicapped adults demonstrated hand positioning of wrist and finger flexion due to spasticity that was so severe it made palmar hygiene difficult, which made splinting a necessity. However, this patient was not fond of splints and went to extreme measures to remove and/or destroy them. The typical splints fabricated out of a rubber-based thermoplastic with Velcro and webbing D-ring strapping were literally eaten one small piece at a time. After a great deal of trial and error, splints fabricated out of elastic-based thermoplastic (because of its durability) with leather D-ring straps and luggage locks were successful.

The following are a variety of pediatric splints with directions for patterns and fabrication as well as a variety of adaptations for each splint. Reference can be made to Table 18-1 for assistance in splint selection. Splinting equipment previously described in this book is needed for fabrication of most thermoplastic splints. A sewing machine with a very sharp size 11 or 14 stretch needle, or a needle and thread for hand sewing, is necessary for fabrication of most neoprene splints. An alternative method to sewing neoprene is to use commercially available products, such as neoprene glue, iron-on seam tape, and iron-on Velcro hook and loop, for creating custom neoprene splints without having to sew a single stitch.[5,8]

Detailed fabrication instructions for 15 splints that are commonly used with pediatric patients are presented in the next section of this chapter. Each splint is named according to the ESCS; its colloquial name is identified; pattern, construction, and fit details are

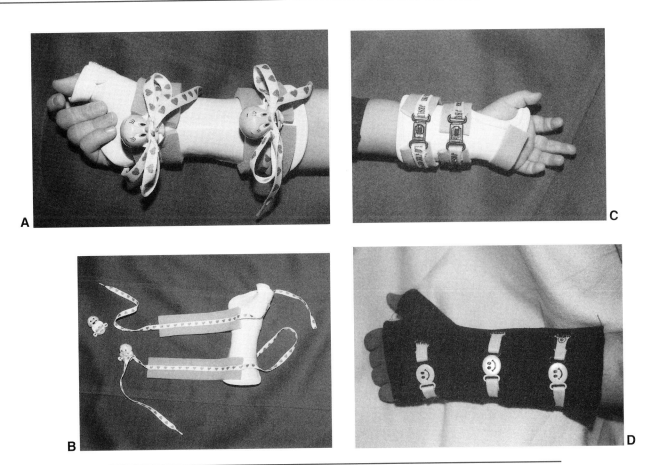

Fig. 18-4   A, Wrist, extension, thumb CMC palmar abduction and MP extension mobilization splint, type 0 (3) B, Wrist extension, thumb CMC palmar abduction and MP extension mobilization splint, type 0 (3) C, Wrist extension mobilization splint, type 0 (1) D, Wrist extension, thumb CMC radial abduction and MP extension mobilization splint, type 0 (3)
Children are great escape artists when it comes to removing splints. A creative therapist may add **(A,B)** shoelaces with Bow Biters **(C,D)** push down/pull out type fasteners to secure the straps in place.

provided; and common variations of the splint are illustrated. The 15 splints are organized according to the Splint Sequence Ranking Index (SSRI), in which the most proximal primary joint or segment influenced by the splint defines its entry position in the SSRI. Presence of more distal primary joints in the splint further refines the splint's ranking order.

Ranking categories for these splints include thumb, wrist, wrist–thumb, wrist fingers thumb, forearm wrist thumb, elbow, and elbow wrist fingers. Description of various grasp assists is included at the end of the fabrication section of this chapter. Appendix F contains larger-scale versions of all the patterns illustrated in this chapter.

■ ARTICULAR SPLINTS

Thumb Splints

Thumb CMC

Fig. 18-5A *Thumb CMC radial abduction mobilization splint, type 0 (1)*
Fig. 18-5B *Thumb CMC radial abduction mobilization splint, type 0 (1)*

Thumb CMC, MP

Fig. 18-5D *Thumb CMC radial abduction and MP extension mobilization splint, type 0 (2)*

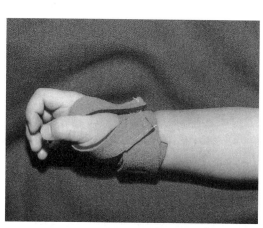
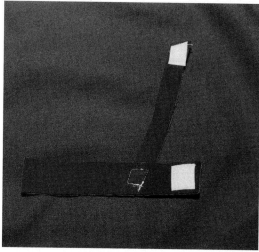

Fig. 18-5A   Fig. 18-5B

(Fig. 18-5A,B) A "thumb loop splint" brings the thumb into radial abduction. These splints are typically used with patients who have mild to moderate tone pulling the thumb into the palm but these splints usually do not provide enough support for individuals with high tone.

Materials needed include neoprene $\frac{1}{8}$ to $\frac{1}{4}$ inch thick, depending on the size of the patient, and Velcro.

Pattern and Fabrication Sequence

(Fig. 18-5C)

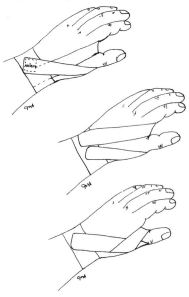

Fig. 18-5C

1. Cut a strip of neoprene $\frac{1}{2}$ to $1\frac{1}{2}$ inches wide (the width will vary with the size of the hand) at a length that will wrap around the wrist and overlap enough to add a Velcro attachment.
2. Sew Velcro onto the underside of the strap end. The Velcro will be positioned at the ulnar wrist.
3. Cut another strap $\frac{1}{2}$ to 1 inch wide at a length that will begin at the proximal edge of the wrist strap at the center of the dorsal wrist, wrap through the web space, around the thenar eminence, and end at the proximal edge of the wrist strap just radial to the attachment of the other end.
4. Sew one end of this strap to the wrist strap at the center of the dorsal wrist.
5. Sew Velcro onto the other end. If a neoprene that is not Velcro-sensitive is being used, Velcro loop will need to be sewn at the points of attachment.
6. When applying to the patient, the wrist strap is attached at the ulnar side. The thumb loop is brought over the dorsum of the hand, through the web space, around the thenar eminence proximal to the thumb MP joint so as not to cause hyperextension, and attached to the wrist cuff just proximal to the other end. The line of pull should bring the thumb out of the palm into radial abduction.
7. It is important that specific instruction in splint application be provided to the patient and caregivers because correct application of this is important to achieve optimal function.

Adaptations

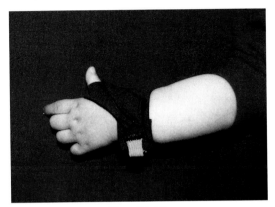

Fig. 18-5D

- (Fig. 18-5D) To further insure correct application, both ends of the thumb loop may be sewn onto the wrist strap and instructions given to position the Velcro at the ulnar side of the wrist and attach.
- Instead of sewing, the thumb loop strap may be attached on both ends by Velcro.[12]
- The thumb loop may be glued or sewn to itself more distally with a single point of attachment at the wrist.
- The "thumb loop splint" may be fabricated out of cotton webbing material. The webbing can be trimmed with a scissor to contour around the web space and then wrapped with moleskin to increase comfort. Softer strapping materials may also be used but are not as durable.[3]
- A neoprene supination strap may be added.

Thumb Splints—cont'd

Thumb CMC, MP

Fig. 18-6A *Thumb CMC radial abduction and MP extension mobilization splint, type 0 (2)*
Fig. 18-6D *Thumb CMC radial abduction and MP extension mobilization splint, type 0 (2)*
Fig. 18-6E *Thumb CMC radial abduction and MP extension mobilization splint, type 0 (2) \\ Thumb CMC palmar abduction mobilization splint, type 0 (1)*

Forearm, Wrist, Thumb CMC, MP

Fig. 18-6J *Forearm supination, wrist extension, thumb CMC radial abduction and MP extension mobilization splint, type 0 (4)*

Wrist, Thumb CMC, MP

Fig. 18-6F *Wrist extension, thumb CMC radial abduction and MP extension mobilization splint, type 0 (3)*
Fig. 18-6G *Wrist extension, thumb CMC radial abduction and MP extension mobilization splint, type 0 (3)*

Wrist, Finger MP, PIP, Thumb CMC, MP

Fig. 18-6H *Wrist extension, index finger MP-PIP extension, thumb CMC radial abduction and MP extension mobilization splint, type 0 (5); with grasp assist*
Fig. 18-6I *Wrist extension, index finger MP-PIP extension, thumb CMC radial abduction and MP extension mobilization splint, type 0 (5); with grasp assist*

(Fig. 18-6A) The neoprene "thumb abduction splint", is an excellent alternative to hard thermoplastic materials. Its mobilization action assists in thumb radial abduction and MP joint extension, while the circumferential design provides support to the thumb MP joint and neutral warmth for some relaxation. It works nicely to decrease thumb-in-palm positioning in patients with mild to moderate spasticity and can be adapted for use with patients who exhibit extreme spasticity.

Materials needed include neoprene, preferably in the patient's favorite color, $\frac{1}{8}$ to $\frac{1}{4}$ inch thick, depending on the size of the patient and the spasticity present. The greater the patient's size and spasticity, the thicker the neoprene needed. Attach Velcro or alternative strapping.

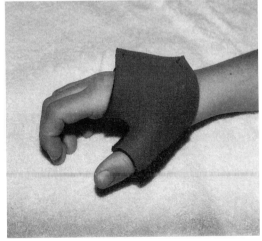

Fig. 18-6A

Pattern and Fabrication Sequence

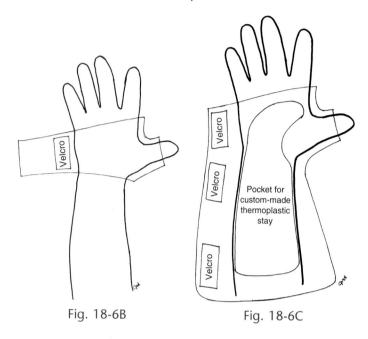

Fig. 18-6B   Fig. 18-6C

(Fig. 18-6B,C)

1. Trace the hand (and forearm if the splint will be lengthened).
2. Mark the finger MP joints, thumb IP joint, and wrist crease.
3. Draw a line across the wrist crease, the MP joints, and the thumb IP joint.
4. Measure the distance that will bring the splint halfway around the thumb, usually $\frac{1}{4}$ inch in small children to $\frac{1}{2}$ to $\frac{3}{4}$ inch in adults, and add that distance along the side from the thumb IP joint to the wrist crease and around the thenar web space.
5. Extend the ulnar side approximately $\frac{3}{4}$ the width of the palm.
6. Try the pattern on the patient to check fit.
7. Trace the pattern onto the neoprene to make the volar piece. Flip the pattern and cut off or fold at the point where it would lie over the fifth metacarpal. Trace in this flipped position for the dorsal piece; the pieces should be mirror images of one another.
8. Cut out the neoprene.
9. Glue or sew the radial side of the thumb and the thumb web space.
10. Try on the patient to check fit. If needed, trim the distal end so it clears the distal palmar crease and the thumb so the IP joint is clear for motion.
11. The volar piece wraps gently around the ulnar side over the dorsum of the hand. Attach Velcro onto the dorsal piece so that when it attaches with Velcro over the fifth digit the thumb is pulled into abduction.

Adaptations

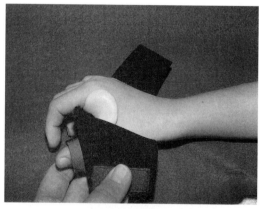

Fig. 18-6D

- The thumb may be lengthened to include the IP joint.
- The splint may be lengthened to include the wrist.
- Another thumb loop may be added to further encourage abduction.
- The splint could also include another finger if support is desired for computer access or if protection against self-abusive behavior is needed.
- (Fig. 18-6D) The splint may be worn over an elastomer web space insert for extra support and positioning in the web space.

- (Fig. 18-6E) The splint may be used in combination with a "wrist cock-up" *(Wrist extension mobilization splint, type 0 (1))*, "ulnar gutter" *(Wrist extension mobilization / ulnar deviation restriction splint, type 0 (1))*, or "thumb C-bar splint" *(Thumb CMC palmar abduction mobilization splint, type 0 (1))*.
- Iron-on neoprene tape can be added over the seam in the thumb web space for added support.
- Extra support may be added to the radial/dorsal thumb in the form of a pocket with a stay of leather or thermoplastic.

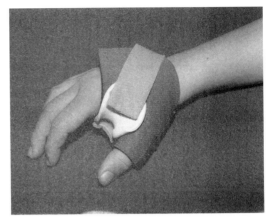

Fig. 18-6E

- (Fig. 18-6F) A pocket may be added to the volar or dorsal side of the lengthened splint to accommodate a customized thermoplastic stay to control wrist position.
- A pocket and stay may be added to the ulnar side of the lengthened splint to prevent ulnar deviation.

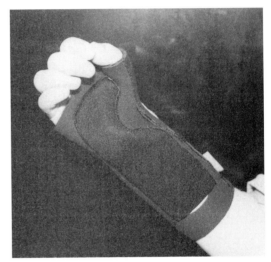

Fig. 18-6F

- (Fig. 18-6G) For extra wrist support, an additional length or strap wrapping around the wrist may be added to the splint.

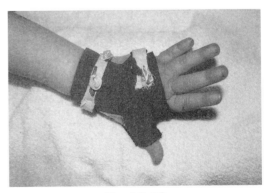

Fig. 18-6G

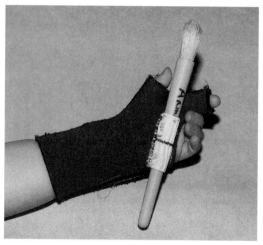

Fig. 18-6H

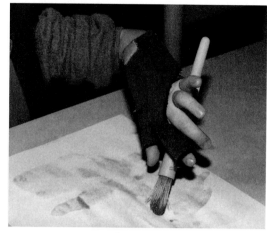

Fig. 18-6I

- (Fig. 18-6H,I) If a child has difficulty maintaining grasp, an elastic pocket or neoprene grasp assist (rubber-backed piece of neoprene with Velcro hook sewn on one end that may be wrapped around an object and then attached to the splint with Velcro) may be added to the palm. (Refer to "Neoprene Grasp Assist" at the end of this chapter.)

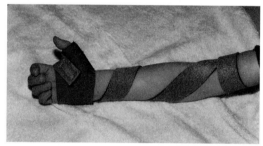

Fig. 18-6J

- (Fig. 18-6J) A serpentine strap attached at the volar base and wrapped laterally up the forearm may be added to assist in supination.[4] This strap thickness may be doubled to increase the supination pull.

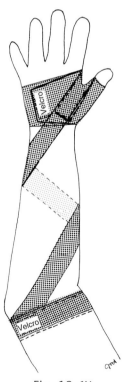

Fig. 18-6K

- (Fig. 18-6K) To add the serpentine strap do the following:
  1. Using a flexible tape measure, measure the length from the palm, through the web space, around the wrist and forearm, wrapping around just proximal to the elbow.
  2. Cut a strip of neoprene the length measured. The width will vary depending on the size of the patient, but will typically be a width slightly smaller than the width of the web space (usually between $\frac{1}{2}$ and 2 inches).
  3. Sew Velcro on the bottom surface of each end of the strap. Also sew Velcro in the palm of the splint perpendicular to the web space for strap attachment if the neoprene used is not Velcro sensitive.
  4. Attach the strap to the splint at the palm and wrap around the forearm and upper arm as directed in the pattern. Secure the strap to itself with the Velcro proximal to the elbow.
  5. The strap may be attached and wrapped in reverse if pronation is desired.
  6. Neoprene can be a difficult material with which to work, especially when using double thickness or adding Velcro. Some hints that may help include the following:
  7. Using permanent marker to trace the pattern onto the neoprene.
  8. Using a very sharp stretch needle in the sewing machine. A smaller needle, size 11 or 14 stretch needle, has worked well. However, each sewing machine will handle differently.
  9. If you choose to sew rather than glue a double layer of neoprene, position it in the machine so that it is stitching over the edge.

Although like most prefabricated splints they do not have the advantages of a custom fit, there are a variety of prefabricated neoprene thumb abduction splints available through therapy catalogs.

Wrist Splints

Wrist

Fig. 18-7A   *Wrist extension mobilization splint, type 0 (1)*

Wrist, Thumb CMC

Fig. 18-7C   *Wrist extension, thumb CMC radial abduction mobilization splint, type 1 (3)*
Fig. 18-7D   *Wrist extension, thumb CMC radial abduction mobilization splint, type 1 (3)*

(Fig. 18-7A) The "wrist cock-up splint" is used to stabilize the wrist typically in extension. With this stabilization, an increase in coordinated activity specifically involving grasp and pinch is often seen more distally. It is often used with children who have hypertonia in the flexion synergy pattern, but also for children who have a decrease in muscle tone to maintain wrist extension and facilitate hand use.

Materials needed include a low-temperature thermoplastic and strapping of choice.

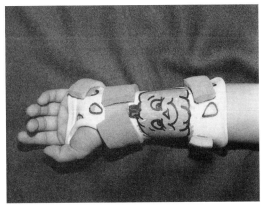

Fig. 18-7A

Pattern and Fabrication Sequence

(Fig. 18-7B)
1. Trace the hand and forearm $\frac{3}{4}$ the distance to the elbow.
2. Mark the MP joints.
3. Draw a line across the MP joints.
4. Draw along the thenar crease.
5. Draw the web space bar at a 45° angle from the web space, widening and rounding the end to support the palmar arches if it will be fitted dorsally. It should be a length that when wrapped around the hand will end over the fourth metacarpal.
6. Draw the width of the forearm trough by measuring the distance that would bring it halfway up the forearm when fabricated.
7. Round all corners.
8. Try the pattern on the patient to check fit.
9. Trace the pattern onto the thermoplastic, heat, and cut out.
10. Form the splint on either the volar or dorsal side in the amount of wrist extension desired. The radial bar is wrapped around the radial side and over the dorsal or volar side depending on splint choice for support. On a volar splint make certain to roll the distal end back to the distal palmar crease so that the MP joints are clear for movement.
11. Strap at the wrist, ulnar hand, and proximal forearm.

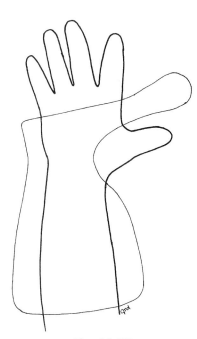

Fig. 18-7B

Adaptations

- A "thumb-hole wrist cock-up" *(Wrist extension mobilization splint, type 0 (1))* could also be used to achieve wrist extension.
- The "wrist cock-up" *(Wrist extension mobilization splint, type 0 (1))* could also be made without a radial bar.
- (Fig. 18-7C,D) A neoprene "thumb loop" *Thumb CMC radial abduction mobilization splint, type 0 (1))* could be added for thumb abduction.
- The "wrist cock-up" could be used in combination with other splints such as the neoprene "thumb abduction splint."

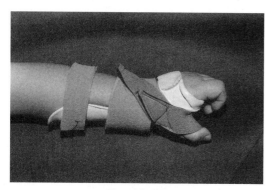

Fig. 18-7C

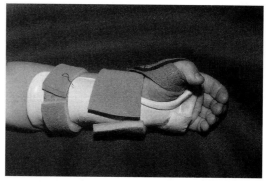

Fig. 18-7D

Wrist Splints—cont'd

Wrist

Fig. 18-8A   *Wrist extension mobilization splint, type 0 (1)*
Fig. 18-8C   *Wrist extension mobilization splint, type 0 (1)*

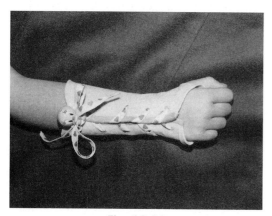

Fig. 18-8A

(Fig. 18-8A) The circumferential "thumb hole wrist cock-up splint" is used to position and stabilize the wrist in extension. It is a good splinting choice for patients with a high degree of spasticity where control is desirable from all sides, as well as for individuals who have so much tone they tend to pop out of the wrist strap or for those who tend to remove splints. By maintaining wrist extension, grasp and pinch patterns may be enhanced distally.

Materials needed include low-temperature thermoplastic at $\frac{1}{16}$- or $\frac{1}{12}$-inch perforated elastic-based material, which provides good conformability while still remaining lightweight and flexible enough for donning and removing, and strapping material of choice. Shoelaces work nicely on this splint for children who remove splints as soon as they are applied.

Pattern and Fabrication Sequence

(Fig. 18-8B)

1. Trace the hand and forearm.
2. Mark the MP joints and the thumb web space.
3. Draw a line across the MP joints and extend ulnarly the distance that when wrapped around would come to the dorsal long finger metacarpal. This can be measured with a flexible tape measure around the arm.
4. Draw a line radially at about the same angle extending to the distance that when wrapped around would come to the dorsal ring finger metacarpal.
5. Extend the line proximally about $\frac{2}{3}$ the distance up the forearm and round the corners.
6. Cut a small hole at the base of the thumb web space.
7. Try the pattern on the patient to check fit.
8. Trace onto the thermoplastic and cut out.
9. Form the splint by positioning the wrist in the desired amount of extension, putting the thumb through the thumb hole, and wrapping the material circumferentially around the forearm. Overlap the material on the top. Roll back the material to clear the distal palmar crease so MP joint motion is not blocked. Smooth around the thumb hole.
10. Strap at the dorsal hand, wrist, and proximal end of the splint.

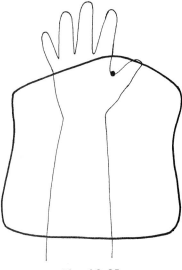

Fig. 18-8B

Adaptations

- (Fig. 18-8B) Shoelaces may be used for strapping by punching holes in the thermoplastic on either side with a hole punch then lacing the shoelace through. A double bow or a "Bow Biter" may help to further secure the hand in the splint..
- (Fig. 18-8C) Moleskin may be applied around the edge of the splint for comfort.

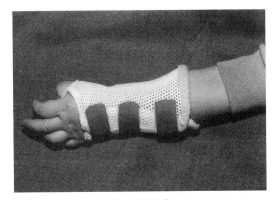

Fig. 18-8C

Wrist Splints—cont'd

Wrist

Fig. 18-9A *Wrist extension mobilization / ulnar deviation restriction splint, type 0 (1)*
Fig. 18-9B *Wrist extension mobilization / ulnar deviation restriction splint, type 0 (1)*

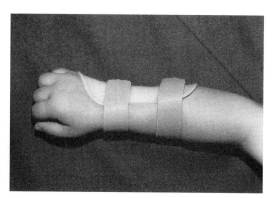

Fig. 18-9A

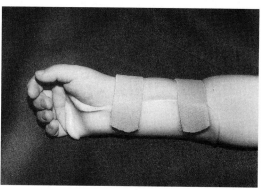

Fig. 18-9B

(Fig. 18-9A,B) The "ulnar gutter splint" positions the wrist in neutral, preventing ulnar deviation.

Materials needed include low-temperature thermoplastic and strapping of choice.

Pattern and Fabrication Sequence

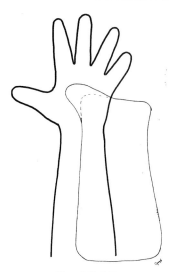

Fig. 18-9C

(Fig. 18-9C)
1. Trace the hand and the forearm.
2. Mark the distal palmar crease on the ulnar side and the web space between the ring and middle fingers.
3. Draw a line from the mark between the ring and middle fingers down the center of the hand and forearm. If extra support to the palmar arches is desired, add contour to the palm, staying clear of the thenar and distal palmar creases.
4. Draw the ulnar side the distance that would bring it around the ulnar side of the wrist and forearm to the center of the dorsal wrist and forearm.
5. Try the pattern on the patient for size.
6. Trace onto the thermoplastic, heat, and cut out.
7. Form the splint with the wrist in neutral.
8. Strap at the wrist and proximal forearm.

Adaptations

• This splint may be inserted into a long neoprene "thumb abduction splint" *(Wrist extension, thumb CMC radial abduction and MP extension mobilization / wrist ulnar deviation restriction splint, type 0 (3))* to stabilize and mobilize the wrist out of ulnar deviation.

• This splint works well used with a short neoprene "thumb abduction splint." The neoprene may actually be attached to the splint with Velcro, making a distal strap unnecessary.

Wrist Splints—cont'd

Wrist, Thumb CMC, MP

Fig. 18-10A   *Wrist extension, thumb CMC palmar abduction and MP flexion mobilization splint, type 0 (3)*

Wrist, Finger MP, PIP, Thumb CMC, MP

Fig. 18-10D   *Wrist, extension, index finger MP flexion and IP extension, thumb CMC palmar abduction and MP extension mobilization splint, type 0 (5)*

Fig. 18-10E   *Wrist, extension, index finger MP flexion and IP extension, thumb CMC palmar abduction and MP extension mobilization splint, type 0 (5)*

(Fig. 18-10A) The long "thumb opponens" maintains the thumb in a position of palmar abduction and opposition. It is typically used with patients that have difficulty with thumb-in-palm positioning but also may be used with patients with hypotonia and poor thumb joint stability for stabilization and positioning during activity performance. It assists in maintaining web space length and may also be used if there is scarring in the web space area following injury.

Materials needed include low-temperature thermoplastic and strapping of choice.

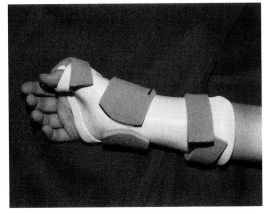

Fig. 18-10A

Pattern and Fabrication Sequence

(Fig. 18-10B)
1. Measure the distance from the thumb web space to the dorsal fifth metacarpal. This will be the length of the dorsal piece (a).
2. Measure the distance from the thumb web space around the palm to the dorsal fifth metacarpal. This will be the length of the volar piece (b).
3. Measure the distance from the dorsal index metacarpal through the web space to the center of the palm. This will be the width of the thumb piece (c).
4. Measure the distance from the volar thumb IP joint crease to the volar index MP joint crease. This will be the length of the thumb piece (d).
5. Draw the pattern with the measurements according to the accompanying diagram. The width of the dorsal and volar pieces is usually equal to the distance from the distal palmar crease to the thumb metacarpal.[6]
6. Try the pattern on the patient to check the fit.
7. Trace the pattern onto thermoplastic, heat, and cut out.
8. Fabricate the splint with the thumb in a position of palmar abduction and opposition with the thumb in slight flexion (position may be varied according to patient needs). Form the web space first making certain edges are smooth and rounded, and then bring the strap pieces around the end with the volar piece just proximal to the distal palmar crease. Round strap corners.
9. Stabilize ends with a Velcro strap or ends may be lengthened and attached with self-adhesive Velcro.

Fig. 18-10B

Alternate Pattern Sequence

(Fig. 18-10C) This pattern is preferred if stretch and support through the palmar arches are also desired. It may be made in the short or long forms.

1. Trace the hand and forearm $\frac{2}{3}$ the distance to the elbow if the long splint is desired.
2. Draw a line across the MP joints and the thumb IP joint.
3. Extend the lines to meet with contour distal to the web space area.
4. Draw a line along the radial side of the thumb at a distance that will allow it to wrap around the thumb metacarpal.
5. Extend the ulnar side on the short splint so that when wrapped around to the dorsal side it will come to approximately the ring finger metacarpal.
6. Form the splint in a position of wrist extension if long and thumb opposition and abduction. Contour the material to the palmar arches, around the thumb and through the web space, rolling back at the distal palmar crease and the thumb IP joint to allow flexion.
7. Strap around the thumb, dorsal hand, wrist, and proximal forearm on the long splint.

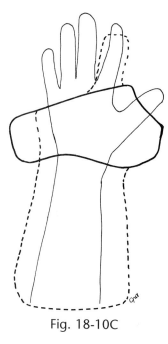

Fig. 18-10C

Adaptations

- Thumb position may be adjusted to allow more radial abduction.
- Thumb positioning may also be achieved using a C-bar through the thumb web space when strapped in a figure-eight pattern around the wrist to secure.
- (Fig. 18-10D,E) A gutter extension may be added to the index finger (usually allowing the tip to be free for sensory input) in order to assist in finger isolation for improving computer or communication board access.

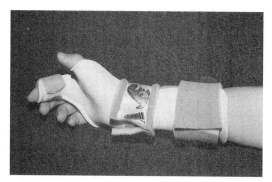

Fig. 18-10D

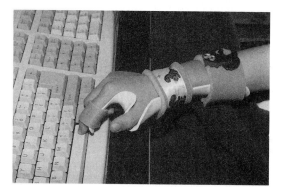

Fig. 18-10E

Wrist Splints—cont'd

Wrist, Finger MP, Thumb CMC, MP

Fig. 18-11A *Wrist extension, index-small finger MP extension, thumb CMC radial abduction and MP extension mobilization splint, type 0 (7)*

(Fig. 18-11A) The "MacKinnon splint" is designed under the principle that pressure applied to the metacarpal heads with stretch to the intrinsics causes relaxation of flexor spasticity. With this relaxation, increased wrist and finger extension and thumb abduction are sometimes seen. This results in less fisting with an increase in hand use. Improvements are seen primarily in grasp and hand use for bimanual activities.[9,11,14] In the literature this splint has been shown to be effective with patients who have limited hand use due to moderate or severe spasticity that is either constant or is increased on initiation of movement.[7]

Materials needed include low-temperature thermoplastic, plastic tubing (surgical or aquarium), and strapping of choice.

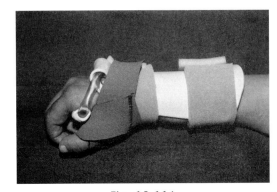

Fig. 18-11A

Pattern and Fabrication Sequence

(Fig. 18-11B)
1. Trace the hand and forearm marking the wrist crease, the metacarpal heads, and $\frac{2}{3}$ the distance up the forearm.
2. Draw the forearm piece by measuring the distance that would bring it halfway up the side of the forearm when formed. Extend the forearm piece about 2 inches beyond the wrist so there is enough material to roll back and secure the tubing.
3. Cut a piece of thermoplastic the width of the palm at the metacarpal heads and about 2 inches wide.
4. Cut a length of tubing that is equal to the distance from the center of the dorsal wrist across the volar metacarpal heads, and then back to the center of the dorsal wrist. It is easier to cut the tubing a little long initially and then shorten it as it is measured on the patient after the palmar piece is fabricated.
5. Fabricate the palmar piece by rolling the thermoplastic around the center of the tubing. The diameter of this will depend on the size of the patient, typically $\frac{1}{2}$ to $\frac{3}{4}$ inch.
6. Position the palmar piece so it conforms at the volar heads of the metacarpals and attach the tubing to the distal end of the splint by securing with the extra thermoplastic in a position of slight wrist extension.
7. Strap across the wrist and proximal forearm.

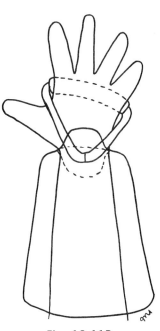

Fig. 18-11B

Adaptations

* The original pattern for the "MacKinnon splint" used a dowel with nails to attach the tubing to the dowel and the forearm piece consisted of a small piece of San-splint with a Velcro strap. Eliminating the use of sharp nails and increasing the proximal stability of the forearm piece has modified the directions provided here.
* The splint may be lined with padding or a piece of Dycem to assist in preventing distal migration.
* The metacarpal piece may be modified to include the thumb web space to increase thumb abduction.
* Exercise tubing may be used in place of the plastic tubing if the individual has some active wrist extension.

Wrist Splints—cont'd

Wrist, Finger, MP, PIP, DIP, Thumb CMC, MP, IP

Fig. 18-12A *Wrist extension, index–small finger extension, thumb CMC palmar abduction and MP-IP extension mobilization splint, type 0 (16)*

Fig. 18-12C *Wrist extension, index–small finger extension, thumb CMC palmar abduction and MP-IP extension mobilization splint, type 0 (16)*

Fig. 18-12F *Wrist extension, index, ring–small finger MP abduction, index-small finger extension, thumb CMC radial abduction and MP-IP extension mobilization splint, type 0 (16)*

Fig. 18-12G *Wrist extension, index, ring–small finger MP abduction, index-small finger extension, thumb CMC radial abduction and MP-IP extension mobilization splint, type 0 (16)*

Fig. 18-12H *Wrist extension, index, ring–small finger MP abduction, index-small finger extension, thumb CMC radial abduction and MP-IP extension mobilization splint, type 0 (16)*

Wrist, Finger

Fig. 18-12D *Wrist extension, index-small finger extension mobilization splint, type 0 (13)*

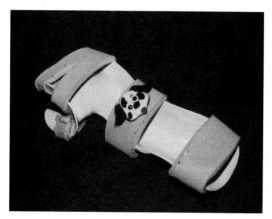

Fig. 18-12A

(Fig. 18-12A) The "resting hand splint" is a commonly used splint in adult as well as pediatric splinting to place and maintain the hand in a position of rest or function. In pediatrics, it is often used when extensive muscle tone is present to correct or prevent loss of range of motion and contracture formation. It may also be used with hypotonic hands to maintain ideal positioning at rest.

Materials needed include a low-temperature thermoplastic (it is the preference of this author to use a rubber-based thermoplastic for the desired control) and a choice of strapping.

Pattern and Fabrication Sequence

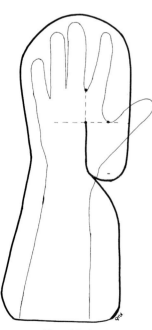

Fig. 18-12B

(Fig. 18-12B)
1. Trace the hand and forearm ($\frac{3}{4}$ the distance to the elbow) in palm down position on a piece of paper.
2. Mark the thumb web space and the web space between the index and middle fingers.
3. Draw a line around the perimeter of the hand drawing, rounding all corners. The distance is determined by measuring how much material would bring the splint halfway around the forearm and to the top of the fingers when the splint is formed.
4. Draw a line from the thumb web space dot horizontally and from the finger web space dot vertically. The point where these lines intersect is the point where the thumb piece begins.
5. Measure the length of the thumb and draw the thumb piece that length with the sides being the radial side of the splint and the line down from the finger web space mark.
6. Cut out the pattern and try it on the patient for size.
7. Trace the pattern onto the thermoplastic, heat, and cut out.
8. Position the patient comfortably with gravity assisting. Make certain the arm is in a position of pronation rather than supination, because pronation is the position that the hand will be in when the splint is worn. If formed in supination there will be a twist in the forearm of the splint with resulting improper fit.

9. Form the splint on the volar side, placing the wrist in extension, thumb in abduction, and fingers in slight flexion. Concentrate initially on the wrist, thenar crease, and thumb web space.
10. Apply strapping over the wrist, proximal forearm, and fingers. A thumb strap may also be needed.

Adaptations

- (Fig. 18-12C,D) A neoprene sheet strap may be used when it is very difficult to maintain hand position. The neutral warmth provided by the neoprene may also help to decrease spasticity.
- (Fig. 18-12E) As shown in this pattern the position of the wrist, fingers, and thumb may need to be adapted to accommodate for contracture formation or spasticity.
- Because hypertonia causes a significant amount of stress on the splint material, reinforcing the material may prevent stress fractures and increase the life of the splint. This may be done by (1) adding a reinforcing bar along the center of the splint under the wrist and finger pan, making certain that the reinforcement is contoured and attached well, (2) adding a thumb reinforcement underneath the thumb piece to prevent stress fracture in the thumb web space, and (3) folding back extra thermoplastic when forming around the thenar eminence to reinforce this area.

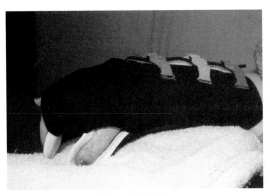

Fig. 18-12C

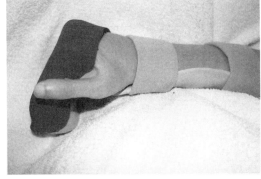

Fig. 18-12D

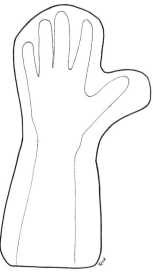

Fig. 18-12E

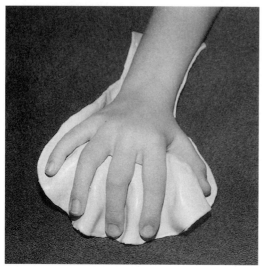

Fig. 18-12F

- (Fig. 18-12F) The "resting hand splint" may be fabricated from a traced palm (mitt) pattern if the thumb will be held in a position of more radial than palmar abduction.

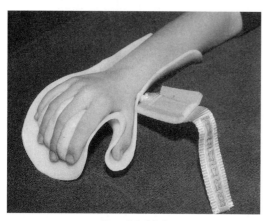

Fig. 18-12G

- (Fig. 18-12G) Finger spacers may be added using thermoplastic, foam, Velfoam, or elastomer.

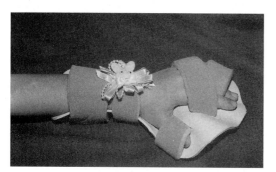

Fig. 18-12H

- (Fig. 18-12H) Fingers can be held in position with strapping that is brought up between the fingers.
- When splinting to increase range of motion, position at maximum range and then when tissue length and relaxation have improved, change the splint to increase the range. Continue with these serial changes until maximum ROM goals are achieved.

Wrist Splints—cont'd

Wrist, Finger MP, PIP, DIP, Thumb CMC, MP, IP

Fig. 18-13A *Wrist extension, index–small finger extension, thumb CMC palmar abduction and MP-IP extension mobilization splint, type 0 (16)*

Fig. 18-13B *Wrist extension, index–small finger extension, thumb CMC palmar abduction and MP-IP extension mobilization splint, type 0 (16)*

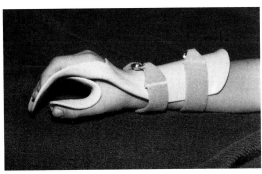

Fig. 18-13A

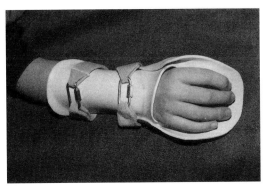

Fig. 18-13B

(Fig. 18-13A,B) The "antispasticity splint" maintains the hand in a reflex inhibitory posture of wrist extension, finger and thumb extension, and CMC palmar abduction and is typically used with patients who have flexor spasticity. The forearm piece is dorsally based to eliminate any stimulation to the flexors.[13]

Materials needed include a low-temperature rubber-based thermoplastic (the author's choice for desired control) and choice of strapping.

Pattern and Fabrication Sequence

(Fig. 18-13C, D)
1. Trace the hand in a palm-down position.
2. Mark the MP joints of the fingers and thumb.
3. Draw a line around the perimeter of the hand drawing. The distance away is determined by measuring how much material would bring the splint halfway around the forearm and to the top of the fingers when the splint is formed. Add an extra fold of thermoplastic at the MPs on either side to use for reinforcement.
4. Draw a line across the MP joints of the fingers and across the MP joint of the thumb. Widen slightly and round corners.
5. Try the pattern on the patient to check the fit.
6. Trace onto the thermoplastic, heat, and cut out.
7. Form the splint placing the forearm section dorsally. Bring the fingers and thumb through the MP joint slots with the fingers supported in the volar finger pan.
8. Strap at the wrist, proximal forearm, fingers, and thumb; sometimes thumb and finger strapping is not needed.
9. It is particularly important with this splint to provide the patient or caregivers with detailed instruction and demonstration regarding splint application.

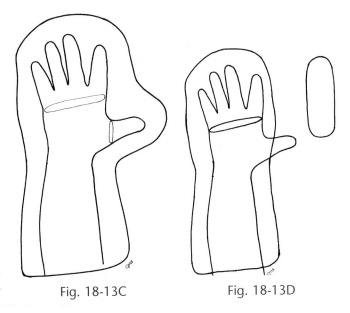

Fig. 18-13C   Fig. 18-13D

Adaptations

- (Fig. 18-13D) Make the pattern without the thumb piece and form the wrist and finger pan first. Then add a separate thumb piece by attaching to the finger pan. This method allows further reinforcement at the sides of the MP joints to prevent stress fracture and the thumb piece can be fabricated to conform well around the thumb providing improved support to the thumb MP joint and web space.
- Add a thumb post for reinforcement.
- Foam or elastomer finger separators may be added after the finger pan is formed.

Wrist Splints—cont'd

Wrist, Finger MP, PIP, DIP, Thumb CMC, MP, IP

Fig. 18-14A   *Wrist extension, index–small finger MP extension and IP flexion, thumb CMC radial abduction and MP-IP extension mobilization splint, type 0 (16)*

Fig. 18-14B   *Wrist extension, index–small finger MP extension and IP flexion, thumb CMC radial abduction and MP-IP extension mobilization splint, type 0 (16)*

Fig. 18-14C   *Wrist extension, index–small finger MP extension and IP flexion, thumb CMC radial abduction and MP-IP extension mobilization splint, type 0 (16); right \\ Wrist extension, index–small finger MP extension and IP flexion, thumb CMC radial abduction and MP-IP extension mobilization splint, type 0 (16); left*

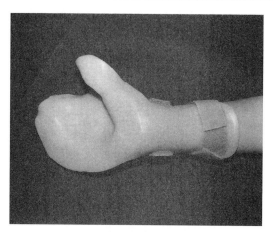

Fig. 18-14A

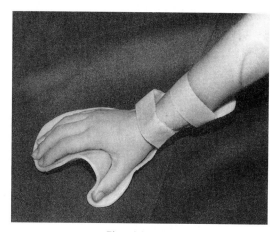

Fig. 18-14B

(Fig. 18-14A,B) The "weight-bearing splint" positions the hand in a normal weight-bearing posture of wrist extension, with the weight supported on the base and lateral side of the palm with slight flexion of the IP joints (increasing to the radial side). It is typically used with children who demonstrate excess tone pulling the extremity into a flexion synergy pattern of wrist and elbow flexion.[10]

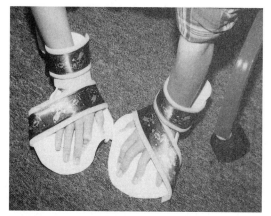

Fig. 18-14C

(Fig. 18-14C) This splint is most often used as a therapy tool during weight-bearing activities (a therapist's third hand) to maintain ideal hand position.

Materials needed include low-temperature thermoplastic (elastic-based is preferable due to its durability) and strapping of choice.

Pattern and Fabrication Sequence

(Fig. 18-14D)
1. Trace the hand and continue halfway up the forearm.
2. Draw around the hand approximately $\frac{1}{2}$ to 1 inch from the perimeter depending on patient size, closing the web spaces at the top in a continuous line. The distance around the perimeter of the forearm is measured so that it will wrap halfway around.
3. Check the pattern for fit.
4. Trace the pattern onto the thermoplastic, heat, and cut out.
5. Form the splint on the volar hand with the wrist in 45-50° extension, thumb in slight radial abduction, and finger PIP joints and DIP joints in slight flexion. As the weight-bearing should occur on the heel and lateral sides of the hand, place the patient in this position as much as possible after the initial forming to assure proper weight-bearing position.
6. Strap over the wrist and distal end of the splint. Straps over the fingers and thumb may be necessary for ideal positioning.

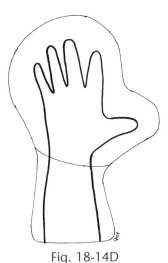

Fig. 18-14D

Adaptations

- The forearm piece can be extended for greater control. This is particularly beneficial if a significant amount of ulnar deviation is present. The splint may be made for the hand only to support finger extension. An elastic figure-eight strap works well for attachment at the wrist.
- A cut may be made between the thumb and index finger for strap application; however, with this some splint strength is lost.
- This splint may be used in combination with a "pneumatic (air) splint" *(Elbow extension mobilization splint, type 0 (1))* for control of elbow extension. Inexpensive "air splints" that work well are children's "water wings" or "swimmies" available at most discount stores.

Forearm Splints

Forearm, Wrist, Thumb CMC

Fig. 18-15B *Forearm supination, wrist extension, thumb CMC radial abduction mobilization splint, type 0 (3)*

Forearm, Wrist, Thumb, CMC, MP, IP

Fig. 18-15C *Forearm supination, wrist extension, thumb CMC palmar abduction and MP-IP extension mobilization splint, type 0 (5)*

The "serpentine splint" assists thumb palmar abduction, wrist extension, and supination. It facilitates good position and functional use of the hand, without inhibiting sensory input. This splint is typically used with children who have mild hypertonia, but it may also be used to improve hand position and function in children with hypotonia to assist in and decrease fatigue during activity. This splint may be modified for use with children who have higher (moderate) tone by adding a thumb C-bar or thumb post. However, it is not typically appropriate for children with high tone because it does not provide adequate wrist support.

Materials needed include low-temperature thermoplastic.

Pattern and Fabrication Sequence

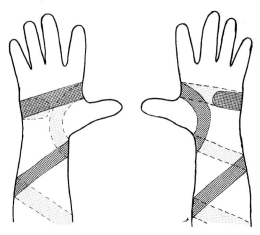

Fig. 18-15A

(Fig. 18-15A)

1. Cut a strip of thermoplastic approximately 1 inch wide, thinner for a very small hand and thicker for larger hands or hands that have increased tone. Measure the length by wrapping a flexible tape measure around the hand as the pattern suggests.
2. Heat the splinting material until soft and roll into a log, and then flatten slightly.
3. When wrapping the material, keep the seam side up away from the skin. Begin wrapping by placing the end of the material just below the distal palmar crease of the ring finger. Wrap around the ulnar side of the hand and across the dorsum of the hand through the thumb web space. Bring it around the thenar eminence just radial to the thenar crease. For the short serpentine splint, end the splint as it wraps over the dorsal hand across the metacarpals just distal to the wrist joint. For the long serpentine splint, continue wrapping $2\frac{1}{2}$ times around the forearm being careful to avoid the ulnar styloid and ending on the dorsal forearm just distal to the elbow with the wrist positioned in extension.

4. Hold in place until completely cooled.
5. Round and smooth the ends.
6. Teaching proper application is important with this splint; it may be confusing initially

Adaptations

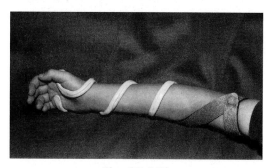

Fig. 18-15B

- (Fig. 18-15B) Addition of a neoprene strap to the proximal end of the long "serpentine splint" *(Forearm supination, wrist extension, thumb CMC radial abduction mobilization splint, type 0 (3))*, attached just proximal to the elbow, will stabilize the splint to prevent distal migration as well as maximize the serpentine function to further increase supination (almost always used by the author).

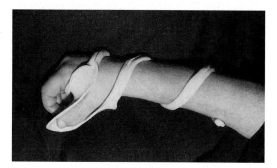

Fig. 18-15C

- (Fig. 18-15C) A thumb web space bar or thumb post may be added to maintain better thumb position. If greater material length is needed, it may be gained by using a plastic-based thermoplastic, cutting it thicker and stretching it.

Elbow Splints
Elbow
Fig. 18-16A *Elbow extension mobilization splint, type 0 (1)*
Fig. 18-16B *Elbow extension mobilization splint, type 0 (1)*
Fig. 18-16C *Elbow extension mobilization splint, type 0 (1)*

(Fig. 18-16A) The "elbow extension splint" is used to maintain elbow extension when there is extreme hypertonus in the flexion synergy pattern, which makes elbow extension difficult to achieve or maintain. It may be used serially to increase elbow extension when a flexion contracture is present.

Materials needed include low-temperature thermoplastic and strapping of choice, preferably wide and soft.

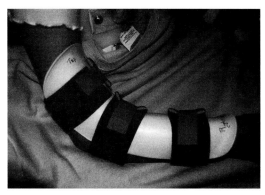

Fig. 18-16A

Pattern and Fabrication Sequence

1. Measure the distance from $\frac{2}{3}$ proximal to the elbow to $\frac{2}{3}$ distal to the elbow. This is the length of the splint.
2. Measure the distance around the biceps, elbow, and forearm and divide in half. This is the width of the splint at the various positions.
3. Draw the pattern using the above measurements.
4. Try the pattern on the patient for size.
5. Trace onto the thermoplastic, heat, and cut out.
6. Form the splint with good contour on the volar side of the elbow and flare ends.
7. Strap on the proximal and distal segments. A soft wide strap provides for the best comfort and stability.

Adaptations

- The splint could be positioned dorsally or volarly.
- Two splints can be fabricated, one dorsally and one volarly, and bivalved for extra support.
- A circumferential splint could be fabricated out of thin Aquaplast.
- (Fig. 18-16B) The splint may be secured in a pocket of a neoprene sleeve to achieve neutral warmth for increased muscle relaxation.

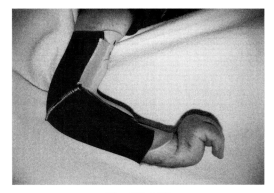

Fig. 18-16B

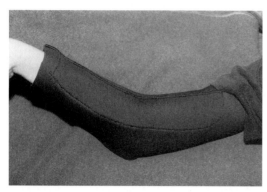

Fig. 18-16C

- (Fig. 18-16C) A neoprene sheet strap best distributes the pressure, securing position well into the splint. The neutral warmth of the neoprene also tends to facilitate increased relaxation of muscle tone.

Elbow Splints—cont'd

Elbow

Fig. 18-17A *Elbow extension mobilization splint, type 0 (1)*

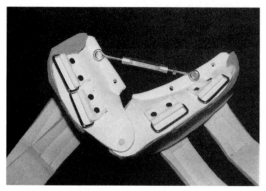

Fig. 18-17A

(Fig. 18-17A) The "turnbuckle elbow extension splint" is an inelastic mobilization splint used to increase elbow extension. Tension into extension may be increased gradually by positioning or turning the turnbuckle.

Materials needed include low-temperature thermoplastic, self-adhesive padding, turnbuckle, two screws with screw posts, two rivets (plastic finger rivets work well), soft wide strapping, Velcro, D-rings.

Pattern and Fabrication Sequence

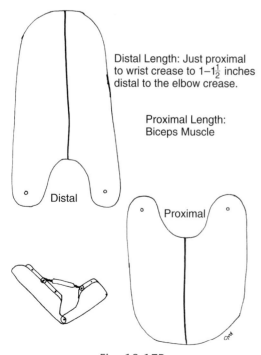

Distal Length: Just proximal to wrist crease to 1–1½ inches distal to the elbow crease.

Proximal Length: Biceps Muscle

Distal

Proximal

Fig. 18-17B

(Fig. 18-17B)
1. Measure the length of the forearm from just proximal to the wrist crease to 1 to 1½ inches distal to the elbow. This is the length of the distal piece. Measure the length of the upper arm from 1 to 1½ inches proximal to the elbow to approximately 2 inches distal to the axilla. This will cover the biceps. Measure the width of each piece so that it will wrap halfway around the arm.
2. Draw the pattern with the above measurements.
3. Draw a line down the middle of the pattern lengthwise.
4. Cut along the line, dividing the pattern in half.
5. When placing the pattern on the thermoplastic, place the pieces 1½ to 2 inches apart so there is material to pinch up and make the center bar for the turnbuckle attachment.
6. Heat thermoplastic and cut out.
7. Form the pieces so they contour around the volar arm and articulate at the elbow, pinching the middle bar up prior to forming.
8. Punch holes and rivet at the elbow joint.
9. Pad both pieces completely.
10. Add soft wide strapping (a D-ring strap works best).
11. Punch holes in the middle bar.
12. Attach the turnbuckle to the holes using screws and screw posts.

13. The turnbuckle may be moved to the different holes and adjusted by turning to change the degrees of extension.

Adaptations

• The turnbuckle may be padded with a foam tube.

Elbow Splints—cont'd

Elbow

Fig. 18-18A   *Elbow extension mobilization splint, type 0 (1) \\ Wrist extension mobilization splint, type 0 (1)*

Fig. 18-18C   *Elbow extension mobilization splint, type 0 (1) \\ Wrist extension mobilization splint, type 0 (1)*

(Fig. 18-18A) The elastic and nonelastic segments of the "orthokinetic cuff "stimulate and inhibit the underlying muscles respectively when placed over antagonistic muscle pairs. The word *orthokinetic*, which is Greek in origin, means righting of motion: *orthos* meaning right, and *kinetic* meaning motion. This happens through facilitation or inhibition of the exterocepter and proprioceptors of the nervous system, which excite or inhibit the underlying muscles.[2]

The "orthokinetic cuff" may assist in normalizing tone in the upper extremity without restricting movement, and facilitates more normal movement patterns. When used with a patient that exhibits a typical flexor synergy pattern, the cuffs are applied to facilitate the triceps and wrist extensors while inhibiting the biceps and wrist flexors.

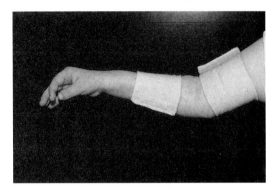

Fig. 18-18A

Materials needed include elastic wrap between $2\frac{1}{2}$ and 6 inches wide (depending on patient size), Velcro hook and loop, and cotton/polyester blend material.

Pattern and Fabrication Sequence

(Fig. 18-18B)

1. Measure the circumference of the arm at the point where the cuff will be applied.
2. Cut a piece of elastic wrap three times that length plus about $\frac{1}{2}$ inch for the seam.
3. Fold the material over so there are three layers of material of equal lengths.
4. Measure the width of the muscle belly that you wish to facilitate and subtract 1 inch. This will be the length of the elastic portion.
5. Subtract this length from the total length of the cuff circumference of the arm. Divide by two. Add one inch to allow for Velcro overlap. This will be the length of each inelastic portion.
6. Cut two pieces of cotton/polyester material this length and the width of the cuff.
7. Insert one piece on either end of the cuff between the layers of elastic bandage.
8. Sew these into place by sewing around the edge, and then stabilizing with an X sewn across the center.

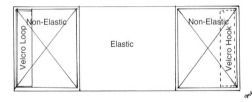

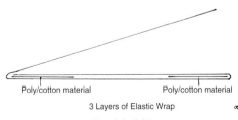

3 Layers of Elastic Wrap

Fig. 18-18B

9. Sew Velcro onto each end of the cuff hook on the topside and loop on the underside so that the cuff may be secured when wrapped around the arm.
10. Apply the elastic field over the muscle to be facilitated and the inelastic field over the muscle belly to be inhibited.
11. Provide patients and caregivers with instruction in proper application; the cuff needs to be applied appropriately to achieve the proper stimulation and inhibition desired.

Adaptations

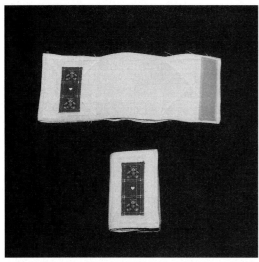

Fig. 18-18C

- The orthokinetic cuff may be made by another pattern where the inelastic field consists of four layers of elastic wrap stitched multiple times to make it inelastic.[1]
- (Fig. 18-18C) Fabric appliqués may be added over the inelastic field for decoration.

■ OTHER

Splints with Grasp Assist ("The Truly Universal, Universal Cuff!")

Thumb CMC, MP

Fig. 18-19D   *Thumb CMC radial abduction and MP extension mobilization splint, type 0 (2); with grasp assist*

Fig. 18-19E   *Thumb CMC radial abduction and MP extension mobilization splint, type 0 (2); with grasp assist*

Fig. 18-19F   *Thumb CMC radial abduction and MP extension mobilization splint, type 0 (2); with grasp assist*

Wrist

Fig. 18-19G   *Wrist extension mobilization splint, type 0 (1); with grasp assist*

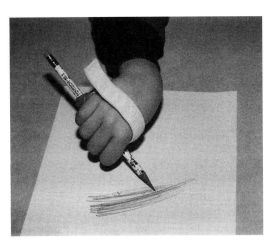

Fig. 18-19A

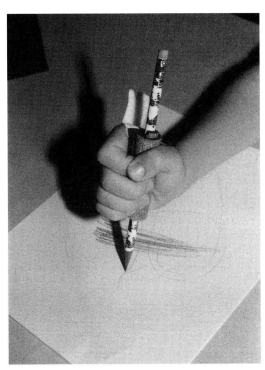

Fig. 18-19B

(Fig. 18-19A,B) The neoprene grasp assist is a very effective tool for maintaining grasp of an object in the palm of the hand for individuals who are unable to maintain grasp independently, such as children with fluctuating tone or individuals with limited grasp due to nerve or spinal cord injury. The assist may be attached to the hand with an elastic strap as described in the accompanying figures or an alternate strapping design may be used. It may also be attached easily to a splint with Velcro hook. As the design of the assist has the rubber-backed neoprene against the object surface, the object does not slide around but remains stable in the palm of the hand. Due to the open-ended design and length of the neoprene, objects of a variety of sizes may be held and orientation may be changed to be in a radial or ulnar direction (Armstrong, patent pending).

Materials needed include neoprene that is rubber-backed and Velcro-sensitive, Velcro hook, Velcro loop, and $\frac{3}{4}$-inch elastic.

Pattern and Fabrication Sequence

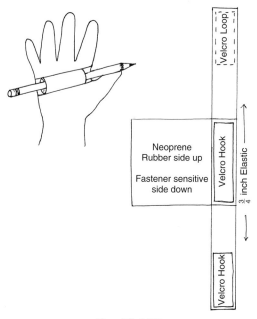

Velcro Loop

Neoprene
Rubber side up

Fastener sensitive
side down

Velcro Hook

¾ inch Elastic

Velcro Hook

Fig. 18-19C

(Fig. 18-19C)
1. Measure the width of the palm at the distal palmar crease. The neoprene is cut this width. The length may be varied, depending on the size of tools the individual anticipates using; 3 to 5 inches is adequate for most writing instruments and tools.
2. Cut a piece of Velcro 1-inch hook the width of the neoprene and stitch onto the end of the neoprene on the rubber-backed side.
3. Fabricate the strap by cutting a piece of the elastic the length equal to the distance around the hand with an overlap over the dorsum of the hand for Velcro attachment.
4. Attach the neoprene onto the center of the strap by stitching through the Velcro.
5. Sew the Velcro hook onto one end of the elastic on the same side as the neoprene was sewn (in this position it will not come into contact with the hand).
6. Sew the Velcro loop on the end of the elastic on the opposite side so that when it wraps around the end it will connect with the Velcro hook.
7. Wrap any utensil in the neoprene, and then attach the elastic strap around the hand with the utensil pointing either radial or ulnar depending on the desired use.

Adaptations

- Cotton webbing strapping or Velcro loop could be used instead of the elastic.
- The strap could be made of continuous elastic rather than using the Velcro closure.
- (Fig. 18-19D-F) The neoprene could be attached to the strap at a different angle if an alternate grasp pattern is desired.
- (Fig. 18-19G) The grasp assist may be attached directly to a splint (thermoplastic or neoprene) that has a piece of Velcro hook in the palm.
- The length of the neoprene may be increased to accommodate tools of a much wider diameter such as a broom handle, dowel, or rolling pin.

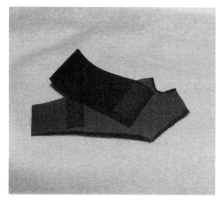

Fig. 18-19D

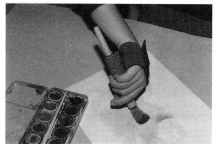

Fig. 18-19E

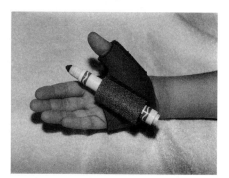

Fig. 18-19F

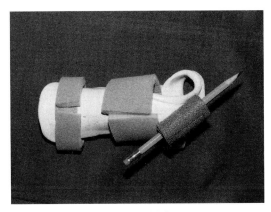

Fig. 18-19G

SUMMARY

Pediatric splinting can be challenging and incredibly fun. It requires clinical problem-solving skills to choose the ideal splint with the appropriate adaptation for each patient, as well as technical abilities in construction and design. Although splint effectiveness in the pediatric population is observed clinically, the lack of objective research, including a larger number of patients and a strong study design, continues to make splinting with the pediatric population a controversial treatment technique. It will be a challenge to all therapists using splinting as a pediatric treatment technique to increase the research through strong research design, reporting not only changes in range of motion and muscle tone but also in overall hand function (see Chapter 19).

REFERENCES

1. Armstrong J. Personal Communication, EE Fess, 1996.
2. Blashy M, Fuchs R: Orthokinetics: a new receptor facilitation method, *Am J Occup Ther* 13(5):226-34, 1959.
3. Boehme R: *Improving upper body control: an approach to assessment and treatment of tonal dysfunction*, Therapy Skill Builders, 1988, Tucson.
4. Casey CA, Kratz EJ: Soft splinting with neoprene: the thumb abduction supinator splint, *Am J Occup Ther* 42(6):395-8, 1988.
5. Colditz, JC, *Splinting with neoprene*, North Coast Medical, 1999, Morgan Hill, Cal.
6. Duvall-Riley B: *Splinting for infants and young children*, John Hopkins Hospital, 1995, Baltimore.
7. Exner C, Bonder B: Comparative effects of three hand splints of bilateral hand use, grasp and arm-hand posture in hemiplegic children, *Occup Ther J Res* 3(2):75-92, 1983.
8. Hogan L, Uditsky, T: *Pediatric splinting selection, fabrication and clinical application of upper extremity splints*, Therapy Skill Builders, 1999, San Antonio, Tex.
9. Langlois S, MacKinnon J, et al: Hand splints and cerebral spasticity: a review of the literature, *Canadian J Occup Ther* 56(3):113–19, 1989.
10. Lindholm L: Weight bearing hand splint: a method of managing upper extremity spasticity, *Phys Ther Forum* 5, 1986.
11. MacKinnon J, Sanderson E, et al: The MacKinnon splint: a functional hand splint, *Canadian J Occup Ther* 42(40):157-58, 1975.
12. Reymann J: The soft-splint and wonder strap, *Occup Ther Forum* 1988.
13. Snook JH: Spasticity reduction splint, *Am J Occup Ther* 33(10):648-51, 1979.
14. Thompson T, Tobin A: The modified MacKinnon, a low temperature approach to pediatric splinting. *Adv Occup Ther* 1997.

SUGGESTED READING

Achenbach C: A rule of thumb: age-proofing static splints, *Occup Ther Forum* March, 1993.
Bellefeuille-Reid DT: Aid to independence: hand splint for cerebral palsied children, *Canadian J Occup Ther* 51(1):37-9, 1984.
Brennan J: Response to stretch of hypertonic muscle groups in hemiplegia, *Br Med J* 1:1504-7, 1959.
Charait SE: A comparison of volar and dorsal splinting of the hemiplegic hand, *Am J Occup Ther* 22(4):319-21, 1968.
Coppard B, Lohman H: *Introduction to splinting: a critical-thinking and problem-solving approach*, Mosby, 1996, St. Louis.
Hagerstedt J: Splint adaptation encourages functional activity, *OT Week*, 1993.
Hettinger J: Pediatric splinting: expect the unexpected, *OT Week*, 1996.
Hogan L, Uditsky T: *Splinting the pediatric upper extremity*, AOTA National Conference, 1996.
Jamison SL, Dayhoff N: A hard hand positioning device to decrease wrist and finger hypertonicity: a sensorimotor approach for the patient with non-progressive brain damage, *Nurs Res* 29(5):285-9, 1980.
Kaplan N: Effect of splinting on reflex inhibition and sensorimotor stimulation in treatment of spasticity, *Arch Phys Med Rehab* 43:565-9, 1962.
Kiel J: *Basic hand splinting: a pattern design approach*, Little, Brown, 1983, Boston.
Mack S: Multi-handicapped splinting hints, *Occup Ther Forum*, 1992.
Malik M: *Manual of static hand splinting*, Hamarville Rehabilitation Center, 1976, Pittsburgh.
McPherson JJ: Objective evaluation of a splint designed to reduce hypertonicity, *Am J Occup Ther* 35(3):189-94, 1981.
McPherson JJ, Kreimeyer D, Aalderks M, et al: (1982). A comparison of dorsal and volar resting hand splints in the reduction of hypertonus, *Am J Occup Ther* 36(10):664-70, 1982.

Neeman L: Treatment of pain by orthokinetic orthosis (cuffs), *Occup Ther Forum* 11, 1986.

Neuhaus BE, Ascher ER, Coullon BA, et al: A survey of rationales for and against hand splinting in hemiplegia, *Am J Occup Ther* 35(2):83-90, 1981.

Reid DT: A survey of Canadian Occupational Therapists' use of hand splints for children with neuromuscular dysfunction, *Canadian J Occup Ther* 59(1):16-27, 1992.

Reid DT, Sochaniwskyj A: (1992). Influences of a hand positioning device on upper-extremity control of children with cerebral palsy, *Int J of Rehabil Res* 15(1):15-29, 1992.

Smith S: Splinting the severely involved hand, *Occup Ther Forum*, 1990.

Thompson T, Malloy M: The computer access splint, *Adv Occup Ther*, 1997.

Thompson-Rangel T: The mystery of the serpentine splints, *Occup Ther Forum*, 1991.

Whelan J: Effects of orthokinetics on upper extremity function of the adult hemiplegia patient, *Am J Occup Ther* 18(4):141-3, 1964.

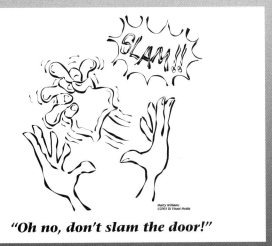

"Oh no, don't slam the door!"

CHAPTER 19

Splinting for Patients with Upper Extremity Spasticity*,†,‡

Chapter Outline

This chapter follows the expanded ASHT Splint Classification System[2] (ESCS) format by first dividing splints into articular or nonarticular categories. In the articular category, splints are next grouped according to the primary joint or joints they influence. Splints in the nonarticular category are defined by the anatomic segments upon which they are based.

Once articular splints are grouped according to their primary joints, they are further defined by direction of force application and then divided according to one of four purposes: immobilization, mobilization, restriction, or torque transmission. ESCS names for the splints illustrated in this chapter are in boldface type at the beginning of each of the figure captions. For clarification, colloquial splint names also are included along with the ESCS nomenclature in the text.

When applying the ESCS to splints described in this chapter, the assumption was made that splints were fitted to patients with upper motor neuron problems to counter the commonly observed clinical patterns of shoulder adduction and internal rotation, elbow flexion, forearm pronation, wrist flexion, finger

*The authors wish to acknowledge the work of Anita McAfee, MS, OTR, Zionsville, Ind., for developing the format and providing the initial information included in the Splinting and Upper Extremity Spasticity Studies Table.

†This chapter is part of a literature review that is submitted for journal publication.

‡For additional splint designs, patterns, and fabrication instructions, see Chapter 18, Splinting the Pediatric Patient.

517

flexion, and thumb adduction and flexion.[44] Working with this assumption, it quickly became apparent that the majority of splints in the chapter were classified as *type 0*, indicating that for this select group of patients, the vast majority of joints that are splinted are defined as primary joints.

INTRODUCTION

Splinting patients with spastic upper extremity problems continues to remain an enigma in upper extremity rehabilitation. Unlike orthopedic conditions that frequently have predictable courses of recovery, which allow development, testing, and generalization of treatment methodologies, the inherently complex nature of spasticity confounds study and subsequent development of splinting treatment guidelines.

The purpose of this chapter is to present a literature review of splint designs used in the conservative management of upper extremity spasticity. Table 19-1 at the end of this chapter summarizes information from published studies about splints used in the management of upper extremity spasticity. This table includes primary joint(s), author, year, title, splint, sample size, presence of statistical analysis, and whether improvement was noted for each article cited. Inhibitory casts, air pressure splints, and splints used in the postoperative phases of surgeries performed on spastic joints are not within the scope of this chapter.

Spasticity is defined by Lance as "a motor disorder characterized by a velocity-dependent increase in tonic stretch reflexes ('muscle tone') with exaggerated tendon jerks, resulting from hyperexcitability of the stretch reflex, as one component of the upper motor neuron syndrome."[33] Commonly encountered problems in the upper extremity secondary to spasticity include increased muscle tone, lack of smooth coordination, joint contractures, hygiene problems, decreased functional ability, pain, and potential nerve compression.[23,43,52] Splinting, especially for prevention and correction of contractures, along with other treatment methods including facilitation and inhibition techniques, conventional rehabilitation techniques, biofeedback, electrical stimulation, and other physical modalities traditionally have been used in the management of these secondary problems.[7,54,55]

Purposes of splints used in the management of upper extremity spasticity include prevention or correction of contractures, facilitation of normal movement, enhancement of function, inhibition of spasticity, and diminution of pain.[1,48] With advances in tone modifying chemical agents such as the administration of botulinum toxin, joint spasticity may be

decreased to allow splint fitting especially in situations where prior splint application was impossible.[1,55] Splints also may be used in conjunction with constraint-induced therapy (CIT). In CIT, splints or slings may be used to immobilize the nonaffected extremity to "force" functional use of the affected extremity and to influence the central nervous system through motor relearning.[14,25,67]

GENERAL LITERATURE REVIEW

Historically, the subject of splinting the spastic upper extremity has been riddled with controversy.* Some physicians and therapists feel strongly that the spastic extremity should not be splinted, whereas others are equally adamant that splinting has beneficial results. Even among proponents of splinting, numerous disagreements exist concerning splint design, inelastic versus elastic mobilization methods, surface of splint application, joints to be splinted, specific construction materials for splints and splint components, and wearing times and schedules. For example, in the debate regarding surface application of splints, dorsal application of splints has been encouraged to minimize sensory stimulation of spastic flexor muscle groups. Several authors have pointed out that splints cannot be truly volar or dorsal due to the circumferentially applied straps or elastic wraps necessary to secure the splint to the arm.[37,62,72]

Although numerous splints have been advocated to combat the effects of deforming forces to the upper extremity from upper motor neuron (UMN) lesions, few, if any, have been shown to produce consistently satisfactory results. The literature abounds with treatises on the technique and ramifications of splinting the spastic hand, but close examination reveals a surprising paucity of supporting data based on solid scientific research design and statistically significant analysis. Problems with studies reported in the literature include weak or limited research design, extremely small population samples, invalid and unreliable methods of measuring spasticity, lack of variable control, and lack of consistent methodology.[21,22,47,53]

Aside from the inadequacy of research data, one of the most glaring omissions seems to be a fundamental lack of understanding that the upper extremity (UE) is an open-ended intercalated articular chain. Some of the most frequently used splints are designed to position spastic digits in extension without controlled wrist position or they influence the wrist without affecting the fingers and thumb. These splints

---

*References 12, 21, 22, 27, 35, 51, 62.

produce a consistent sequence of events that are both predictable and immediately evident. Either the wrist assumes a compensatory flexed attitude as the fingers and thumb are brought into extension, or the unsplinted digits assume a greater attitude of flexion as the wrist is extended. This compensatory chain of events occurs because the tendons of the extrinsic finger flexors cross and affect not only the digital joints but the wrist as well.[21,22]

With prolonged progressive mobilization splinting of both digital and wrist joints, a spastic hand may be slowly brought into a more functional position, and spasticity seems to decrease.[9,29] However, when corrective splinting is discontinued, if the source of the deforming forces has not been altered, the hand and wrist will gradually return to a position of deformity.[45] To date no study has shown through good research design and appropriate statistical analysis that splinting will permanently control or diminish spasticity in the upper extremity.

Factors influencing the use of splinting as a treatment intervention in upper extremity spasticity include therapist training, familiarity and expertise in fabrication of splints used in the treatment of upper extremity spasticity, availability of resources, including time, equipment, materials, and patient compliance.[57] Additionally, Wilton noted "the fact that expertise in splint design and fabrication is the domain of the hand therapist who rarely treats clients with neurological dysfunction, while therapists who have experience and expertise in addressing issues related to spasticity often do not have the same expertise in splint fabrication."[73]

Based on an extensive literature review encompassing 125 years, Neuhaus and associates identified two basic treatment theories influencing splinting of the spastic upper extremity: the biomechanical approach, which emphasizes mechanical techniques to combat deformity, and the neurophysiologic approach that was introduced in the 1950s, which uses movement and handling techniques to reduce spasticity.[51] In many of the early neurophysiologic theories rigid, nonarticulated splinting was either omitted or contraindicated.

In a survey of the use of 12 different splints employed in the treatment of neuromuscular dysfunction by pediatric occupational therapists, greater than half of the 174 therapists surveyed reported regularly using the following splints: "resting palmar hand," "thumb," and "hard cone" splints.[57] Factors influencing therapist use of these three splints included instruction in fabrication of these splints in an occupational therapy course, effectiveness of the splints, patient comfort, and ease of fabrication. Citing a "lack of familiarity" as the primary reason, 65% of

the therapists surveyed had never used the other nine splints surveyed, including the "MacKinnon," "thumb abduction supination splint (TASS)," "orthokinetic cuff," "spasticity reduction," "finger abduction," "J-splint," "orthokinetic wrist," "inflatable," and "functional hand splint."[57]

Traditionally, splints from a wide range of categories have been used in the management of upper extremity spasticity, including inhibitory casting, inflatable pressure splints (air splints), custom-fabricated low-temperature thermoplastic splints, prefabricated or preformed splints, and splints custom fabricated by orthotists. Materials used in the construction of these splints include, but are not limited to, low- and high-thermoplastic materials, plaster, fiberglass, flexible plastic (air splints), neoprene, leather, Velcro strapping, cloth toweling, foam, Lycra, elastic bandages, elastic gloves, and wooden dowels.

■ SPECIFIC LITERATURE REVIEW: SPLINTS USED IN THE CONSERVATIVE TREATMENT OF UPPER EXREMITY SPASTICITY

Articular Splints

Shoulder, Elbow Splints

In a study by Neeman and Neeman of the effects of "orthokinetic cuffs" on a hemiparetic upper extremity, one of three cuffs applied to the subject included a proximally placed cuff to "enhance shoulder flexion and abduction and elbow extension."[50] Although the effects of the "orthokinetic cuff" on shoulder motion were not evaluated in their pilot study, the authors reported improvement in "active shoulder mobility" after a longer duration of treatment.

Further, researchers studying the effects of other splint designs on spasticity in joints distal to the shoulder have anecdotally noted improvement in shoulder spasticity during or post splinting of distal upper extremity joints.[45,64,74] Researchers studying the effects of elastic garments on elbow, forearm, wrist and hand spasticity also have reported improvement in shoulder spasticity.[26,68]

Elbow Splints

A variety of materials with different levels of rigidity have been used in the construction of splints designed to manage elbow spasticity (Fig. 19-1). In the literature reviewed, the mechanism attributed to improvement of elbow range of motion is the beneficial effect of low-load prolonged stretch to local tissues according to some researchers.*

---

*References 9, 38, 39, 49, 69, 70.

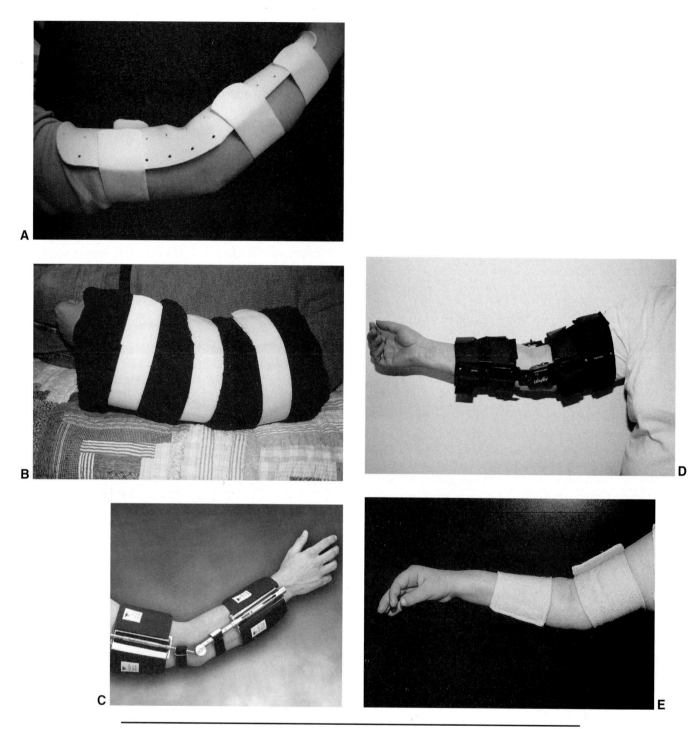

Fig. 19-1   A, Elbow extension mobilization splint, type 2 (3) B, Elbow extension mobilization splint, type 0 (1) C, Elbow extension mobilization splint, type 0 (1) D, Elbow extension mobilization splint, type 0 (1) E, Elbow extension mobilization splint, type 0 (1) \\ Wrist extension mobilization splint, type 0 (1)
Custom (A,B,E) and prefabricated (C,D) splints used to treat elbow spasticity and secondary contractures. B, Similar to the "soft splint" described by Wallen and O'Flaherty, this splint is constructed of foam and covered with a terry cloth towel. It is wrapped around the elbow to provide a gentle elbow extension mobilization force. E, An "orthokinetic cuff" with its inelastic field over the biceps to inhibit elbow flexion and the elastic field over the triceps facilitates elbow extension. (The second splint is an "orthokinetic cuff" for wrist extension.) [Courtesy (C) Dynasplint Systems, Inc., Severna Park, Md.; (D) Ultraflex Systems, Downington, Pa.; (E) Joni Armstrong, OTR, CHT, Bemidji, Minn.]

In contrast, "orthokinetic cuffs" (Fig. 19-1, *E*) are purported to facilitate paretic agonistic muscles and inhibit antagonistic muscles affecting joint motion through a neurophysiological mechanism.[50] "Orthokinetic cuffs" were developed to minimize the potentially adverse effects of joint immobilization caused by upper motor neuron problems.[4,20] These splints have an elastic field (facilitory) and an inelastic field (inhibitory). The elastic field portion of the cuff is positioned over the muscle(s) to be facilitated. Blashy and Fuchs reported clinical observations of "diminishing or disappearance of spasticity in muscles covered by the inelastic part of the segment, its reappearance in muscles under the elastic part."[4] These authors also noted that the use of an elastic bandage alone does not produce the desired effect. Positive outcomes have been reported by researchers studying the effects of "orthokinetic cuffs" on elbow spasticity.[4,50,71]

Elbow, Forearm, Wrist, Finger MP, PIP, DIP, Thumb CMC, MP, IP Splints

Positive findings were reported in upper extremity function of children with cerebral palsy using a treatment protocol of neuromuscular electrical stimulation and a custom-fabricated mobilization splint to reduce upper extremity spasticity (Fig. 19-2).[60] In a follow-up study, the authors concluded that neuromuscular electrical stimulation and mobilization bracing were more effective than neuromuscular electrical stimulation or splinting alone.[56] Additionally the investigators acknowledged that the treatment program may be lifelong for continued benefits.[60]

Elbow, Forearm, Wrist, Thumb CMC Splints

Fabricated to improve the functional ability of a child with cerebral palsy, the "Switzer splint" was designed to position the child's elbow, forearm, wrist, and thumb to allow the child to engage in functional hand activities (Fig. 19-3).[66]

Forearm, Wrist, Thumb CMC, MP Splints

The neoprene "thumb abduction supinator splint" (TASS) positions the spastic forearm in supination and the thumb in abduction. This splint was developed to decrease spasticity and increase function in bilateral and fine motor activities (Fig. 19-4).[11]

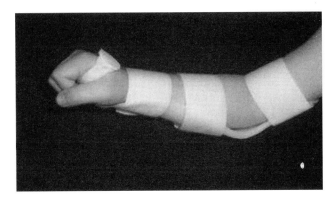

Fig. 19-3   Elbow extension, forearm pronation, wrist extension, thumb CMC radial abduction mobilization splint, type 0 (4) Described by Switzer, this splint was constructed to facilitate functional use in a child with moderate to severe flexor spasticity.

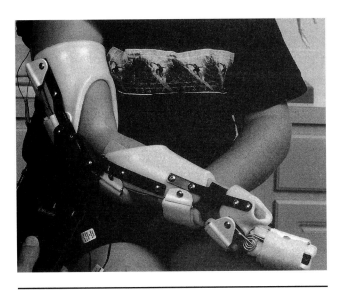

Fig. 19-2   Elbow extension, forearm supination, wrist extension, index–small finger extension, thumb CMC radial abduction and MP-IP extension mobilization splint, type 0 (18) Custom-designed splint used in the FirstFlex program by Ultraflex Systems, Inc. based on the original two-part splint in Scheker, Chesher, and Ramirez's study which consisted of a wrist, finger, and thumb extension mobilization splint and an Ultraflex elbow and forearm supination mobilization splint. (Courtesy Ultraflex Systems, Inc., Downington, Pa.)

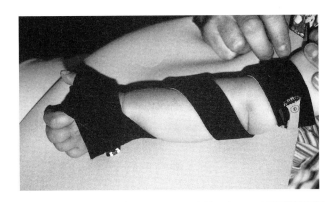

Fig. 19-4   Forearm supination, wrist extension, thumb CMC radial abduction and MP extension mobilization splint, type 0 (4) Constructed of neoprene, a thumb abduction supinator splint (TASS) was described by Casey & Kratz. (Courtesy Joni Armstrong, OTR, CHT, Bemidji, Minn.)

Wrist Splints

In studies focusing on wrist splinting, the primary purposes of wrist extension mobilization splinting were to stabilize the wrist to increase finger function using a dorsal application,[10] to mobilize spastic wrist joints[9,13] and to assess EMG changes in wrist flexor activity during splinted and nonsplinted conditions using circumferential splints and/or elastic wrap to secure splints to the extremity.[49] In Brennan's (1959) study,[9] although numerous authors have reported a volar surface of splint application, in reviewing the original article, no specific information by Brennan regarding the surface of application was found. However, in an earlier article by Brennan (1954),[8] several wrist splints are illustrated with volar surfaces of application.

Wrist, Finger MP Splints

The "MacKinnon splint" was designed to facilitate hand function in children with spastic cerebral palsy by positioning the wrist and finger MP joints in extension (Fig. 19-5).[27,40] Although results were not statistically significant, in Exner and Bonder's study,[18] the "MacKinnon splint" along with the "orthokinetic cuff" (positioned on the forearm to facilitate wrist and finger extension) were associated with improvement in bilateral hand use and the "MacKinnon splint" was associated with the greatest improvement in grasp skill. Furthermore, it was reported that the subjects and their parents tended to prefer the "MacKinnon splint."

Wrist, Finger MP, PIP, DIP Splints

EMG activity of spastic forearm flexor muscles was compared under three conditions: (1) no splint, (2) a

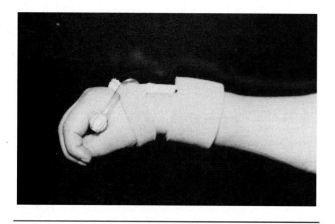

Fig. 19-5   Wrist extension, index–small finger MP extension mobilization splint, type 0 (5)
The theoretic rationale supporting the "MacKinnon splint" is based on Rood's neurophysiological theory of deep pressure to facilitate finger extension. The splint is used to increase function during hand use. (Courtesy Joni Armstrong, OTR, CHT, Bemidji, Minn.)

dorsally applied splint with Velcro straps that positioned the wrist in extension, finger MP joints in extension and adduction, and finger IP joints in extension (the thumb was not included in this dorsal splint), and (3) a volarly applied splint secured with a circumferentially wrapped elastic bandage that positioned the wrist in extension, finger MP joints in extension and abduction, and finger IP joints in extension. The thumb was not included in the volar splint.[76] Flexor EMG activity was reported to be lowest with the volarly applied splint and greatest with the dorsally applied splint.

Blashy and Fuchs[4] reported positive clinical results in a hemiplegic patient with spasticity wearing "orthokinetic cuffs" applied to facilitate wrist and finger flexion (inactive fields positioned over the "brachioradialis-extensor group"). The authors also reported positive responses to orthokinetics in 26 of 37 patients with central nervous system involvement whose diagnoses included hemiplegia, paraplegia, post-polio, multiple sclerosis, and Parkinson's disease, who were treated with upper and lower extremity orthokinetic cuffs.[4]

Wrist, Thumb CMC Splints

Designed by Hill to enhance functional use by positioning the wrist in extension and the thumb in radial abduction, the "J-splint" was named for the shape of its palmar metacarpal bar (Fig. 19-6).[27] The author acknowledged the tendency of the forearm bar to migrate distally due to the acute angle of application of the rubber band.

Wrist, Finger MP, Thumb CMC Splints

Neeman and Neeman[50] studied the effects of application of three "orthokinetic cuffs" to a hemiplegic patient. To enhance wrist extension, finger extension, and thumb radial abduction the active field of the "orthokinetic cuff" was positioned over the ECRL, ECRB, ECU, EDC, and APL. During the clinical treatment period that followed their pilot study, gains in the subject's active range of motion and function were reported.

Wrist, Finger MP, Thumb CMC, MP Splints

A splint design incorporating wrist extension, finger MP abduction, and thumb CMC palmar abduction and MP extension, described by Woodson, was reported to be beneficial.[75] The splint used a unique application of finger dividers to achieve finger MP joint abduction without impeding finger MP, PIP, and DIP extension and flexion.

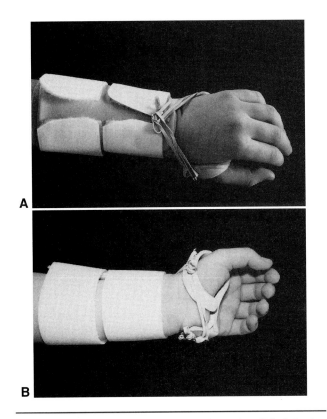

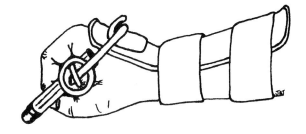

Fig. 19-7   Wrist extension, index–small finger extension, thumb CMC palmar abduction mobilization splint, type 0 (14); with grasp assist
Based on the "MacKinnon splint," a "functional splint" described by Bellefeuille-Reid includes a "grasp assist," consisting of a hole drilled in the palmar dowel to hold crayons, paint brushes, etc. to enhance functional hand and extremity use.

Fig. 19-6   A,B, Wrist extension, thumb CMC radial abduction mobilization splint, type 0 (2)
Based on the "MacKinnon splint," this "J-splint" was designed and described by Hill. It is intended for use only during functional activities. This classroom demonstration splint shows dorsal (A) and palmar (B) views. The palmar view shows the J-shaped bar that begins on the ulnar side of the palm, crosses the palm proximal to the palmar flexion crease, wraps around the thumb and thenar eminence where it imparts a radial abduction force to the CMC joint of the thumb.

Wrist, Finger MP, PIP, DIP, Thumb CMC Splints

Bellefeuille-Reid[3] created a splint design similar to the "MacKinnon splint" to increase independent hand function in children with spastic cerebral palsy (Fig. 19-7).

Wrist, Finger MP, PIP, DIP, Thumb CMC, MP, IP Splints

In the management of spasticity, splints incorporating the wrist, fingers, and thumb differ mainly in surface of application, finger and thumb joint positioning, and use of inelastic or elastic traction mobilization (Fig. 19-8).* Aside from a few elastic traction mobilization splints, the majority of these splints employ inelastic traction to mobilize joints. Their colloquial

*References 12, 29, 41, 42, 45-47, 59, 61, 64, 74, 76.

names include "resting pans," "resting," "functional position," "neutral position," "submaximal range," "antispasticity," and "antispasticity ball" splints.

The "spasticity reduction splint" designed by Snook and later empirically studied by McPherson positions the wrist in 30° of extension, finger MP joints in abduction and 45° of MP flexion, IP joints in extension, and the thumb in abduction (Fig. 19-8, A).[27,45,64] Snook reported that an "immediate and marked reduction of tone in the hand as well as in the entire upper extremity was observed in all cases."[64] McPherson reported statistically significant results in the reduction of wrist flexor spasticity with the use of Snook's "spasticity reduction splint."[45]

A study comparing the effects of splint surface of application, specifically dorsal and volar "resting pan splints" on spastic wrist flexors, found no significant differences between the splints, but both produced statistically significant findings in the reduction of spasticity.[47]

Authors using splint designs that included elastic traction in the form of elastic strapping and flexible metal stays have reported beneficial results in decreasing spasticity (Fig. 19-8, I,J).[46,61,74] McPherson et al. compared mobilization splinting with elastic traction versus passive range of motion and found a statistically significant reduction of spasticity in the splinted group. Comparing data from another study, McPherson et al.[47] reported a statistically significant difference in the reduction of spasticity among elastic mobilization, inelastic mobilization, and PROM groups with the highest mean reduction of spasticity in the elastic mobilization group and the lowest in the PROM group.

In a combination splint design, Wolcott designed an elastic mobilization splint that incorporated the wrist,

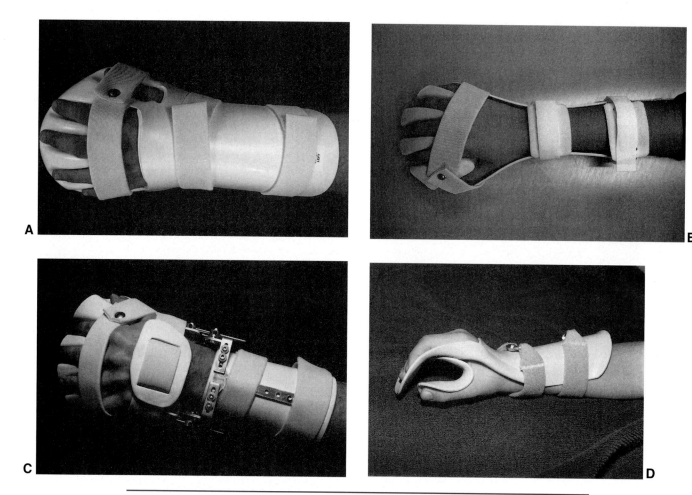

Fig. 19-8   A, Wrist extension, index, ring–small finger MP abduction, index–small finger extension, thumb CMC radial abduction and MP-IP extension mobilization splint, type 0 (16) B, Wrist extension, index, ring–small finger MP abduction, index–small finger extension, thumb CMC radial abduction and MP-IP extension mobilization splint, type 0 (16) C, Wrist extension, index, ring–small finger MP abduction, index–small finger extension, thumb CMC radial abduction and MP-IP extension mobilization splint, type 0 (16) D, Wrist extension, index–small finger extension, thumb CMC palmar abduction and MP-IP extension mobilization splint, type 0 (16) E, Wrist extension, index–small finger extension, thumb CMC palmar abduction and MP-IP extension mobilization splint, type 0 (16) F, Wrist extension, index–small finger extension, thumb CMC palmar abduction and MP-IP extension mobilization splint, type 0 (16) G,H, Wrist extension, index–small finger extension, thumb CMC palmar abduction and MP-IP extension mobilization splint, type 0 (16) I, Wrist extension, index–small finger extension, thumb CMC palmar abduction and MP-IP extension mobilization splint, type 0 (16) J, Wrist extension, index–small finger extension, thumb CMC radial abduction and MP-IP extension mobilization splint, type 0 (16) K, Wrist extension, index–small finger extension, thumb CMC palmar abduction and MP-IP extension mobilization splint, type 0 (16)

A-K, Demonstrating the diversity of splints that incorporate the wrist, finger, and thumb joints, differences in these splints involve joint positioning, materials, methods of mobilization, and surfaces of application. Splints A-C incorporate finger MP joint abduction whereas splints D-K position finger MP joints in adduction. A, Prefabricated version of Snook's "spasticity reduction splint" design that incorporates finger MP abduction, along with other prefabricated versions: volar (B) and dorsal (C) with an articulated wrist hinge. Designs using different methods of elastic mobilization: elastic straps (I) and flexible stays* (J). K, An "orthokinetic wrist splint" described by Farber et al. [Courtesy (A-C,E,F,I) Smith & Nephew Rolyan, Inc., Menomonee Falls, Wis.; (D) Joni Armstrong, OTR, CHT, Bemidji, MN; (G,H) Expansao, Sao Paulo, Brazil; (J) From Feldman P: Upper extremity casting and splinting. In Glenn M, Whyte J: *The practical management of spasticity in children and adults*, Lea & Felbiger, 1990, Philadelphia.]

*In conversation with Becker (5/17/2003), the original "Becker splint" design incorporated flexible metal stays (see McPherson J, Becker A, Franszczak N, 1985). A modification of this design uses a flexible polycarbonate material (Fig. 19-8J).

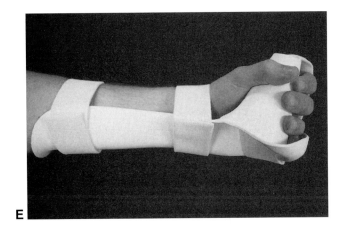

E

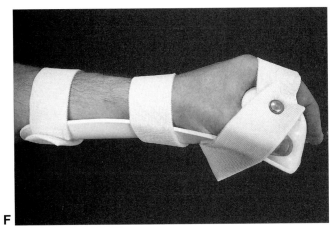

F

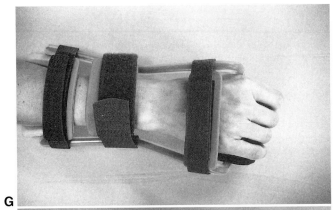

G

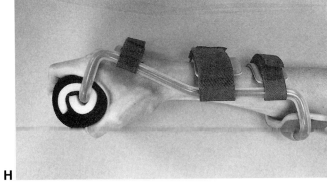

H

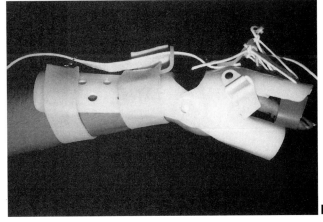

I

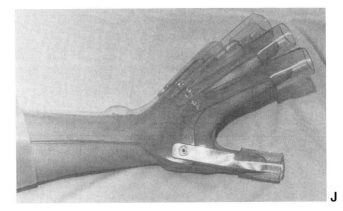

J

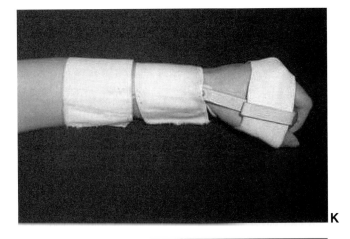

K

Fig. 19-8, cont'd
For legend see p. 524.

fingers, and thumb for day wear and, with the addition of an attachable nonelastic splint, could be transformed to inelastic traction for night wear.[74]

A splint incorporating several neurophysiologic concepts within its design is the "orthokinetic wrist splint" (Fig. 19-8, *K*).[19,20,27,30,31] Theorized to facilitate extension, the "orthokinetic wrist splint" has a wooden palmar dowel, which is similar in concept to a firm cone, an articulated wrist joint that is restricted in flexion by an extension of the volar forearm trough crossing the wrist joint, and instead of conventional strapping uses "orthokinetic cuffs" with their elastic fields positioned dorsally to facilitate extrinsic wrist and digital extensor muscles. No studies involving this splint were found in the literature.

Finger MP, PIP, Thumb CMC, MP, IP Splints

Doubilet and Polkow reported a moderate reduction in the spasticity of patients wearing their adapted "finger spreader" constructed from low-temperature thermoplastic (Fig. 19-9, *A*).[16,27] A statistically insignificant trend in wrist flexor spasticity was noted with longer wearing times of the "finger spreader splint" studied by Langlois, Pederson, and MacKinnon.[36]

Finger MP, PIP, DIP, Thumb CMC, MP, IP Splints

Incorporating Bobath's "key points of control," the original "finger spreader splint" designed by Bobath was constructed of foam and positioned the finger MP joints in extension and abduction and the thumb CMC joint in abduction (Fig. 19-9, *B*).[6,27]

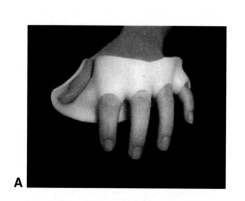
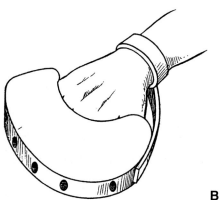

Fig. 19-9   A, Index, ring–small finger MP abduction, index–small finger MP extension, thumb CMC radial abduction and MP-IP extension mobilization splint, type 0 (7) B, Index, ring–small finger MP abduction, index–small finger extension, thumb CMC radial abduction and MP-IP extension mobilization splint, type 0 (15) C,D, Index–small finger extension, thumb CMC radial abduction and MP-IP extension mobilization splint, type 0 (15) E, Soft palm protector F, Index–small finger extension, thumb CMC palmar abduction and MP-IP extension mobilization splint, type 0 (15) G, Index–small finger extension, thumb CMC palmar abduction and MP-IP extension mobilization splint, type 0 (15) H, Index–small finger extension, thumb CMC palmar abduction and MP-IP extension mobilization splint, type 0 (15) I, Index–small finger extension, thumb CMC radial abduction and MP-IP extension mobilization splint, type 0 (15) J, Index–small finger extension, thumb CMC radial abduction and MP-IP extension mobilization splint, type 0 (15) K, Index, ring–small finger MP abduction, index–small finger extension, thumb CMC radial abduction and MP-IP extension mobilization splint, type 0 (15)

A-K, A variety of hand-based splints designed to increase finger and thumb extension. "Finger spreader splints": **A,** A durable design by Doubilet and Polkow based on Bobath's original design **(B).** Cone positioning in the hand: **C,** Traditional placement of a firm cone with the narrow end placed radially and ulnarly **(D)** as suggested by Milazzo and Gillen. **E,** Soft palm protectors inherently lack the ability to provide an extension mobilization force, but may be indicated in some instances. **F-H,** Similar to a cone, these splints are fabricated from the foam "noodles" used for play in swimming pools. **I,** Bloch and Evans described a glove attached to an air bladder, which was inflated and deflated by a sphygmomanometer bulb to increase finger extension and thumb abduction. **J,** Commercially available, the air bladder within this splint also allows varying levels of inflation depending on finger and thumb tightness. **K,** Putting into practice Bobath's neurophysiological theory, this splint is often used during weight-bearing activities/exercises. [**(B)** from Milazzo S, Gillen G: Splinting applications. In Gillen G, Burkhardt A: *Stroke rehabilitation: a function-based approach,* Mosby, 1998, St. Louis. Courtesy **(E,J,K)** Smith & Nephew Rolyan, Inc., Menomonee Falls, Wis.; **(F-H)** Joni Armstrong, OTR, CHT, Bemidji, Minn.; **(I)** adapted from Bloch R, Evans MG: *An inflatable splint for the spastic hand,* Arch Phys Med Rehab 58(4):179-80, 1977.]

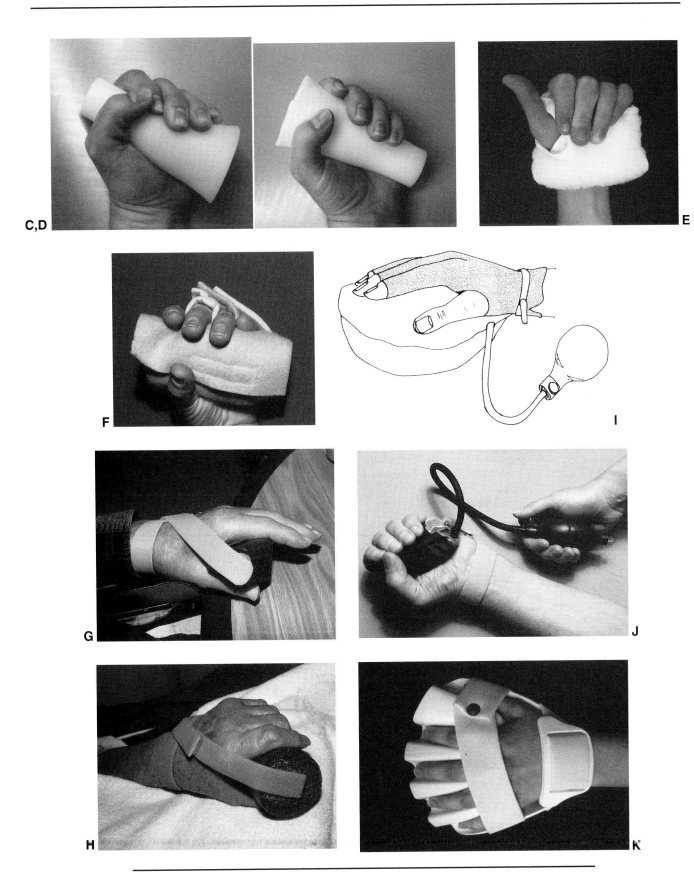

Fig. 19-9, cont'd
For legend see p. 526.

The use of a "firm cone" to apply pressure to the palm of the hand to facilitate digital extension is based on neurophysiological theory developed by Rood.[58,65] Since its introduction in the early 1950s, the "cone splint" has achieved wide acceptance. Use of a "firm cone" with the larger diameter end positioned ulnarly within the hand has been advocated to reduce hand and wrist spasticity (Fig. 19-9, C).[16,19,28,65] Milazzo and Gillen question this ulnar placement acknowledging that in tightly clenched fisted hands the traditional positioning may be initially more ideal. However, as finger and thumb extension improves, placement of the cone would appear to be more biomechanically correct with the larger diameter end of the cone placed radially within the first web space (Fig. 19-9, D).[48] Studies evaluating the use of a "hard cone" versus the traditional soft rolls used in nursing care to prevent hand flexion deformities are inconclusive. Dayhoff, as well as Jamison and Dayhoff, reported that a "soft hand-positioning device may contribute to flexion of the hand."[16,28] Further hypothesizing that soft hand-positioning devices facilitate the palmar grasp reflex which may reappear in brain-damaged individuals, Dayhoff noted improvement in passive digital extension with the wrist in flexion and less improvement with the wrist in neutral.[16]

Advocating muscle inhibition through application of pressure at the muscle's insertion, Farber, as well as Farber and Huss, promoted the use of hard materials rather than soft materials to obtain the inhibitory pressure necessary to avoid a grasping response, and to avoid facilitation of the muscles in contact with the soft materials.[19,20] In the debate regarding the use of a hard or soft device/material in the palm to increase finger extension and thumb abduction, it is important to consider the dissimilar material properties between the splints. Splints made of soft deformable materials will inherently not prevent finger and thumb flexion into the palm, but may be useful for hygiene purposes when indicated (Fig. 19-9, E). Other materials such as cylindrical foam plastics possess varying degrees of resistance and may be used to biomechanically mobilize the digits (Fig. 19-9, F-H).

Similar to the concept of a "hard cone," an inflatable pneumatic hand splint developed by Bloch and Evans was reported to produce good results in reducing severe finger flexion contractures and spasticity (Fig. 19-9, I,J).[5] The pneumatic hand splint is gradually inflated to the patient's tolerance and once an acceptable amount of extension is achieved, a rigid mobilization splint may be applied.

"Weight-bearing splints" that position the fingers and thumb in extension and abduction are typically used in conjunction with the neurodevelopmental treatment (NDT) approach during weight-bearing exercises to inhibit spasticity (Fig. 19-9, K).[32,63] In some cases the wrist may be included in the splint's design.[27]

Thumb CMC Splints

Several designs that mobilize the thumb out of an adducted and flexed posture were described in the literature, including the "cortical thumb orthosis," "soft-splint," and the "thumb loop."[15,27] These splints are constructed from a variety of materials including strapping, neoprene, and strips of low-temperature thermoplastic (Fig. 19-10, A).

Thumb CMC, MP Splints

Incorporating the thumb CMC and MP joints, the "short opponens splint" mobilizes the thumb out of an adducted and flexed posture (Fig. 19-10, B,C).[24,34,41] Exner and Bonder did not find the "short opponens splint" to neurophysiologically influence spasticity; however, they reported it may biomechanically increase hand function in children with adducted thumbs.[18] Another study reported statistically significant improvements clinically in thumb abduction, thumb opposition, lateral pinch, Box and Block Test performance, cube stacking, and grip strength in a child with cerebral palsy using a "short opponens splint."[24]

■ SUMMARY

Splinting the spastic upper extremity is a challenge even for the most experienced of therapists. While the neurophysiological effects of splinting are not fully understood, the biomechanical effects are clearly evident in preventing or correcting contractures and in the positioning of the upper extremity to enhance function. The dynamic and inconsistent nature of spasticity itself presents daunting and seemingly endless arrays of difficult-to-control variables that make research in this area extremely complex. Quantification of muscle tone continues to remain elusive,[53] making other accepted forms of assessment unreliable and invalid for evaluating the effects of particular treatment interventions including that of splinting upper extremity spasticity. Future research efforts should employ repeatable standardized test instruments combined with multiple measures assessment and statistical analyses. Allowing carefully delineated and focused questions to be addressed, controllable variables must be equal so that "apples are not compared to oranges." For example, in a study comparing differences in splint designs that affect the thumb CMC joint, all other joints incorporated by the

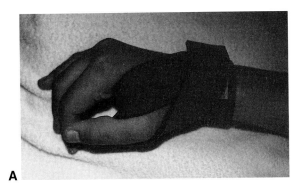

A

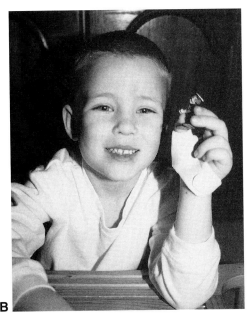

B

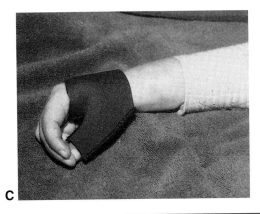

C

comparison splints should be positioned in a similar manner to each other. Specific joints and number of joints included in the splints also should be consistent, in addition to splint wearing times. It is also important that researchers carefully describe splints providing the ESCS name, details of joint positioning, surface of application, construction materials, and any other noteworthy features. Splints used in research studies should encompass excellent mechanics, use of outriggers and mobilization assists, design, construction, and fit principles. For example, it is a waste of critical resources to study wrist immobilization splint designs if the proximal ends of the splints studied end mid-forearm, resulting in poor mechanical advantage for controlling wrist position! Regardless of how well intended, the combination of poor splint design and poor research design is not helpful to expanding professional knowledge. Two times zero is still zero. In truth, the single greatest obstacle to good research studies in this area is finding sufficient numbers of like subjects to achieve statistical significance. If small numbers of subjects are used, research designs must be carefully chosen and results from these studies interpreted with caution and analytical perspective. Through consistent and improved research approaches, studies may be replicated, more easily compared, and meta-analyses may be performed, eventually fortifying the body of knowledge in this area.

The successful use of splints as a therapeutic modality in the management of upper extremity spasticity requires an individualized approach tailored to the specific needs of each patient. Splints used in conjunction with other treatment interventions can contribute to maximizing the best possible outcome for each patient. It is important to keep in mind that splints do not treat the source of upper extremity spasticity, but manage the symptoms of the spasticity: to prevent or correct contractures, facilitate normal movement, enhance function, inhibit spasticity, and decrease pain.

Fig. 19-10   A, Thumb CMC palmar abduction mobilization splint, type 0 (1) B, Thumb CMC palmar abduction and MP extension mobilization splint, type 0 (2) C, Thumb CMC palmar abduction and MP-IP extension mobilization splint, type 0 (3)
Including one or more joints, splints used to position the thumb for functional use may be constructed from a variety of materials including neoprene (A,C) and thermoplastic (B). [Courtesy (A,C) Joni Armstrong, OTR, CHT, Bemidji, Minn.]

TABLE 19-1   Splinting and Upper Extremity Spasticity Studies

Primary Joint(s)	Author*	Year	Title	Expanded Splint Classification System (ASHT)	Colloquial Name	Sample Size	Inferential Statistical Analysis	Reported Improvement
Shoulder, elbow	Neeman, RL Neeman, M	1992	Rehabilitation of a post-stroke patient with upper extremity hemiparetic movement dysfunctions by orthokinetic orthoses	†1. Shoulder flexion and abduction, elbow extension mobilization splint, type 0 (2) 2. Elbow extension mobilization splint, type 0 (1) 3. Wrist extension, index–small finger MP extension, thumb CMC radial abduction mobilization splint, type (0) 6	Orthokinetic cuffs	1	No (shoulder)	Yes
Elbow	Mackay, S Wallen, M	1996	Re-examining the effects of the soft splint on acute hypertonicity at the elbow	Elbow extension mobilization splint, type 0 (1)	Soft splint	1	No	Yes
Elbow	Wallen, M Mackay, S	1995	An evaluation of the soft splint in the acute management of elbow hypertonicity	Elbow extension mobilization splint, type 0 (1)	Soft splint	1	No	Yes
Elbow	Neeman, RL Neeman, M	1992	Rehabilitation of a post-stroke patient with upper extremity hemiparetic movement dysfunctions by orthokinetic orthoses	1. Shoulder flexion and abduction, elbow extension mobilization splint, type 0 (2) †2. Elbow extension mobilization splint, type 0 (1) 3. Wrist extension, index–small finger MP extension, thumb CMC radial abduction mobilization splint, type (0) 6	Orthokinetic cuffs	1	Yes (elbow)	Yes
Elbow	Wallen, M O'Flaherty, S	1991	The use of the soft splint in the management of spasticity of the upper limb	Elbow extension mobilization splint, type 0 (1)	Soft splint	1	No	Yes
Elbow	MacKay-Lyons, M	1989	Low-load, prolonged stretch in treatment of elbow flexion contractures secondary to head trauma: A case report	Elbow extension mobilization splint, type 0 (1)	Dynasplint	1	No	Yes
Elbow	Mills, VM	1984	Electromyographic results of inhibitory splinting	Insufficient information—unable to provide complete ESCS name	Bivalve plaster splints or Orthoplast splints secured with circumferential elastic wrap (Splint details not provided)	8 (2 wrists, 2 elbows, 4 ankles)	Yes	Yes
Elbow	Whelan, JK	1964	Effect of orthokinetics: on upper extremity function of the adult hemiplegic patient	Elbow extension mobilization splint, type 0 (1)	Orthokinetic cuff	20	Yes	Yes (ROM and "postural carriage")
Elbow	Blashy, MR Fuchs, RL	1959	Orthokinetics: A new receptor facilitation method	†1. Elbow extension mobilization splint, type 0 (1) 2. Wrist flexion, index–small finger flexion mobilization splint, type 0 (13)	Orthokinetic cuff	1	No	Yes
Elbow	Brennan, JB	1959	Response to stretch of hypertonic muscle groups in hemiplegia	Insufficient information—unable to provide complete ESCS name	Not provided	14 (3 elbows, 10 wrists, 5 fingers)	No	Yes

TABLE 19-1   Splinting and Upper Extremity Spasticity Studies—cont'd

Primary Joint(s)	Author*	Year	Title	Expanded Splint Classification System (ASHT)	Colloquial Name	Sample Size	Inferential Statistical Analysis	Reported Improvement
Elbow, forearm, wrist, finger, thumb	Ramirez, S Chesher, S Scheker, LR	1999	Evaluation of combined neuromuscular electrical stimulation and dynamic orthotic management of children with hemiplegic spastic cerebral palsy	Elbow extension, forearm supination mobilization splint, type 0 (2) (Ultraflex) \\ Wrist extension, index-small finger extension, thumb CMC radial abduction and MP extension mobilization splint, type 0 (15)	Two part: wrist-hand unit & elbow unit (Ultraflex)	21 (7 NMES only, 7 splint only & 7 NMES & splint)	No	Yes
Elbow, forearm, wrist, finger, thumb	Scheker, LR Chesher, SP Ramirez, S	1999	Neuromuscular electrical stimulation and dynamic bracing as a treatment for upper-extremity spasticity in children with cerebral palsy	Elbow extension, forearm supination mobilization splint, type 0 (2) (Ultraflex) \\ Wrist extension, index-small finger extension, thumb CMC radial abduction and MP extension mobilization splint, type 0 (15)	Two part: wrist-hand unit & elbow unit (Ultraflex)	19	No	Yes
Elbow, forearm, wrist, thumb	Switzer, S	1980	The Switzer splint	Elbow extension, forearm pronation, wrist extension, thumb CMC radial abduction mobilization splint, type 0 (4)	Switzer splint	1	No	Yes
Forearm, wrist, thumb	Casey, CA Kratz, EJ	1988	Soft splinting with neoprene: the thumb abduction supinator splint	Forearm supination, wrist extension, thumb CMC radial abduction and MP extension mobilization splint, type 0 (4)	TASS: Thumb abduction supinator splint	>50	No	Yes
Wrist	Carmick, J	1997	Use of neuromuscular electrical stimulation and a dorsal wrist splint to improve the hand function of a child with spastic hemiparesis	Wrist extension mobilization splint, type 0 (1)	Dorsal wrist splint	1	No	Yes
Wrist	Collins, K Oswald, P Burger, G Nolden, J	1985	Customized adjustable orthoses: their use in spasticity	Wrist extension mobilization splint, type 0 (1)	Customized adjustable wrist orthosis	1	No	Yes
Wrist	Mills, VM	1984	Electromyographic results of inhibitory splinting	Insufficient information—unable to provide complete ESCS name	Bivalve plaster splints or Orthoplast splints secured with circumferential elastic wrap (splint details not provided)	8 (2 wrists, 2 elbows, 4 ankles)	Yes	Yes
Wrist	Brennan, JB	1959	Response to stretch of hypertonic muscle groups in hemiplegia	Insufficient information—unable to provide complete ESCS name	Not provided	14 (3 elbows, 10 wrists, 5 fingers)	No	Yes
Wrist, finger	Exner, CE Bonder, BR	1983	Comparative effects of three hand splints on bilateral hand use, grasp, and arm-hand posture in hemiplegic children: a pilot study	[†]1. Wrist extension, index–small finger MP extension mobilization splint, type 0 (5) 2. Thumb CMC palmar abduction and MP extension mobilization splint, type 0 (2) [†]3. Wrist extension, index–small finger MP extension mobilization splint, type 0 (5)	1. Orthokinetic cuff 2. Short opponens thumb splint 3. MacKinnon splint	12	Yes	Yes, but not statistically significant
Wrist, finger	MacKinnon, J Sanderson, E Buchanan, J	1975	The MacKinnon splint-a functional hand splint	Wrist extension, index–small finger MP extension mobilization splint, type 0 (5)	MacKinnon splint	31	No	Yes

TABLE 19-1 Splinting and Upper Extremity Spasticity Studies—cont'd

Primary Joint(s)	Author*	Year	Title	Expanded Splint Classification System (ASHT)	Colloquial Name	Sample Size	Inferential Statistical Analysis	Reported Improvement
Wrist, finger	Zislis, JM	1964	Splinting of hand in a spastic hemiplegic patient	1. Wrist extension, index–small finger extension mobilization splint, type 0 (13) (Dorsal) 2. Wrist extension, index, ring–small finger MP abduction, index–small finger extension mobilization splint, type 0 (13) (Volar)	1. Dorsal splint 2. Volar splint	1	No	Yes, Volar splint
Wrist, finger	Blashy, MR Fuchs, RL	1959	Orthokinetics: A new receptor facilitation method	1. Elbow extension mobilization splint, type 0 (1) †2. Wrist flexion, index–small finger flexion mobilization splint, type 0 (13)	Orthokinetic cuff	1	No	Yes
Wrist, finger	Brennan, JB	1959	Response to stretch of hypertonic muscle groups in hemiplegia	Insufficient information— unable to provide complete ESCS name	Not provided	14 (3 elbows, 10 wrists, 5 fingers)	No	Yes
Wrist, finger, thumb	Neeman, RL Neeman, M	1992	Rehabilitation of a post-stroke patient with upper extremity hemiparetic movement dysfunctions by orthokinetic orthoses	1. Shoulder flexion and abduction, elbow extension mobilization splint, type 0 (2) 2. Elbow extension mobilization splint, type 0 (1) †3. Wrist extension, index–small finger MP extension, thumb CMC radial abduction mobilization splint, type (0) 6	Orthokinetic cuffs	1	Yes	Yes
Wrist, finger, thumb	Scherling, E Johnson, H	1989	A tone-reducing wrist-hand orthosis	Wrist extension, index-small finger extension, and thumb CMC palmar abduction and MP-IP extension mobilization splint, type 0 (16)	Tone-reducing Wrist-Hand Orthosis	18	No	Yes
Wrist, finger, thumb	Woodson, AM	1988	Proposal for splinting the adult hemiplegic hand to promote function	Wrist extension, index, ring–small finger MP abduction, thumb CMC palmar abduction and MP extension mobilization splint, type 0 (6) (Dorsal)	Static dorsal hand splint with finger separators	2	No	Yes
Wrist, finger, thumb	Rose, V Shah, S	1987	A comparative study on the immediate effects of hand orthoses on reducation of hypertonus	1. Wrist extension, index–small finger extension, thumb CMC palmar abduction and MP-IP extension mobilization splint, type 0 (16) (Dorsal) 2. Wrist extension, index–small finger extension, thumb CMC palmar abduction and MP-IP extension mobilization splint, type 0 (16) (Volar)	1. Dorsal static orthosis 2. Volar static orthosis	30 (3 groups: dorsal splint, volar splint, & no splint)	Yes	Yes, significant hypertonicity reduction with volar and dorsal splints
Wrist, finger, thumb	McPherson, JJ Becker, AH Franszczak, N	1985	Dynamic splint to reduce the passive component of hypertonicity	Wrist extension, index–small finger extension, thumb CMC radial abduction and MP-IP extension mobilization splint, type 0 (16)	Becker splint	8	Yes	Yes
Wrist, finger, thumb	Mathiowetz, V Bolding, DJ Trombly, CA	1983	Immediate effects of positioning devices on the normal and spastic hand measured by electromyography	†1. Index–small finger extension, thumb CMC palmar abduction and MP-IP extension mobilization splint, type 0 (16) 2. Index–small finger extension, thumb CMC palmar abduction mobilization splint, type 0 (13) 3. Index, ring–small finger MP abduction, index–small finger extension, thumb CMC radial abduction and MP-IP extension mobilization splint, type 0 (15)	1. Volar resting splint 2. Firm cone splint 3. Finger spreader splint	12 (4 spastic, 8 normal)	Yes	No significant difference between splints 1–3 during grasping and post-grasp period

TABLE 19-1   Splinting and Upper Extremity Spasticity Studies—cont'd

Primary Joint(s)	Author*	Year	Title	Expanded Splint Classification System (ASHT)	Colloquial Name	Sample Size	Inferential Statistical Analysis	Reported Improvement
Wrist, finger, thumb	McPherson, JJ Kreimeyer, D Aalderks, M Gallagher, T	1982	A comparison of dorsal and volar resting hand splints in the reduction of hypertonus	1. Wrist extension, index, ring–small finger MP abduction, index–small finger extension, thumb CMC radial abduction and MP-IP extension mobilization splint, type 0 (16) (Dorsal) 2. Wrist extension, index, ring–small finger MP abduction, index–small finger extension, thumb CMC radial abduction and MP-IP extension mobilization splint, type 0 (16) (Volar)	1. Dorsal resting hand splint 2. Volar resting hand splint	10 (5 dorsal, 5 volar)	Yes	No significant difference between dorsal and volar splints; significant reduction in hypertonicity in younger subjects
Wrist, finger, thumb	McPherson, JJ	1981	Objective evaluation of a splint designed to reduce hypertonicity	Wrist extension, index, ring–small finger MP abduction, index–small finger extension, thumb CMC radial abduction and MP-IP extension mobilization splint, type 0 (16)	Spasticity reduction splint (Snook, 1979)	5 (7 wrists)	Yes	Yes
Wrist, finger, thumb	Snook, JH	1979	Spasticity reduction splint	Wrist extension, index, ring–small finger MP abduction, index–small finger extension, thumb CMC radial abduction and MP-IP extension mobilization splint, type 0 (16)	Spasticity reduction splint	18	No	Yes
Wrist, finger, thumb	Charait, SE	1968	A comparison of volar and dorsal splinting of the hemiplegic hand	1. Wrist extension, index–small finger extension, thumb CMC palmar abduction and MP-IP extension mobilization splint, type 0 (16) (Volar) 2. Wrist extension, index–small finger extension, thumb CMC palmar abduction and MP-IP extension mobilization splint, type 0 (16) (Dorsal)	Functional position splint-static type	20 (10 dorsal, 10 volar)	No	Yes with dorsal splint
Wrist, finger, thumb	Wolcott, LE	1966	Orthotic management of the spastic hand	Insufficient information—unable to provide complete ESCS name	Static splint, dynamic functional splint	16	No	Yes
Wrist, finger, thumb	Kaplan, N	1962	Effect of splinting on reflex inhibition and sensorimotor stimulation in treatment of spasticity	Wrist extension, index–small finger extension, thumb CMC radial abduction and MP-IP extension mobilization splint, type 0 (16) (Dorsal)	Dorsal splint	10	No	Yes
Finger, thumb	Kinghorn, J Roberts, G	1996	The effect of an inhibitive weight-bearing splint on tone and function: A single-case study	Index–small finger extension, thumb CMC radial abduction and MP-IP extension mobilization splint, type 0 (15)	Weight-bearing splint	1	Yes	No significant effects
Finger, thumb	Langlois, S Pederson, L MacKinnon, J	1991	The effects of splinting on the spastic hemiplegic hand: report of a feasibility study	Index, ring–small finger MP abduction, index–small finger MP-PIP extension, thumb CMC radial abduction and MP-IP extension mobilization splint, type 0 (11)	Finger abduction splint (finger spreader)	9	Yes	Not significant in spasticity reduction
Finger, thumb	Smelt, HR	1989	Effect of an inhibitive weight-bearing mitt on tone reduction and functional performance in a child with cerebral palsy	Index–small finger extension, thumb CMC radial abduction and MP-IP extension mobilization splint, type 0 (15)	Weight-bearing mitt	1	?	Yes

TABLE 19-1 Splinting and Upper Extremity Spasticity Studies—cont'd

Primary Joint(s)	Author*	Year	Title	Expanded Splint Classification System (ASHT)	Colloquial Name	Sample Size	Inferential Statistical Analysis	Reported Improvement
Finger, thumb	Mathiowetz, V Bolding, DJ Trombly, CA	1983	Immediate effects of positioning devices on the normal and spastic hand measured by electromyography	1. Index–small finger extension, thumb CMC palmar abduction and MP-IP extension mobilization splint, type 0 (16) †2. Index–small finger extension, thumb CMC palmar abduction mobilization splint type 0 (13) †3. Index, ring–small finger MP abduction, index–small finger extension, thumb CMC radial abduction and MP-IP extension mobilization splint, type 0 (15)	1. Volar resting splint 2. Firm cone splint 3. Finger spreader splint	12 (4 spastic, 8 normal)	Yes	No significant difference between splints 1-3 during grasping and post-grasp period Significant increase in EMG activity with finger spreader
Finger, thumb	Jamison, SL Dayhoff, NE	1980	A hard hand-positioning device to decrease wrist and finger hypertonicity: A sensorimotor approach for the patient with nonprogressive brain damage	Index–small finger extension, thumb CMC palmar abduction mobilization splint, type 0 (13)	Firm cone splint	11	Yes	Yes
Finger, thumb	Doubilet, L Polkow, LS	1977	Theory and design of a finger abduction splint for the spastic hand	Index, ring–small finger MP abduction, index–small finger MP-PIP extension, thumb CMC radial abduction and MP-IP extension mobilization splint, type 0 (11) (Difficult to determine splint's positioning of MP and PIP joints)	Finger abduction splint (finger spreader)	15	No	Yes
Finger, thumb	Bloch, R Evans, MG	1977	An inflatable splint for the spastic hand	Index–small finger extension, thumb CMC radial abduction and MP-IP extension mobilization splint, type 0 (15)	Pneumatic glove splint	1	No	Yes
Finger, thumb	Dayhoff, N	1975	Soft or hard devices to position hands?	Index–small finger extension, thumb CMC palmar abduction and MP-IP extension mobilization splint, type 0 (13)	Firm cone splint	3	No	Yes
Thumb	Goodman, S Bazyk, S	1991	The effects of a short thumb opponens splint on hand function in cerebral palsy: a single-subject study	Thumb CMC palmar abduction mobilization splint, type 0 (2)	Short opponens thumb splint	1	Yes	Yes
Thumb	Currie, DM Mendiola, A	1987	Cortical thumb orthosis for children with spastic hemiplegic cerebral palsy	Thumb CMC radial abduction mobilization splint, type 0 (1)	Cortical thumb orthosis	5	No	Yes
Thumb	Exner, CE Bonder, BR	1983	Comparative effects of three hand splints on bilateral hand use, grasp, and arm-hand posture in hemiplegic children: a pilot study	1. Wrist extension, index–small finger extension mobilization splint, type 0 (5) †2. Thumb CMC palmar abduction and MP extension mobilization splint, type 0 (2) 3. Wrist extension, index–small finger MP extension mobilization splint, type 0 (5)	1. Orthokinetic cuff 2. Short opponens thumb splint 3. MacKinnon splint	12	Yes	Yes, not statistically significant

*Full citations for studies cited are found in reference section.
†Splint is included in the Primary Joint section.

REFERENCES

1. Albany K: Physical and occupational therapy considerations in adult patients receiving botulinum toxin injections for spasticity, *Muscle Nerve Suppl* 20(Supplement 6):S221-31, 1997.
2. ASHT: *American Society of Hand Therapists splint classification system*, ed 1, Ed. Bailey et al, The American Society of Hand Therapists, 1992, Chicago.
3. Bellefeuille-Reid D: Aid to independence—hand splint for cerebral palsied children, *Canadian J Occup Ther* 51(1):37-9, 1984.
4. Blashy M, Fuchs R: Orthokinetics: a new receptor facilitation method, *Am J Occup Ther* 13(5):226-34, 1959.
5. Bloch R, Evans MG: An inflatable splint for the spastic hand, *Arch Phys Med Rehab* 58(4):179-80, 1977.
6. Bobath B: *Adult hemiplegia: evaluation and treatment*, ed 2, William Heinemann Medical Books Ltd, 1978, London.
7. Brand P, Hollister A: *Clinical biomechanics of the hand*, ed 3, Mosby, 2000, St. Louis.
8. Brennan J: Moulding polythene plastic splints direct to patient, a safe and practical method, *Lancet* pp. 948-51, 1954.
9. Brennan J: Response to stretch of hypertonic muscle groups in hemiplegia, *Br Med J* 1:1504-7, 1959.
10. Carmick J: Use of neuromuscular electrical stimulation and a dorsal wrist splint to improve the hand function of a child with spastic hemiparesis, *Phys Ther* 77(6):661-71, 1997.
11. Casey C, Kratz E: Soft splinting with neoprene: the thumb abduction supinator splint, *Am J Occup Ther* 42(6):395-8, 1988.
12. Charait S: A comparison of volar and dorsal splinting of the hemiplegic hand, *Am J Occup Ther* 22(4):319-21, 1968.
13. Collins K, Oswald P, Burger G, Nolden J: Customized adjustable orthoses: Their use in spasticity, *Arch Phys Med Rehab* 66:397-8, 1985.
14. Crocker M, MacKay-Lyons M, McDonnell E: Forced use of the upper extremity in cerebral palsy: a single-case design, *Am J Occup Ther* 51(10):824-33, 1997.
15. Currie DM, Mendiola A: Cortical thumb orthosis for children with spastic hemiplegic cerebral palsy, *Arch Phys Med Rehab* 68(4):214-6, 1987.
16. Dayhoff N: Soft or hard devices to position hands? *Am J Nurs* 75(7):1142-4, 1975.
17. Doubilet L, Polkow L: Theory and design of a finger abduction splint for the spastic hand, *Am J Occup Ther* 31(5):320-2, 1977.
18. Exner C, Bonder B: Comparative effects of three hand splints on bilateral hand use, grasp, and arm-hand posture in hemiplegic children: a pilot study, *Occup Ther J Res* 3(2):75-92, 1983.
19. Farber S: *Neurorehabilitation: a multisensory approach*, WB Saunders, 1982, Philadelphia.
20. Farber S, Huss A: *Sensorimotor evaluation and treatment procedures for allied health personnel*, ed 2, The Indiana University Foundation, 1974, Indianapolis.
21. Fess EE, Gettle K: *Hand splinting: principles and methods*, Mosby, 1981, St. Louis.
22. Fess EE, Philips C: *Hand splinting: principles and methods*, ed 2, Mosby, 1987, St. Louis.
23. Gelber D, Jozefczyk P: Therapeutics in the management of spasticity, *Neurorehab Neural Repair* 13(5):5-14, 1999.
24. Goodman G, Bazyk S: The effects of a short thumb opponens splint on hand function in cerebral palsy: a single-subject study, *Am J Occup Ther* 45(8):726-31, 1991.
25. Gourley M: Regaining upper-extremity function through constraint-induced movement therapy. OT Practice 7(3), 2002.
26. Gracies J, Marosszeky JE, Renton R, et al: Short-term effects of dynamic Lycra splints on upper limb in hemiplegic patients, *Arch Phys Med Rehab* 81(12):1547-55, 2000.
27. Hill S: Current trends in upper-extremity splinting. In Boeheme R: *Improving upper body control: an approach to assessment and treatment of tonal dysfunction*, Therapy Skill Builders, 1988, Tucson.
28. Jamison S, Dayhoff N: A hard hand-positioning device to decrease wrist and finger hypertonicity: a sensorimotor approach for the patient with nonprogressive brain damage, *Nurs Res* 29(5):285-9, 1980.
29. Kaplan N: Effect of splinting on reflex inhibition and sensorimotor stimulation, *Arch Phys Med Rehab* 43:565-9, 1962.
30. Kiel J: Making the dyamic orthokinetic wrist splint for flexor spasticity in hand and wrist. In Farber S, Huss A: *Sensorimotor evaluation and treatment procedures for allied health personnel*, ed 2, The Indiana University Foundation, 1974, Indianapolis.
31. Kiel J: Orthokinetic wrist splint for flexor spasticity: construction methods. In Farber S: *Neurorehabilitation: a multisensory approach*, WB Saunders, 1982, Philadelphia.
32. Kinghorn J, Roberts G: The effect of an inhibitive weight-bearing splint on tone and function: a single-case study, *Am J Occup Ther* 50(10):807-15, 1996.
33. Lance J: Symposium synopsis. In Feldman R, Young R, Koella W: *Spasticity: disordered motor control*, Year Book Medical Publishers, 1980, Chicago, page 485.
34. Landmesser W, McCrum R, Allen J: The opponens spacer, *Am J Occup Ther* 9(3):112-14,39, 1955.
35. Langlois S, MacKinnon J, Pederson L: Hand splints and cerebral spasticity: a review of the literature, *Canadian J Occup Ther* 56(3):113-9, 1989.
36. Langlois S, Pederson L, MacKinnon J: The effects of splinting on the spastic hemiplegic hand: report of a feasibility study, *Canadian J Occup Ther* 58(1):17-25, 1991.
37. Louis W: Hand splinting, effect on the afferent system, *Am J Occup Ther* 16(3):143-5, 1962.
38. Mackay S, Wallen M: Re-examining the effects of the soft splint on acute hypertonicity at the elbow, *Austr Occup Ther J* 43:51-9, 1996.
39. MacKay-Lyons M: Low-load, prolonged stretch in treatment of elbow flexion contractures secondary to head trauma: a case report, *Phys Ther* 69(4):292-6, 1989.
40. MacKinnon J, Sanderson E, Buchanan J: The MacKinnon splint—a functional hand splint, *Canadian J Occup Ther* 42(40):157-8, 1975.
41. Malick M: *Manual on static hand splinting*, Harmarville Rehabilitation Center, 1970, Pittsburgh.
42. Mathiowetz V, Bolding D, Tromby C: Immediate effects of positioning devices on the normal and spastic hand measured by electromyography, *Am J Occup Ther* 37(4):247-54, 1983.
43. Mayer N: Clinicophysiologic concepts of spasticity and motor dysfunction in adults with an upper motor neuron lesion, *Muscle Nerve Suppl* 20(Supplement 6):S1-13, 1997.
44. Mayer N, Esquenazi A, Childers M: Common patterns of clinical motor dysfunction, *Muscle Nerve Suppl* 20(Supplement 6):S21-35, 1997.
45. McPherson J: Objective evaluation of a splint designed to reduce hypertonicity, *Am J Occup Ther* 35(3):189-94, 1981.
46. McPherson J, Becker A, Franszczak N: Dynamic splint to reduce the passive component of hypertonicity, *Arch Phys Med Rehab* 66(4):249-52, 1985.
47. McPherson JJ, Kreimeyer D, Aalderks M, et al: A comparison of dorsal and volar resting hand splints in the reduction of hypertonus, *Am J Occup Ther* 36(10):664-70, 1982.
48. Milazzo S, Gillen G: Splinting applications. In Gillen G, Burkhardt A: *Stroke rehabilitation: a function-based approach*, Mosby, 1998, St. Louis.

49. Mills V: Electromyographic results of inhibitory splinting, *Phys Ther* 64(2):190-3, 1984.

50. Neeman R, Neeman M: Rehabilitation of a post-stroke patient with upper extremity hemiparetic movement dysfunction by orthokinetic orthoses, *J Hand Ther* 3(5):147-55, 1992.

51. Neuhaus B, Ascher ER, Coullon BA, et al: A survey of rationales for and against hand splinting in hemiplegia, *Am J Occup Ther* 35(2):83-90, 1981.

52. Orcutt S, Kramer WG III, Howard MW, et al: Carpal tunnel syndrome secondary to wrist and finger flexor spasticity, *J Hand Surg [Am]* 15(6):940-4, 1990.

53. Pierson S: Outcome measures in spasticity management, *Muscle Nerve Suppl* 20(Supplement 6):S36-60, 1997.

54. Pierson S: Physical and occupational approaches. In Jeffrey D: *Clinical evaluation and management of spasticity*, Humana Press, 2002, Totowa, NJ.

55. Preston L, Hecht J: *Spasticity management, rehabilitation strategies*, The American Occupational Therapy Association, Inc, 1999, Bethesda, MD.

56. Ramirez S, Chesher S, Scheker L: Evaluation of combined neuromuscular electrical stimulation and dynamic orthotic management of children with hemiplegic spastic cerebral palsy. In *American Academy of Cerebral Palsy Developmental Medicine*, 1999.

57. Reid D: A survey of Canadian occupational therapists' use of hand splints for children with neuromuscular dysfunction, *Canadian J Occup Ther* 59(1):16-27, 1992.

58. Rood M: Neurophysiological reactions as a basis for physical therapy, *Phys Ther Rev* 34(9):444-9, 1954.

59. Rose V, Shah R: A comparative study on the immediate effects of hand orthoses on reducation of hypertonus, *Austr Occup Ther J* 34(2):59-64, 1987.

60. Scheker L, Chesher S, Ramirez S: Neuromuscular electrical stimulation and dynamic bracing as a treatment for upper-extremity spasticity in children with cerebral palsy, *J Hand Surg [Br]* 24(2):226-32, 1999.

61. Scherling E, Johnson H: A tone-reducing wrist-hand orthosis, *Am J Occup Ther* 43(9):609-11, 1989.

62. Shah S: Hand orthosis for upper motor neuron paralysis, *Austr Occup Ther J* 29(3):97-101, 1982.

63. Smelt H: Effect of an inhibitive weight-bearing mitt on tone reduction and functional performance in a child with cerebral palsy, *Phys Occup Ther Pediatr* 9(2):5380, 1989.

64. Snook J: Spasticity reduction splint, *Am J Occup Ther* 33(10):648-51, 1979.

65. Stockmeyer S: An interpretation of the approach of Rood to the treatment of neuromuscular dysfunction, *Am J Phys Med* 46(1):900-61, 1967.

66. Switzer S: The Switzer splint, *Br J Occup Ther* 43:63-4, 1980.

67. Taub E, et al: Technique to improve chronic motor deficit after stroke, *Arch Phys Med Rehab* 74:347-54, 1993.

68. Twist D: Effects of a wrapping technique of passive range of motion in a spastic upper extremity, *Phys Ther* 65(3):299-304, 1985.

69. Wallen M, O'Flaherty S: The use of the Soft Splint in the management of spasticity of the upper limb, *Austr Occup Ther J* 38(1):227-231, 1991.

70. Wallen M, Mackay S: An evaluation of the Soft Splint in the acute management of elbow hypertonicity, *Occup Ther J Res* 15(1):3-16, 1995.

71. Whelan J: Effects of orthokinetics on upper extremity function of the adult hemiplegic patient, *Am J Occup Ther* 18(4):141-3, 1964.

72. Wilson D, Caldwell C: Central control insufficiency: III. Disturbed motor control and sensation: a treatment approach emphasizing upper extremity orthoses, *Phys Ther* 58(3):313-20, 1978.

73. Wilton J: *Hand splinting: principles of design and fabrication*, WB Saunders, 1997, Philadelphia.

74. Wolcott L: Orthotic management of the spastic hand, *South Med J* 59(8):971-4, 1966.

75. Woodson A: Proposal for splinting the adult hemiplegic hand to promote function. In Cromwell F, Bear-Lehman J: *Hand Rehabilitation In Occupational Therapy*, Haworth Press Inc., 1987, New York.

76. Zislis J: Splinting of hand in a spastic hemiplegic patient, *Arch Phys Med Rehab*, pp. 41-3, 1964.

SUGGESTED READING

Milazzo S, Gillen G: Splinting applications. In Gillen G, Burkhardt A: *Stroke rehabilitation, a function-based approach*, Mosby, 1998, St. Louis.

RESOURCE

A website of interest for healthcare professionals and patients is WEMOVE: Worldwide Education and Awareness for Movement Disorders at www.wemove.org.

PART SIX

Application

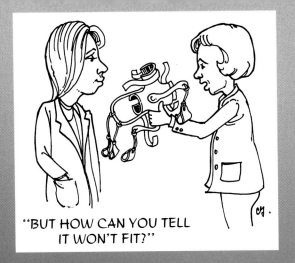

"BUT HOW CAN YOU TELL IT WON'T FIT?"

CHAPTER 20

Analysis of Splints

Chapter Outline

Generally speaking, most of the mistakes made in hand splinting are caused by inattention to detail. The splints chosen are correct according to the circumstances presented. However, they fail to be effective because of relatively minor design or adjustment flaws that cause discomfort, mechanical inefficiency, or poor appearance. Each splint fitted on a patient must be thoroughly evaluated according to the principles of mechanics, outriggers and mobilization assists, design, construction and fit. Immobilization, mobilization, restriction, and torque transmission splints have differing kinesiologic and kinematic effects, and these also must be correlated to patients' specific requirements. Failure to do so may not only produce poor results but also may compound or cause additional deformity.

The purpose of this chapter is to provide the reader with an opportunity to apply the theoretical material presented in the previous chapters and to allow for immediate independent assessment through self-evaluation techniques. Although there is no substitute for actual practical learning experience, it is hoped that this chapter will initiate, facilitate, and strengthen sound analytical thinking in regard to splint design and fabrication.

On the following pages illustrations of improperly constructed splints are presented and analyzed according to the expanded ASHT Splint Classification System purpose of application, clinical problems, solutions to the problems, and design options. The splints, although generally constructed correctly, incorporate one or more common mistakes that clinically produce diminished results. The reader is asked to assess these illustrations using the information in the preceding chapters of this book as a theoretical framework. Application of the ESCS facilitates analysis of the splints. Comparison of one's results with those presented here will provide a standard for self-evaluation.

While most of the mistakes illustrated in this chapter relate to fit problems, a few figures depict inherent splint design errors. It is important to understand that a flawed design may be reflected by an accompanying illogical ESCS designation. In other words, faulty designs frequently beget faulty ESCS terminology. Look carefully at the ESCS type and total number of joints for illustrations A, B, C, and D within each figure. Generally speaking, if the errors involve fit problems, the ESCS type and total number of joints remain reasonably consistent for all the splints included in the figure although the splint configurations themselves may differ considerably. In contrast, design problems often produce widely discrepant ESCS type and total joint descriptors between the incorrect illustrations, the corrected drawing, and the various design options for each figure.

So that the reader may more easily adapt this chapter to a personal level of expertise, the format of splint illustrations and their accompanying assessments is presented consistently. Selected sections may be blocked out to reduce the amount of background information given about each splint illustrated, making analysis more difficult or less difficult. For example, the novice may choose not to block any of the sections, allowing open comparison of the classification, problems, and solutions of each example, whereas someone with intermediate experience may identify the blocked-out problems and solutions knowing only the classification of the splints. Finally, the blocking of all sections and the "incorrect/correct" drawings requires the reader to independently identify the classification, problems, and solutions of each splint picture. Use of a splint checkout form may be helpful in providing an organizational basis for splint analysis. For immediate feedback, we recommend that readers compare their conclusions with those accompanying each illustration before proceeding to the next splint picture. Blue indicates areas of changes in the correct drawings.

This chapter consists of eighteen splint analysis units, which are presented in distal to proximal order, according to the Sequenced Splint Ranking Index. Each splint analysis unit is presented in a consistent order: ESCS Classification, incorrect splint photograph, drawing of the incorrect splint,* clinical problems, corrected drawing, and Clinical Solutions. Lastly, various design options with the ESCS Classification are provided for alternatives to the clinical solution. The ESCS name provided for splints A and B in each analysis unit defines the correct, original intent of the splint, as opposed to the ESCS name that would be associated with the illustrated splint as it was made incorrectly.

■ FINGER MP SPLINTS

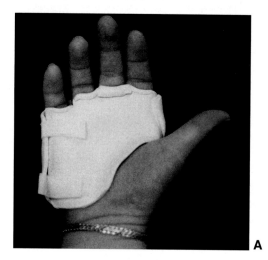

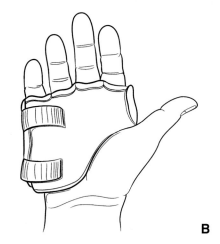

Fig. 20-1   A,B, Index–small finger MP extension immobilization splint, type 0 (4)

---

*Drawings by Craig Gosling and Christopher M. Brown, Medical Illustrators, Indianapolis, Ind.

Clinical Problem

1. Inhibits PIP joint flexion.

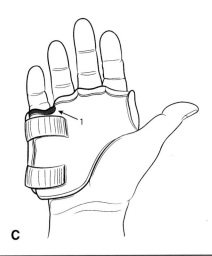

Fig. 20-1   C, Index–small finger MP extension immobilization splint, type 0 (4)

Clinical Solutions

1. Adjust distal end of the palmar phalangeal bar to allow small finger PIP joint to flex without impingement.
2. For total MP joint immobilization, splint requires dorsal metacarpal and dorsal phalangeal bars in addition to the palmar phalangeal bar.

Design Options

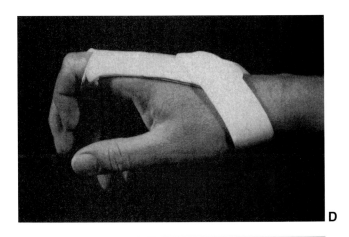

Fig. 20-1   D, Index finger MP extension immobilization splint, type 0 (1)

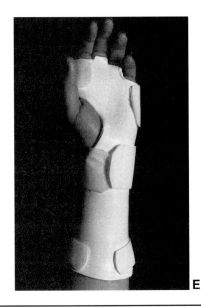

Fig. 20-1   E, Index–small finger MP extension immobilization splint, type 1 (5)

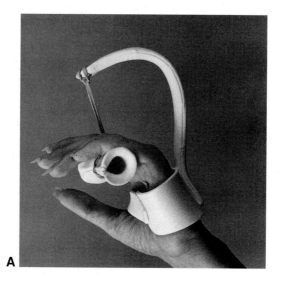

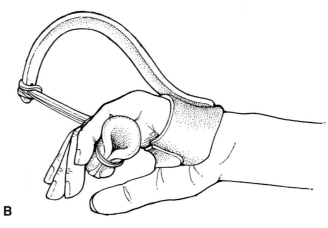

Fig. 20-2   A,B, Index–small finger MP extension mobilization splint, type 0 (4)

Clinical Problems

1. Distal aspect of the dorsal metacarpal bar is causing pressure on the dorsum of the hand.
2. Flexion of ring and small PIP joints is limited by the palmar phalangeal bar.
3. Transverse arch is not supported at the phalangeal level.
4. Second to fifth MP joints are mobilized in unison.
5. The acute angle of force application of the elastic traction to proximal phalanges causes the palmar phalangeal bar to slip distally.
6. Radial aspect of the palmar metacarpal bar is too wide, impinging thumb motion.

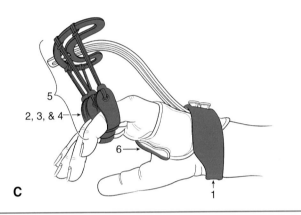

Fig. 20-2   C, Index–small finger MP extension mobilization splint, type 0 (4)

Clinical Solutions

1. Add a wrist strap to the proximal aspect of the dorsal metacarpal bar with clearance for the thumb CMC joint or include the wrist in the splint for increased purchase.
2-4. Add individual MP joint extension finger cuffs.
5. Design and adjust the extension outrigger to provide a 90° angle of approach of the elastic traction to the proximal phalanges that also provides a perpendicular force to the flexion/extension axis of motion of each MP joint.
6. Trim radial aspect of palmar metacarpal bar to allow unimpeded thumb motion.

Design Options

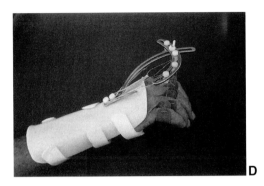

Fig. 20-2   D, Index–small finger MP extension mobilization splint, type 1 (5)
(Courtesy Helen Marx, OTR, CHT, Human Factors Engineering of Phoenix, Wickenburg, Ariz.)

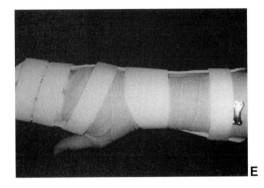

Fig. 20-2   E, Long–small finger MP extension mobilization splint, type 3 (10)

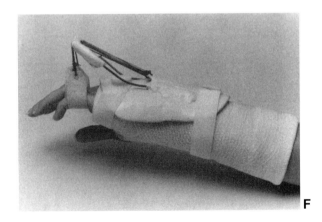

Fig. 20-2   F, Index–small finger MP extension mobilization splint, type 1 (5)
(Courtesy Barbara (Allen) Smith, OTR, Oklahoma City, Okla.)

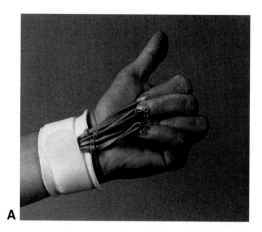

A

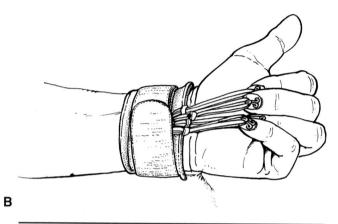

B

Fig. 20-3   A,B, Index–small finger MP flexion mobilization
splint, type 2 (12)

Clinical Problems

1. In each individual finger, the least stiff joint (MP, PIP, or DIP) alters the mobilization force, causing less force to be applied to the stiffer joints within the articulated finger chain.
2. The single finger convergence hole causes fingers to "bunch" when flexed simultaneously.
3. If extrinsic tendons are involved, wrist flexion or extension will decrease or increase rubber band tension, respectively. Patient's habitual posturing in wrist flexion limits splint's effectiveness.

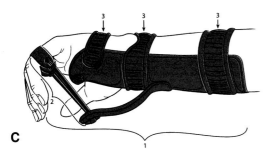

Fig. 20-3   C, Index–small finger MP flexion mobilization splint, type 1 (5)

Clinical Solutions

1. For maximum effectiveness, use a volarly designed splint with separate MP joint finger cuffs with a 90° angle of approach.
2. Add a high-profile outrigger with individual finger cuffs for a 90° angle of approach of the elastic traction to the proximal phalanges to prevent bunching of the fingers when mobilization assists are attached to a single point on the outrigger.
3. Strap placement applies three-point pressure for optimal immobilization of wrist.

Design Options

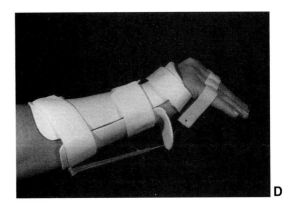

Fig. 20-3   D, Index–small finger MP flexion mobilization splint, type 1 (5)
(Courtesy Rachel Dyrud Ferguson, OTR, CHT, Taos, N.M.)

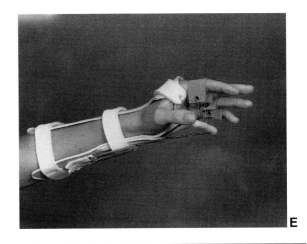

Fig. 20-3   E, Index–small finger MP flexion mobilization splint, type 1 (5)
(Courtesy Barbara [Allen] Smith, OTR, Edmond, Okla.)

■ FINGER MP, PIP SPLINTS

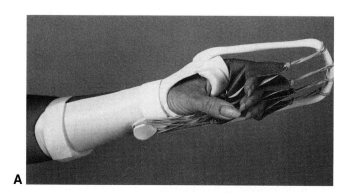

A

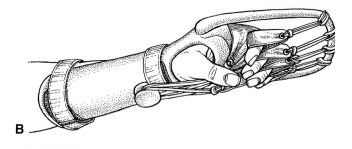

B

Fig. 20-4   A,B, Index–small finger MP flexion, PIP extension mobilization splint, type 1 (9)

Clinical Problems

1. Antagonistic elastic traction on consecutive longitudinal joints results in application of diminished flexion and extension forces.
2. Distal end of the splint inhibits flexion of the MP joints.
3. Acute angle of force application of elastic flexion traction to the proximal phalanges results in MP joint compression.
4. Angle of elastic extension traction to the middle phalanges results in diminished rotational force and may cause MP joint hyperextension.
5. Finger cuffs inhibit IP joint flexion.
6. Ends of the straps have sharp corners.

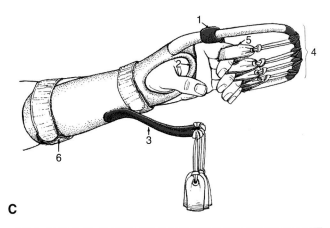

C

Fig. 20-4   C, Index–small finger PIP extension mobilization splint, type 2 (9) or Index–small finger MP flexion mobilization splint, type 1 (5)

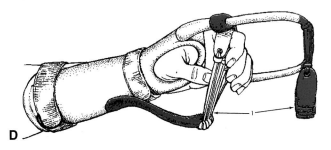

D

Fig. 20-4   D, Index–small finger MP flexion mobilization splint, type 1 (5) or Index–small finger PIP extension mobilization splint, type 2 (9)

Clinical Solutions

1. If the MP joints exhibit full flexion, add an immobile dorsal phalangeal bar to stabilize the proximal phalanges and prevent MP joint hyperextension. If the MP joints lack flexion, separate wearing times for MP flexion and PIP extension, and add a dorsal phalangeal bar to prevent MP hyperextension while in the extension cuffs.

2. Adjust the distal end of the splint proximal to the distal palmar flexion crease.
3. Add a volar outrigger to provide a 90° angle of force application of the elastic traction to the proximal phalanges for MP flexion.
4. Adjust the dorsal outrigger to provide a 90° angle of force application of the elastic traction to the middle phalanges for PIP extension.
5. Contour the extension finger cuffs.
6. Round the ends of the straps.

Design Options

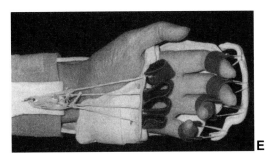

E

Fig. 20-4   E, Index–small finger PIP extension mobilization splint, type 2 (9) or Index–small finger MP flexion mobilization splint, type 1 (5)
(Courtesy Diana Williams, MBA, OTR, CHT, Macon, Ga.)

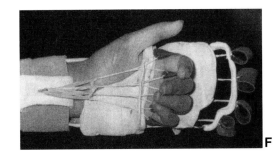

F

Fig. 20-4   F, Index–small finger MP flexion mobilization splint, type 1 (5) or Index–small finger PIP extension mobilization splint, type 2 (9)
(Courtesy Diana Williams, MBA, OTR, CHT, Macon, Ga.)

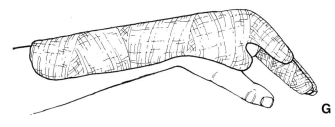

G

Fig. 20-4   G, Index–small finger MP flexion mobilization splint, type 1 (5) \\ Finger MP flexion torque transmission finger PIP extension mobilization splint, type 1 (2); 4 splints @ finger separate
(Courtesy Judith Bell-Krotoski, OTR, FAOTA, CHT, Baton Rouge, La.)

■ FINGER MP, PIP, DIP SPLINTS

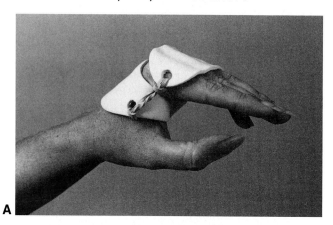

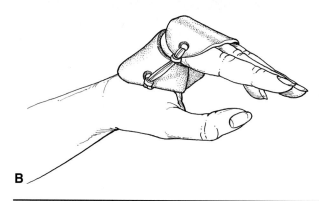

Fig. 20-5 A,B, Index–small finger MP extension restriction / IP extension torque transmission splint, type 0 (12)

Clinical Problems

1. Pressure exists in the thumb web space from the palmar metacarpal bar.
2. Dorsal phalangeal bar migrates proximally.
3. Metacarpal bars migrate distally.
4. Acute angle of force application of elastic traction to the proximal phalanges results in diminished rotational force on the MP joints.

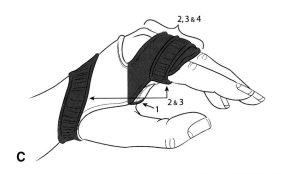

Fig. 20-5   C, Index–small finger MP extension restriction / IP extension torque transmission splint, type 0 (12)

Clinical Solutions

1. Flange proximal aspect of the palmar metacarpal bar edge.
2-3. Add proximal phalangeal strap and wrist strap.
2-4. Redesign splint to provide a 60°-70° angle of restriction to proximal phalanges, which is also perpendicular to the axis of sagittal rotation. Eliminate elastic traction.

Design Options

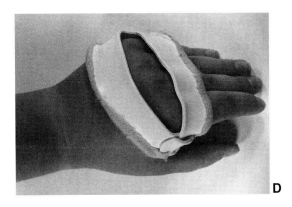

Fig. 20-5   D, Index–small finger MP extension restriction / IP extension torque transmission splint, type 0 (12) (Courtesy Ruth Coopee, MOT, OTR, CHT, Athol, Mass.)

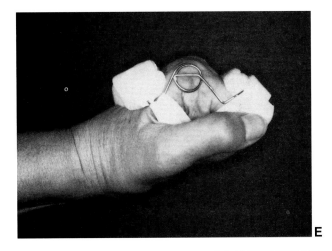

Fig. 20-5   E, Index–small finger MP extension restriction / IP extension torque transmission splint, type 0 (12)

■ FINGER PIP SPLINTS

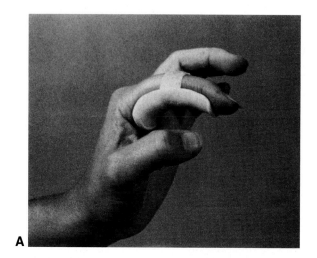

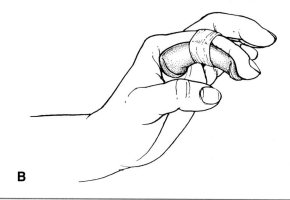

Fig. 20-6   A,B, Index finger PIP flexion immobilization splint, type 0 (1)

Clinical Problems

1. Distal end of the splint limits DIP joint flexion.
2. Splint is unstable on the finger.

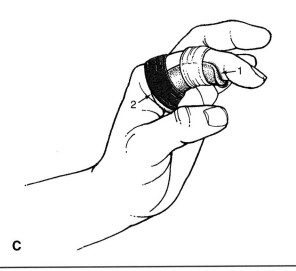

C

Fig. 20-6   C, Index finger PIP flexion immobilization splint, type 0 (1)

Clinical Solutions

1. Shorten the distal splint edge to end proximal to the DIP joint flexion crease.
2. Add proximal strap.

Design Options

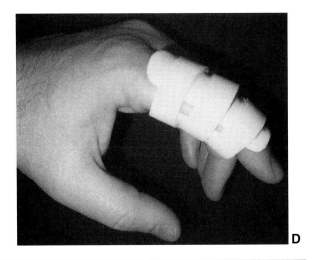

D

Fig. 20-6   D, Index finger PIP flexion immobilization splint, type 0 (1)

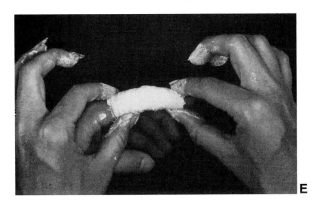

E

Fig. 20-6   E, Index finger PIP flexion immobilization splint, type 1 (2)

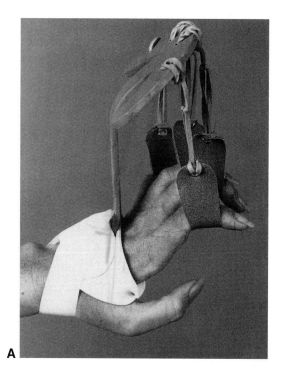

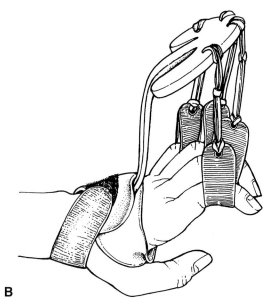

Fig. 20-7   A,B, Index–small finger PIP extension mobilization
splint, type 0 (8)

Clinical Problems

1. The more mobile finger MP joints are hyperextended.
2. Angle of elastic traction to the proximal phalanges enhances MP joint hyperextension.
3. Finger cuffs prevent full IP joint flexion.
4. Uncovered Velcro hook fastener is abrasive to clothing.

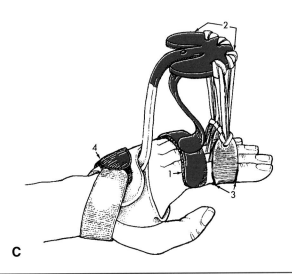

C

Fig. 20-7   C, Index–small finger PIP extension mobilization splint, type 1 (8)

Clinical Solutions

1. Add a dorsal phalangeal bar to prevent MP joint hyperextension.
2. Adjust outrigger to provide a 90° angle of the elastic traction to middle phalanges.
3. Trim the proximal and distal edges of the finger cuffs to allow for IP joint flexion.
4. Lengthen the wrist strap to completely cover hook Velcro
5. Wrist may need to be immobilized in some instances.

Design Options

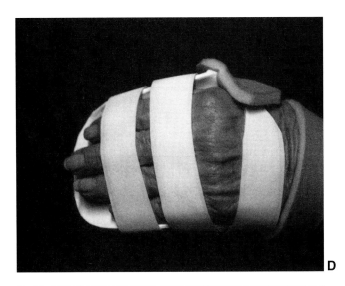

D

Fig. 20-7   D, Index–small finger PIP extension mobilization splint, type 2 (12)

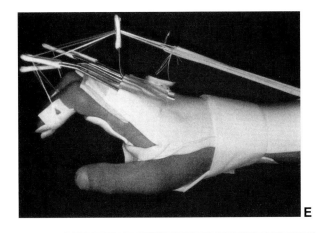

E

Fig. 20-7   E, Index–small finger PIP extension mobilization splint, type 3 (13) \\ Finger PIP extension torque transmission splint, type 1 (2); 4 splints @ finger separate
(Jill Francisco, OTR, CHT, Cicero, Ind.)

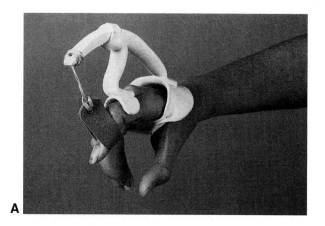

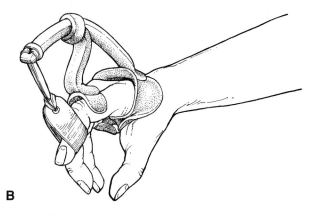

Fig. 20-8   A,B, Index finger PIP extension mobilization splint, type 1 (2)

Clinical Problems

1. Dorsal and palmar metacarpal bars are loose and allow splint to rotate.
2. Proximal edge of the dorsal phalangeal bar creates pressure on the dorsum of the proximal phalanx.
3. Dorsal phalangeal bar does not prevent subluxation of the MP joint.
4. Angle of the elastic traction to the middle phalanx diminishes the magnitude of the rotational force and compresses the PIP joint surfaces.
5. Finger cuff inhibits DIP joint flexion.

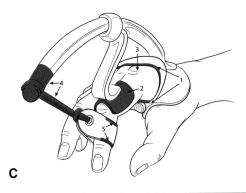

C

Fig. 20-8   C, Index finger PIP extension mobilization splint, type 1 (2)

Clinical Solutions

1. Adjust the dorsal and palmar metacarpal bars to provide continuous circumferential contact.
2. Adjust the dorsal phalangeal bar to provide equal pressure on the dorsum of the phalanx. To further disseminate pressure, add foam padding to the palmar aspect of the dorsal phalangeal bar.
3. Increase MP joint flexion of the dorsal phalangeal bar to prevent subluxation of the MP joint. If MP subluxation occurs, add a volar component to the dorsal phalangeal bar for added stability in positioning the MP joint.
4. Adjust the outrigger to provide a 90° angle of force application of the elastic traction to the middle phalanx. This traction should also be perpendicular to the axis of the joint rotation.
5. Trim the proximal and distal edges of the finger cuff.

Design Options

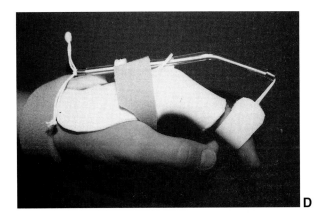

D

Fig. 20-8   D, Index finger PIP extension mobilization splint, type 1 (2)
(Courtesy Paul van Lede, OT, MS, Orfit Industries, Wijnegem, Belgium.)

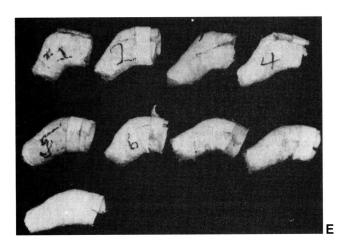

E

Fig. 20-8   E, Index finger PIP extension mobilization splint, type 1 (2)

▤ FINGER PIP, DIP SPLINTS

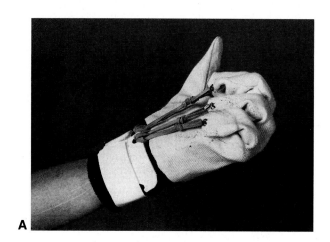

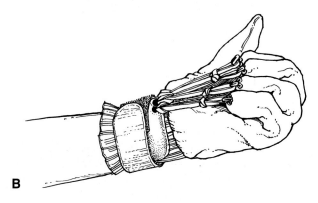

Fig. 20-9   A,B, Index–small finger IP flexion mobilization splint, type 1 (12)

Clinical Problems

1. Traction does not adequately affect the stiffer IP joints.
2. Glove decreases sensory feedback, is bulky, hot, and retains moisture and dirt.

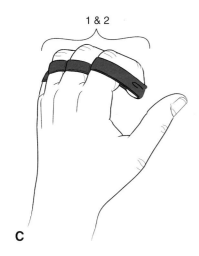

Fig. 20-9   C, Finger IP flexion mobilization splint, type 0 (2); 4 splints @ finger separate

Clinical Solutions

1. Change design to apply elastic traction for PIP and DIP joint flexion.
2. Use of a non-glove design allows sensory feedback and ventilation.

Design Options

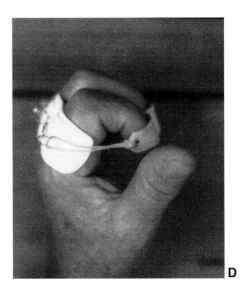

Fig. 20-9   D, Index–small finger IP flexion mobilization splint, type 0 (8)
(Courtesy Kathryn Schultz, OTR, CHT, Orlando, Fla.)

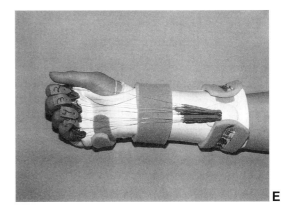

Fig. 20-9   E, Index–small finger IP flexion mobilization splint, type 2 (13)
(Courtesy Joni Armstrong, OTR, CHT, Bemidji, Minn.)

◼ THUMB CMC SPLINTS

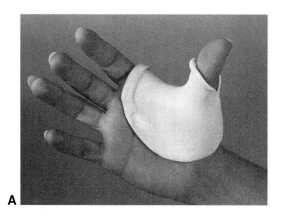

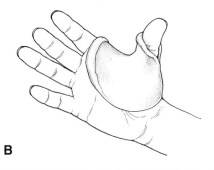

Fig. 20-10 A,B, Thumb CMC palmar abduction mobilization splint, type 2 (3)

Clinical Problems

1. Distal end of the splint inhibits flexion of the index and long finger MP joints.
2. Distal end of the thumb post limits thumb IP joint flexion.
3. Distal migration of the splint results in application of the rotational force to the proximal phalanx of the thumb with potential stretching of the MP joint ulnar collateral ligament.
4. Pressure at wrist.
5. Pressure in palm.
6. Lack of proper thumb positioning. Splint was intended to position thumb CMC joint in palmar abduction.

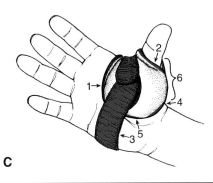

C

Fig. 20-10   C, Thumb CMC palmar abduction mobilization splint, type 1 (2)

Clinical Solutions

1. Adjust the distal edge of the splint to end proximal to the distal palmar flexion crease.
2. Adjust the distal edge of the thumb post to end proximal to the flexion crease of the thumb IP joint.
3. Add a strap for stabilization of the splint in the web space. May need wrist strap for additional stabilization.
4. Roll back the proximal edge of the splint to prevent pressure at the wrist.
5. Trim ulnar border.
6. Serially adjust splint into palmar abduction.

Design Options

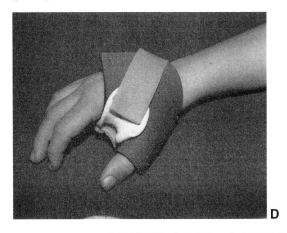

D

Fig. 20-10   D, Thumb CMC palmar abduction mobilization splint, type 1 (2); \\ Thumb CMC palmar abduction mobilization splint, type 0 (1)
(Courtesy Joni Armstrong, OTR, CHT, Bemidji, Minn.)

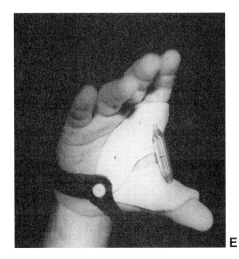

E

Fig. 20-10   E, Thumb CMC palmar abduction mobilization splint, type 3 (4)
(Courtesy Daniel Lupo, OTR, CHT, Ventura, Calif.)

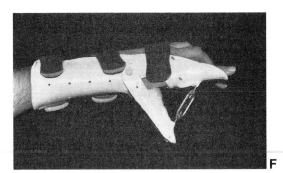

F

Fig. 20-10   F, Thumb CMC palmar abduction mobilization splint, type 6 (7)
(Courtesy Daniel Lupo, OTR, CHT, Ventura, Calif.)

THUMB IP SPLINTS

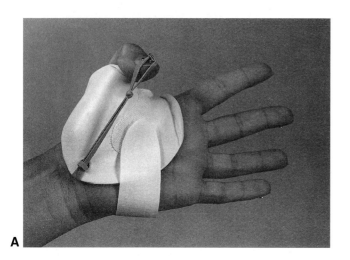

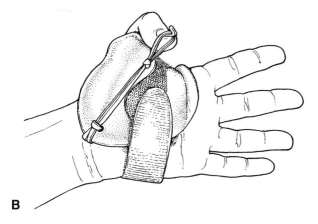

Fig. 20-11   A,B, Thumb IP flexion mobilization splint, type 2 (3)

Clinical Problems

1. Because the angle of the mobilization traction is not perpendicular to the axis of rotation of the IP joint, unequal stress is applied to the collateral ligaments and may result in ulnar collateral ligament attenuation.
2. Distal end of the splint inhibits index and long finger MP joint flexion.
3. MP joint is not adequately immobilized to stabilize the thumb for distally applied traction.

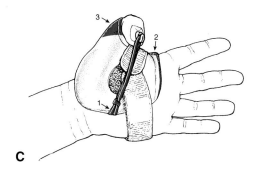

Fig. 20-11   C, Thumb IP flexion mobilization splint, type 2 (3)

Clinical Solutions

1. Adjust the elastic traction to provide a perpendicular angle of force application to the IP joint axis of rotation.
2. Roll the distal edge of the splint proximally. It should not extend beyond the distal palmar flexion crease.
3. Continue splint material to cover dorsal aspect of thumb for greater stability.

Design Options

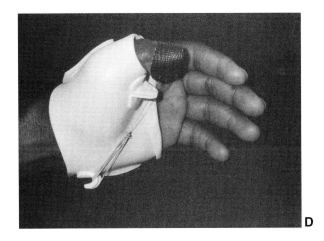

Fig. 20-11   D, Thumb IP flexion mobilization splint, type 2 (3) (Courtesy Peggy McLaughlin, OTR, CHT, San Bernardino, Calif.)

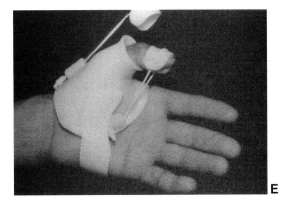

Fig. 20-11   E, Thumb IP flexion or extension mobilization splint, type 2 (3) (Courtesy Kathryn Schultz, OTR, CHT, Orlando, Fla.)

■ FINGER MP, PIP, DIP, THUMB CMC, MP SPLINTS

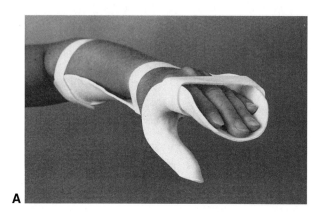

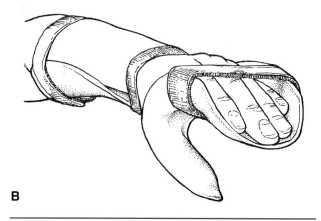

Fig. 20-12   A,B, Index–small finger flexion, thumb CMC palmar abduction immobilization splint, type 3 (16)

Clinical Problems

1. Proximal end of the splint limits elbow joint flexion and causes edge pressure.
2. Transverse arch is not supported at the phalangeal level.
3. High deviation bars of the finger pan prevent finger positioning by the finger straps.
4. Distal end of the thumb post is too long.
5. Straps do not adequately secure the hand and wrist.
6. Distal end of splint does not protect the hand from further injury.

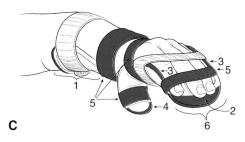

C

Fig. 20-12   C, Index–small finger flexion, thumb CMC palmar abduction immobilization splint, type 3 (16)

Clinical Solutions

1. Shorten the forearm trough to two-thirds the length of the anterior forearm and flange the proximal end of the splint.
2. Continue the transverse arch the length of the finger pan.
3. Decrease the height of the lateral and medial borders of the finger pan to provide continuous contact of the strap across the dorsal aspect of the fingers.
4. Decrease the distal length of the thumb post.
5. Add straps to the dorsal MP and IP joints of the digits, and the IP joint of the thumb. Widen the wrist strap.
6. Lengthen the distal end of the splint to protect the digits from injury.

Design Options

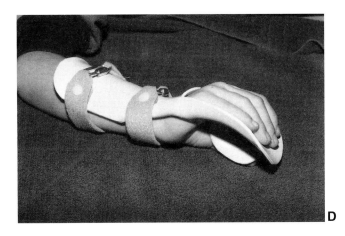

D

Fig. 20-12   D, Index–small finger flexion, thumb CMC palmar abduction immobilization splint, type 3 (16)
(Courtesy Joni Armstrong, OTR, CHT, Bemidji, Minn.)

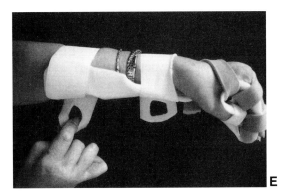

E

Fig. 20-12   E, Index–small finger flexion, thumb CMC palmar abduction immobilization splint, type 3 (16)

FINGER PIP, THUMB CMC, MP SPLINTS

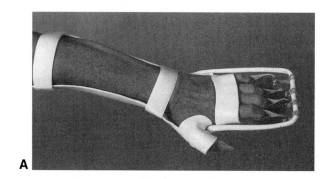

A

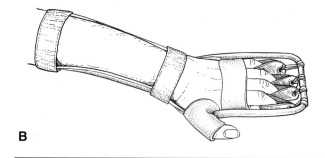

B

Fig. 20-13   A,B, Index–small finger PIP extension, thumb CMC radial abduction and MP extension mobilization splint, type 3 (15)

Clinical Problems

1. Ulnar aspect of forearm trough causes pressure on the ulnar border of the forearm.
2. Distal edge of thumb post limits the thumb interphalangeal joint.
3. Finger metacarpophalangeal joints are hyperextended.
4. Angle of force of application of elastic traction to the middle phalanges causes the finger cuffs to migrate distally.
5. Outrigger is too short to allow full rotational effect of the elastic traction.

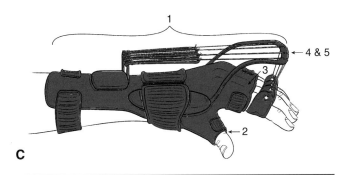

C

Fig. 20-13   C, Index–small finger PIP extension, thumb CMC radial abduction and MP extension mobilization splint, type 2 (11)

Clinical Solutions

1. Change splint design to a contoured dorsal-based splint to decrease pressure.
2. Shorten distal thumb post to allow IP joint flexion.
3. Incorporation of a dorsal phalangeal bar positioning MP joints in flexion prevents MP joint hyperextension.
4-5. Adjust outrigger to achieve 90° angle of force application.

Design Options

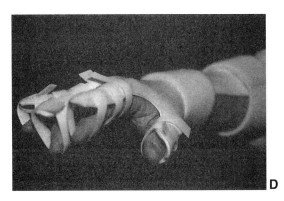

D

Fig. 20-13   D, Index–small finger PIP extension, thumb CMC radial abduction and MP extension mobilization splint, type 4 (16)
(Courtesy Elizabeth Spencer Steffa, OTR/L, CHT, Seattle, Wash.)

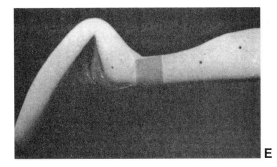

E

Fig. 20-13   E, Index–small finger PIP extension, thumb CMC radial abduction and MP-IP extension mobilization splint, type 3 (16)

■ WRIST SPLINTS

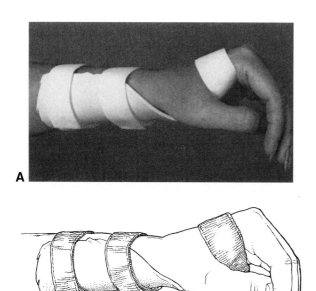

Fig. 20-14   A,B, Wrist extension immobilization splint, type 0 (1)

Clinical Problems

1. Splint length is too short, causing increased pressure on the forearm.
2. Wrist is not fully immobilized.
3. Strap in the thumb web space causes discomfort and the splint impedes MP joint flexion.
4. Appearance of splint is poor.

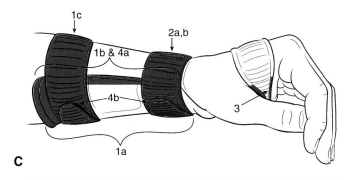

Fig. 20-14   C, Wrist extension immobilization splint, type 0 (1)

Clinical Solutions

1a. Increase the length of the forearm trough to two-thirds the length of the anterior forearm and flange the proximal end.
1b. Decrease the width of the forearm trough to one-half the circumference of the forearm.
1c. Move proximal forearm strap proximally to end of splint.
2a. Move wrist strap distally over wrist joint.
2b. Widen the wrist strap and avoid the ulnar styloid process and thumb CMC joint area.
3. Contour distal palmar edge of strap and splint in the thumb web space.
4a. Cut splint edges smoothly.
4b. Round the strap ends.

Design Options

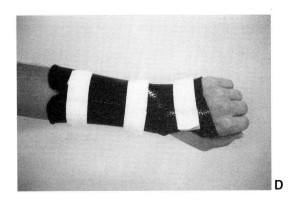

Fig. 20-14   D, Wrist extension immobilization splint, type 0 (1) (Courtesy Paul van Lede, OT, MS, Orfit Industries, Wijnegem, Belgium.)

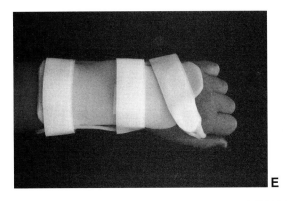

Fig. 20-14   E, Wrist extension immobilization splint, type 0 (1)

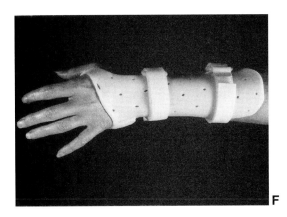

Fig. 20-14   F, Wrist neutral immobilization splint, type 0 (1) (Courtesy Sharon Flinn, MEd, OTR/L, CHT, Cleveland, Ohio.)

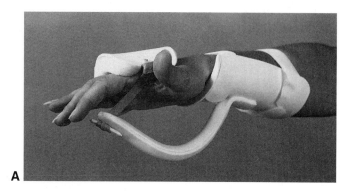

A

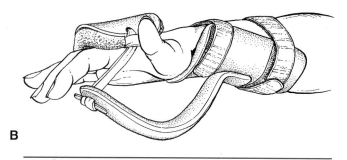

B

Fig. 20-15 A,B, Wrist flexion mobilization splint, type 0 (1)

Clinical Problems

1. Radial aspect of the forearm trough is too wide.
2. Wrist bar impinges wrist flexion.
3. Lateral and medial borders of the dorsal metacarpal cuff may cause pressure areas on the dorsum of the hand.
4a. Dorsal metacarpal cuff migrates distally.
4b. Angle of force of application of the elastic traction to the metacarpals diminishes the magnitude of the rotational force.
5. Pressure exists under the splint's distal and proximal straps.

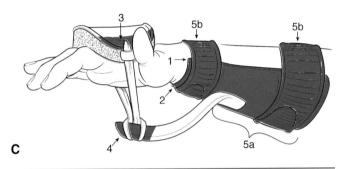

Fig. 20-15   C, Wrist flexion mobilization splint, type 0 (1)

Clinical Solutions

1. Decrease the radial border of the forearm trough to half the width of the forearm.
2. Shorten the distal end of the wrist bar to prevent impingement of the wrist.
3. Widen the dorsal metacarpal cuff.
4. Adjust outrigger to provide a 90° angle of the elastic traction to the metacarpals.
5a. Lengthen the forearm trough and move the strap proximally.
5b. Apply wider straps distally and proximally to decrease pressure and increase comfort.

Design Options

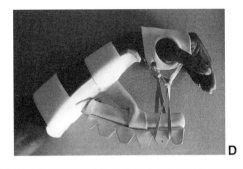

Fig. 20-15   D, Wrist flexion mobilization splint, type 0 (1)

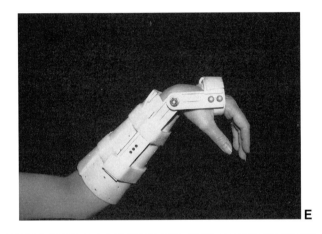

Fig. 20-15   E, Wrist flexion mobilization splint, type 0 (1) (Courtesy Shelli Dellinger, OTR, CHT, San Diego, Calif.)

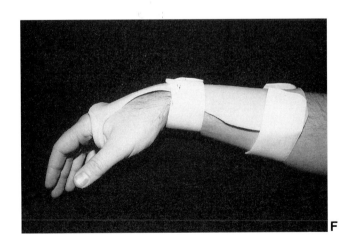

Fig. 20-15   F, Wrist flexion mobilization splint, type 0 (1)

WRIST, THUMB CMC SPLINTS

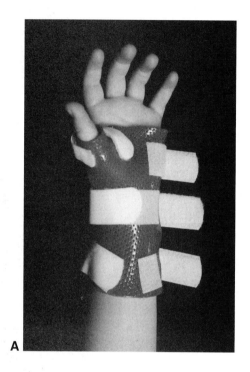

A

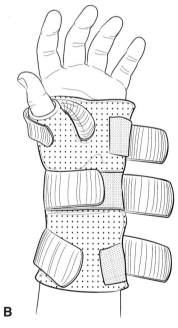

B

Fig. 20-16   A,B, Wrist extension, thumb CMC palmar abduction
immobilization splint, type 1 (3)

Clinical Problems

1a. Forearm trough—has finger indentation marks from therapist grasping too firmly during fabrication, causing uneven pressure.

1b. Thumb CMC joint is not positioned in palmar abduction.

2. Thumb post is too low, doesn't adequately immobilize MP joint.

3. Ulnar aspect of the distal end of the splint impinges finger MP joint flexion.

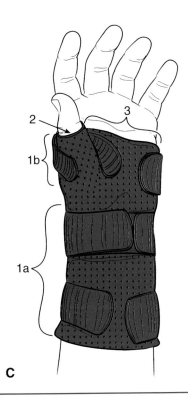

Fig. 20-16   C, Wrist extension, thumb CMC palmar abduction immobilization splint, type 1 (3)

Design Options

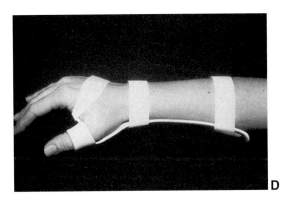

Fig. 20-16   D, Wrist extension, thumb CMC palmar abduction immobilization splint, type 1 (3)

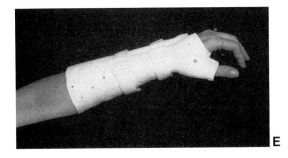

Fig. 20-16   E, Wrist neutral, thumb CMC palmar abduction immobilization splint, type 1 (3)
(Courtesy Shelli Dellinger, OTR, CHT, San Diego, Calif.)

Clinical Solutions

1. Reheat entire splint to:
   a. Achieve contiguous fit along forearm trough and eliminate finger indentations.
   b. Position thumb CMC joint in increased palmar abduction.
2. Lengthen thumb post to properly immobilize thumb MP joint and clear thumb IP joint extension and flexion creases.
3. Trim distal end of splint to allow unimpeded finger MP joint flexion.

■ ELBOW SPLINTS

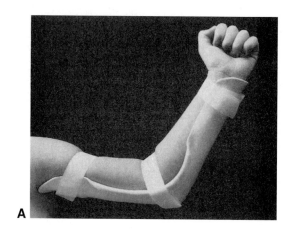

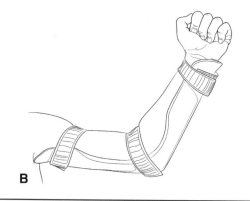

Fig. 20-17   A,B, Elbow flexion immobilization splint, type 0 (1)

Clinical Problems

1. Elbow positioned in less than the intended 90° of flexion.
2. Strapping too narrow to adequately disperse pressure.
3. Forearm trough too high and narrow.
4. Distal end of splint impinges wrist.
5. Proximal end of splint impinges axilla.
6. Pressure exists over the bony prominences of the olecranon and medial and lateral epicondyles.

Design Options

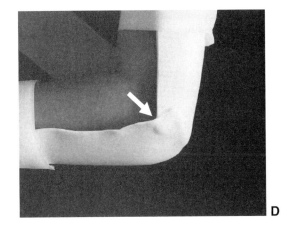

Fig. 20-17   D, Elbow flexion immobilization splint, type 0 (1); with tuck

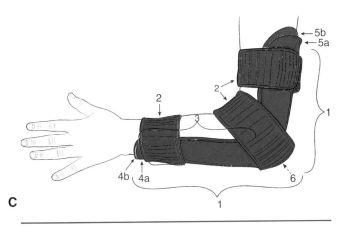

Fig. 20-17   C, Elbow flexion immobilization splint, type 0 (1)

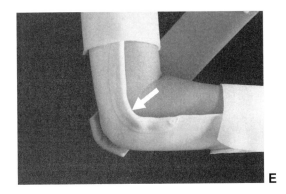

Fig. 20-17   E, Elbow flexion immobilization splint, type 0 (1); with roll

Clinical Solutions

1. Refit to obtain 90° angle of elbow flexion.
2. Increase strap width and add soft strapping at elbow flexion crease for greater comfort.
3. Decrease width of forearm trough to half the circumference of the forearm.
4a. Remove length from distal end of splint to avoid impingement of wrist motion.
4b. Add soft padding to interior splint at the distal end for comfort.
5a. Remove length from proximal end of splint to avoid impingement of shoulder motion.
5b. Add soft padding to interior splint at the proximal end for comfort.
6. Pad elbow to decrease pressure at bony prominences.

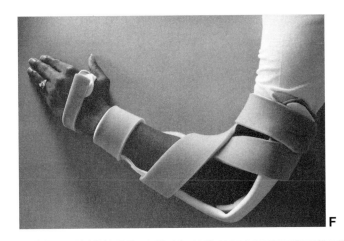

Fig. 20-17   F, Elbow flexion immobilization splint, type 2 (3)

■ EFFECTS OF HEAT ON THERMOPLASTICS

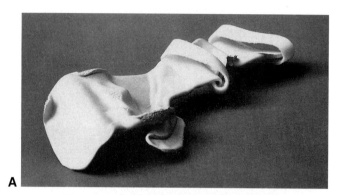

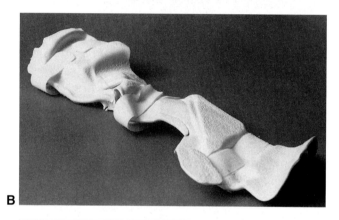

Fig. 20-18   A,B, Index–small finger flexion, thumb CMC palmar abduction immobilization splint, type 3 (16)

Clinical Problem

1. Splint was left in a closed car on a hot day, which resulted in numerous fit problems and over-stretching of thermoplastic material.

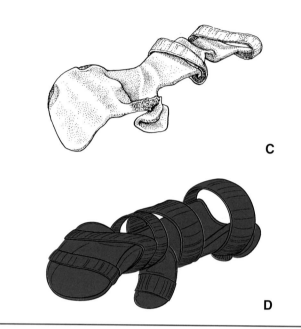

Fig. 20-18   C,D, Index–small finger flexion, thumb CMC palmar abduction immobilization splint, type 3 (16)

Clinical Solution

1. Start over.

PART SEVEN

Technique

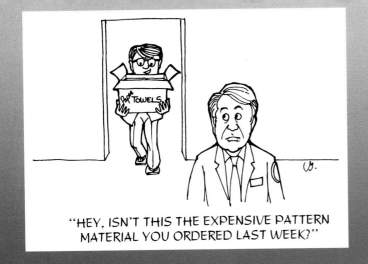

"HEY, ISN'T THIS THE EXPENSIVE PATTERN MATERIAL YOU ORDERED LAST WEEK?"

Patterns

Chapter Outline

The transition from the cognitive design process to the actual construction of tangible splint patterns is facilitated by the progression through the hierarchy of design principles. Once the design process is traversed, construction of a workable pattern is simplified. Pattern assembly and connection of the various splint parts may then be carried out until the ultimate configuration of the splint becomes apparent. This allows alterations of shape and size to be governed by individual specifications of the extremity being splinted before actual fabrication of splint materials commences.

In the pattern stage, simple splints with uncomplicated objectives allow for rather routine application of design principles, whereas in the presence of unusually difficult problems a more innovative approach is required. Nevertheless, a progression through the design principles facilitates a more efficient, organized thought process from which practical variations may be made.

The rigid use of standard, unmodified, commercially available patterns is not recommended because this may result in the preparation of a splint without the appropriate adaptation necessary to accommodate individual anatomic variations. With experience comes the knowledge of where and how to incorporate changes in these dye patterns, and the potential hazards of using commercial patterns are diminished considerably (Fig. 21-1). All patterns, whether individually constructed or adapted from a commercial design, should be fitted and checked on the patient before construction of the splint begins, since a poorly conceived or fitted pattern almost always leads to frustration and failure during the subsequent stages of construction, fit, and use.

SPLINT PATTERN FABRICATION

The fabrication of splint patterns is defined according to the construction methods employed: (1) combining

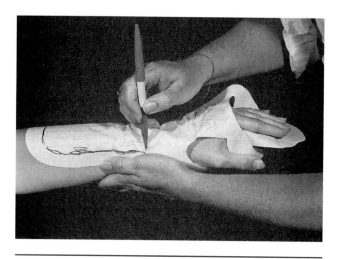

Fig. 21-1   A commercial pattern must be adapted to the variations of the individual hand before it is used.

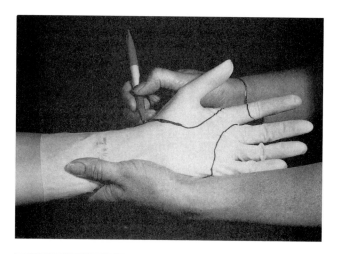

Fig. 21-2   Outline pattern construction is more expedient for uncomplicated designs.

of individual splint parts, (2) outlining of the total splint configuration, or (3) taking of specific measurements to form a general pattern shape.

All patterns, like the splints they represent, consist of individual parts that, when combined, form a whole.[5] For the beginner or for the experienced individual attempting to translate a difficult splint design into pattern form, taping and combining cutout paper splint parts on the patient's extremity may ease pattern construction. An alternative technique of pattern fabrication, the drawing of an outline of a splint, is more efficient when dealing with familiar, uncomplicated splint designs. The uncut pattern material is first applied to the extremity, and the configuration of the proposed splint outlined according to anatomic landmarks and mechanical considerations (Fig. 21-2).[6-9] These two methods of pattern construc-

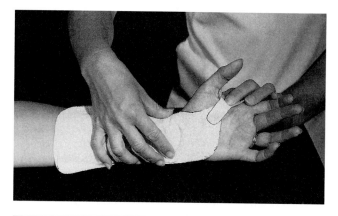

Fig. 21-3   Individual components may be added to a basic outline pattern.

tion may be effectively combined to blend the efficiency of the outline method with the specificity of the parts technique (Fig. 21-3). The third method of pattern construction is appropriate only when a stretchable/drapable splinting material is to be used. This less exacting technique of pattern preparation results in a pattern that bears little resemblance to the finished splint. Length and width measurements are frequently the only requirements for this kind of pattern construction because the splint material is draped, stretched, molded, and trimmed during the fitting phase of fabrication (Fig. 21-4).

Experienced clinicians often save special "generic" splint patterns that are easily adapted to a wide range of hand sizes, evolving over time a practical pattern file that increases splint fabrication efficiency. Use of a photocopier allows splint pattern size to be proportionally increased or decreased depending on the hand size. Tracing precut splints is another option to make generic patterns. If a patient is particularly difficult to fit and replacement splints will be needed in the future, it is helpful to save the original splint pattern in the patient's therapy chart. Unfortunately, this may not be possible in some facilities where only approved items are permitted in patient charts.

■ PATTERN MATERIALS AND EQUIPMENT

Although pattern materials are of seemingly infinite variety, they possess some common properties. They should be readily available, inexpensive, flexible, clean, and allow easy marking, taping, and cutting. Examples are paper towels, x-ray film, cloth, light cardboard, cellophane, plastic wrap, clear plastic bags, and surgical gloves. The choice of pattern material may be influenced by the splint design, pathologic condition of the extremity, material accessibility,

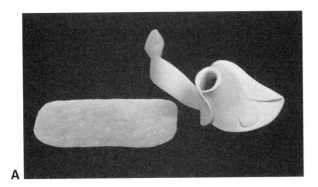

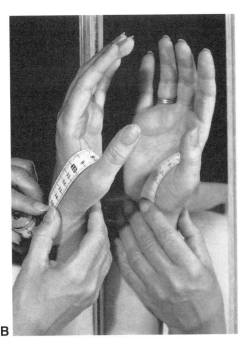

therapist preference or environmental factors. A pattern for a splint requiring contour would be difficult to make from light cardboard because of its mildly rigid properties and, in contrast, a bar configuration splint pattern out of plastic wrap would be flimsy and could allow alteration of the splint form during transfer to the final splint material. Paper towels are available in most medical offices and therapy departments and are flexible enough to allow contouring. Even the wax papers that separate sheets of boxed thermoplastic materials can be used for pattern construction.[10] Cellophane, plastic bags, and plastic wrap provide the unique property of transparency, giving full visibility to underlying anatomic structures, and a surgical glove allows three-dimensional perspective. Paper towels that are provided with sterile surgical gloves also make excellent pattern materials when working in isolation conditions.

Positioning devices[1,2] have been advocated in some circumstances when making a single plane pattern proves to be difficult. These devices allow various segments of the extremity to be placed in the desired position, theoretically making tracings and fitting more accurate. However, the final configurations of patterns made with and without a positioning device are similar enough that the addition of the extraneous piece of equipment is usually unwarranted except for special circumstances where the patient is unable to maintain a needed position even for the short time it takes to make a pattern (Fig. 21-5).[3,4]

If it appears that the amount of hand movement required to construct a pattern will be poorly tolerated by a patient, a pattern may be traced from the

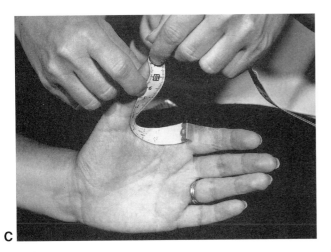

Fig. 21-4   A. Thumb CMC palmar abduction immobilization splint, type 1 (2)
A. As seen in this thumb CMC immobilization pattern design by Kay Carl, OTR, Indianapolis, Ind., measurement patterns often bear little resemblance to the final splint configuration. B. The length between dorsal and volar wrist flexion creases through the first web space is the pattern length. C. The length from the index proximal digital flexion crease to the thumb interphalangeal joint equals the width.

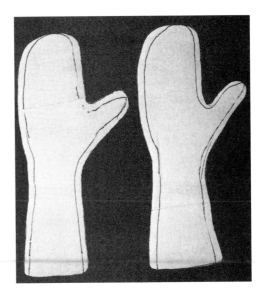

Fig. 21-5   Wrist, finger, and thumb splint pattern made with (A) and without (B) a positioning device.

opposite, unaffected hand, allowing for individual variations such as edema or amputation. This pattern should then be reversed and checked for fit on the injured extremity. If the pathologic condition disallows pattern construction on either extremity as with some burn patients or patients with bilateral injuries, longitudinal and horizontal measurements may be taken (Fig. 21-6), and a hand of similar size located on which a pattern may be made.

SPECIFIC PATTERNS

Although exceptions exist, patterns are generally employed when constructing those major sections of a splint that directly contact the extremity. These constituent elements may function independently or they may form the foundation for attachment of other splint components. With experience, clinicians develop individualized methods of constructing patterns and preferences for certain pattern materials. While no two clinicians may make patterns exactly alike and designs for hand/upper extremity splints are seemingly endless, the process of constructing patterns depends on a thorough knowledge of anatomy, an understanding of the principles of mechanics, using outriggers and mobilization assists, design, construction, and fit, and familiarity with the physical properties of available splinting materials.[11]

Many patterns for hand/upper extremity splints are derived from one of four basic configurations consisting of specialized components which provide transverse or longitudinal positioning: (1) metacarpal shell, (2) metacarpal/wrist/forearm shell (dorsal), (3) metacarpal/wrist/forearm shell (volar), and (4) forearm/elbow/humerus shell. Although inclusion of all the potential variations is impractical, descriptions of these basic patterns and some of their more common adaptations are briefly outlined and illustrated in this chapter. It is important to remember that although these patterns reflect basic configurations, they must be specifically adapted to individual patients before being used in the clinic setting. Rote application without consideration of the variations in

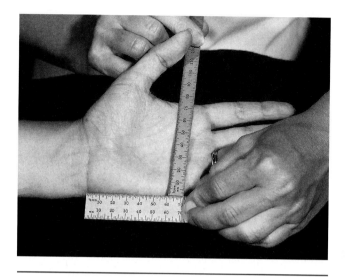

Fig. 21-6   The width of the hand at the metacarpophalangeal flexion crease and the length from the wrist flexion crease to the metacarpophalangeal flexion crease on the ulnar aspect of the palm are the two most important measurements to take when attempting to locate a similar-sized hand for pattern construction.

patient anatomy and pathology would be shortsighted and is definitely contraindicated.

To provide readers with more options, other chapters are referenced when alternate pattern designs are available to those shown in the following sections. Also, many innovative splint patterns for children are included in Chapter 18, Splinting the Pediatric Patient. In the next section of this chapter, commonly used splints are converted into their respective component shells and patterns. Providing visual diversity, anatomic landmarks for each splint illustrated are shown either on the hand/extremity or on the paper pattern. Adaptations to the basic shells and separate component patterns are also illustrated. So that pattern size may be readily adapted, all patterns are photographed on a 4×4 square $= \frac{1}{2}$ inch background. Appendix F presents larger-scale versions of all of the patterns illustrated in this chapter. Shells, splints, anatomic landmarks, patterns, and shell adaptations are presented according to the following order and format:

Metacarpal Shell

PURPOSES (Fig. 21-7, *A,B*)

1. Supports the transverse metacarpal arch via dorsal and palmar metacarpal bars and hypothenar bar.
2. Provides a base of attachment for finger or thumb phalangeal bars and for outrigger components.

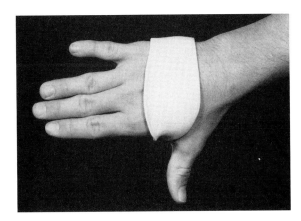

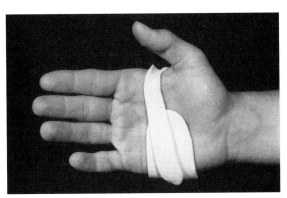

Fig. 21-7A,B

Splint: *Index finger PIP extension mobilization splint, type 1 (2)* (Fig. 21-7, *C*)

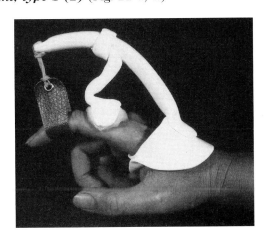

Fig. 21-7C   *Example of completed splint.*

ANATOMIC LANDMARKS

1. Dorsal (Fig. 21-7, *D*)
   a. Index finger PIP joint
   b. Index–small finger MP joints
   c. First web space
   d. Extensor pollicis longus tendon
   e. Distal wrist extension crease
2. Palmar (Fig. 21-7, *E*)
   a. Distal palmar flexion crease
   b. Opponens crease
   c. Distal wrist flexion crease ulnar side

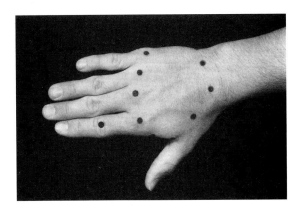

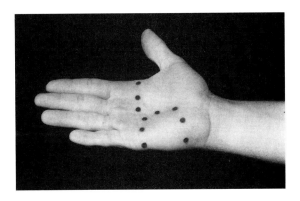

Fig. 21-7D,E

COMPLETED PATTERN (Fig. 21-7, *F*)

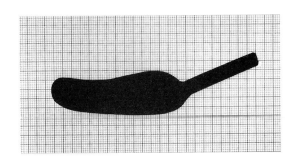

Fig. 21-7F

Metacarpal/Wrist/Forearm Shell (Dorsal)

PURPOSES (Fig. 21-8, *A,B*)

1. Supports the transverse metacarpal arch via dorsal and palmar metacarpal bars.
2. Positions the wrist.
3. Provides a base of attachment for finger or thumb phalangeal bars and for outrigger components.

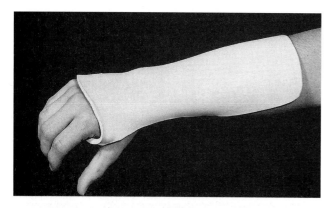

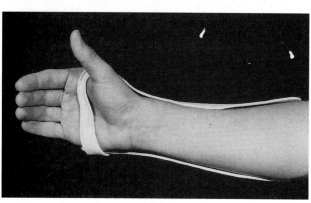

Fig. 21-8A,B

Splint: ***Index–small finger MP extension and radial deviation mobilization splint, type 1 (5)*** (Fig. 21-8, *C*)

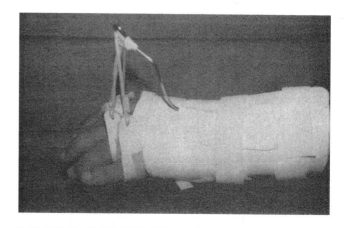

Fig. 21-8C   *Example of completed splint.*

ANATOMIC LANDMARKS

1. Dorsal (Fig. 21-8, *D,E*)
   a. Index–small finger MP joints
   b. First web space
   c. Two-thirds distal length of forearm
2. Palmar (Fig. 21-8, *F*)
   a. First web space
   b. Distal palmar flexion crease
3. Medial and lateral (Fig. 21-8, *D,E*)
   a. Half thickness fifth metacarpal
   b. Half thickness ulnar and radial wrist
   c. Half thickness ulnar and radial forearm

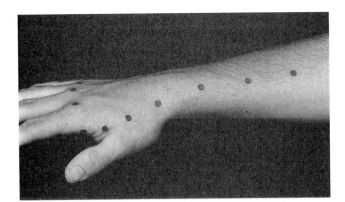

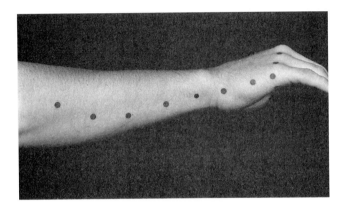

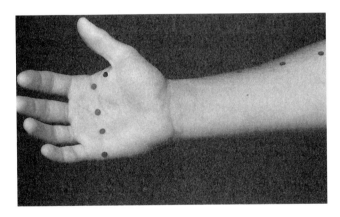

Fig. 21-8D,E,F

COMPLETED PATTERN (Fig. 21-8, G)

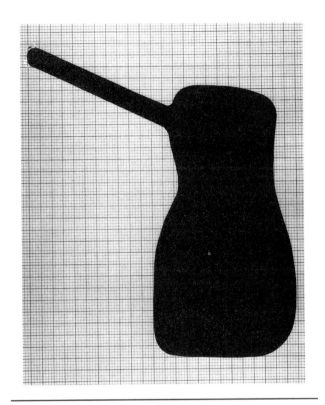

Fig. 21-8G

Metacarpal/Wrist/Forearm Shell (Volar)

PURPOSES (Fig. 21-9, *A*)

1. Supports the transverse metacarpal arch via palmar and dorsal radial metacarpal bars.
2. Positions the wrist.
3. Provides a base of attachment for finger or thumb phalangeal bars and for outrigger components.

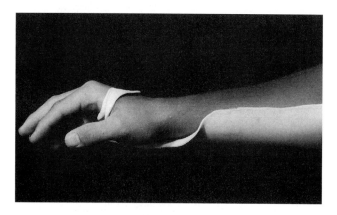

Fig. 21-9A

Splint: ***Ring–small finger MP flexion mobilization splint, type 1 (3)*** (Fig. 21-9, *B*)

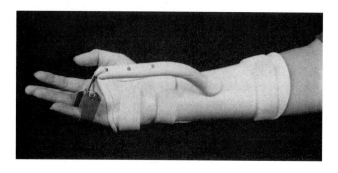

Fig. 21-9B   *Example of completed splint*

ANATOMIC LANDMARKS

1. Dorsal
   a. First web space
   b. Third metacarpal
2. Palmar (Fig. 21-9, *C*)
   a. Distal palmar crease
   b. Opponens crease
   c. First web space
   d. Two-thirds distal length of forearm
3. Medial and lateral (Fig. 21-9, *C,D*)
   a. Half thickness fifth metacarpal
   b. Half thickness ulnar and radial wrist
   c. Half thickness ulnar and radial forearm

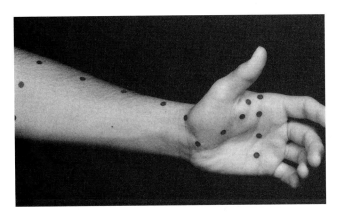

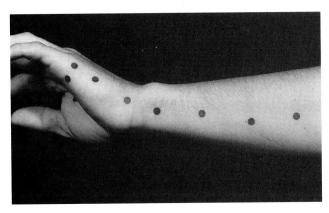

Fig. 21-9C,D

COMPLETED PATTERN (Fig. 21-9, *E*)

Other pattern design options include Figs. 18-7, *B*, 18-8, *B*, and 18-9, *C*.

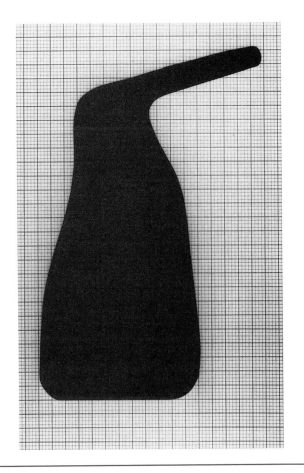

Fig. 21-9E

Forearm/Elbow/Humerus Shell

PURPOSE (Fig. 21-10, *A*)

1. Positions the elbow joint.

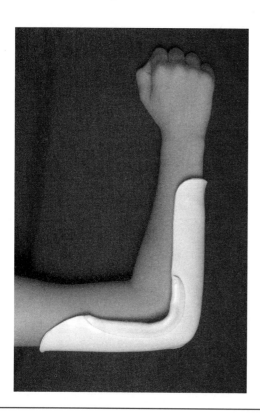

Fig. 21-10A

Splint: ***Elbow flexion immobilization splint, type 1 (2)*** (Fig. 21-10, *B*)

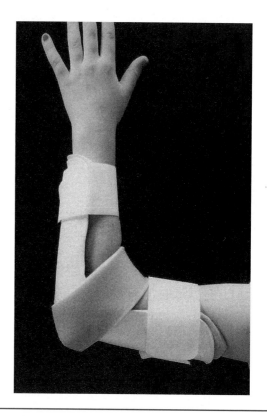

Fig. 21-10B   *Example of completed splint.*

ANATOMIC LANDMARKS

1. Dorsal (Fig. 21-10, *C*)
   a. Two-thirds distal length of forearm
   b. Two-thirds proximal length of upper arm
2. Volar (Fig. 21-10, *D*)
   a. Two-thirds distal length of forearm
   b. Two-thirds proximal length of upper arm
3. Medial and lateral (Fig. 21-10, *C,D*)
   a. Half thickness forearm
   b. Half thickness upper arm

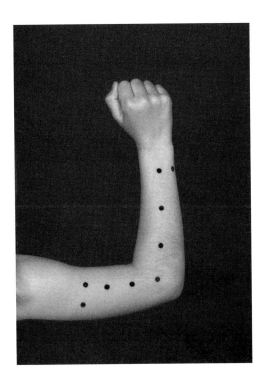

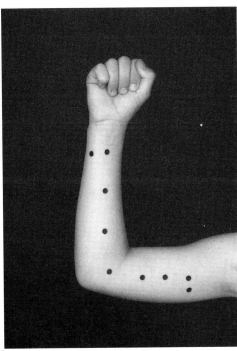

Fig. 21-10C,D

COMPLETED PATTERN (Fig. 21-10, *E*)

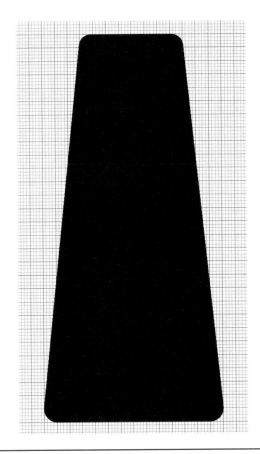

Fig. 21-10E

■ CONTIGUOUS ADAPTATIONS OF BASIC PATTERNS

Proximal Phalangeal/Metacarpal/Wrist/Forearm Shell

PURPOSES (Fig. 21-11, *A*)

1. Positions index–small finger MP joints in predetermined amount of flexion.
2. Supports the transverse metacarpal arch via dorsal and palmar metacarpal bars.
3. Positions the wrist.
4. Provides a base of attachment for thumb phalangeal bar and for outrigger components.

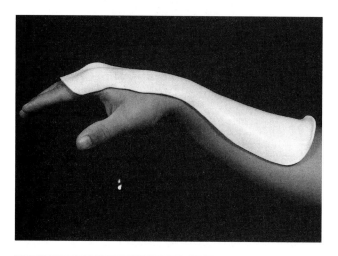

Fig. 21-11A

Splint: *Index finger PIP extension mobilization splint, type 2 (3)* (Fig. 21-11, *B*)

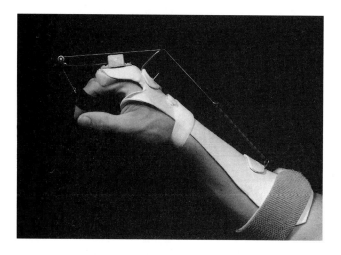

Fig. 21-11B *Example of completed splint.*

ANATOMIC LANDMARKS

1. Dorsal (Fig. 21-11, *C,D*)
   a. Index–small finger PIP joints
   b. First web space
   c. Two-thirds distal length of forearm
2. Palmar (Fig. 21-11, *E*)
   a. First web space
   b. Distal palmar flexion crease
3. Medial and lateral (Fig. 21-11, *C,D*)
   a. Half thickness second and fifth proximal phalanges
   b. Half thickness fifth metacarpal
   c. Half thickness ulnar and radial wrist
   d. Half thickness ulnar and radial forearm

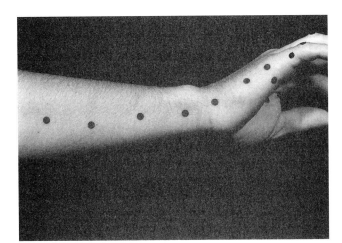

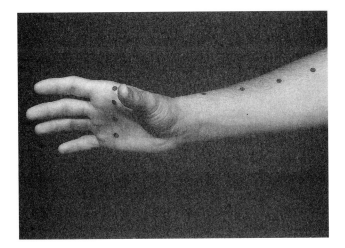

Fig. 21-11C,D,E

COMPLETED PATTERN (Fig. 21-11, *F*)

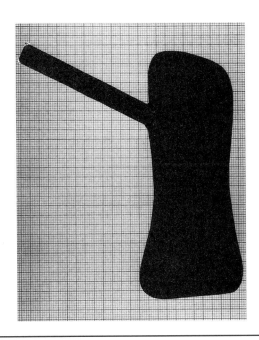

Fig. 21-11F

Finger/Metacarpal/Wrist/Forearm Shell (Dorsal)

PURPOSES (Fig. 21-12, *A*)

1. Positions MP, PIP, and DIP joints of index, long, ring, and small fingers.
2. Supports the transverse metacarpal arch via dorsal metacarpal bar.
3. Positions the wrist.

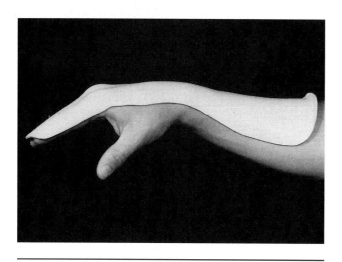

Fig. 21-12A

Splint: *Index–small finger MP flexion and IP extension immobilization splint, type 1 (13)* (Fig. 21-12, *B*)

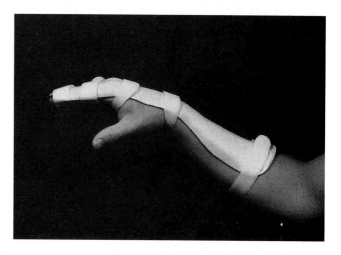

Fig. 21-12B *Example of completed splint.*

ANATOMIC LANDMARKS (on paper pattern)

1. Dorsal (Fig. 21-12, *C*)
   a. Distal ends of fingers
   b. First web space
   c. Two-thirds distal length of forearm
2. Medial and lateral (Fig. 21-12, *C*)
   a. Half thickness second and fifth rays
   b. Half thickness ulnar and radial wrist
   c. Half thickness ulnar and radial forearm

Fig. 21-12C

COMPLETED PATTERN (Fig. 21-12, *D*)

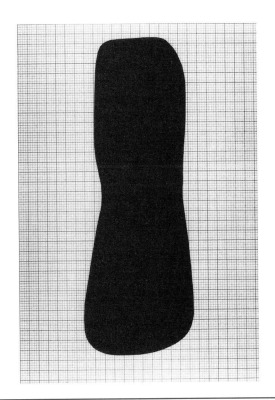

Fig. 21-12D

Finger/Metacarpal/Wrist/Forearm Shell (Volar)

PURPOSES (Fig. 21-13, *A,B*)

1. Positions MP, PIP, and DIP joints of fingers.
2. Positions CMC, MP, and IP joints of thumb. Specific CMC joint ligaments are either taut or relaxed, depending on CMC joint positioning.
3. Supports the transverse metacarpal arch via palmar metacarpal bar.
4. Positions wrist

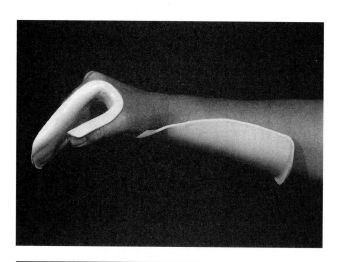

Fig. 21-13A

Splint: *Index–small finger MP flexion and IP extension, thumb CMC palmar abduction and MP-IP extension mobilization splint, type 1 (16)* (Fig. 21-13, *A*)

Splint: *Index–small finger MP flexion and IP extension, thumb CMC radial abduction and MP-IP extension mobilization splint, type 1 (16)* (Fig. 21-13, *B*)

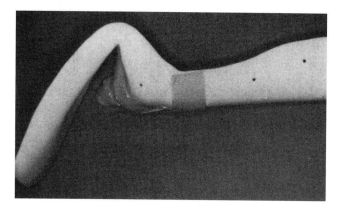

Fig. 21-13B *Example of completed splint.*

ANATOMIC LANDMARKS (on paper pattern)

1. Dorsal (Fig. 21-13, *C*)
   a. Distal ends of fingers and thumb
   b. First web space
   c. Two-thirds distal length of forearm
2. Medial and lateral (Fig. 21-13, *D*)
   a. Half thickness second and fifth metacarpals and phalanges
   b. Half thickness ulnar and radial thumb
   c. Half thickness ulnar and radial wrist
   d. Half thickness ulnar and radial forearm

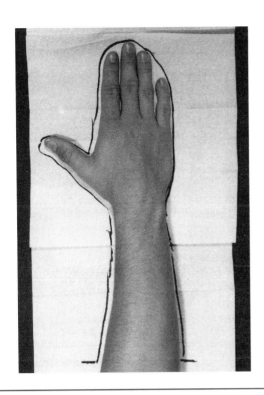

Fig. 21-13C

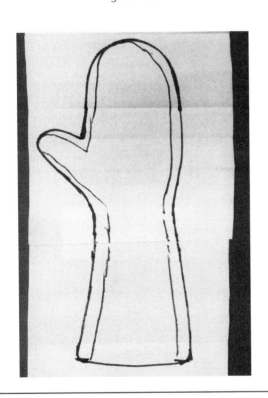

Fig. 21-13D

COMPLETED PATTERN (Fig. 21-13, *E*)

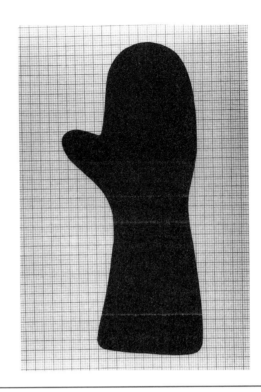

Fig. 21-13E

Other pattern design options include Figs. 18-12, *B,E*, and 18-13, *C,D*.

■ **SEPARATE COMPONENT PATTERNS**

Phalangeal Bar

PURPOSES (Fig. 21-14, *A*)

1. Positions MP joints in predetermined amount of flexion.
2. Prevents hyperextension of MP joints.
3. Maintains transverse metacarpal arch.

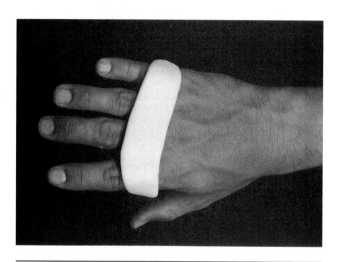

Fig. 21-14A

Splint: *Index–small finger MP extension restriction / IP extension torque transmission splint, type 0 (12)* (Fig. 21-14, *B*)

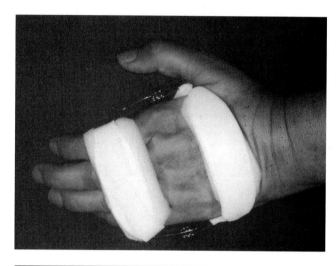

Fig. 21-14B *Example of completed splint.*

ANATOMIC LANDMARKS

1. Dorsal (Fig. 21-14, *C,D*)
   a. Index–small finger MP joints
   b. Index–small finger PIP joints
2. Medial and lateral (Fig. 21-14, *C,D*)
   a. Half thickness second proximal phalanx
   b. Half thickness fifth proximal phalanx

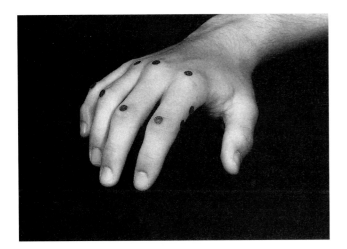

COMPLETED PATTERN (Fig. 21-14, *E*)

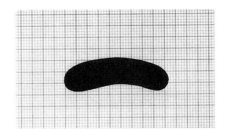

Fig. 21-14E

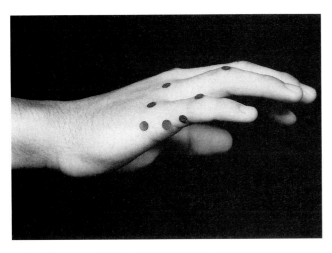

Fig. 21-14C,D

Four-Finger Outrigger
PURPOSE (Fig. 21-15, *A,B*)

1. Provides a base of attachment or fulcrum for mobilization assist component.
2. Controls direction of force application.

Splints: ***Index–small finger MP extension mobilization splint, type 1 (5)*** (Fig. 21-15, *C*)

Index–small finger PIP extension mobilization splint, type 2 (9) (Fig. 21-15, *D*)

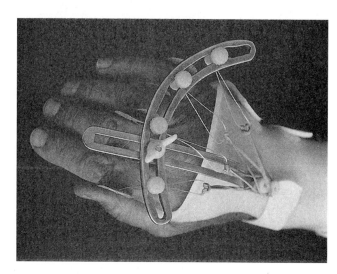

Fig. 21-15C   *Example of completed splint.*
(Courtesy Helen Marx, OTR, CHT, Human Factors Engineering of Phoenix, Wickenburg, Ariz.)

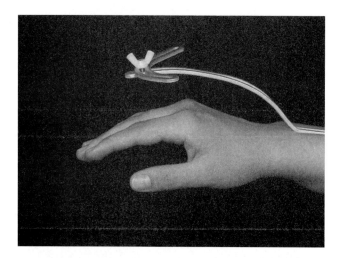

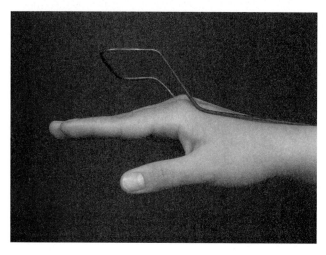

Fig. 21-15A,B

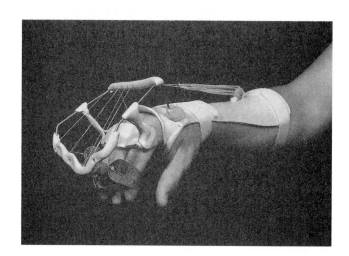

Fiig. 21-15D   *Example of completed splint.*

POSITIONING DORSAL OUTRIGGERS

1. MP joint outrigger (Fig. 21-15, *A,C,E*)
2. PIP joint outrigger (Fig. 21-15, *B,D,F*)

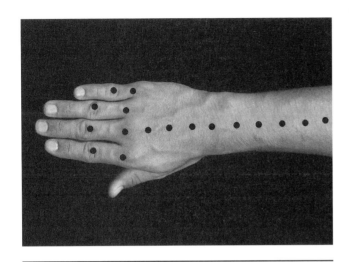

Fig. 21-15E

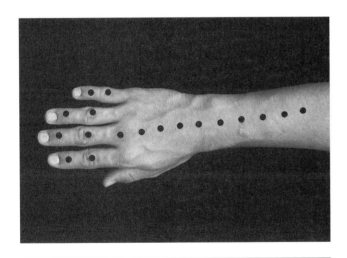

Fig. 21-15F

COMPLETED PATTERN (Fig. 21-15, *G*)

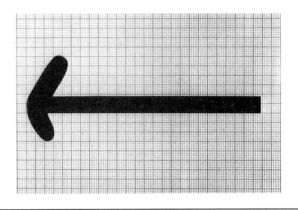

Fig. 21-15G

■ SUMMARY

Constructed to meet anatomic variations and to comply with basic splinting principles, patterns provide visual guidelines during the initial stages of splint fabrication. Employment of patterns diminishes chances for design error and facilitates optimum use of materials and time. Generally speaking, patterns are constructed by assembling separate components, by outlining the configuration of the shell or splint, or by taking specific measurements. Even though all patterns must be adapted to individual patient requirements, many splint designs originate from one of four basic patterns.

REFERENCES

1. Barr N, Swan D: *The hand: principles and techniques of splintmaking,* ed 2, Butterworth-Heinemann, 1988, Boston.
2. Barr NR: *The hand: principles and techniques of simple splintmaking in rehabilitation,* Butterworth, 1975, Boston.
3. Fess EE, Philips C: *Hand splinting: principles and methods,* ed 2, Mosby, 1987, St. Louis.
4. Fess EE, Gettle K, Strickland J: *Hand splinting principles and methods,* Mosby, 1981, St. Louis.
5. Kiel J: *Basic hand splinting: a pattern designing approach,* Little, Brown & Company, 1983, Boston.
6. Malick M: *Manual on static hand splinting,* vol 1, Harmarville Rehabilitation Center, 1970, Pittsburgh.
7. Malick M: *Manual on static hand splinting,* vol 1, Rev ed, Harmarville Rehabilitation Center, 1972, Pittsburgh.
8. Malick M: *Manual on dynamic hand splinting with thermoplastic materials,* Harmarville Rehabilitation Center, 1974, Pittsburgh.
9. Tenney C, Lisak J: *Atlas of hand splinting,* Little, Brown & Company, 1986, Boston.
10. Wallen S: Personal communication, 1998.
11. Ziegler E: *Current concepts in orthotics—a diagnosis-related approach to splinting,* Rolyan Medical Products, 1984, Chicago.

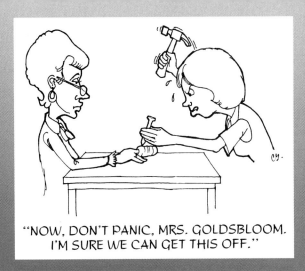

"NOW, DON'T PANIC, MRS. GOLDSBLOOM. I'M SURE WE CAN GET THIS OFF."

CHAPTER 22

Plaster Serial Casting for the Remodeling of Soft Tissue, Mobilization of Joints, and Increased Tendon Excursion

Judith Bell Krotoski, OTR, FAOTA, CHT

Chapter Outline

MOBILIZATION SPLINTING

In the Splint Classification System (SCS) implemented in 1992, the term *static splint* was recognized as misleading and has been discarded in view of better understanding of hand biomechanics (see Chapter 4, Classification and Nomenclature of Splints and Splint Components). A splint often thought to be static and immobilizing is not always static in its function. A splint that holds a joint in one position can (1) dynamically remodel and mobilize the joint and soft tissue being held, (2) mobilize proximal and distal joints through transfer of moment, and (3) mobilize the muscle tendon units that act on the joint. The described soft tissue remodeling technique is made possible by a splint that holds a joint at one position. But the purpose of using the splint in treatment is for tissue mobilization and for the rebalancing of forces acting on and around the joint. The splint is thus a mobilization splint, rather than one for immobilization.

Paul W. Brand first conceived the casting for joint remodeling technique in the late 1940s, when he observed a need for correction of clubfoot deformity in children without all of the joint destruction and stiffness observed after treatment with traditional "wedge casting."[4,19] The common method of treatment for clubfoot deformity required force to be used in

599

serial plaster correction of an ankle into improved positions. Brand recognized that an unwanted end result of a foot corrected with traditional "wedge casting" was that the ankle joint would be stiff, whereas adults with the deformity who were never treated with wedge casting still had mobile joints (see Chapter 1, Section II, Lessons from Hot Feet).[22]

■ "INEVITABILITY OF GRADUALNESS" IN THE REMODELING OF SOFT TISSUE

Brand envisioned the "inevitability of gradualness" in the correction of joint and soft tissue deformity.[10,21,22] He developed a casting for soft tissue and joint remodeling technique using gentle positioning under slight tension to encourage soft tissue growth as opposed to forceful stretching of the tissue (see Chapter 3, Biomechanics of Splinting, Section II). The technique was so successful in providing correction while maintaining joint mobility that Brand tried it for patients with joint stiffness thought at the time to be permanent, and by all but Brand to be beyond any possibility of correction. After successful remodeling of feet of Hansen's disease (leprosy) patients, the technique was applied extensively to the hands of patients with joint stiffness in order to help reverse the internal ravages of the joints and tissue that resulted from peripheral nerve damage.

The author of this chapter learned of the casting for remodeling technique directly from Brand while he was a surgical consultant to the former United States Public Health Service Hospital, New Orleans, La. This technique was used with success for patients with joint contracture where other forms of treatment failed. Seamen and military personnel were treated who had multiple types of joint and soft tissue contracture of the hand from disease and injury. The remodeling concept was introduced to the Hand Rehabilitation Center, Ltd., in Philadelphia, Pa., in 1976, when the author joined its staff. It was presented by the author and by Dr. Brand at the first Rehabilitation of the Hand Correlated with Hand Surgery meeting sponsored by the Center, and was subsequently published in the first edition of the classic book, *Rehabilitation of the Hand*.[1] Brand introduced the concept to many other surgeons and rehabilitation programs, and has published in detail on the technique and the biomechanics of deformity and correction.[5-17] The casting for remodeling technique is well described and widely used to remodel joint deformity and tissue contracture resulting from a variety of disease and injury conditions.[2,3] Today, it is understood that this technique works for any joint or soft tissue contracture unless bony restriction is present and that the principles that enable remodeling can be applied to any soft tissue of the body. Techniques such as tissue expansion with balloon implants and bone lengthening in response to stress traction have in recent years become common and take advantage of the same tissue remodeling principles. For the purposes of this chapter, the remodeling technique is primarily described for mobilization of the fingers, hand, and upper extremity.

■ CASTING TECHNIQUE
Special Considerations

The plaster cast splint described primarily casts the proximal interphalangeal joint, beginning at the metacarpophalangeal joint and extending distally to or beyond the distal interphalangeal joint. When the proximal interphalangeal joint of the finger is casted, the distal interphalangeal joint is often included in the cast. A therapist may intentionally leave out the distal interphalangeal joint for exercise if adhesions of the flexor profundus prevent full flexion of the distal interphalangeal joint. It would most certainly be included if, in addition to a joint contracture at the proximal interphalangeal joint or distal interphalangeal joint, there was contracture of the extrinsic flexor profundus muscle tendon unit. The casting would then not only reduce the interphalangeal joint contracture(s) but would also encourage lengthening of the musculotendinous contracture when the hand is used, particularly with full extension of the wrist and fingers.

The plaster cast technique for remodeling and mobilization of joints holds a joint or muscle tendon unit at one position at its maximum resting length, for a given length of time, in the direction required for correction. This selective holding of tissue under slight tension induces tissue growth, not just stretch, as the tissue responds to a slight increase in stress by growing new cells in an attempt to restore a more relaxed resting state. The new growth allows increased extension of the tissue, and greater flexion or extension of the joint or muscle tendon unit casted. Repeated serial casting with successive periods of tissue growth remodels the soft tissue over time. One has to discard the previous conception that the plaster is only forming a mold around the part. One also has to abandon the conception that force while the plaster is setting is what is required to reposition the joint and soft tissue into correction. The saving of plaster casts or a tracing of them serves as a demonstrative record of improvement for the patient. Torque angle measurements showing increased angle with reduced force for extension or flexion serve as permanent records.[18,20]

Exercise between castings is necessary to maintain active range of motion. The casts are changed for exercise at least every other day, or a minimum of twice a week. Depending on individual requirements, patients may be instructed to remove their casts for 10 to 15 minutes of exercise as often as every 3 to 4 hours. Exercise for as long as 30 minutes has been observed to result in slower improvement than when the cast is removed for only a few minutes. The remodeling process is dependent on enough time at maximum resting length to encourage regrowth of tissue.[21]

Force required to extend a normal supple finger is small and seldom requires measuring because the finger is simply positioned in the desired posture. In contrast, the force required to begin to remodel a finger with contracted joints varies between 100 and 300 grams of force at the distal interphalangeal joint; this small amount of force is all that is necessary for elongating a contracted joint into a corrected position for progressive mobilization. The force used with gentle positioning for progressive casting is not enough stress to cause tissue damage. A therapist can gain an idea of how minimal this force is by using a strain gauge to apply this amount of force to a distal interphalangeal joint and observing the movement of the other joints.[18]

Plaster is used for corrective splinting because it conforms to the finger so precisely and allows pressure to be dissipated along the length of the finger rather than at specific points. In contrast, rubber band tension used to improve a contracted joint by elastic traction is often measured at 450 grams/cm^2 applied at 2-3 cm from the axis of the joint.[2,18] The same amount of force has an increasing torque on the joint the longer the distance from the joint axis the force is applied and a rubber band cuff concentrates pressure in a small area under the cuff. The most damaging force to skin is not direct pressure but sheer, or translational, forces. Because the plaster conforms so precisely, sheer force from movement of the finger under the cast is eliminated or reduced, whereas sheer stress from elastic traction splints can be damaging to tissue.

Plaster can be relied on to maintain the joint and skin at a chosen position near the ends of their elastic limit. Other materials, such as thermoplastics, do not conform as effectively. Since only 1-2° of change is expected with each cast change, a material that allows some play or does not secure the soft tissue may not achieve the same result. Plaster allows skin underneath to breathe somewhat. In contrast to other materials such as plastic, it does not macerate the skin if applied directly next to the skin. Thermoplastic splints can be used if desired as retainer splints once

correction has been achieved, but do not work as well for correction.

Swelling is never increased by plaster casting unless the cast is wrapped too tightly and becomes constrictive; swelling is most often decreased because the cast keeps the joint or part quiet for periods of rest. The patient can be instructed to remove a cast if it appears too tight, but this is not usually found necessary. The casting is not often used in situations of fresh injury. Even when used in the first few postoperative days, such as following a collateral ligament release to gain a few degrees more extension, swelling is not usually a problem. Swelling from joint dislocations tends to decrease under the cast due to restriction of mechanical irritation. Even swelling from infections tends to decrease under the cast due to the restriction of mechanical irritation.

The casting technique is indicated in treatment of any joint or soft tissue contracture where there is not a bony block and the joint has internal integrity (as determined by x-ray of the joint). If for any reason a joint would be unstable or painful if range of motion were increased, one would not want to use the method. While casting can be used to help reduce some subluxed arthritic joints for reconstructive surgery, often the joint surfaces and lack of structural support for arthritic joints make it inadvisable to attempt mobilization by any method. Casting does not improve irregular joint surfaces damaged by fractures, but these may remodel themselves through movement over time. Casting with exercise in between casts is sometimes used in the resolution of joint stiffness following fracture.

Materials and Application

Fabrication of Proximal Interphalangeal Joint Casts

Materials include the following:
- Quick-setting specialist plaster
- Paper towel
- Water (sterile if desired)
- Bandage scissors (to cut plaster)
- Curved scissors, wire cutters, suture removal scissors (for removal and trimming of cast)
- Lanolin (optional)

Procedure
1. Cut plaster gauze strips 2.5 cm wide and 18 cm long.
2. Wet plaster gauze and dry excess on a paper towel (if Specialist fast-setting plaster; do not dry if gypsona plaster).

3. Fold edge slightly (0.5 cm for the first 2.5 cm) to make a smooth edge for the cast against the skin (Fig. 22-1, *A*).

4. Begin wrapping the plaster strip on the finger, placing the smooth edge under the palmar metacarpophalangeal crease (interphalangeal crease in distal interphalangeal joint casting) and continue in an overlapping fashion to the tip of the finger, leaving only the fingertip exposed (Fig. 22-1, *B*).

5. Prepare a second strip, as in step 3. Place the edge on the tip of the finger and wrap in a figure-eight fashion in the opposite direction (Fig. 22-1, *C*). Trim excess length. (The cast may be made from only one strip, but wrapping from proximal to distal, then distal to proximal, allows the last length of material to be available where most needed, usually for additional strength under the palmar surface of the proximal interphalangeal joint.) The cast should be about two layers thick at every point. A figure-eight wrap provides the best strength for the thin eggshell-type plaster cast; completely circular wraps can have weak points.

6. Once the finger is wrapped, use continuous finger movement to smooth the cast, supporting the finger until the plaster becomes warm and sets firmly. The plaster makes a firm cast in a few minutes. It does not reach maximum strength until completely dry in several hours, so instruct the patient to be careful until then (Fig. 22-1, *D*).

7. Change the cast every other day, or at least once a week, and have the patient exercise the joint for a short period. If the cast is left off for long periods, the tissue is not held continuously at the ends of its elastic limits, and progress is compromised. The cast is removed with suture scissors, wire cutters (with elongated and filed tips), curved scissors, or is soaked and unwrapped off the finger.

Casting should never compromise blood supply to the skin or part. An opening left at the tip of the finger as a precaution allows therapist and patient recognition of circulation problems. The circulation of the finger or part is checked after cast application to make sure the vascular supply is not compromised. The finger should not feel to the patient like it is throbbing. Excessive force during casting may compromise circulation in the cast, and sometimes a finger must be recast with less tension. Blood vessels also become shortened in contracted tissue and may shut down if a contracted joint is extended too fast. Blood vessels remodel and elongate with the growth of other soft tissue if time to remodel is allowed.

The patient can cover the hand and cast with a plastic bag for bathing. Plaster of Paris casts should not become wet. If a cast becomes damp, it should be removed. It does not always lose its correction if wet, but if it softens and changes position, pressure can be increased at specific sites, such as the dorsum of a proximal interphalangeal joint, causing redness and, potentially, tissue damage. Removable casts can be removed for washing of the digit.

Although it is always preferable for the therapist to change the cast, casting is such a relatively safe and noninvasive way of remodeling the joint that, when distance to therapy clinic is a problem, recasting may occasionally be done by another family member who has been carefully instructed (and observed using the technique). If something goes wrong, the patient can always soak the cast and remove it, and it can be reapplied at a later date.

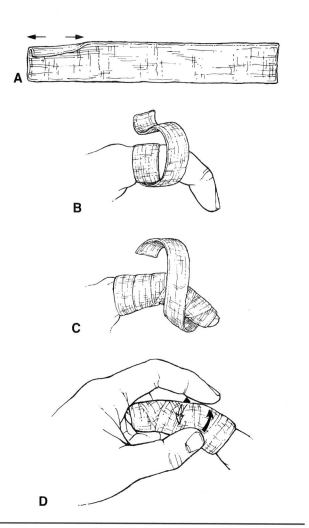

Fig. 22-1   **D, Index finger IP extension mobilization splint, type 0 (2)**
Technique for proximal interphalangeal cylinder casts.

Lack or Minimal Use of Padding

Padding under plaster shifts and repositions as the hand is used, allowing soft tissue being corrected to return slightly toward the direction of contracture (Fig. 22-2). The plaster casting technique originally described by Brand does not use padding, and padding is not recommended except in rare cases. The use of padding changes the technique and thus may not achieve the same results. The cast itself distributes pressure if molded correctly. If padding is used, it should be kept to a minimum, and used where most needed. A small piece of cotton fluff over the dorsal interphalangeal joint and under the edge of the cast seems to work best. The fluff tends to expand and relieve the cast slightly at the desired site (Fig. 22-3).

■ REMOVABLE CASTS

A cast can be made easily removable for exercise if loosened slightly along its length and removed once just after it has become firm, and then replaced. Lanolin or other oil is not always necessary but helps to prepare a finger for a removable cast. A small spot

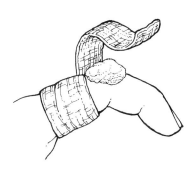

Fig. 22-2   Padding under the cast can shift slightly or compact, allowing pressure to be concentrated at specific points.

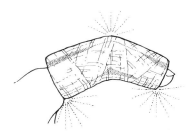

Fig. 22-3   **Index finger PIP extension mobilization splint, type 1 (2)**
When padding is used, a small piece of cotton fluff may be placed over the dorsum of an interphalangeal joint or where the cast makes an edge against the finger. As explained in this chapter, padding is not required except in cases of specific need.

of lanolin placed inside the cast assists replacement on the finger.

Casts for Severe Contracture

If the finger is too severely flexed for the cast to be easily removed, the cast could cause shear stress at the dorsum of the proximal interphalangeal joint on replacement. A small cut made along the proximal lateral dorsal surface of the cast may be all that is needed (Fig. 22-4, A) or this can be extended in a U-shape and top flap cut or removed from the cast (Fig. 22-4, B). The cut cast can be secured back on the finger with paper tape. It should be noted that the cast is more secure without the cuts and correction is achieved faster if the casts do not have to be removed.

■ OTHER JOINTS AND TENDONS

The technique of casting other parts and areas is based on the same principles as casting for finger interphalangeal joint contractures. A minimal amount of padding or no padding is used, and point pressure is avoided. For forearm casts, including the fingers and wrist, casting is best accomplished in two stages: (1) a slab thickness that fits volarly (Fig. 22-5, A) and (2) a thin circular wrap of plaster that secures the slab and distributes pressure along the length of the forearm (Fig. 22-5, B).

The forearm and hand are first prepared with a very light cotton Webril-like dressing, and a volar slab (six layers of plaster), which has been cut to approximate the length and shape of the fingers and forearm, is placed on the hand while it is held gently in its maximum position of correction. Once this sets, a 2- to 3-inch plaster roll is then wrapped around the forearm and hand volar slab to secure the slab. Only a thin cast is needed to secure the volar slab—one or two

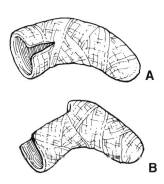

Fig. 22-4   Cutting to relieve a cast for removable casting. **A,** A small cut can be made in the proximal dorsum of the cast. **B,** A window can be cut in the cast and the top removed.

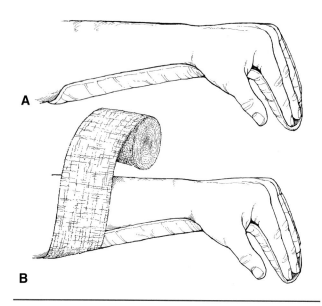

Fig. 22-5   A,B, Wrist extension mobilization splint, type 3 (13) In this removable casting for extrinsic musculotendinous contractures, a minimal amount of padding is used, and a circular plaster bandage is wrapped around a plaster slab.

layers. The circular plaster can be smoothed along the length of the forearm and hand, particularly over the fingers (plaster bandage will dimple in finger creases and stick to the fingers to secure their position).

Zero or minimal padding is necessary over the fingers or fingers with casts in the two-part forearm cast because the thin layer of plaster conforms well to the curvatures of the fingers and joints, minimizing shear stress. Most of the pressure sores that occur with casts from other forms of casting are from point pressure under the cast, causing ischemia, and from shear stress where the cast moves and rubs against the tissue. Without padding, the cast is more secure. The thin layer of cast made to secure the cast on the forearm can easily be cut with scissors to remove the cast.

Caution: A cast cutter (circular saw) *should not be used* on the thin plaster because it has little or no padding.

■ CASTING IN TWO DIRECTIONS

Some joint contractures of the hand require casting in two directions. In proximal interphalangeal joint contractures, regaining extension of the fingers is usually more difficult than regaining flexion. The finger flexor muscles through location and positioning have a mechanical advantage over the extensors. Often during casting to increase joint extension, flexion range of motion may be increased by exercise in between casting. This is true particularly in joints that

have been recently subluxed, where stiffness is often present during both flexion and extension of the involved joint. When gains in flexion are not satisfactory, the casting may be alternated for periods of both flexion and extension. Approximately every 2 days the casting direction may be alternated. Some of the benefits of casting in one direction might initially be lost when this is done. However, the casting does effect a change in the tissue, and progress can be seen when the casting is continued for a week or more.

■ TWO-STAGE CASTING

Boutonniere and swan neck deformities require two-stage casting because of the joint forces they produce in opposite directions. Casting with one stage usually is not successful and may actually be harmful because cast pressures are concentrated where they could cause damage.

Boutonniere Deformity

In patients with boutonniere deformity, migration of the lateral bands has occurred so that they have become flexors of the proximal interphalangeal joint and extensors of the distal interphalangeal joint (Fig. 22-6, A). Casting does not usually correct the underlying problem, only the joint stiffness, and the patient requires surgical correction. Casting is done first for the DIP joint with the PIP joint in full flexion (Fig. 22-6, B). This reduces the tension on the lateral bands. At the first casting, flexion of the DIP joint may seem impossible. But as cast changes are made, improvement in flexion of this joint can be demonstrated. Once the plaster has set firmly around the DIP joint, the PIP joint can be extended and a second cast made (Fig. 22-6, C), beginning at the metacarpophalangeal joint crease. Casting of both joints at the same time is impossible because the very short lever arm of the distal phalanx makes it difficult to control this joint and the PIP joint in the opposite direction. By casting the distal interphalangeal joint into flexion first, one has a longer and more powerful lever arm to extend the proximal interphalangeal joint. Although the force to extend the PIP joint is only that at the end of its elastic limit, one is able to accomplish this more effectively once the DIP joint is casted. Gradually, the lateral bands causing the deformity relax, and casting in opposite directions becomes easier.

The joint stiffness returns quickly if casting is discontinued and surgery is not performed. If the deformity is recognized early and casting in the described fashion is done, occasionally the migration of the lateral bands may be arrested. This is probably due to an incomplete division of the dorsal hood supporting

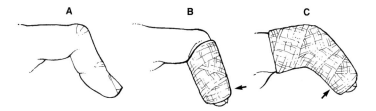

Fig. 22-6   B, Finger DIP flexion mobilization splint, type 0 (1) C, Finger PIP extension mobilization splint, type 1 (2)
A, Two-stage casting of a boutonniere deformity. B, With proximal interphalangeal joint fully flexed, cast distal interphalangeal joint into flexion. C, Once cast is firm, cast proximal interphalangeal joint into extension.

the lateral bands. If the finger is not casted for a while after injury, active flexion of the PIP joint increases tension on the dorsal hood and the migration of the lateral bands. The finger then quickly develops fixed joint contractures.

Two to three weeks after surgical correction of the underlying problem, a cylinder cast of only the proximal interphalangeal joint may be made, leaving the distal interphalangeal joint free to maintain extension of the joint. Restriction of the proximal interphalangeal joint maintains this joint in extension and allows early protected gliding of the dorsal hood repair as the distal joint moves. The cast may be removed for gentle controlled flexion of the proximal interphalangeal joint. Forced flexion is avoided for several weeks until the surgical repair has matured and the deformity is less likely to recur.

Swan Neck Deformity

The swan neck deformity is similar to the boutonniere deformity in that it quickly becomes a fixed contracture and usually requires surgical correction of the underlying problem to prevent contractures from recurring (Fig. 22-7, A). Rupture of the lateral bands at their attachment on the distal interphalangeal joint or disruption of the palmar plate at the proximal interphalangeal joint can cause the deformity. If recognized and casted or splinted early, deformity might be arrested or prevented.

The distal interphalangeal joint is first casted into extension, beginning with a plaster wrap at the proximal interphalangeal joint (Fig. 22-7, B). With other forms of splinting the distal phalanx is such a short lever arm that it is sometimes impossible to extend this joint after a swan neck injury without causing more injury. The dispersion of the pressure of the cast over the length of the distal end of the finger helps prevent localized pressure to the dorsum of the distal interphalangeal joint, where injury often occurs.

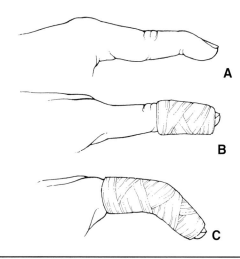

Fig. 22-7   B, Index finger DIP extension mobilization splint, type 0 (1) C, Index finger PIP flexion mobilization splint, type 1 (2)
A, Two-stage casting of a swan neck deformity. B, Cast distal interphalangeal joint into extension. C, Once cast is firm, cast proximal interphalangeal joint into flexion.

Once the distal joint is casted, the lever arm is increased, and when the cast is firm, the finger can be gently flexed at the proximal interphalangeal joint and casted with a second cast, beginning at the metacarpophalangeal joint (Fig. 22-7, C).

■ CASTING COMBINED WITH ELASTIC TRACTION MOBILIZATION SPLINTING

There are times when casting as a technique can be combined with elastic traction mobilization splinting to reduce the amount of splinting necessary and to allow for correction of multiple problems at the same time. An example is correcting stiff interphalangeal joints into extension and metacarpophalangeal joints into flexion. If casting is done to correct interphalangeal joint problems, these casts, by stabilizing the

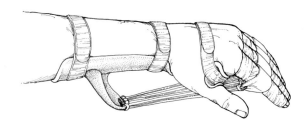

Fig. 22-8 Finger IP extension mobilization splint, type 0 (2), 4 splints @ finger separate \\ Index–small finger MP flexion mobilization splint, type 2 (6)

Casting of the interphalangeal joints in extension allows rubber band traction to the metacarpophalangeal joint at a position of mechanical advantage. Possibilities of tissue injury are minimized by the cast displacement of pressure on the dorsum of the fingers.

interphalangeal joints, transfer power of the finger flexors proximal to the metacarpophalangeal joint. If this is not enough to accomplish increases in flexion range of motion at the metacarpophalangeal joint, an elastic traction mobilization splint can be used with the casts to augment the flexion. Since the casts stabilize the interphalangeal joints, they provide a longer lever arm for traction to be distributed over the length of the finger. In this way more tension of the rubber bands can be used to provide more flexion at the metacarpophalangeal joints, while the possibilities of tissue injury and circulation compromise from the elastic traction are minimized (Fig. 22-8).

The mobilization assist cuff then produces more tension at a better mechanical advantage because the tension of the rubber band can be farther away from the joint axis, for example, over the dorsum of the proximal interphalangeal joint, where it could not be if the fingers were not casted. Other combinations of cylinder casting and elastic traction splinting are, of course, possible.

■ SUMMARY

Casting for soft tissue remodeling as originally conceived by Brand is an effective tool. It may be used in a variety of clinical situations where joint and soft tissue increases in range of motion are desired. The technique does not require force other than that required to gently position soft tissue near the ends of its elastic limit, allowing regrowth and remodeling of the tissue to occur. Although described mostly at the interphalangeal joints of the fingers, the biomechanical principles of tissue growth and remodeling remain the same for remodeling other joints and soft tissues. Plaster of Paris has unique properties that make it an ideal choice for the remodeling of tissue. Very little if any padding is used in the processes to avoid shifting

of padding and increases of pressure, and to ensure positioning of tissues near the ends of their elastic limits. The casting for remodeling splint is a mobilization splint or a torque transmission splint. The splints that hold a joint in one position can induce tension for remodeling of the joint held, transfer force for mobilization of other joints, and mobilize extrinsic muscle tendon units.

REFERENCES

1. Bell JA: Plaster cylinder casting for contractures of the interphalangeal joints. In Hunter J, et al: *Rehabilitation of the hand*, ed 1, Mosby, 1978, St. Louis.
2. Bell-Krotoski J, Breger DE, Beach RB: Biomechanics and evaluation of the hand. In Mackin E, et al: *Rehabilitation of the hand*, ed 5, Mosby, 2002, St. Louis.
3. Bell-Krotoski J, Figarola JH: Biomechanics of soft-tissue growth and remodeling with plaster casting, *J Hand Ther* 8(2):131-7, 1995.
4. Brand PW: Lessons from hot feet: a note on tissue remodeling, *J Hand Ther* 15(2):133-5, 2002.
5. Brand PW: Rehabilitation of the hand with motor and sensory impairment, *Orth Clin North Am* 4:1135-9, 1973.
6. Brand PW: The reconstruction of the hand in leprosy, *Ann Royal College of Surg* 11:350, 1952.
7. Brand PW, Beach RB, Thompson DE: Relative tension and excursion of muscles in the forearm and hand, *J Hand Surg* [Am] 6(3):209-19, 1981.
8. Brand PW, Cranor KC, Ellis JC: Tendons and pulleys at the metacarpophalangeal joint of a finger, *J Bone Joint Surg Am* 57A:779-84, 1975.
9. Brand PW, Hollister A: External stress: effect at the surface. In *Clinical mechanics of the hand*, Mosby, 1999, St. Louis.
10. Brand PW, Hollister A: Hand stiffness and adhesions. In *Clinical mechanics of the hand*, Mosby, 1999, St. Louis.
11. Brand PW, Hollister A: How joints move. In *Clinical mechanics of the hand*, Mosby, 1999, St. Louis.
12. Brand PW, Hollister A: Mechanics of individual muscles at individual joints. In *Clinical mechanics of the hand*, Mosby, 1999, St. Louis.
13. Brand PW, Hollister A: Muscles: the motors of the hand. In *Clinical mechanics of the hand*, Mosby, 1999, St. Louis.
14. Brand PW, Hollister A: Operations to restore muscle balance to the hand. In *Clinical mechanics of the hand*, Mosby, 1999, St. Louis.
15. Brand PW, Hollister A, Agee JM: Transmission. In *Clinical mechanics of the hand*, Mosby, 1999, St. Louis.
16. Brand PW, Hollister A, Giurintano D: External stress: forces that effect joint action. In *Clinical mechanics of the hand*, Mosby, 1999, St. Louis.
17. Brand PW, Hollister A, Thompson D: Mechanical resistance. In *Clinical mechanics of the hand*, Mosby, 1999, St. Louis.
18. Breger-Lee DE, Bell-Krotoski J, Brandsma JW: Torque range of motion in the hand clinic, *J Hand Ther* 3:7-13, 1990.
19. Fess EE: A history of splinting: to understand the present, view the past, *J Hand Ther* 15(2):97-132, 2002.
20. Flowers K, Pheasant S: Use of torque angle curves in the assessment of digital joint stiffness, *J Hand Ther* 1(2):69-75, 1988.
21. Kolumban SL: The role of static and dynamic splints, physiotherapy techniques and time in straightening contractures of the interphalangeal joints, *Lepr India* Oct:323-8, 1969.
22. Wilson DC: Sahib doctor: the healing surgeon of Vellore, *Reader's Digest*, 1966.

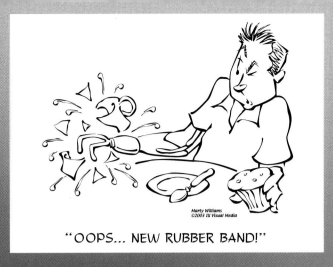

"OOPS... NEW RUBBER BAND!"

Marty Williams
©2003 IU Visual Media

CHAPTER 23

Cast, Splint, and Design Prostheses for Patients with Total or Partial Hand Amputations

Judith Bell Krotoski, OTR, FAOTA, CHT

Chapter Outline

INTRODUCTION

As surgeons and therapists understand what is necessary to reconstruct a functioning hand after traumatic injury, the same concepts and principles need to be applied to prosthetic hand design.

Countless times, a decision is made that a patient with a total or partial hand amputation would not benefit from a prosthesis. But hands are critical for everyday life skills. The patient needs the missing function, but available prostheses have limited capacity to replicate a hand. Traditional prosthetic designs often enclose and restrict motion of remaining joints or digits, covering up skin areas critical for sensibility during active use of the extremity. "Passive" (nonoperational) hands are totally cosmetic. "Active" hands, including newer "soft hands," are severely limited in function. And all of these are expensive. Partial hands

or special need prosthetics must be custom designed, molded, and redesigned for need at still additional costs. The traditionally metal terminal device is both functional and durable, but not at all cosmetic. A good argument can be made for the use of trial prostheses, where designs can be tried and problems solved before incorporation into a final prosthesis by a prosthetic company. More patients would benefit from total or partial hand prostheses if they were function enhancing, generally available, and cost-effective.

A VIEW OF THE PROBLEM

Increased attention needs to be given to the design of a prosthetic hand that works. Knowledge and understanding of the biomechanics of the "normal" hand have outpaced what is available in prosthetic

607

replacement in general. Existing knowledge in biomechanics and hand function developed by hand surgeons and therapists can enhance prosthetic design today.

Bunnell, the "father of hand surgery," emphasized that rehabilitation of hand injuries includes custom prosthetic fitting of the partially or totally amputated hand.[1,4] His comprehensive paper on surgical planning for prosthetics[7] was republished in the first edition of *Rehabilitation of the Hand*.[5,6] Moberg advocated the need for a key-pinch prosthesis. Hand surgeons understand that when muscle power is limited in reconstruction of a hand, a key-pinch is optimum over a tip-pinch for hand function.[9] Moberg also suggested that proprioception of the thumb and fingers could be provided from surrounding skin areas of cutaneous sensation. Yet conventional hand prostheses continue to use a tip-pinch design, and few attempts are made to provide any sensory feedback. Even an otherwise normal hand may be of little use if it has no tactile feedback.

◼ A CHANGING FUTURE

Cast, splint, and design prostheses made with Plaster of Paris and/or thermoplastic materials offer a key in the advancement of hand prosthetics for patients with total or partial hand amputations. As in splinting for other hand injuries, trials can be quickly and easily fashioned in temporary materials, discarded, or refashioned without prohibitive costs. Temporary materials used by therapists make allowances for patient changes in postinjury wounds, tissue swelling, joint contractures, and healing during treatment, before a patient is ready for a final prosthesis. Patient compliance is enhanced with early fit, trial of options according to need, and training in prosthetic use during therapy. The patient and the insurance company are then assured that the permanent prosthesis ordered will meet the need and will be used.

Prosthetic companies also stand to benefit by a collaborative approach to the problems. More business is generated, the patient is referred when healed and ready for a final prosthesis, and the prosthetist has fewer fitting headaches during costly fabrication time. A close affiliation of therapists with a prosthetic company willing to reproduce the temporary preparatory prosthesis in permanent materials is essential. Direct explanation of program intentions and assurance that a prosthetist who is skilled in producing designs in lasting materials will fabricate the final prostheses help develop bilateral collaboration. Some local prosthetic companies have made parts available to therapists as needed or have extra parts useful for trials. Parts can be obtained ahead of time for early fit designs. Advanced education promotes common language and understanding of therapists and prosthetists and is available to therapists through courses such as those offered by Northwestern University Medical School, Chicago, Ill.

◼ PLASTER OF PARIS CAST EARLY FIT PROSTHESIS

Burkhalter emphasized the psychological advantages of prostheses' immediate fit. He envisioned that, rather than wake up with a missing extremity, the patient would instead find a terminal device or mechanical hand that immediately becomes part of his or her life and recovery.[8] While making a plaster of Paris cast over an amputation in the operating room, he attached a conventional metal terminal device and cable anchor. Later added to this was a conventional cable and nylon webbing harness. Plaster of paris is used rather than thermoplastics because plaster allows access of some air to the wound. Thermoplastic can be used over the plaster of Paris cast to secure cable attachments and for later cast socket versions with bandage wrapping, to help shape a stump for final prostheses. No stress on the wound or scar should be allowed with active pull on the cable, and casts are used over bandages or for stump sockets until the wounds are healed.

◼ PARTIAL HAND SPLINT PROSTHESIS

Through availability of thermoplastic, and applications at the Hand Rehabilitation Center, Ltd., in Philadelphia, in 1977, and the National Hansen's Disease Center, in Carville, La., in 1978, a basic splint prosthesis design evolved for patients with partial or stiff hands where heavy use of the extremity is needed.[2,3] This design covers only what has to be covered to provide optimal stability for a terminal device, and avoids encapsulating the remaining hand in a prosthetic socket or sleeve. Remaining hand digits are free for movement and, if functioning, for use and tactile feedback (Fig. 23-1).

Aquaplast* or Reveal† thermoplastics (sticky preferred) assure a near perfect fit, secure metal parts, and necessary strength for areas of small diameter.[5] Prosthetic parts have been ordered directly, or

---

*Originally trademarked by WFR Corporation; sold to Smith Nephew Corporation 1992; acquired by Ability One Sammons Preston, 2002, Germantown, WI.
†WFR Corporation, 30 Lawlins Park, Wyckoff, NJ, 07481.

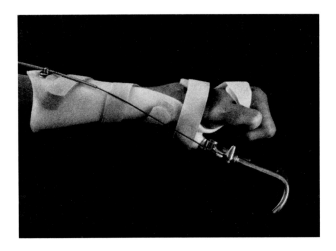

Fig. 23-1   Shoulder flexion, elbow extension, forearm pronation: [finger TD open] / shoulder extension, elbow flexion,
forearm supination: [finger TD close] torque transmission splint-
prosthesis, type 1 (4)
Partial hand splint-prosthesis; a radial view of volar splint with base
plate attachment and cable.

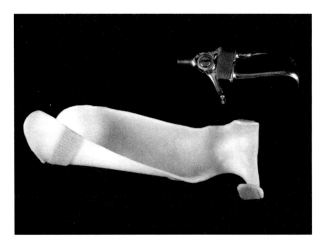

Fig. 23-2   Dorsal view, with unattached metal terminal device.
The open design allows a stiff or partial hand to slip in and out with
ease.

through local prosthetic companies.[‡] Two 1- or 2-hour
fittings are recommended.

FABRICATION OF PARTIAL HAND SPLINT PROSTHESES

Step 1

A thermoplastic wrist splint is made with careful
attention to curves in molding the palmar eminence
and metacarpal arch, to provide anatomic support
and splint strength (Fig. 23-2). The distal thumb and
metacarpophalangeal (MP) crease edges can be folded
and add to strength with minimal coverage. Tongue
extensions (radial and ulnar deviation bars) around
the thumb web space and at the ulnar border of the
metacarpals add to splint stabilization on the arm
during active use of the prosthesis. The forearm
portion is made approximately three-quarters of the
forearm, with an ulnar tongue wrapping around onto
the dorsal forearm for a cable attachment. The final
splint mold should allow the patient's forearm and
hand to slide in and out easily. It should also allow full
forearm pronation and supination (Fig. 23-1).

Step 2

A terminal device (hook) 5X or 5XA is screwed into a
small metal APRL forearm lengthener (FL-749) (Fig.
23-3, *A*). The terminal device is aligned in position

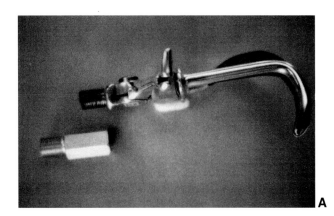

A

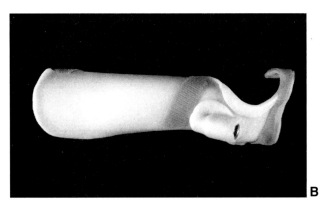

B

Fig. 23-3   **A,** Close view of components. **B,** Volar view, with added
forearm lengthener.

by placing the metal parts just proximal to the wrist
(Fig. 23-1). The terminal device should angle slightly
away from the splint to allow it to be unscrewed. It
should simulate the thumb, index and long finger, but
be slightly radial, so that the patient can easily view

[‡]Hosmer Dorrance Corp, 561 Division St., P.O. Box 37, Campbell,
CA 95008.

objects. The patient should be able to supinate the terminal device to reach his mouth and pronate to reach objects on a table.

Once alignment is determined, the forearm lengthener is secured on the volar portion of the splint by a small piece of thermoplastic that has been heated until clear with a heat gun (Fig. 23-3, *B*). The piece is placed over the forearm lengthener and pressed against the splint. Once cool, the plastic addition and lengthener will break apart from the splint. The lengthener is permanently bonded to the splint by heating thermoplastic contact areas until they are tacky and then pressed together. (For coated material, remove coating on contact surfaces before heating.)

Step 3

Velcro straps add stability dorsally across the hand, radial and ulnar deviation bars, and at the wrist. A long, continuous strap around the splint and forearm further enhances stability on the forearm critical to prevent shifting during patient operation of the cable attachment (Fig. 23-1, radial view; Fig. 23-4, ulnar view).

Step 4

A cable and housing assembly is prepared using a standard "cable kit" (Fig. 23-1); this can be preassembled by the prosthetic company in approximate lengths. The kit (Kable Kit No. 6 1/16") comes with a diagram and the following parts: control cable C-100, cable housing CH-100, retainer C-709, base plate with rubber backing C-708, terminal device swivel ball

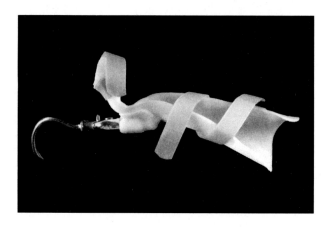

Fig. 23-4   Shoulder flexion, elbow extension: [finger TD open] / shoulder extension, elbow flexion: [finger TD close] torque transmission splint-prosthesis, type 1 (3)
Ulnar view, with terminal device in place. Note traditional hand splint strap and addition of forearm wrap-around strap.

attachment C-701 with rubber grommet C-759, cable housing cross-bar assembly C-710, and cable-to-harness-hanger attachment C-11. A cable cutter and swaging tool, CST-100, cuts the woven metal cable, and crimp on end attachments.

Step 5

The metal base plate with rubber backing is attached to the splint proximal forearm extension with small pieces of thermoplastic (Fig. 23-1). The retainer (screwed onto the cable housing) slips into the base plate and turns 90° to lock (or unlock). These anchor the cable housing on the splint for the cable to slide through and operate the terminal device.

Step 6

A thermoplastic triceps cuff is made for the patient's posterior humerus (Fig. 23-5). To this is added a leather strap and metal backing plate (included in cable kit). One strong rivet is necessary through the provided hole in the leather and the backing plate, and the hole made through the triceps cuff (head of rivet is outside cuff). Adhesive-backed Velcro hook (with nonadhesive pile) straps placed over the edges of the metal plate further secure it to the triceps cuff. A layer of felt padding is made for inside the cuff. These anchor the cable housing where it extends around the posterior humerus.

Step 7

The cable housing is assembled (adjusted with splint on the patient). One end of the housing is cut with wire cutters (sharp edges filed). This is screwed through the splint (base plate) retainer and extended toward the terminal device to protect the cable (stops before it eliminates full opening of the terminal device). The other end is cut just beyond the triceps cuff attachment (and filed). A removable cross-bar is screwed onto the end of the cable housing and inserts into the precut slit in the leather strap (previously attached to the cuff). Once assembled, the housing can be adjusted for length by rotation (screwing) at attachments.

Step 8

The cable is assembled through the housing. The swivel ball and grommet for distal cable attachment to thumb of the terminal device is crimped onto the cable using a swaging tool (Fig. 23-1). The proximal opposite cable end is threaded through the cable housing on the splint and triceps cuff and is cut to

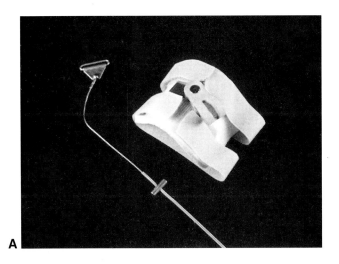

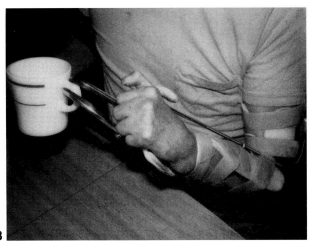

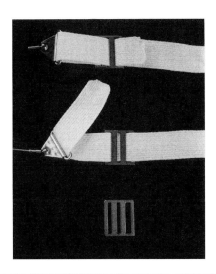

Fig. 23-6   A harness buckle allows cable tension adjustments.

Fig. 23-5   **B, Shoulder flexion, elbow extension: [finger TD open] / shoulder extension, elbow flexion: [finger TD close] torque transmission splint-prosthesis, type 1 (3)**
A, Triceps cuff and assembly to secure housing for cable to patient's posterior humerus. **B,** Splint-prosthesis positioned on patient.

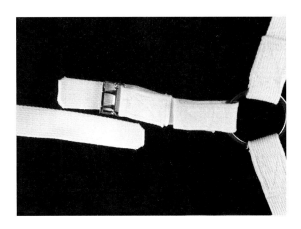

Fig. 23-7   Northwestern ring: The straps on the right loop around the patient's shoulder opposite the prosthesis.

extend a few inches beyond where it exits the housing at the posterior elbow. The cable should be made long enough so that it does not disappear into the housing when the terminal device is closed and the arm is extended. A cable-to-harness hanger attachment is crimped onto the cable with the crimping tool (or may be soldered on) (Fig. 23-5, *B*).

Step 9

A conventional harness is made of nylon webbing. A one-inch, four-bar harness buckle, FBB-10, is used for securing the hanger attachment of the cable to the harness (Fig. 23-6). A second buckle is added to secure the continuing harness strap (Fig. 23-7). Adding this a few inches beyond the cable hanger

makes the harness and cable tension adjustable. The strap is folded around the buckle and sewn to itself. An extension of the strap is made for padding behind the buckle. The other end of the strap is sewn to itself around a metal Northwestern ring, NRH-8 (Fig. 23-7). The ring should fall between the scapulae, at the mid-scapular level and slightly to the opposite side. The remaining harness consists of a shoulder strap looped around the patient's shoulder opposite to the prosthesis, with felt padding added.

Step 10

Prosthetic rubber bands add closure tension to the terminal device. Use a hook tension tool, BZ 1512. Only one or two bands are used for closure tension until usual adjustments are made and the patient becomes accustomed to the prosthesis.

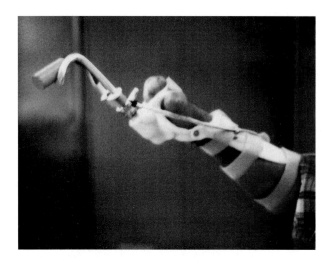

Fig. 23-8   Shoulder flexion, elbow extension, forearm pronation, wrist extension: [finger TD open] / shoulder extension, elbow
flexion, forearm supination, wrist flexion: [finger TD close] torque
transmission splint-prosthesis, type 1 (5)
Making a hinge to allow movement of an active wrist and dorsal
splint prosthesis is an alternative.

Considerations and Variations

- The splint design final can be fabricated in fiberglass
  or cast-molded in skin colors by local prosthetic
  companies.
- A metal or brace-type appearance is avoided as it is
  undesirable to many patients.
- The distal splint can be extended in a platform to
  support flaccid fingers.
- A wrist-hinge joint can be included, and the splint
  made to be dorsal (Fig. 23-8).
- Unconditional routing of the cable helps some
  patients. Routing the cable around the medial side
  of the elbow restores pronation in a patient absent
  these muscles and stabilizes the forearm for operation of the terminal device.
- Computer technology offers untapped and unlimited possibilities in functional hand designs and
  applications.

■ DUAL-OPERATED LATERAL THUMB DESIGN PROSTHESIS

Based on Moberg concepts, and neglected forearm
pronation and supination for prosthetic hand operation, the author used Aquaplast covered with skin-
toned thermoplastics to design a Dual-Operated
Lateral Thumb Hand Prosthesis (U.S. Patent No.
4,258,441, 1980) (Fig. 23-9). This design received first
place in the Maddak Award for competition at the
American Occupational Therapy Association Annual
Conference, 1980. Trials were first made for subjects

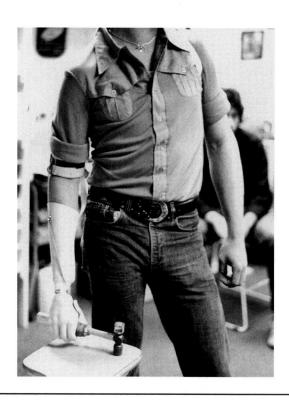

Fig. 23-9   Shoulder flexion, elbow extension, forearm pronation: [thumb lateral abduction, finger flexion fixed] / shoulder
extension, elbow flexion, forearm supination: [thumb lateral
adduction, finger flexion fixed] torque transmission prosthesis,
type 1 (4)
Dual-Operated Lateral Thumb Design Prosthesis (U.S. Patent No.
4,258,441) uses humeral flexor or forearm pronation for opening.

with normal hands, using a hinge joint for the thumb,
and thermoplastic shells fitted separately over the
fingers and thumb. A cable was attached to the base
of the thumb and routed anteriorly and over the
forearm to the posterior elbow and then to a cuff.
Forearm pronation selectively opens the thumb in
resistance to an internal spring at the base of the
thumb, which closes the thumb against the fingers.
Increased pressure on the back of the elbow relative
to forearm pronation and thumb opening translated
into subject understanding the degree of thumb
opening or closing. Following demonstrations to
James Hunter, MD, at the Hand Rehabilitation Center,
Ltd., in Philadelphia, he agreed to reattach forearm
pronation and supination muscles to the distal
forearm of a patient with a traumatic wrist amputation already selected for an early fit prosthesis. (Reat-
tachment is possible but not often considered
necessary in amputations.)

The subsequent trial was an immediate success and
the design was recognized as an improvement over the
operation of conventional hand prostheses by therapist, surgeon, and patient. The patient wanted a prosthesis that looked like a hand, but could be used for

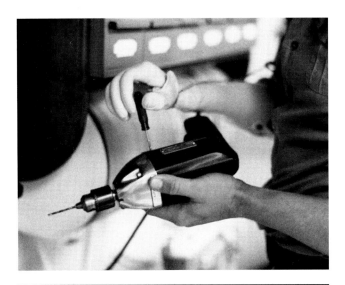

Fig. 23-10   Shoulder flexion, elbow extension, forearm prona-tion: [thumb lateral abduction, finger flexion fixed] / shoulder extension, elbow flexion, forearm supination: [thumb lateral adduction, finger flexion fixed] torque transmission prosthesis, type 1 (4)

A prosthetic hand needs to be able to operate tools safely and effi-ciently, and it should allow some degree of sensory feedback, per-mitting visual focus on objects rather than focusing on operation of the prosthesis.

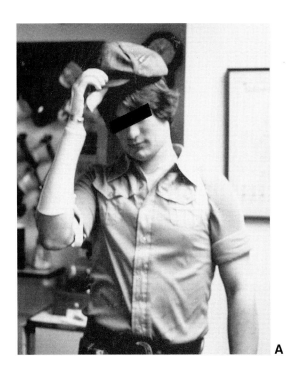

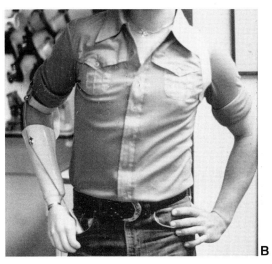

Fig. 23-11   A,B, Shoulder flexion, elbow extension, forearm pronation: [thumb lateral abduction, finger flexion fixed] / shoul-der extension, elbow flexion, forearm supination: [thumb lateral adduction, finger flexion fixed] torque transmission prosthesis, type 1 (4)

A,B, A lateral thumb design is functional in many planes.

work, particularly to hold or operate tools; thus the prosthesis was designed as such (Fig. 23-10). It could provide the patient with a sense of thumb position and anchored tool handles in the palm through the broad support of four fingers opposing the thumb. It securely operated in otherwise difficult over-the-head (Fig. 23-11, A), toward-the-back, and other positions (Fig. 23-11, B). The addition of standard harnessing provided dual-control for operation, humeral flexion or forearm pronation for opening. This design works because, mechanically, the thumb functions as only one lever arm working against the flat plane in its lateral approach to the fingers in a key-pinch. Pronation for thumb opening, with degrees of return to supination for thumb closing, is physiologic to the way one uses an extremity when approaching and handling objects, as when picking up an object from the table, or when bringing food to the mouth. The hand was cosmeti-cally pleasing and designed for work, thus was not covered with a cosmetic glove, but could be if so desired.

■ SUMMARY

Plaster of Paris and thermoplastic temporary materi-als allow early and trial fittings of cast, splint, or design prostheses for immediate fit, problem solving, and trial designs before a final prosthesis is ordered.

Knowledge of hand biomechanics and the under-standing of function that has evolved among surgeons and therapists can play an important role in the cre-ation of prosthetic hands that work and can be used for life activities. Where reconstruction is not possi-ble, surgeons can optimize surgery for prosthetic use. Therapist creation of design prostheses according to the patient's rehabilitation possibilities and work requirements is ideal, as therapists provide direct treatment of patients with disease and injury. Through the use of splinting and adaptive devices, therapists provide restoration of function in patients in rehabilitation and are the professionals who provide training in prosthetic use.

REFERENCES

1. Alldredge R, Murphy E: *Prosthetic research and the amputation surgeon*. In Bunnell S: *Artificial limbs*, Krigor Publishing Company, 1956, Huntington, NY.
2. Bell J: *Preparatory design splint prosthesis*, Third Congress of the International Societies for Surgery of the Hand, Therapist Section, 1986.
3. Bell J, Freeman M: Preparatory design splint prosthesis. In *The Star*, 1986.
4. Bunnell S: *Surgery of the hand*, ed 3, JB Lippincott, 1956, Philadelphia.
5. Bunnell S: The management of the non-functional hand: reconstruction vs. prosthesis. In Hunter J, et al: *Rehabilitation of the hand*, Mosby, 1978, St. Louis.
6. Bunnell S: The management of the non-functional hand: reconstruction vs. prosthesis. In Hunter J, et al: *Rehabilitation of the hand*, ed 2, Mosby, 1983, St. Louis.
7. Bunnell S: *Artificial limbs*, Krigor Publishing Company, 1956, Huntington, NY.
8. Burkhalter WE, Mayfield G, Carmona LS: The upper extremity amputee. Early and immediate post-surgical prosthetic fitting, *J Hand Joint Surg* [Am] 58(1):46-51, 1976.
9. Moberg E: Hand surgery and the development of hand prosthesis, *Scand J Plastic Reconstr Surg* 9:227-30, 1975.

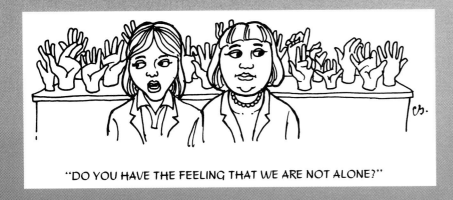

CHAPTER 24

Replicasting: Making Molds of the Hand

Chapter Outline

▨ INTRODUCTION

Prepared directly on a subject's hand, a negative mold provides the external frame or shell for a positive reproduction or mold* of the hand in plaster, dental acrylic, or similar casting material. After removal, the negative mold is filled with a liquid material that, through an endogenous heat process, dries and hardens. When this material is completely solid, the negative mold is peeled away, revealing a positive three-dimensional "copy" of the hand. A positive mold may be used for a variety of purposes, including fabrication of patient splints for special situations; as educational tools for students, therapists, patients, or other healthcare professionals; as a keepsake; or as a work of art. The intent of this chapter is to acquaint the reader with the rationale for using negative and positive molds and to briefly describe three methods for constructing these molds.

Historically, early splint materials were often too rigid, too caustic, or too hot in their malleable forms to be placed directly on a patient's skin. Positive molds

were indispensable in providing inert replicas upon which splints made from metal, solvent-based materials, or high-temperature plastics could be fitted without harm to the patient.[8] Unfortunately, the construction of negative and positive molds added considerably to splint fabrication time. Also, since molds produced rigid duplications of normally mobile structures, splints shaped to the molds frequently required further refinement to accommodate active hands, again adding to total fabrication time. With the advent of low-temperature thermoplastics, splint materials could be fitted directly to the patient and the need to produce positive molds for splint fabrication has all but disappeared. Current splinting materials allow efficient splint fabrication, and the idea of making a negative/positive mold system for every patient requiring a hand splint seems far-fetched indeed! There are, however, particular situations when positive molds are important.

Positive molds of the hand are invaluable for teaching patients, students, and other professionals (Fig. 24-1). For example, studying a splint without the corresponding anatomic landmarks can confuse and mislead even the most experienced clinician, to say

---

*Also described as a cast, casting, or positive mold.

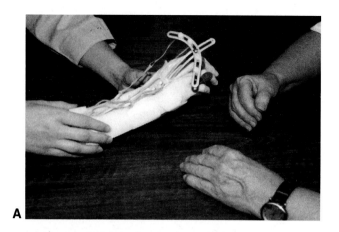

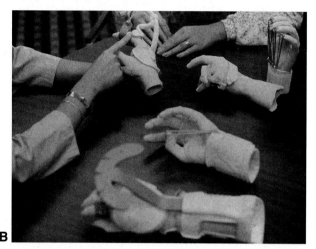

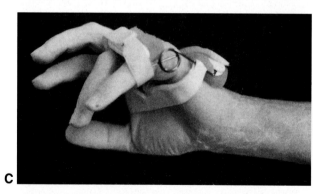

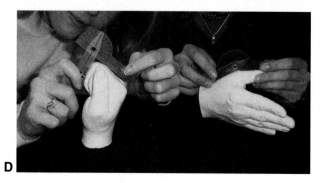

nothing of its effect on an apprehensive patient who has never encountered such a device. However, when the splint is placed on a positive mold of a hand, familiar points of reference are readily apparent, allowing the patient or student to direct full attention to the instructions or explanation being given, instead of groping for spatial orientation. Serial positive molds also provide a permanent three-dimensional record of postural changes of the hand as a result of therapeutic or surgical intervention or through a pathologic process occurring over a period of time (Fig. 24-2). In addition to providing permanent records of the changes in deformity in a given hand, these serial casts may be of considerable assistance in general patient counseling and teaching. Further, there are specific occasions when a positive mold may be helpful because of unusual patient circumstances, either environmental or medical. For instance, patients who will need periodic splint replacement but do not have ready access to the hand clinic may have additional splints fabricated by having permanent positive molds available at the clinic.[1]

Although medical circumstances necessitating construction of positive molds are rare, they can and do occur. Overly anxious, hypersensitive, or hyperactive individuals comprise the majority of challenging patients in this area, sometimes requiring some means of anesthesia for the fabrication of the negative mold. A final situation requiring the preparation of negative/positive molds is when high-temperature plastics, caustic materials, or metal must be used for splint construction. The use of a positive mold during the construction and fitting processes of these types of splints frees the patient from involvement in tedious hours of splint fabrication.

■ MATERIAL SELECTION*

A range of materials and methods is available to create negative and positive molds of the hand and upper extremity. When selecting materials and methods that are appropriate to the situation, several factors must be considered: level of detail desired in the finished positive mold, material availability, material characteristics and safety of use, hand size, cost, fabrication time, and therapist experience level.

---

*See the list of resources at the end of this chapter.

Fig. 24-1 **A-C,** Positive molds used as visual aids may be of considerable assistance in the education of patients or students. **D,** Occupational therapy students in a kinesiology course develop skill in goniometry by measuring joint range of motion on plaster and dental acrylic hand models.

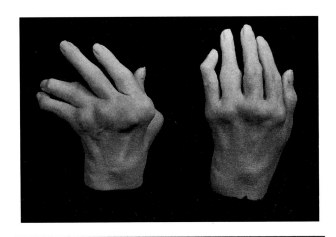

Fig. 24-2   Molds may provide a permanent record of postural changes in the hand, as does this set of preoperative **(left)** and postoperative **(right)** molds.

The purpose of the final positive hand mold determines the amount of detail required in the negative mold (Fig. 24-3, *A-C*). For example, if the objective is to replicate the form of the hand along with its intricate topographical details, including fingerprints, skin creases, superficial vein patterns, and fingernails, a molding alginate or skin-safe silicone rubber is preferable. When only the overall form of the hand is desired, and detail is less important, or when molding alginate or skin-safe silicone rubber materials are inaccessible, plaster bandages may be used to fabricate the negative mold. This method yields a positive mold of the hand that reflects only the shape, but not the intimate topographical details of the hand from which it was cast.

Different types of materials are required for making negative molds and for making positive molds. The negative mold or shell must first be fabricated on the subject. Once the negative mold is dry or set, depending on the material, the subject's hand is removed, leaving the empty negative mold. The completed negative mold is patched if needed and a high-quality plaster, dental acrylic, or similar material in liquid form is then poured into the negative mold, filling the void left by the subject's hand. When the poured material solidifies, the surrounding negative mold is removed to reveal the final positive mold of the hand.

In choosing materials, one of the most important material characteristics to consider is setting time. This is the time it takes for the material to convert from a liquid mixture to its final form as a flexible solid (molding alginate and silicone rubber) or a hard solid (plaster bandages, plaster, and dental acrylic). Setting times may be affected by component mixing ratios and temperatures. For example, setting times of molding alginates are variable with some products ranging from

3-5 minutes to 8-9 minutes. In general, a 3-5 minute setting time is appropriate for the hand. Cooler temperatures and thinner mixtures slow the set time and higher temperatures and thicker mixtures accelerate the set time.[10] It is important to avoid a setting time that is too rapid, resulting in material that sets up before it can be used. Conversely, an extended set-up time is inefficient and may cause the subject discomfort and fatigue from having to hold a hand position or posture for an extended period of time.

When using chemical compounds, especially within a clinical setting, it is essential that all involved in the mold-making process be familiar with the product's material safety data sheet. The importance of this information regarding a product's potential risks, storage, proper use, disposal, and emergency guidelines cannot be disregarded. For example, molding alginate and plaster products are in powdered forms and must be mixed with water prior to use. During the mixing process, these materials may become airborne, irritating the respiratory system and/or eyes. To minimize exposure, use of eye goggles and breathing masks for protection is advised.

While the actual process of creating a negative mold on a subject's hand may take several minutes, depending on the setting time of the negative molding material used, the entire process including preparation, pouring and setting of the molds, and cleanup may involve 1-2 hours. In addition, 1-2 days are needed to allow for complete drying of plaster positive molds.

Commercially available hand casting kits are an easy and relatively inexpensive way to gain experience in fabricating hand molds. These kits range in cost from $20-$60 and may be purchased online through lifecasting and art company websites* or locally through retail hobby or art stores. Non-kit materials used in the fabrication of negative and positive molds may be purchased individually from lifecasting, art, theatrical, medical, or dental supply companies. Cost of materials is dependent on product quality, quantity, and individual vendors. Molding alginate and plaster are among the least expensive and most commonly used materials in the fabrication of negative and positive hand molds. Other materials used in creating casts of the hand include, but are not limited to, skin-safe silicone rubber for negative mold fabrication and dental acrylic for fabrication of the positive mold or hand cast. For positive molds, dental acrylic is the most durable material. Several positive dental acrylic molds that belong to one of the authors have been used without chipping or breaking for more than 25 years for therapy students to practice measuring range of motion.

---

*Keywords: lifecasting, hand casting.

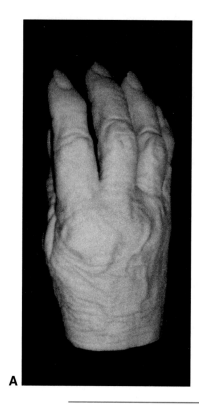
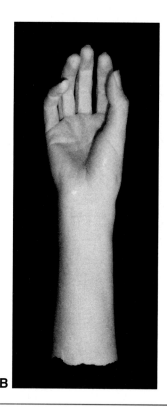
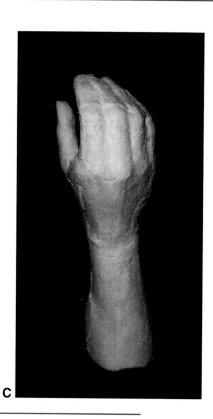

A   **B**   **C**

Fig. 24-3   Comparison of positive molds fabricated from different negative molding techniques: matrix method using molding alginate (**A**), brush-on method using silicone rubber (**B**), and the plaster bandage wrap method (**C**). These positive molds are made of plaster (**A,C**) and dental acrylic (**B**). **A,B,** Note the high level of hand topographical detail.

▩ FABRICATION METHODS

With unique advantages and disadvantages inherent to each technique, this chapter describes three basic methods of negative mold fabrication: (1) the matrix method using molding alginate, (2) the brush-on method using silicone rubber, and (3) the wrap method using plaster bandage. All three of the negative mold techniques share a similar method for making the associated positive molds: the pour method, using plaster or dental acrylic. Of the three systems, the matrix method of negative mold fabrication using molding alginate and the pour method of positive mold fabrication using a high-quality plaster are generally a good place for beginners to start. This system commonly is used and it is inexpensive, simple, and yields highly detailed reproductions of the hand.

General Concepts of Mold Fabrication

Precautions

Before starting on any mold-making project, always ask the subject and all others who will be in the immediate area, including staff and patient family members,

if they have allergies to any of the products to be used. If someone is allergic to one or more of the materials, the person must leave the area or the project must be discontinued. Although infrequent, allergic reactions to materials range from a mild rash to serious respiratory problems.

Preparation

The work area must be well ventilated, and both therapist and patient should wear dust masks and eye protection because of the tendency for these materials to become airborne during the process of pouring and mixing. A ventilation hood is recommended when working with dental acrylic. Consulting the MSDS* information about the products to be used is a prerequisite to getting started. For efficiency and to reduce clutter, all materials and equipment for the preparation of hand molds should be organized before initiating work. Therapist, subject, and work area, including the floor, should have protective coverings. If the subject is unable to independently maintain the

---

*MSDS information is available upon request from suppliers and/or manufacturers.

hand posture required, an assistant should be present to help.

Mold Fabrication Tips[9]

The following practical suggestions pertain to all three techniques described and, to avoid redundancy, are presented here before reviewing the individual methods of mold fabrication.

Air bubbles. During mixing and pouring of materials, care must be taken to minimize the opportunity for air bubbles to form. Air bubbles create surface irregularities in the final positive cast in the form of various sized craters and trapped air also may prevent liquid plaster or dental acrylic from reaching the fingertips during pouring into the negative mold, resulting in a positive mold that lacks fingertips (Fig. 24-4).

Tips to minimize air bubbles include the following:

- Add dry materials to wet materials when mixing.
- Use a wire whisk for mixing alginate and plaster materials.
- Tap the outer walls of the mixing container to encourage air bubbles to rise to the surface.
- Choose a hand position that minimizes air entrapment at the fingertips, e.g., a hook grasp hand position is more prone to trapping air bubbles at the fingertips.
- Coat subject's hand with a small amount of water prior to immersion into the negative mold (for matrix method only).
- Upon submersion into molding alginate/water mixture, encourage the subject to quickly rub hand against the sides of the container and to rub fingers together before assuming desired hand position (for matrix method only).
- Tap the outer walls of the negative mold container as the material sets (for matrix method only).
- When creating the positive mold, pour material into the negative mold in small incremental amounts as the mold is rotated and tapped.

Fingernails

- To minimize unsightly broken fingernails in the final positive mold, long fingernails should be trimmed or reinforced with putty or modeling clay prior to fabrication of the negative mold (Fig. 24-5).

Objects

- When casting a hand holding an object, it is important that the object is gripped in a manner that allows part of the object to be embedded within the

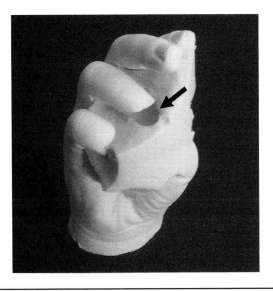

Fig. 24-4   The distal phalanx of the positive mold ring finger is lost due to a trapped air bubble during fabrication of the positive plaster mold. Replacing the dorsal portion of the negative mold, covering part of the missing distal phalanx, and adding freshly mixed plaster to form a new fingertip repaired the defect.

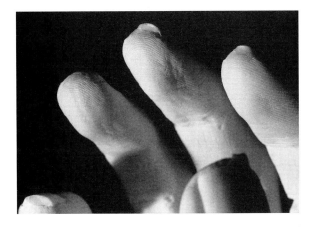

Fig. 24-5   The inherent thinness of long fingernails makes their reproduction in plaster or similar material difficult. Long plaster fingernails can easily fracture during removal of the negative mold. Note the fractured thumbnail.

mold. This allows removal of the hand from the negative mold while the object remains secured in place in the negative mold.

- For objects that may become damaged from exposure to the wet mixtures, tightly wrap the object in plastic wrap prior to mold fabrication.

Negative Hand Mold Fabrication

Matrix Method Using Molding Alginate[7,9-12,14]

General Considerations

The matrix method of negative mold fabrication requires a waterproof container, called the *matrix*, the size of which will accommodate the width and length of the hand. Depth of the container should allow hand immersion to a maximum proximal level of the wrist or mid-forearm. Premixed molding alginate and water is poured into the container and the subject's hand is submersed into the molding mixture until the material sets, becoming firm enough to withstand removal of the hand without damaging the mold. During this process it is important that the subject maintain the desired hand position and avoid touching the inner walls of the container. Once the material is set or cures, the hand is removed by having the subject gently wiggle his or her digits to release the suction that may occur. Once the suction is released the hand can be carefully pulled out of the mold. Many of the commercially available hand casting kits use this method to fabricate negative molds. Once the negative mold is completed, plaster is poured into the mold and allowed to harden. Due to material incompatibility, do not use dental acrylic or other resins in alginate negative molds.[5,6,12] Upon hardening, the negative mold is carefully peeled away to reveal the positive plaster mold.

For fabricating longer molds, including the hand and more proximal structures such as the elbow, alternative methods of negative mold fabrication should be employed. It is beyond the scope of this chapter to cover all the materials and methods of hand mold fabrication. Interested readers are encouraged to contact vendors specializing in mold-making materials for additional information.

Materials

The materials needed include the following:
- Aprons and/or old lab coats
- Newspapers, plastic sheeting
- Dust mask
- Protective eyewear
- Molding alginate (~1 lb. for an adult hand with setting time of ~5-7 minutes)
- Water (amount and temperature per alginate manufacturer's recommendation)
- Thermometer
- Matrix (container) (Fig. 24-6)
- Measuring cups
- Gram scale (required if alginate is measured according to weight)
- Large mixing bowl
- Wire whisk
- Large spoon

Procedure

1. Cover self, subject, and work area with protective garments or materials.
2. Use a matrix (container) of sufficient height to prevent overflow of displaced alginate mixture when hand is submersed.
3. Determine desired hand position. Have subject practice placing hand into empty matrix (container) while avoiding resting hand against the inner walls. Check to ensure correct hand position.
4. Consult manufacturer recommendations for mixing ratios and the quantity of molding alginate required to fabricate negative mold.
5. Measure water and place into mixing bowl or directly into the matrix.
6. Add premeasured alginate to water and quickly mix using a wire whisk (refer to section on tips to minimize air bubbles).
7. Keep in mind the setting time of the alginate and work accordingly.
8. Pour mixture into the matrix and quickly place subject's hand into the mixture (alternately, mixing may be directly performed within the matrix).
9. Subject's hand must remain motionless until mixture sets, becoming firm to the touch.

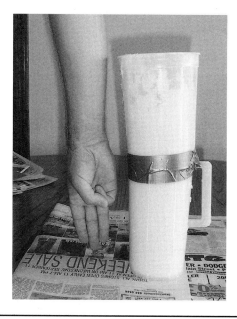

Fig. 24-6   To minimize waste of alginate material, choose an appropriate sized plastic matrix (container) that is slightly wider and longer than the hand and forearm to be molded. Plastic containers work well and clean easily and may be adapted as shown to accommodate longer hands and forearms. To fabricate a mold for an award trophy, subject's hand is positioned in the scout sign of the Boy Scouts of America.

10. Once mold is set, instruct subject to gently rotate hand and wiggle fingers to release suction and facilitate removal from mold.

11. Inspect inner area of the mold and remove any alginate debris (Fig. 24-7).

12. Turn mold upside down and allow it to drain for about one hour. Caution: Due to drying and shrinking of the alginate negative mold after setting, do not wait much longer than an hour or two before pouring the positive plaster mold. (If desired, may skip draining the mold and immediately pour the positive plaster mold with good results.)

13. Proceed to the section titled "Positive Hand Mold Fabrication: Plaster."

Warning: Never use liquid plaster to create a negative mold using the matrix method. The direct application of liquid plaster surrounding a subject's hand within a container may result in burning of the skin, as well as potential limb entrapment within the hardened plaster.[13]

Brush-On Method Using Silicone Rubber[3,4,12]

General Considerations
It is important that silicone rubber negative molds are fabricated in well-ventilated areas because of noxious fumes produced by catalytic reaction. Silicone rubber requires addition of a separate catalyst to create the endogenous heat necessary for the conversion from a liquid to solid state. When purchasing silicone rubber for fabricating negative hand molds, ensure that the product is safe for direct skin application. In addition to choosing a safe product, select a product with a catalyst that has a reasonable setting time (~5-7 minutes) for hand molding purposes. After thoroughly mixing the silicone rubber and catalyst, the silicone rubber is

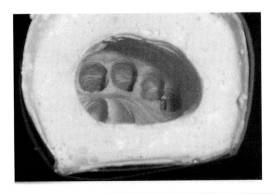

Fig. 24-7   Inner view of an alginate negative mold after removal of the subject's hand shows excellent detail. Any excess or loose pieces of alginate are carefully removed to minimize defects in the positive mold.

applied to the hand and wrist using a tongue depressor or similar tool in a manner similar to that of icing a cake (hence, the "brush-on" method). Any silicone rubber that runs off the hand and onto the wax paper is scraped up and reapplied to the hand until a surface layer of about 5-7 mm is achieved and the silicone rubber becomes unworkable. Once set, the silicone rubber negative mold is slightly flexible, allowing for removal of the subject's hand from the mold.

Materials
The materials needed include the following:
- Aprons and/or old lab coats
- Newspapers, plastic sheeting
- Wax paper
- Nonsterile gloves (wear during mixing of silicone rubber and catalyst)
- Dust mask
- Protective eyewear
- Petroleum jelly
- Silicone rubber and catalyst (~1 lb., skin-safe)
- Tongue depressors
- Mixing bowl

Procedure
1. Cover self, subject, and work area with protective garments or materials.
2. Coat skin and any hair with a thin layer of petroleum jelly. Avoid using too much petroleum jelly as it may decrease the final amount of surface detail in the final positive mold (Fig. 24-8).
3. Set aside a small amount of silicone rubber along with a proportional amount of catalyst for later use to repair cuts made in the negative mold.
4. Mix silicone rubber and catalyst per manufacturer's directions with tongue depressor.
5. Position hand.
6. Pour mixture slowly over subject's hand as the subject gradually rotates hand. Scrape excess material from wax paper and reapply to hand. Cover all desired areas evenly with a thick layer (~5-7 mm thick) of silicone rubber (Fig. 24-9).
7. Subject's hand must remain motionless until silicone rubber cures, becoming firm to the touch.
8. Small cuts may be created in the tip of each digit to aid in releasing suction.
9. Instruct subject to gently rotate hand and wiggle digits to facilitate removal from mold.
10. If the negative mold includes the forearm, it may be necessary to make a small cut in the mold at the radial wrist level to allow hand to be removed from mold, depending on individual hand size and configuration.

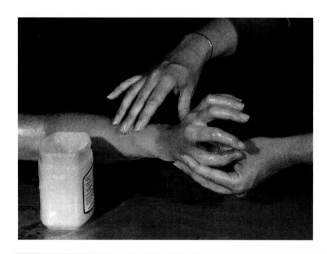

Fig. 24-8 Skin and hair should be thoroughly covered with a thin coating of petroleum jelly to prevent adherence to the inner surfaces of the negative mold.

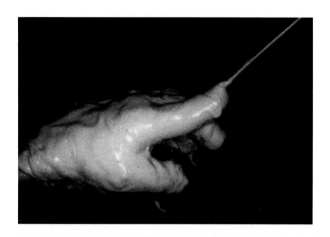

Fig. 24-9 To ensure adequate coverage, careful attention should be directed to the web spaces and adjacent finger surfaces.

11. Remove mold from hand by gently pulling in a distal direction.
12. Inspect inner area of the mold and remove any loose debris (Fig. 24-10).
13. Externally repair any cuts or tears in the negative mold with additional silicone rubber or tape.
14. Proceed to the section entitled "Positive Hand Mold Fabrication." Plaster or dental acrylic may be used for casting the positive mold.

Plaster Bandage Method[1,3,4,8]

General Considerations

An alternative method of negative mold fabrication is the plaster bandage wrap method. This method may be used in situations where detail-producing negative

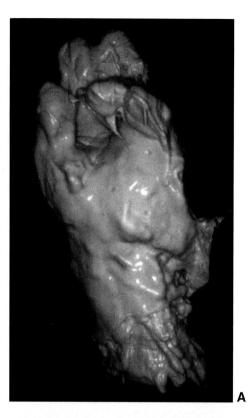

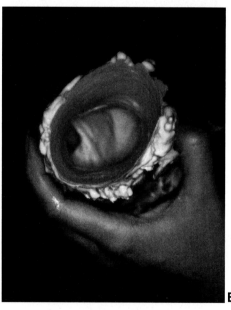

Fig. 24-10 External (A) and internal (B) views of a silicone rubber negative mold show excellent detail.

mold fabrication materials are scarce or cost prohibitive and/or only a positive mold of the aggregate form of the hand is desired.

Plaster cures through an endogenous heat process created by a catalytic reaction between water and crystallized gypsum. The strength of plaster is proportionate to the ratio of plaster and water as well as the type of plaster used. Adjusting the water temperature may to some extent regulate curing time of the plaster. An increased temperature externally augments the catalytic heat response and decreases the curing time. Plaster-impregnated bandage is available in a range of approximate setting times and should be selected according to the specific task and the expertise of the clinician. When applied, wet layers of plaster bandage should be worked until the plaster layers are integrated and smooth. Adjustments during the curing time for most plaster bandage molds should be kept to a minimum because disruption of the plaster molecules at this stage may cause weakness in the mold. Plaster bandages are applied to the hand and forearm in a series of layers thick enough to maintain dimensional stability upon removal of the plaster bandage negative mold. During the removal process, cuts are made in the negative mold to facilitate removal of the hand. After repair of these cuts, a mold release agent is used to coat the inner surface of the plaster bandage negative mold. This coating prevents adherence of the negative and positive molds, both of which are made of homogeneous plaster. Once the plaster positive hardens, the negative mold is carefully removed.

Materials
The materials needed include the following:
- Aprons and/or old lab coats
- Newspapers, plastic sheeting
- Dust mask
- Protective eyewear
- Nonsterile gloves (plaster may cause skin irritation)
- Plaster bandage, 2-inch width, fast-curing (about three rolls to cover hand and forearm)
- Pan of water
- Bandage scissors
- Petroleum jelly
- Mold release agent (options: commercially available mold release agents, paraffin wax, or a mixture of 1:1 kerosene to liquid soap)
- Paper towels

Procedure
1. Cover subject and work area with protective garments or materials.
2. Precut plaster bandage strips according to the length of intended mold and size of the hand and forearm. Following are measurements for a forearm and hand mold on an adult subject:
    a. 12 to 15 14-inch lengths (includes 2-inch distal overlap) for forearm/hand
    b. Several $\frac{1}{2}$-inch widths 8 inches long for reinforcement of thumb, first web space, and fingers.
    c. One 18- to 24-inch length for the final spiraling wrap.
3. Evenly coat subject's hand and forearm skin and hair with a thin layer of petroleum jelly (Fig. 24-8).
4. Position digits and wrist.
5. Roll strips, and as needed dip into water, gently wringing to remove excess water.
6. Apply wet strips, longitudinally to forearm and hand, alternating dorsally and volarly. The 2-inch additional length of each strip is brought around fingertips and run in a proximal direction to provide overlapping of strip ends (if desired, fingertips may be wrapped separately). Work around forearm with overlapping strips until two or three layers have been worked together (Fig. 24-11).
7. Use narrower bandage strips when working on thumb and reinforcing first web space and fingers.
8. Spiral the final strip around the extremity to provide circumferential stability.
9. Allow plaster to set approximately 10-15 minutes.
10. Loosen the negative mold by having subject rotate forearm.
11. Cut mold with bandage scissors to allow extraction of hand. Cut should be in the shape of an elongated Y following radial aspect of forearm and first and second metacarpals. For patient comfort, at the level of the wrist, the cut should be routed dorsal to the head of the radius (Fig. 24-12, *A-C*).
12. Remove negative mold by pulling gently in a distal direction.
13. Close the radial cut and externally reinforce weak areas in the negative mold with additional strips of plaster bandage (Fig. 24-13).
14. When using plaster to create the positive mold, it is necessary to coat the inner surfaces of the negative mold with a mold release agent to prevent adherence of the plaster positive mold to the plaster bandage negative mold. Mold release agents include specific products designed and labeled as such, paraffin wax (using a heat gun for melting), or a 1:1 mixture of kerosene (purchased from a hardware store) and liquid soap.
15. Proceed to the next section.

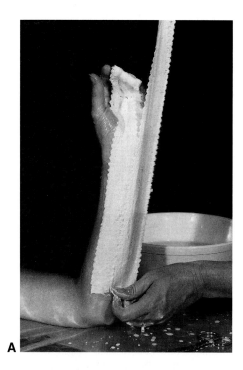

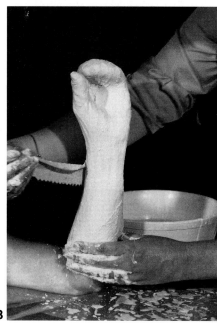

Fig. 24-11 A-B, Plaster strips are applied to alternate surfaces of the hand and thumb until a thickness of three layers is reached. Because of the potential for collapse at the time of removal, care should be taken to reinforce the thumb, first web space, and fingers.

Positive Hand Mold Fabrication

Pour Method Using Plaster[1,3,4,8]

General Considerations

The pour method simply involves mixing plaster with water until a consistency of heavy cream is achieved and pouring the liquid plaster, in stages, directly into

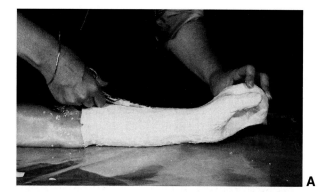

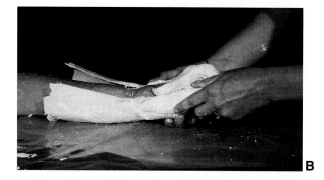

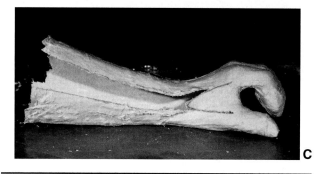

Fig. 24-12 A-C, The radial Y-shaped opening allows extraction of the hand from the plaster negative mold. Because of pressure from the scissors on underlying tissue, the course of the cut should run slightly dorsal to the prominences of the head of the radius and first metacarpal and slightly palmar to the lateral aspect of the second metacarpal. Once the cut is complete, the negative mold is removed from the hand by gently pulling distally.

the negative mold. Plaster cures through an endogenous heat process created by a catalytic reaction between water and crystallized gypsum. The strength of plaster is proportionate to the ratio of plaster and water as well as the type of plaster used. Adjusting the water temperature may to some extent regulate curing time of plaster. An increased temperature externally augments the catalytic heat response and decreases the curing time. A high-quality plaster rather than ordinary plaster of Paris is recommended for the casting material used in the negative mold due to its greater strength and impression ability.[11] *Warning:*

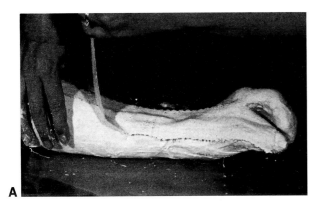

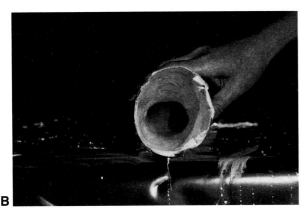

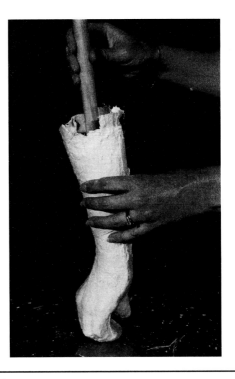

Fig. 24-14   A dowel rod or similar object incorporated into the positive mold at the time of pouring allows the finished mold to be secured in a vise, display stand, etc.

Fig. 24-13   **A,** The radial cut is closed with additional layers of plaster bandage. **B,** Visual examination of the internal surfaces of the mold by holding it to a light source will reveal weak areas in the layers of plaster.

Because of the endogenous heat created by a catalytic reaction between water and crystallized gypsum during the curing process of plaster, liquid plaster must not be used for direct fabrication of negative hand molds (i.e., poured around a subject's hand within a container) due to its potential for causing a burn injury to the skin as well as entrapment of the hand.[13]

During incremental pouring of the plaster into the negative mold, the mold is tapped and rotated to minimize air bubble production. Once the negative mold is completely filled, wait 2 hours before its removal to minimize risk of breaking digits. At this point, the plaster is still not fully dry allowing for cosmetic touch-up if needed. Two to three days are required for the plaster positive to completely dry before applying a finish.

Materials
- The materials needed include the following:
- Aprons and/or old lab coats
- Newspapers, plastic sheeting
- Dust mask
- Protective eyewear
- Gloves, if desired (plaster may cause drying of the skin)
- High-quality plaster for positive mold-making
- Water (temperature per plaster manufacturer's recommendation)
- Measuring cups
- Gram scale (required if plaster is measured according to weight)
- Large mixing bowl
- Cake spatula
- Mixing spoon
- Thermometer

Procedure
1. Cover self, subject, and work area with protective garments or materials.
2. Consult manufacturer's recommendations for mixing ratios and quantity of plaster required to fabricate an adult-sized positive hand mold.
3. Set aside a small amount of unmixed, dry plaster for later use to repair defects in the final positive mold.
4. Mix plaster into water by hand (with donned glove) or use cake spatula. Mix until the consistency of heavy cream is achieved (refer to the section on tips to minimize air bubbles).

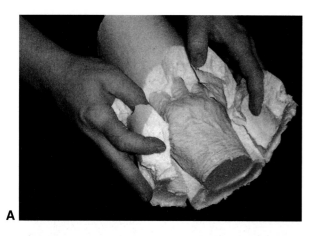

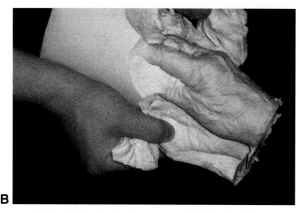

Fig. 24-15   **A,B,** Once plaster sets, the negative mold is carefully peeled away to reveal the beautifully detailed positive mold; removal of a negative mold fabricated using the matrix method with molding alginate.

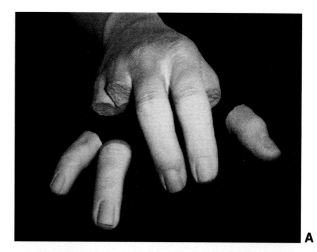

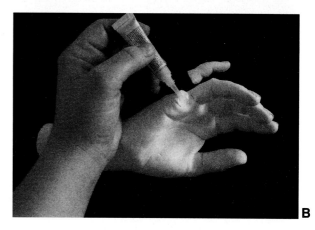

Fig. 24-16   **A,** Aggressive demolding may result in unintentional breaking of positive mold fingers. **B,** Once plaster fully dries, broken fingers may be reattached using cyanoacrylate glue.

5. Pour a small amount of the plaster mixture into negative mold, rotating and shaking mold gently to allow plaster to flow into the more distal crevices. (Note: When pouring liquid plaster into a plaster bandage negative mold, be sure to carefully support the negative mold. Avoid resting the distal end of the mold on a hard surface as the weight of poured plaster may cause collapse of this area. After the plaster hardens, the plaster bandage mold may be laid flat on a table surface.)

6. Slowly fill negative mold with plaster mixture, continuing to rotate and shake mold gently to dislodge air bubbles.

7. Optional: If desired, a dowel rod or similar object may be incorporated into the positive mold (Fig. 24-14).

8. When the plaster is completely solid and cool to the touch, gently peel away and dispose of the negative mold to reveal the plaster positive hand mold (Fig. 24-15). If necessary, a knife may be used to carefully cut away the negative

mold while avoiding cutting the surface of the underlying positive mold. During this process, special care must be taken when removing the negative mold from around the thumb and any isolated digits to prevent accidental breakage of these structures (Fig. 24-16).

9. Allow one to two days for the plaster to completely dry (check with plaster manufacturer regarding oven heating to decrease drying time).

10. Repair holes etc. with freshly mixed plaster.

11. Remove surface irregularities using fine sandpaper or a dull knife.

12. Seal plaster with a lacquer, acrylic, or shellac.

13. Finish as desired.

Pour Method Using Dental Acrylic[2,3,4,8]

General Considerations

The pour method involves preparing the dental acrylic by mixing in its catalyst and pouring it, in stages, directly into the negative mold. During pouring, the

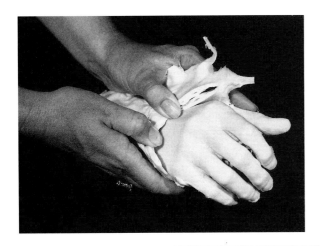

Fig. 24-17   Because the materials are heterogeneous, the silicone rubber negative mold is easily peeled from the positive without the need for an intervening separator substance.

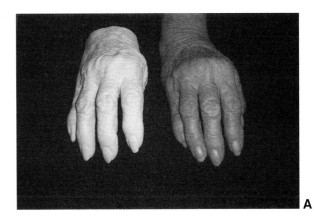

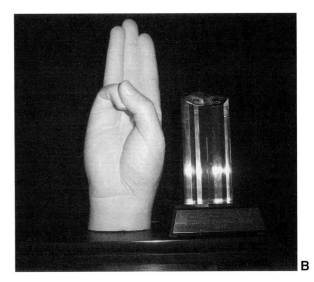

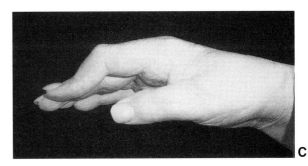

Fig. 24-18   A, Detailed plaster mold of an osteoarthritic hand along with the hand from which it was cast. B, Hand reproductions may serve as works of art as shown in this award. The trophy displays the Boy Scouts of America's scout sign. C, This positive mold of a rheumatoid hand is used for teaching to demonstrate a boutonniere deformity.

negative mold is rotated and tapped to minimize production of air bubbles. After the fingers in the negative mold have been filled with dental acrylic, the mold may be rotated during pouring of the proximal wrist and forearm areas so that a thinner outer layer of dental acrylic is formed creating a hollow center of the positive mold, if desired.

Because of noxious fumes produced by catalytic reaction, the fabrication of hand casts from dental acrylic must be carried out in a well-ventilated area, ideally under a ventilation hood to ensure maximum safety. Dental acrylic requires the addition of a separate catalyst to create the endogenous heat necessary for the conversion from a liquid to solid state. In comparison to positive molds made with plaster, acrylic molds are lighter, more durable, and have an appealing plastic-like appearance. Additionally, dental acrylic positive molds allow artists to achieve a more lifelike appearance when painted than that obtainable with plaster.[2]

Materials
The materials needed include the following:
- Aprons and/or old lab coats
- Newspapers, plastic sheeting
- Dust mask
- Protective eyewear
- Gloves
- Dental acrylic or similar substance and catalyst
- Tongue depressor
- Mixing container

Procedure
1. Cover self, subject, and work area with protective garments or materials.
2. Prepare dental acrylic according to manufacturer's specifications.
3. Mix acrylic until the consistency of heavy cream is achieved (refer to the section on tips to minimize air bubbles).
4. Pour a small amount of acrylic into the negative mold, rotating and shaking mold gently to allow the dental acrylic to flow into the more distal crevices.

5. Slowly fill negative mold with acrylic, continuing to rotate and shake mold gently to dislodge air bubbles.

6. The proximal end (i.e., wrist or forearm portion) of the mold does not have to be completely filled with acrylic. By continuing to rotate the negative mold, a thick layer of acrylic will form, leaving a hollow center.

7. When the acrylic is completely solid and cool to the touch, gently peel away and dispose of the silicone rubber negative mold to reveal the acrylic positive hand mold (Fig. 24-17). If necessary, a knife may be used to carefully cut away the negative mold while avoiding cutting the surface of the underlying positive mold. During this process, special care must be taken when removing the negative mold from around the thumb and any isolated digits to prevent accidental breakage of these structures.

8. Sand or file any surface irregularities.

9. Finish as desired.

■ SUMMARY

Although negative/positive molds are not used as they formerly were, a definite place remains for the methods described in this chapter in certain clinical situations. In addition, accurate hand reproductions created by these methods may be of considerable value in teaching students and clinicians, educating patients, providing a permanent record of a particular hand or changes in deformity, a keepsake, or simply to serve as a work of art (Fig. 24-18).

REFERENCES

1. Barr NR: *The hand: principles and techniques of simple splint-making in rehabilitation*, Butterworth, 1975, London.
2. Beck J: Personal communication to R. Janson, 2003, Indianapolis.
3. Fess EE, Gettle K, Strickland J: *Hand splinting: principles and methods*, Mosby, 1981, St. Louis.
4. Fess EE, Philips C: *Hand splinting: principles and methods*, ed 2, Mosby, 1987, St. Louis.
5. Kerr Dental, *Kerr Dental formatray liquid material safety data sheet*, 2003.
6. Kerr Dental, *Kerr Dental formatray powder material safety data sheet*, 2003.
7. Malick M: *Manual on dynamic hand splinting with thermoplastic materials*, Harmarville Rehabilitation Center, 1974, Pittsburgh.
8. Malick M: *Manual on static hand splinting*, vol 1, Harmarville Rehabilitation Center, 1970, Pittsburgh.
9. McCormick E: *Alginate—lifecasters' gold*, Art Casting J Assoc Lifecasters Int, 2001.
10. McCormick E: *Lifecasting hands and feet*, ArtMolds Sculpture Studio, 2001, Summit, NJ.
11. McCormick E: Personal communication to R. Janson, 2002.
12. McCormick E: Personal communication to R. Janson, 2003.
13. United States Gypsum Company: *Material safety data sheet USG Hydrocal White Gypsum Cement*, 2002, United States Gypsum Company (1999).
14. Winn Creative Corporation: *Body parts LifeCast kit step-by-step instructions*, section I: basic LifeCast design, Winn Creative Corporation.

RESOURCES*

ArtMolds Sculpture Studio, LLC, www.artmolds.com, 18 Bank Street, Summit, NJ 07901, 866-ARTMOLDS.

LifeCast, www.lifecast.net, Winn Creative Corp, PO Box 5886 Incline Village, NV 89450, 866-278-6653.

Special Effect Supply Corporation, www.fxsupply.com, 164 East Center Street, North Salt Lake, UT 84054, (801) 936-9762.

The Casting Kit Company, www.castingkits.com, 6648 South Highway 89, Unit 8, Ogden, UT, 84405, 1-800-211-2741.

NOTES

Products advertised as skin-safe are available through vendors listed. (Note: Authors have not tested all of the products listed.) Listed resources are not all inclusive of products available. Quality of products and/or service is not implied. Company and product information subject to change without notice.

SILICONE RUBBER PRODUCTS

- Dow Corning silicone rubber 3110 & catalyst no. 4 (Dow Corning: Midland, Michigan 48686, www.dow-corning.com, 989-496-7881) has been used by the authors without incident for negative mold fabrication. Setting time of approximately 3-20 minutes depending on mixing ratio. Note: Dow Corning does not endorse this product for mold making directly on the skin.

- When using RTV11 (1 pound), you may use STO catalyst (purchased separately) to speed up setting time.

- Sammons Preston Rolyan elastomer (Sammons Preston Rolyan: Bolingbrook, Illinois, 800-323-5547). Decrease manufacturer's recommended amount of catalyst to increase working time.

DENTAL ACRYLIC

- Kerr Formatray (Kerr Dental: Orange, California, www.kerrdental.com, 800-537-7123)

---

*Supplies, kits, instructional materials, and material safety data sheets

Splint Room Organization*

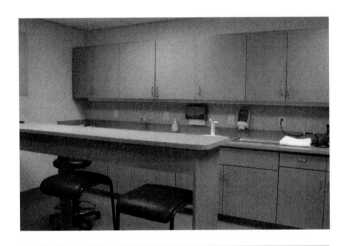

Fig. A-1 This efficiently designed splint room incorporates a raised worktable to simplify and speed splint fabrication. The worktable is elevated slightly to adapt ergonomically to therapists' heights and its narrow width allows easy access to patients' upper extremities, decreasing potential for therapist arm and back fatigue. Therapists may stand or sit between the table and the conveniently situated cabinets that are within easy reach.

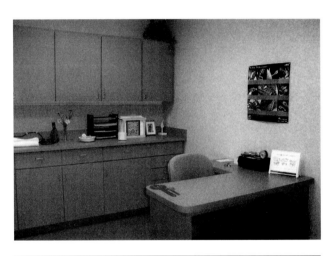

Fig. A-2 A therapy treatment table is located within the same room to allow evaluation and treatment of patients without leaving the splint area. The majority of patients in this particular clinic are referred for splint fabrication; therefore, more square footage is dedicated to that purpose. The splint fabrication worktable may also be used as a hand therapy table if needed.

*Clinic design by Cheri Alexy, OTR, CHT, Methodist Sports Medicine Clinic, Indianapolis, IN.

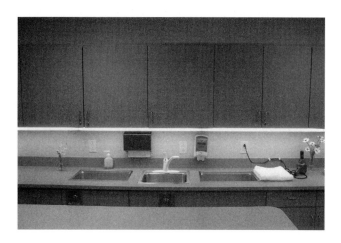

Fig. A-3 A counter insert for a hot water pan is strategically placed close to the splint fabrication worktable, providing an efficient workspace where water is maintained at a constant temperature appropriate for low-temperature splinting materials. The expanded size of the inserted pan allows immersion of larger pieces of materials or splints and a valve situated beneath the pan facilitates drainage. Positioned adjacent to the insert pan, a faucet simplifies quick cooling of heated materials and filling of the pan. On the opposite side of the pan, a heat gun and a towel for cooling and drying materials prior to fitting are situated.

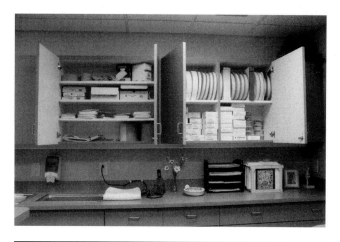

Fig. A-5 Cabinets behind the worktable are within easy reaching distance. They contain low-temperature thermoplastics, strapping materials, tools, and hand therapy supplies. Ergonomic modifications and the working efficiency afforded by this excellently designed splint room reflect the skill and expertise of a highly experienced therapist specializing in hand/upper extremity rehabilitation.

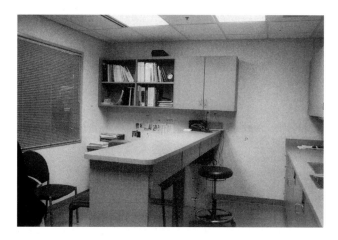

Fig. A-4 Drawers in the worktable allow effortless retrieval of equipment and tools that may be required during splint fabrication. The left corner of the splint room keeps books and files accessible so therapists do not have to leave the main work area.

Forms

Forms Included in This Appendix

RANGE OF MOTION
HAND

DATE: _____	THUMB	CHANGE +/−	INDEX	CHANGE +/−	LONG	CHANGE +/−	RING	CHANGE +/−	SMALL	CHANGE +/−
MP	( ) ( )		( ) ( )		( ) ( )		( ) ( )		( ) ( )	
PIP	IP ( ) ( )		( ) ( )		( ) ( )		( ) ( )		( ) ( )	
DIP	CMC ( ) ( )		( ) ( )		( ) ( )		( ) ( )		( ) ( )	
TAM (TPM)	( ) ( )		( ) ( )		( ) ( )		( ) ( )		( ) ( )	

DATE: _____	THUMB	CHANGE +/−	INDEX	CHANGE +/−	LONG	CHANGE +/−	RING	CHANGE +/−	SMALL	CHANGE +/−
MP	( ) ( )		( ) ( )		( ) ( )		( ) ( )		( ) ( )	
PIP	IP ( ) ( )		( ) ( )		( ) ( )		( ) ( )		( ) ( )	
DIP	CMC ( ) ( )		( ) ( )		( ) ( )		( ) ( )		( ) ( )	
TAM (TPM)	( ) ( )		( ) ( )		( ) ( )		( ) ( )		( ) ( )	

DATE: _____	THUMB	CHANGE +/−	INDEX	CHANGE +/−	LONG	CHANGE +/−	RING	CHANGE +/−	SMALL	CHANGE +/−
MP	( ) ( )		( ) ( )		( ) ( )		( ) ( )		( ) ( )	
PIP	IP ( ) ( )		( ) ( )		( ) ( )		( ) ( )		( ) ( )	
DIP	CMC ( ) ( )		( ) ( )		( ) ( )		( ) ( )		( ) ( )	
TAM (TPM)	( ) ( )		( ) ( )		( ) ( )		( ) ( )		( ) ( )	

KEY:
   Active: extension/flexion
   Passive: (extension/flexion)
   Thumb CMC: adduction/abduction
   Change: record in red

Name: _____

Number: _____

Hand: _____

RANGE OF MOTION
WRIST, FOREARM, ELBOW, SHOULDER

		DATE: _____		DATE: _____		DATE: _____	
			CHANGE +/−		CHANGE +/−		CHANGE +/−
W R I S T	EXTENSION	( ) ( )		( ) ( )		( ) ( )	
	FLEXION	( ) ( )		( ) ( )		( ) ( )	
	RADIAL DEVIATION	( ) ( )		( ) ( )		( ) ( )	
	ULNAR DEVIATION	( ) ( )		( ) ( )		( ) ( )	
F O R E A R M / E L B O W	SUPINATION	( ) ( )		( ) ( )		( ) ( )	
	PRONATION	( ) ( )		( ) ( )		( ) ( )	
	EXTENSION	( ) ( )		( ) ( )		( ) ( )	
	FLEXION	( ) ( )		( ) ( )		( ) ( )	
S H O U L D E R	EXTENSION	( ) ( )		( ) ( )		( ) ( )	
	FLEXION	( ) ( )		( ) ( )		( ) ( )	
	ABDUCTION	( ) ( )		( ) ( )		( ) ( )	
	INTERNAL ROTATION	( ) ( )		( ) ( )		( ) ( )	
	EXTERNAL ROTATION	( ) ( )		( ) ( )		( ) ( )	

KEY:
  Active: #0
  Passive: (#0)
  Change: Record in red

Name: _____
Number: _____
Extremity: _____

EXAMPLE OF COMPLETED ROM FORM

DATE: _____	THUMB	CHANGE +/−	INDEX	CHANGE +/−	LONG	CHANGE +/−	RING	CHANGE +/−	SMALL	CHANGE +/−
MP	( ) ( )		30/70 (0/90) ( )	+10	10/30 ( ) ( )		( ) ( )		( ) ( )	
PIP	IP ( ) ( )		45/60 (0/90) ( )	+15	30/45 ( ) ( )		( ) ( )		( ) ( )	
DIP	CMC ( ) ( )		10/80 (0/90) ( )	+5	0/75 ( ) ( )		( ) ( )		( ) ( )	
TAM (TPM)	( ) ( )		125 (270) ( )		110 ( ) ( )		( ) ( )		( ) ( )	

Total motion provides a single numerical value for composite digital motion: summation of digit flexion (30 + 45 + 75 = 150); summation of digit extension deficits (10 + 30 + 0 = 40); flexion sum minus extension deficit sum (150 − 40 = 110); total active motion of digit equals 110.
(Long Finger)

SUMMARY SHEET
TOTAL ACTIVE MOTION/TOTAL PASSIVE MOTION

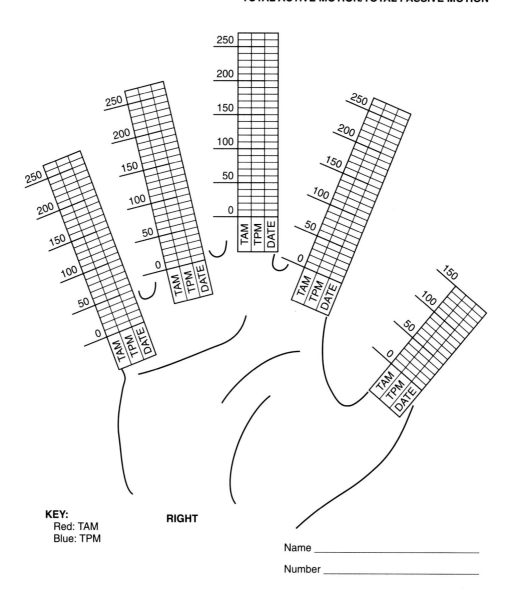

KEY:
Red: TAM
Blue: TPM

RIGHT

Name _____

Number _____

VOLUME

VOLUMETER MEASUREMENTS:

	Date	Date	Date	Date	Date	Date
800 ml						
700 ml						
600 ml						
500 ml						
400 ml						
300 ml						
200 ml						

NORMAL VOLUME (opposite hand): _____ ml.

CIRCUMFERENCE/DIAMETER[c]:

Biceps*	_____	_____	_____	_____	_____	_____
Forearm*	_____	_____	_____	_____	_____	_____
DPC	_____	_____	_____	_____	_____	_____
Digit (_____)	_____	_____	_____	_____	_____	_____

NORMAL MEASUREMENT (opposite hand):

Biceps _____ Forearm _____ DPC _____ Digit _____

c Circle method used.

* 10 cm. above/below the medial
   epicondyle of the humerus

Name: _____

Number: _____

Hand: _____

GRIP STRENGTH

JAYMAR DYNAMOMETER # _____

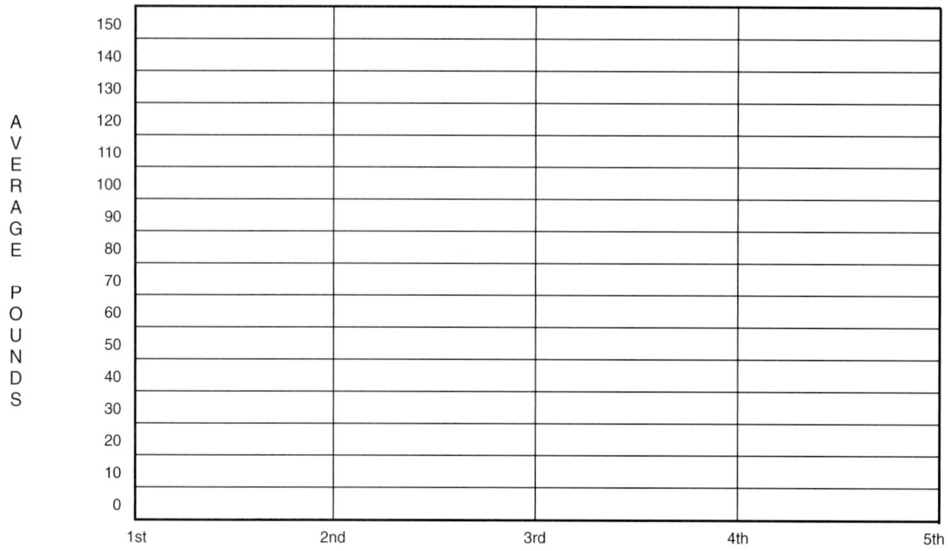

A
V
E
R
A
G
E

P
O
U
N
D
S

150				
140				
130				
120				
110				
100				
90				
80				
70				
60				
50				
40				
30				
20				
10				
0				

1st   2nd   3rd   4th   5th

TRIALS: HANDLE POSITION

N
O
R
M
A
L

DATE _____ (———)

	1st	2nd	3rd	4th	5th
(1)	_____	_____	_____	_____	_____
(2)	_____	_____	_____	_____	_____
(3)	_____ *	_____ *	_____ *	_____ *	_____
Average:	_____	_____	_____	_____	_____

DATE _____ (· · · · ·)

	1st	2nd	3rd	4th	5th
(1)	_____	_____	_____	_____	_____
(2)	_____	_____	_____	_____	_____
(3)	_____ *	_____ *	_____ *	_____ *	_____
Average:	_____	_____	_____	_____	_____

DATE _____ (· · · · ·)

	1st	2nd	3rd	4th	5th
(1)	_____	_____	_____	_____	_____
(2)	_____	_____	_____	_____	_____
(3)	_____ *	_____ *	_____ *	_____ *	_____
Average:	_____	_____	_____	_____	_____

DATE _____ (xxxxx)

	1st	2nd	3rd	4th	5th
(1)	_____	_____	_____	_____	_____
(2)	_____	_____	_____	_____	_____
(3)	_____ *	_____ *	_____ *	_____ *	_____
Average:	_____	_____	_____	_____	_____

*5-minute rest period

Name: _____

Number: _____

Hand: _____

NERVE-MUSCLE EXAMINATION

DATE	DATE	DATE	
			Upper
			Middle trapezius (Accessory, C_3 and C_4)
			Lower
			Rhomboids
			Supraspinatus
			Infraspinatus
			Serratus anterior
			Teres major
			Clavicle }Pectoralis major
			Sternum
			Latissimus dorsi
			Biceps and brachialis
			Coracobrachialis
			Anterior
			Middle
			Posterior }Deltoid
			Teres minor
			Pronator quadratus
			Pronator teres
			Flexor carpi radialis
			Flexor digitorum profundus 1, 2
			Flexor digitorum superficialis
			Palmaris longus
			Flexor pollicis longus
			Flexor pollicis brevis (superficial head)
			Abductor pollicis brevis
			Opponens pollicis
			Lumbricals 1, 2
			Triceps
			Supinator
			Brachioradialis
			Extensor carpi radialis
			Extensor carpi ulnaris
			Extensor digitorum communis
			Extensor digiti quinti
			Extensor indicis proprius
			Extensor policis longus
			Extensor policis brevis
			Abductor policis longus
			Flexor carpi ulnaris
			Flexor digitorum profundus 3, 4
			Abductor digiti quinti
			Abductor pollicis
			Opponens digiti quinti
			1
			2 Dorsal
			3 interossei
			4
			1 Volar
			2 interossei
			3
			Lumbricals 3, 4
			Flexor pollicis brevis (deep head)

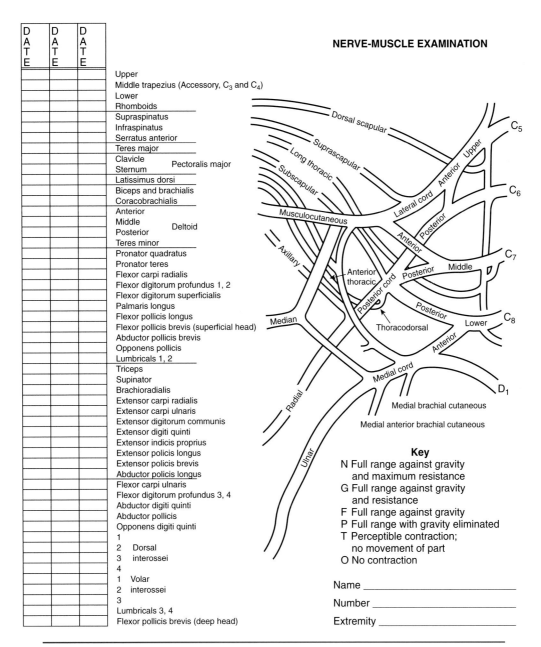

Key

N Full range against gravity
   and maximum resistance
G Full range against gravity
   and resistance
F Full range against gravity
P Full range with gravity eliminated
T Perceptible contraction;
   no movement of part
O No contraction

Name _____

Number _____

Extremity _____

Adapted from form by Lorraine F. Lake, Ph.D.

SENSIBILITY AND PAIN

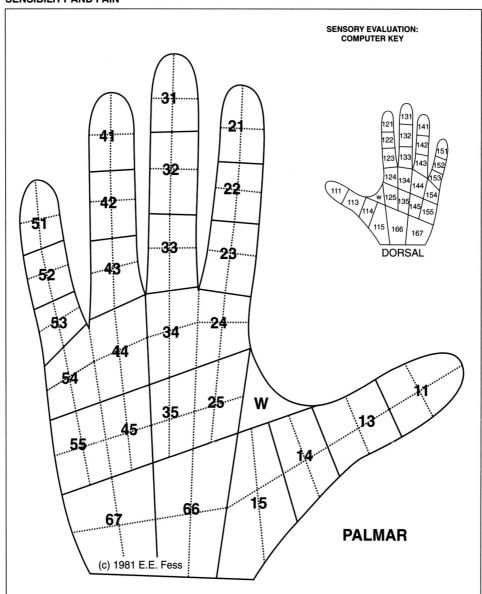

SENSORY EVALUATION:
COMPUTER KEY

DORSAL

PALMAR

(c) 1981 E.E. Fess

Longitudinal:
10s = Thumb ray
20s = Index ray
30s = Long ray
40s = Ring ray
50s = Small ray
60s = Carpus*

Transverse:
1s = Distal phalanx
2s = Middle phalanx
3s = Proximal phalanx
4s = Distal palm
5s = Mid palm
6/7s = Proximal palm*

Anterior/Posterior
10s = Volar
100s = Dorsal

Subdivisions:
D = Distal
P = Proximal
R = Radial
U = Ulnar

*Modification suggested by J. Bell, 1982.

SENSORY EVALUATION:
SEMMES-WEINSTEIN CALIBRATED MONOFILAMENTS

PALMAR/DORSAL   (circle):

Date:	Thumb __1__		Index __2__		Long __3__		Ring __4__		Small __5__	
	U	R	U	R	U	R	U	R	U	R
__1										
__2										
__3										
__4										
__5										
__6/__7	/////		__6__				__6__			

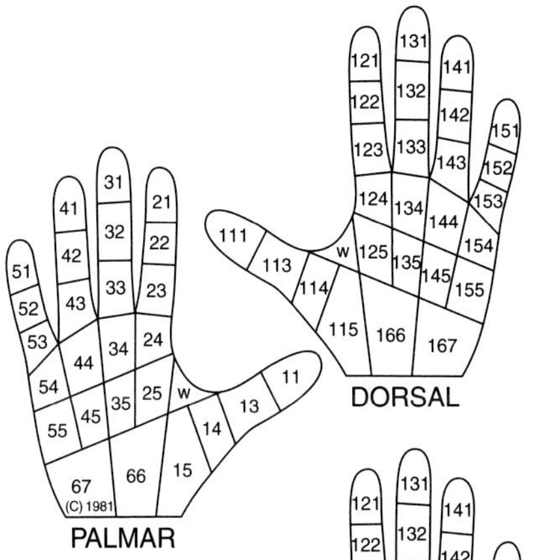

PALMAR/DORSAL   (circle):

Date:	Thumb __1__		Index __2__		Long __3__		Ring __4__		Small __5__	
	U	R	U	R	U	R	U	R	U	R
__1										
__2										
__3										
__4										
__5										
__6/__7	/////		__6__				__6__			

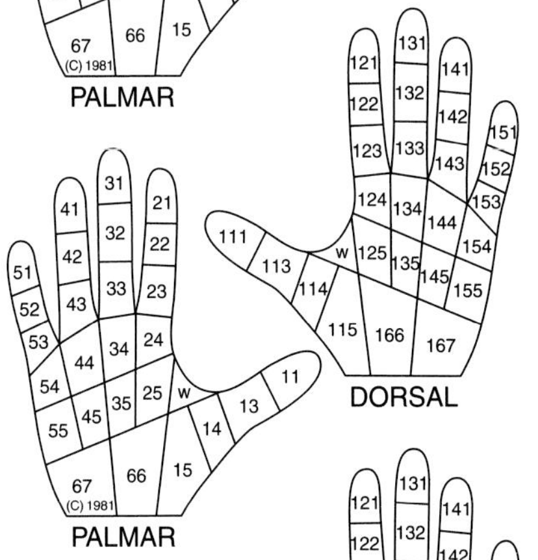

PALMAR/DORSAL   (circle):

Date:	Thumb __1__		Index __2__		Long __3__		Ring __4__		Small __5__	
	U	R	U	R	U	R	U	R	U	R
__1										
__2										
__3										
__4										
__5										
__6/__7	/////		__6__				__6__			

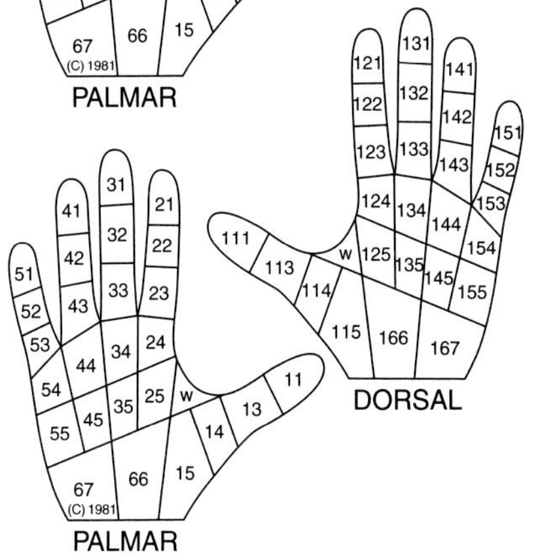

KEY:*

		Filament	Pressure
	Normal	1.65-2.83	1.45-4.86
Blue	Diminished light touch	3.22-3.61	11.1-17.7
Purple	Diminished protective sensation	3.84-4.31	19.3-33.1
Red	Loss of protective sensation	4.56-6.65	47.3-439.0
Red-lined	Untestable	6.65	439.0
Levine, S., Pearsall, G., & Ruderman, R.: J Hand Surg., 3:211,1978.			(gm/mm²)

Name: _____

Number: _____

Hand: _____

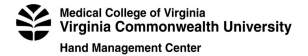

Medical College of Virginia
Virginia Commonwealth University
Hand Management Center

PAIN EVALUATION

Name _____   Date _____

Right Arm

Intensity

Unpleasantness

DORSAL

PALMAR

Courtesy Karen Hull Lauckardt, M.A., R.P.T.

REFERRAL

SPLINT REFERRAL FORM

DATE: _____

PATIENT NAME: _____

DIAGNOSIS: _____

_____

      DATE OF INJURY _____

      PRECAUTIONS: _____

      HAND/EXTREMITY INJURED *(CIRCLE):*   R   L

Using the chart and abbreviations below, please indicate the primary joint(s), purpose(s), and direction(s) of splint. See following page for examples of completed referral form.

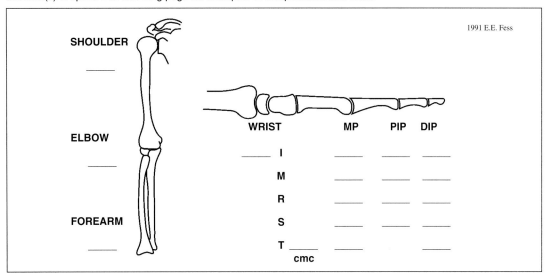

1. PRIMARY JOINTS: circle
                            (primary joints only)

2. PURPOSE:
    Immobilization   X
    Mobilization: →
    Restriction: (X)
        Specific degrees: *(write as needed)*

    Torque Transmission: ≥

3. DIRECTION:
    Abduction   <>
    Abduction, Palmar   PA
    Abduction, Radial   RA
    Adduction   ><

Circumduction   C
Deviation, Ulnar   UD
Deviation, Radial   RD
Distraction   D
Extension   ↑
Flexion   ↓
Pronation   P
Rotation, Internal   IR
Rotation, External   ER
Supination   S
Other: _____

4. Nonarticular splint _____
             _____
             _____

SIGNATURE: _____

Examples of completed referral forms:

Index-small finger MP flexion mobilization splint, type 1 (5)

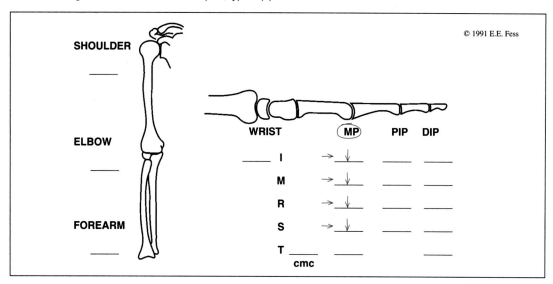

Wrist immobilization splint, type 0 (1)

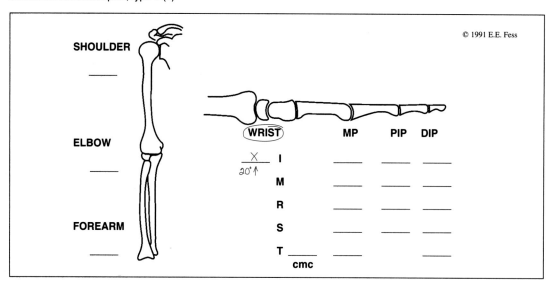

American Society for Surgery of the Hand Total Active Motion/Total Passive Motion*

█ MOTION

1. Total passive motion (TPM): Sum of angles formed by metacarpal (MIP), proximal interphalangeal (PIP), and distal interphalangeal (DIP) joints in maximum passive flexion minus the sum of angles of deficit from complete extension at each of these three joints: (MP + PIP + DIP) − (MP + PIP + DIP) = Total flexion − Total extensor lag = TPM.

2. Total active motion (TAM): Sum of angles formed by MP, PIP, and DIP joints in maximum active flexion; that is, fist position, minus total extension deficit at the MP, PIP, and DIP joints with active finger extension. Significant hyperextension at any joint, particularly the PIP and DIP joints, is recorded as a deficit in extension and is included in the total extension deficit. Hyperextension must be considered an abnormal value in swan neck (PIP) and boutonniere deformities (DIP). Comparison of pretreatment and post-treatment TAM values will be significant; however, comparison as a percentage of normal value is invalid. TAM is a term applied to one finger and is as follows:

   a. Sum of active MP flexion plus active PIP flexion plus active DIP flexion

   b. Minus sum of incomplete active extension if any is present (Figs. C-1 to C-3).

---

*From the American Society for Surgery of the Hand: *The hand examination and diagnosis*, ed 2, Churchill Livingstone, 1983, New York.

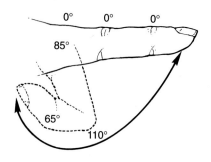

Fig. C-1 Normal range of motion.

Active	Flexion	Extension lack
MP	85°	0°
PIP	110°	0°
DIP	65°	0°
Totals	260°	0°

TAM = 260° − 0° = 260°

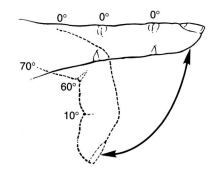

Fig. C-3 Limited metacarpophalangeal and proximal interphalangeal joint flexion with good extension.

Active	Flexion	Extension lack
MP	70°	0°
PIP	60°	0°
DIP	10°	0°
Totals	140°	0°

TAM = 140° − 0° = 140°

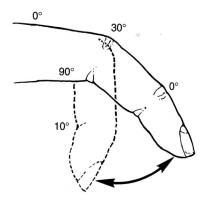

Fig. C-2 Stiff metacarpophalangeal and limited proximal interphalangeal joint extension.

Active	Flexion	Extension lack
MP	0°	0°
PIP	90°	30°
DIP	10°	0°
Totals	100°	30°

TAM = 100° − 30° = 70°

Brachial Plexus Mnemonic

"53-year-old Robert Taylor"© is a simple memory device for learning the nomenclature and form of the brachial plexus.[1] It is not intended to replace formal study of the brachial plexus.

The mnemonic "**Robert Taylor Drinks Coffee Black**" has been used to recall the nomenclature of the levels of the brachial plexus: (proximal to distal) **R** = Rami, **T** = Trunks, **D** = Divisions, **C** = Cords, and **B** = Branches.

The rationale for Robert Taylor's age of 53 years is that the structures at each of the levels are in groups of five and three throughout the brachial plexus: beginning with C5 of the five anterior rami of spinal nerves C5, C6, C7, C8, and T1; three trunks (superior, middle, and inferior); three anterior and three posterior divisions, three cords (lateral, posterior, and medial), and five terminal branches (musculocutaneous, axillary, radial, median, and ulnar nerves).

After learning the mnemonic and the number of structures at each level of the brachial plexus, the next step is to learn to draw the form of the brachial plexus.

The right anterior view is the view most frequently depicted in anatomy texts illustrating the brachial plexus (Fig. D-1). In learning to draw "53-year-old Robert Taylor," the instructional orientation will change from a right anterior view to that of a vertical view. From this view, the anterior rami of the spinal nerves are oriented horizontally, with the nerves of the brachial plexus "hanging" vertically. From this orientation, the brachial plexus will be drawn in a form that resembles a human body. Once completed, rotate the drawing 90° clockwise to re-approximate the conventional right anterior brachial plexus view.

■ DRAWING "53-YEAR-OLD ROBERT TAYLOR"©

Materials needed include a blank sheet of paper oriented in a portrait view, pencil, and eraser.

Follow the written directions below along with the corresponding illustrations (Figs. D-2 through D-11) in learning to draw "53-year-old Robert Taylor."

1. Draw the 5 spinal nerves on a sign held by Robert Taylor: C5, C6, C7, C8, and T1. Note that the segments begin with C5 and have 5 segments. Add Robert Taylor's face (Fig. D-2).
2. Draw two V-shaped adducted arms with flexed elbows connecting C5 to C6 and C8 to T1 to hold the spinal nerve sign. Add his hands (Fig. D-3).
3. From the point of the flexed elbows, draw the right and left sides of Robert Taylor's body. Label the right and left sides of his body, referencing anatomic position (Fig. D-4).
4. Draw a "V" at the level of the lower abdomen to create hip flexion creases (Fig. D-5).
5. From the point of the "V" (drawn in Fig. D-5), draw a line that divides his lower body into two legs (Fig. D-6).
6. Draw V-shaped pectoralis muscles at his chest level (Fig. D-7).
7. Beginning at spinal nerve C7, draw a line that descends down the middle of the chest, abdomen,

---

©J. Robin Janson, OTR, CHT, 2001.
[1]Authors' note: Many variations of this mnemonic may be found in colloquial usage. This instructional technique does not include the nerve branches originating from the structures proximal to the terminal branches of the brachial plexus.

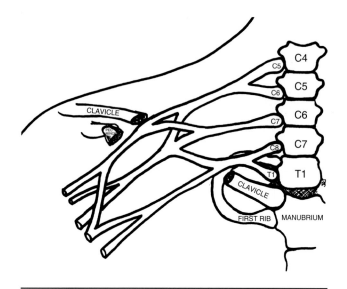

Fig. D-1 Brachial plexus, right anterior view.

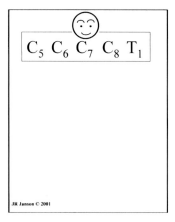

Fig. D-2

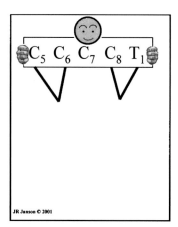

Fig. D-3

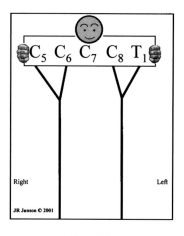

Fig. D-4

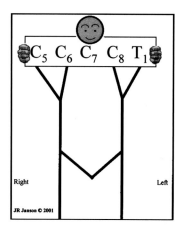

Fig. D-5

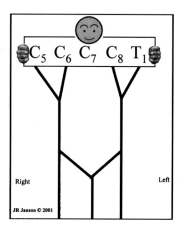

Fig. D-6

and over the middle of Robert Taylor's right leg (Fig. D-8).

8. Draw a line from the center mid-line of his chest that crosses over the right pectoralis muscle line and connects to his right side line just above his waist (Fig. D-9).

9. At the about the center of his abdomen, draw a branch coming off the abdominal mid-line (drawn in Fig. D-8) descending down the lateral portion of his right thigh (Fig. D-10).

10. Rotate drawing 90° clockwise to re-approximate the normal orientation of the right anterior view of the brachial plexus and label structures (Fig. D-11).

11. Practice drawing and labeling "53-year-old Robert Taylor" until committed to memory.

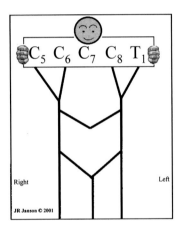

Fig. D-7

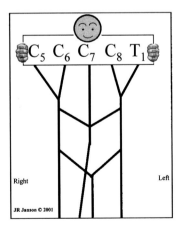

Fig. D-8

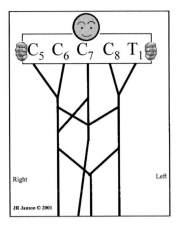

Fig. D-9

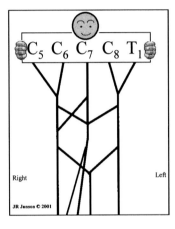

Fig. D-10

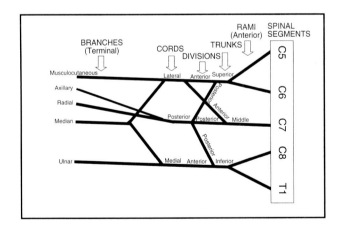

Fig. D-11

SUGGESTED READING

Agur AMR, *Grant's atlas of anatomy*, ed 9, Williams & Wilkins, 1991, Baltimore.

Balke S, *Clinical anatomy made ridiculously simple*, MedMaster, Inc, 1997, Miami.

Netter FH, *Atlas of human anatomy*, CIBA-GEIGY Corporation, 1989, Summit, NJ.

Mathematic Equations for Chapter 6,
Mechanical Principles

Fig. 6-12, *A-C*: $F \times FA = R \times RA$
$F \times 3 = 0.9 \times 2.5$
$F \times 3 = 2.25$
$F = 0.75$

$F \times 5 = 0.9 \times 2.5$
$F \times 5 = 2.25$
$F = 0.45$

$F \times 7 = 0.9 \times 2.5$
$F \times 7 = 2.25$
$F = 0.32$

Scale: 1 cm = 0.5 pound

Fig. 6-13, *A-C*: $F \times FA = R \times RA$
$F \times 1.5 = 4(0.5) \times 5$
$F1.5 = 10$
$F = 6.67$

$F \times 3.75 = 4(0.5) \times 5$
$F3.75 = 10$
$F = 2.67$

$F \times 5.75 = 4\,(0.5) \times 5$
$F5.75 = 10$
$F = 1.74$

Scale: 1 cm = 1 pound

Fig. 6-15:   Sine $= \dfrac{\text{Opposite side}}{\text{Hypotenuse}} = \dfrac{O}{H}$

30° $\quad\quad 0.5 = \dfrac{O}{8}$

$\quad\quad\quad 4.0 = O$

45° $\quad\quad 0.707 = \dfrac{O}{8}$

$\quad\quad\quad 5.656 = O$

60° $\quad\quad 0.866 = \dfrac{O}{8}$

$\quad\quad\quad 6.928 = O$

90° $\quad\quad 1 = \dfrac{O}{8}$

$\quad\quad\quad 8 = O$

120° $\quad\quad$ *See 60°*

135° $\quad\quad$ *See 45°*

150° $\quad\quad$ *See 30°*

Cosine $= \dfrac{\text{Adjacent side}}{\text{Hypotenuse}} = \dfrac{A}{H}$

$0.866 = \dfrac{A}{8}$

$6.928 = A$

$0.707 = \dfrac{A}{8}$

$5.656 = A$

$0.5 = \dfrac{A}{8}$

$4.0 = 8$

$0.0 = \dfrac{A}{8}$

$0.0 = A$

Fig. 6-19, *A-B*:   Sine $= \dfrac{\text{Opposite side}}{\text{Hypotenuse}} = \dfrac{O}{H}$

30° $\quad\quad 0.3420 = \dfrac{O}{4}$

$\quad\quad\quad 1.37 = O$

45° $\quad\quad 0.4226 = \dfrac{O}{4}$

$\quad\quad\quad 1.69 = O$

60° $\quad\quad 0.5446 = \dfrac{O}{4}$

$\quad\quad\quad 2.18 = O$

Cosine $= \dfrac{\text{Adjacent side}}{\text{Hypotenuse}} = \dfrac{A}{H}$

$0.9848 = \dfrac{A}{4}$

$3.9392 = A$

$0.9063 = \dfrac{A}{4}$

$3.63 = A$

$0.8387 = \dfrac{A}{4}$

$3.35 = A$

Fig. 6-21:   Torque $=$ Force $\times$ length
$T = 8 \times 1$
$T = 8$ inch-ounces

$T = 8 \times 2.25$
$T = 18$ inch-ounces

Fig. 6-28, *A*: $F \times 3.5 = 0.9 \times 3$
$F3.5 = 2.7$
$F = 0.77$
$0.77 = 0.9 = 1.67$

Fig. 6-28, *B*: $F \times FA = R \times RA$
$F \times 9 = 0.9 \times 3$
$F9 = 2.7$
$F = 0.3$
$0.3 + 0.9 = 1.2$

Fig. 6-28, *C*:   6.67 from Fig. 6-13
$2 + 6.67 = 8.67$

Fig. 6-28, *D*:   1.74 from Fig. 6-13
$2 + 1.74 = 3.74$

Scale: 1 cm = 1 pound

Patterns for Splinting from Chapters 18 and 21

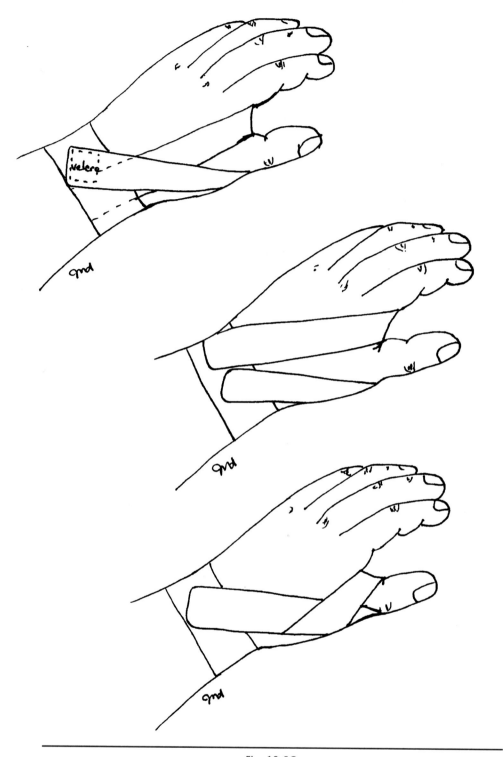

Fig. 18-5C

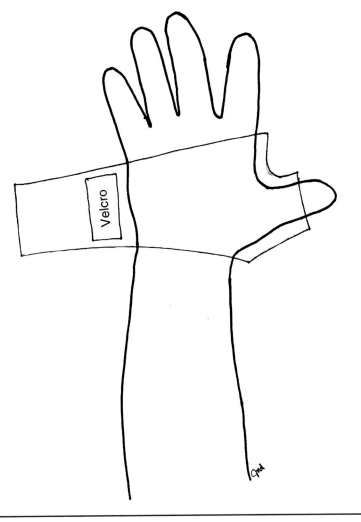

Velcro

Fig. 18-6B

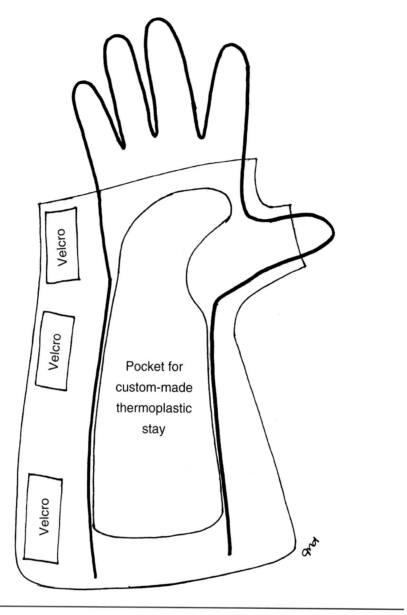

Fig. 18-6C

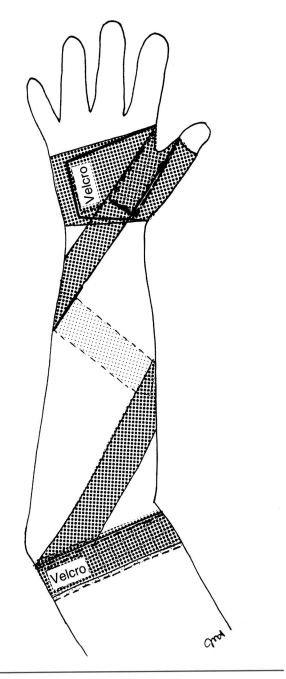

Fig. 18-6K

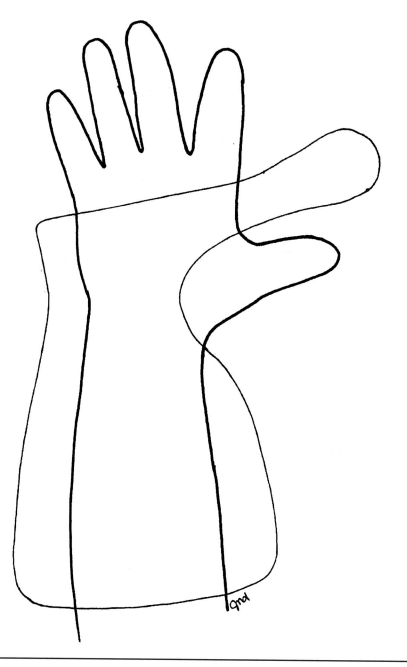

Fig. 18-7B

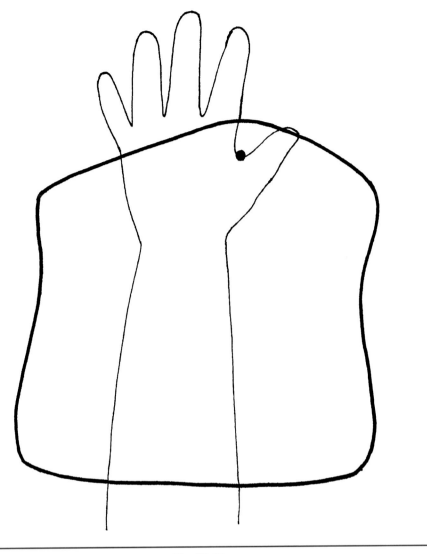

Fig. 18-8B

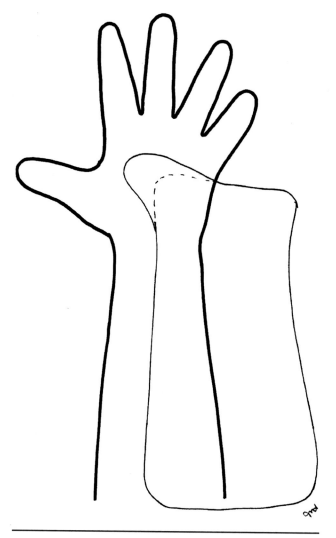

Fig. 18-9C

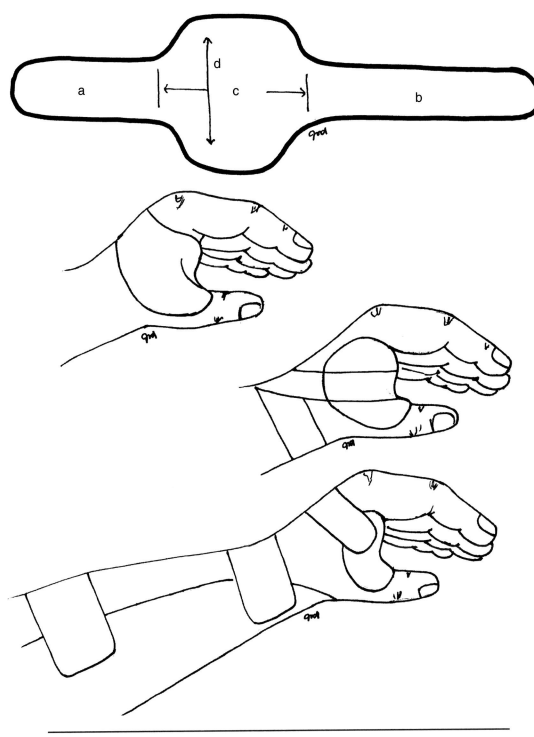

Fig. 18-10B

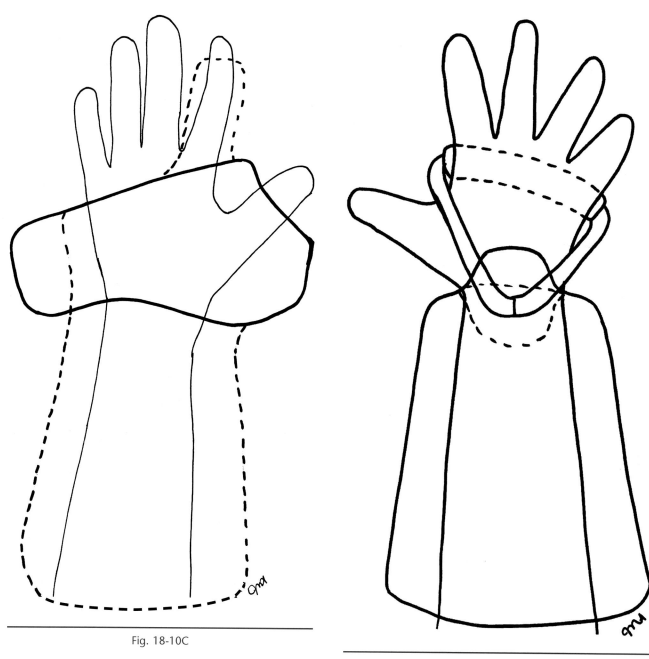

Fig. 18-10C

Fig. 18-11B

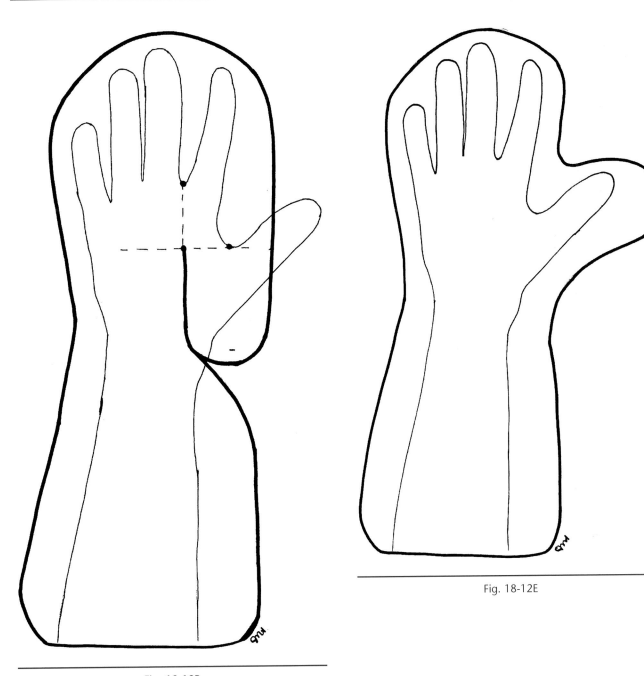

Fig. 18-12B

Fig. 18-12E

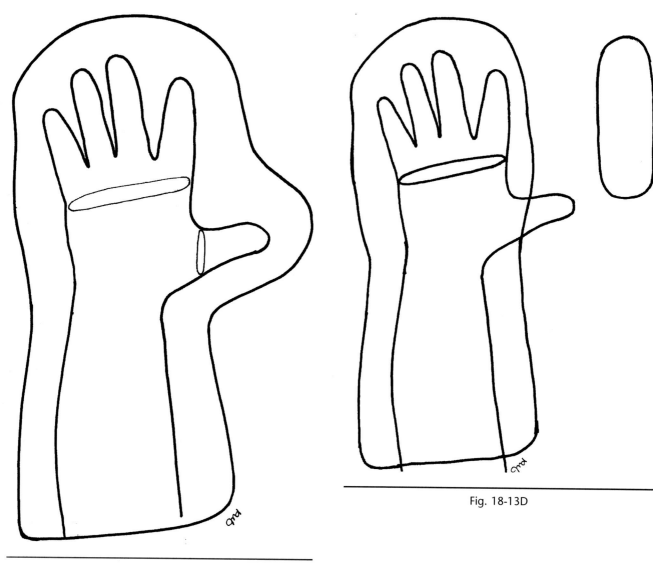

Fig. 18-13C

Fig. 18-13D

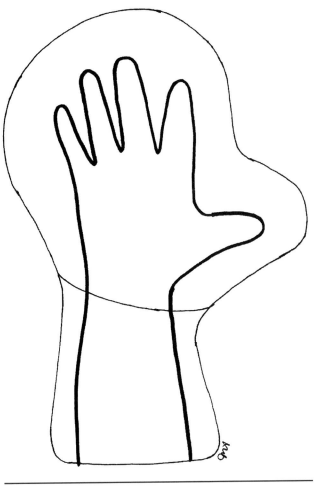

Fig. 18-14D

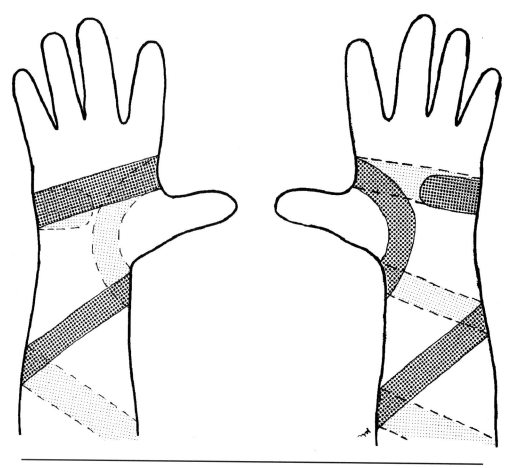

Fig. 18-15A

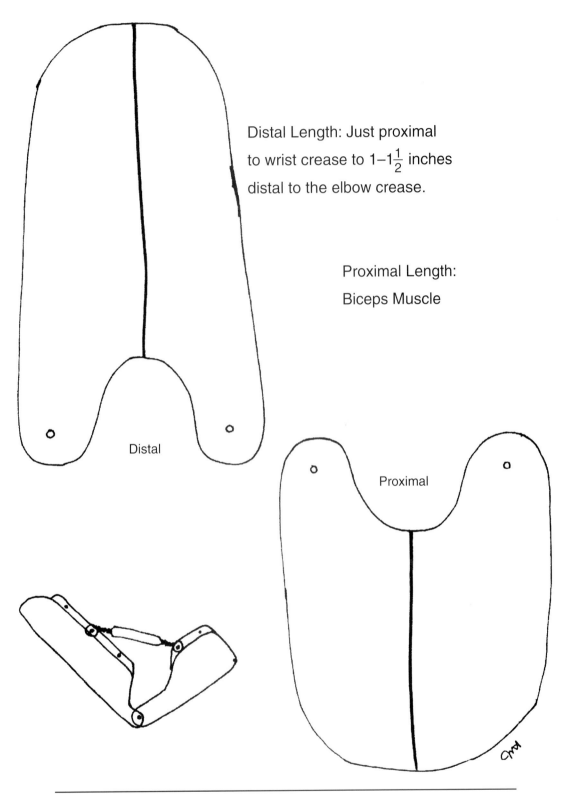

Distal Length: Just proximal to wrist crease to $1-1\frac{1}{2}$ inches distal to the elbow crease.

Proximal Length: Biceps Muscle

Distal

Proximal

Fig. 18-17B

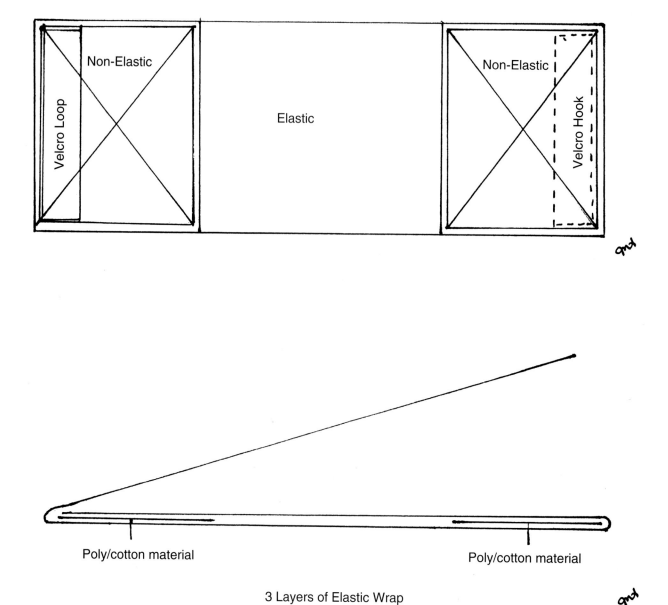

Poly/cotton material   Poly/cotton material

3 Layers of Elastic Wrap

Fig. 18-18B

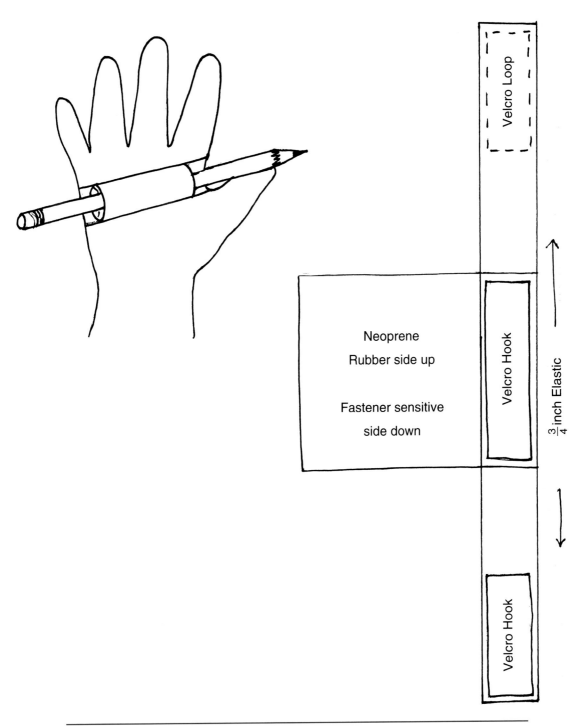

Fig. 18-19C

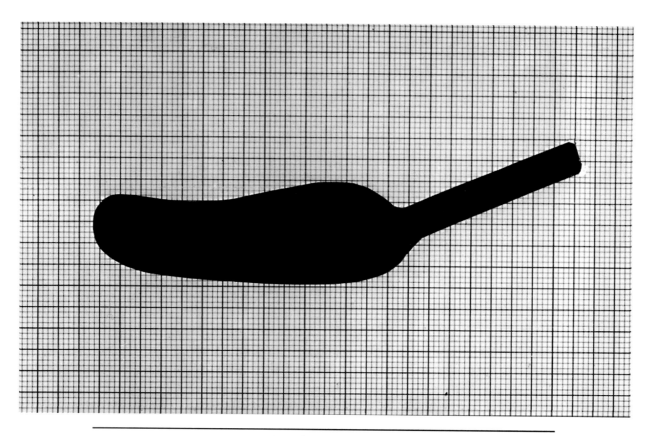

Fig. 21-7F

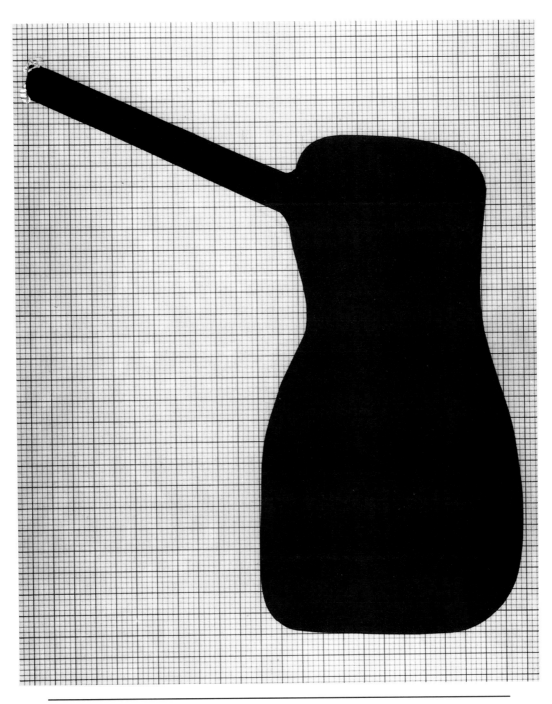

Fig. 21-8G

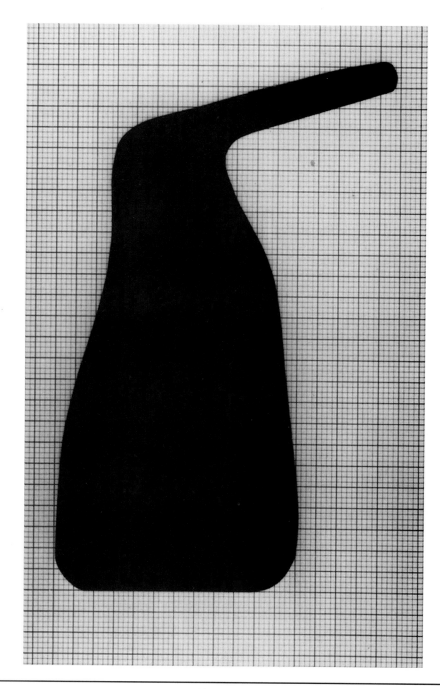

Fig. 21-9E

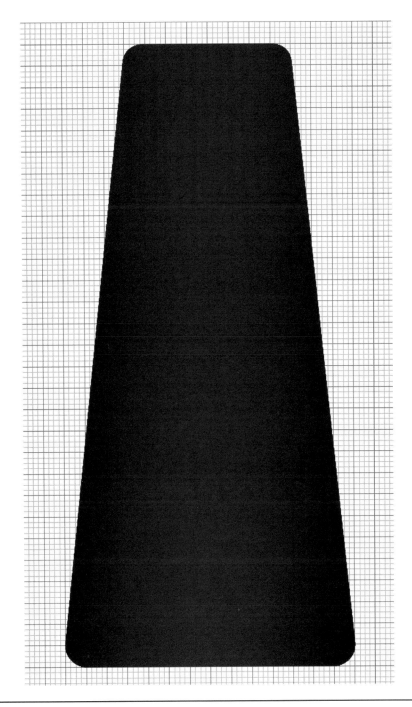

Fig. 21-10E

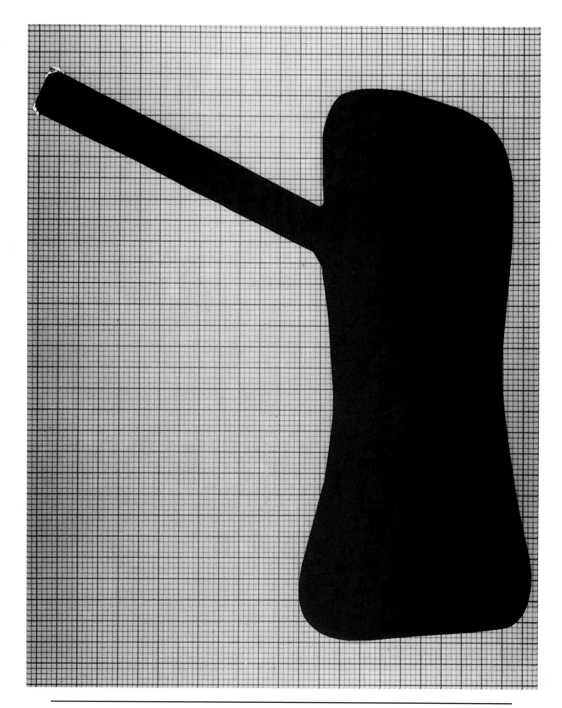

Fig. 21-11F

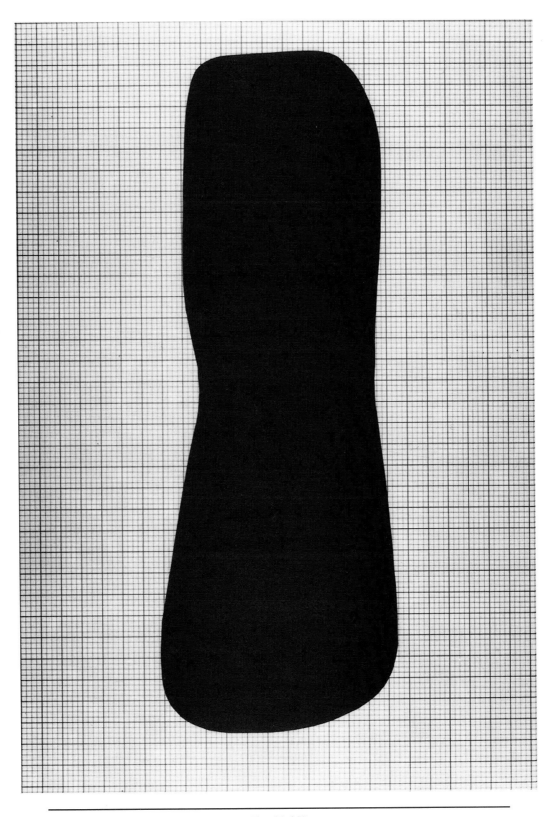

Fig. 21-12D

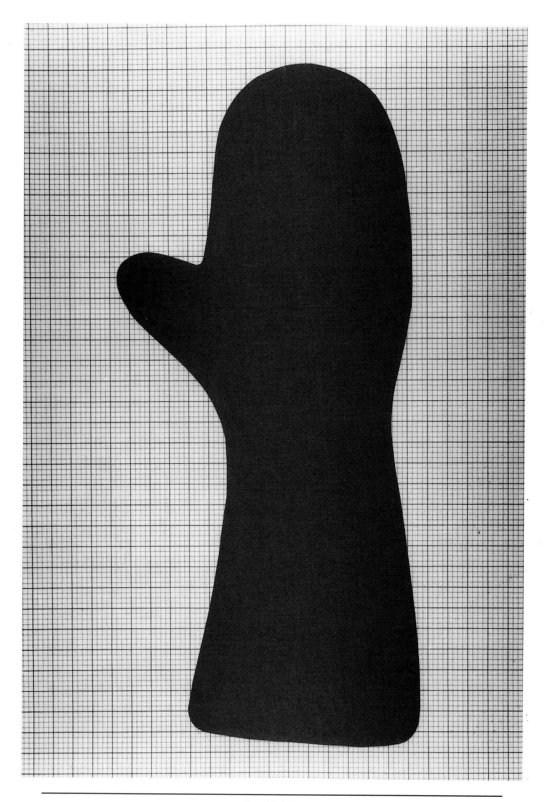

Fig. 21-13E

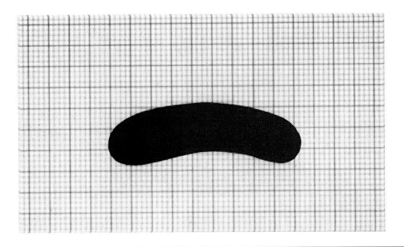

Fig. 21-14E

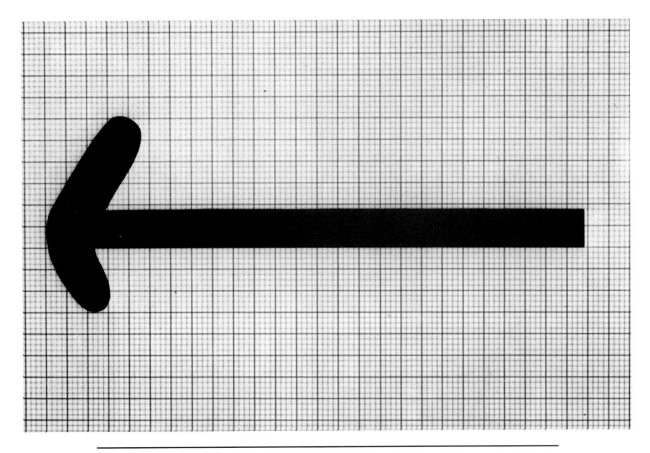

Fig. 21-15G

Splint[1] Index (SSRDI©)

Articular/Nonarticular Joint/Segment Purpose	Direction	Type	Joints	Digits	ESCS Name	Figure

Articular

Shoulder

Immobilization

Purpose	Direction	Type	Joints	Digits	ESCS Name	Figure
	Abduction, external rotation	3	(04)		Shoulder abduction and external rotation immobilization splint, type 3 (4)	4-12 B
	Abduction, external rotation	3	(04)		Shoulder abduction and external rotation immobilization splint, type 3 (4)	14-14 B
	Abduction, neutral rotation	1	(02)		Shoulder abduction and neutral rotation immobilization splint, type 1 (2)	14-14 A
	External rotation	3	(04)		Shoulder external rotation immobilization splint, type 3 (4)	14-15 A
	External rotation	3	(04)		Shoulder external rotation immobilization splint, type 3 (4)	14-15 B
	Flexion, internal rotation	3	(04)		Shoulder flexion and internal rotation immobilization splint, type 3 (4)	14-15 C-D

Mobilization

Purpose	Direction	Type	Joints	Digits	ESCS Name	Figure
	Abduction, external rotation	7	(14)		Shoulder abduction and external rotation mobilization splint, type 7 (14)	14-18 A
	Abduction, external rotation	3	(04)		Shoulder abduction and external rotation mobilization splint, type 3 (4)	7-1 Q
	Abduction, external rotation	3	(04)		Shoulder abduction and external rotation mobilization splint, type 3 (4)	14-17 A-B
	Abduction, external rotation	3	(04)		Shoulder abduction and external rotation mobilization splint, type 3 (4)	14-17 D
	Abduction, external rotation	7	(14)		Shoulder abduction and external rotation mobilization splint, type 7 (14)	14-18 B
	Abduction, neutral rotation	3	(04)		Shoulder abduction and neutral rotation mobilization splint, type 3 (4); left	14-17 C
	Abduction, neutral rotation	3	(04)		Shoulder abduction and neutral rotation mobilization splint, type 3 (4); right	14-17 C
	Abduction, neutral rotation	3	(04)		Shoulder abduction and neutral rotation mobilization splint, type 3 (4); left	15-25 B
	Abduction, neutral rotation	3	(04)		Shoulder abduction and neutral rotation mobilization splint, type 3 (4); right	15-25 B
	Coaptation	1	(02)		Shoulder coaptation mobilization splint, type 1 (2)	14-16 A-C
	Flexion	3	(04)		Shoulder flexion mobilization splint, type 3 (4)	14-17 E

Shoulder, Elbow, Forearm, Wrist, Finger MP, Thumb CMC

Immobilization

Purpose	Direction	Type	Joints	Digits	ESCS Name	Figure
	Abduction, neutral rotation, supination, flexion, extension, palmar abduction	0	(10)	Index-small, thumb	Shoulder abduction and neutral rotation, elbow flexion, forearm supination, wrist extension, index-small finger MP extension, thumb CMC palmar abduction and MP extension immobilization splint, type 0 (10)	1-5

Shoulder, Elbow, Forearm, Wrist, Finger MP, PIP, DIP, Thumb CMC, MP, IP

Immobilization

Purpose	Direction	Type	Joints	Digits	ESCS Name	Figure
	Abduction, neutral rotation, flexion, extension, palmar abduction	0	(19)	Index-small, thumb	Shoulder abduction and neutral rotation, elbow flexion, forearm neutral, wrist extension, index-small finger MP flexion, thumb CMC palmar abduction and MP-IP extension immobilization splint, type 0 (19)	1-6 A

Shoulder, Elbow: [finger splint-prosthesis]

Transmission

Purpose	Direction	Type	Joints	Digits	ESCS Name	Figure
	Extension, flexion [open, close]	1	(03)		Shoulder flexion, elbow extension: [finger TD open] / shoulder extension, elbow flexion: [finger TD close] torque transmission splint-prosthesis, type 1 (3)	23-4
	Extension, flexion [open, close]	1	(03)		Shoulder flexion, elbow extension: [finger TD open] / shoulder extension, elbow flexion: [finger TD close] torque transmission splint-prosthesis, type 1 (3)	23-5 B

Shoulder, Elbow, Forearm: [finger splint-prosthesis]

Purpose	Direction	Type	Joints	Digits	ESCS Name	Figure
	Extension, flexion, pronation, supination [open, close]	1	(04)		Shoulder flexion, elbow extension, forearm pronation: [finger TD open] / shoulder extension, elbow flexion, forearm supination: [finger TD close] torque transmission splint-prosthesis, type 1 (4)	23-1

Shoulder, Elbow, Forearm, Wrist: [finger splint-prosthesis]

Transmission

Extension, flexion, pronation, supination [open, close]	1	(05)	Shoulder flexion, elbow extension, forearm pronation, wrist extension: [finger TD open] / shoulder extension, elbow flexion, forearm supination, wrist flexion: [finger TD close] torque transmission splint-prosthesis, type 1 (5)	23-8

Shoulder, Elbow, Forearm: [thumb, finger prosthesis]

Transmission

Extension, flexion, pronation, supination [lateral abduction, lateral adduction]	1	(04)	Shoulder flexion, elbow extension, forearm pronation: [thumb lateral abduction, finger flexion fixed] / shoulder extension, elbow flexion, forearm supination: [thumb lateral adduction, finger flexion fixed] torque transmission prosthesis, type 1 (4)	23-9
Extension, flexion, pronation, supination [lateral abduction, lateral adduction]	1	(04)	Shoulder flexion, elbow extension, forearm pronation: [thumb lateral abduction, finger flexion fixed] / shoulder extension, elbow flexion, forearm supination: [thumb lateral adduction, finger flexion fixed] torque transmission prosthesis, type 1 (4)	23-10
Extension, flexion, pronation, supination [lateral abduction, lateral adduction]	1	(04)	Shoulder flexion, elbow extension, forearm pronation: [thumb lateral abduction, finger flexion fixed] / shoulder extension, elbow flexion, forearm supination: [thumb lateral adduction, finger flexion fixed] torque transmission prosthesis, type 1 (4)	23-11 A-B

Elbow

Immobilization

Flexion	0	(01)	Elbow flexion immobilization splint, type 0 (1)	20-17 C
Flexion	0	(01)	Elbow flexion immobilization splint, type 0 (1); with tuck	20-17 D
Flexion	0	(01)	Elbow flexion immobilization splint, type 0 (1); with roll	20-17 E
Flexion	1	(02)	Elbow flexion immobilization splint, type 1 (2)	14-1 A
Flexion	1	(02)	Elbow flexion immobilization splint, type 1 (2)	14-1 B
Flexion	1	(02)	Elbow flexion immobilization splint, type 1 (2)	21-10 B
Flexion	2	(03)	Elbow flexion immobilization splint, type 2 (3)	14-2 A
Flexion	2	(03)	Elbow flexion immobilization splint, type 2 (3)	14-2 B
Flexion	2	(03)	Elbow flexion immobilization splint, type 2 (3)	17-28
Flexion	2	(03)	Elbow flexion immobilization splint, type 2 (3)	20-17 F

Mobilization

Extension	0	(01)	Elbow extension mobilization splint, type 0 (1)	8-25 A
Extension	0	(01)	Elbow extension mobilization splint, type 0 (1)	14-3 A-B
Extension	0	(01)	Elbow extension mobilization splint, type 0 (1)	18-16 A
Extension	0	(01)	Elbow extension mobilization splint, type 0 (1)	18-16 B
Extension	0	(01)	Elbow extension mobilization splint, type 0 (1)	18-16 C
Extension	0	(01)	Elbow extension mobilization splint, type 0 (1)	18-17 A
Extension	0	(01)	Elbow extension mobilization splint, type 0 (1)	18-18 A
Extension	0	(01)	Elbow extension mobilization splint, type 0 (1)	18-18 C
Extension	0	(01)	Elbow extension mobilization splint, type 0 (1)	19-1 B
Extension	0	(01)	Elbow extension mobilization splint, type 0 (1)	19-1 C
Extension	0	(01)	Elbow extension mobilization splint, type 0 (1)	19-1 D-E
Extension	1	(02)	Elbow extension mobilization splint, type 1 (2)	1-2
Extension	1	(02)	Elbow extension mobilization splint, type 1 (2)	14-4 A

1. Includes splints, orthoses, braces, casts, splint-prostheses, and other related devices.
© Elaine E. Fess, Karan S. Gettle, Cynthia A. Philips, J. Robin Janson, 2005.

Continued

Splint[1] Index (SSRDI©)

Articular/Nonarticular Joint/Segment Purpose	Direction	Type	Joints	Digits	ESCS Name	Figure
Extension		1	(02)		Elbow extension mobilization splint, type 1 (2)	14-4 B
Extension		1	(02)		Elbow extension mobilization splint, type 1 (2)	14-4 C
Extension		1	(02)		Elbow extension mobilization splint, type 1 (2)	15-32 A
Extension		2	(03)		Elbow extension mobilization splint, type 2 (3)	14-6 A
Extension		2	(03)		Elbow extension mobilization splint, type 2 (3)	19-1 A
Extension or flexion		2	(03)		Elbow extension or flexion mobilization splint, type 2 (3)	14-6 E
Flexion		0	(01)		Elbow flexion mobilization splint, type 0 (1)	7-2 D
Flexion		0	(01)		Elbow flexion mobilization splint, type 0 (1)	7-15 D
Flexion		1	(02)		Elbow flexion mobilization splint, type 1 (2)	14-5 A
Flexion		1	(02)		Elbow flexion mobilization splint, type 1 (2)	14-5 B
Flexion		1	(02)		Elbow flexion mobilization splint, type 1 (2)	14-5 C
Flexion		1	(02)		Elbow flexion mobilization splint, type 1 (2)	14-5 D
Flexion		1	(02)		Elbow flexion mobilization splint, type 1 (2)	14-5 E
Flexion		2	(03)		Elbow flexion mobilization splint, type 2 (3)	14-6 B
Flexion		2	(03)		Elbow flexion mobilization splint, type 2 (3)	14-6 C
Flexion or extension		2	(03)		Elbow flexion or extension mobilization splint, type 2 (3)	14-6 D
Restriction						
Extension		1	(02)		Elbow extension restriction splint, type 1 (2)	14-8 A-B
Extension		2	(03)		Elbow extension restriction splint, type 2 (3)	10-38
Extension, flexion		0	(01)		Elbow extension and flexion restriction splint, type 0 (1)	14-7
Extension, flexion		1	(02)		Elbow extension and flexion restriction splint, type 1 (2)	5-5 A
Extension, flexion		1	(02)		Elbow extension and flexion restriction splint, type 1 (2)	14-10
Extension, flexion		2	(03)		Elbow extension and flexion restriction splint, type 2 (3)	17-26 B
Flexion		0	(01)		Elbow flexion restriction splint, type 0 (1)	14-9
Flexion		0	(01)		Elbow flexion restriction splint, type 0 (1)	17-22
Lateral deviation, medial deviation		1	(02)		Elbow lateral and medial deviation restriction splint, type 1 (2)	14-11
Lateral deviation, medial deviation		2	(03)		Elbow lateral and medial deviation restriction splint, type 2 (3)	17-26 A

Elbow, Forearm

Mobilization

Purpose	Direction	Type	Joints	Digits	ESCS Name	Figure
Flexion, neutral		1	(03)		Elbow flexion, forearm neutral mobilization splint, type 1 (3)	14-12 A-B

Restriction/Immobilization

Purpose	Direction	Type	Joints	Digits	ESCS Name	Figure
Extension, supination		1	(03)		Elbow extension restriction / forearm supination immobilization splint, type 1 (3)	14-13

Restriction/Mobilization/Immobilization

Purpose	Direction	Type	Joints	Digits	ESCS Name	Figure
Extension, flexion, neutral		0	(02)		Elbow extension restriction / elbow flexion mobilization / forearm neutral immobilization splint, type 0 (2)	15-21 A-B

Elbow, Forearm, Wrist, Finger MP, PIP, DIP, Thumb CMC, MP, IP

Mobilization

Purpose	Direction	Type	Joints	Digits	ESCS Name	Figure
Extension, supination, radial abduction		0	(18)	Index-small, thumb	Elbow extension, forearm supination, wrist extension, index-small finger extension, thumb CMC radial abduction and MP-IP extension mobilization splint, type 0 (18)	19-2

Elbow, Forearm, Wrist, Thumb CMC

Mobilization

			Splint	Digit	Figure
Extension, pronation, radial abduction	0	(04)	Elbow extension, forearm pronation, wrist extension, thumb CMC radial abduction mobilization splint, type 0 (4)		19-3

Forearm

Immobilization

			Splint	Figure
Neutral	1	(02)	Forearm neutral immobilization splint, type 1 (2)	13-23 A-B
Neutral	2	(03)	Forearm neutral immobilization splint, type 2 (3)	6-33 B
Neutral	2	(03)	Forearm neutral immobilization splint, type 2 (3)	8-17 A
Neutral	2	(03)	Forearm neutral immobilization splint, type 2 (3)	9-17 B
Neutral	2	(03)	Forearm neutral immobilization splint, type 2 (3)	13-23 C-D
Neutral	2	(03)	Forearm neutral immobilization splint, type 2 (3)	13-23 E-F

Mobilization

			Splint	Figure
Coaptation	0	(01)	Forearm coaptation mobilization splint, type 0 (1)	13-24
Pronation	2	(03)	Forearm pronation mobilization splint, type 2 (3)	13-25 B-C
Pronation	2	(03)	Forearm pronation mobilization splint, type 2 (3)	13-26 A
Pronation	2	(03)	Forearm pronation mobilization splint, type 2 (3)	13-27 A-B
Pronation	4	(08)	Forearm pronation mobilization splint, type 4 (8)	13-29 B
Pronation or supination	2	(03)	Forearm pronation or supination mobilization splint, type 2 (3)	8-4 F
Supination	2	(03)	Forearm supination mobilization splint, type 2 (3)	7-2 E
Supination	2	(03)	Forearm supination mobilization splint, type 2 (3)	8-11 B
Supination	2	(03)	Forearm supination mobilization splint, type 2 (3)	13-25 A
Supination	2	(03)	Forearm supination mobilization splint, type 2 (3)	13-26 B
Supination	2	(03)	Forearm supination mobilization splint, type 2 (3)	13-27 C-D
Supination	2	(03)	Forearm supination mobilization splint, type 2 (3)	13-27 E
Supination	2	(03)	Forearm supination mobilization splint, type 2 (3)	13-28 A-B
Supination	2	(03)	Forearm supination mobilization splint, type 2 (3)	13-28 C
Supination	2	(03)	Forearm supination mobilization splint, type 2 (3)	13-28 D-E
Supination	4	(08)	Forearm supination mobilization splint, type 4 (8)	13-29 A
Supination or pronation	2	(03)	Forearm supination or pronation mobilization splint, type 2 (3)	8-4 G

Forearm, Wrist, Finger MP

Mobilization

			Splint	Digit	Figure
Supination, extension	1	(07)	Forearm supination, wrist extension, index-small finger MP extension mobilization splint, type 1 (7)	Index-small	1-19

Mobilization/Restriction

			Splint	Digit	Figure
Pronation	1	(06)	Forearm pronation mobilization / index-small finger MP extension restriction splint, type 1 (6)	Index-small	13-30

Forearm, Wrist, Thumb CMC

Mobilization

			Splint	Digit	Figure
Supination, extension, palmar abduction	0	(03)	Forearm supination, wrist extension, thumb CMC palmar abduction mobilization splint, type 0 (3)	Thumb	13-31
Supination, extension, radial abduction	0	(03)	Forearm supination, wrist extension, thumb CMC radial abduction mobilization splint, type 0 (3)	Thumb	18-15 B

Continued

Splint[1] Index (SSRDI©)

Articular/Nonarticular Joint/Segment Purpose	Direction	Type	Joints	Digits	ESCS Name	Figure
Forearm, Wrist, Thumb CMC, MP						
Mobilization						
Supination, extension, radial abduction	0	(04)	Thumb	Forearm supination, wrist extension, thumb CMC radial abduction and MP extension mobilization splint, type 0 (4)	19-4
Supination, extension, radial abduction	0	(04)	Thumb	Forearm supination, wrist extension, thumb CMC radial abduction and MP extension mobilization splint, type 0 (4)	18-6 J
Forearm, Wrist, Thumb CMC, MP, IP						
Mobilization						
Supination, extension, palmar abduction	0	(05)	Thumb	Forearm supination, wrist extension, thumb CMC palmar abduction and MP-IP extension mobilization splint, type 0 (5)	18-15 C
Wrist						
Immobilization						
Extension	0	(01)		Wrist extension immobilization splint, type 0 (1)	4-13 B
Extension	0	(01)		Wrist extension immobilization splint, type 0 (1)	4-22
Extension	0	(01)		Wrist extension immobilization splint, type 0 (1)	6-11
Extension	0	(01)		Wrist extension immobilization splint, type 0 (1)	6-12 A
Extension	0	(01)		Wrist extension immobilization splint, type 0 (1)	6-12 B
Extension	0	(01)		Wrist extension immobilization splint, type 0 (1)	6-12 C
Extension	0	(01)		Wrist extension immobilization splint, type 0 (1)	8-2 C-D
Extension	0	(01)		Wrist extension immobilization splint, type 0 (1)	8-8 F
Extension	0	(01)		Wrist extension immobilization splint, type 0 (1)	8-26 A
Extension	0	(01)		Wrist extension immobilization splint, type 0 (1)	10-13 A
Extension	0	(01)		Wrist extension immobilization splint, type 0 (1)	13-2 A
Extension	0	(01)		Wrist extension immobilization splint, type 0 (1)	13-2 D
Extension	0	(01)		Wrist extension immobilization splint, type 0 (1)	15-19 G-H
Extension	0	(01)		Wrist extension immobilization splint, type 0 (1)	16-7
Extension	0	(01)		Wrist extension immobilization splint, type 0 (1)	17-4 A
Extension	0	(01)		Wrist extension immobilization splint, type 0 (1)	17-12 A
Extension	0	(01)		Wrist extension immobilization splint, type 0 (1)	17-12 B-C
Extension	0	(01)		Wrist extension immobilization splint, type 0 (1)	17-23
Extension	0	(01)		Wrist extension immobilization splint, type 0 (1)	17-20
Extension	0	(01)		Wrist extension immobilization splint, type 0 (1)	20-14 C
Extension	0	(01)		Wrist extension immobilization splint, type 0 (1)	20-14 D
Extension	0	(01)		Wrist extension immobilization splint, type 0 (1)	20-14 E
Extension	1	(02)		Wrist extension immobilization splint, type 1 (2)	13-3
Extension	2	(03)		Wrist extension immobilization splint, type 2 (3)	13-4 A-B
Flexion	0	(01)		Wrist flexion immobilization splint, type 0 (1)	13-2 E
Neutral	0	(01)		Wrist neutral immobilization splint, type 0 (1)	4-19
Neutral	0	(01)		Wrist neutral immobilization splint, type 0 (1)	4-20
Neutral	0	(01)		Wrist neutral immobilization splint, type 0 (1)	6-8
Neutral	0	(01)		Wrist neutral immobilization splint, type 0 (1)	6-9
Neutral	0	(01)		Wrist neutral immobilization splint, type 0 (1)	6-10 A

Neutral	0	(01)	Wrist neutral immobilization splint, type 0 (1)	6-10 B
Neutral	0	(01)	Wrist neutral immobilization splint, type 0 (1)	10-5 B
Neutral	0	(01)	Wrist neutral immobilization splint, type 0 (1)	10-16 B
Neutral	0	(01)	Wrist neutral immobilization splint, type 0 (1)	10-16 C
Neutral	0	(01)	Wrist neutral immobilization splint, type 0 (1)	10-17
Neutral	0	(01)	Wrist neutral immobilization splint, type 0 (1)	13-1
Neutral	0	(01)	Wrist neutral immobilization splint, type 0 (1)	13-2 B
Neutral	0	(01)	Wrist neutral immobilization splint, type 0 (1)	13-2 C
Neutral	0	(01)	Wrist neutral immobilization splint, type 0 (1)	17-25 A
Neutral	0	(01)	Wrist neutral immobilization splint, type 0 (1)	20-14 F
Neutral	2	(03)	Wrist neutral immobilization splint, type 2 (3)	13-4 C-D
Neutral	2	(03)	Wrist neutral immobilization splint, type 2 (3)	13-4 E

Mobilization

Dorsal, extension	0	(01)	Pisiform dorsal, proximal carpal row extension mobilization splint, type 0 (1)	13-7 E-F
Extension	0	(01)	Wrist extension mobilization splint, type 0 (1)	1-20 A
Extension	0	(01)	Wrist extension mobilization splint, type 0 (1)	1-20 B
Extension	0	(01)	Wrist extension mobilization splint, type 0 (1)	1-20 C
Extension	0	(01)	Wrist extension mobilization splint, type 0 (1)	4-30 C
Extension	0	(01)	Wrist extension mobilization splint, type 0 (1)	6-2 B
Extension	0	(01)	Wrist extension mobilization splint, type 0 (1)	6-15 B
Extension	0	(01)	Wrist extension mobilization splint, type 0 (1)	6-27 A
Extension	0	(01)	Wrist extension mobilization splint, type 0 (1)	6-28 A
Extension	0	(01)	Wrist extension mobilization splint, type 0 (1)	6-28 B
Extension	0	(01)	Wrist extension mobilization splint, type 0 (1)	7-1 P
Extension	0	(01)	Wrist extension mobilization splint, type 0 (1)	8-6 A
Extension	0	(01)	Wrist extension mobilization splint, type 0 (1)	8-8 A-B
Extension	0	(01)	Wrist extension mobilization splint, type 0 (1)	8-10 F
Extension	0	(01)	Wrist extension mobilization splint, type 0 (1)	10-8 B
Extension	0	(01)	Wrist extension mobilization splint, type 0 (1)	10-21
Extension	0	(01)	Wrist extension mobilization splint, type 0 (1)	13-5 A
Extension	0	(01)	Wrist extension mobilization splint, type 0 (1)	13-5 B
Extension	0	(01)	Wrist extension mobilization splint, type 0 (1)	13-5 C
Extension	0	(01)	Wrist extension mobilization splint, type 0 (1)	13-6 A
Extension	0	(01)	Wrist extension mobilization splint, type 0 (1)	13-6 B
Extension	0	(01)	Wrist extension mobilization splint, type 0 (1)	13-6 C
Extension	0	(01)	Wrist extension mobilization splint, type 0 (1)	13-6 D
Extension	0	(01)	Wrist extension mobilization splint, type 0 (1)	13-6 E
Extension	0	(01)	Wrist extension mobilization splint, type 0 (1)	13-6 G
Extension	0	(01)	Wrist extension mobilization splint, type 0 (1)	13-6 H
Extension	0	(01)	Wrist extension mobilization splint, type 0 (1)	13-6 J
Extension	0	(01)	Wrist extension mobilization splint, type 0 (1)	13-7 A
Extension	0	(01)	Wrist extension mobilization splint, type 0 (1)	13-7 B
Extension	0	(01)	Wrist extension mobilization splint, type 0 (1)	13-8
Extension	0	(01)	Wrist extension mobilization splint, type 0 (1)	13-9 A
Extension	0	(01)	Wrist extension mobilization splint, type 0 (1)	13-9 B
Extension	0	(01)	Wrist extension mobilization splint, type 0 (1)	14-19 A
Extension	0	(01)	Wrist extension mobilization splint, type 0 (1)	15-14 A
Extension	0	(01)	Wrist extension mobilization splint, type 0 (1); with grasp assist	15-17 A

Continued

Splint Index

Splint[1] Index (SSRDI©)

Continued

Splint[1] Index (SSRDI)©

Articular/Nonarticular Joint/Segment Purpose	Direction	Type	Joints	Digits	ESCS Name	Figure
Extension, palmar abduction	1	(03)	Thumb	Wrist extension, thumb CMC palmar abduction immobilization splint, type 1 (3)	20-16 D
Neutral, palmar abduction	1	(03)	Thumb	Wrist neutral, thumb CMC palmar abduction immobilization splint, type 1 (3)	20-16 E
Mobilization					
Extension, palmar abduction	0	(02)	Thumb	Wrist extension, thumb CMC palmar abduction mobilization splint, type 0 (2)	15-17 C
Extension, radial abduction	0	(02)	Thumb	Wrist extension, thumb CMC radial abduction mobilization splint, type 0 (2)	19-6 A-B
Extension, radial abduction	1	(03)	Thumb	Wrist extension, thumb CMC radial abduction mobilization splint, type 1 (3)	18-7 C-D
Restriction					
Circumduction	1	(03)	Thumb	Wrist circumduction, thumb CMC circumduction restriction splint, type 1 (3)	8-26 B
Restriction/Immobilization					
Radial deviation, ulnar deviation, palmar abduction	1	(03)	Thumb	Wrist radial and ulnar deviation restriction / thumb CMC palmar abduction immobilization splint, type 1 (3)	13-19 A-C

Wrist, Thumb CMC, MP

Immobilization

Extension, palmar abduction	0	(03)	Thumb	Wrist extension, thumb CMC palmar abduction and MP flexion immobilization splint, type 0 (3)	17-17 A
Extension, palmar abduction	0	(03)	Thumb	Wrist extension, thumb CMC palmar abduction and MP flexion immobilization splint, type 0 (3)	17-20
Extension, radial abduction, extension	0	(03)	Thumb	Wrist extension, thumb CMC radial abduction and MP extension immobilization splint, type 0 (3)	9-18
Extension, radial abduction, flexion	0	(03)	Thumb	Wrist extension, thumb CMC radial abduction and MP flexion immobilization splint, type 0 (3)	4-3
Immobilization/Restriction					
Extension, palmar abduction	0	(03)	Thumb	Wrist extension, thumb CMC palmar abduction immobilization / MP flexion restriction splint, type 0 (3)	17-17 B
Mobilization					
Extension, flexion, palmar abduction	0	(03)	Thumb	Wrist extension, thumb CMC palmar abduction and MP flexion mobilization splint, type 0 (3)	18-10 A
Extension, palmar abduction	0	(03)	Thumb	Wrist extension, thumb CMC palmar abduction and MP extension mobilization splint, type 0 (3)	15-4 A
Extension, palmar abduction	0	(03)	Thumb	Wrist extension, thumb CMC palmar abduction and MP extension mobilization splint, type 0 (3)	18-4 A-B
Extension, radial abduction	0	(03)	Thumb	Wrist extension, thumb CMC radial abduction and MP extension mobilization splint, type 0 (3)	18-6 F
Extension, radial abduction	0	(03)	Thumb	Wrist extension, thumb CMC radial abduction and MP extension mobilization splint, type 0 (3)	18-6 G
Extension, radial abduction	0	(03)	Thumb	Wrist extension, thumb CMC radial abduction and MP extension mobilization splint, type 0 (3)	18-4 D
Restriction					
Circumduction, flexion	0	(03)	Thumb	Wrist circumduction, thumb CMC circumduction and MP flexion restriction splint, type 0 (3)	17-18 A

Continued

Splint[1] Index (SSRDI©)

Articular/Nonarticular Joint/Segment Purpose	Direction	Type	Joints	Digits	ESCS Name	Figure
	Neutral, flexion, palmar abduction	0	(16)	Index-small, thumb	Wrist neutral, index-small finger flexion, thumb CMC palmar abduction and MP-IP flexion immobilization splint, type 0 (16)	16-2 C
Mobilization						
	Extension, abduction, radial abduction	0	(16)	Index-small, thumb	Wrist extension, index, ring-small finger MP abduction, index-small finger extension, thumb CMC radial abduction and MP-IP extension mobilization splint, type 0 (16)	18-12 F
	Extension, abduction, radial abduction	0	(16)	Index-small, thumb	Wrist extension, index, ring-small finger MP abduction, index-small finger extension, thumb CMC radial abduction and MP-IP extension mobilization splint, type 0 (16)	18-12 G
	Extension, abduction, radial abduction	0	(16)	Index-small, thumb	Wrist extension, index, ring-small finger MP abduction, index-small finger extension, thumb CMC radial abduction and MP-IP extension mobilization splint, type 0 (16)	18-12 H
	Extension, abduction, radial abduction	0	(16)	Index-small, thumb	Wrist extension, index, ring-small finger MP abduction, index-small finger extension, thumb CMC radial abduction and MP-IP extension mobilization splint, type 0 (16)	10-2 B
	Extension, abduction, radial abduction	0	(16)	Index-small, thumb	Wrist extension, index, ring-small finger MP abduction, index-small finger extension, thumb CMC radial abduction and MP-IP extension mobilization splint, type 0 (16)	19-8 A
	Extension, abduction, radial abduction	0	(16)	Index-small, thumb	Wrist extension, index, ring-small finger MP abduction, index-small finger extension, thumb CMC radial abduction and MP-IP extension mobilization splint, type 0 (16)	19-8 B
	Extension, abduction, radial abduction	0	(16)	Index-small, thumb	Wrist extension, index, ring-small finger MP abduction, index-small finger extension, thumb CMC radial abduction and MP-IP extension mobilization splint, type 0 (16)	19-8 C
	Extension, abduction, radial abduction	0	(16)	Index-small, thumb	Wrist extension, index, ring-small finger MP abduction, index-small finger extension, thumb CMC radial abduction and MP-IP extension mobilization splint, type 0 (16)	10-5 A
	Extension, flexion, palmar abduction	0	(16)	Index-small, thumb	Wrist extension, index-small finger flexion, thumb CMC palmar abduction and MP-IP extension mobilization splint, type 0 (16)	18-14 A-B
	Extension, flexion, radial abduction	0	(16)	Index-small, thumb	Wrist extension, index-small finger MP extension and IP flexion, thumb CMC radial abduction and MP-IP extension mobilization splint, type 0 (16)	18-14 C
	Extension, flexion, radial abduction	0	(16)	Index-small, thumb	Wrist extension, index-small finger MP extension and IP flexion, thumb CMC radial abduction and MP-IP extension mobilization splint, type 0 (16); left	18-14 C
	Extension, flexion, radial abduction	0	(16)	Index-small, thumb	Wrist extension, index-small finger MP extension and IP flexion, thumb CMC radial abduction and MP-IP extension mobilization splint, type 0 (16); right	18-14 C
	Extension, palmar abduction	0	(16)	Index-small, thumb	Wrist extension, index-small finger extension, thumb CMC palmar abduction and MP-IP extension mobilization splint, type 0 (16)	18-12 A
	Extension, palmar abduction	0	(16)	Index-small, thumb	Wrist extension, index-small finger extension, thumb CMC palmar abduction and MP-IP extension mobilization splint, type 0 (16)	18-12 C
	Extension, palmar abduction	0	(16)	Index-small, thumb	Wrist extension, index-small finger extension, thumb CMC palmar abduction and MP-IP extension mobilization splint, type 0 (16)	18-13 A-B
	Extension, palmar abduction	0	(16)	Index-small, thumb	Wrist extension, index-small finger extension, thumb CMC palmar abduction and MP-IP extension mobilization splint, type 0 (16)	19-8 D
	Extension, palmar abduction	0	(16)	Index-small, thumb	Wrist extension, index-small finger extension, thumb CMC palmar abduction and MP-IP extension mobilization splint, type 0 (16)	19-8 E
	Extension, palmar abduction	0	(16)	Index-small, thumb	Wrist extension, index-small finger extension, thumb CMC palmar abduction and MP-IP extension mobilization splint, type 0 (16)	19-8 F
	Extension, palmar abduction	0	(16)	Index-small, thumb	Wrist extension, index-small finger extension, thumb CMC palmar abduction and MP-IP extension mobilization splint, type 0 (16)	19-8 G-H
	Extension, palmar abduction	0	(16)	Index-small, thumb	Wrist extension, index-small finger extension, thumb CMC palmar abduction and MP-IP extension mobilization splint, type 0 (16)	19-8 I
	Extension, palmar abduction	0	(16)	Index-small, thumb	Wrist extension, index-small finger extension, thumb CMC palmar abduction and MP-IP extension mobilization splint, type 0 (16)	19-8 K
	Extension, radial abduction	0	(16)	Index-small, thumb	Wrist extension, index-small finger extension, thumb CMC radial abduction and MP-IP extension mobilization splint, type 0 (16)	19-8 J

Wrist: Finger MP
Transmission

Motion			Digits	Splint	Figure
Flexion extension	0	(05)	Index-small	Wrist flexion: index-small finger MP extension / index-small finger MP flexion: wrist extension torque transmission splint, type 0 (5)	1-12 A
Flexion extension	0	(05)	Index-small	Wrist flexion: index-small finger MP extension / index-small finger MP flexion: wrist extension torque transmission splint, type 0 (5)	1-12 B
Flexion extension	0	(05)	Index-small	Wrist flexion: index-small finger MP extension / index-small finger MP flexion: wrist extension torque transmission splint, type 0 (5)	1-12 F
Flexion extension	0	(05)	Index-small	Wrist flexion: index-small finger MP extension / index-small finger MP flexion: wrist extension torque transmission splint, type 0 (5)	1-12 F
Flexion extension	0	(05)	Index-small	Wrist flexion: index-small finger MP extension / index-small finger MP flexion: wrist extension torque transmission splint, type 0 (5)	1-12 G
Flexion extension	0	(05)	Index-small	Wrist flexion: index-small finger MP extension / index-small finger MP flexion: wrist extension torque transmission splint, type 0 (5)	4-5 A
Flexion extension	0	(05)	Index-small	Wrist flexion: index-small finger MP extension / index-small finger MP flexion: wrist extension torque transmission splint, type 0 (5)	6-33 A
Flexion extension	0	(05)	Index-small	Wrist flexion: index-small finger MP extension / index-small finger MP flexion: wrist extension torque transmission splint, type 0 (5)	8-16 B
Flexion extension	0	(05)	Index-small	Wrist flexion: index-small finger MP extension / index-small finger MP flexion: wrist extension torque transmission splint, type 0 (5)	9-11
Flexion extension	0	(05)	Index-small	Wrist flexion: index-small finger MP extension / index-small finger MP flexion: wrist extension torque transmission splint, type 0 (5)	9-12 A
Flexion extension	0	(05)	Index-small	Wrist flexion: index-small finger MP extension / index-small finger MP flexion: wrist extension torque transmission splint, type 0 (5)	9-13 B
Flexion extension	0	(05)	Index-small	Wrist flexion: index-small finger MP extension / index-small finger MP flexion: wrist extension torque transmission splint, type 0 (5)	10-39 D
Flexion extension	0	(05)	Index-small	Wrist flexion: index-small finger MP extension / index-small finger MP flexion: wrist extension torque transmission splint, type 0 (5)	13-20 A-B
Flexion extension	0	(05)	Index-small	Wrist flexion: index-small finger MP extension / index-small finger MP flexion: wrist extension torque transmission splint, type 0 (5)	15-14 E
Flexion extension	0	(05)	Index-small	Wrist flexion: index-small finger MP extension / index-small finger MP flexion: wrist extension torque transmission splint, type 0 (5)	15-14 F
Flexion extension	0	(05)	Index-small	Wrist flexion: index-small finger MP extension / index-small finger MP flexion: wrist extension torque transmission splint, type 0 (5)	15-14 G-I

Wrist: Finger MP, PIP, DIP
Restriction/Mobilization

Motion			Digits	Splint	Figure
Extension: flexion	0	(07)	Index-small	Wrist extension: index-small finger MP extension restriction and index finger flexion mobilization / wrist flexion: index-small finger MP extension restriction and index finger IP extension mobilization splint, type 0 (7)	15-20 A
Extension: flexion	0	(13)	Index-small	Wrist extension restriction: index-small finger flexion mobilization / index-small finger extension restriction / wrist flexion: index-small finger extension restriction splint, type 0 (13); with wrist locking device	8-10 A
Extension: flexion	0	(13)	Index-small	Wrist extension restriction: index-small finger flexion mobilization / index-small finger extension restriction / wrist flexion: index-small finger extension restriction splint, type 0 (13)	15-20 B-D
Extension: flexion	0	(13)	Index-small	Wrist extension restriction: index-small finger flexion mobilization / index-small finger extension restriction / wrist flexion: index-small finger extension restriction splint, type 0 (13)	15-20 E

Continued

Splint Index

Splint[1] Index (SSRDI[©])

Wrist: Finger MP, Thumb CMC
Transmission/Mobilization

Articular/Nonarticular Joint/Segment Purpose	Direction	Type	Joints	Digits	ESCS Name	Figure
Flexion: extension, radial abduction		0	(06)	Index-small, thumb	Wrist flexion: index-small finger MP extension / index-small finger MP flexion: wrist extension torque transmission / thumb CMC radial abduction mobilization splint, type 0 (6)	1-12 E
Flexion: extension, radial abduction		0	(06)	Index-small, thumb	Wrist flexion: index-small finger MP extension / index-small finger MP flexion: wrist extension torque transmission / thumb CMC radial abduction mobilization splint, type 0 (6)	1-12 C

Wrist: Finger MP, Thumb CMC, MP
Transmission/Mobilization

Flexion: extension, radial abduction		0	(07)	Index-small, thumb	Wrist flexion: index-small finger MP extension / index-small finger MP flexion: wrist extension torque transmission / thumb CMC radial abduction and MP extension mobilization splint, type 0 (7)	1-12 D
Flexion: extension, radial abduction		0	(07)	Index-small, thumb	Wrist flexion: index-small finger MP extension / index-small finger MP flexion: wrist extension torque transmission / thumb CMC radial abduction and MP extension mobilization splint, type 0 (7)	8-6 B
Flexion: extension, radial abduction		0	(07)	Index-small, thumb	Wrist flexion: index-small finger MP extension / index-small finger MP flexion: wrist extension torque transmission / thumb CMC radial abduction and MP extension mobilization splint, type 0 (7)	15-14 B-D

Wrist: Finger MP, Thumb CMC, MP, IP
Transmission/Immobilization

Extension: flexion, palmar abduction		2	(10)	Index-long; thumb	Wrist extension: index-long finger flexion / wrist flexion: index-long finger extension torque transmission / thumb CMC palmar abduction and MP-IP extension immobilization splint, type 2 (10)	4-5 B
Extension: flexion, palmar abduction		2	(10)	Index-long; thumb	Wrist extension: index-long finger flexion / wrist flexion: index-long finger extension torque transmission / thumb CMC palmar abduction and MP-IP extension immobilization splint, type 2 (10)	13-21 A-B
Extension: flexion, palmar abduction		2	(10)	Index-long; thumb	Wrist extension: index-long finger flexion / wrist flexion: index-long finger extension torque transmission / thumb CMC palmar abduction and MP-IP extension immobilization splint, type 2 (10)	15-18 B-C
Extension: flexion, palmar abduction		2	(10)	Index-long; thumb	Wrist extension: index-long finger flexion / wrist flexion: index-long finger extension torque transmission / thumb CMC palmar abduction and MP-IP extension immobilization splint, type 2 (10)	15-18 D

Wrist: [finger splint-prosthesis]
Transmission

Extension, flexion		0	(01)		Wrist extension: [finger prosthesis flexion] / wrist flexion: [finger prosthesis extension] torque transmission splint-prosthesis, type 0 (2)	10-34 A
Extension, flexion		0	(01)		Wrist extension: [finger prosthesis flexion] / wrist flexion: [finger prosthesis extension] torque transmission splint-prosthesis, type 0 (2)	15-31 H

Finger MP

Immobilization

Mobilization

Continued

Splint[1] Index (SSRDI©)

Articular/Nonarticular Joint/Segment — Purpose	Direction	Type	Joints	Digits	ESCS Name	Figure
Extension, radial deviation		3	(07)	Index-small	Index-small finger MP extension and radial deviation mobilization splint, type 3 (7)	16-4 F
Extension, radial deviation, supination		3	(07)	Index-small	Index-small finger MP extension and radial deviation, index finger MP supination mobilization splint, type 3 (7)	16-4 C-D
Extension, radial deviation, supination		3	(08)	Index-ring	Index-ring finger MP extension and radial deviation, index-long finger MP supination mobilization splint, type 3 (8)	16-4 E
Extension, radial deviation, supination		3	(11)	Index-small	Index-small finger MP extension and radial deviation, index-ring finger MP supination mobilization splint, type 3 (11)	16-19 A-B
Flexion		0	(01)	Small	Small finger MP flexion mobilization splint, type 0 (1)	6-16 D
Flexion		0	(01)	Small	Small finger MP flexion mobilization splint, type 0 (1)	7-1 C
Flexion		0	(01)	Small	Small finger MP flexion mobilization splint, type 0 (1)	8-24 E
Flexion		0	(01)	Small	Small finger MP flexion mobilization splint, type 0 (1)	11-2 D
Flexion		0	(01)	Small	Small finger MP flexion mobilization splint, type 0 (1)	14-16 A-B
Flexion		0	(01)	Ring	Ring finger MP flexion mobilization splint, type 0 (1)	7-1 D-G
Flexion		0	(01)	Ring	Ring finger MP flexion mobilization splint, type 0 (1)	11-2 E
Flexion		0	(02)	Ring-small	Ring-small finger MP flexion mobilization splint, type 0 (2)	11-2 C
Flexion		1	(02)	Long	Long finger MP flexion mobilization splint, type 1 (2); with triceps cuff	4-14
Flexion		1	(02)	Small	Small finger MP flexion mobilization splint, type 1 (2)	6-16 E
Flexion		1	(02)	Small	Small finger MP flexion mobilization splint, type 1 (2)	11-3 F
Flexion		1	(03)	Ring-small	Ring-small finger MP flexion mobilization splint, type 1 (3)	10-35 A
Flexion		1	(03)	Ring-small	Ring-small finger MP flexion mobilization splint, type 1 (3)	21-9 B
Flexion		1	(04)	Index-ring	Index-ring finger MP flexion mobilization splint, type 1 (4)	11-3 G-H
Flexion		1	(05)	Index-small	Index-small finger MP flexion mobilization splint, type 1 (5)	7-25 A
Flexion		1	(05)	Index-small	Index-small finger MP flexion mobilization splint, type 1 (5)	10-31
Flexion		1	(05)	Index-small	Index-small finger MP flexion mobilization splint, type 1 (5)	11-3 I
Flexion		1	(05)	Index-small	Index-small finger MP flexion mobilization splint, type 1 (5)	11-3 J
Flexion		1	(05)	Index-small	Index-small finger MP flexion mobilization splint, type 1 (5)	20-3 C
Flexion		1	(05)	Index-small	Index-small finger MP flexion mobilization splint, type 1 (5)	20-3 D
Flexion		1	(05)	Index-small	Index-small finger MP flexion mobilization splint, type 1 (5)	20-3 E
Flexion		2	(06)	Index-small	Index-small finger MP flexion mobilization splint, type 2 (6)	20-4 G
Flexion		2	(09)	Index-small	Index-small finger MP flexion mobilization splint, type 2 (9)	22-8
Flexion		3	(13)	Index-small	Index-small finger MP flexion mobilization splint, type 3 (13)	11-4 C
Flexion		1	(05)	Index-small	Index-small finger MP flexion mobilization splint, type 1 (5)	1-22 B
Flexion or extension		1	(05)	Index-small	Index-small finger MP flexion mobilization splint, type 1 (5) or Index-small finger PIP extension mobilization splint, type 2 (9)	11-42 A
Flexion or extension		1	(05)	Index-small	Index-small finger MP flexion mobilization splint, type 1 (5) or Index-small finger PIP extension mobilization splint, type 2 (9)	20-4 D
Flexion or extension		1	(05)	Index-small	Index-small finger MP flexion mobilization splint, type 1 (5) or Index-small finger PIP extension mobilization splint, type 2 (9)	20-4 F
Supination		3	(04)	Index	Index finger MP supination mobilization splint, type 3 (4)	11-5 B
Supination		3	(04)	Index	Index finger MP supination mobilization splint, type 3 (4)	16-4 P
Supination		5	(06)	Ring	Ring finger MP supination mobilization splint, type 5 (6)	11-5 D-E

690

Splint[1] Index (SSRDI©)

Articular/Nonarticular Joint/Segment Purpose	Direction	Type	Joints	Digits	ESCS Name	Figure
Extension or flexion		1	(03)	Small, index, long	Small finger MP-PIP extension mobilization splint, type 1 (3) or Index-long finger MP-PIP flexion mobilization splint, type 1 (6)	1-22 D
Flexion		0	(02)	Small	Small finger MP-PIP flexion mobilization splint, type 0 (2)	11-8 A
Flexion		1	(03)	Ring	Ring finger MP-PIP flexion mobilization splint, type 1 (3)	11-8 B
Flexion		1	(06)	Ring-small	Ring-small finger MP-PIP flexion mobilization splint, type 1 (6)	11-8 C-D
Restriction/Mobilization						
Extension, flexion		1	(07)	Index-small	Index-small finger MP extension restriction / long-ring PIP flexion mobilization splint, type 1 (7)	8-13 B
Extension, flexion		2	(07)	Index-small	Index-small finger MP extension restriction / long finger MP-PIP flexion mobilization splint, type 2 (7)	11-8 E
Transmission						
Extension, Flex on		2	(04)	Long	Long finger MP-PIP extension and flexion torque transmission splint, type 2 (4)	4-8 B
Extension, flexion		2	(04)	Index	Index finger MP-PIP extension and flexion torque transmission splint, type 2 (4)	10-9
Extension, flexion		2	(04)	Long	Long finger MP-PIP extension and flexion torque transmission splint, type 2 (4)	11-9 A
Extension, flexion		2	(04)	Long	Long finger MP-PIP extension and flexion torque transmission splint, type 2 (4)	11-9 B
Extension, flexion		2	(04)	Long	Long finger MP-PIP extension and flexion torque transmission splint, type 2 (4)	11-9 C
Extension, flexion		2	(04)	Index	Index finger MP-PIP extension and flexion torque transmission splint, type 2 (4)	15-22 A
Supination, extension, flexion		2	(04)	Small	Small finger MP supination, PIP extension and flexion torque transmission splint, type 2 (4)	6-5 A
Supination, extension, flexion		2	(04)	Small	Small finger MP supination, PIP extension and flexion torque transmission splint, type 2 (4)	8-8 E
Transmission/Immobilization						
Extension, flexion		1	(03)	Index	Index finger MP extension and flexion torque transmission / PIP extension immobilization splint, type 1 (3)	8-9 E-F
Transmission/Mobilization						
Extension		1	(03)	Index-small	Finger MP flexion torque transmission / PIP extension mobilization splint type 1 (3): 4 splints @ finger separate	20-4 G

Finger MP, PIP, DIP

Purpose	Direction	Type	Joints	Digits	ESCS Name	Figure
Immobilization						
Extension		0	(03)	Ring	Ring finger extension immobilization splint, type 0 (3)	11-10 A
Extension		1	(07)	Ring-small	Ring-small finger extension immobilization splint, type 1 (7)	11-10 C
Extension		1	(10)	Long, small	Long-small finger extension immobilization splint, type 1 (10)	11-10 D
Flexion, extension		0	(12)	Index-small	Index-small finger MP flexion and IP extension immobilization splint, type 0 (12)	11-10 B
Flexion, extension		1	(13)	Index-small	Index-small finger MP 20° flexion and IP extension immobilization splint, type 1 (13)	4-25 C
Flexion, extension		1	(13)	Index-small	Index-small finger extension restriction / index-ring finger flexion mobilization splint, type 1 (13)	8-10 B-C
Flexion, extension		1	(13)	Index-small	Index-small finger MP flexion and IP extension immobilization splint, type 1 (13)	21-12 B
Flexion, extension		4	(16)	Index-small	Index-small finger MP flexion and IP extension immobilization splint, type 4 (16)	8-13 A
Mobilization						
Extension		0	(03)	Ring	Ring finger extension mobilization splint, type 0 (3)	1-22 F
Extension		0	(05)	Ring	Ring finger, small finger MP-PIP extension mobilization splint, type 0 (5)	7-15 C
Extension		0	(05)	Ring-small	Ring finger MP-PIP, small finger extension mobilization splint, type 0 (5)	11-11 A

Splint Index

Splint[1] Index (SSRDI©)

Articular/Nonarticular Joint/Segment Purpose	Direction	Type	Joints	Digits	ESCS Name	Figure
Extension, flexion	1	(13)	Index-small	Index-small finger extension restriction / index-ring finger flexion mobilization splint, type 1 (13)	5-5 B
Extension, flexion	1	(13)	Index-small	Index-small finger extension restriction / ring finger flexion mobilization splint, type 1 (13)	6-20
Extension, flexion	1	(13)	Index-small	Index-small finger extension restriction / index-ring finger flexion mobilization splint, type 1 (13)	8-10 B-C
Extension, flexion	1	(13)	Index-small	Index-small finger extension restriction / index-small finger flexion mobilization splint, type 1 (13)	11-12 A-D
Extension, flexion	1	(13)	Index-small	Index-small finger MP extension restriction / index-small finger flexion mobilization splint, type 1 (13)	15-20 M-N
Restriction/Mobilization/Immobilization						
Extension, flexion	1	(13)	Index-small	Index-long finger extension restriction / index-long finger flexion mobilization / ring-small finger MP flexion, IP extension immobilization splint, type 1 (13)	8-16 E-F
Extension, flexion	1	(13)	Index-small	Index-long finger extension restriction / index-long finger flexion mobilization / ring-small finger MP flexion, IP extension immobilization splint, type 1 (13)	15-20 O-P
Restriction/Transmission						
Extension	0	(06)	Ring-small	Ring-small finger MP extension restriction / IP extension torque transmission splint, type 0 (6)	4-25 A
Extension	0	(06)	Ring-small	Ring-small finger MP extension restriction / IP extension torque transmission splint, type 0 (6)	8-5 C
Extension	0	(06)	Ring-small	Ring-small finger MP extension restriction / IP extension torque transmission splint, type 0 (6)	8-12 B-C
Extension	0	(06)	Ring, small	Ring-small finger MP extension restriction / IP extension torque transmission splint, type 0 (6)	8-16 D
Extension	0	(06)	Ring-small	Ring-small finger MP extension restriction / IP extension torque transmission splint, type 0 (6)	10-40
Extension	0	(06)	Ring-small	Ring-small finger MP extension restriction / IP extension torque transmission splint, type 0 (6)	15-15 A
Extension	0	(06)	Ring-small	Ring-small finger MP extension restriction / IP extension torque transmission splint, type 0 (6)	15-15 C-D
Extension	0	(06)	Ring-small	Ring-small finger MP extension restriction / IP extension torque transmission splint, type 0 (6)	15-15 E
Extension	0	(06)	Ring-small	Ring-small finger MP extension restriction / IP extension torque transmission splint, type 0 (6)	15-15 F-G
Extension	0	(12)	Index-small	Index-small finger MP extension restriction / IP extension torque transmission splint, type 0 (12)	7-2 F
Extension	0	(12)	Index-small	Index-small finger MP extension restriction / IP extension torque transmission splint, type 0 (12)	8-26 D
Extension	0	(12)	Index-small	Index-small finger MP extension restriction / IP extension torque transmission splint, type 0 (12)	15-16 A
Extension	0	(12)	Index-small	Index-small finger MP extension restriction / IP extension torque transmission splint, type 0 (12)	15-16 B
Extension	0	(12)	Index-small	Index-small finger MP extension restriction / IP extension torque transmission splint, type 0 (12)	20-5 C
Extension	0	(12)	Index-small	Index-small finger MP extension restriction / IP extension torque transmission splint, type 0 (12)	20-5 D

Continued

Splint[1] Index (SSRDI©)

Articular/Nonarticular Joint/Segment Purpose	Direction	Type	Joints	Digits	ESCS Name	Figure
Extension		0	(01)	Small	Small finger PIP extension mobilization splint, type 0 (1)	16-9 D
Extension		1	(02)	Index	Index finger PIP extension mobilization splint, type 1 (2)	4-2
Extension		1	(02)	Index	Index finger PIP extension mobilization splint, type 1 (2)	4-10 A
Extension		1	(02)	Long	Long finger PIP extension mobilization splint, type 1 (2)	4-10 B
Extension		1	(02)	Index	Index finger PIP extension mobilization splint, type 1 (2)	6-16 A
Extension		1	(02)	Index	Index finger PIP extension mobilization splint, type 1 (2)	6-18
Extension		1	(02)	Index	Index finger PIP extension mobilization splint, type 1 (2)	6-23 A
Extension		1	(02)	Ring	Ring finger PIP extension mobilization splint, type 1 (2)	6-26
Extension		1	(02)	Index	Index finger PIP extension mobilization splint, type 1 (2)	6-29
Extension		1	(02)	Index	Index finger PIP extension mobilization splint, type 1 (2)	7-6
Extension		1	(02)		Finger PIP extension mobilization splint, type 1 (2)	7-11 A-B
Extension		1	(02)	Small	Small finger PIP extension mobilization splint, type 1 (2)	7-17 B
Extension		1	(02)	Index	Index finger PIP extension mobilization splint, type 1 (2)	8-20 D
Extension		1	(02)	Long	Long finger PIP extension mobilization splint, type 1 (2)	10-32
Extension		1	(02)	Index	Index finger PIP extension mobilization splint, type 1 (2)	10-35 D-F
Extension		1	(02)	Small	Small finger PIP extension mobilization splint, type 1 (2)	11-17 A-B
Extension		1	(02)	Small	Small finger PIP extension mobilization splint, type 1 (2)	11-17 C
Extension		1	(02)	Index	Index finger PIP extension mobilization splint, type 1 (2)	11-17 D
Extension		1	(02)	Index	Index finger PIP extension mobilization splint, type 1 (2)	11-17 E
Extension		1	(02)	Index	Index finger PIP extension mobilization splint, type 1 (2)	11-17 F-G
Extension		1	(02)	Index	Index finger PIP extension mobilization splint, type 1 (2)	11-17 H
Extension		1	(02)		Finger PIP extension mobilization splint, type 1 (2)	15-12 B
Extension		1	(02)	Index	Index finger PIP extension mobilization splint, type 1 (2)	20-8 C
Extension		1	(02)	Index	Index finger PIP extension mobilization splint, type 1 (2)	20-8 D
Extension		1	(02)	Index	Index finger PIP extension mobilization splint, type 1 (2)	20-8 E
Extension		1	(02)	Index	Index finger PIP extension mobilization splint, type 1 (2)	21-7 C
Extension		1	(02)	Index	Index finger PIP extension mobilization splint, type 1 (2)	22-3
Extension		1	(04)	Long-ring	Long-ring finger PIP extension mobilization splint, type 1 (4)	7-2 P
Extension		1	(04)	Index-long	Index-long finger PIP extension mobilization splint, type 1 (4)	11-17 I
Extension		1	(06)	Index-ring	Index-ring finger PIP extension mobilization splint, type 1 (6)	11-17 J
Extension		1	(08)	Index-small	Index-small finger PIP extension mobilization splint, type 1 (8)	7-3 D
Extension		1	(08)	Index-small	Index-small finger PIP extension mobilization splint, type 1 (8)	11-17 K
Extension		1	(08)	Index-small	Index-small finger PIP extension mobilization splint, type 1 (8)	20-7 C
Extension		2	(03)	Small	Small finger PIP extension mobilization splint, type 2 (3)	4-10 C
Extension		2	(03)	Index	Index finger PIP extension mobilization splint, type 2 (3)	7-2 H
Extension		2	(03)	Small	Small finger PIP extension mobilization splint, type 2 (3)	7-2 J-K
Extension		2	(03)	Long	Long finger PIP extension mobilization splint, type 2 (3)	7-3 B
Extension		2	(03)	Index	Index finger PIP extension mobilization splint, type 2 (3)	7-26 B
Extension		2	(03)	Long	Long finger PIP extension mobilization splint, type 2 (3)	10-8 A
Extension		2	(03)	Index	Index finger PIP extension mobilization splint, type 2 (3)	11-18 A
Extension		2	(03)	Long	Long finger PIP extension mobilization splint, type 2 (3)	11-18 F
Extension		2	(03)	Long	Long finger PIP extension mobilization splint, type 2 (3)	11-18 G
Extension		2	(03)	Long	Long finger PIP extension mobilization splint, type 2 (3)	11-18 H-I
Extension		2	(03)	Index	Index finger PIP extension mobilization splint, type 2 (3)	21-11 B
Extension		2	(06)	Long-ring	Long-ring finger PIP extension mobilization splint, type 2 (6)	7-3 A
Extension		2	(13)	Index-small	Index-small finger IP extension mobilization splint, type 2 (13)	7-1 B
Extension		2	(06)	Long	Long finger PIP extension mobilization splint, type 2 (6)	8-24 A

Motion	Digit	No.	Code	Splint	Figure
Extension	Long-ring	2	(06)	Long-ring finger PIP extension mobilization splint, type 2 (6)	11-18 B
Extension	Long-ring	2	(06)	Long-ring finger PIP extension mobilization splint, type 2 (6)	6-3
Extension	Ring-small	2	(06)	Ring-small finger PIP extension mobilization splint, type 2 (6)	11-18 C
Extension	Index-small	2	(09)	Index-small finger PIP extension mobilization splint, type 2 (9)	4-25 B
Extension	Index-small	2	(09)	Index-small finger PIP extension mobilization splint, type 2 (9)	6-16 B
Extension	Index-small	2	(09)	Index-small finger PIP extension mobilization splint, type 2 (9)	6-30 B
Extension	Index-small	2	(09)	Index-small finger PIP extension mobilization splint, type 2 (9)	6-30 D
Extension	Index-small	2	(09)	Index-small finger PIP extension mobilization splint, type 2 (9)	7-2 A
Extension	Index-small	2	(09)	Index-small finger PIP extension mobilization splint, type 2 (9)	7-17 A
Extension	Index-small	2	(09)	Index-small finger PIP extension mobilization splint, type 2 (9)	7-19 A
Extension	Index-small	2	(09)	Index-small finger PIP extension mobilization splint, type 2 (9)	9-6
Extension	Index-small	2	(09)	Index-small finger PIP extension mobilization splint, type 2 (9)	7-24 A-B
Extension	Index-small	2	(09)	Index-small finger PIP extension mobilization splint, type 2 (9)	11-18 J
Extension	Index-small	2	(09)	Index-small finger PIP extension mobilization splint, type 2 (9)	21-15 D
Extension	Index-small	2	(13)	Index-small finger PIP extension mobilization splint, type 2 (13)	6-17 A-C
Extension	Long	3	(04)	Long finger PIP extension mobilization splint, type 3 (4)	11-19 A
Extension	Index-small	3	(09)	Index-small PIP extension mobilization splint, type 3 (10)	1-22 I
Extension	Index-small	3	(13)	Index-small finger PIP extension mobilization splint, type 3 (13)	11-19 B
Extension	Index-small	3	(13)	Index-small finger PIP extension mobilization splint, type 3 (13)	20-7 E
Extension or flexion	Long	1	(02)	Long finger PIP flexion or extension mobilization splint, type 1 (2)	8-16 C
Extension or flexion	Index-small	2	(09)	Index-small finger PIP extension mobilization splint, type 2 (9) or Index-small finger MP flexion mobilization splint, type 1 (5)	11-42 B
Extension or flexion	Index-small	2	(09)	Index-small finger PIP extension mobilization splint, type 2 (9) or Index-small finger MP flexion mobilization splint, type 1 (5)	20-4 C
Extension or flexion	Index-small	2	(09)	Index-small finger PIP extension mobilization splint, type 2 (9) or Index-small finger MP flexion mobilization splint, type 1 (5)	20-4 E
Extension, flexion	Index-small	2	(12)	Index-small finger PIP extension or flexion mobilization splint, type 2 (12)	11-18 D-E
Extension, distraction	Small	1	(02)	Small finger middle phalanx distraction, PIP extension and distraction mobilization splint, type 1 (2)	11-20 A
Extension, distraction	Small	3	(04)	Small finger middle phalanx distraction, PIP extension and distraction mobilization splint, type 3 (4)	11-20 B-C
Flexion	Ring	1	(02)	Ring finger PIP flexion mobilization splint, type 1 (2)	8-4 A
Flexion	Index	1	(02)	Index finger PIP flexion mobilization splint, type 1 (2)	11-21 A-C
Flexion	Long	1	(02)	Long finger PIP flexion mobilization splint, type 1 (2)	11-21 D-G
Flexion	Small	1	(02)	Small finger PIP flexion mobilization splint, type 1 (2)	11-21 H-I
Flexion	Small	1	(02)	Small finger PIP flexion mobilization splint, type 1 (2)	17-7
Flexion	Index	1	(02)	Index finger PIP flexion mobilization splint, type 1 (2)	22-7 C
Flexion	Index-long, small	1	(09)	Index-long finger IP, small finger PIP flexion mobilization splint, type 1 (9)	11-21 J
Flexion	Index	2	(03)	Index finger PIP flexion mobilization splint, type 2 (3)	6-23 B
Flexion	Ring	2	(03)	Ring finger PIP flexion mobilization splint, type 2 (3)	11-22 B
Flexion	Long	2	(03)	Long finger PIP flexion mobilization splint, type 2 (3)	11-22 C
Flexion	Index-small	2	(08)	Index-small finger PIP flexion mobilization splint, type 2 (8)	11-22 A
Flexion, extension	Index-small	2	(12)	Index-small finger PIP extension mobilization splint, type 2 (12)	20-7 D
Radial deviation	Ring	1	(02)	Ring finger PIP radial deviation mobilization splint, type 1 (2)	10-34 C-D
Ulnar deviation, extension	Ring	0	(01)	Ring finger PIP ulnar deviation and extension mobilization splint, type 0 (1)	11-23 B
Ulnar deviation, extension	Ring	1	(02)	Ring finger PIP ulnar deviation and extension mobilization splint, type 1 (2)	11-23 C

Restriction

Motion	Digit	No.	Code	Splint	Figure
Extension	Index-small	0	(01)	Finger PIP extension restriction splint, type 0 (1); 4 splints @ finger separate	8-3 A-B
Extension	Index	0	(01)	Index finger PIP extension restriction splint, type 0 (1)	8-25 B
Extension	Index	0	(01)	Index finger PIP extension restriction splint, type 0 (1)	11-24 A

Continued

Splint Index

Splint[1] Index (SSRDI©)

Articular/Nonarticular Joint/Segment Purpose	Direction	Type	Joints	Digits	ESCS Name	Figure
Extension		0	(01)	Index-small	Finger PIP extension restriction splint, type 0 (1); 4 splints @ finger separate; left	11-24 B
Extension		0	(01)	Index-small	Finger PIP extension restriction splint, type 0 (1); 4 splints @ finger separate; right	11-24 B
Extension		0	(01)	Index	Index finger PIP extension restriction splint, type 0 (1)	11-24 C-D
Extension		0	(01)	Index-small	Finger PIP extension restriction splint, type 0 (1); 4 splints @ finger separate; left	16-9 B
Extension		0	(01)	Index-small	Finger PIP extension restriction splint, type 0 (1); 4 splints @ finger separate; right	16-9 B
Extension		0	(01)	Long	Long finger PIP extension restriction splint, type 0 (1)	11-25 C
Extension		0	(01)	Index-small	Finger PIP extension restriction splint, type 0 (1); 4 splints @ finger separate	8-5 G-H
Extension		1	(02)	Ring	Ring finger PIP extension restriction splint, type 1 (2)	10-33
Extension, flexion		0	(01)	Index	Index finger PIP extension and flexion restriction splint, type 0 (1)	11-25 A-B
Extension, radial deviation		1	(02)	Index	Index finger PIP extension and radial deviation restriction splint, type 1 (2)	11-25 C
Radial deviation, ulnar deviation		2	(03)	Long	Long finger PIP radial and ulnar deviation restriction splint, type 2 (3)	8-15 B
Radial deviation, ulnar deviation		2	(03)	Long	Long finger PIP radial and ulnar deviation restriction splint, type 2 (3)	11-26 A-C

Restriction/Mobilization

Purpose	Direction	Type	Joints	Digits	ESCS Name	Figure
Extension, distraction		3	(04)	Index	Index finger PIP extension restriction / distraction mobilization splint, type 3 (4)	11-27 A-B

Transmission

Purpose	Direction	Type	Joints	Digits	ESCS Name	Figure
Extension		1	(02)	Index-small	Finger PIP extension torque transmission splint, type 1 (2); 4 splints @ finger separate	6-17 B-C
Extension		1	(02)	Index-small	Finger PIP extension torque transmission splint, type 1 (2); 4 splints @ finger separate	7-17 A
Extension		1	(02)	Index-small	Finger PIP extension torque transmission splint, type 1 (2); 4 splints @ finger separate	11-18 J
Extension		1	(02)	Index-small	Finger PIP extension torque transmission splint, type 1 (2); 4 splints @ finger separate	20-7 E
Extension, flexion		2	(04)	index-long	Long finger PIP extension and flexion torque transmission splint, type 2 (4)	17-6
Flexion or extension		1	(02)	Long	Long finger PIP flexion or extension torque transmission splint, type 1 (2)	8-16 C

Finger PIP, DIP

Immobilization

Purpose	Direction	Type	Joints	Digits	ESCS Name	Figure
Extension		0	(02)	Ring	Ring finger IP extension immobilization splint, type 0 (2)	11-18 G
Extension		0	(02)	Small	Small finger IP extension immobilization splint, type 0 (2)	11-18 G
Flexion		0	(02)	Ring	Ring finger IP flexion immobilization splint, type 0 (2)	16-18
Flexion		0	(02)	Small	Small finger IP flexion immobilization splint, type 0 (2)	16-18
Flexion		0	(02)	Ring	Ring finger IP flexion immobilization splint, type 0 (2)	16-19 A-B
Flexion		0	(02)	Small	Small finger IP flexion immobilization splint, type 0 (2)	16-19 A-B

Mobilization

Purpose	Direction	Type	Joints	Digits	ESCS Name	Figure
Extension		0	(02)	Small	Small finger IP extension mobilization splint, type 0 (2)	6-6 A
Extension		0	(02)	Ring	Ring finger IP extension mobilization splint, type 0 (2)	6-6 A
Extension		0	(02)	Small	Small finger IP extension mobilization splint, type 0 (2)	6-6 B
Extension		0	(02)	Ring	Ring finger IP extension mobilization splint, type 0 (2)	6-6 B
Extension		0	(02)	Index	Index finger IP extension mobilization splint, type 0 (2)	22-1 D
Extension		0	(02)	Index-small	Finger IP extension mobilization splint, type 0 (2); 4 splints @ finger separate	22-8
Extension		1	(03)	Small	Small finger IP extension mobilization splint, type 1 (3)	10-28
Extension		2	(10)	Index-ring	Index-ring finger IP extension mobilization splint, type 2 (10)	11-30 B
Extension		2	(13)	Index-small	Index-small finger IP extension mobilization splint, type 2 (13)	4-24
Extension		2	(13)	Index-small	Index-small finger IP extension mobilization splint, type 2 (13)	7-1 B
Extension, flexion		0	(02)	Index	Index-small finger PIP extension, DIP flexion mobilization splint, type 0 (2)	11-28 G

Motion			Finger	Splint	Reference
Extension, flexion	0	(02)	Index	Finger PIP extension, DIP flexion mobilization splint, type 0 (2)	22-6 C
Extension, flexion	2	(13)	Index-small	Index-small finger IP extension and flexion mobilization splint, type 2 (13)	15-10 B
Flexion	0	(02)	Index	Index finger IP flexion mobilization splint, type 0 (2)	6-2 A
Flexion	0	(02)	Index-small	Finger IP flexion mobilization splint, type 0 (2); 4 splints @ finger separate	8-4 B
Flexion	0	(02)	Index	Index finger IP flexion mobilization splint, type 0 (2)	8-24 C
Flexion	0	(02)	Index	Index finger IP flexion mobilization splint, type 0 (2)	11-28 A
Flexion	0	(02)	Index-small	Finger IP flexion mobilization splint, type 0 (2); 4 splints @ finger separate	11-28 B
Flexion	0	(02)	Index-small	Finger IP flexion mobilization splint, type 0 (2); 4 splints @ finger separate	20-9 C
Flexion	0	(08)	Index-small	Index-small finger IP flexion mobilization splint, type 0 (8)	11-28 C-D
Flexion	0	(08)	Index-small	Index-small finger IP flexion mobilization splint, type 0 (8)	20-9 D
Flexion	1	(03)	Index	Index finger IP flexion mobilization splint, type 1 (3)	4-9
Flexion	1	(03)	Index	Index finger IP flexion mobilization splint, type 1 (3)	8-20 A
Flexion	1	(03)	Index	Index finger IP flexion mobilization splint, type 1 (3)	11-29 A
Flexion	1	(03)	Index	Index finger IP flexion mobilization splint, type 1 (3)	11-29 B
Flexion	1	(03)	Ring	Ring finger IP flexion mobilization splint, type 1 (3)	11-29 C-D
Flexion	1	(09)	Index, long, small	Index-long finger IP, small finger PIP flexion mobilization splint, type 1 (9)	7-19 D
Flexion	2	(04)	Small	Small finger IP flexion mobilization splint, type 2 (4)	7-19 C
Flexion	2	(04)	Small	Small finger IP flexion mobilization splint, type 2 (4)	11-30 C
Flexion	2	(13)	Index-small	Index-small finger IP flexion mobilization splint, type 2 (13)	8-24 F-H
Flexion	2	(13)	Index-small	Index-small finger IP flexion mobilization splint, type 2 (13)	11-30 A
Flexion	2	(13)	Index-small	Index-small finger IP flexion mobilization splint, type 2 (13)	11-30 D
Flexion	2	(13)	Index-small	Index-small finger IP flexion mobilization splint, type 2 (13)	11-30 E
Flexion	2	(13)	Index-small	Index-small finger IP flexion mobilization splint, type 2 (13)	15-12 C
Flexion	2	(13)	Index-small	Index-small finger IP flexion mobilization splint, type 2 (13)	20-9 E
Flexion or extension	1	(03)	Long	Long finger IP flexion or extension mobilization splint, type 1 (3)	8-20 B-C

Mobilization/Restriction/Transmission

Motion			Finger	Splint	Reference
Extension, flexion	0	(02)	Long	Long finger PIP extension mobilization / DIP extension restriction / DIP flexion torque transmission splint, type 0 (2)	11-31 A-B
Extension, flexion	0	(02)	Index	Index finger PIP extension mobilization / DIP extension restriction / DIP flexion torque transmission splint, type 0 (2)	11-31 C-D
Extension, flexion	2	(04)	Index	Index finger IP extension mobilization / PIP flexion restriction / DIP flexion torque transmission splint, type 2 (4)	15-19 I-J

Mobilization/Transmission

Motion			Finger	Splint	Reference
Extension, flexion	0	(02)	Index	Index finger PIP extension mobilization / DIP flexion torque transmission splint, type 0 (2)	17-3

Restriction

Motion			Finger	Splint	Reference
Flexion	0	(02)	Index	Index finger IP flexion restriction splint, type 0 (2)	11-32

Restriction/Immobilization

Motion			Finger	Splint	Reference
Extension	0	(02)	Long	Long finger PIP extension restriction / DIP extension immobilization splint, type 0 (2)	11-33 A-B

Transmission

Motion			Finger	Splint	Reference
Extension, flexion	1	(03)	Long	Long finger IP extension and flexion torque transmission splint, type 1 (3)	15-5 B
Extension, flexion	1	(03)	Index	Index finger IP extension and flexion torque transmission splint, type 1 (3)	15-8 A
Extension, flexion	1	(12)	Index-small	Index-small finger IP extension and flexion torque transmission splint, type 1 (12)	15-5 C
Extension, flexion	2	(13)	Index-small	Index-small finger IP extension and flexion torque transmission splint, type 2 (13)	11-43 A
Extension, flexion	2	(13)	Index-small	Index-small finger IP extension and flexion torque transmission splint, type 2 (13)	15-5 D

Continued

Splint[1] Index (SSRDI©)

Articular/Nonarticular Joint/Segment Purpose	Direction	Type	Joints	Digits	ESCS Name	Figure
Finger DIP						
Immobilization						
Extension	0	(01)	Long, ring	Finger DIP extension immobilization splint, type 0 (1); 2 splints long and ring @ finger separate	8-13 B
Extension	0	(01)	Index	Index finger DIP extension immobilization splint, type 0 (1)	10-23
Extension	0	(01)	Ring	Ring finger DIP extension immobilization splint, type 0 (1)	11-34 A
Extension	0	(01)	Index	Index finger DIP extension immobilization splint, type 0 (1)	11-34 B
Extension	0	(01)	Index	Index finger DIP extension immobilization splint, type 0 (1)	11-34 D
Extension	0	(01)	Ring	Ring finger DIP extension immobilization splint, type 0 (1)	15-28 A
Extension	0	(01)	Index-small	Finger DIP extension immobilization splint, type 0 (1); 4 splints @ finger separate	15-30 B
Hyperextension	0	(01)	Index	Index finger DIP hyperextension immobilization splint, type 0 (1)	11-34 C
Hyperextension	0	(01)	Index	Index finger DIP hyperextension immobilization splint, type 0 (1)	17-1
Hyperextension	0	(01)	Index	Index finger DIP hyperextension immobilization splint, type 0 (1)	17-2
Mobilization						
Extension	0	(01)	Small	Small finger DIP extension mobilization splint, type 0 (1)	11-35
Extension	0	(01)	Index	Index finger DIP extension mobilization splint, type 0 (1)	22-7 B
Extension	1	(02)	Long	Long finger DIP extension mobilization splint, type 1 (2)	11-36 A
Extension	1	(02)	Long	Long finger DIP extension mobilization splint, type 1 (2)	11-36 B
Extension	2	(03)	Index	Index finger DIP extension mobilization splint, type 2 (3)	11-37 A
Flexion	0	(01)		Finger DIP flexion mobilization splint, type 0 (1)	11-28 F
Flexion	0	(01)		Finger DIP flexion mobilization splint, type 0 (1)	22-6 B
Flexion	1	(02)	Index	Index finger DIP flexion mobilization splint, type 1 (2)	11-36 C
Flexion	2	(03)	Small	Small finger DIP flexion mobilization splint, type 2 (3)	11-37 B
Flexion	2	(03)	Small	Small finger DIP flexion mobilization splint, type 2 (3)	11-37 C-D
Transmission						
Extension, flexion	2	(12)	Index-small	Index-small finger DIP extension and flexion torque transmission splint, type 2 (12)	7-1 M
Extension, flexion	3	(13)	Index-small	Index-small finger DIP extension and flexion torque transmission splint, type 3 (13)	3-26
Flexion	1	(02)	Index	Index finger DIP flexion torque transmission splint, type 1 (2)	10-1
Thumb CMC						
Immobilization						
Palmar abduction	0	(01)	Thumb	Thumb CMC palmar abduction immobilization splint, type 0 (1)	12-2 A-C
Palmar abduction	1	(02)	Thumb	Thumb CMC palmar abduction immobilization splint, type 1 (2)	12-2 D-E
Palmar abduction	1	(02)	Thumb	Thumb CMC palmar abduction immobilization splint, type 1 (2)	12-2 F-G
Palmar abduction	1	(02)	Thumb	Thumb CMC palmar abduction immobilization splint, type 1 (2)	21-4 A
Palmar abduction	2	(03)	Thumb	Thumb CMC palmar abduction immobilization splint, type 2 (3)	4-11
Palmar abduction	2	(03)	Thumb	Thumb CMC palmar abduction immobilization splint, type 2 (3)	4-23
Palmar abduction	2	(03)	Thumb	Thumb CMC palmar abduction immobilization splint, type 2 (3)	5-2
Palmar abduction	2	(03)	Thumb	Thumb CMC palmar abduction immobilization splint, type 2 (3)	8-19 A
Palmar abduction	2	(03)	Thumb	Thumb CMC palmar abduction immobilization splint, type 2 (3)	12-2 H
Palmar abduction	2	(03)	Thumb	Thumb CMC palmar abduction immobilization splint, type 2 (3)	16-10
Palmar abduction	3	(04)	Thumb	Thumb CMC palmar abduction immobilization splint, type 3 (4)	4-27
Radial abduction	3	(04)	Thumb	Thumb CMC radial abduction immobilization splint, type 3 (4)	12-2 I

Mobilization

Palmar abduction	0	(01)	Thumb	Thumb CMC palmar abduction mobilization splint, type 0 (1)	8-5 A-B
Palmar abduction	0	(01)	Thumb	Thumb CMC palmar abduction mobilization splint, type 0 (1)	18-6 E
Palmar abduction	0	(01)	Thumb	Thumb CMC palmar abduction mobilization splint, type 0 (1)	19-10 A
Palmar abduction	0	(01)	Thumb	Thumb CMC palmar abduction mobilization splint, type 0 (1)	20-10 D
Palmar abduction	1	(02)	Thumb	Thumb CMC palmar abduction mobilization splint, type 1 (2)	1-24
Palmar abduction	1	(02)	Thumb	Thumb CMC palmar abduction mobilization splint, type 1 (2)	8-14
Palmar abduction	1	(02)	Thumb	Thumb CMC palmar abduction mobilization splint, type 1 (2)	12-3 A-B
Palmar abduction	1	(02)	Thumb	Thumb CMC palmar abduction mobilization splint, type 1 (2)	12-4 C
Palmar abduction	1	(02)	Thumb	Thumb CMC palmar abduction mobilization splint, type 1 (2)	15-13
Palmar abduction	1	(02)	Thumb	Thumb CMC palmar abduction mobilization splint, type 1 (2)	20-10 C
Palmar abduction	1	(02)	Thumb	Thumb CMC palmar abduction mobilization splint, type 1 (2)	20-10 D
Palmar abduction	3	(04)	Thumb	Thumb CMC palmar abduction mobilization splint, type 3 (4)	4-13 A
Palmar abduction	3	(04)	Thumb	Thumb CMC palmar abduction mobilization splint, type 3 (4)	6-36 C
Palmar abduction	3	(04)	Thumb	Thumb CMC palmar abduction mobilization splint, type 3 (4)	7-2 Q
Palmar abduction	3	(04)	Thumb	Thumb CMC palmar abduction mobilization splint, type 3 (4)	12-5 A-B
Palmar abduction	3	(04)	Thumb	Thumb CMC palmar abduction mobilization splint, type 3 (4)	20-10 E
Palmar abduction	6	(07)	Thumb	Thumb CMC palmar abduction mobilization splint, type 6 (7)	8-17 B
Palmar abduction	6	(07)	Thumb	Thumb CMC palmar abduction mobilization splint, type 6 (7)	20-10 F
Radial abduction	0	(01)	Thumb	Thumb CMC radial abduction mobilization splint, type 0 (1)	12-4 A-B
Radial abduction	0	(01)	Thumb	Thumb CMC radial abduction mobilization splint, type 0 (1)	18-5 A-B
Radial abduction	5	(06)	Thumb	Thumb CMC radial abduction mobilization splint, type 5 (6)	12-5 C

Restriction

Adduction	0	(01)	Thumb	Thumb CMC adduction restriction splint, type 0 (1)	12-6 A-B
Adduction	1	(02)	Thumb	Thumb CMC adduction restriction splint, type 1 (2)	12-6 C-D
Circumduction	1	(02)	Thumb	Thumb CMC circumduction restriction splint, type 1 (2)	8-15 A
Circumduction	1	(02)	Thumb	Thumb CMC circumduction restriction splint, type 1 (2)	12-6 E-F
Circumduction	1	(02)	Thumb	Thumb CMC circumduction restriction splint, type 1 (2)	12-6 G-H
Circumduction	2	(03)	Thumb	Thumb CMC circumduction restriction splint, type 2 (3)	12-6 I

Transmission

Circumduction	2	(03)	Thumb	Thumb CMC circumduction torque transmission splint, type 2 (3)	12-6 J-K
Circumduction	3	(04)	Thumb	Thumb CMC circumduction torque transmission splint, type 3 (4)	12-6 L

Thumb CMC [thumb splint-prosthesis]

Circumduction [flexion]	0	(01)	Thumb	Thumb CMC circumduction / [thumb MP-IP flexion fixed] torque transmission splint-prosthesis, type 0 (1)	15-31 B-C
Circumduction [flexion]	0	(01)	Thumb	Thumb CMC circumduction / [thumb MP-IP flexion fixed] torque transmission splint-prosthesis, type 0 (1)	15-31 D

Thumb CMC, MP

Immobilization

Palmar abduction, extension	0	(02)	Thumb	Thumb CMC palmar abduction and MP extension immobilization splint, type 0 (2)	12-7 A
Palmar abduction, extension	1	(03)	Thumb	Thumb CMC palmar abduction and MP extension immobilization splint, type 1 (3)	1-4 A
Palmar abduction, extension	1	(03)	Thumb	Thumb CMC palmar abduction and MP extension immobilization splint, type 1 (3)	1-4 B
Palmar abduction, flexion	0	(02)	Thumb	Thumb CMC palmar abduction and MP flexion immobilization splint, type 0 (2)	12-7 B
Palmar abduction, flexion	1	(03)	Thumb	Thumb CMC palmar abduction and MP flexion immobilization splint, type 1 (3)	9-5 B
Radial abduction, flexion	0	(02)	Thumb	Thumb CMC palmar abduction and MP flexion immobilization splint, type 0 (2)	9-14 B

Continued

Splint[1] Index (SSRDI©)

Articular/Nonarticular Joint/Segment Purpose	Direction	Type	Joints	Digits	ESCS Name	Figure
Mobilization						
Palmar abduction, extension		0	(02)	Thumb	Thumb CMC palmar abduction and MP extension mobilization splint, type 0 (2)	19-10 B
Palmar abduction, extension		0	(02)	Thumb	Thumb CMC palmar abduction and MP extension mobilization splint, type 0 (2)	15-31 A
Palmar abduction, flexion		0	(02)	Thumb	Thumb CMC palmar abduction and MP flexion mobilization splint, type 0 (2)	12-8 A-B
Palmar abduction, flexion		0	(02)	Thumb	Thumb CMC palmar abduction and MP flexion mobilization splint, type 0 (2)	12-8 C
Radial abduction, extension		0	(02)	Thumb	Thumb CMC radial abduction and MP extension mobilization splint, type 0 (2)	18-5 D
Radial abduction, extension		0	(02)	Thumb	Thumb CMC radial abduction and MP extension mobilization splint, type 0 (2)	18-6 A
Radial abduction, extension		0	(02)	Thumb	Thumb CMC radial abduction and MP extension mobilization splint, type 0 (2)	18-6 D
Radial abduction, extension		0	(02)	Thumb	Thumb CMC radial abduction and MP extension mobilization splint, type 0 (2)	18-6 E
Radial abduction, extension		0	(02)	Thumb	Thumb CMC radial abduction and MP extension mobilization splint, type 0 (2); with grasp assist	18-19 D
Radial abduction, extension		0	(02)	Thumb	Thumb CMC radial abduction and MP extension mobilization splint, type 0 (2); with grasp assist	18-19 E
Radial abduction, extension		0	(02)	Thumb	Thumb CMC radial abduction and MP extension mobilization splint, type 0 (2); with grasp assist	18-19 F
Mobilization/Immobilization						
Palmar abduction, flexion		0	(02)	Thumb	Thumb CMC palmar abduction mobilization / thumb MP flexion immobilization splint, type 0 (2)	12-9 B
Radial abduction, flexion		0	(02)	Thumb	Thumb CMC radial abduction mobilization / thumb MP flexion immobilization splint, type 0 (2)	12-9 A

Thumb CMC, MP, IP

Purpose	Direction	Type	Joints	Digits	ESCS Name	Figure
Immobilization						
Palmar abduction, extension		1	(04)	Thumb	Thumb CMC palmar abduction and MP-IP extension immobilization splint, type 1 (4)	1-11
Radial abduction, extension		1	(04)	Thumb	Thumb CMC radial abduction and MP-IP extension immobilization splint, type 1 (4)	12-10 A
Radial abduction, extension		1	(04)	Thumb	Thumb CMC radial abduction and MP-IP extension immobilization splint, type 1 (4)	12-10 B
Mobilization						
Palmar abduction and opposition		0	(03)	Thumb	Thumb CMC palmar abduction and opposition mobilization splint, type 0 (3)	4-28
Palmar abduction, extension		0	(03)	Thumb	Thumb CMC palmar abduction and MP-IP extension mobilization splint, type 0 (3)	8-26 C
Palmar abduction, extension		0	(03)	Thumb	Thumb CMC palmar abduction and MP-IP extension mobilization splint, type 0 (3)	19-10 C
Palmar abduction, flexion		0	(03)	Thumb	Thumb CMC palmar abduction and MP-IP flexion mobilization splint, type 0 (3)	12-11 A-B
Mobilization/Immobilization						
Radial abduction, extension		0	(03)	Thumb	Thumb CMC radial abduction mobilization / MP-IP extension immobilization splint, type 0 (3)	10-6 B
Restriction/Mobilization						
Radial abduction, extension, palmar abduction, flexion		1	(04)	Thumb	Thumb CMC radial abduction and MP-IP extension restriction / thumb CMC palmar abduction and MP-IP flexion mobilization splint, type 1 (4)	12-12 A-B
Radial abduction, extension, palmar abduction, flexion		1	(04)	Thumb	Thumb CMC radial abduction and MP-IP extension restriction / thumb CMC palmar abduction and MP-IP flexion mobilization splint, type 1 (4)	15-20 Q-R

Thumb CMC, IP

Mobilization

Motion	Splint				Figure
Palmar abduction, flexion	Thumb CMC palmar abduction and IP flexion mobilization splint, type 1 (3)	1	(03)	Thumb	8-23
Palmar abduction, flexion	Thumb CMC palmar abduction and IP flexion mobilization splint, type 1 (3)	1	(03)	Thumb	12-13

Thumb MP

Immobilization

Motion	Splint				Figure
Extension	Thumb MP extension immobilization splint, type 1 (2)	1	(02)	Thumb	16-12 A-B
Flexion	Thumb MP flexion immobilization splint, type 0 (1)	0	(01)	Thumb	15-3
Flexion	Thumb MP flexion immobilization splint, type 0 (1)	0	(01)	Thumb	12-14 A
Flexion	Thumb MP flexion immobilization splint, type 0 (1)	0	(01)	Thumb	12-14 B
Flexion	Thumb MP flexion immobilization splint, type 0 (1)	0	(01)	Thumb	16-11
Flexion	Thumb MP flexion immobilization splint, type 1 (2)	1	(02)	Thumb	12-14 C
Flexion	Thumb MP flexion immobilization splint, type 1 (2)	1	(02)	Thumb	12-14 E
Flexion	Thumb MP flexion immobilization splint, type 2 (3)	2	(03)	Thumb	8-18 D

Mobilization

Motion	Splint				Figure
Distraction, flexion	First metacarpal distraction, thumb MP distraction and flexion mobilization splint, type 2 (3)	2	(03)	Thumb	12-15 D
Flexion	Thumb MP flexion mobilization splint, type 1 (2)	1	(02)	Thumb	12-15 A
Flexion	Thumb MP flexion mobilization splint, type 1 (2)	1	(02)	Thumb	12-15 B
Flexion	Thumb MP flexion mobilization splint, type 1 (2)	1	(02)	Thumb	12-15 C

Restriction

Motion	Splint				Figure
Extension	Thumb MP extension restriction splint, type 1 (2)	1	(02)	Thumb	12-16 A-B
Extension	Thumb MP extension restriction splint, type 1 (2)	1	(02)	Thumb	12-16 C
Radial deviation, ulnar deviation	Thumb MP radial and ulnar deviation restriction splint, type 0 (1)	0	(01)	Thumb	17-11 B
Radial deviation, ulnar deviation	Thumb MP radial and ulnar deviation restriction splint, type 1 (2)	1	(02)	Thumb	17-10 A
Radial deviation, ulnar deviation	Thumb MP radial and ulnar deviation restriction splint, type 1 (2)	1	(02)	Thumb	17-10 B
Radial deviation, ulnar deviation	Thumb MP radial and ulnar deviation restriction splint, type 1 (2)	1	(02)	Thumb	17-10 C
Radial deviation, ulnar deviation	Thumb MP radial and ulnar deviation restriction splint, type 1 (2)	1	(02)	Thumb	12-16 D-E
Radial deviation, ulnar deviation	Thumb MP radial and ulnar deviation restriction splint, type 1 (2)	1	(02)	Thumb	17-11 A

Thumb MP, IP

Immobilization

Motion	Splint				Figure
Extension	Thumb MP-IP extension immobilization splint, type 0 (2)	0	(02)	Thumb	10-8 C
Extension	Thumb MP-IP extension immobilization splint, type 0 (2)	0	(02)	Thumb	12-17 A
Extension	Thumb MP-IP extension immobilization splint, type 1 (3)	1	(03)	Thumb	12-17 B

Continued

Splint[1] Index (SSRDI©)

Articular/Nonarticular Joint/Segment Purpose	Direction	Type	Joints	Digits	ESCS Name	Figure
Immobilization/Restriction						
Extension	0	(02)	Thumb	Thumb MP extension immobilization / IP extension restriction splint, type 0 (2)	8-5 E
Extension	0	(02)	Thumb	Thumb MP extension immobilization / IP extension restriction splint, type 0 (2)	10-4 D
Extension, ulnar deviation	1	(02)	Thumb	Thumb MP extension immobilization / IP ulnar deviation restriction splint, type 1 (2)	12-17 C
Flexion, extension	0	(02)	Thumb	Thumb MP flexion immobilization / IP extension restriction splint, type 0 (2)	16-18
Flexion, extension	0	(02)	Thumb	Thumb MP flexion immobilization / IP extension restriction splint, type 0 (2)	16-19 A-B
Flexion, extension	1	(03)	Thumb	Thumb MP flexion immobilization / IP extension restriction splint, type 1 (3)	8-18 C
Flexion, extension	1	(03)	Thumb	Thumb MP flexion immobilization / IP extension restriction splint, type 1 (3)	12-17 D
Mobilization						
Extension	2	(04)	Thumb	Thumb MP-IP extension mobilization splint, type 2 (4)	6-16 C
Flexion	0	(02)	Thumb	Thumb MP-IP flexion mobilization splint, type 0 (2)	6-22
Restriction/Transmission						
Extension, flexion	2	(04)	Thumb	Thumb MP flexion restriction / MP-IP extension and flexion torque transmission splint, type 2 (4)	12-17 E
Thumb IP						
Immobilization						
Extension	0	(01)	Thumb	Thumb IP extension immobilization splint, type 0 (1)	12-18 A
Extension	0	(01)	Thumb	Thumb IP extension immobilization splint, type 0 (1)	12-18 B
Extension	0	(01)	Thumb	Thumb IP extension immobilization splint, type 0 (1)	16-13 A
Mobilization						
Extension	0	(01)	Thumb	Thumb IP extension mobilization splint, type 0 (1)	7-2 L-M
Extension	3	(04)	Thumb	Thumb IP extension mobilization splint, type 3 (4)	12-19 F
Extension	3	(04)	Thumb	Thumb IP extension mobilization splint, type 3 (4)	12-19 G
Extension or flexion	2	(03)	Thumb	Thumb IP extension or flexion mobilization splint, type 2 (3)	7-2 C
Extension or flexion	2	(03)	Thumb	Thumb IP extension or flexion mobilization splint, type 2 (3)	10-39 C
Extension or flexion	2	(03)	Thumb	Thumb IP extension or flexion mobilization splint, type 2 (3)	12-19 D-E
Flexion	2	(03)	Thumb	Thumb IP flexion mobilization splint, type 2 (3)	12-19 A-B
Flexion	2	(03)	Thumb	Thumb IP flexion mobilization splint, type 2 (3)	12-19 C
Flexion	2	(03)	Thumb	Thumb IP flexion mobilization splint, type 2 (3)	20-11 C
Flexion	2	(03)	Thumb	Thumb IP flexion mobilization splint, type 2 (3)	20-11 D
Flexion or extension	2	(03)	Thumb	Thumb IP flexion or extension mobilization splint, type 2 (3)	7-15 F
Flexion or extension	2	(03)	Thumb	Thumb IP flexion or extension mobilization splint, type 2 (3)	8-10 D
Flexion or extension	2	(03)	Thumb	Thumb IP flexion or extension mobilization splint, type 2 (3)	20-11 E
Restriction						
Extension	0	(01)	Thumb	Thumb IP extension restriction splint, type 0 (1)	16-13 B
Extension	0	(01)	Thumb	Thumb IP extension restriction splint, type 0 (1)	16-15 B
Extension	1	(02)	Thumb	Thumb IP extension restriction splint, type 1 (2)	16-15 C, D
Transmission						
Extension, flexion	3	(04)	Thumb	Thumb IP extension and flexion torque transmission splint, type 3 (4)	12-20
Extension, flexion	12	(13)	Thumb	Thumb IP flexion and extension torque transmission splint, type 12 (13)	8-21

[Thumb splint-prosthesis]

Immobilization

Motion		Type	Code	Digits	Splint name	Figure
[Radial abduction, flexion]		0	(00)	[Thumb]	[Thumb CMC radial abduction, MP-IP flexion fixed] splint-prosthesis, type 0 (00)	15-31 E

Finger Metacarpal, Thumb Metacarpal

Mobilization

Motion		Type	Code	Digits	Splint name	Figure
Distraction		7	(16)	Index, thumb	Index finger metacarpal, thumb metacarpal distraction mobilization splint, type 7 (16)	1-23 B

Finger MP, Thumb CMC

Restriction/Mobilization

Motion		Type	Code	Digits	Splint name	Figure
Extension palmar abduction		1	(06)	Index-small, thumb	Index-small finger MP extension restriction / thumb CMC palmar abduction mobilization splint, type 1 (6)	3-24 C

Finger MP, Thumb CMC, MP

Mobilization

Motion		Type	Code	Digits	Splint name	Figure
Extension, palmar abduction		1	(03)	Ring, thumb	Ring finger MP extension, thumb CMC palmar abduction and MP extension mobilization splint, type 1 (3)	10-2 C
Extension, radial abduction		1	(07)	Index-small, thumb	Index-small finger MP extension, thumb CMC radial abduction and MP extension mobilization splint, type 1 (7)	15-14 J
Extension, radial abduction		1	(07)	Index-small, thumb	Index-small finger MP extension, thumb CMC radial abduction and MP extension mobilization splint, type 1 (7)	15-14 K-M
Extension, radial deviation, supiration, radial abuction		3	(09)	Index-small, thumb	Index-small finger MP extension and radial deviation, index finger MP supination, thumb CMC radial abduction and MP extension mobilization splint, type 3 (9)	16-4 O
Flexion, palmar abduction		1	(07)	Index-small, thumb	Index-small finger MP flexion, thumb CMC palmar abduction and MP flexion mobilization splint, type 1 (7)	10-25

Restriction/Immobilization

Motion		Type	Code	Digits	Splint name	Figure
Extension, radial abduction		1	(04)	Index, thumb	Index finger MP extension restriction / thumb CMC radial abduction and MP extension immobilization splint, type 1 (4)	9-17 A
Flexion, palmar abduction, extension		0	(06)	Index-small, thumb	Index-small finger MP flexion restriction / thumb CMC palmar abduction and MP extension immobilization splint, type 0 (6); right	1-7 B

Finger MP, Thumb CMC, MP, IP

Immobilization/Restriction

Motion		Type	Code	Digits	Splint name	Figure
Flexion, radial abduction, extension		1	(08)	Index-small, thumb	Index-small finger MP flexion, thumb CMC radial abduction and MP flexion immobilization / thumb IP extension restriction splint, type 1 (8)	6-5 A
Flexion, radial abduction, extension		1	(08)	Index-small, thumb	Index-small finger MP flexion, thumb CMC radial abduction and MP flexion immobilization / thumb IP extension restriction splint, type 1 (8)	8-8 E

Mobilization

Motion		Type	Code	Digits	Splint name	Figure
Flexion, radial abduction, extension		1	(08)	Index-small, thumb	Index-small finger MP flexion, thumb CMC radial abduction and MP-IP extension mobilization splint, type 1 (8), with triceps strap	1-8
Abduction, extension, radial abduction		0	(07)	Index-small, thumb	Index, ring-small finger MP abduction, index-small finger MP extension, thumb CMC radial abduction and MP-IP extension mobilization splint, type 0 (7)	19-9 A

Mobilization/Immobilization

Motion		Type	Code	Digits	Splint name	Figure
Extension, radial deviation, supination, radial abduction, flexion		3	(10)	Index-small, thumb	Index-small finger MP extension and radial deviation, index finger MP supination mobilization / thumb CMC radial abduction and MP-IP flexion immobilization splint, type 3 (10)	16-4 N

Continued

Splint[1] Index (SSRDI©)

Articular/Nonarticular Joint/Segment Purpose	Direction	Type	Joints	Digits	ESCS Name	Figure
Finger MP, PIP, DIP, Thumb CMC						
Immobilization						
Flexion, extension, palmar abduction		1	(13)	Index-small, thumb	Index-small finger MP flexion and IP extension, thumb CMC palmar abduction immobilization splint, type 1 (13)	11-38 A-B
Flexion, extension, palmar abduction		3	(16)	Index-small, thumb	Index-small finger MP 70° flexion and IP extension, thumb CMC palmar abduction immobilization splint, type 3 (16)	4-30 A-B
Flexion, palmar abduction		3	(16)	Index-small, thumb	Index-small finger flexion, thumb CMC palmar abduction immobilization splint, type 3 (16)	8-9 C
Flexion, palmar abduction		3	(16)	Index-small, thumb	Index-small finger flexion, thumb CMC palmar abduction immobilization splint, type 3 (16)	20-12 C
Flexion, palmar abduction		3	(16)	Index-small, thumb	Index-small finger flexion, thumb CMC palmar abduction immobilization splint, type 3 (16)	20-12 D
Flexion, palmar abduction		3	(16)	Index-small, thumb	Index-small finger flexion, thumb CMC palmar abduction immobilization splint, type 3 (16)	20-12 E
Flexion, palmar abduction		3	(16)	Index-small, thumb	Index-small finger flexion, thumb CMC palmar abduction immobilization splint, type 3 (16)	20-18 A-D
Mobilization						
Flexion, palmar abduction, extension		1	(5)	Index, ring-small, thumb	Index-small finger flexion, thumb CMC palmar abduction mobilization splint, type 1 (5) or Index, ring-small finger extension, thumb CMC palmar abduction and MP flexion mobilization splint, type 1 (12)	11-42 D
Flexion, palmar abduction		1	(13)	Index-small, thumb	Index-small finger flexion, thumb CMC palmar abduction mobilization splint, type 1 (13)	11-44
Finger MP, PIP, DIP, Thumb CMC, MP						
Immobilization						
Flexion, palmar abduction, extension		1	(15)	Index-small, thumb	Index-small finger 20° flexion, thumb CMC palmar abduction and MP extension immobilization splint, type 1 (15)	4-4
Mobilization						
Extension or flexion, palmar abduction		1	(12)	Index, ring-small, thumb	Index, ring-small finger extension, thumb CMC palmar abduction and MP flexion mobilization splint, type 1 (12) or Index finger flexion, thumb CMC palmar abduction mobilization splint, type 1 (5)	10-6 A
Flexion or extension, palmar abduction		1	(15)	Index-small, thumb	Index-small finger flexion, thumb CMC palmar abduction and MP flexion mobilization splint, type 1 (15); or index-small finger MP extension mobilization splint, type 1 (5)	8-9 A
Restriction/Transmission/Mobilization						
Flexion, extension, palmar abduction		0	(14)	Index-small, thumb	Index-small finger MP extension restriction / IP extension torque transmission / thumb CMC palmar abduction and MP extension mobilization splint, type 0 (14)	15-16 C
Finger MP, PIP, DIP, Thumb CMC, MP, IP						
Immobilization						
Abduction, flexion, palmar abduction, extension		1	(16)	Index-small, thumb	Index, ring-small finger MP abduction, index-small finger flexion, thumb CMC palmar abduction and MP-IP extension immobilization splint, type 1 (16)	1-9 A-B
Flexion, extension, palmar abduction		1	(16)	Index-small, thumb	Index-small finger MP flexion and IP extension, thumb CMC palmar abduction and MP-IP extension immobilization splint, type 1 (16)	11-39 B

Continued

707

Splint[1] Index (SSRDI©)

Articular/Nonarticular Joint/Segment Purpose / Direction	Type	Joints	Digits	ESCS Name	Figure
Flexion, extension, radial abduction	1	(16)	Index-small, thumb	Index-small finger MP flexion and IP extension, thumb CMC radial abduction and MP-IP extension mobilization splint, type 1 (16)	15-25 A
Flexion, extension, radial abduction	1	(16)	Index-small, thumb	Index-small finger MP flexion and IP extension, thumb CMC radial abduction and MP-IP extension mobilization splint, type 1 (16)	21-13 B
Finger MP, PIP, DIP, Thumb MP *Mobilization*					
Flexion or extension	2	(16)	Index-small, thumb	Index-small finger flexion, thumb MP extension mobilization splint, type 2 (16) or Index-small finger extension, thumb MP flexion mobilization splint, type 2 (16)	11-42 C
Finger MP, PIP, DIP, Thumb MP, IP *Immobilization*					
Extension, flexion	4	(16)	Index-small, thumb	Index-small finger MP extension, long finger PIP extension, ring-small finger IP flexion, thumb MP-IP flexion immobilization splint, type 4 (16)	16-20
Finger MP: Finger PIP *Transmission*					
Flexion: flexion	0	(08)	Index-small	Index-small finger MP flexion: index-small finger PIP flexion / index-small finger MP extension: index-small finger PIP extension torque transmission splint, type 0 (8)	1-22 C
Finger PIP, Thumb CMC, MP *Mobilization*					
Extension, radial abduction	2	(11)	Index-small, thumb	Index-small finger PIP extension, thumb CMC radial abduction and MP extension mobilization splint, type 2 (11)	20-13 C
Extension, radial abduction	4	(16)	Index-small, thumb	Index-small finger PIP extension, thumb CMC radial abduction and MP extension mobilization splint, type 4 (16)	20-13 D
Finger PIP, Thumb CMC, MP, IP *Mobilization*					
Extension, radial abduction	3	(16)	Index-small, thumb	Index-small finger PIP extension, thumb CMC radial abduction and MP-IP extension mobilization splint, type 3 (16)	20-13 E
Femur, knee *Immobilization*					
Extension	0	(01)		Femur, knee extension immobilization splint, type 0 (1)	1-1
Nonarticular **Humerus**					
	0	(00)		Nonarticular humerus splint	14-19 A-B
	0	(00)		Nonarticular humerus splint	17-27

Subject Index